Trauma Anesthesia

Second Edition

Trauma Anesthesia

Second Edition

Edited by

Charles E. Smith MD

Professor of Anesthesia, Case Western Reserve University School of Medicine, Director of Cardiothoracic and Trauma
Anesthesia, MetroHealth Medical Center, Cleveland, Ohio, USA

Associate editor

John J. Como MD, MPH, FACS

Associate Professor of Surgery, Case Western Reserve University School of Medicine, Associate Trauma Director, MetroHealth Medical Center, Cleveland, Ohio, USA

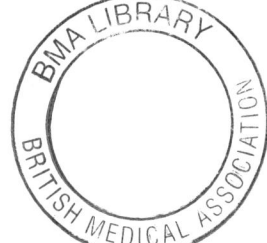

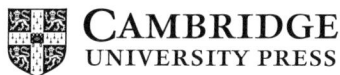

CAMBRIDGE
UNIVERSITY PRESS

University Printing House, Cambridge CB2 8BS, United Kingdom

Cambridge University Press is part of the University of Cambridge.

It furthers the University's mission by disseminating knowledge
in the pursuit of education, learning and research at the highest
international levels of excellence.

www.cambridge.org
Information on this title: www.cambridge.org/9781107038264

First published: 2008
Second edition 2015

Printed in the United Kingdom by TJ International Ltd. Padstow
Cornwall

*A catalogue record for this publication is available from the British
Library*

Library of Congress Cataloging-in-Publication Data
Trauma anesthesia (Smith)
Trauma anesthesia / edited by Charles E. Smith. – Second edition.
    p. ; cm.
Includes bibliographical references and index.
ISBN 978-1-107-03826-4 (Hard back : alk. paper)
I. Smith, Charles E., 1956– , editor.   II. Title.
[DNLM: 1. Anesthesia.   2. Wounds and Injuries.   3. Critical
Care.   4. Perioperative Care.   WO 200]
RD93.93
617.9′604–dc23   2015004553

ISBN 978-1-107-03826-4 Hardback

Contents

v

Section 4 – Special populations

Section 5 – Organization of trauma management

Contributors

Cecil S. Ash, DDS, MS
Private Practice, Walla Walla, WA, and Department of
Surgery, MetroHealth Medical Center, Case Western Reserve
University School of Medicine, Cleveland, OH, USA

Paul Barach, BSc, MD, MPH
Institute of Health Management and Health Economics,
University of Oslo, Oslo, Norway

Ulrike Buehner, MBBS, FRCA
Department of Anaesthesiology and Intensive Care,
Rotorua Hospital, Rotorua, New Zealand

M. Ross Bullock, MD, PhD
Department of Neurosurgery, University of Miami Miller
School of Medicine, Miami, FL, USA

Leonardo Canale, MD
Division of Cardiothoracic Surgery, Department of Surgery,
Cleveland Clinic Foundation, Cleveland, OH, USA

Henry G. Chou, MD
Department of Anesthesia, Cedars Sinai Medical Center, Los
Angeles, CA, USA

Jeffrey A. Claridge, MD
Division of Trauma, Critical Care and Burns, Department of
Surgery, MetroHealth Medical Center, Cleveland, OH, USA

John J. Como, MD, MPH, FACS
Department of Surgery, Case Western Reserve University
School of Medicine and Trauma Services, MetroHealth
Medical Center, Cleveland, OH, USA

Armagan Dagal, MD, FRCA
Department of Anesthesiology and Pain Medicine,
Department of Orthopedics and Sport Medicine, Department
of Neurological Surgery (Adj.), Harborview Medical Center,
University of Washington, Seattle, WA, USA

Martin Dauber, MD
Department of Anesthesia and Critical Care, University of
Chicago, Chicago, IL, USA

James S. Davis, MD
DeWitt Daughtry Family Department of Surgery, University of
Miami Miller School of Medicine, Miami, FL, USA

Shalini Dhir, MD, FRCPC
Department of Anesthesia and Perioperative Medicine,
Schulich School of Medicine and Dentistry, Western
University, and St Joseph's Hospital, London, ON, Canada

François Donati, MD, PhD
Department of Anesthesiology, University of Montreal,
Montreal, QC, Canada

Roman Dudaryk, MD
Departments of Anesthesiology and Critical Care Medicine,
University of Miami Miller School of Medicine, Ryder Trauma
Center, Miami, FL, USA

Richard P. Dutton, MD, MBA
Anesthesia Quality Institute, Park Ridge, IL, and Clinical
Associate, Department of Anesthesia, University of Chicago,
Chicago, IL, USA

Talmage D. Egan, MD
University of Utah School of Medicine, Salt Lake City, UT,
USA

Yashar Eshraghi, MD
Department of Anesthesiology, Case Western Reserve
University, Metrohealth Medical Center, Cleveland, OH, USA

John R. Fisgus, MD
Division of Obstetrical Anesthesia, AtlantiCare Regional
Medical Center, Pomona, NJ, USA

Jeff Gadsden, MD, FRCPC, FANZCA
Department of Anesthesiology, Duke University, Durham, NC,
USA

Sugantha Ganapathy, FRCPC
London Health Sciences Center, University Hospital, London,
ON, Canada

Mark A. Gerhardt, MD, PhD
Department of Anesthesiology, Ohio State University Wexner Medical Center, Columbus, OH, USA

Inderjit Gill, MD
Division of Cardiothoracic Surgery, Department of Surgery, Metrohealth Medical Center, Cleveland, OH, USA

Joseph F. Golob Jr., MD
Division of Surgical Critical Care, Metrohealth Medical Center, Cleveland, OH, USA

Glenn P. Gravlee, MD
Department of Anesthesia, University of Colorado School of Medicine, Denver, CO, USA

Marcello Guglielmi, DDS
Oral and Maxillofacial Surgery, Bronx Lebanon Hospital Center, New York, NY, USA

Jana Hambley, MD
Department of Surgery, Case Western Reserve University, Cleveland, OH, USA

Peter Hebbard MBBS, FANZCA, PG Dip Echo
Department of Anaesthesia, North East Health, Wangaratta, Australia

Elena J. Holak, MD, PharmD
Department of Anesthesiology, Medical College of Wisconsin, Froedtert Memorial Lutheran Hospital, Milwaukee, WI, USA

Khadil Hosein, BA
Department of Neurosurgery, University of Miami Miller School of Medicine, Miami, FL, USA

Ken Johnson, MD
Department of Anesthesiology, University of Utah Hospital, Salt Lake City, UT, USA

Matthew A. Joy, MD
Department of Anesthesiology, MetroHealth Medical Center, Cleveland, OH, USA

George W. Kanellakos, MD, FRCPC
Division of Thoracic Anesthesia, Department of Anesthesia, Dalhousie University, Halifax, NS, Canada

Olga Kaslow, MD, PhD
Trauma Anesthesiology Service, Department of Anesthesiology, Medical College of Wisconsin, Froedtert Memorial Lutheran Hospital, Milwaukee, WI, USA

Arthur M. Lam, MD
Department of Anesthesiology, Swedish Neuroscience Institute, Seattle, WA, USA

Vanetta Levesque, MD
Department of Anesthesiology, Maimonides Medical Center, Brooklyn, NY, USA

Jessica Anne Lovich-Sapola, MD, MBA
Department of Anesthesiology and Pain Management, Case Western Reserve University School of Medicine, and Metrohealth Medical Center, Cleveland, OH, USA

M. Jocelyn Loy, MD
Department of Anesthesiology, MetroHealth Medical Center, Cleveland, OH, USA

Peter F. Mahoney, OBE, MBA, FRCA, FIMC, FFICM
Royal Centre for Defence Medicine, Queen Elizabeth Hospital, Birmingham, and Centre for Blast Injury Studies, Imperial College, London, UK

Donn Marciniak, MD
Department of Cardiothoracic Anesthesia, Cleveland Clinic Foundation, Cleveland, OH, USA

Maureen McCunn, MD, MIPP, FCCM
Departments of Anesthesiology and Critical Care Medicine, University of Pennsylvania, Philadelphia, PA, USA

Craig C. McFarland, MD
Department of Anesthesia and Operative Services, San Antonio Military Medical Center, Fort Sam Houston, TX, and United States Army Research Laboratory, Adelphi, MD, USA

Maroun J. Mhanna, MD
Department of Pediatrics, MetroHealth Medical Center, Cleveland, OH, USA

Timothy Moore, MD
Departments of Orthopedic Surgery and Neurosciences, Director of Spine Trauma, MetroHealth Medical Center, and Case Western Reserve University School of Medicine, Cleveland, OH, USA

Cynthia Nguyen, MD
Department of Orthopedic Surgery, Case Western Reserve University School of Medicine, Cleveland, OH, USA

Maxim Novikov, MD
Promedica Physician Group, Promedica Anesthesiology Consultants, Toledo, OH, USA

E. Orestes O'Brien, MD
Department of Anesthesiology, UCSD School of Medicine, San Diego, CA, USA

Ketan P. Parekh, DDS
Pinnacle Oral & Facial Surgery, Rockwall, TX, USA

Claire L. Park, MBE, FRCA, FFICM, RCS(Ed), RAMC
Department of Critical Care, King's College Hospital, London, UK

Michael J. A. Parr, MBBS, FRCP, FRCA, FANZCA, FJFICM
Department of Intensive Care, Liverpool Hospital, University of New South Wales, Sydney, NSW, Australia

Elie Rizkala, MD
Division of Pediatric Neurology, Metrohealth Medical Center, Cleveland, OH, USA

Steven Roth, MD
Department of Anesthesia and Critical Care, University of Chicago, Chicago, IL, USA

Alistair Royse, MBBS, MD, FRACS, FCSANZ
Department of Surgery, University of Melbourne, and Department of Cardiothoracic Surgery, The Royal Melbourne Hospital, Melbourne, VIC, Australia

Colin Royse, MBBS, MD, FANZCA
Department of Surgery, University of Melbourne, and Department of Anaesthesia and Pain Management, The Royal Melbourne Hospital, Melbourne, VIC, Australia

Kasia Petelenz Rubin, MD
Departments of Anesthesiology and Pediatrics, Case Western Reserve University School of Medicine, Cleveland, OH, USA

David Ryan, MD
Department of Anesthesiology, MetroHealth Medical Center, Cleveland, OH, USA

Claire Sandstrom, MD
Department of Radiology, University of Washington School of Medicine, and Section of Emergency and Trauma Radiology at Harborview Medical Center, Seattle, WA, USA

Carl I. Schulman, MD, PhD, MSPH, FACS
DeWitt Daughtry Family Department of Surgery, University of Miami Miller School of Medicine, Miami, FL, USA

Rishad Shaikh, DMD
Division of Maxillofacial Surgery, Department of Surgery, Case Western Reserve University, Cleveland, OH, USA

Ranjita Sharma, FANZCA
Department of Anaesthesia, St. Joseph's Hospital, London, ON, Canada

Jeffrey H. Silverstein, MD
Departments of Anesthesiology, Surgery and Geriatrics and Palliative Care, Mount Sinai School of Medicine, New York, NY, USA

Peter Slinger, MD, FRCPC
Department of Anesthesia, University of Toronto and Toronto General Hospital, Toronto, ON, Canada

Charles E. Smith, MD
Department of Anesthesiology, MetroHealth Medical Center, Case Western Reserve University School of Medicine, Cleveland, OH, USA

Christopher Smith, MD
St. John Medical Center, University Hospitals Case Medical Center, Westlake, OH, USA

Paul Soeding, PhD, MBBS, FANZCA, DDU
Department of Anaesthesia and Pain Management, Royal Melbourne Hospital, Melbourne, VIC, Australia

Rakesh V. Sondekoppam, MD
Department of Anesthesia and Perioperative Medicine, Schulich School of Medicine and Dentistry, Western University, London, ON, Canada

P. David Soran, MD
Department of Anesthesiology, Perioperative and Pain Medicine, Stanford Hospital and Clinics, Stanford, CA, USA

Eldar Søreide, MD PhD
Intensive Care Unit, Department of Anaesthesiology and Intensive Care, Stavanger University Hospital, Stavanger, Norway

Elizabeth A. Steele, MD
Department of Anesthesiology, University of New Mexico, Albuquerque, NM, USA

Kristian Strand, MD PhD
Department of Anesthesiology, Stavanger University Hospital, Stavanger, Norway

Dennis M. Super, MD, MPH, FAAP
Department of Pediatric Critical Care Medicine, MetroHealth Medical Center, Cleveland, OH, USA

Kutaiba Tabbaa, MD
Metrohealth Pain Management Service, Department of Anesthesiology, MetroHealth Medical Center, Cleveland, OH, USA

Nicholas T. Tarmey, FRCA, FFICM, DipIMC, RCS(Ed), RAMC
Academic Department of Critical Care, Ministry of Defence Hospital Unit, Portsmouth, UK

Joshua M. Tobin, MD
Division of Trauma Anesthesiology, Department of Anesthesiology, Keck School of Medicine at USC, Los Angeles, CA, USA

Kalpana Tyagaraj, MD
Department of Obstetric Anesthesia, Maimonides Medical Center, Brooklyn, NY, USA

Heather A. Vallier, MD
Department of Orthopedic Surgery, Case Western Reserve University, and Department of Orthopedic Surgery, MetroHealth Medical Center, Cleveland, OH, USA

Sandra Werner, MD, MA, FACEP
Department of Emergency Medicine, MetroHealth Medical Center, Cleveland, OH, USA

Earl Willis Weyers, MD
Department of Anesthesiology, University of Miami Miller School of Medicine, Ryder Trauma Center, Miami, FL, USA

William C. Wilson, MD, MA
Departments of Anesthesiology and Surgery, University of California, Irvine Medical Centre, Irvine, CA, USA

Shoji Yokobori, MD, PhD
Department of Neurosurgery, University of Miami Miller School of Medicine, Miami, FL, USA and Department of Emergency and Critical Care Medicine, Nippon Medical School, Tokyo, Japan

Charles J. Yowler, MD, FACS
Department of Surgery, Case Western Reserve University, Cleveland, OH, USA

Foreword to the second edition

Trauma represents one the most serious threats to public health in developed countries. In the United States, trauma represents a broad spectrum of disease and is the leading cause of death and disability among young patients. Trauma claims more lost quality life years than cancer or cardiovascular disease and sadly often robs a society of its youth. However, each and every day through the thoughtful and dedicated effort of many skilled trauma providers working in complex systems we have successfully mitigated the impact of injury on countless numbers of the seriously injured. Lives are saved, limbs are preserved, and function is restored at a level considered unreachable less than a decade ago. Many of the advancements upon which these gains have been achieved rest upon improvements in resuscitation, anesthesia, advanced monitoring, and timely surgical intervention.

Modern trauma care has evolved since the last edition of this valued textbook, and the editors and authors have further defined and updated the role of anesthesia and anesthesiologists in the expert management of patients with major injury. As the rearing of children "takes a village," the care of major trauma "takes a system." Care of the seriously injured requires a team of providers working in a hospital that is part of a complex larger system. System thinking within and beyond the hospital setting is essential for the management of trauma care.

The role of the anesthesiologist in trauma care has expanded over the past several years with the development of early appropriate care protocols and the emphasis on timely surgery. Early appropriate care establishes a framework for decision making across multiple disciplines engaged in trauma care and highlights the importance for ongoing resuscitation from induction of anesthesia, through time-sensitive surgery and transfer from the operating suite to the surgical intensive care unit. The anesthesiologist also plays a central role in pain management in the early postoperative period, one of the most challenging and important issues in the patient experience. This text addresses the important and ever-changing issues in the management of trauma patients. The chapters herein comprehensively address a broad range of clinical conditions and the complexity of anesthesia-related care of trauma patients.

This book provides expert insight into the many facets of trauma anesthesia, trauma surgery, pain management, and coordinated care of the injured in complex systems and across the continuum from accident through recovery. The editors and the authors promote best practice as it is currently done in the most influential trauma centers. The text is an indispensable resource for those with an interest in the care of injury, be it an isolated fracture or a patient with multisystem injury.

Brendan M. Patterson, MD, MBA
Professor, Orthopedic Surgery, Case Western Reserve University School of Medicine

Executive Director, Surgical Services, The MetroHealth System

Foreword to the second edition

In his foreword for *Trauma Anesthesia*, Adolph H. (Buddy) Giesecke, MD opened with the following statement: "Dr. Charles E. Smith has been inspiring improved anesthesia for the victims of traumatic injuries for many years..." This premise rings as true now as it did then. Based at Metro Health Medical Center and Case Western Reserve University School of Medicine in Cleveland, Ohio, Dr. Smith continues to be a respected lecturer and prolific author of trauma-related studies and publications. His expertise in the anesthesia care of the trauma patient supports his reputation and is well exemplified by his major contributions to this book. As with the original volume, he has chosen a group of highly respected authors who add significant substance to this new edition. *Trauma Anesthesia, Second Edition* is an engaging and informative read. It should become part of the armamentarium of all those who aspire to better care for the patient who has suffered a traumatic injury.

Appropriately, this book begins by providing the reader with an overview of the epidemiology of trauma. We quickly understand the cost of trauma, not only to the individual patient, but also to society in general. The book then moves from this broad topic to those which are more specific, allowing the reader the opportunity to review particular aspects of traumatic injury and then to see specific examinations of how one may best provide anesthetic care for these patients. It is accepted that anesthesia care for the patient with traumatic injuries has continued to evolve since the first edition of *Trauma Anesthesia*. Mirroring this evolution of anesthesia care, the information provided within this book has kept pace with those changes. Examinations of fluid resuscitation of the trauma patient, the continued fine-tuning of massive transfusion protocols, and an ongoing analysis of damage control in severe trauma are all included here. Another hot topic included in this book is monitoring of the trauma patient. There continues to be considerable morbidity associated with traumatic injuries. Besides discussions of chronic pain in the trauma survivor, the science of injury prevention is presented.

One aspect of this book that especially appeals to me is the pairing of discussions of trauma to a particular organ system or region of the body, and the subsequent presentation of anesthetic considerations for patients with that particular pattern of injury. Because of this presentation of the information, there is something in this book that will be of interest to every student of trauma care. Included are chapters on pediatric trauma, cardiac injury, head, brain and spinal cord trauma, as well as coverage of the anesthetic care for these patients. There are discussions for those whose interests lie more towards postoperative critical care (pulmonary care of the severely injured patient, operations of a trauma unit) or using simulation in education. There is an update on military injuries, and field anesthesia for treating these patients. There are chapters on burn injuries and anesthesia, as well as sections on anesthesia for the elderly patient with trauma.

When Dr. Smith first asked me to write this foreword, it was an unexpected request. Why would he want me, an unknown name in the trauma anesthesiology world, to prepare readers who open this book? My reading of the pages that follow brought back to me the presence of my father, A.H. "Buddy" Giesecke, MD. It enabled me to reflect on his career in trauma anesthesiology, and on the support he gave to those who shared his interest in trauma, in general, and in the specialty of trauma anesthesiology, in particular. Studying these pages made me more fully understand the particular attractions of trauma anesthesia, and of its physicians. Dr. Smith and my father are examples who truly fit that model of the teaching anesthesiologist.

In *Trauma Anesthesia, Second Edition*, Dr. Smith and his invited authors have once again produced an eloquently readable book. The information held within will allow the reader to better understand the nature of traumatic injuries and the relationship that the practicing trauma anesthesiologist plays in producing the best outcomes in this patient population. Though written with anesthesiologists in mind, this book will be particularly useful to any student, physician, or other health professional who spends time caring for the patient with traumatic injury. It is my desire to echo my father's closing statement in his foreword from the original edition. Congratulations to Dr. Smith and the entire authorship for a job well done!

Martin Giesecke, MD
M.T. "Pepper" Jenkins Professor and Vice Chairman

Anesthesiology and Pain Management
University of Texas Southwestern Medical Center
Dallas, Texas

Foreword to the first edition

Dr. Charles E. Smith has been inspiring improved anesthesia for the victims of traumatic injury for many years, having spent the majority of his career at MetroHealth Medical Center, Cleveland, Ohio, which is the city's major trauma center. He has regularly served as lecturer in refresher courses for the International Trauma Anesthesia and Critical Care Society (now called International TraumaCare). He is a productive author of innovative research in the care of the traumatized patient. These attributes easily qualify him to be editor of a multi-authored comprehensive book on trauma anesthesia, to which he is also a major contributor. His invited chapter authors are similarly qualified. The result is an authoritative, readable, and educational resource for the student, resident, or practitioner wishing to stay abreast of a rapidly changing field.

Epochal changes have occurred in the practice of anesthesiology in the last ten years. Improved monitors, safer drugs, and better-trained anesthesiologists, nurse anesthetists, and anesthesia assistants have all reduced the morbidity and mortality of anesthesia. Anesthesia has become safer. Safer anesthesia improves the outcome of traumatic injuries. Our surgical colleagues have contributed to the improvements in trauma care. Innovations in the care of serious fractures, use of damage control in abdominal injuries, and improved care of burns have reduced morbidity and mortality. Dr. Smith has included all of the latest innovations in this text. Despite the advances, the importance of trauma as a cause of disability and lost life remains and, in fact, when expressed as a proportion to overall mortality in young people, is increasing in importance.

Throughout history significant advances have been made in anesthetic care during times of war. The war in Iraq is no exception, and the lessons learned in that conflict are included. The technology of vascular access has greatly improved. Ultrasonic localization of major veins for central access is a major advance greatly enhancing safety for the patient. The technique of intraosseous infusion was once painful and cumbersome to establish, such that it was considered a circus stunt and not of much practical value. Newly designed equipment has revolutionized the technique. It is now fast, painless, convenient, and effective in any patient with difficult IV access. Having established vascular access, the choice and volume of fluid therapy is critical to survival and outcome of the traumatized patient.

This book discusses the established and the controversial concepts. Also discussed is a new protocoldriven, multidisciplinary approach to massive transfusion. This approach, which requires cooperation between the blood bank, the traumasurgeons, and anesthesiologists, takes the guesswork out of massive transfusion. No longer do we have to stand at the OR table and ponder, "Is it time for platelets and fresh frozen plasma?" These collaborative decisions have been made in advance, and all we have to do is to activate the protocol and administer whatever comes in the incremental allotments.

Patients now expect to be relieved of significant pain, and pain is considered the fifth vital sign. Significant advances have been made in the techniques for relief of acute traumatic and postoperative pain. Entire teams of people are now dedicated to this practice. Nobody questions the value of pain relief, but it comes with some risk. A multimodal approach appears to accomplish the goal and simultaneously minimize the risks.

Thermal injuries, brain injuries, and spinal cord injuries are specialized forms of trauma that are occasionally neglected. Not so in this text. The public health implications are presented along with the practical considerations for safe clinical management. The practical considerations are important because, for example, drugs and procedures that may be beneficial in the management of orthopedic injuries are contraindicated in neurologic injuries. We must be able to recognize these conflicts when they occur together in the same patient and create an anesthetic plan that will benefit the patient.

Dr. Smith and his invited authors have done a magnificent job of pulling together the diverse concepts of the management of the traumatized patient and presenting us with a valuable resource for the anesthesiologist. Although directed at the anesthesiologist, the text is useful for emergency medicine physicians, surgeons, orthopedists, and, in fact, any health care professional who deals with trauma. Congratulations to the entire group of authors!

Adolph H. (Buddy) Giesecke MD, Emeritus Professor

Anesthesiology and Pain Management
University of Texas Southwestern Medical Center
Dallas, Texas

Foreword to the first edition

The challenge of managing seriously injured patients encompasses an expanse of issues linked by a common factor – trauma. In these critical situations, anesthesiologists are often faced with the need to simultaneously address emergent airway management, resuscitation, massive blood loss, acidemia, coagulopathy, hypothermia, and the consequences of damage to various organs. The management of each of these conditions alone can be essential for survival, and their convergence presents a unique situation in which the likelihood of death or a bad outcome is real. Success in this stressful situation requires a sophisticated understanding of basic sciences and expertise in the clinical and technical skills of anesthetic management. Together, the anesthesiologist and trauma surgeon must orchestrate the human and physical resources of the trauma center with a patient's life on the line.

Recent advances in the field of trauma anesthesiology parallel those in other related medical disciplines. Concepts promulgated by experiences in recent military conflicts have affected resuscitation and the use of blood products. The adoption of damage control operations and the use of simultaneous surgical teams to address multiple critical injuries have improved survival. Rules regarding the transfusion of blood and blood components and the use of recombinant clotting factors such as Factor VII concentrate have led to a "sea change" in trauma management that has resulted in the survival of soldiers and others injured under war conditions beyond what was possible just a few years ago. These concepts have been readily adopted in civilian trauma centers. The intensity associated with their use has placed an increased demand on anesthesiologists who are already taxed in their care for the critically injured.

This excellent book addresses these important and evolving changes in management of the injured patient as well as more traditional issues in trauma anesthesia. The breadth of topics addressed by the authors reflects the challenges and complexities of anesthesia-related care for victims of traumatic injury.

Trauma surgeons realize the tremendous importance of coordinated care promulgated at trauma centers and by trauma systems. Injury accounts for more lost productive years of life than any other disease; therefore, survival and ultimate returnto an acceptable level of function are important outcome parameters both for the patient, their loved ones, and our society. Because many seriously injured patients will require an operation, the anesthesiologist is an important link in the coordinated approach to trauma care andmust be aware of the unique problems related to managing injury. That is why this book is such an important contribution for anesthesiologists who care for trauma patients.

Mark A. Malangoni, MD
Surgeon-in-Chief

Chairperson, Department of Surgery
MetroHealth Medical Center
Professor of Surgery
CaseWestern Reserve University School of Medicine
Cleveland, Ohio

Preface

Trauma is a leading cause of death and disability in modern society. Trauma will continue to be a leading cause of death well into the future. We are all vulnerable to traumatic injury. Managing adult and pediatric victims of major trauma and burns continues to be a great challenge requiring a tremendous amount of dedication and resources. As with the first edition, the overall aim of this textbook is to review the anesthesia considerations for trauma patients and to provide a rational approach to the choice of anesthetic techniques and drugs. Nearly all authors from the first edition were asked to review and revise their chapters in order to reflect recent changes in the field of trauma anesthesiology. In addition, six new chapters have been added to make a total of 43 chapters, and the second edition of *Trauma Anesthesia* has been reorganized into five sections as follows: (1) *Initial management of the trauma patient*, which includes a new chapter on trauma in the prehospital environment and the emergency department; (2) *Techniques for monitoring, imaging, and pain relief*, including a new chapter highlighting major advances in diagnostic and interventional radiology for victims of blunt and penetrating trauma; (3) *Anesthetic considerations*, including new chapters on surgical issues in head trauma, anesthesia for oral and maxillofacial trauma, and surgical considerations in abdominal trauma; (4) *Special populations*; and (5) *Organization of trauma management*, which includes a new chapter on prevention of injuries.

I have been fortunate in assembling an outstanding group of clinicians who regularly care for trauma patients at major trauma centers. The authors provide an in-depth discussion of their areas of expertise, and concentrate on clinical aspects of trauma management. I have selected members of my hospital to assist with this textbook, as well as notable contributors from other major centers around the globe. The 43 chapters deal in detail with pertinent areas of trauma care such as airway and shock management, monitoring, vascular access, pharmacology of anesthetic drugs, fluid and blood resuscitation, and the treatment of acute and chronic pain after injury. For several patterns of injuries, including head, spinal cord, oral and maxillofacial, extremity and pelvis, abdomen, cardiac and great vessel, and burns, surgical considerations and management principles are presented to the reader in the chapter preceding the one dealing with anesthetic considerations. Specific chapters review the anesthesia considerations of vulnerable patient populations such as elderly, pediatric, pregnant, and military patients. Other sections deal with important issues of trauma care including damage control in severe trauma, hypothermia in trauma, mechanical ventilation following traumatic injury, and use of echocardiography and ultrasound in trauma. Training for trauma, including the use of simulation, and the role of trauma care systems in facilitating the allocation of resources for optimally managing injured patients, are also covered.

As with the first edition, I hope that this text will be of use for anesthesia care providers who are faced with caring for trauma patients at all hours of the day and night. I am certain that the text will benefit anesthesia residents and staff of major trauma centers, help pave the way to improved care of the injured, and stimulate future advances in trauma care.

Acknowledgments

I would like to thank my mentors in anesthesia from McGill University, David Bevan, François Donati, Earl Wynands, and Jamie Ramsey, for providing teaching and inspiration, instilling in me the confidence to manage complex patients, and stimulating my interest in clinical research. I am indebted to all the staff at MetroHealth Medical Center who work long and hard to transport, stabilize, diagnose, treat, and rehabilitate victims of blunt and penetrating injury. Thanks to my associate editor and colleague, John Como, and to the many contributors to this book for sharing their experience and knowledge. I am grateful to the staff of Cambridge University Press for their tireless efforts in seeing this book through to publication: Nisha Doshi, Joanna Chamberlin, Deb Russell, Beata Mako, Hugh Brazier, Ross Higman, and Divya Mathesh. I would also like to thank my colleagues at the Trauma Anesthesiology Society and Committee on Trauma and Emergency Preparedness for their friendship, support, and vision in caring for trauma patients: Albert Varon, Rick Dutton, Marc Steurer, Maureen McCunn, Jean-François Pittet, Arman Dagal, Olga Kaslow, Mike Murray, Josh Tobin, Carin Hagberg, Uday Jain, Jay McIsaac, Tony Chang, Bert Pierce. I also note the passing of one of the greatest trauma anesthesiologists of our time, Buddy Giesecke, who inspired me to learn more about trauma, and was a source of strength, guidance, friendship, and support. The love and encouragement of my parents Thelma and David, my children Adrienne, Emily, and Rebecca, and my granddaughter Sweet Baby Jane was ever present and much appreciated.

Charles E. Smith, MD

Mechanisms and demographics

Joseph F. Golob Jr. and John J. Como

Objectives

(1) Describe the epidemiology and clinical importance of trauma in the United Sates and worldwide.

(2) Describe the epidemiology of the most common traumatic mechanisms of injury.

(3) Describe the injury patterns seen within these common traumatic mechanisms of injury.

Introduction

Trauma is defined as bodily damage as a result of mechanical, chemical, thermal, electrical, or other energy that exceeds the tolerance of the body. Although trauma is often seen as "accidental," in reality it should be viewed as a "disease" with modifiable risk factors (see Chapter 41). Data have shown that ~25% of trauma patients evaluated at a busy academic trauma center experienced a prior traumatic event and required evaluation in a hospital setting within the previous five years.[1] Statistics such as these confirm that trauma is not a random event affecting random people.

In 2009, within the United States, injury was the leading cause of death in people between the ages of 1 and 44. Overall, traumatic injury was the fifth leading cause of death for all age groups (Fig. 1.1).[2] Worldwide, an estimated 5 million people died from injuries in 2000 – a mortality rate of 83.7 per 100,000 population.[3] This mortality rate accounted for 9% of the world's deaths. Traffic injuries accounted for 25% of these deaths, with homicide and suicide accounting for an additional 26% of deaths (Fig. 1.2).[3] The financial burden of trauma can also not be overlooked. In 2005, within the United States, fatal injuries resulted in $1.6 billion in medical costs and a staggering $164 billion in loss of work to society (Fig. 1.3).[4]

Traumatic injuries are often divided into unintentional and intentional mechanisms. Examples of unintentional mechanisms include motor vehicle and motorcycle collisions, pedestrians struck by a vehicle, and falls. Examples of intentional mechanisms include suicide and homicide. Both unintentional and intentional mechanisms can include penetrating causes such as gunshot wounds and stab wounds.

Unfortunately, both these unintentional and intentional injuries often involve substance abuse. Alcohol has been cited as a contributory factor in nearly 50% of traumatic injury deaths. The combination of drugs and alcohol with access to a deadly weapon often results in death or serious injury. Traumatic injuries can also cause posttraumatic stress disorder and result in initiation or worsening of substance abuse practices. Many trauma centers have recognized the association of substance abuse and traumatic injury and have implemented programs to assist with patient rehabilitation, but better data are needed to see if these programs actually decrease trauma recidivism.

Trauma mechanisms

Motor vehicle collisions

Motor vehicle collisions are the leading cause of death due to injury. In 2008, just over 100 people per day died on United States roads. Drivers under the influence of alcohol and drugs are significantly more likely to be involved in a motor vehicle collision and subsequently die from their injuries.[5] Estimates show that 32% of all fatal motor vehicle crashes involve alcohol. This number increases to 65% in fatal crashes between 12 a.m. and 3 a.m.[6] More recently, driver distractions from cellular phone and global positioning system (GPS) technology have been implicated in motor vehicle collisions. A Harris Interactive Health Day poll of 2810 adults conducted in November 2011 demonstrated that 37% had sent or received cellular text messages while driving, and 18% said they did so regularly.[7] This has prompted some states to introduce legislation to prohibit cellular phone text messaging while driving, in hopes of decreasing the number of motor vehicle collisions (see Chapter 41).

Injury patterns depend on the location of the impact and the presence or absence of protective devices. Frontal impacts of the down-and-under type result in lower extremity and pelvic fractures. The up-and-over type of frontal impact often results in chest, spine, and traumatic brain injuries. Lateral impact causes injuries to the chest and upper abdomen such as liver and spleen. Rear impact often results in cervical spine

Trauma Anesthesia, 2nd Edition, ed. Charles E. Smith. Published by CAMBRIDGE UNIVERSITY PRESS. © Charles E. Smith, 2015.

10 Leading Causes of Death by Age Group, United States – 2009

Rank	<1	1-4	5-9	10-14	15-24	25-34	35-44	45-54	55-64	65+	Total
				Age Groups							
1	Congenital Anomalies 5,319	Unintentional Injury 1,466	Unintentional Injury 773	Unintentional Injury 916	Unintentional Injury 12,458		Unintentional Injury 15,102	Malignant Neoplasms 50,616	Malignant Neoplasms 106,829	Heart Disease 479,150	Heart Disease 599,413
2	Short Gestation 4,538	Congenital Anomalies 464	Malignant Neoplasms 477	Malignant Neoplasms 419	Homicide 4,862	Suicide 5,320	Malignant Neoplasms 12,519	Heart Disease 36,927	Heart Disease 67,261	Malignant Neoplasms 391,035	Malignant Neoplasms 567,628
3	SIDS 2,226	Homicide 376	Congenital Anomalies 195	Suicide 259	Suicide 4,371	Homicide 4,222	Heart Disease 11,081	Unintentional Injury 19,974	Chronic Low. Respiratory Disease 14,160	Chronic Low Respiratory Disease 117,098	Chronic Low. Respiratory Disease 137,353
4	Maternal Pregnancy Comp. 1,608	Malignant Neoplasms 350	Homicide 119	Homicide 186	Malignant Neoplasms 1,636	Malignant Neoplasms 3,659	Suicide 6,677	Suicide 8,598	Unintentional Injury 12,933	Cerebro-vascular 109,238	Cerebro-vascular 128,842
5	Unintentional Injury 1,181	Heart Disease 154	Influenza & Pneumonia 106	Congenital Anomalies 169	Heart Disease 1,035	Heart Disease 3,174	Homicide 2,762	Liver Disease 8,377	Diabetes Mellitus 11,361	Alzheimer's Disease 78,168	Unintentional Injury 118,021
6	Placenta Cord . Membranes 1,064	Influenza & Pneumonia 146	Heart Disease 97	Influenza & Pneumonia 122	Congenital Anomalies 457	HIV 881	Liver Disease 2,481	Cerebro-vascular 6,163	Cerebro-vascular 10,523	Diabetes Mellitus 48,944	Alzheimer's Disease 79,003
7	Bacterial Sepsis 652	Septicemia 71	Chronic Low. Respiratory Disease 64	Heart Disease 120	Influenza & Pneumonia 418	Influenza & Pneumonia 807	HIV 2,425	Diabetes Mellitus 5,725	Liver Disease 9,154	Influenza & Pneumonia 43,469	Diabetes Mellitus 68,705
8	Respiratory Distress 595	Chronic Low. Respiratory Disease 66	Benign Neoplasms 40	Chronic Low. Respiratory Disease 59	Complicated Pregnancy 227	Diabetes Mellitus 604	Cerebro-vascular 1,916	Chronic Low. Respiratory Disease 4,664	Suicide 5,808	Nephritis 40,465	Influenza & Pneumonia 53,692
9	Circulatory System Disease 581	Perinatal Period 58	Septicemia 33	Benign Neoplasms 45	Cerebro-vascular 193	Cerebro-vascular 537	Diabetes Mellitus 1,872	HIV 3,388	Nephritis 4,792	Unintentional Injury 39,111	Nephritis 48,935
10	Neonatal Hemorrhage 517	Benign Neoplasms 53	Cerebro-vascular 32	Cerebro-vascular 42	Chronic Low. Respiratory Disease 187	Liver Disease 459	Influenza & Pneumonia 1,314	Influenza & Pneumonia 2,918	Septicemia 4,628	Septicemia 26,763	Suicide 36,909

Data Source: National Vital Statistics System, National Center for Health Statistics, CDC.
Produced by: Office of Statistics and Programming, National Center for Injury Prevention andControl, CDCusing WISQARS™.

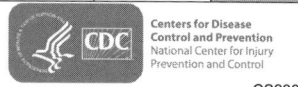

Centers for Disease Control and Prevention National Center for Injury Prevention and Control

CS230409

Figure 1.1 Ten leading causes of death by age group. (From CDC Vital Statistics: http://www.cdc.gov/Injury/wisqars/pdf/10LCD-Age-Grp-US-2009-a.pdf.[2])

injuries. Seatbelts and airbags have been shown to decrease mortality, but they can also cause significant injuries. Lap belts have been implicated in Chance fractures of the lumbar spine and perforations of hollow viscus organs, as well as in pancreatic injuries. Airbags can cause corneal, facial, and neck trauma.

Motorcycle collisions

In 2010, within the United States, there were 4502 fatalities as a result of motorcycle collisions.[6] Motorcyclists are about 34 times more likely than passenger car occupants to die in a vehicular crash.[6] The potential for injury in a motorcycle collision is high because of the massive amount of energy transferred to the motorcyclist, who is then usually ejected from the bike, as well as because of the lack of protection from the vehicle itself. Motorcycle helmets are designed to reduce the direct force to the head and disperse it over the entire foam padding of the helmet. Helmets have been shown to decrease risk of death by 37% and serious injury by 67%.[8] Despite the proven benefit of motorcycle helmets, only 19 states have mandatory helmet laws for riders of all ages.

Similar to motor vehicle crashes, motorcycle crash injury patterns depend on the location and speed of impact. Frontal impact with ejection can lead to injury to the head, chest, abdomen, or long bones. Lateral impact often results in closed and open fractures of the extremities. Soft tissue injuries and abrasions such as "road rash" are common in all impact patterns.

Pedestrian struck

It is estimated that nearly two people for every 100,000 in the population will die as a result of being struck by a motor vehicle. Nearly 46% of pedestrian fatalities are alcohol-related either in the pedestrian or in the driver. January 1st and October 31st are the most common dates for being struck by a vehicle. Pedestrians are more likely to be killed between the hours of 3 a.m. and 6 a.m. on Saturday or Sunday. Males are more likely to be struck than females. On average, a pedestrian is killed every 108 minutes and injured every eight minutes.[9]

The pattern of injury depends on the height of the person and the vehicle involved. A bumper impact to the lower extremities results in closed and open fractures, knee dislocations, and pelvic fractures. Impact with the hood or windshield can cause head and torso injuries. Impact with the ground after being struck can cause head injuries and soft tissue injury (road rash). Children who are struck by a car are often knocked down and subsequently run over by the vehicle (see Chapters 34 and 35). This can result in an array of injuries to the torso, extremities, and head.

Falls

In the United States, falls are the most common unintentional cause for nonfatal injuries. As our population continues to age, falls are becoming even more common (see Chapter 36). Elderly patients can sustain significant injury even with a low impact fall from standing. Medical comorbidities and medications such as anticoagulants and antiplatelet agents all contribute to elderly fall patient injuries. The Centers for Disease Control and Prevention (CDC) estimate that one in three adults over 65 years old fall each year. Older adults are hospitalized five times more often as a result of a fall than any other injury mechanism. In 2009, United States emergency departments treated 2.2 million elderly fall patients, with more than 582,000 of these requiring hospital admissions. Treatment costs for elderly fall patients are staggering. In 2000, over $19 billion was spent treating falls in patients over 65 years old.[10]

Younger patients are more likely to fall from heights such as a ladder or scaffold while working. The median lethal distance for falls (LD50) is four stories or 48 feet (15 meters). This means that 50% of patients who fall four stories will die.

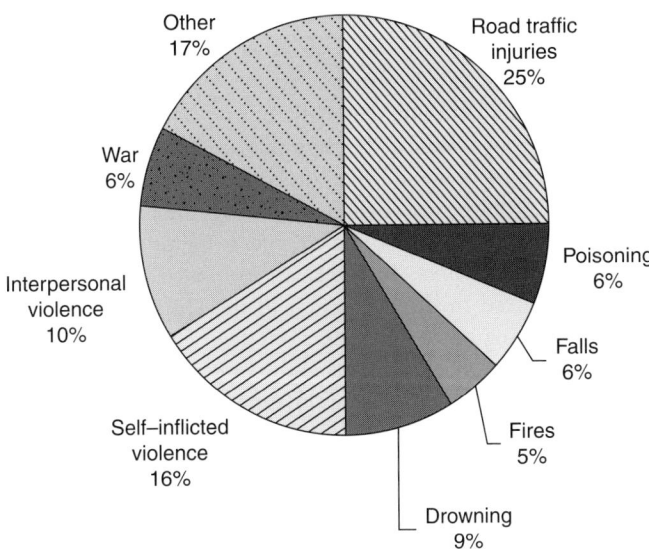

Distribution of global injury mortality by cause, 2000

Figure 1.2 Distribution of global injury mortality by cause. (From Peden M, McGee K, Sharma G. *The injury Chart Book: a Graphical Overview of the Global Burden of Injuries.* Geneva: World Health Organization, 2002.[3]) *A black and white version of this figure will appear in some formats. For the color version, please refer to the plate section.*

Number of Deaths and Estimated Average and Total Lifetime Costs Classified by Mechanism and Intent
Costs Expressed in 2005 U.S. Prices

Death and Type of Cost			Intent			
			Unintentional	Suicide	Homicide	Total
Mechanism						
	Deaths	–	117 809	32 637	18 124	168 570
	Medical Cost	Average	$11 670	$3 056	$6 265	$9 421
		Total	$1 374 873 000	$99 733 000	$113 552 000	$1 588 159 000
All Mechanisms	Work Loss Cost	Average	$890 723	$1 058 114	$1 390 878	$976 907
		Total	$104 935 229 000	$34 533 683 000	$25 208 272 000	$164 677 183 000
	Combined Cost	Average	$902 394	$1 061 170	$1 397 143	$986 328
		Total	$106 310 102 000	$34 633 416 000	$25 321 824 000	$166 265 342 000

Figure 1.3 2005 economic burdens of unintentional and intentional (suicide and homicide) injuries. (From the Web-based Injury Statistics Query and Reporting System: http://www.cdc.gov/injury/wisqars.[4])

Mortality increases to 90% when the fall is seven stories.[11] In addition to height, other prognostic factors include the impact surface and which body part makes first contact.[12] Patients who land on their feet sustain injuries to the calcaneus, tibia, femoral neck, and spine. Both solid and/or hollow viscus injuries are also common. Fall victims who land on their back see significant spine, pulmonary, and cardiac injuries. Patients who land on their head may suffer significant brain and cervical spine injuries.

Suicide

Suicide is a major public health concern. In 2009, suicide was the tenth most common cause of death within the United States, with 36,909 fatalities (Fig. 1.1). An estimated 11 suicide attempts occur for every suicide death.[4] Risk factors for suicide include depression and other mental disorders, substance abuse, family history of mental disorders, history of previous suicide attempts, history of family violence, and presence of firearms in the home. Firearms are involved in 54% of all suicides in the United States.[13] Significant money and research has been dedicated to suicide prevention. Suicide programs focus on modifying risk factors and treating the underlying mental and substance-abuse disorders.

Homicide

In 2010, there were 12,996 murder victims in the United States. Seventy-seven percent of these were male, 50% were black, and 47% were white. Sixty-eight percent of the homicides included the use of a firearm, and 53% were conducted by someone the victim knew (family member, friend, acquaintance, significant other).[14] Unfortunately, homicide rates are not decreasing and homicide victims will continue to be a common patient population in trauma centers.

Penetrating trauma

Injuries due to firearms and stab wounds continue to plague younger, inner-city, African-American males. As stated above, firearms are very common in both suicide and homicide. Nonfatal firearm injuries are also common. In 2004, there were 64,389 persons treated in American hospitals for nonfatal gunshot injuries.[13] Males comprised 89% of these nonfatal injuries. Over 1.2 billion healthcare dollars were spent treating these injuries. Eighty percent of this money was borne by the public because the injured patient was not insured.[13]

Firearm-related injuries are determined by several factors. One of the main factors is the velocity of the bullet. High-velocity bullets (rifles) compared to low-velocity bullets (handguns) tend to cause more injury because of the amount of kinetic energy within the moving projectile being transferred to the tissues. Individual bullet ballistics (full metal jacket, hollow points, soft points) and trajectory can also help predict the injury severity. Blast injury away from the penetrating bullet must also be considered when evaluating a gunshot wound patient.

Although not as deadly as gunshot wounds, stab wounds carry a mortality of 1.5%. Stab wounds produce damage locally by blunt force and sharp cutting edges. Surrounding tissue damage is minimal. In 2007, approximately 2600 Americans died from violence-related stab wounds.[8]

Burn wounds

Burns remain a common traumatic injury, often requiring the extensive care of a dedicated burn unit (see Chapters 39 and 40). Most victims of fires die from smoke and toxic gas inhalation rather than from burns. Cigarette smoking remains a common cause of fire-related deaths, and cooking is the primary cause of residential house fires. In 2011, an estimated 450,000 burn patients received medical attention in the United States, with 45,000 requiring admission, and 3500 died. Forty-four percent of these burns were from flame and 33% were scalds. In 2005, burn injuries and deaths cost approximately $4 billion.[15]

Summary

Trauma should be viewed as a disease rather than a random accidental event. Traumatic injury continues to be the leading cause of death in patients aged 1–44. Worldwide, injury is responsible for 9% of deaths. Injuries also create a significant financial burden due to direct costs as well as the loss of productivity and wages from the permanently injured or deceased patient. Traumatic injuries can be broken down into unintentional (e.g., motor vehicle collisions, falls) and intentional (suicide and homicide) mechanisms. Injury patterns within these various mechanisms depend on the kinetic energy absorbed by the body and the direction the energy travels through the body. Motor vehicle collisions are the most common mechanism for traumatic fatalities, and falls are the most common mechanism for nonfatal injuries. Suicide and homicide continue to be important mechanisms of trauma, accounting for 26% of global mortality. A basic understanding of the epidemiology of traumatic disease is imperative if we wish to decrease the burden of this illness through education, legislation, and research.

Questions

(1) True or false? In 2009, injury was the leading cause of death for people aged 1–44 years.
(2) Which of the following is responsible for the greatest number of traumatic deaths?
   a. Suicide
   b. Firearm-related mortality
   c. Motor vehicle collisions
   d. Falls
(3) Approximately what percentage of all fatal motor vehicle collisions involve alcohol consumption?

a. 10%
b. 30%
c. 50%
d. 70%

(4) **In the United States, what is the most common cause of nonfatal injuries?**
a. Suicide attempts
b. Motor vehicle collisions
c. Falls
d. Firearms

(5) **What is the median lethal distance for falls (i.e., the fall height at which 50% of patients will die)?**
a. 1 story (12 feet)
b. 2 stories (24 feet)
c. 3 stories (36 feet)
d. 4 stories (48 feet)

(6) **Regarding suicide, which of the following is *false*?**
a. In 2009, suicide was the tenth most common cause of death within the United States
b. Substance abuse is a risk factor for suicide
c. Firearms are involved in 80% of suicide attempts
d. There are 11 suicide attempts for every 1 suicide death

(7) **True or false? Females are more likely to be killed in a homicide-related death than males.**

(8) **Which of the following are important considerations when determining injury patterns from firearm injuries?**
a. Velocity of the bullet
b. Trajectory of the bullet
c. Individual bullet ballistics
d. All of the above

(9) **The mortality of stab wounds is approximately:**
a. 1.5%
b. 5.5%
c. 10.5%
d. 25.5%

(10) **True or false? Most victims of fires die from smoke and toxic gas inhalation rather than from burns.**

Answers

(1) True
(2) c
(3) b
(4) c
(5) d
(6) c
(7) False
(8) d
(9) a
(10) True

References

1. McCoy AM, Como JJ, Greene G, Laskey SL, Claridge JA. A novel prospective approach to evaluate trauma recidivism: the concept of the past trauma history. *J Trauma Acute Care Surg* 2013; **75**: 116–21.

2. Centers for Disease Control and Prevention. 10 leading causes of death by age group, United States – 2009. National Vital Statistics System. Atlanta, GA: US Department of Health and Human Services, CDC, National Center for Injury Prevention and Control. http://www.cdc.gov/Injury/wisqars/pdf/10LCD-Age-Grp-US-2009-a.pdf (accessed July 2014).

3. Peden M, McGee K, Sharma G. *The Injury Chart Book: a Graphical Overview of the Global Burden of Injuries.* Geneva: World Health Organization. 2002.

4. Centers for Disease Control and Prevention. Web-based Injury Statistics Query and Reporting System (WISQARS). Atlanta, GA: US Department of Health and Human Services, 2002. http://www.cdc.gov/injury/wisqars (accessed July 2014).

5. Peden M. *World Report on Road Traffic Injury Prevention: Summary.* Geneva: World Health Organization, 2004.

6. US Department of Transportation. National Highway Traffic Safety Administration. Fatality Analysis Reporting System (FARS). http://www.nhtsa.gov/FARS (accessed July 2014).

7. Harris Interactive Health Day Poll. Most U.S. drivers engage in "distracting" behaviors: poll. November 30, 2011. http://www.harrisinteractive.com/vault/HI-HealthDay-Distracted-Driving-2011-11-30.pdf (accessed July 2014).

8. Varon AJ, Smith CE, eds. *Essentials of Trauma Anesthesia.* Cambridge: Cambridge University Press, 2012.

9. US Department of Transportation. National Highway Traffic Safety Administration. *National Pedestrian Crash Report*, 2008. http://www-nrd.nhtsa.dot.gov/Pubs/810968.pdf (accessed July 2014).

10. Centers for Disease Control and Prevention. Costs of falls among older adults. http://www.cdc.gov/HomeandRecreationalSafety/Falls/fallcost.html (accessed July 2014).

11. Rosen P, ed. *Emergency Medicine: Concepts and Clinical Practice*, 4th edition. St. Louis, MO: Mosby-Year Book, 1998: 352.

12. Lapostolle F, Gere C, Borron SW, *et al.* Prognostic factors in victims of falls from height. *Crit Care Med* 2005; **33**: 1239–42.

13. Feliciano DV, Mattox KL, Moore EE, eds. *Trauma*, 6th edition. New York, NY: McGraw Hill, 2008.

14. Federal Bureau of Investigation. Crime in the United States 2010. http://www.fbi.gov/about-us/cjis/ucr/crime-in-the-u.s/2010/crime-in-the-u.s.-2010/offenses-known-to-law-enforcement/expanded/expandhomicidemain (accessed July 2014).

15. American Burn Association. Burn incidence and treatment in the United States: 2013 fact sheet. http://www.ameriburn.org/resources_factsheet.php (accessed July 2014).

Chapter

2

Trauma in the prehospital environment and the emergency department

Sandra Werner

Objectives

(1) Describe the role of prehospital providers in the initial assessment/stabilization of trauma patients.

(2) List criteria for initial patient transport to a trauma center versus non-trauma-center emergency department (ED).

(3) Determine which patients in non-trauma-center EDs should be transferred to trauma centers.

(4) Describe the initial assessment and resuscitation of trauma patients in the ED.

(5) Discuss pain management and procedural sedation strategies for trauma patients in the ED.

Introduction

Injury mortality is classically described as having a trimodal distribution, with immediate deaths at the scene, early deaths due to airway obstruction and hemorrhage, and late deaths from organ failure. The second peak of trauma deaths occurs minutes to hours after the injury. Care given in the prehospital setting and in the emergency department (ED) is critical to reducing trauma mortality during this period (Fig. 2.1).

For most trauma victims, patient care commences with activation of the emergency medical services (EMS). Emergency medical responders are dispatched, arrive at the scene, and provide initial patient assessment and stabilization. Using protocols based on local and state trauma system requirements, patients are treated and transported to a local ED or trauma center.

Once in the ED, patients are reassessed and stabilized. Resuscitation measures are commenced or continued. For those trauma patients treated initially at freestanding EDs, or in EDs at smaller hospitals without the ability to provide trauma care, rapid transfer to a trauma center is usually indicated.

At the trauma center, patients are systematically reassessed in the ED by a dedicated trauma team. Airway management and initial resuscitation measures are continued, and the patient's further care is determined by the trauma team. Unstable patients requiring immediate surgical intervention go directly to the operating room (OR). However, most

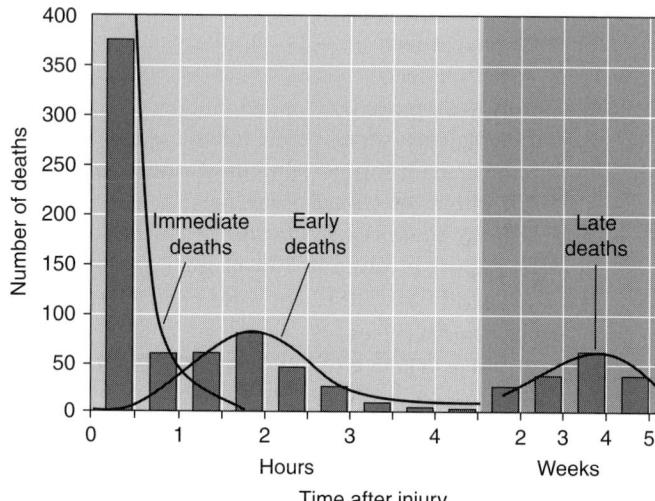

Figure 2.1 Graph demonstrating the three peaks of trauma deaths. (Reproduced with permission from American College of Surgeons. *Advanced Trauma Life Support, Student Manual*, 9th edition, 2012.[1])

trauma patients will require imaging and consultation by specialty surgeons prior to disposition. Of the patients who do not require immediate operative intervention, some are admitted to the intensive care unit (ICU), some to the floor, and some are discharged to home. A number of patients will undergo additional procedures or imaging requiring sedation in the ED, or requiring transport and sedation in the interventional radiology suite.

This chapter provides an overview of prehospital and ED trauma patient assessment and management.

Prehospital trauma care

Historical perspective

The white paper *Accidental Death and Disability: the Neglected Disease of Modern Society*, written by the Committee on Trauma and Committee on Shock of the National Academy of Sciences in 1966, identified injury as the leading cause of death in young persons, and pointed out serious weaknesses in the American EMS system, including the fact that half of the nation's ambulance services were provided by morticians. The paper made 29 recommendations for improving prehospital care.[2]

In the same year, the 1966 Highway Safety Act established the foundation for the United States' modern emergency medical system.[3] The newly created Department of Transportation was given authority to improve EMS, including establishing standards of training for prehospital providers, development of regional EMS systems, and requirements for ambulance equipment. Training for prehospital providers today is based on standard curricula provided by the National Highway Administration. Prehospital care of the trauma patient is also based on guidelines developed by the American College of Surgeons (ACS) and taught in prehospital trauma life support courses.

EMS systems have evolved differently in other countries. In the US, prehospital care is provided nearly exclusively by emergency medical technicians (EMTs) and paramedics. In contrast, in the European model, physicians often make up part of the prehospital care team.

In the US, there are four levels of prehospital providers, first responder, EMT-basic, EMT-intermediate/advanced, and paramedic. Most ambulances are staffed primarily by EMTs or paramedics. Many rural EMS services are provided solely by volunteer basic EMTs. Most urban systems are staffed primarily by paramedics. A brief summary of the allowable scope of practice of EMTs versus paramedics is provided in Table 2.1.[4]

The exact scope of practice for prehospital providers is defined by a physician medical director, under whose license they practice. Advanced airway management and medication administration must be sanctioned by the medical director.

The goals of prehospital trauma care are the rapid assessment, stabilization, and transport of patients with potentially serious traumatic injuries to the appropriate trauma facility for definitive care. The steps of prehospital care are briefly outlined below.

On-scene trauma care

In some cases, care of the trauma patient commences upon the arrival of EMS. However, there are often delays in the initiation of care due to scene safety and patient access issues. If a patient is accessible but requires extrication, resuscitative measures including basic airway intervention, hemorrhage control, immobilization, administration of fluids and pain medication, and prevention of hypothermia may be attempted.

Table 2.2 lists some of the causes of delay in reaching the trauma patient in common trauma scenarios.

Once the scene has been deemed safe and the patient has been reached, prehospital providers rapidly assess, provide critical interventions, and transfer the patient to an appropriate facility in accordance with prehospital trauma life support principles. Basic and advanced prehospital interventions are discussed below.

Table 2.1 Basic emergency medical technician (EMT) and paramedic interventions

Intervention	Basic EMT	Additional paramedic interventions
Airway	Assessment Suction Bag valve mask ventilation Oral and nasal airway adjuncts Supplemental oxygen	Noninvasive positive-pressure ventilation Tracheal intubation Alternative airways Percutaneous cricothyroidotomy Needle chest decompression
Resuscitation	Hemorrhage control	IV access IO access IV fluid administration
Immobilization	Cervical collar Spinal immobilization Extremity and/or pelvic splinting Emergency patient moves	
Medications	Assist patient with own medications Administer oral glucose	Parenteral administration of ACLS medications, opioids, and antiepileptic medications, as well as anxiolytics RSI drugs in some cases
Defibrillation	Automated external defibrillation	Manual defibrillation 12-lead ECG acquisition Cardioversion Pacing

ACLS, advanced cardiac life support; ECG, electrocardiogram; IO, intraosseous; IV, intravenous; RSI, rapid sequence induction/intubation.

Airway

Prehospital providers initiate basic airway measures, including oxygenation and ventilation, suction, and oral/nasal airways as needed (see Chapter 3). In-line stabilization of the cervical spine is maintained when indicated. Prehospital providers may also perform life-saving measures including needle decompression of tension pneumothoraces, placement of chest seals for open pneumothoraces, and stabilization of flail chest segments.

Advanced airway management may be initiated in the prehospital environment. The current Eastern Association for the Surgery of Trauma (EAST) level 1 guidelines for emergency endotracheal intubation in trauma patients are listed in Table 2.3.[5]

Studies of prehospital trauma intubations have yielded mixed results. Some studies have reported very high success rates in prehospital intubations, especially when paralytics are routinely used.[6,7] An early study in 1997 demonstrated

Table 2.2 Factors contributing to delayed initiation of patient care in the field

Mechanism	Causes of delay
Motor vehicle collision	Fire Power wires/poles Prolonged vehicle extrication Location of vehicle in unsafe area Weather extremes
Falls in outdoor areas	Location of fall Accessing area Equipment set-up Specialty rescue teams Weather extremes
Industrial or construction injuries	Chemical contamination Physical/equipment hazards Need for specialized rescue equipment Weather extremes
Terrorist incident	Scene safety Secondary device Patient contamination
Mass casualty incidents	Multiple patient access Triage of multiple patients Availability of transportation resources Coordination of patient disposition

Table 2.3 Eastern Association for the Surgery of Trauma (EAST) level 1 indications for emergency tracheal intubation of the trauma patient

Airway obstruction
Hypoventilation
Persistent hypoxemia ($SaO_2 < 90$ despite supplemental oxygen)
Severe cognitive impairment (GCS $\leq$ 8)
Severe hemorrhagic shock
Cardiac Arrest

GCS, Glasgow Coma Scale (see Table 35.1); SaO_2, oxygen saturation.

improved outcomes in patients with severe head injury intubated in the field,[8] but several other studies demonstrated increased mortality in moderately and severely head-injured patients intubated during the prehospital phase of care.[9–11] The single study using computed tomography (CT) criteria for determination of head injury found that there was no difference in outcome in patients with Glasgow Coma Scale score (GCS) < 8, head injury on CT, and intubation in the field or ED (see Chapter 35, Table 35.1 for GCS).[12] The only prospective study of prehospital intubations was done in the pediatric population and demonstrated no improvement in outcomes in trauma patients intubated in the field.[13]

All of these studies have significant limitations, and there is no conclusive evidence to recommend for or against prehospital trauma intubation. Systems with the highest success rates have in common stringent training and skill maintenance requirements, including live OR intubations.[14] Prehospital trauma airway protocols should include the use of rescue airways such as the King LT, laryngeal mask airway, or Combitube.

Hemorrhage control

Uncontrolled hemorrhage is the second leading cause of death for civilian trauma and the leading cause of combat mortality.[15] Immediate identification and control of external hemorrhage is a major goal of prehospital trauma care.

Basic hemorrhage control in the prehospital environment consists of application of direct pressure, use of pressure points, and application of pressure dressings. Hemorrhage control is also achieved through reduction of angulated fractures and binding of open-book pelvic fractures.

Tourniquet use in civilian EMS systems is not common, because of concerns of increased morbidity and mortality. However, recent combat studies have demonstrated that tourniquets have low morbidity and improve outcomes when applied early (see Chapter 38).[16,17] Current Prehospital Trauma Life Support treatment guidelines recommend tourniquet use prior to extrication and transport if direct pressure and a pressure dressing fail to control bleeding.[18] A number of commercially available pelvic binders exist for compression of open-book pelvic fractures.

Resuscitation

Resuscitation measures initiated in the field depend on level of training and local protocols. Most trauma protocols currently call for initiation of two large-bore IVs and administration of crystalloid fluid (see Chapters 4 and 5). However, evidence is emerging that administration of crystalloid solely to maintain blood pressure (BP), particularly in penetrating trauma, may be harmful.[19,20] The most recent revision of the Advanced Trauma Life Support (ATLS) guidelines for prehospital treatment has reduced the amount of crystalloid to be infused from 2 L to 1 L.[1]

Current ATLS guidelines call for initial resuscitation with lactated Ringer's (LR) with 0.9% saline (NS) as an alternative.[21] However, many EMS systems use 0.9% NS exclusively, as it is compatible with medication administration and reduces costs associated with deploying two types of crystalloid.

Colloids are not generally administered in the prehospital environment. In addition, while the use of hypertonic saline (HTS) in early resuscitation showed initial promise, two large studies were stopped early due to lack of benefits, and the ninth-edition ATLS guidelines do not recommend HTS.[1,21,22]

Because of the strict storage and administration requirements, blood products are not commonly administered in the prehospital environment. However, a growing number of aeromedical transport services are carrying O negative blood, and a few carry plasma. Third-generation hemoglobin-based oxygen carriers have been studied in the prehospital environment, but none has been shown to improve outcomes.[23]

Immobilization

All prehospital providers are trained in spinal, pelvis, and extremity immobilization. Most blunt trauma patients will be fully immobilized with C-collar and long backboard for transport. Airway control is accomplished with manual in-line C-spine control. Patients arriving in the ED must be removed from long spine boards as soon as possible to prevent skin breakdown.

Additional EMS interventions

History taking is critical in the prehospital phase of trauma care. EMTs or paramedics may be the only healthcare providers with the opportunity to obtain the patient's medical history, allergies, and medications in a deteriorating trauma patient.

In addition, prehospital providers obtain critical information about the mechanism of injury. In falls, this information may include the height of the fall, position of patient, and type of surface struck. For motor vehicle collisions (MVCs), critical information includes vehicle speed, vehicle damage, position of the patient in the vehicle, restraints, and if the patient was ejected. Many EMS units carry cameras and provide scene photos.

Pain management may be initiated in the prehospital environment. Paramedics may administer narcotics in accordance with local protocols, and many services carry morphine or fentanyl.

Prehospital termination of efforts

The American College of Surgeons (ACS) Committee on Trauma (COT) and National Association of EMS Physicians (NAEMSP) developed a joint guideline for the withholding and terminating resuscitation in trauma patients who are in cardiopulmonary arrest (see Chapter 42, Table 42.4).[24] Most EMS systems have developed local protocols implementing these guidelines.

Initial transport of the trauma patient

Prehospital providers must field triage patients for transport to the closest hospital or to a trauma center based on patient condition, mechanism of injury, distance, road and air conditions, and additional factors. The ACS COT, in conjunction with the Centers for Disease Control and Prevention (CDC), has developed guidelines to assist prehospital providers with these decisions. The 2011 prehospital guidelines for triage to a trauma center are provided in Figure 2.2.[25]

Patients may be transported by ground unit or by aeromedical services. In most urban areas, ground units transport directly to the nearest trauma center. For remote trauma, EMS may transport to the closest local hospital, where the patient can be stabilized before transport to a trauma center, or,

alternatively, the patient may be transported directly from the scene by an aeromedical transport team.

Aeromedical transport, particularly by helicopter, has become more common in the past 20 years. Helicopter medical crews are usually experienced paramedics and/or nurses, and sometimes a physician. Crews are often trained in advanced airway management, including rapid sequence induction/ intubation (RSI) and cricothyroidotomy. They may be trained in tube thoracostomy, limited ultrasound, central line placement, and administration of blood products. A number of studies, including a recent very large retrospective study, have found that helicopter transport of trauma patients reduces mortality, except in cases of traumatic cardiac arrest.[26,27]

Aeromedical transport is both expensive and a limited resource. Determining the appropriateness of ground versus helicopter transportation of trauma patients should take into account logistical and patient conditions. Helicopter transport may be indicated when ground transport times are lengthy and when extrication times exceed 20 minutes. The NAEMSP guidelines for patient conditions warranting consideration of aeromedical transport are provided in Table 2.4.[28]

Emergency department care

Trauma patients may initially be transported either to a trauma-center ED or to a non-trauma-center ED. Patients with minor trauma may be fully treated at non-trauma centers. However, in patients with significant traumatic injuries that have the potential to exceed the capabilities of the non-trauma hospital, expeditious transfer to a trauma center is indicated. One recent study found that mortality is improved with transfer to a Level I rather than Level II center.[29] The ACS COT criteria for inter-facility transfer are provided in Table 2.5.

Assessment and treatment of the trauma patient in non-trauma-center EDs should be in guided by the principles of ATLS, with rapid assessment and stabilization, including essential airway, hemorrhage control, and resuscitative measures. For patients meeting trauma-center transfer criteria, imaging and laboratory studies should be minimized and should not delay transfer to the trauma center. The emergency physician (EP) at the outlying facility must communicate pertinent information, including exam findings and any interventions performed, to the receiving trauma center.

Trauma-center emergency department initial assessment

Dedicated ED trauma teams are generally composed of trauma surgeons, anesthesiologists, EPs, and other surgical subspecialties, as well as nurses, technicians, and ancillary personnel. Many trauma centers are academic hospitals, and residents in emergency medicine, surgery, surgery subspecialties, and anesthesiology may be make up the majority of the trauma team.

Advanced planning, preparation, and anticipation of patient conditions and injuries are critical to optimal

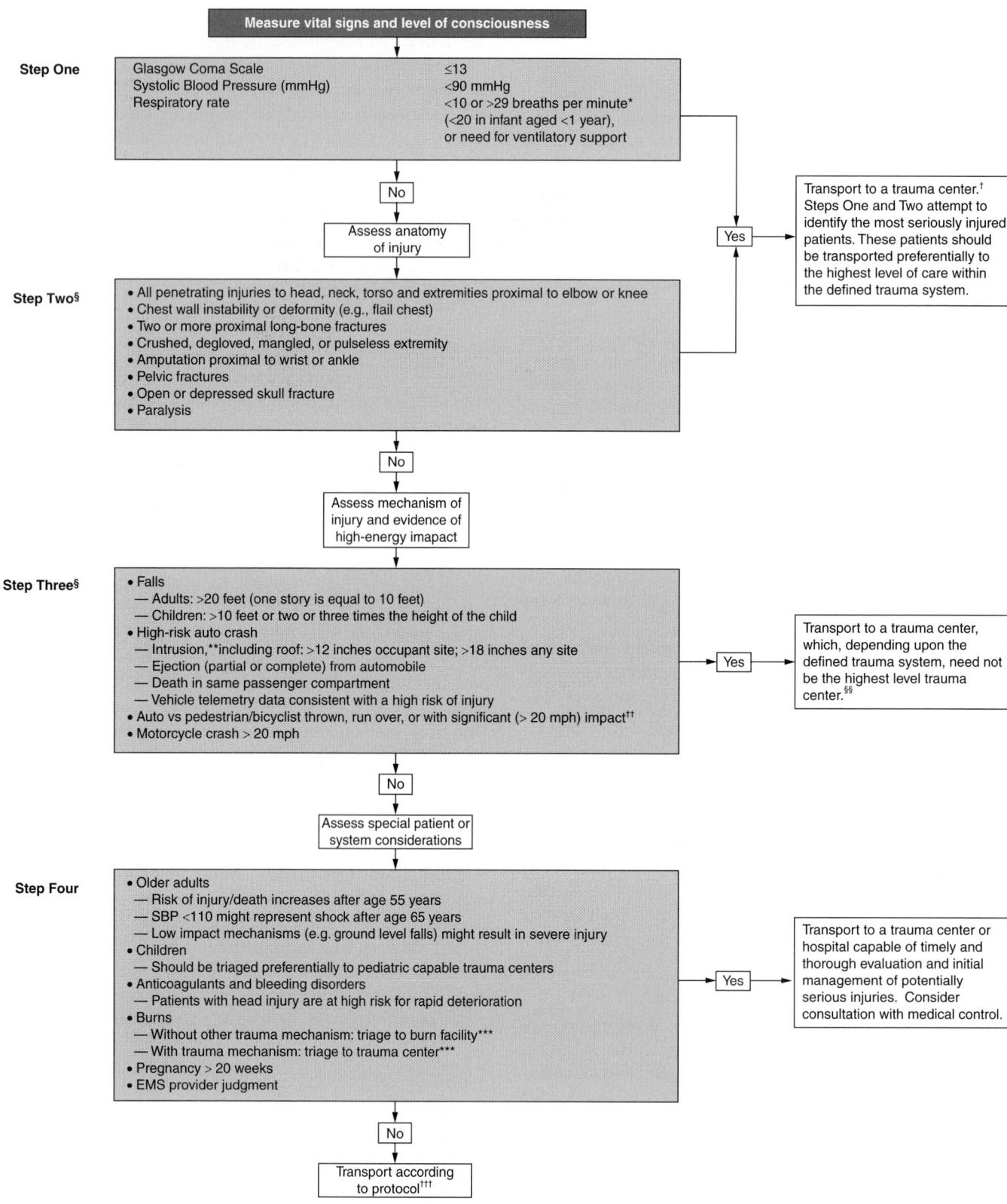

Measure vital signs and level of consciousness

Step One

Glasgow Coma Scale	≤13
Systolic Blood Pressure (mmHg)	<90 mmHg
Respiratory rate	<10 or >29 breaths per minute* (<20 in infant aged <1 year), or need for ventilatory support

No → Assess anatomy of injury

Yes → Transport to a trauma center.† Steps One and Two attempt to identify the most seriously injured patients. These patients should be transported preferentially to the highest level of care within the defined trauma system.

Step Two§

- All penetrating injuries to head, neck, torso and extremities proximal to elbow or knee
- Chest wall instability or deformity (e.g., flail chest)
- Two or more proximal long-bone fractures
- Crushed, degloved, mangled, or pulseless extremity
- Amputation proximal to wrist or ankle
- Pelvic fractures
- Open or depressed skull fracture
- Paralysis

No → Assess mechanism of injury and evidence of high-energy imapact

Step Three§

- Falls
  — Adults: >20 feet (one story is equal to 10 feet)
  — Children: >10 feet or two or three times the height of the child
- High-risk auto crash
  — Intrusion,** including roof: >12 inches occupant site; >18 inches any site
  — Ejection (partial or complete) from automobile
  — Death in same passenger compartment
  — Vehicle telemetry data consistent with a high risk of injury
- Auto vs pedestrian/bicyclist thrown, run over, or with significant (> 20 mph) impact††
- Motorcycle crash > 20 mph

Yes → Transport to a trauma center, which, depending upon the defined trauma system, need not be the highest level trauma center.§§

No → Assess special patient or system considerations

Step Four

- Older adults
  — Risk of injury/death increases after age 55 years
  — SBP <110 might represent shock after age 65 years
  — Low impact mechanisms (e.g. ground level falls) might result in severe injury
- Children
  — Should be triaged preferentially to pediatric capable trauma centers
- Anticoagulants and bleeding disorders
  — Patients with head injury are at high risk for rapid deterioration
- Burns
  — Without other trauma mechanism: triage to burn facility***
  — With trauma mechanism: triage to trauma center***
- Pregnancy > 20 weeks
- EMS provider judgment

Yes → Transport to a trauma center or hospital capable of timely and thorough evaluation and initial management of potentially serious injuries. Consider consultation with medical control.

No → Transport according to protocol†††

When in doubt, transport to a trauma center

Figure 2.2 Flow chart for prehospital trauma triage. (Reproduced with permission from the Centers for Disease Control and Prevention, 2012.[25])

Table 2.4 Considerations for aeromedical transport (NAEMSP)

General considerations	Trauma score < 12 Unstable vital signs Significant trauma < 12 or > 55 years Pregnancy Multisystem injuries
Mechanistic considerations	Ejection from vehicle Pedestrian or cyclist struck Falls from significant heights
Injury types	Penetrating trauma to chest, abdomen, pelvis, neck or head Crush injuries to the abdomen, chest or head
Additional considerations	Significant damage to passenger compartment Death in same passenger compartment

Table 2.5 Interhospital trauma transfer criteria

Category	Specific injury or other criteria
Central nervous system	Head injury: penetrating wound, depressed skull fracture, open injury with or without CSF leak, GCS < 15 or neurologically abnormal, lateralizing signs Spinal cord injury or major vertebral injury
Chest	Widened mediastinum or other indication of great vessel injury, major chest wall injury or pulmonary contusion, cardiac injury, patients who may require prolonged ventilation
Abdomen/pelvis	Unstable pelvic ring disruption, pelvic ring disruption with shock or evidence of ongoing hemorrhage, open pelvic injury, solid organ injury
Extremities	Severe open fractures, traumatic amputation with possibility of replantation, complex articular fractures, major crush injuries, ischemia
Multisystem injuries	Head injury with face, chest, abdominal or pelvic injury, Injury to more than two body regions, major burns or burns with associated injuries, multiple proximal long-bone fractures
Comorbid factors	Age > 55 or < 5 years, cardiac or respiratory disease, insulin-dependent diabetes, morbid obesity, pregnancy, immunosuppression
Secondary deterioration (late sequelae)	Mechanical ventilation required, respiratory disease, single or multiple organ system failure (deterioration in CNS, cardiac, pulmonary, hepatic, renal or coagulation systems), major tissue necrosis

CNS, central nervous system; CSF, cerebrospinal fluid; GCS, Glasgow Coma Scale.
Adapted with permission from American College of Surgeons Committee on Trauma. *Resources for Optimal Care of the Injured Patient: 2006.* Chicago, IL: ACS, 2006.

resuscitation of the trauma patient. A trauma surgeon or EP is generally the trauma team leader. Roles, responsibilities, and tasks of each trauma team member should be defined prior to the patient's arrival. Personnel and all necessary equipment and medications should be in place prior to the patient's arrival as well. Table 2.6 provides a list of supplies that should be in the resuscitation area or readily available.

Transfer of care: the handoff

The handoff is a brief but critical exchange of crucial patient information between the prehospital and ED trauma teams. Key information provided includes: time and mechanism of the injury, extrication time, initial patient condition, prehospital interventions and patient response, treatment at an outside hospital, the patient's past medical history, and medications/allergies. The information must be accurately delivered and received (Fig. 2.3).

Patient assessment

Whether in a trauma center or rural ED, trauma patient assessment generally follows ATLS guidelines. The primary survey is a rapid evaluation of the ABCs, which is interrupted only for critical interventions.

Primary survey

Airway – The airway is assessed for patency, facial trauma, secretions, and neck trauma, as well as expected difficulties with intubation or ventilation. If the trachea is already intubated, tube placement must be confirmed by direct visualization or quantitative end-tidal carbon dioxide (CO_2) measurement and assessment of lung sounds.

Breathing – The adequacy of ventilation is assessed, including auscultation, inspection of the chest wall for contusions, crepitation, penetrating trauma, symmetry, and adequacy of chest rise. If intubated, adequacy of oxygenation and ventilation should be confirmed.

Circulation – Circulation is assessed including central and peripheral pulses, skin color, temperature, BP, and pulse rate. The focused assessment with sonography for trauma (FAST) exam may be completed during the initial assessment of circulation in unstable patients to determine the source of bleeding (see Chapter 10).

Disability – Disability is assessed by the GCS (see Chapter 35, Table 35.1), pupillary response, and movement/ sensation in all extremities, to the extent testable.

Exposure – The patient is fully exposed to briefly inspect for additional severe injuries, including evaluation of the back, particularly in penetrating trauma.

Table 2.6 Recommended supplies immediately available for trauma patient care

Airway	Standard airway box Oxygen masks, tubing Difficult airway cart/box Suction NG/OG tubes
Resuscitation	Warmed crystalloid IV fluids and tubing Large-bore angiocatheters, IV start kits, blood tubes Blood/plasma Rapid infuser
Procedural supplies	Thoracostomy Thoracotomy Trauma central line Sterile towels Betadine/chlorhexidene Sutures/staples/Raney clips
Medications	RSI medications Narcotic pain medications Nalaxone Antiemetic Antiepileptic Sedatives
Additional supplies	Portable ultrasound Warm blankets Convective warming system Foley catheter (temperature-sensing if available)

IV, intravenous; NG, nasogastric; OG, orogastric; RSI, rapid sequence induction/intubation

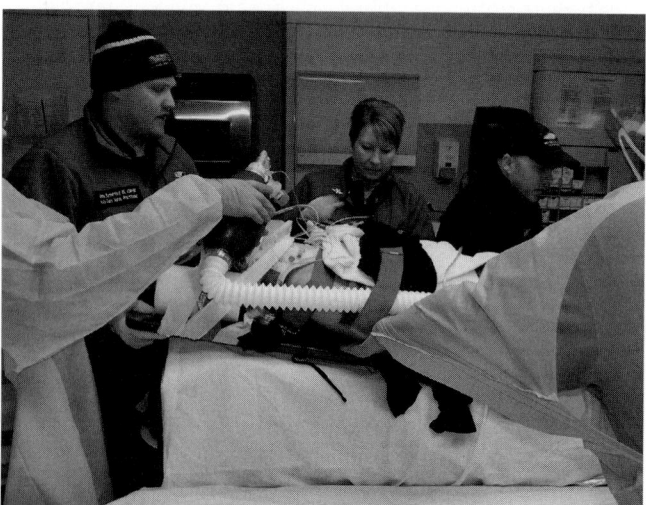

Figure 2.3 The handoff: prehospital providers give report as a patient's care is transitioned to the trauma team.

Only life-saving interventions are performed in the primary survey. Table 2.7 lists the interventions indicated during the primary survey.

Table 2.7 Interventions performed in the primary survey

Survey component	Intervention
Airway	Oxygen, suction, oral airway, tracheal intubation if immediately indicated (see Tables 2.3 and 2.8)
Breathing	Ventilatory assistance Needle chest decompression (followed by chest tube after primary survey) Occlusion of open pneumothorax Flail chest stabilization
Resuscitation	Intravenous access Fluid/blood administration Hemorrhage control Pericardiocentesis Emergency department thoracotomy

Unstable patients with obvious thoraco-abdominal bleeding may be taken directly to the OR without completion of the secondary survey. The patient must be completely examined by the admitting team once surgical control of hemorrhage has been achieved.

In patients with suspected severe traumatic brain injury (TBI) with GCS ≤ 8, especially with signs of impending herniation, procedures that do not specifically correct a problem identified in the primary survey should be deferred until after CT of the head is obtained. This allows for early identification of patients who will benefit from surgical intracerebral hematoma evacuation.

Secondary survey

The secondary survey is a head-to-toe examination of the trauma patient to evaluate for further evidence of trauma. Specific physical findings of trauma, listed by anatomic region, may include:

Head – scalp and facial lacerations, skull and facial fractures, oral and dental trauma, evidence of basilar skull fractures such as raccoon eyes and battle signs (bruising behind the ears), hemotympanum, or cerebrospinal fluid (CSF) rhinorrhea/otorrhea.

Neck – hematomas, crepitance, lacerations, cervical spine tenderness, or step-offs. (The neck is briefly examined with the cervical collar open while a member of the trauma team holds in-line stabilization.)

Chest – lack of chest wall excursion, asymmetry, ecchymosis, open wounds, crepitance, subcutaneous air, decreased lung sounds.

Abdomen – contusions – including of the flank, erythema, open wounds, tenderness, peritoneal signs.

Back – ecchymosis, open wounds, spinal tenderness. (In order to assess the back, the patient is log-rolled, maintaining in-line stabilization.)

Extremities – deformities, tenderness, lacerations, evidence of open fractures, edema, diminished or unequal pulses.

Genitourinary (GU) – genital bruising, lacerations, blood at the urethral meatus. A rectal exam is done in unresponsive patients to evaluate for reflexes and tone and to evaluate for a high-riding prostate. A Foley catheter may be placed at this time, if there is no suspicion of urethral injury.

Central nervous system (CNS) – unequal or absent pupillary response, focal neurologic deficits, loss of reflexes. In patients with suspected spinal injury, the level of sensory and motor deficits should be documented.

At the conclusion of the primary survey, trauma labs may be sent, as indicated. For most trauma patients this includes type and screen, complete blood count, electrolytes, renal function, and coagulation panel. A beta human chorionic gonadotropin (β-hCG) is indicated in women of childbearing age. A hepatic function panel and amylase/lipase should be obtained for suspected abdominal trauma. An arterial blood gas (ABG) should be sent for intubated patients. An alcohol level and toxicology screen as well as blood glucose level is indicated for patients with altered mental status. An initial lactate is useful to guide resuscitation efforts. Of note, bloods drawn in the field can be used for most laboratory studies but will result in a falsely elevated lactate. Cardiac enzymes and an electrocardiogram (ECG) are indicated in the elderly, and in patients with chest trauma.

Limited plain film imaging in the trauma bay may be obtained, if indicated (e.g., chest and pelvic x-rays). At the completion of the secondary survey, further imaging and testing, consultations, and patient disposition are determined by the trauma team. Tetanus status is updated and IV antibiotics given as indicated for open fractures.

Interventions during the ED assessment

Airway management

Supplemental oxygen is indicated for all trauma patients. The EAST level 1 recommendations for immediate intubation are provided in Table 2.3. Additional indications (level 3) are provided in Table 2.8.[5]

RSI is the preferred method for ED trauma intubations. Until recently, direct laryngoscopy (with manual in-line stabilization as indicated) was recommended as the first line for trauma intubations. However, recent studies have concluded that video laryngoscopy improves glottic visualization with stabilization, and may be preferred over direct laryngoscopy.[5] Awake fiberoptic intubation may be indicated (see Chapter 3).

Succinylcholine is currently recommended as the first-line paralytic for RSI, except in cases where hyperkalemia is likely, in which case rocuronium is the drug of choice (see Chapter 13).[5] There is no current recommendation for sedative medication. Etomidate or ketamine are good choices in hypotensive patients (see Chapter 7). Midazolam and propofol should be used with caution in hypovolemic patients.

Table 2.8 Additional indications for emergency tracheal intubation

Facial or neck injury with potential airway obstruction
Moderate cognitive impairment (GCS 9–12)
Persistent combativeness refractory to pharmacologic agents
Respiratory distress
Preoperative management (i.e., patients with painful injuries or undergoing painful procedures before nonemergent operation)
Spinal cord injury with evidence of respiratory insufficiency
Burns with evidence of inhalation injury, facial, chest, and neck burns interfering with ventilation

GCS, Glasgow Coma Scale.

Utilization of a standard RSI protocol with limited medication choices has been shown to decrease the time to intubation and increase success.[30]

Airway management in trauma centers may be the responsibility of anesthesiologists or EPs, both of whom have been shown to be proficient at trauma airway management.[31–33]

The keys to successful airway management in the trauma patient are: anticipation of the difficult airway, adequate assessment and preparation, proficiency in direct laryngoscopy (DL) and alternative techniques, including video-assisted intubation, use of a gum elastic bougie, placement and exchange of rescue airways with endotracheal tube (ETT), and cricothyroidotomy.

Coordination of the timing of trauma intubations in centers where anesthesiologists are not present in the trauma bay during the initial resuscitation is essential. For patients requiring operative care but without an urgent indication for intubation, it may be preferable to delay intubation until the patient is in the OR suite.

Hemorrhage control and resuscitation

Control of external hemorrhage, if not achieved in the prehospital phase, must be immediately accomplished in the ED. Primary sites of external hemorrhage include scalp lacerations, neck wounds, and arterial or venous extremity bleeding. Significant hemorrhage is possible from scalp lacerations with arterial or venous bleeding, and this should be controlled early in the resuscitation. Temporary control of arterial bleeding from extremities can usually be achieved with a manual BP cuff. Once hemostasis is achieved, the source of bleeding can be identified and ligated in the ED, or the tourniquet may be left on until the patient is in the OR.

Primary sources of internal hemorrhage are the thoracic and abdominal cavities, pelvis, and femur fractures. Unstable patients with thoraco-abdominal bleeding are best treated with immediate operative intervention. Open-book pelvic fractures (Fig. 2.4) should be bound with either a commercial device or a properly applied sheet secured with a large hemostat or clamp.

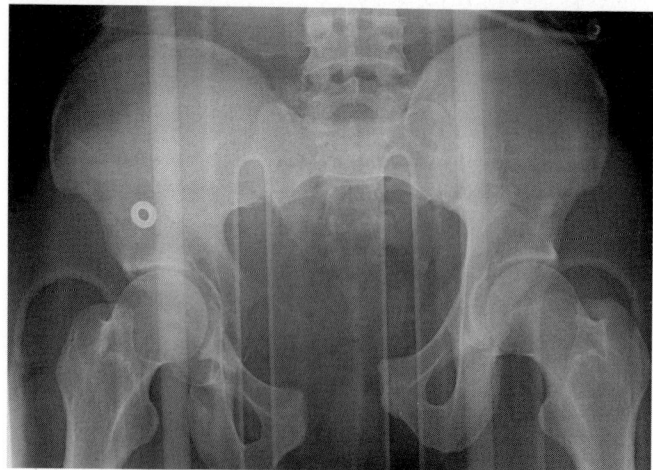

Figure 2.4 AP pelvis film demonstrating open-book pelvis fracture.

If not already accomplished in the prehospital environment, adequate vascular access must be obtained. Two short, large-bore peripheral intravenous catheters placed in the antecubital fossa are the preferred access for initial resuscitation. If peripheral access is not possible, large-bore central lines may be placed (see Chapter 5). Femoral line placement should be avoided if inferior vena cava (IVC) injury is suspected. In children under 6 years of age, intraosseous (IO) access is preferred to central line placement if peripheral access is not rapidly obtained (see Chapter 34).[1] IO access may also be temporarily used in adult patients.

The goal of ED resuscitation is to restore organ perfusion. ATLS currently recommends 1 L (20 mL/kg in pediatric patients) of warmed crystalloid solutions for initial resuscitation.[1] *This total includes fluid given in the prehospital environment.* Early administration of blood products in the ED is recommended for patients who do not respond or who respond only transiently to limited crystalloids.

In blunt trauma with suspected head injury, the goal is to prevent hypotension and thus cerebral hypoperfusion. However, recent studies in patients with penetrating trauma suggest that delayed or limited fluid resuscitation until the source of hemorrhage is controlled may prevent rebleeding and decrease mortality.[34,35] In addition, rapid transfusion protocols, including fresh frozen plasma (FFP) and platelets as well as red blood cells, have been shown to increase survival in patients with massive hemorrhage (see Chapter 6).[36,37]

A recently developed fibrinolytic agent, tranexamic acid (TXA), has shown promise in the reduction of mortality if it is administered within an hour after the onset of hemorrhage.[38,39] Tranexamic acid is easy to administer, does not have strict storage requirements, and has its greatest benefit if administered within the first hour. The presence of anticoagulants may complicate hemorrhage control and resuscitation efforts. Many patients over age 50 are on antiplatelet therapy or warfarin. While platelets and plasma/vitamin K may be useful in reversing the effects of these medications, the introduction of new anticoagulants, including direct thrombin inhibitors and factor Xa inhibitors, presents a challenge to resuscitation efforts in the immediate care of the trauma patient.

Identification and treatment of life-threatening thoracic injuries

Immediately life-threatening thoracic injuries include tension pneumothorax, massive hemothorax, and pericardial tamponade. Early ED treatment of each of these conditions is discussed below.

Tension pneumothorax

Identification and treatment of tension pneumonthorax during the primary survey is critical. Physical exam findings include decreased breath sounds and hyperresonance on the affected side, shock, distended neck veins, respiratory distress, tracheal deviation away from the injury, or increased resistance to ventilatory support. Immediate treatment of the tension pneumothorax is needle decompression with placement of a long, large-bore needle in the second intercostal space at the midclavicular line. Needle decompression must be followed by chest tube placement.

Open pneumothorax

Open chest wounds as small as 2–3 cm in diameter may result in a sucking chest wound. Closing the wound with a three-sided occlusive dressing will prevent formation of a tension pneumothorax. A large-bore chest tube should be placed at a location away from the injury site.

Massive hemothorax

Hemothorax identified by chest x-ray, extended FAST (EFAST) exam (see Chapter 10), or physical exam should prompt placement of a chest tube in the trauma bay. Immediate output of 1500 mL constitutes a massive hemothorax, and preparations should be made for immediate operative repair. If available, the blood may be collected in a cell-saver for autotransfusion (Fig. 2.5).

Pericardial tamponade

The pericardial sac is tough and fibrous, and even a small amount of blood can significantly compromise cardiac function. Penetrating trauma is the most common cause of pericardial tamponade, but it can occur with blunt thoracic trauma (see Chapters 29 and 30). Physical findings include the classic Beck's triad – hypotension, distended neck veins, and muffled heart tones. However, neck veins may be flat in the presence of hypovolemia, and muffled heart sounds may be difficult to detect in the trauma bay. Ultrasound has been shown to be 90–95% sensitive in detecting pericardial effusion and is indicated if pericardial effusion/tamponade is suspected (see Chapter 10).[40]

Definitive treatment of tamponade is evacuation of the pericardial blood and repair of the injury, preferably in the

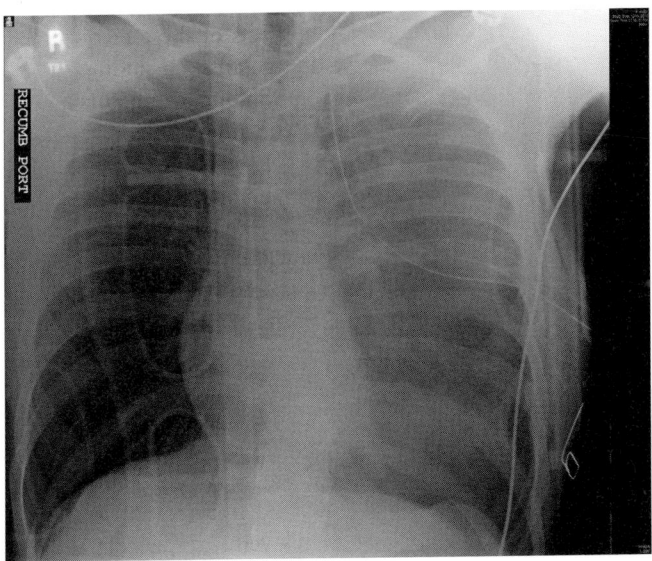

Figure 2.5 AP chest x-ray demonstrating massive left sided hemothorax with chest tube in place.

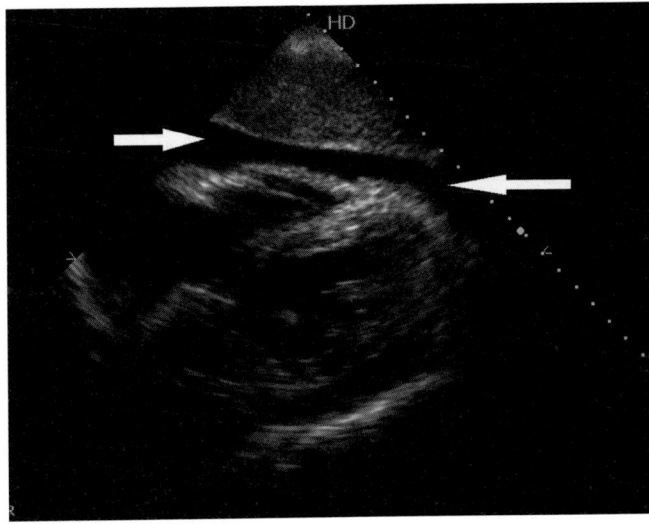

Figure 2.6 Cardiac FAST window with large pericardial effusion (arrows).

OR. If a qualified surgeon is not available, pericardiocentesis can be performed as a temporizing measure. ED thoracotomy may be required if the pericardial fluid is clotted or the patient deteriorates rapidly (Fig. 2.6).

Traumatic arrest

Most EMS systems have protocols for field pronouncement protocols for pulseless trauma patients with obvious nonsurvivable injuries. However, occasionally trauma patients will lose vital signs with paramedics on scene, en route to the hospital, or in the emergency department.

ED thoracotomy is indicated for only a select few of these patients and should only be conducted if a qualified surgeon is present at the time of the patient's arrival in the ED and an OR is immediately available. According to ATLS guidelines, only patients with penetrating traumatic injuries receiving cardiopulmonary resuscitation (CPR) should be evaluated for thoracotomy. Only patients with signs of life and/or cardiac activity are candidates for thoracotomy.[1] The Western Trauma Society expands slightly on these indications, and includes blunt trauma patients with < 10 minutes of CPR as potential candidates for ED thoracotomy.[41]

Immediate tracheal intubation and ventilation as well as volume resuscitation are essential during the thoracotomy. Massive transfusion protocols (MTPs) should be initiated if the decision is made to proceed with thoracotomy. Measures taken during resuscitative thoracotomy include evacuation of pericardial blood, cardiac massage, cardiac or thoracic vessel hemorrhage control, and crossclamping of the aorta to prevent infradiaphragmatic blood loss. Once damage control has been achieved in the ED, the OR must be ready to receive the patient for further surgical treatment.

Imaging and additional testing during the ED trauma evaluation (see also Chapter 11)

Imaging during the ED evaluation of trauma patients may include the use of plain films, ultrasound, CT, and occasionally magnetic resonance imaging (MRI), angiography, and additional imaging modalities.

Plain films

Plain films which may be obtained in the trauma bay include anterior–posterior (AP) chest and pelvic x-rays, cervical spine (C-spine) x-rays, and scout films of fractured extremities. Films may be obtained after the primary or secondary survey.

C-spine plain films may be obtained in the trauma bay but have been shown to miss at least 15% of fractures,[42] and imaging of the C-spine is often deferred until the patient is in CT.

Chest x-ray may be helpful in identifying pneumo- or hemothorax, pulmonary contusions, evidence of aortic rupture, and endotracheal and nasogastric tube placement. Ultrasound is superior to supine chest x-ray for detection of pneumothorax.[43]

AP pelvis films are indicated in polysystem trauma, especially in patients who were not ambulatory on scene to diagnose unstable pelvic fractures and proximal femur fracture and dislocation.

In penetrating trauma, plain films are often useful to help locate bullets/bullet fragments and assist with prediction of the bullet track. In stable patients, initial films of deformed extremities may be obtained to evaluate the extent of a fracture and delineate further imaging requirements.

Ultrasound (see also Chapter 10)

Ultrasound may be used during the primary survey or secondary survey, and for procedural guidance. During the primary survey, the EFAST exam may identify causes of profound shock including tamponade, large-volume hemothorax or hemoperitoneum, and tension pneumothorax. In stable patients, the FAST exam may be deferred until the secondary survey, or may not be utilized if CT is readily available. In stable patients, EFAST results may be useful in triaging patients awaiting CT scan or identification of occult pneumothoraces. Ultrasound is recommended for central line placement as well.

Computed tomography (see also Chapter 11)

Most polysystem trauma patients not requiring immediate operative intervention undergo extensive CT scanning as part of the ED evaluation. Helical CT scanners in most trauma centers are within or adjacent to the ED, but they still require patients to leave the trauma bay. Patients going to CT scan must have a secure airway and be sedated if appropriate. Qualified staff, including a physician for critical patients, should be immediately available during CT. Patients with suspected closed head injury should have end-tidal CO_2 monitoring.

Additional modalities

Occasionally, ED trauma patients require imaging outside the ED but not in the OR, including MRI or endoscopy. Patients must be accompanied by appropriate staff, and agreements for patient responsibility during trips out of the ED should be formalized prior to the occurrence.

Pain management

Pain management is an important aspect of early trauma care (see Chapter 15). Pain management must be considered in all patients, including those who are tracheally intubated and sedated. Agitation, tachycardia, hypertension, and high doses of sedatives may be indications of pain in these patients.

Parenteral narcotic pain medications are generally recommended as first-line agents. Nonsteroidal anti-inflammatory drugs (NSAIDs) should be avoided because of bleeding complications and potential renal failure in hypovolemic patients. Fentanyl is a good choice for initial pain medication because of its short half-life and minimal hemodynamic effects. Morphine and hydromorphone may also be used in hemodynamically stable patients.

Regional anesthesia should be considered for extremity injuries and rib fractures, and for joint or fracture reduction, or for soft tissue wound debridement and repair.

Opioid addiction is often encountered in the ED setting and must be considered in trauma patients. Narcotic overdose may cause injuries, patients with opioid addictions may be refractory to pain management, and some patients may feign injury in order to obtain opioids. Indications of opioid addiction are summarized in Table 2.9.

Table 2.9 Indications of heroin or opioid dependence

Overdose	CNS and respiratory depression, miosis, hypoperistalsis
Withdrawal	Restlessness, tachycardia, hypertension, diaphoresis, piloerection, hyperperistalsis
Physical findings of heroin use	Track marks Multiple skin abscesses Poor nutrition/hygiene
History	Requests for narcotic pain medications by name Multiple NSAID allergies Multiple ED and/or PCP visits for painful conditions Multiple narcotic prescriptions Use of aliases during registration
Indications during treatment	Pain refractory to normal doses of narcotics Pain out of proportion to physical findings No overdose symptoms with high doses of narcotics

CNS, central nervous system; ED, emergency department; NSAID, nonsteroidal anti-inflammatory drug; PCP, primary care provider.

Procedural sedation

After the initial evaluation of the trauma patient who does not require immediate operative intervention, certain procedures, including reduction of fractures and joint dislocations and soft tissue injury repair, may be conducted in the ED. Procedural sedation may be indicated. The appropriateness of these patients for ED sedation must be determined. **Joint reductions are time-sensitive, but patients with abnormal vital signs or potential significant head or intraabdominal injuries should have appropriate imaging studies performed prior to procedural sedation to ensure they are stable for sedation.** Brief sedation for soft tissue injury repair may be conducted in the ED, but expected lengthy procedures are best performed in the OR. Procedural sedation is appropriate in patients meeting the American College of Emergency Physicians (ACEP) guidelines for sedation in adult and pediatric patients.[44]

Management of specific injuries in the emergency department

Traumatic brain injury

In the initial approach to traumatic brain injury (TBI), the severity, rather than the specific type of injury, is used to guide treatment. TBI is divided into mild (GCS 14–15), moderate (GCS 9–13), and severe (GCS ≤8). Eighty percent of TBI presenting to the ED is mild. Moderate and severe TBI are associated with high mortality and long-term morbidity.

While the GCS may be affected by intoxication, TBI must be assumed as the cause of altered mental status in trauma patients until proven otherwise. Intoxicated trauma patients with normal head CTs should be observed until returned to normal mental status.

Management of the moderate and severely brain-injured patient is focused on identifying patients requiring prompt surgical evacuation through early CT and preventing secondary insult. Patients with severe TBI should have their tracheas intubated and be mechanically ventilated to prevent hypoxia and hypercarbia. Hyperventilation is no longer recommended for TBI, and PCO_2 should be maintained at 35–40 mmHg. Patients with moderate TBI must be closely monitored for signs of deterioration (see Chapters 20 and 21).

Reversal of anticoagulants may limit the extent of initial bleeding. FFP and vitamin K should be given to patients on warfarin. **Prothrombin complex** concentrate (four-factor) has recently been approved for urgent reversal of warfarin in patients with acute major bleeding. Platelets are often administered to patients on antiplatelet agents such as aspirin and clopidogrel, although there is no strong evidence for this treatment. There are no known direct reversal agents for newer anticoagulants, including direct thrombin inhibitors and factor Xa inhibitors.

Avoidance of hypotension is the single most critical step in preventing secondary injury. **A single instance of hypotension in patients with severe head injury has been shown to double mortality.**[45] Maintaining a systolic BP of at least 90 mmHg, a mean arterial pressure (MAP) of 80 mmHg, and hematocrit of ≥ 30 is recommended.

Increasing intracranial pressure (ICP) may be manifested by worsening headache, vomiting, seizures, and decreasing mental status. Cushing's triad – hypertension, bradycardia, and alterations in respiratory pattern – may be present. Treatment of increased ICP includes adequate sedation and pain control, and elevation of the head of the bed to 30 degrees. Seizure prophylaxis with phenytoin may be indicated, but should be done in consultation with neurosurgery. Impending signs of herniation (posturing, unilateral dilated pupil, or rapidly declining neurologic status) may be treated with an osmotic diuretic such as mannitol, provided the patient is not hypotensive. A very brief period of hyperventilation with a PCO_2 of 30 mmHg may be helpful.

Open skull fractures should be treated with antibiotics, and depressed fractures must be assessed for the need for operative management. Nasogastric tubes should not be placed in patients with suspected basilar skull fractures.

CT scanning is recommended for all adults with GCS less than 15. Patients with isolated head trauma and a normal head CT, who return to baseline, may be discharged from the ED. These patients must be given concussion instruction and appropriate close follow-up.

Facial fractures and injuries

Facial fractures and dental trauma are common in assaults and MVCs. Treatment generally includes antibiotics for open facial fractures, including mandible fractures. Wounds should be carefully cleaned and assessed for foreign bodies. Unstable maxilla and facial fractures (Le Fort fractures) and orbital fractures with evidence of extraocular muscle entrapment require early oral and maxillofacial surgery consultation (see Chapter 24). Orbital fractures without extraocular muscle entrapment may be seen in close follow-up. Avulsed teeth may be salvaged if immediately replaced, but are often not present in the trauma bay. Subluxed teeth may be splinted and referred for early dental follow-up.

During the secondary survey, the eyes should be evaluated for evidence of globe rupture, retrobulbar hematomas, and the presence of foreign bodies/abrasions. If retrobulbar hematoma is diagnosed, immediate lateral canthotomy is indicated and can be vision-saving. Ocular trauma may require urgent operative repair, which may need to be coordinated with other planned surgical procedures.

Nasal bone fractures rarely require ED intervention, but the secondary survey should include evaluation for septal hematomas, which should be drained if present.

Spine and spinal cord injury

Spine injury, with or without neurologic compromise, must be considered in all multiply injured trauma patients. Most spinal trauma is the result of blunt trauma, but penetrating injury, particularly gunshot wounds (GSWs), may also result in spine and spinal cord injury.

Patients with altered mental status must be considered to have cervical spine injuries until proven otherwise. Approximately 5% of patients with TBI have associated spinal trauma, and 25% of patients with a cervical spine injury have TBI. Over half of spinal injuries occur in the cervical spine, and about 10% of patients with cervical spine fractures have additional, noncontiguous spinal fractures.[1]

ED management of spinal injuries includes identification of neurological deficits indicating spinal cord damage, airway and ventilator support for cervical cord injuries, identification and treatment of neurogenic shock, maintenance of spinal immobilization until the spine is cleared, appropriate spinal imaging to evaluate for fractures and cord damage, and urgent consultation where early surgical intervention is indicated. Steroids were initially thought to improve outcomes in patients with spinal cord injuries but are no longer recommended by the American Association of Neurological Surgeons.[46]

Cervical spine

In polytrauma patients, the cervical spine remains immobilized in a rigid collar until it can be radiographically and clinically cleared. Immediate tracheal intubation is indicated for high cervical spine trauma with respiratory compromise. Even without cord compromise, prevertebral edema may necessitate emergent intubation. Current recommendations for intubation are to maintain manual in-line immobilization during intubation with either DL or video assistance. Recent evidence indicates that early intervention for lower cervical cord injuries is beneficial.[47] Awake fiberoptic intubation, when

Table 2.10 NEXUS criteria for clinical C-spine clearance

No midline cervical spine tenderness
No evidence of intoxication
Normal mental status
No neurologic deficits
No painful distracting injuries

Table 2.11 Canadian C-spine rules

High-risk factors: presence of ANY mandates imaging	Low-risk factors: allows safe assessment of range of motion
Age ≥ 66 Dangerous mechanism Extremity paresthesias	Simple rear-end motor vehicle collision Sitting position in emergency department Ambulatory at any time Delayed onset of neck pain Absence of midline C-spine tenderness

feasible, may be the best option. Neurologic assessment of function before intubation is recommended, if possible.

In general, plain films of the cervical spine are no longer indicated in most patients. CT is generally accepted as the initial screening modality of choice. CT scanning has been shown to be more specific for cervical spine injuries, and it is often far more expeditiously obtained than plain films.[42,48] All patients with cervical spine fractures should be seen by spine consult, although many fractures will be managed conservatively.

Not all trauma patients require cervical spine imaging. Two clinical decision rules exist to identify awake, alert low-risk trauma patients who do not require imaging:

- The NEXUS rule (National Emergency X-Radiography Utilization Study) identifies five negative predictors of bony cervical spine injury with a 99.6% sensitivity and 99.9% negative predictive value for the presence of fractures. Awake, adult patients meeting the criteria in Table 2.10 are at extremely low risk of cervical spine injury and may not require imaging.[49]
- The Canadian C-spine rule is a decision tool that incorporates mechanistic factors and examination findings and has demonstrated slightly higher predictive value than the NEXUS criteria with validation.[50] Patients with *none* of the high-risk factors and one of the low-risk factors shown in Table 2.11 are allowed to range the neck, and if pain-free in 45 degrees of rotation, do not require imaging.

Many clinicians use a combination of these rules to determine when cervical spine imaging may safely be omitted.

Thoracic, lumbar, and sacral spine

The remainder of the spine is less frequently injured, but physicians should have a high index of suspicion in patients with significant mechanisms of injury and in patients with cervical spine fractures. Regular hospital beds provide adequate support for the remainder of the spine in the supine position. Patients should be removed from hard backboards during the initial assessment in order to prevent skin breakdown. Patients can be transferred to the scanner and other beds using a sliding board. Imaging guidelines similar to those for cervical spine imaging can be followed for thoracic and lumbar spine imaging. Polytrauma patients undergoing CT scanning of the chest, abdomen, and pelvis should have spinal reconstructions performed.

Neurogenic and spinal shock

Neurogenic shock should be differentiated from spinal shock. Neurogenic shock, manifested by bradycardia, hypotension, and peripheral vasodilatation, may occur within hours of upper thoracic or cervical cord injury. Other causes of shock must be ruled out before neurogenic shock is diagnosed. ED treatment includes IV fluids, atropine for extreme bradycardia, and possibly inotropic agents.

Spinal shock refers to the loss of spinal reflexes below the level of cord injury, and it can make it difficult to differentiate between incomplete and complete cord injury on initial presentation. The bulbocavernosus reflex is among the first to return with resolution of spinal shock. Priapism on initial presentation is indicative of complete cord injury.

Penetrating injuries

Penetrating spinal cord injury is usually the result of a gunshot wound (GSW). Patients with spinal cord injuries who have sustained wounds transecting the abdomen should receive IV antibiotics in the ED and be treated operatively. For patients without abdominal involvement, management will vary depending on CT findings and neurologic presentation.

Neck trauma

The most critical element of ED management of neck trauma is the recognition and immediate treatment of impending airway and circulatory compromise. Respiratory distress, subcutaneous emphysema, expanding neck hematoma, or tracheal shift requires immediate intubation. Even without clear signs of respiratory distress, early intubation should be considered. The risks of a possibly unnecessary intubation likely outweigh the risks of delayed intubation, or attempt at surgical airway, when external and internal landmarks are distorted or obliterated.

The neck has classically been divided into three zones. Structures in each zone are shown in Table 2.12. Traditional teaching is that zone II injuries require surgical evaluation. However, recent evidence has changed this practice. The 2008 EAST clinical practice guidelines for penetrating neck

Table 2.12 Neck zone boundaries and structures of concern within each zone

Zone	Boundaries	Structures
I	Clavicles to cricoid cartilage	Vertebral and proximal carotid arteries Major thoracic vessels Superior mediastinum Upper lungs Trachea and esophagus Thoracic duct Spinal cord
II	Inferior margin of the cricoid cartilage to the angle of the mandible	Vertebral and carotid arteries Jugular veins Trachea and esophagus Larynx Spinal cord
III	Angle of the mandible to the base of the skull	Distal vertebral and carotid arteries Pharynx Spinal cord

Table 2.13 Hard and soft signs of neck trauma

Hard signs: require operative management	Soft signs: selective management
Emergency department hypotension Arterial bleeding Decreased carotid pulse Bruit Expanding hematoma Lateralizing neurologic deficits Air bubbling from wound Hemoptysis or hematemesis Large hemothorax	Field reported hypotension Field reported arterial bleeding Stridor or hoarseness Apical cap on chest x-ray Bradycardia Isolated seventh nerve palsy

trauma state that "selective operative management and mandatory exploration of penetrating injuries to zone II of the neck are equally justified and safe."[51] In penetrating trauma, if the platysma muscle has been violated, surgical consultation is indicated. If the patient is at a non-trauma center, transfer should be considered.

Current practice is based on the presence of hard or soft signs in order to determine the need for emergent operative treatment versus selective imaging in penetrating neck trauma in any zone. Hard signs are predictive of the need for operative intervention.[51] Table 2.13 lists both hard and soft signs associated with neck trauma.

In stable patients with soft signs, a combination of imaging studies may be required to evaluate for potential injuries, depending on the zone involved. Chest x-ray is useful in zone I injuries (may identify pneumothorax or hemothorax), but helical CT is often the initial imaging study in zones II and III. Additional imaging may include angiography, esophagography, esophagoscopy, bronchoscopy, and laryngoscopy as indicated.[51]

These studies necessitate that the patient be transported outside the ED. The patient must be monitored and accompanied by qualified staff. Before transporting the patient from the ED, the airway should be reevaluated and the trachea intubated if there is concern for deterioration.

If helical CT imaging clearly demonstrates a superficial trajectory, no further imaging is indicated, and the patient is usually discharged home from the ED.

Thoracic trauma

In addition to life-threatening injuries identified during the primary survey, potentially life-threatening injuries may be identified in the secondary survey and by ED imaging. The only signs and symptoms of thoracic injury may be dyspnea and tachypnea. Potential injuries include aortic disruption, pneumothorax, hemothorax, pulmonary contusions, and cardiac contusions (see also Chapters 30 and 31)

Great vessel injury

Approximately half of all patients who survive an aortic or other great vessel injury long enough to arrive at the ED have no external evidence of trauma.[52] Significant mechanisms of injury, such as high-speed MVC with rapid deceleration, should prompt imaging to evaluate for this injury. Chest x-ray findings, including a widened mediastinum, apical cap and tracheal deviation, may be present, but CT is more sensitive. CT angiography (CTA) or conventional angiography is usually necessary to fully evaluate the extent of the injury. Operative repair is often indicated, although some minor injuries may be observed. Vascular or cardiothoracic consultation is recommended.

Pneumo- and hemothorax

Pneumothorax seen on chest x-ray generally requires placement of a chest tube in the ED. Small pneumothoraces seen only on CT may require only observation. Chest tubes are usually placed, even for small pneumothoraces, if the patient is receiving positive-pressure ventilation; however, one recent study suggests that this may not be necessary, and may increase length of stay and complications.[53] Persistent pneumothorax despite adequate chest tube placement is indicative of tracheobronchial injury.

Rib fractures

First and second rib fractures are associated with a high incidence of great vessel injury. Multiple fractures should raise concerns for flail segments. Lower rib fractures may be associated with renal, splenic, and liver injuries. Isolated fractures in young people often require only pain control. Multiple rib fractures are usually associated with significant respiratory compromise and pulmonary contusions. Admission for pain control is usually required.

Pulmonary contusions

Pulmonary contusions are common. The initial ED chest x-ray may demonstrate only small infiltrates, but contusions generally blossom over 6 hours, so observation for progression of respiratory compromise is indicated. Large pulmonary contusions often require intubation and ventilatory support.

Diaphragm injuries

These injuries are frequently not diagnosed in the ED. The trauma team must have a high index of suspicion based on mechanism. Diaphragm injuries may be missed on both chest x-ray and CT. Laparoscopy may be required to make the diagnosis, although even this technique is not perfect. Laparoscopy is warranted in patients at risk for diaphragm injury, as unrepaired injuries may result in a remote presentation of herniated bowel.

Abdominal trauma

Blunt abdominal injuries are not always detected by exam. The initial ED exam in patients with visceral injuries is often benign, but up to 35% of patients with an initially "benign" exam are later found to have significant abdominal injuries requiring laparotomy.[54] Retroperitoneal injuries are also notoriously difficult to diagnose. Patients with pancreatic and visceral injuries may be nontender and have no external evidence of trauma (see also Chapters 31 and 32).

Abdominal ecchymosis often indicates significant abdominal trauma. Flank contusions are associated with retroperitoneal injuries.

Blunt trauma

The FAST exam may be performed in the ED as a screening exam for hemoperitoneum but does *not* rule out intraabdominal trauma. CT is the gold standard for diagnosing visceral and solid organ injury. However, radiation and contrast administration risks should be considered in determining whether to obtain CT scans in stable patients. Observation with repeat exams may be indicated in stable patients. For solid organ injuries identified on CT, patients with active bleeding may go to angiography rather than the OR. Many liver and splenic lacerations are now managed nonoperatively, but must be admitted to the appropriate level of care.

Penetrating trauma

Transabdominal GSW is usually an indication for operative intervention. Stable patients may be CT scanned at the surgeon's discretion, for delineation of injuries (see Chapter 11). The management of penetrating trauma has changed in recent years, and many patients without evidence of visceral injury can be managed conservatively, with CT scanning and observation, in accordance with the EAST algorithm for the management of penetrating abdominal trauma.[55]

Genitourinary injuries

Renal injuries should be suspected with the presence of frank hematuria. These injuries are best evaluated with CT using delayed contrast imaging. If urethral injury is suspected, a retrograde urethrogram must be performed prior to Foley catheter placement. Suspected bladder injuries are evaluated with a retrograde cystogram. Urological consult is required to determine the appropriate management of these injuries, which may include Foley placement, suprapubic catheter placement, or operative repair.

Extremity and soft tissue trauma

Except for pelvic fractures, orthopedic injuries are rarely immediately life-threatening, but may be limb-threatening. The ED role in extremity care is to limit further damage by immobilization, expeditiously reduce fractures or dislocations compromising circulation, evaluate for vascular compromise and compartment syndrome, and identify open fractures. Joint and fracture reduction as well as soft tissue injury repair may be conducted in ED with sedation but may be best accomplished in the OR, depending on the patient's condition, the expected time of the procedure, and the status of the ED.

Extremes of age

Trauma assessment and treatment of patients at the extremes of age can be complicated by physiologic and anatomic factors, as well as by communication issues. Special considerations for ED management of pediatric and geriatric trauma patients are outlined below.

Pediatrics

Preparation

Pediatric patients require appropriate equipment, and personnel specifically trained in pediatric trauma (see Chapter 34). Appropriately sized C-collars and spinal immobilization devices must be utilized. Use of resuscitation tapes with length-based determination of tube sizes and medication dosages is highly recommended.

Initial assessment and resuscitation

Airway positioning is key in the young child. Immobilization in an in-line position must take into account the relatively large occiput in younger children, and support under the shoulders is often required. RSI is still the preferred method for intubation. Cuffed or uncuffed ETT may be used.[1] Appropriately sized bag-mask devices must be utilized in order to prevent overdistention of the lungs and pneumothorax. Gastric decompression should be done to prevent abdominal distension. Needle cricothyroidotomy is not recommended in children under age 6.

Vital signs can be deceptive. An elevated heart rate may indicate emotional stress, pain, and/or hypovolemia. In children, decreased BP is seen only in very late shock. Vascular access may be challenging, and intraosseus access is

Table 2.14 Anatomic considerations in pediatric trauma

Anatomic feature	Exam and treatment considerations
Large head-to-body ratio	Head injury very common in polysystem trauma Scalp wounds cause significant blood loss Patient must be positioned with support under shoulders
Weak neck muscles	Upper C-spine injuries much more common
Smaller airway structures	Airway easily obstructed by tongue, slight hyperflexion or extension
Cartilaginous ribs	Can have significant chest trauma, especially pulmonary contusions, in the absence of rib fractures
Abdominal organs	Abdominal and pelvic organs more frequently injured as less well protected by ribs and pelvic bones
Extremities	Fractures may extend into growth plates, causing significant abnormalities in future growth without proper care

recommended rather than central line placement. Scalp wounds can cause significant blood loss. The FAST exam is less well researched in the pediatric population, but a positive FAST in a hemodynamically unstable child is still predictive of the need for operative management.[1] Hypothermia is more likely to occur, due to the larger body surface area to mass ratio. Specific anatomic considerations are listed in Table 2.14.

Imaging and ancillary testing

Radiation exposure is more of a concern in the pediatric population and must be considered in imaging decisions. The American Academy of Pediatrics (AAP) has established guidelines for head CT in pediatric patients.[56] Initial imaging of the cervical spine in children is generally plain film, followed by CT or MRI of specific areas of concern. CT of the head, neck, chest, abdomen, and pelvis imparts a significant dose of radiation to the thyroid, and should be avoided when possible.[57] In stable patients with no evidence of abdominal trauma, consideration should be given to observing the child instead of CT. Standard trauma labs are generally indicated for pediatric patients. In addition, while microscopic blood in urine is not helpful for adults, its presence in pediatric patients may be indicative of renal injury.

Elderly

Preparation

Significant trauma from relatively minor mechanisms should be anticipated in the elderly patient, as patients may be anticoagulated, may have multiple underlying medical conditions and medications, and may have baseline dementia (see

Chapter 36). The antecedent event leading to trauma (e.g., acute myocardial infarction causing fall or MVC) should be considered. Obtaining past medical history and current medications is critically important in these patients.

Initial assessment and resuscitation

Vital signs may be deceptive. A "normal" BP of 110/50 may indicate relative hypotension for a patient with a "usual" BP of 170/80. In blunt trauma patients 65 years and older, there is an association between hypotension and mortality starting with systolic BP below 110 mmHg and heart rates above 90 bpm.[58] In addition, a systolic BP < 90 mmHg in the elderly blunt trauma patient is associated with a mortality between 82% and 100%.[59]

An initial respiratory rate < 10 breaths/minute in geriatric trauma patients is also highly predictive of mortality.[60] In addition, rib fractures in the elderly are associated with mortality. Rates of pneumonia and mortality in patients 65 years old are twice those in younger patients, with the rates increasing with each additional fractured rib.[61] Table 2.15 lists specific considerations in geriatric trauma patients.

Trauma in pregnant patients

Trauma in pregnancy is common. Death of the mother is the leading cause of fetal mortality, followed by placental abruption and uterine rupture. Optimal care for the fetus is excellent care for the mother (see Chapter 37).

Specific physiologic changes occur during pregnancy which may complicate ED evaluation and treatment of the trauma patient. Table 2.16 lists these changes and their impact on trauma care of the pregnant patient.

Initial assessment and resuscitation

Supplemental oxygen should be applied to all pregnant trauma patients. Fluid resuscitation should follow the guidelines for nonpregnant trauma patients. History and uterine size should be used to estimate gestational age. Obstetrics should be consulted, or be part of the initial trauma team, for any patient with a potentially viable fetus. Patients beyond 18–20 weeks gestational age must be stabilized in a semi-lateral position in order to displace the uterus from the IVC. Type and screen should be sent on all pregnant trauma patients, and $Rh_0(D)$ immune globulin administered, if indicated. The Kleihauer–Betke test for maternal–fetal hemorrhage should be sent, but results are not immediately available.

Ultrasound and tocographic monitoring should be initiated in the ED. Ultrasound is useful for fetal dating and assessing fetal well-being but is not sensitive enough to rule out abruption or uterine rupture. CT imaging should be carried out as indicated in multisystem trauma patients. Minor trauma patients cleared by the trauma team are generally admitted for fetal monitoring. All pregnant trauma patients should be screened for domestic violence.

Table 2.15 Specific considerations in geriatric trauma patients

Airway	Cervical fusion or mandibular arthritis Poor dentition or foreign body obstruction with dentures/bridges
Respiratory	Decreased reserve with age Presence of pulmonary disease Fragile rib cage
Cardiovascular	Decreased cardiac reserve with age Presence of flow/pressure-sensitive CAD Presence of underlying CHF Cardiac medications blunt sympathetic response Diuretic medications causing relative hypovolemia
Head and neck	Increased frequency of subdural hematomas due to smaller brain, delicate bridging veins – often delayed presentation Preexisting cervical stenosis increases risk of central cord syndrome with hyperextension
Gastrointestinal/renal	Poor motility Decreased esophageal tone Decreased GFR increases risk of contrast nephropathy
CNS/mental status	Baseline may not be known Hearing loss may confound assessment
Hematologic	Presence of antiplatelet medications, warfarin, direct thrombin inhibitors compounds hemorrhage control May have anemia at baseline
Musculoskeletal	Increased bone fragility leads to severe fractures Fusion of vertebrae increases risk of multiple fractures

CAD, coronary artery disease; CHF, congestive heart failure; CNS, central nervous system; GFR, glomerular filtration rate.

Table 2.16 Physiologic considerations in emergency department treatment of pregnant trauma patients

Physiologic change	Considerations
Blood volume increased	Delayed manifestation of shock
Early constriction of fetal/placental vessels	Fetal injury prior to maternal
Displacement of abdominal organs	Unusual injury patterns Delayed diagnosis of injuries Delayed gastric emptying
Displacement of diaphragm superiorly	Decreased tidal volume and respiratory reserve
Uterine compression of inferior vena cava	Shock without volume depletion if uterus is not displaced laterally Increased hemorrhage from lower extremity injuries

benzodiazepines, opioids, cannabis, or other intoxicants. Table 2.17 lists some common intoxicants, and considerations in the ED management of intoxicated trauma patients. The ED diagnosis of intoxication/abuse must be communicated to the OR and admitting teams, as withdrawal may develop over the course of treatment.

Abuse and nonaccidental trauma

Abuse or nonaccidental trauma is more common in pregnant, elderly, and pediatric patients but should be considered in the evaluation of every trauma patient. EMS providers often pick up initial clues to abuse and neglect, and these should be noted by ED personnel (e.g., social workers) as well as the trauma team. Table 2.18 lists factors which should raise suspicion for nonaccidental trauma

Summary

The role of prehospital and ED trauma care is to identify and provide initial intervention for immediately life-threatening traumatic injuries. Appropriate care during this interval reduces mortality in the second peak of trauma deaths, and may reduce morbidity. Short on-scene times, immediate resuscitation, appropriate immobilization, and timely transfer or transport to an appropriate facility are key factors in the provision of prehospital trauma care.

In the ED, rapid but thorough assessment with critical interventions and immediate operative care when indicated is critical to the survival of unstable trauma patients. Initially stable patients require diligence to ensure that complete assessment with appropriate imaging is undertaken in order to avoid missing potential injuries. Trauma patients initially assessed in non-trauma-center EDs should be transferred whenever the resources required to care for the patient may exceed the facility's capabilities. In trauma-center EDs, teamwork, coordination of expert consultation, imaging, observation, and

Perimortem cesarean section

Perimortem cesarean section (C-section) is indicated when a pregnant patient with a potentially viable fetus loses pulse in ED. The best predictor of fetal viability is the time from loss of pulses to delivery.[62] The patient should not be moved to the OR, as valuable time will be lost. Maternal resuscitative measures should be continued during the operation. The procedure may be performed by EP, surgeon, or obstetrician with anesthesiologist involvement. A separate neonatal resuscitation team should be in the trauma bay as soon as possible to take over care of the infant.

Substance abuse and the trauma patient

Many traumatic injuries directly or indirectly involve the use of intoxicants. Initial evaluation of the trauma victim may be complicated by the presence of stimulants, alcohol,

Table 2.17 Common drugs of abuse: effects and considerations

Class	Typical drugs	Effects	Treatment and considerations
Stimulants	Cocaine Methamphetamine Designer stimulants (MDMA, ecstasy)	Agitation or aggression Hypertension Vasospasm Tachycardia Diaphoresis Dilated pupils	IV benzodiazepines Quiet environment Consider sedation/paralysis/RSI if patient is in danger of further harm to self
Hallucinogens	Phencyclidine (PCP) Lysergic Acid (LSD)	AMS Hallucinations Extreme aggression/pain tolerance (PCP)	Close monitoring necessary Benzodiazepines Consider sedation/paralysis/RSI if patient is in danger of further harm to self (PCP)
CNS depressants	Alcohol Benzodiazepines Barbiturates	AMS – varies from mild to unresponsive Respiratory depression Hypotension	Airway intervention as needed – nasal airway, intubation depending on LOC IV fluids Flumazenil is not recommended for benzodiazepine overdose
	Chronic alcoholism	Coagulopathy Brain atrophy Electrolyte derangements Hypoglycemia Malnutrition	High risk for SDH Consider K^+ and mg^+ replacement Glucose, consider thiamine Consider multivitamin
Opioids	Heroin Narcotic pain medications	Reduced LOC Decreased respiratory drive Decreased GI motility Pinpoint pupils	Respiratory assistance Naloxone – given in small increments Consider NG tube placement

AMS, altered mental status; CNS, central nervous system; GI, gastrointestinal; IV, intravenous; K, potassium; LOC, loss of consciousness; mg, magnesium; NG, nasogastric; RSI, rapid sequence induction/intubation; SDH, subdural hematoma.

Table 2.18 Potential indicators of nonaccidental trauma

History	Injuries inconsistent with history Patient with history of physical or mental impairment Delayed presentation for injury
Chart review	Multiple ED visits for injuries Escalating injury pattern Multiple ED visits for other minor complaints
Physical exam	Multiple injuries in various stages of healing Injuries in defensive pattern – nightstick fractures, hand injuries Injuries to protected body locations – inner thighs, genitalia, axilla Burns of entire hand or foot or buttocks Lighter or cigarette burns Evidence of neglect, malnutrition, developmental delay
Psychosocial	Hovering spouse, significant other, parent or child Developmental delay Pregnancy History of abuse in past Recent stressors

ED, emergency department.

appropriate disposition are critical components of successful trauma care.

Questions

(1) Which of the following is *not* considered a skill of a basic EMT?
   a. C-spine immobilization
   b. Assistance with patient medications
   c. IV access
   d. Ventilation with bag-mask

(2) Which of the following is true regarding patient immobilization?
   a. The cervical spine must be immobilized for all trauma patients
   b. Young children often require support under the head in order to maintain the C-spine in neutral position
   c. Trauma patients should remain immobilized on boards until they are safely transferred to the OR or the hospital bed
   d. Reduction and immobilization of fractures may reduce hemorrhage

(3) Which of the following patients would *not* be considered appropriate for aeromedical transport?
   a. 32-year-old female ejected from a car

b. 30-year-old male with penetrating trauma to the forearm

c. 5-year-old female following a fall of 18 feet (5.5 m)

d. 20-year-old pregnant female involved in a moderate speed MVC with abdominal pain and a seatbelt sign

(4) Which of the following is true?

a. Paramedics may make the decision to withhold or terminate resuscitation efforts in trauma patients in cardiac arrest

b. All penetrating trauma patients in cardiac arrest should undergo resuscitation efforts

c. Resuscitation efforts, including ED thoracotomy, are indicated for blunt trauma patients in cardiac arrest on the arrival of EMS

d. EMS providers cannot withhold treatment for trauma patients in cardiac arrest

(5) Which of the following interventions is *not* appropriately performed during the primary survey?

a. Airway suctioning

b. Blood pressure cuff tourniquet application to arterial bleeding from an upper extremity wound

c. Plaster splinting of a suspected lower extremity fracture

d. Administration of warm IV fluids

(6) Regarding hemothoraces, which of the following is true?

a. The treatment for a massive hemothorax is immediate operation

b. Blood from a hemothorax cannot be collected with a cell-saver and autotransfused

c. A massive hemothorax is defined as 2000 mL of blood output at the time the chest tube is placed

d. Hemothorax cannot be diagnosed with ultrasound

(7) The most important aspect to treating severe TBI in the ED is:

a. Preventing seizures

b. Elevation of the head of the bed 30 degrees

c. Hyperventilation

d. Preventing hypotension

(8) Which of the following is *not* a "hard" sign of significant neck trauma?

a. ED hypotension

b. Hemoptysis

c. Stridor

d. Lateralizing neurologic deficits

(9) Regarding pediatric trauma, which of the following is true?

a. Head injuries are less common in small children

b. Upper C-spine injuries are more frequent in children than adults

c. Pulmonary contusions rarely occur without rib fractures

d. Fracture considerations are the same as for adults

(10) Which of the following is *not* generally an indicator of nonaccidental trauma?

a. Multiple recent ED visits

b. Spiral fractures of humerus or tibia in young children

c. Burns of chest/abdomen in toddlers

d. Delayed presentation of injury

Answers

(1) c
(2) d
(3) b
(4) a
(5) c
(6) a
(7) d
(8) c
(9) b
(10) c

References

1. American College of Surgeons. *Advanced Trauma Life Support, Student Manual*, 9th edition. Chicago, IL: ACS, 2012.

2. Institute of Medicine of the National Academies. *Emergency Medical Services at the Crossroads*. Washington, DC: National Academies Press, 2006. http://books.nap.edu/openbook.php?record_id=11629 (accessed July 2014).

3. *The Highway Safety Act of 1966* (P.L. 89–564, 80 Stat. 731).

4. *National EMS Scope of Practice Model*. DOT HS 810 657, September 2006.

5. Mayglothling J, Duane TM, Gibbs M, *et al.* Emergency tracheal intubation immediately following traumatic injury: an Eastern Association for the Surgery of Trauma practice management guideline. *J Trauma Acute Care Surg* 2012; **73**: S333–40.

6. Bulger EM, Nathens AB, Rivara FP, *et al.* National variability in out-of-hospital treatment after traumatic injury. *Ann Emerg Med* 2007; **49**: 293–301.

7. Davis DP, Ochs M, Hoyt DB, *et al.* Paramedic-administered neuromuscular blockade improves prehospital intubation success in severely head-injured patients. *J Trauma* 2003; **55**: 713–19.

8. Winchell RJ, Hoyt DB. Endotracheal intubation in the field improves survival in patients with severe head injury. Trauma Research and Education of San Diego. *Arch Surg* 1997; **132**: 592–7.

9. Davis DP, Peay J, Sise MJ, *et al.* The impact of prehospital endotracheal intubation on outcome in moderate to severe traumatic brain injury. *J Trauma* 2005; **58**: 933–9.

10. Bochicchio GV, Ilahi O, Joshi M, *et al.* Endotracheal intubation in the field does not improve outcome in trauma patients who present without an acutely lethal traumatic brain injury. *J Trauma* 2003; **54**: 307–11.

11. Wang HE, Peitzman AB, Cassidy LD, et al. Out-of-hospital endotracheal intubation and outcome after traumatic brain injury. *Ann Emerg Med* 2004; **44**: 439–50.

12. Vandromme MJ, Melton SM, Griffin R, et al. Intubation patterns and outcomes inpatients with computed tomography-verified traumatic brain injury. *J Trauma* 2011; **71**: 1615–19.

13. Gausche M, Lewis RJ, Stratton SJ, et al. Effect of out-of-hospital pediatric endotracheal intubation on survival and neurological outcome: a controlled clinical trial. *JAMA* 2000; **283**: 783–90.

14. Kerby JD, Cusick MV. Prehospital emergency trauma care and management. *Surg Clin North America* 2012; **92**: 823–41.

15. Stewart RM, Myers JG, Dent DL, et al. Seven hundred fifty-three consecutive deaths in a level I trauma center: the argument for injury prevention. *J Trauma* 2003; **54** (1): 66–70.

16. Kragh JF, Walters TJ, Baer DG, et al. Practical use of emergency tourniquets to stop bleeding in major limb trauma. *J Trauma* 2008; **64** (Suppl 2): S38–49.

17. Kragh JF, Walters TJ, Baer DG, et al. Survival with emergency tourniquet use to stop bleeding in major limb trauma. *Ann Surg* 2009; **249**: 1–7.

18. NAEMT. *PHTLS: Prehospital Trauma Life Support*, 6th edition. St. Louis, MO: Mosby; 2007.

19. Stern SA, Wang X, Mertz M, et al. Under-resuscitation of near-lethal uncontrolled hemorrhage: effects on mortality and end-organ function at 72 hours. *Shock* 2001; **15**: 16–23.

20. Mapstone J, Roberts I, Evans P. Fluid resuscitation strategies: a systematic review of animal trials. *J Trauma* 2003; **55**; 571–89.

21. Bulger EM, May S, Brasel KJ, et al. Out-of-hospital hypertonic resuscitation following severe traumatic brain injury: a randomized controlled trial. *JAMA* 2010; **304**: 1455–64.

22. Bulger EM, May S, Kerby JD, et al. Out-of-hospital hypertonic resuscitation after traumatic hypovolemic shock: a randomized, placebo controlled trial. *Ann Surg* 2011; **253**: 431–41.

23. Moore EE, Moore FA, Fabian TC, et al. Human polymerized hemoglobin for the treatment of hemorrhagic shock when blood is unavailable: the USA multicenter trial. *J Am Coll Surg* 2009; **208**: 1–13.

24. Hopson LR, Hirsch E, Delgado J, et al. Guidelines for withholding or termination of resuscitation in prehospital traumatic cardiac arrest: joint position paper of the National Association of EMS Physicians and the American College of Surgeons Committee on Trauma. *Prehosp Emerg Care* 2003: 7; 141–6.

25. Sasser SM, Hunt RC, Faul M, et al. Guidelines for field triage of injured patients: recommendations of the National Expert Panel on Field Triage, 2011. Centers for Disease Control and Prevention. *MMWR Recomm Rep* 2012: **61**; 1–20.

26. Di Bartolomeo S, Sanson G, Nardi G, Michelutto V, Scian F. HEMS vs. ground-BLS care in traumatic cardiac arrest. *Prehosp Emerg Care* 2005; **9**: 79.

27. Brown JB, Stassen NA, Bankey PE, et al. Helicopters and the civilian trauma system: national utilization patterns demonstrate improved outcomes after traumatic injury. *J Trauma* 2010; **69**: 1030–4.

28. American College of Emergency Physicians, National Association of EMS Physicians. *Guidelines for Air Medical Dispatch*. http://www.acep.org/uploadedFiles/ACEP/Practice_Resources/issues_by_category/Emergency_Medical_Services/GuidelinesForAirMedDisp.pdf (accessed July 2014).

29. Cudnik MT, Newgard CD, Sayre MR, Steinberg SM. Level I versus level II trauma centers: an outcomes-based assessment. *J Trauma* 2009; **66**: 1321–6.

30. Ballow SB, Kaups KL, Anderson S, Chang M. A standardized rapid sequence intubation protocol facilitates airway management in critically injured patients. *J Trauma Acute Care Surg* 2012; **73**: 1401–5.

31. Omert L, Yeaney W. Role of the emergency medicine physician in airway management of the trauma patient. *J Trauma* 2001; **51**: 1065–8.

32. Stephens CT, Kahntroff S, Dutton RP. The success of emergency endotracheal intubation in trauma patients: a 10-year experience at a major adult trauma referral center. *Anesth Analg* 2009; **109**: 866–72.

33. Walls RM, Brown CA, Bair AE, Pallin DJ; NEAR II Investigators. Emergency airway management: a multi-center report of 8937 emergency department intubations. *J Emergency Med* 2011; **41**: 347–54.

34. Bickell WH, Wall MJ, Pepe PE, et al. Immediate versus delayed fluid resuscitation for hypotensive patients with penetrating torso injuries. *N Engl J Med* 1994; **331**: 1105–9.

35. Dutton RP, Mackenzie CF, Scalea TM. Hypotensive resuscitation during active hemorrhage: impact on in-hospital mortality. *J Trauma* 2002; **52**: 1141–6.

36. Dente CJ, Shaz BH, Nicholas JM, et al. Improvements in early mortality and coagulopathy are sustained better in patients with blunt trauma after institution of a massive transfusion protocol in a civilian level I trauma center. *J Trauma* 2009; **66**: 1616–24.

37. Cotton BA, Au BK, Nunez TC, et al. Predefined massive transfusion protocols are associated with a reduction in organ failure and post injury complications. *J Trauma* 2009; **66**: 41–9.

38. CRASH-2 trial collaborators. Effects of tranexamic acid on death, vascular occlusive events, and blood transfusion in trauma patients with significant haemorrhage (CRASH-2): a randomised, placebo-controlled trial. *Lancet* 2010; **376**: 23–32.

39. CRASH-2 collaborators. The importance of early treatment with tranexamic acid in bleeding trauma patients: an exploratory analysis of the CRASH-2 randomised controlled trial. *Lancet* 2011; **377**: 1096–101.

40. Rozycki GS, Feliciano DV, Ochsner MG, et al. The role of ultrasound in patients with possible penetrating cardiac wounds: a prospective multicenter study. *J Trauma* 1999; **46**: 543–51.

41. Burlew CC, Moore EE, Moore FA, et al. Western Trauma Association critical decisions in trauma: resuscitative thoracotomy. *J Trauma Acute Care Surg* 2012; **73**: 1359–63.

42. Holmes JF, Akkinepalli R. Computed tomography versus plain radiography to screen for cervical spine injury: a meta-analysis. *J Trauma* 2005; **58**: 902–7.

43. Ding W, Shen Y, Yang J, He X, Zhang M. Diagnosis of pneumothorax by

radiography and ultrasonography. *Chest* 2011; **140**: 859–66.

44. American College of Emergency Physicians. Clinical policy: procedural sedation and analgesia in the emergency department. *Ann Emerg Med* 2005; **45**: 177–84.

45. Chesnut RM, Marshall LF, Klauber MR, *et al.* The role of secondary brain injury in determining outcome from severe head injury. *J Trauma* 1993; **34**: 216–22.

46. Hadley MN, Walters BC, Grabb PA, *et al.* Guidelines for the management of acute cervical spine and spinal cord injuries. *Clin Neurosurg* 2002; **49**: 407–15.

47. Hassid VJ, Schinco MA, Tepas JJ, *et al.* Definitive establishment of airway control is critical for optimal outcome in lower cervical spinal cord injury. *J Trauma* 2008; **65**: 1328–32.

48. Baron BJ, McSherry KJ, Larson JL, Scalea TM. Spine and spinal cord trauma. In Tintinalli JE, Kelen GD, Stapczynski JS, eds., *Tintinalli's Emergency Medicine: a Comprehensive Study Guide*, 7th edition. New York, NY: McGraw-Hill; 2011.

49. Hoffman JR, Mower WR, Wolfson AB, *et al.* Validity of a set of clinical criteria to rule out injury to the cervical spine in patients with blunt trauma. *N Engl J Med* 2000; **343**: 94–9.

50. MacDonald RL, Schwartz ML, Mirich D, *et al.* The Canadian C-spine rule for radiography in alert and stable trauma patients. *JAMA* 2001; **286**: 1841–6.

51. Tisherman SA, Bokhari F, Collier B, *et al. Clinical Practice Guidelines: Penetrating Neck Trauma.* Chicago, IL: Eastern Association for the Surgery of Trauma, 2008.

52. Ross C, Schwab TM. Cardiac trauma. In Tintinalli JE, Kelen GD, Stapczynski JS, eds., *Tintinalli's Emergency Medicine: a Comprehensive Study Guide*, 7th edition. New York, NY: McGraw-Hill; 2011.

53. Moore F, Goslar P. Blunt traumatic occult pneumothorax: is observation safe? Results of a prospective, AAST multicenter study. *J Trauma* 2011; **70**: 1019–25.

54. Arikan S, Kocakusak A, Yucel AF, Adas G. A prospective comparison of the selective observation and routine exploration methods for penetrating abdominal stab wounds with organ or omentum evisceration. *J Trauma* 2005; **58**: 526–30.

55. Como JJ, Bohkari F, Chiu WC, *et al. Practice Management Guidelines for the Nonoperative Management of Penetrating Abdominal Trauma.* Chicago, IL: Eastern Association for the Surgery of Trauma, 2007.

56. Kuppermann N, Holmes JF, Dayan PS, *et al.* Identification of children at very low risk of clinically-important brain injuries after head trauma: a prospective cohort study. *Lancet* 2009; **374**: 1160–70.

57. Mueller DL, Hatab M, Al-Senan R, *et al.* Pediatric radiation exposure during the initial evaluation for blunt trauma. *J Trauma* 2011; **70**: 724–31.

58. Heffernan DS, Thakkar RK, Monaghan SF, *et al.* Normal presenting vital signs are unreliable in geriatric blunt trauma victims. *J Trauma* 2010; **69**: 813–18.

59. Knudson MM, Lieberman J, Morris JA, *et al.* Mortality factors in geriatric blunt trauma patients. *Arch Surg* 1994; **129**: 448–55.

60. Horst HM, Obeid RN, Sorensen VJ, *et al.* Factors influencing survival of elderly trauma patients. *Crit Care Med* 1986; **14**: 681–6.

61. Bulger EM, Arneson MA, Mock CN, Jukovich GJ. Rib fractures in the elderly. *J Trauma* 2000; **48**: 1040–4.

62. Oates S, Williams GL, Rees GA. Cardiopulmonary resuscitation in late pregnancy. *BMJ* 1988; **297**: 404–5.

Chapter

3

Trauma airway management

E. Orestes O'Brien and William C. Wilson

Objectives

(1) Review the major considerations and tools needed for trauma airway management.
(2) Characterize the difficult airway in trauma.
(3) Evaluate the American Society of Anesthesiologists (ASA) difficult airway algorithm with regard to trauma.
(4) Provide a plan for managing common difficult airway scenarios in the trauma patient.

Introduction

Airway management disasters account for a large proportion of malpractice lawsuits in the American Society of Anesthesiologists (ASA) closed claims database.[1] Airway loss is a major cause of preventable prehospital death in trauma patients. Trauma airway management is complicated because of associated pathology and suboptimal intubating conditions, and also because complete preintubation evaluation and planning is rarely possible. Furthermore, trauma patients are at increased risk for hypoxia, airway obstruction, hypoventilation, hypotension, and aspiration.

A significant reduction in airway management claims has occurred over the past decade due to the introduction of the ASA difficult airway algorithm, which institutionalized the need for airway evaluation, awake intubation techniques, and the use of back-up rescue modalities such as laryngeal mask airway (LMA), esophageal-tracheal combitube (Combitube), and transtracheal jet ventilation (TTJV).[1] It is therefore logical that incorporation of the ASA difficult airway algorithm, with certain minor modifications, can likewise improve safety during trauma airway management.

This review of airway management for trauma begins with a survey of the equipment and drugs that should be prepared ahead of time, defines and characterizes the "difficult airway," and describes the principles of airway evaluation and management for the trauma patient under both elective and emergency conditions. Proper evaluation and prioritization of treatment are emphasized throughout this chapter, with awake intubation techniques recommended for difficult airway management in cooperative, stable trauma patients. Emergency airway adjuncts such as the LMA and Combitube may be required to rescue the cannot intubate–cannot ventilate situation. Specific tips are provided regarding the successful techniques and pitfalls of fiberoptic bronchoscopy, and the fiberoptic bronchoscopy technique is emphasized where appropriate.

After providing a survey of the major considerations and tools useful in trauma airway management, the ASA difficult airway algorithm is formally reviewed, along with the suggested modifications required for trauma situations. With this foundation, the management of five common trauma difficult airway scenarios is reviewed. Important trauma airway complications are then summarized. Finally, new concepts and techniques that are currently being developed to improve trauma airway management are described.

Equipment and drug preparation

Regardless of the urgency associated with any particular intubation event, several key drugs and airway management tools are universally required; these should be available (and guaranteed to be in working order) for the physician providing airway management for the trauma patient. Essential emergency airway equipment items are listed in Table 3.1 and include: (1) an oxygen (O_2) source and various types of administration devices; (2) an assortment of oral and nasal airways, along with a bag-mask ventilation device capable of applying positive-pressure ventilation (and able to deliver 100% O_2); (3) intubation equipment (including laryngoscopes, styletted and pretested endotracheal tubes [ETTs]); (4) suction tubing and a tonsil-tipped suction device; (5) a functioning intravenous (IV) catheter; (6) prelabeled syringes containing induction and resuscitation drugs including vasopressors and inotropes; (7) appropriate monitors and intubation detectors (as will be described shortly). All of the aforementioned equipment (except for the O_2 source) should fit into a portable storage unit (i.e., code bag) for trauma resuscitation. In austere environments, small tanks of O_2 will also need to be transported to the site of emergency airway management. The importance of each of these essential airway management devices and drugs will be reviewed in this section.

Trauma Anesthesia, 2nd Edition, ed. Charles E. Smith. Published by Cambridge University Press. © Charles E. Smith, 2015.

Table 3.1 Essential emergency airway equipment contained in portable storage unit for trauma resuscitation

Equipment category	Specific emergency airway device
Oxygen	Oxygen (O_2) inflow tubing and O_2 source
Ventilation	Bag-mask device (connect to O_2 source) Soft nasal airway Rigid oral airway Transtracheal jet ventilation equipment Laryngeal mask airway Esophageal-tracheal Combitube
Intubation	Laryngoscope, with new tested batteries #3 and #4 Macintosh blades, with functioning light bulbs #2 and #3 Miller blades, with functioning light bulbs Endotracheal tubes – various sizes, styletted, with balloon tested Tracheal tube guides (gum elastic bougie, semi-rigid stylets, ventilating tube changer, light wand) Flexible fiberoptic intubation equipment Retrograde intubation equipment Adhesive tape or umbilical tape for securing endotracheal tube
Suction	Yankauer, endotracheal suction
Monitor	Capnograph/capnometer, pulse oximeter, esophageal detector device
Drugs	Intravenous induction and paralytic medication Topicalization drugs DeVilbiss sprayer for application of topical drugs Resuscitation drugs (epinephrine, atropine, etc.)
Miscellaneous	Various syringes, needles, stopcocks, intravenous connector tubes

Oxygen: critical during trauma airway management

Advanced Trauma Life Support (ATLS) begins with assessment and management of the airway and breathing, the top two priorities in the ABCDEs of the primary survey. As soon as a trauma patient is encountered in the field or in the trauma bay, O_2 is immediately applied. Furthermore, O_2 should be administered throughout the trauma assessment and treatment phase.

Hypoxemia is a constant threat in trauma and critical illness, because of disease processes that cause respiratory failure and those associated with injury. In addition, 100% O_2 should be administered for 3–5 minutes immediately preceding airway management (i.e., preoxygenation) to increase the duration of adequate O_2 saturation during the period of post-induction apnea.

Treatment of hypoxemia

Clinically, the term hypoxia denotes decreased O_2 tension at the tissue level. Hypoxemia is defined as decreased O_2 tension in the arterial blood (PaO_2). In trauma scenarios, when tissue hypoxia occurs, hypoxemia is nearly always present.

Hypoxemia has eight major causes. The first five etiologies are related to the atmosphere (low partial pressure of inspired O_2) or the lungs (hypoventilation, ventilation/perfusion mismatch, right-to-left transpulmonary shunt, and diffusion abnormalities). The next two causes of hypoxemia involve delivery of O_2 to the tissues (low oxyhemoglobin or low cardiac output). The final cause of hypoxemia is termed *histo-cytic*, denoting a problem in O_2 utilization at the tissue level, usually due to the poisoning of the mitochondrial electron transport chain, as seen with cyanide or carbon monoxide toxicity. Patients suffering from any of these eight causes of hypoxemia will benefit from the administration of 100% O_2.

Preoxygenation: maximizing arterial saturation during apnea

During trauma airway management, O_2 is administered prior to intubation in a process called preoxygenation. Optimum preoxygenation requires that 100% O_2 be delivered by a tight-fitting mask during spontaneous ventilation for 3–5 minutes prior to administering drugs that cause apnea. If the time does not allow for a full 5 minutes of preoxygenation, the patient should be instructed to take 4–8 vital capacity breaths; this will increase O_2 stores, though not to the same level as a full 5 minutes of preoxygenation. The goal of preoxygenation is the replacement of nitrogen with O_2 (denitrogenation), thereby increasing the O_2 stores in the lungs, in arterial and mixed venous blood, and in the tissues. Consequently, the duration that apnea can be tolerated, without causing arterial O_2 desaturation, is prolonged.

Preoxygenation is an essential component of any intubation technique that might involve a period of apnea. Preoxygenation is especially important for a rapid sequence induction and intubation (RSI). When a patient is rendered apneic, the patient has a finite period of time prior to the onset of arterial desaturation. This time period is directly related to the reservoir of O_2 in the lungs at end exhalation during normal tidal breathing (the functional residual capacity [FRC]), and inversely related to the oxygen consumption (approximately 250 mL/minute in a 70 kg patient) (Fig. 3.1).

Preoxygenation with 100% O_2 allows for up to 10 minutes of oxygen reserve following apnea in a normal patient at rest with healthy lungs and a normal FRC (approximately 2.5 L). The same patient when breathing room air (21% O_2) would theoretically have about one-fifth the time (only two minutes) prior to arterial desaturation. Furthermore, trauma patients frequently have a decreased FRC due to numerous causes (e.g., pneumothorax, hemothorax, rib fractures, diaphragmatic hernia, abdominal injuries, and intraabdominal blood), and will desaturate earlier than normal patients following apnea. Patients in respiratory failure from pulmonary edema,

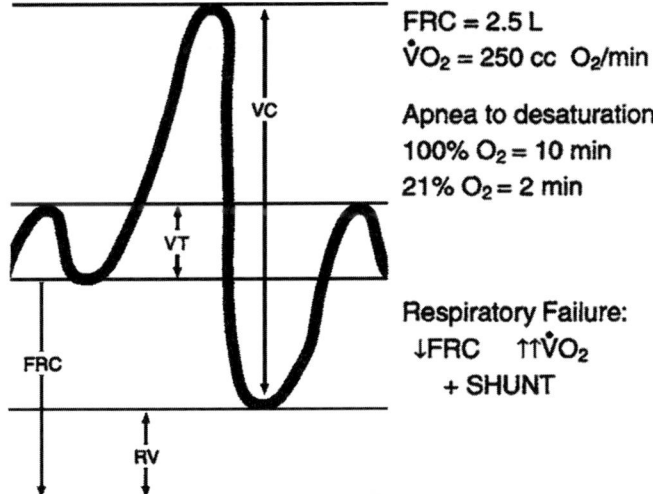

FRC = 2.5 L

$\dot{V}O_2$ = 250 cc O_2/min

Apnea to desaturation
100% O_2 = 10 min
21% O_2 = 2 min

Respiratory Failure:
$\downarrow$FRC $\uparrow\uparrow\dot{V}O_2$
+ SHUNT

Figure 3.1 Functional residual capacity (FRC) and relationship of oxygen reserve. This figure illustrates the factors that determine the time from apnea until desaturation including the FRC, the concentration of oxygen in this reservoir (FiO_2), and the oxygen consumption ($\dot{V}O_2$) of the patient. The spirometric trace on the left side of the figure depicts the relative volumes of the FRC, tidal volume (VT), residual volume (RV), and vital capacity (VC). The reservoir of oxygen in the lungs at end exhalation (FRC) in a normal 70 kg patient is approximately 2.5 L, and the resting ($\dot{V}O_2$) is approximately 250 mL per minute. If the patient is breathing 100% O_2 then there are theoretically 10 minutes prior to desaturation. Whereas if the patient is breathing room air (21% O_2) there are only 2 minutes prior to desaturation. Furthermore, ICU patients are typically sicker, with lower FRCs, increased ($\dot{V}O_2$), and increased shunting, all of which can cause more rapid desaturation following apnea. (Reproduced with permission from Wilson, 1996.[5])

pneumonia, or pulmonary contusion will desaturate even sooner due to increased O_2 consumption, increased right-to-left transpulmonary shunting, and further decreased FRC (atelectasis, lobar collapse) (Fig. 3.2).

Ventilation and intubation equipment

An assortment of face masks should be available; and an appropriately sized mask should be attached to the manual ventilation device. The mask should be pre-tested for integrity and ability to generate positive pressure without leaks and should be capable of delivering 100% O_2 at high flow rates. In austere environments, where O_2 supplies are intermittent, a self-inflating device such as a bag-mask is recommended.

Rigid oral and soft nasal airways should be available in small, medium, and large sizes for the adult patient. If managing pediatric airways, a pediatric kit with appropriately sized equipment must also be available (see Chapter 34).

Styletted ETTs of various sizes, with pretested balloons, should be prepared as follows. An adult-sized ETT (size 7.0 or 8.0) should have a malleable stylet passed through its interior to a position just short (5–10 mm) of the tip. The malleable stylet allows the distal end of the ETT to be molded into a configuration that will most easily pass through the patient's vocal cords. In addition, a styletted 6.0 ETT (or 5.0 ETT) should be prepared as a backup for patients who have small glottic openings and/or difficult airways (smaller ETTs pass more easily into the trachea through swollen or edematous glottic openings).

The rigid direct laryngoscope, with several blades, is the central piece of intubation equipment. The laryngoscope

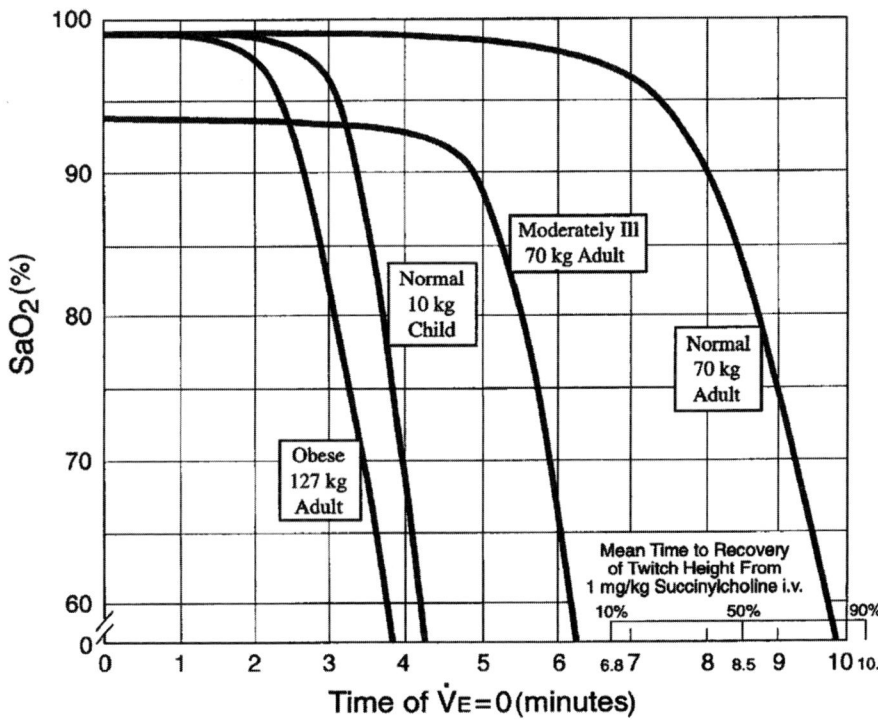

Figure 3.2 Oxygen saturation (SaO_2) versus time of apnea for various types of patients. Time to hemoglobin desaturation with initial $FiO_2 = 0.87$. The SaO_2 versus time curves were produced by the computer apnea model. The mean times to recovery from 1 mg/kg IV succinylcholine are shown in the lower right-hand corner. (Modified from Benumof JL. Critical hemoglobin desaturation will occur before return to an unparalyzed state following 1 mg/kg IV succinylcholine. *Anesthesiology* 1997; **87**: 979–82.)

handle should be clean, and all electrical connections must be free of corrosion or debris. The batteries should be fully charged, and one should verify that a bright beam of light is generated when the blade is attached and extended into the working position. At least two sizes of Miller (#2 and #3) and two sizes of Macintosh blades (#3 and #4) should be provided in the kit, as each has advantages in certain types of airway problems. All of the items listed in Table 3.1 are essential and constitute the minimum airway equipment that should be contained in the portable storage unit.

Suction

Trauma patients, like other patients in respiratory failure, can have thick, tenacious, or bloody secretions, or they may have regurgitated. To minimize the risk of aspiration and to maximize visualization of the laryngeal anatomy, suctioning of the airway is frequently required during a trauma intubation.

The suction apparatus should provide a continuous vacuum of sufficient force to rapidly clear oropharyngeal secretions or vomitus. During initial airway management, a large tonsil-type suction tip (e.g., Yankauer) is best suited for suction of debris out of the oropharynx. After tracheal intubation, long, soft endotracheal suction catheters are most capable of clearing tracheobronchial secretions and aspirated material from the airways. Alternatively, a fiberoptic bronchoscope (FOB) can be used after intubation to remove plugs and secretions from specific lung segments under direct vision. The FOB can also be used to diagnose existing airway pathology and to confirm ETT position. Small, portable, battery-powered FOB devices are now available.

Functioning intravenous catheter

The ability to administer fluids, cardiovascular support drugs, and other medications is essential in urgent and emergent conditions. Thus, after applying O_2 by mask, assessing the airway, and ensuring ventilation, an IV should be established prior to airway manipulation whenever time allows. If confronted with a patient in full arrest, IV access is secured immediately after initiating chest compressions and bag-mask ventilation according to Advanced Cardiac Life Support (ACLS) protocols.

Note that most ACLS protocol drugs can be administered via the ETT except for high-concentration ionic compounds such as calcium, bicarbonate, and magnesium. The intraosseous route can be used as well. If access cannot be obtained, a central venous catheter should be placed (see Chapter 5).

Monitoring and ETT confirmation devices

Pulse oximetry, blood pressure (BP), and continuous electrocardiogram (ECG) constitute the appropriate minimal noninvasive monitoring that should be applied prior to attempting tracheal intubation (see Chapter 9). A complete set of vital signs is obtained when time allows. Vital sign stability and adequate SaO_2 are the goals prior to, during, and after intubation of the trachea. Immediately following placement of the ETT, the partial pressure of CO_2 at the end of the exhaled breath ($P_{ET}CO_2$) should be monitored. A number of devices and techniques for measuring $P_{ET}CO_2$ are available and can be used to confirm intratracheal ETT position and subsequently to assess ongoing ventilation adequacy. In situations with low or no cardiac output, an esophageal detector device is used to confirm ETT position. Both of these items should be contained in the portable storage unit (Table 3.1).

Vasopressors and inotropes

Vasopressors must be available for immediate use, because hypotension is a frequent accompaniment of trauma and critical illness. In addition, the administration of anesthetic drugs and the use of positive-pressure ventilation can exacerbate or initiate hypotension in hypovolemic patients. Furthermore, premorbid conditions in previously ill or elderly patients will further increase the likelihood of hypotension following intubation.

Portable storage unit for trauma resuscitation equipment

Commercially available toolboxes or soft duffel bags can be used for portable storage units. In addition to the aforementioned items, the adjunct equipment needed for assistance in managing the difficult airway should be available. Each portable storage unit should be customized to meet the specific needs and preferences of the practitioner as well as the healthcare facility, and it should be stored in the trauma bay or brought there by the airway expert.[2]

Definition of the difficult airway

Airway difficulty can occur during bag-mask ventilation or during endotracheal intubation. The two are not synonymous; indeed, some patients who are difficult to ventilate (e.g., edentulous, bearded, large jaw) may be quite easy to intubate. Others who are difficult to ventilate (e.g., obstructive sleep apnea, abnormal neck anatomy) may be both difficult to bag-mask ventilate and to intubate. The difficulty of maintaining gas exchange by using bag-mask ventilation can range from a zero degree of difficulty to infinite (Fig. 3.3).

Difficulty of intubation using direct laryngoscopy also proceeds along a similar continuum from easy to nearly impossible (Fig. 3.3). Difficult intubation has been defined as requiring multiple attempts with multiple maneuvers including external laryngeal manipulation, multiple laryngoscope blades, and/or multiple endoscopists.[2] The ASA difficult airway guidelines define difficult laryngoscopy as the impossibility of visualizing any portion of the vocal cords after multiple attempts using a conventional laryngoscope.[3]

Probably the best definition of difficult intubation for documentation from one clinician to another and for research

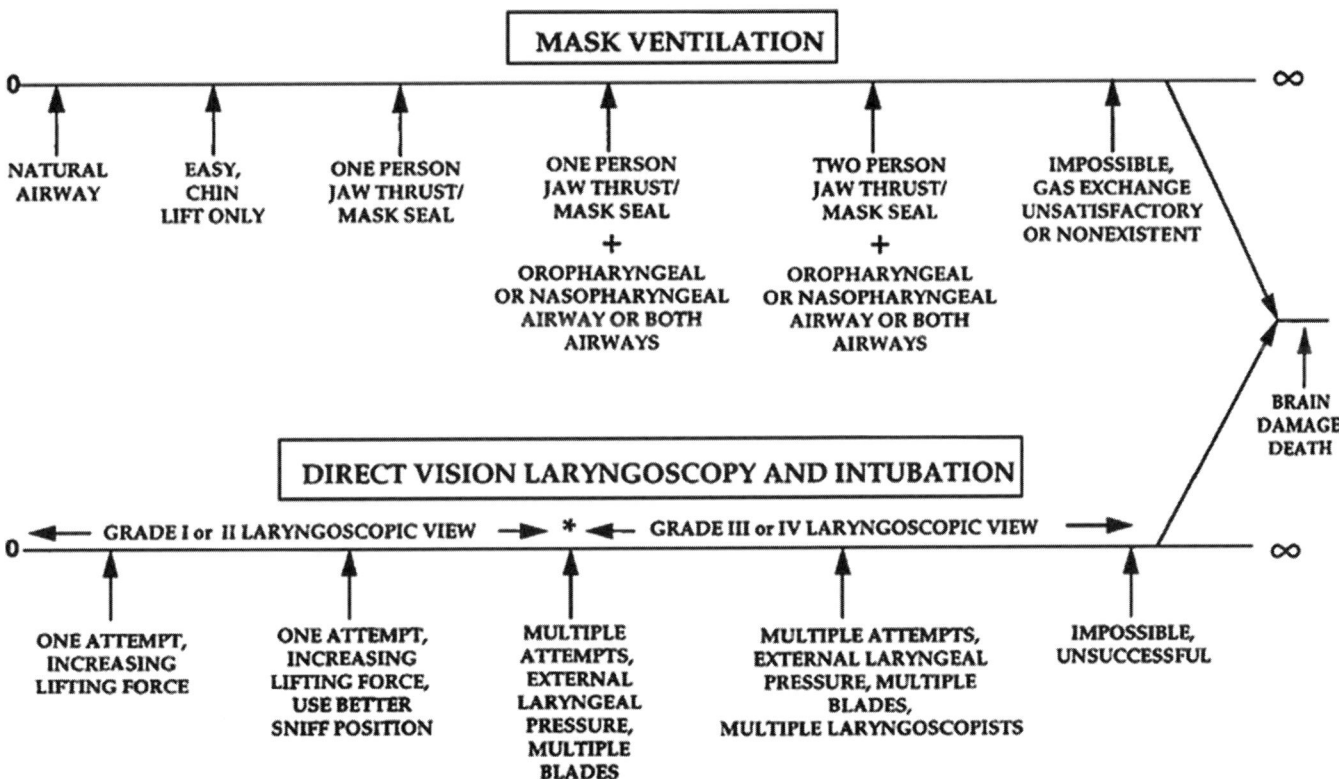

Figure 3.3 Degree of airway difficulty continuum for mask ventilation and direct-vision laryngoscopy at intubation. This illustration provides a conceptual framework for the definition of airway difficulty with mask ventilation (top) and direct vision laryngoscopy (bottom). The degree of difficulty ranges from zero to the impossible or infinitely difficult airway. The amount of difficulty can vary in the same patient with different anesthesiologists using various techniques. The grade of laryngoscopic view refers to grades defined by Cormack and Lehane (Fig. 3.4).

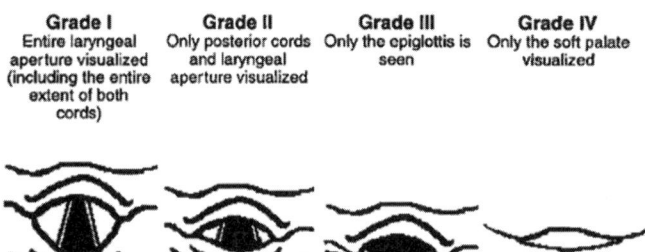

Figure 3.4 Four grades of laryngoscopic view. The grading is based upon the anatomic features that are visualized during the performance of direct laryngoscopy. (Courtesy of medical illustrator at MetroHealth Medical Center; redrawn from Cormack and Lehane, 1984.[4])

purposes involves the grading of the laryngoscopic views as defined by Cormack and Lehane.[4] In the Cormack and Lehane classification (Fig. 3.4), grade 1 denotes visualization of the entire laryngeal aperture, grade 4 is visualization of soft palate only, and grades 2 and 3 are intermediate views.[5] Grade 3 or 4 laryngoscopic views correlate well with difficult intubations in the vast majority of patients.[6] However, there are some clinically relevant situations that provide exceptions to this rule. First, the skill and experience of the endoscopist in manipulating the laryngoscope, the ETT, and the patient's anatomy must be taken into account. Second, a grade 3 laryngoscopic view has been described differently by different investigators.[6,7] Third, the blade attached to the laryngoscope will affect the laryngeal view and therefore the assigned grade. Fourth, the blade selection can solve or exacerbate certain problems. For example, a long floppy epiglottis may yield a high-grade view (3, 4) with a Macintosh blade and a relatively low-grade view (1, 2) if a straight blade is used. Finally, traumatic conditions such as cervical spine (C-spine) injury (i.e., inability to move the neck into a "sniffing position"), laryngeal fractures, or expanding hematomas may disassociate the laryngoscopic view from the difficulty of tracheal intubation. Despite these considerations, the laryngoscopic grading of Cormack and Lehane is used by most authors to define intubation difficulty, and it should be documented for each patient intubated.[2]

Historical indicators of airway difficulty

The intent of obtaining an airway history is to elicit previously known factors indicating that airway management has been difficult in the past. Any patient who is awake and capable of coherent conversation should be asked about prior intubation and ventilation successes or failures. Some patients possess a MedicAlert bracelet indicating a history of difficult intubation or ventilation, and this can be useful in obtunded patients. Regardless of the patient's mental state, if time permits, the physician should review the patient's chart for details of previous intubations and other concurrent problems that may complicate intubation. If an obese patient relays that he or she requires nasal continuous positive airway pressure at night to sleep, this may indicate that mask ventilation and/or intubation will be more difficult than in a thin patient without such history.

Pathologic/anatomic predictors of airway difficulty

In the trauma setting, numerous lesions (e.g., hematoma, foreign body, facial fractures/edema) can pose difficulty for spontaneous ventilation as well as bag-mask ventilation and intubation (Table 3.2). Suspected C-spine injuries pose intubation difficulty due to inability to extend the head on the neck or flex the neck on the chest. Other trauma conditions that make intubation difficult include burns and other inflammatory conditions, where massive edema can impair the laryngoscopic view. Similarly, stab wounds or blunt trauma to the soft tissue in the neck can cause expanding hematomas or airway disruption to occur.

Anatomic predictors (Table 3.2) of difficult mask ventilation and intubation may be evident before formal examination. Morbid obesity poses difficulty with mask ventilation due to inadequate mask fit and difficulty with holding the mask to the massive face with only one hand. In addition, ventilatory efforts are less effective because of the decreased compliance of the chest wall. Obese patients are also problematic because of decreased FRC and the propensity for rapid O_2 desaturation. Furthermore, soft tissues in the obese patient can intrude on the airway above and occasionally below the glottis, further impeding ventilation. Another common mask ventilation problem is the case of sunken cheeks and absent dentition, where the mask fit and subsequent ventilation can be difficult; conversely, intubation of edentulous patients is often less difficult.

Whenever the patient is recognized to have a difficult airway, the clinician should consider securing the airway while the patient is awake. In trauma patients who are uncooperative or hemodynamically unstable (e.g., shock, head injury), an awake technique is usually not practical.

Table 3.2 Anatomic and pathologic predictors of difficult intubation and ventilation

	Difficult ventilation	**Difficult intubation**
Anatomy		
Neck	Bull neck Obesity History of obstructive sleep apnea	Bull neck Obesity Decreased head extension or neck flexion
Tongue	Large tongue	Large tongue
Mandible	Thick beard	Receding mandible Decreased jaw movement
Teeth	Edentulous	Buck teeth
Pathology		
Maxillofacial	Facial fractures Lacerations Facial plethora	Facial fractures Facial plethora
Oropharyngeal	Edema Hematoma Inflammation Foreign body Tumor	Edema Hematoma Inflammation Infection/abscess
Glottis	Edema Vocal cord paralysis Tumor	Edema Vocal cord paralysis Tumor
Neck	Penetrating or blunt injury Subcutaneous emphysema	C-spine injury Neck mass/hematoma Subcutaneous emphysema Ankylosing spondylitis Rheumatoid arthritis

Airway examination principles
The 11-step airway exam of Benumof

Although trauma and other emergency conditions do not always allow the requisite time, an airway physical examination should be conducted prior to the initiation of anesthetic care and airway management in all patients whenever feasible. The intent of the airway examination is to detect anatomic or pathologic physical characteristics indicating that airway management will be difficult. Currently, the ASA difficult airway guidelines have endorsed an easily performed 11-step airway physical examination, as originally proposed by Benumof (Table 3.3).[3] The decision to examine all or some of the components listed in Table 3.3 depends on the clinical context and the judgment of the practitioner. The order of presentation in the table follows the "line of sight" that occurs during conventional oral laryngoscopy and intubation. Of note, several of the examination components listed in Table 3.3 require an awake, cooperative patient (which is not always the case with trauma). For example, the Mallampati classification (Fig. 3.5), relating the size of the tongue to the pharyngeal space, requires the patient to open the mouth maximally and protrude the tongue as far as possible without phonation.[8] In addition, the Mallampati classification is normally performed with the patient sitting upright, whereas trauma patients are often immobilized supine on a spine board. Furthermore, blunt-trauma patients should not be asked to move their neck until the C-spine is cleared, and they should not be asked to sit up until the entire spine is cleared. Because certain elements of this 11-step exam cannot be practically evaluated in the trauma patient, an abbreviated trauma airway examination is recommended.

Table 3.3 Eleven-step airway examination of Benumof

Step	Airway examination component	Non-reassuring findings	Can evaluate in trauma patient
1	Length of upper incisors	Relatively long	YES ✓
2	Maxillary–mandibular incisor relationship	Prominent "overbite"	YES
3	Ability to prognath jaw	Unable	YES
4	Interincisor distance	< 3 cm	YES
5	Visibility of uvula	Mallampati class III/IV	YES
6	Shape of palate	Highly arched or narrow	YES
7	Mandibular space compliance	Stiff, indurated, noncompliant	YES ✓
8	Thyromental distance	< 3 "normal finger" breadths	YES ✓
9	Length of neck	Short	YES ✓
10	Thickness of neck	Thick	YES ✓
11	Range of motion of head and neck (ROM)	Incomplete ROM Assume incomplete ROM in C-spine injured patients	NO, unless C-spine cleared Cannot examine ROM if possible C-spine injury

Steps 1–10 can be evaluated in stable, cooperative trauma patients (even with known or suspected C-spine injury).
✓, can be done, even in patients who are unstable and uncooperative (steps 1, 7–10), and should be examined whenever time allows.

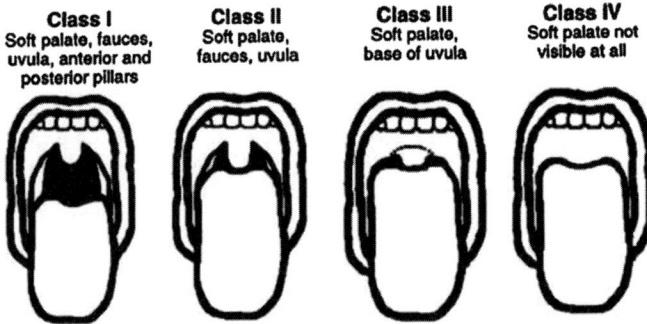

Class I
Soft palate, fauces, uvula, anterior and posterior pillars

Class II
Soft palate, fauces, uvula

Class III
Soft palate, base of uvula

Class IV
Soft palate not visible at all

Figure 3.5 Mallampati classification of the upper airway, relating the size of the tongue to the pharyngeal space based on the anatomic features seen with the mouth open and the tongue extended. (Modified from Mallampati *et al.*, 1985.[8])

Abbreviated trauma airway examination

In an uncooperative and unstable patient, most elements of even an abbreviated exam are impractical. In addition, laryngoscopy would likely be performed regardless of examination results; either an RSI or a modification would be used. If intubation difficulty is encountered, the emergency airway adjuncts recommended in the ASA algorithm should be used. However, in awake, cooperative trauma patients requiring semi-urgent or emergent intubation, steps 1–10 can and should be evaluated (Table 3.3). Step 11, examination of C-spine range of motion, is omitted when C-spine injury is known or suspected. Even with uncooperative patients, and in urgent situations, the airway expert can check the length of the upper incisors, the mandibular space compliance, thyromental distance, neck length, and neck thickness to assess the relative difficulty of intubation, because the aforementioned components do not require patient cooperation.

Conventional trauma airway management
Patient preparation and positioning

Regardless of whether an awake topicalized technique or an RSI technique is chosen, optimum patient positioning and preparation will improve intubation success. If an awake FOB-assisted intubation is planned in a patient capable of flexing the lower back, the head of the patient's bed should be elevated at least 45 degrees to optimize intubating conditions with the FOB. In the setting of C-spine injury, cervical immobilization must also be maintained. However, in conditions where spine injury is likely, the patient must remain supine with the entire spine maintained in anatomic alignment with in-line immobilization. The patient should also be psychologically prepared, and the clinician must be patient in ensuring that the nasopharynx, oropharynx, and larynx are properly anesthetized with topical local anesthesia prior to commencing airway instrumentation.

For patients without concern for C-spine injury, who will undergo RSI, the sniffing position is the optimum orientation for laryngoscopy-assisted orotracheal intubation. The sniffing position involves forward flexion of the neck on the chest and atlantooccipital extension of the head at the neck. This position attempts to create a line-of-sight between the operator's eye and the patient's larynx. The easiest way to accomplish this is to place at least two folded towels under the head of the supine patient. It is recognized, however, that in nonanesthetized volunteers with normal anatomy, neither the sniffing position nor simple head extension provides complete alignment of the laryngeal, pharyngeal, and oral axes.[9]

The sniffing position is contraindicated whenever C-spine injury is suspected. In these patients, the head and neck are maintained in the neutral position, and immobilized throughout airway manipulation.

Mask ventilation

Face masks come in a variety of configurations, but most airway experts prefer anatomically shaped masks because these best fit the patient's face as well as the clinician's hand. Adult masks come in small, medium, and large (sizes 3, 4, and 5). Most adults can be ventilated with a size 4 mask, but occasionally a patient will have a small or large jaw, requiring a size 3 or 5 mask respectively. Children's masks come in newborn, infant, and children's sizes and should be provided in the pediatric code bag (see Chapter 34).

The face mask must be applied firmly to the patient's face, ensuring an adequate seal. Simultaneously, care is taken to not injure the bridge of the nose with excessive pressure. A single-hand technique is acceptable if the airway is easy to ventilate (Fig. 3.6). However, if ventilation is difficult using only one hand, two hands should be used to hold the mask in place while a second person squeezes the bag in a combined effort to ventilate the lungs (Fig. 3.7). Frequently, the application of a chin lift or "jaw thrust" (backward and upward pull of the jaw

in a supine patient) will open an airway and facilitate ventilation. The jaw-thrust maneuver, rather than the chin lift, should be used in patients with suspected C-spine injury.

Oropharyngeal and nasopharyngeal airways

When the tongue and other soft tissues are maintained in the normal forward position, as occurs in the awake patient, the posterior pharyngeal wall remains unobstructed and the airway is generally open. This is particularly the case when the patient is sitting upright. The most common cause of airway obstruction occurs when the tongue and epiglottis fall back in supine, unconscious patients. This can be alleviated by the jaw-thrust maneuver. An oral or nasal airway (if not contraindicated) can be employed as an adjunct to bag-mask ventilation to open up a closed airway. Nasopharyngeal airways are relatively contraindicated in cases of coagulopathy or suspected cribriform plate injury (basilar skull fracture and massive facial injury) due to the increased risk of bleeding and the chance of ETT passage into the cranial vault, respectively (see Chapters 24 and 25).

Both oral and nasal airways restore airway patency by separating the tongue from the posterior pharyngeal wall. A rigid oral airway can elicit a gag response in an awake or semiconscious patient, resulting in increased intracranial pressure or vomiting. The soft nasal airways often provoke less gag response than rigid oral airways and are frequently inserted in patients who are awake and prone to gagging.

Laryngeal mask airway

The most recent revision of the ASA algorithm now places the LMA within the anesthetized limb of the pathway to be used whenever bag-mask ventilation is difficult. Ventilatory obstruction above the level of the vocal cords can often be alleviated by the LMA because of its supraglottic placement (Fig. 3.8). However, the LMA is not an effective ventilatory

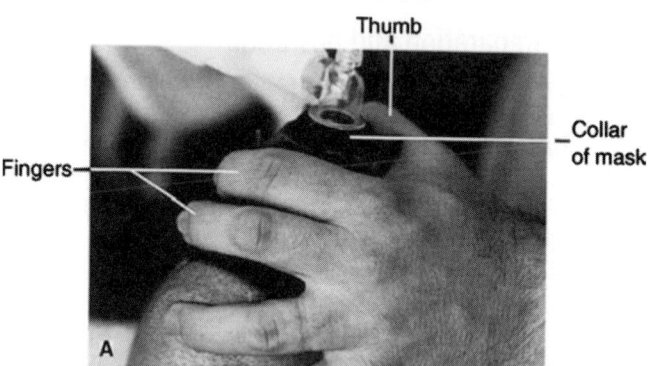

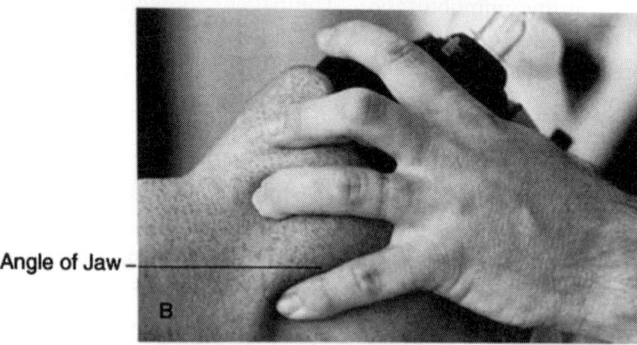

Caudad-side view

Figure 3.6 One-hand mask ventilation technique. This figure shows the one-handed technique for holding a mask properly on a patient's face. The top figure (**A**) demonstrates the standard one-handed grip of the mask on the face. The thumb encircles the upper part of the mask while the second and third fingers are applied to the lower portion of the mask with the fourth and fifth fingers pulling the soft tissue under the mandible up toward the mask. The lower panel (**B**) demonstrates the one-handed mask grip while maintaining jaw thrust. The hand positions are altered such that only the thumb and the second finger encircle the mask, while the third, fourth, and fifth fingers maintain upward and backward pull of the mandible jaw thrust. Typically, an oral airway would have been placed in the patient's oropharynx prior to manipulating the mandible with the jaw-thrust maneuver.

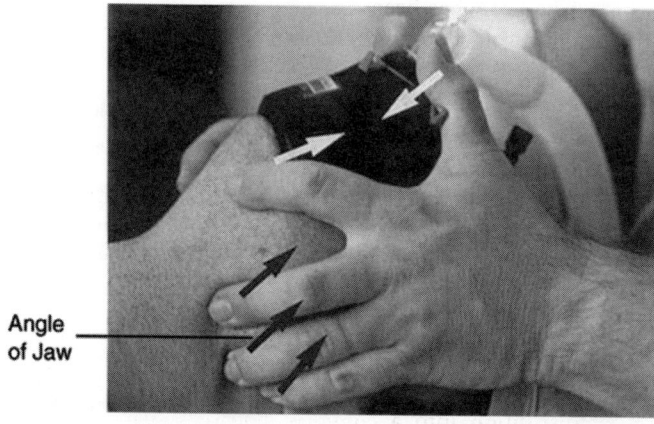

Figure 3.7 Two-hand mask ventilation technique. With the two-handed technique the thumbs are hooked over the collar of the mask while the lower fingers maintain jaw thrust and the upper fingers are pulling the mandible into the mask while extending the head (arrows indicate direction of force).

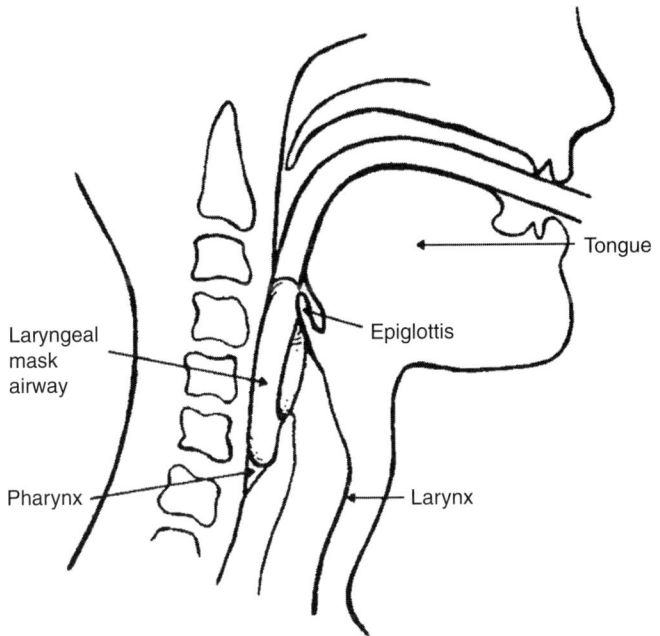

Figure 3.8 Laryngeal mask airway (LMA): normal anatomic position. The proximal portion of the LMA rests on the epiglottis, while the distal end extends into the pharynx at the upper end of the esophagus. The airway opening on the LMA overlies the laryngeal inlet. This figure demonstrates a prototypical LMA and is not meant to represent any particular commercially available device. (Modified from Brain AJJ. The laryngeal mask: a new concept in airway management. *Br J Anaesth* 1983; **55**: 801; with permission.)

device in cases of periglottic or subglottic pathology (e.g., laryngospasm, subglottic obstruction).[10]

The LMA is inserted blindly into the oropharynx, forming a low-pressure seal around the laryngeal inlet and thereby permitting gentle positive-pressure ventilation with a leak pressure in the range of 15–20 cm H_2O. Although the LMA is relatively contraindicated in the presence of a known supraglottic hematoma that might rupture, it can be very useful in other supraglottic obstructive trauma conditions, such as those due to swelling, edema, or redundant tissues. Placement of an LMA requires an anesthetized airway or an anesthetized patient. The LMA has been shown to rapidly restore efficient ventilation in cannot intubate–cannot ventilate situations.[11]

The LMA can be used as an airway intubation "conduit" for various difficult intubation scenarios, in particular for FOB-assisted intubation.[10] Although the LMA usually sits around the larynx, it occupies a perfect central position only 45–60% of the time. Caution should be exercised when attempting to blindly pass an ETT through a functioning LMA, because of the high blind-passage failure rate[12] and the risk of doing harm to a tenuous airway. Blind passage is particularly dangerous in the setting of stridor, known or anticipated partial airway disruption, or obstruction and other conditions where blind passage risks converting a partial airway disruption into a complete one (e.g., partial airway tear). This admonition against blind manipulation in the setting of airway trauma also applies to the Fastrach LMA, despite the fact that this device is marketed for, and has been

successfully used in, other emergency conditions where the risk of airway injury is low.[13] Fiberoptic intubation through a functioning LMA is superior to blind manipulation, because it can be performed under direct vision with almost 100% success through several types of commercially available LMAs, including the Classic, Fastrach, and ILA.[10]

Rigid direct laryngoscopy

Prior to performing laryngoscopy, the blade and handle should be tested to ensure proper function. The laryngoscope is held in the left hand, and the right hand is used to place the styletted ETT through the vocal cords and into the trachea. The mouth is opened by simultaneously extending the head on the neck with the right hand (except in suspected C-spine injury, where in-line immobilization is maintained) and using the small finger of the left hand while holding the laryngoscope to push the anterior part of the mandible in a caudal direction and opening the mouth. As the blade enters the oral cavity gentle pressure is applied on the tongue, sweeping it leftward and anterior, thereby exposing the glottic aperture.

Two basic blade types are commonly used for laryngoscopy: a curved blade (Macintosh) and straight blade (Miller and Wisconsin). The curved Macintosh blade tip is placed in the vallecula after sliding the tongue leftward and anterior, while the laryngoscope handle is lifted in a forward and upward direction, stretching the hyoepiglottic ligament. This causes the epiglottis to move upward out of view, unveiling a view of the arytenoid cartilages and eventually the vocal cords. In contrast, the straight Miller blade is inserted under the epiglottis and then the epiglottis is elevated to expose the glottic aperture.

Six common errors can occur during laryngoscopy using a standard Macintosh or Miller/Wisconsin type blade. First, the blade can be inserted too far into the pharynx, elevating the entire larynx, which exposes the esophagus instead of the glottis. Second, for optimal laryngoscopy, the tongue must be completely swept to the left side of the mouth with the flange on the blade. This is slightly more difficult to accomplish with the Miller blade because the flange is less prominent. Third, novice laryngoscopists frequently rock the laryngoscope in the patient's mouth by using the upper incisor as a fulcrum in a self-defeating attempt to visualize the glottis. This can chip the patient's upper incisors and moves the glottic aperture further anterior out of view. The correct approach is to lift the handle anterior and forward at an approximately 45-degree angle. Fourth, proper sniffing position is not always achieved or indicated. Fifth, in obese, barrel-chested patients and large-breasted women, it can be difficult to insert the blade in the mouth. Use of a short-handled laryngoscope or removal of the blade from the scope handle and reattaching it once the blade is positioned in the mouth helps with this predicament. Finally, improper blade selection may hinder laryngoscopy and intubation. If the patient has a long floppy epiglottis, a Miller blade may be best; a large wide tongue may be best managed using a Macintosh blade.

In-line cervical immobilization

Because of the risk of C-spine injury in severe trauma, all blunt-trauma patients should be suspected of having an unstable C-spine injury until proven otherwise. Rigid cervical collars, sand bags, rigid backboards, and other devices used to immobilize the C-spine can complicate airway management, especially when there is an abrupt and unexpected need for a definitive airway.

Prior to induction and laryngoscopy, the anterior portion of the rigid cervical collar is removed to facilitate intubation. The patient's neck should be prevented from flexing, extending, or rotating during intubation; this is accomplished by in-line immobilization. Rarely, immobilization of the neck may be overridden by the requirement to provide an adequate airway in hypoxemic patients, especially when unable to obtain a surgical airway. However, even under these extreme circumstances, the cervical movement should be limited to the minimum required to achieve airway patency.

RSI principles

Trauma patients and others who require emergency intubation are at increased risk of regurgitation and aspiration because they have not fasted prior to induction. RSI techniques were developed to minimize the likelihood of regurgitation and aspiration. Classically, RSI includes preoxygenation with 100% O_2 for 5 minutes, followed by the application of cricoid pressure, and the IV administration of an induction drug and a rapid-acting neuromuscular blockade drug such as succinylcholine, 1–2 mg/kg, or rocuronium, 1.2 mg/kg, without testing ventilation beforehand (Table 3.4, see Chapter 13). As soon as airway reflexes are lost, the laryngoscope is used to visualize the glottis and facilitate placement of a styletted ETT. Cricoid pressure is maintained until $P_{ET}CO_2$ is detected from the putative ETT, equal bilateral breath sounds are auscultated, and the operator instructs the assistant that it may be released.

Cricoid pressure (Sellick maneuver) denotes downward (posterior) pressure on the neck overlying the cricoid cartilage, which compresses the esophagus, decreasing the likelihood of gastric contents leaking into the pharynx. Occasionally cricoid pressure can impair the laryngoscopic view. "Laryngeal manipulation" is distinct from cricoid pressure and is accomplished by moving the thyroid cartilage posterior, thereby bringing the laryngeal aperture into view. Use of a rigid stylet also increases the likelihood of intubation success in difficult-to-intubate patients.[14] During intubation attempts, the patient should be carefully monitored by pulse oximetry, heart rate, blood pressure, and ECG. Intubation attempts should be interrupted by bag-mask ventilation whenever the procedure takes more than 30 seconds or when O_2 desaturation ($< 90\%$) occurs. If intubation attempts fail and adequate oxygenation cannot be achieved with bag-mask ventilation, an LMA should be considered.[10]

Modified RSI technique

The RSI technique can be modified by instituting bag-mask ventilation prior to placement of the ETT. Bag-mask ventilation during RSI is indicated in instances where apnea is likely to result in rapid desaturation despite properly performed preoxygenation, or if there are preexisting conditions that impair alveolar ventilation and oxygenation (e.g., head injury, respiratory failure). Trauma and critically ill patients often suffer from conditions causing increased right-to-left transpulmonary shunting (e.g., pulmonary contusion, hemothorax, pneumothorax, pneumonia) and thus require additional O_2 and ventilation after induction and prior to full effect of neuromuscular relaxants. This modification to the RSI technique involves gentle bag-mask ventilation with 100% O_2 while maintaining cricoid pressure to prevent gastric insufflation and decrease the risk of regurgitation and/or aspiration.

Drug-assisted intubation with spontaneous ventilation

This technique is employed in situations where apnea is likely to result in the inability to ventilate, such as in patients with partial airway obstruction manifested by audible stridor, and when positive-pressure ventilation might extend a partial airway tear into a complete disruption (e.g., tracheal or main-stem bronchus tears). The maintenance of spontaneous ventilation is also appropriate in a patient who cannot tolerate the hemodynamic consequence of positive-pressure ventilation, such as in decompensated cardiac tamponade. An uncooperative patient with an obvious difficult airway represents another patient condition where the maintenance of spontaneous ventilation is often indicated. In this setting, a small dose of sedation should be administered to gain control of the situation, and spontaneous ventilation is preserved while employing cricoid pressure.

Table 3.4 RSI principles: classic versus modified techniques

Elements	Pre-O_2	Cricoid pressure	Induction drug followed by paralytic	Manual ventilation deferred until ETT confirmed	Confirm ETT with $P_{ET}CO_2$
Classic	+	+	+	+	+
Modified	+	+	+	(−) Ventilate as needed to avoid hypoxemia	+

+, element is utilized during the technique of classic or modified RSI technique; (−), not utilized; ETT, endotracheal tube.

In situations where spontaneous ventilation is maintained and the patient is sedated as needed, the trachea can be intubated by using an FOB through an intubating mask.[15] The proper amount of drugs required to sedate the patient enough to manipulate the airway, without causing apnea, varies based on the size of the patient, the amount of blood loss, and the levels of other drugs already administered.

The difficult trauma airway

Awake techniques

An "awake" intubation technique is recommended for trauma patients with known or anticipated difficult airways, provided they are cooperative, stable, spontaneously ventilating, and as long as time allows. To optimize the conditions for successful intubation, cooperation is enhanced with proper mental and physical preparation. An awake FOB-guided technique is generally safe and appropriate for stable trauma scenarios. Even when a surgical airway is planned, performing an awake FOB-assisted intubation under direct vision is recommended whenever possible to achieve airway protection prior to performing the formal tracheostomy.

Techniques/devices for unstable, uncooperative, or apneic difficult-airway patients

There are three scenarios in which the need arises to intubate the trachea of an unstable, uncooperative, or apneic patient with a preexisting difficult airway. These situations include: (1) when the airway is not recognized to be difficult, (2) when the difficult-airway patient is already unconscious prior to presentation to the trauma bay, and (3) when the difficult-airway patient is hemodynamically unstable or unable to cooperate with an awake technique. In all of these conditions, the guidelines covering the anesthetized limb of the ASA difficult airway algorithm are followed. Whenever intubation cannot be achieved, bag-mask ventilation should be immediately instituted with enriched O_2 while applying cricoid pressure. In the cannot intubate–cannot ventilate patient, the emergency limb of the ASA algorithm is followed. Various airway modalities can be employed to maintain oxygenation and ventilation prior to definitive ETT placement, with the LMA being the first. If ventilation is not successful with the LMA, other secondary emergency airway tools are tried, including the Combitube, TTJV, laryngeal tube airway (LTA), and rigid ventilating bronchoscope. Various surgical airway techniques (cricothyroidotomy, tracheostomy) can also be considered.

Esophageal-tracheal Combitube

The Combitube is a supraglottic device developed specifically for emergency airway management. The Combitube comprises two longitudinally fused tubes made of polyvinyl chloride (PVC), each fastened to a standard 15 mm airway connector at the proximal end. The slightly longer of the two tubes is blue and is the primary (#1) conduit for ventilation in most situations. This longer tube has a blocked distal end with side hole openings at the pharyngeal level. There are two inflatable balloons on the Combitube: a proximal 100 mL latex pharyngeal balloon and a 15 mL PVC esophageal balloon near the distal portion.

Greater than 96% of the time when the Combitube is inserted blindly, esophageal placement results. The tube is inserted until the upper incisors lie between the two proximal black rings etched onto the external surface of the tube. At that point, the proximal cuff is inflated with 100 mL of air via the blue pilot balloon. Next, the distal esophageal cuff is inflated with 15 mL of air via a white pilot balloon. Ventilation is then initiated via the #1 tube (blue) and $P_{ET}CO_2$ should be detected. Detection of $P_{ET}CO_2$ confirms that the Combitube is properly placed in the esophagus, and the ventilation has traveled through the side hole openings between the 100 mL pharyngeal balloon and the 15 mL esophageal balloon then passing through the laryngeal aperture and into the trachea. In rare cases (less than 4%) where the Combitube enters the trachea, applying positive pressure to tube #1 will not ventilate the lungs and CO_2 will not be detected from the exhalate of tube #1. At this point, tube #2 should be ventilated and assessed for $P_{ET}CO_2$.[16]

Laryngeal mask airway

The LMA is not only an emergency aid used to establish ventilation in the cannot intubate–cannot ventilate situation; it can also serve as a conduit for intubation once ventilation has been established. The ASA algorithm and guidelines do not endorse any particular brand or subtype of LMA. However, whenever gastric volumes are expected to be large (e.g., following a large meal, known bowel obstruction), the ProSeal may be superior; and whenever the LMA will likely be used as a conduit for FOB-assisted intubation, the Cookgas ILA (Fig. 3.9) is often best, because the ventilation tube is wider and shorter than in the other conventional LMAs, and the ILA does not include an epiglottis elevating bar, which is present with the Fastrach.

Only in rare trauma situations, where there is absolutely no concern of airway swelling, direct airway injury, stridor, or abscess, should the Fastrach be used with blind ETT insertion. In all of the aforementioned conditions, blind manipulation can convert partial airway obstruction into complete disruption and is therefore contraindicated. The Fastrach LMA is inserted blindly into the pharynx, forming a low seal around the laryngeal inlet just as in the Classic LMA (Fig. 3.8).

The special design features of the Fastrach (Fig. 3.10) include a rigid, anatomically curved conduit that is wide enough to accept an 8.0 ETT with an epiglottic elevating bar to facilitate the blind passage of the special ETT. Once ventilation is confirmed with the Fastrach LMA, the ETT can be blindly passed via the LMA conduit into the trachea. The blind intratracheal placement must be confirmed with $P_{ET}CO_2$.

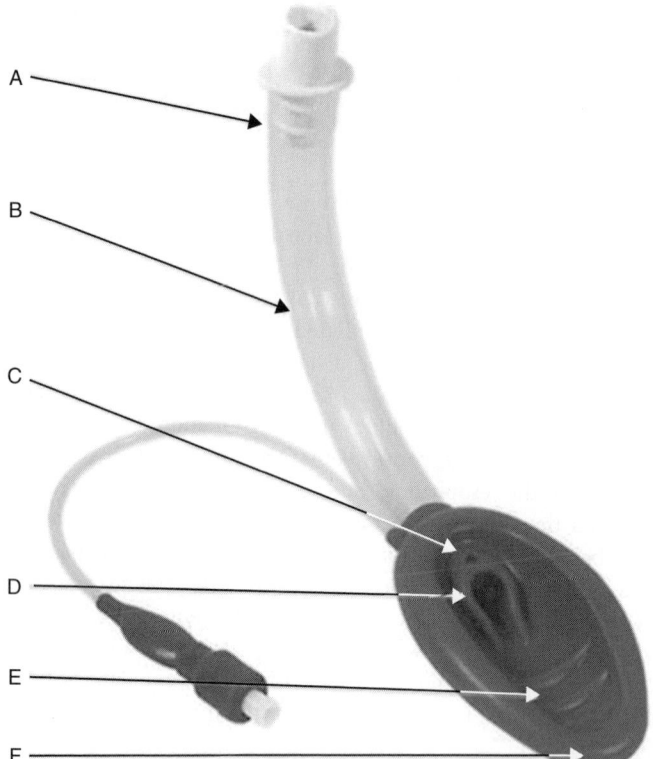

Figure 3.9 Cookgas Intubating Laryngeal Airway (ILA). The Cookgas ILA has several benefits over other LMAs for emergency airway use. (**A**) 15 mm airway connector ridges facilitate easy removal for fiberoptic airway management and improved tube seal upon replacement. (**B**) Oval-shaped hypercurved airway ventilation tube resists kinking. In addition, the relatively large internal diameter accommodates large adult endotracheal tubes (ETTs): 2.5 ILA allows 6.5 ETT, 3.5 ILA allows 7.5 ETT, and 4.5 ILA allows 8.5 ETT. Furthermore, the relatively short length of the ventilation tube facilitates fiberoptic intubation. (**C**) The auxiliary airway hole improves airflow and prevents suction effects from drawing up the epiglottis inside the airway tube. (**D**) The keyhole-shaped airway outlet directs both FOB and ETTs toward the laryngeal inlet and is anatomically engineered to align with the glottic chink. (**E**) The mask ridges move against posterior larynx, improving the anterior seal. (**F**) Recessed front improves posterior pharyngeal fit and ILA stability. (Available through Mercury Medical, Clearwater, FL.)

The LMA can be kept in place until airway stability is achieved. Once successful ETT placement through the LMA is verified, the LMA can be deflated and removed using a push device to help keep the ETT in place. If intubation is not successful, ventilation can occur via the LMA between attempts.

Passage of an FOB through an LMA has a much higher chance of success (nearly 100% successful in most series),[10] compared with blind intubation via the Fastrach. A 6.0 mm internal diameter (ID) cuffed ETT (a nasal RAE tube is most suitable, because of its additional length) may be passed over the fiberoptic bronchoscope and through the shaft of the #3 and #4 sized Classic LMA, whereas a 7.0 mm ID cuffed ETT will only fit through the shaft of the #5 sized Classic LMA. Subsequently, if a larger ETT is required, the 6.0 or 7.0 mm ID cuffed ETT can be exchanged for a larger ETT using an airway exchange catheter.[11] The various-sized ETTs that fit through various-sized "classic" LMAs, and the FOBs that fit through

these ETTs, are listed in Table 3.5. Alternatively, and preferably when the glottis is expected to be of normal size, the authors recommend using the blue intubating LMA (ILA, by Cookgas, Mercury Medical, Clearwater, FL). The large-sized 4.5 will allow passage of an 8.0 or 8.5 ETT (Fig. 3.9).

The LMA, employed as a ventilatory device and/or an intubating conduit, is appropriately used in the ASA algorithm in three different places: (1) on the "awake intubation" limb of the algorithm as a conduit for FOB-guided tracheal intubation, and on the "anesthetized" limb as both (2) a life-saving ventilatory device and (3) a conduit for FOB-assisted tracheal intubation.

In general, the largest FOB that will fit through the ETT is best, to maximize the ability to pass the ETT through a normally sized adult glottis. The possibility of the ETT hanging up at the glottis is more common with the use of the pediatric-sized FOB. However, if the patient has a small glottis, then a smaller FOB and ETT is better. If an FOB of 4.0 mm or less external diameter is used with either the 6.0 mm or the 7.0 mm ID ETT, the lungs can be continuously ventilated around the FOB while it is contained within the ETT by passing the FOB through the self-sealing diaphragm of a bronchoscopy elbow adaptor.

Rigid bronchoscope

A rigid bronchoscope is a straight, metal, lighted tube capable of visualizing the large airways, with ventilatory capacity through the associated ventilating side port (Fig. 3.11). Rigid bronchoscopy is recommended as an emergency airway tool in the cannot intubate–cannot ventilate situation, especially when the LMA has failed or is contraindicated. The rigid bronchoscope is particularly effective in cases of large airway masses and bleeding.

Surgical airway options
Transtracheal jet ventilation

TTJV is another method of gaining emergency ventilation in a cannot intubate–cannot ventilate patient. It is a temporizing life-saving technique that should be considered when the reason for failure to ventilate is supralaryngeal or perilaryngeal (e.g., laryngeal fracture) and the LMA and Combitube have failed.

The TTJV technique involves palpating the cricothyroid membrane and advancing a 14 gauge angiocatheter through the membrane in the midline, aimed at an angle of 30–45 degrees caudally from the perpendicular. The intratracheal position of the catheter must be verified by attaching a syringe to the catheter and attempting to aspirate air. If air is not aspirated, the catheter may not be in the trachea and should be repositioned. Once free flow of air is documented, the syringe is removed from the hub of the IV catheter and replaced by the luer adaptor of a high-pressure TTJV inflation

Table 3.5 Relevant diameters of the different-sized laryngeal mask airways (LMAs), endotracheal tubes (ETTs), and fiberoptic bronchoscopes (FOBs) that fit into the ETTs

LMA	Size	Patient weight (kg)	LMA internal diameter (ID mm)	Cuff volume (mL)	Largest ETT inside LMA (ID mm)	Largest FOB inside ETT (mm)
Classic	1	< 6.5	5.25	2–5	3.5	2.7
Classic	2	6.5–20	7.0	7–10	4.5	3.5
Classic	2.5	20–30	8.4	14	5.0	4.0
Classic	3	30–70	10	15–20	6.0 cuffed	5.0
Classic	4	> 70	10	25–30	6.0 cuffed	5.0
Classic	5	> 90	11.5	25–30	7.0	6.5
Cookgas	2.5	20–50	10	20–25	6.5	6.5
Cookgas	3.5	50–70	12	25–30	7.5	6.5
Cookgas	4.5	> 70	14	25–30	8.5	6.5

Classic LMA (LMA North America, Inc., San Diego, CA.).
Cookgas ILA (Mercury Medical, Clearwater, FL.).

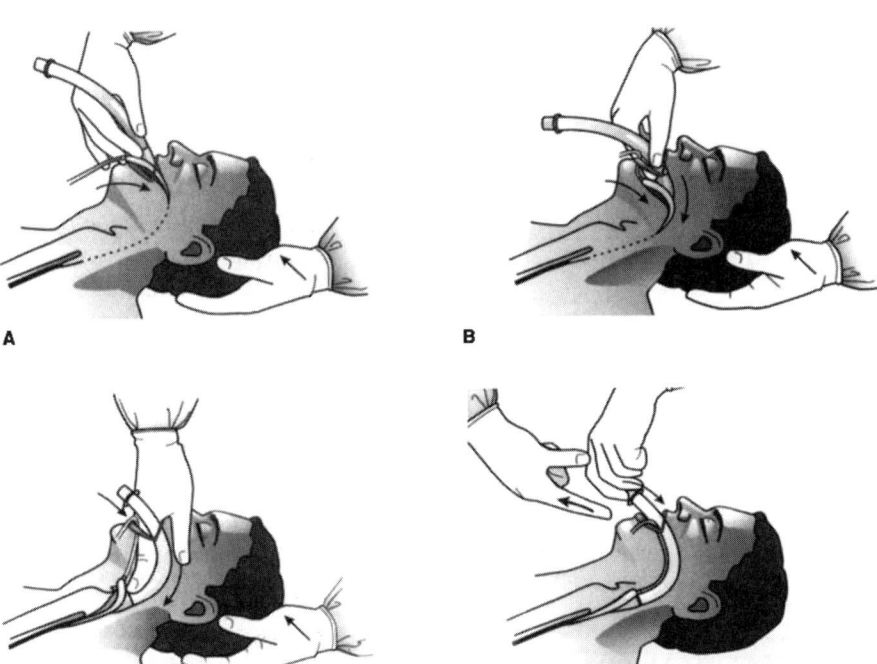

A

B

C

D

Figure 3.10 Fastrach LMA. Intubating laryngeal mask airway (ILMA), illustrating the rigid curve and handle. Notice the different window compared with standard LMA. (Courtesy of LMA North America, Inc., San Diego, CA.)

system. The TTJV inflation system should have 25–50 psi of pressure to allow flow down the small-gauge angiocatheter.

The natural airway must be maintained during exhalation, and occasionally this requires some jaw thrust. TTJV can maintain oxygenation and adequate ventilation for over 40 minutes.[17] Indeed, TTJV can take place while a definitive airway is established by FOB intubation or during the surgical creation of a tracheostomy.

TTJV is an effective means of providing oxygen in the setting where the obstruction to ventilation is at or below the level of the glottis. In airway injuries involving a tear between the glottis and the distal tracheobronchial tree, TTJV is absolutely contraindicated because the positive-pressure ventilation can cause a pneumothorax or pneumomediastinum, or it can even convert a partial airway tear into a complete airway separation.

Cricothyroidotomy: percutaneous

The same technique described for TTJV is used to place a thin-wall (14 gauge or larger) needle into the trachea. Once the needle is confirmed to be intratracheal, a wire is passed

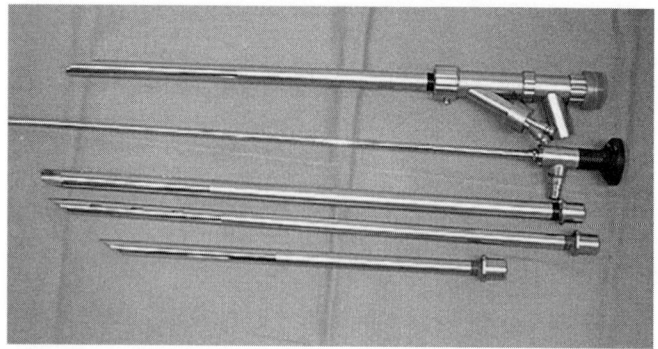

Figure 3.11 Rigid bronchoscope with ventilating side port and optic guide. Several sizes are shown.

through the needle into the trachea by using the Seldinger technique. Maintaining the guidewire several centimeters into the trachea, the cricothyroidotomy site is dilated. Then, using the Seldinger technique, the cricothyroidotomy tube is advanced, confirmed to be intratracheal and secured in place.

Cricothyroidotomy: open

Cricothyroidotomy is the emergency surgical airway of choice (versus tracheostomy) because there is less bleeding and a decreased insertion time due to the ease of determining anatomic landmarks. The thyroid cartilage is stabilized and an incision is made through the skin and subcutaneous tissue overlying the cricothyroid membrane. The membrane is then opened with a stab incision, an ETT or cricothyroidotomy tube is inserted, and placement is confirmed in the usual fashion. Of note, whenever conditions and time allow for a formal tracheostomy, it is favored over the emergency cricothyroidotomy, because of the decreased risk of subglottic stenosis, which more frequently occurs with cricothyroidotomy.

Tracheostomy

Tracheostomy is less desirable in emergency airway scenarios than cricothryoidotomy because it is slower and has greater potential for bleeding. Optimally, a transverse skin incision is made in a midline position for cosmetic and healing purposes. However, in emergency situations with novice surgeons, a vertical incision can be made in the midline of the neck to minimize bleeding and to avoid the anterior jugular veins overlying the trachea (Fig. 3.12). Next, skin and subcutaneous tissue are divided with a scalpel through the platysma, the strap muscles, and potentially the thyroid isthmus. Once the first few tracheal rings are exposed, a horizontal incision is made between the first and second tracheal rings and the tube is introduced into the trachea. Percutaneous placement of a tracheostomy tube can be performed, but bronchoscopic guidance is recommended to reduce the chance of paratracheal insertion and to document real-time intratracheal position of the needle, the wire, the dilators, and the tracheostomy tube.

Blind intubation techniques

Blind intubation techniques are contraindicated in the setting of stridor, known mass-expanding lesions, or known partial airway injuries where blind manipulation can change a partial airway obstruction into a complete obstruction.

Blind nasal intubation

Blind nasal intubation is contraindicated in the presence of maxillofacial trauma, where fracture of the cribriform bone is possible, and in the setting of nasal bleeding or coagulopathy (see Chapters 24 and 25). When performing a blind nasal intubation, the patient should be sitting upright at 45 degrees (rarely appropriate in the acute trauma setting), spontaneously ventilating, and, optimally, awake and cooperative. The ETT is placed in the already dilated and anesthetized nasal passage and the airway expert's ear is placed near the 15 mm connector end of the endotracheal tube.

As the ETT is passed down the nasal passage toward the glottic aperture, the airway sounds from the patient will become louder. When the airway sounds are loudest, the patient should be instructed to pant or take some deep breaths, which then opens the glottic aperture, at which point the ETT should be advanced during inspiration. Using this maneuver, the ETT is most likely to enter the larynx due to the patient's inhalation efforts.

It is occasionally beneficial to use a special flexible-tipped ETT known as an Endotrol tube during blind intubation attempts. The Endotrol tube allows the operator to flex the ETT anteriorly while advancing the tube. Clinical endpoints alerting the physician that the ETT has entered the patient's trachea include: (1) the patient is no longer able to speak, (2) increased secretions are heard emanating from the ETT with exhalation, and (3) coughing is elicited as the ETT passes down the larynx into the trachea. Because clinical endpoints are imprecise, the endotracheal position must be confirmed just as with any other method of intubation, using $P_{ET}CO_2$ and so on.

Light wand

Although the light wand is often used electively in anesthetized patients, it can be used as an adjunct in the cannot intubate–cannot ventilate patient. All commercially available light wands consist of a lighted stylet over which an ETT fits. The patient is anesthetized and the ETT with lighted stylet is passed into the oropharynx. Pulling the tongue out can frequently facilitate passing the light wand into the trachea. Once the ETT passes through the cords and enters into the larynx it produces a "jack-o'-lantern" effect due to transillumination of light. The transillumination is very prominent when the room lights are dimmed but may be difficult to appreciate in bright-light settings. Once the light wand is in the larynx, the ETT is advanced and the stylet is withdrawn. Confirmation that the ETT is in proper tracheal position must then be accomplished

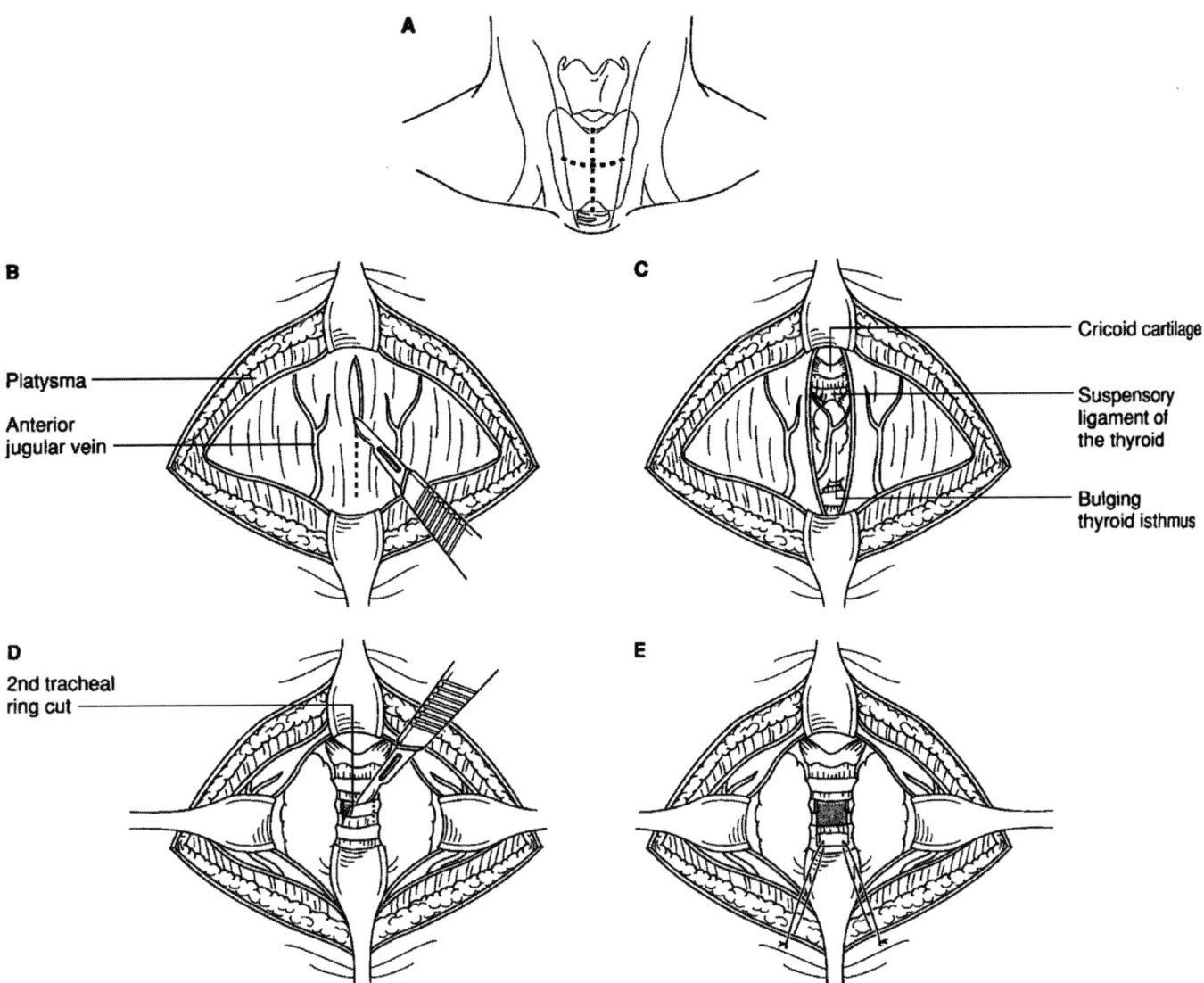

Figure 3.12 Tracheostomy. (**A**) A transverse incision is usually made for elective tracheostomy, but a vertical incision allows for less bleeding in an emergency procedure. (**B**) The strap muscles are separated and (**C, D**) the thyroid isthmus is retracted caudally. (**E**) After the second tracheal ring is cleaned off, an inferiorly based flap is developed in the tracheal wall and sutured to the skin to allow easy access to the trachea while the tract matures. (Reproduced with permission from "Head and neck," in Greenfield LJ, et al., ed., *Surgery: Scientific Principles and Practices*. Philadelphia, PA: Lippincott–Raven, 1997, p. 644.)

using $P_{ET}CO_2$ and other standard means. The light wand technique is widely applicable to many situations and environments. It has been used successfully in patients when conventional laryngoscopy may be difficult, such as small mouth opening, large protruding teeth, and decreased head extension.[18] The light wand is contraindicated in the presence of stridor or obvious airway trauma (as are all "blind" intubation techniques).

Video laryngoscopy

Approximately 2% of patients require three or more attempts or are unable to be successfully intubated with a standard laryngoscope,[19] which can have devastating consequences especially if airway management is not elective. Esophageal and difficult intubation represent the largest source of mortality reported in the ASA's closed claims database, and more than half of these claims resulted in either brain damage or death.[1] Very often, difficult or impossible intubation is due to the inability of the operator to align the oropharyngeal and laryngeal axes and obtain an adequate view of the glottic inlet. Because of this, many novel devices have been introduced commercially, all of which are intended to facilitate endotracheal intubation in the absence of an adequate view of the larynx. These devices have become a popular alternative for airway management in trauma and nontrauma patients.

Video laryngoscopes are a diverse range of devices that use a video camera to image the larynx indirectly. Broadly, they have been divided into three categories based on design: (1) scopes that are optical, lighted stylets, (2) scopes that use an integrated channel to guide the ETT during insertion, and (3) scopes that are modifications of the traditional direct laryngoscopy blades.[20]

Optical stylets are modifications of the light wand described above. They are rigid devices with distal video optics and light sources over which an operator places an ETT. Unlike the light wand, however, optical stylets work by direct video guidance and not transillumination. The stylet is inserted into the larynx and the glottis is visualized as the ETT is slid off past the vocal cords. These devices have a variety of modifications including steep angulation of the distal end, which permits visualization of the larynx through small mouth openings and in patients who have very anteriorly displaced glottic openings. Examples include the Shikani Optical Stylet and the Video RIFL.

Guide-channel video laryngoscope are designed with a distal camera and light source to image the larynx attached to a rigid channel through which an ETT is inserted. The channel guides the ETT into the larynx under direct vision. These devices are available in various sizes designed for adult, pediatric, or double-lumen endobronchial intubation. Some are disposable, and most have connections for external video viewing. Examples of guide-channel devices include the Airtraq and Pentax AWS.

Among the most widely used video laryngoscopes are the devices that incorporate video systems and light bundles into traditional rigid blades. These include the GlideScope, McGrath video laryngoscope, Storz C-Mac video laryngoscope, and others. All of these devices are modifications of the traditional Macintosh or Miller blades incorporating digital cameras and light sources near the distal end of the blade. Some have an attached video screen on the handle of the device, while others use an external video monitor. The GlideScope uses a curved plastic blade over a video and light bundle to improve visualization of the larynx. The blade is curved to approximately 60 degrees and can be either reusable or disposable. The blade has a CMOS (complementary metal oxide semiconductor) camera chip as well as an LED (light-emitting diode) light source, and the image is displayed on a separate view screen. Several different blade sizes are available, and the device comes with a rigid stylet curved at approximately the same angle as the blade. The McGrath video laryngoscope has a similar design but uniquely permits modification of the length of the Macintosh-type blade and incorporates the viewing screen into the device's handle.

In prospective trials, investigators have repeatedly reported that the view of the larynx obtained by a video scope is as good as or superior to the view obtained using traditional laryngoscopy.[21,22] In 2005, Sun and colleagues found that in 200 unselected patients who were randomized to undergo endotracheal intubation with either a traditional Macintosh blade or a GlideScope video laryngoscope, 68% of those who were Cormack and Lehane (C&L) grade 2 or 3 by traditional laryngoscopy demonstrated an improvement in C&L grade with the video laryngoscope.[23] Of note, these investigators

demonstrated that six patients in the GlideScope cohort demonstrated a worsening of their C&L grade, although this did not preclude intubation in any case. Other investigators have shown that, compared to direct laryngoscopy, video laryngoscopy provides an improved laryngeal view in obese patients,[24] patients in whom a difficult airway was predicted,[25] patients requiring in-line neck stabilization during intubation,[26] patients in the ICU,[27] and patients who had failed direct laryngoscopy.[28]

In most instances the improved view results in an increased success rate for intubation. For example, Noppens and colleagues studied 61 patients who had failed direct laryngoscopy and found that video laryngoscopy was able to establish an airway successfully in 95% of the cases. In 5% of the cases, however, endotracheal intubation was not accomplished despite a C&L grade 1 or grade 2 view.[28] This is consistent with other results that demonstrate that video laryngoscopes reliably improve the operator's view but also have a low failure rate for actual intubation.[29] In addition, there is evidence that this rate of failure may increase in settings outside of the operating room. A prospective trial from an academic emergency department reported a failure rate of 14% for video laryngoscopy but only 8% for traditional direct laryngoscopy.[30]

As described above, in-line immobilization of the C-spine is used for patients who require intubation after blunt traumatic injury. Because video laryngoscopes can more often obtain a C&L grade 1 or grade 2 view of the larynx without accessory maneuvers (such as neck extension or anterior laryngeal pressure), a number of authors have investigated whether these devices result in less motion of the cervical vertebrae during laryngoscopy and intubation. Here, findings have been inconsistent, although a majority of studies favor video laryngoscopy. Using video fluoroscopy, Turkstra et al. compared cervical spine motion with manual in-line stabilization during two different types of video laryngoscopy (Lightwand and GlideScope) with direct laryngoscopy.[31] They found a 57% reduction of spine movement with the Lightwand and a 50% reduction with the GlideScope when compared to a Macintosh blade. In their study, intubation with the Lightwand took no longer than with the Macintosh blade, but the GlideScope did require 62% more time. Other investigators, using similar methods, have obtained similar results.[32] Robitaille et al., in contrast, compared cervical spine motion in 20 patients who received direct laryngoscopy with a Macintosh blade and video laryngoscopy with a GlideScope.[33] Using continuous fluoroscopy, they found no difference in C-spine displacement at any level from the skull base to C5. In all studies, visualization of the larynx during in-line stabilization was consistently better with a video laryngoscope than with the traditional Macintosh blade.

Compared with lean subjects, direct laryngoscopy and endotracheal intubation in obese patients is known to be more difficult. Obese patients are more likely to require multiple attempts, require a longer duration to intubation, have a higher incidence of difficult or impossible intubation, and demonstrate poorer tolerance for apnea. Limited oropharyngeal space has been hypothesized to contribute to poor visualization of the larynx and may account for some of the difficulties associated with obese intubations. Video laryngoscopes are known to result in a significantly improved view when compared to traditional Macintosh blades, but their efficacy and safety for intubating the trachea of obese patients is unsettled. Dhonneur et al. studied 318 nonrandomized patients presenting for elective obesity surgery and found that use of the LMA C-Trach and the Airtraq laryngoscope shortened the duration of apnea when compared to a conventional Macintosh blade.[34] They also found that four times as many patients intubated with a Macintosh blade desaturated below 88% as did patients intubated with an Airtraq laryngoscope, and concluded that the LMA C-Trach and Airtraq scopes are superior to the conventional Macintosh blade.

More recent data have not supported these findings. Andersen et al. randomized 100 obese patients scheduled for bariatric surgery to intubation with either a conventional Macintosh laryngoscope or the GlideScope and found that time to intubation was significantly longer in the group intubated with the GlideScope.[24] This was true despite the fact that laryngoscopic views were better in the group assigned to video laryngoscopy. There were no differences in complications between the two groups, and no subjective difference in the difficulty of intubation as estimated by the treating physician was reported. In Andersen's study, all intubations were performed by practitioners familiar with GlideScope and standard Macintosh blades.

Abdallah et al. also studied video laryngoscopy in morbidly obese patients, but compared the Pentax AWS to a conventional Macintosh laryngoscope.[35] They found that use of the Pentax video laryngoscope significantly increased the time to intubation and did not differ from traditional laryngoscopy in the frequency of successful intubation on the first attempt, overall successful intubation, or the number of attempts required. C&L grades were also better in the Pentax group than in controls.

The results of these trials leave unanswered the question as to whether video laryngoscopy makes intubation of obese patients more successful. Duration of apnea is of particular importance in these patients, whose FRC and oxygen reserve is diminished, and prospective trials with remarkably similar designs have yielded conflicting results concerning the effect of video laryngoscopy on duration of apnea. One possible explanation for this difference may be that, in these studies, the subjects' prior experience with video laryngoscopy was poorly controlled. In the data cited above, the authors report that all subjects had extensive experience with both traditional laryngoscopy and video laryngoscopy, but this experience was not quantified. There is some evidence that, in subjects with extensive experience in direct laryngoscopy, the benefits of video laryngoscopy on success rate are significantly smaller. Novices or practitioners with limited experience in traditional laryngoscopy tend to yield the greatest benefit from the video devices. So while it is clear that video laryngoscopes improve the view of the larynx in nearly every case, the extent to which this improved view translates into actual improvement in intubation rate is not yet clear. Some clinical trials of inexperienced trainees have failed to demonstrate any benefit of video laryngoscopy,[36] while others have demonstrated dramatic improvements.[37] In addition, video laryngoscopes confer little advantage to the operator when the cause of a difficult airway is not attributable to a poor view. Poorer success rates caused by pharyngeal or laryngeal edema, airway masses, external compression, poor mouth opening, inadequate anterior neck compliance, or airway distortion or disruption may not be improved with a video-guided laryngeal view. At present, video laryngoscopy seems unlikely to supplant flexible fiberoptic bronchoscopy, which has proven effective for many of these difficulties. Nonetheless, the video laryngoscope has been used either alone or to assist in awake intubation.[38]

But should the video laryngoscope replace the rigid direct laryngoscope, as has been advocated?[39] Recently the ASA published a revision of the difficult airway algorithm, and included video laryngoscopy among the alternative approaches to initial intubation and intubation after one failed attempt.[3] The superior view offered by the video laryngoscope devices will likely expand their role in initial and rescue airway management both in and out of the OR. It seems unlikely that these devices will completely replace the traditional laryngoscope, as their cost and availability remain limiting. In addition, failed video laryngoscopy, either as a primary technique or as a rescue method, has been reported. In one large retrospective study, altered neck anatomy significantly predicted failed video laryngoscopy with the GlideScope.[40] In addition to failure, complications from video laryngoscopy were reported, including palate and tonsillar pillar perforations, vocal cord trauma, and dental injuries. It seems likely that the utilization of video laryngoscope devices will increase, especially among less experienced providers, but maintenance of competence with alternative techniques is recommended.

Retrograde wire

Less commonly performed because of its time requirement, the retrograde technique was first described in 1963 by Ralph Waters, who employed a Tuohy needle to pass through the cricothyroid membrane in a cephalad direction.[41] An epidural catheter was then threaded through the Tuohy needle and the catheter was retrieved from the oropharynx by using a plastic dressmaker's hook. Next, both the tube and the catheter were withdrawn from the nares. In 1967, Powell and Ozdil introduced a wire-through-the-needle technique, and in their modification the wire was placed through the Murphy side hole of the ETT.[42] Placing the wire through the Murphy side hole allowed for the ETT to pass further through the cords than when the wire went out through the tip of the ETT. Other modifications of these techniques have been described, but the basic technique remains the same. Indeed, the Cookgas Critical Care division has developed an emergency retrograde intubation kit (Cookgas Mercury Medical, Clearwater, FL).

Table 3.6 Regional anesthesia and the trauma-related difficult airway

Consideration	Regional anesthesia might be indicated	Regional anesthesia contraindicated
Injury location	Superficial, extremity	Head, chest, abdomen
Mental status	Sober, cooperative, minimal sedation needed	Altered sensorium, decreased mental status
Urgency	Can stop surgery at any time	Unsafe to interrupt surgery to establish a definitive airway
Airway access	Good access to airway	Poor access to airway
Tolerate awake intubation if necessary	Agreed to awake intubation if necessary	Failure to agree on awake intubation if necessary
Hemodynamic status	Hemodynamically stable	Hemodynamically unstable

Regional anesthesia for surgery in the trauma patient with known difficult airway

Occasionally, surgery can be performed without securing the airway of a patient with a known difficult airway. In the cooperative and hemodynamically stable trauma patient with a solitary superficial extremity injury, a regional technique can be utilized so long as the patient understands and agrees to a plan that an awake intubation may need to be done if conditions change and warrant it (Table 3.6). In the patient with head or torso trauma, or an altered sensorium, a regional anesthetic is unwise because airway access is compromised, making a controlled awake intubation impossible.

Fiberoptic bronchoscopy: techniques and pitfalls

An FOB-assisted intubation is optimally performed in awake patients who are breathing spontaneously, but can also be used in anesthetized or apneic patients. There are many recipes for accomplishment of FOB-guided intubation. Success with FOB-guided intubation requires appropriate patient selection and preparation along with appropriate technique and adequate experience, because conditions can vary in different patients, requiring the skill of the endoscopist to achieve success (Table 3.7).

Patient selection

Indications for FOB intubation include (1) situations where alignment of the oral, pharyngeal, and laryngeal axes is diffi-cult or ill-advised (e.g., C-spine injury or neck fixed in halo)

and (2) situations where direct laryngoscopy is expected to be difficult (e.g., hyomental distance [HMD] < 6 cm, Mallampati class III or IV: Fig. 3.5), especially situations with small mouth openings and in temporomandibular disease. Contraindica-tions to FOB intubation include massive oropharyngeal hem-orrhage (unable to adequately see) and conditions where time for adequate topicalization does not exist, such as hemody-namic instability, respiratory distress, or life-threatening airway obstruction.

Relative contraindications for FOB intubation include copious secretions or friable tissues that are difficult to manage with antisialagogues and careful manipulation of the FOB. Oropharyngeal tumors, abscesses, maxillofacial trauma, and most causes of stridor are optimally managed with awake techniques, and should all be considered as good indications for FOB-assisted intubation, providing the endoscopist can avoid blood and see the entire way into the trachea.

Patient preparation
Positioning for FOB

Optimally, the patient is placed into a sitting position; in patients with C-spine injuries, this can be allowed as long as there is no thoracolumbar spine injury. Nasal cannula oxygen is administered, and pulse oximetry and other moni-toring devices are applied. The sitting position allows secre-tions to run down into the esophagus and out of the bronchoscopic view. Gravity also helps direct the fiberoptic bronchoscope toward the larynx better than in the supine position, where gravity tends to favor the posterior esopha-geal orifice.

Analgesia, sedation, and antisialagogue

Patients should receive an antisialagogue (glycopyrrolate, 0.2 mg) and sedation prior to starting the procedure. Opioids, benzodiazepines, dexmedetomidine, ketamine, and droperidol have all been used successfully. However, low-dose opioids alone (fentanyl, 1–2 µg/kg) are usually sufficient in patients who are not opioid-tolerant. Midazolam can cause some patients to become hyperalgesic and uncooperative, but many have used this (and other) benzodiazepines successfully. Fen-tanyl is often adequate as a sole agent because it provides sedation as well as analgesia, both of which are useful while topicalization is occurring. Dexmedetomidine infusion pro-vides excellent sedation, decreases opioid requirements, attenuates tachycardia, and minimally depresses ventilation.

Local anesthesia and vasoconstriction

The described technique of mucosal topicalization and vaso-constriction can be used for FOB-guided ETT placement as well as with other awake airway devices. The patient should receive phenylephrine or oxymetolazone nasal spray applied into both nares prior to initiating topicalization if the nasal

Table 3.7 Causes of failure to intubate with fiberoptic bronchoscope

Cause of failure	Comments and solutions
Patient selection factors	These constitute relative contraindications to FOB.
Massive bleeding	Unable to visualize airway. Small amounts of bleeding can be controlled with frequent suctioning. A vasoconstrictor added to topical agents helps limit bleeding.
Uncooperative patient	Patient will not hold still and or is very belligerent. Rare in elective situations, but common in trauma and emergency scenarios.
Patient too unstable	Does not allow time to properly topicalize airway
Patient preparation factors	
Inadequate topical anesthesia	Be patient, take time to topicalize properly. Dry mucosa (glycopyrrolate), suction secretions from the oropharynx so that topical anesthesia can reach mucosa to work. Anesthetize the nose, nasopharynx, oropharynx, larynx, and trachea. Nerve blocks are usually unnecessary with proper topicalization.
Presence of secretions or small amounts of blood	Treat with proper suctioning, use of an antisialagogue (glycopyrrolate) and a vasoconstricting agent (phenylephrine), or use cocaine. Attach O_2 to suction port of FOB, blowing secretions away.
Patient desaturates during FOB	Patient should be wearing nasal prongs or mask O_2 during FOB. Also, endoscopist can attach O_2 to the suction channel of the FOB and instruct patient to pant (breathe rapidly) during intubation.
Endoscopist experience factors	
Inability to navigate normal anatomy	Most common problem for novice is too little practice with airway models and mannequins prior to attempting to intubate patients.
Distorted anatomy due to tumors or abscess	Use of FOB may be difficult. However, the endoscopist must be well grounded in normal anatomy prior to managing difficult airways.
Inability to visualize cords due to a large floppy epiglottis	Have patient say "Ahh" and or pant "like a puppy." (If patient is anesthetized, assistant can apply jaw thrust or pull the tongue out.)
Fogging of lens	Use a dilute detergent (chlorhexidine) to wipe the FOB lens prior to use, warm the FOB prior to use.
Inability to advance tube into trachea	Inadequate topical anesthesia – perform nerve block or use more topical.
	Large discrepancy between ETT and FOB – use the largest FOB that will fit easily through the ETT yet still allow easy removal with proper lubrication.
	Hung up at glottic opening. Pull back the ETT and rotate 90–180 degrees either right or left to allow the ETT to pass through the cords more easily.
Inability to remove the FOB	Beware the FOB may exit the Murphy eye of the ETT. This can be avoided if the FOB is threaded through the ETT prior to attempting intubation. Some endoscopists will place the lubricated ETT through the nares into the nasopharynx blindly and then pass the FOB through the ETT. This technique has greater risk of FOB exiting the Murphy eye. Also, be sure that the FOB is well lubricated with silicone or Xeroform gauze prior to placing through the ETT.

FOB, fiberoptic bronchoscope; O_2, oxygen; ETT, endotracheal tube.

route is planned. Next, the patient should be asked to report which nares allows for better airflow. This will identify the nares that should be intubated and primarily topicalized. However, both nares should be topicalized to block both the right and left superior laryngeal nerves and more fully anesthetize the supralaryngeal structures.

The nasopharynx, oropharynx, base of the tongue, and larynx should all be anesthetized. The nasopharynx can be anesthetized with either 4% cocaine or 4% lidocaine mixed with dilute phenylephrine. For nasopharyngeal anesthesia, 4% cocaine, although slightly more toxic, can be more efficacious, because of its inherent intense vasoconstriction coupled with a more rapid onset and a longer duration of action than lidocaine. The toxic dose of cocaine is 3 mg/kg, whereas the toxic dose with lidocaine is 7 mg/kg when used with vasoconstriction.

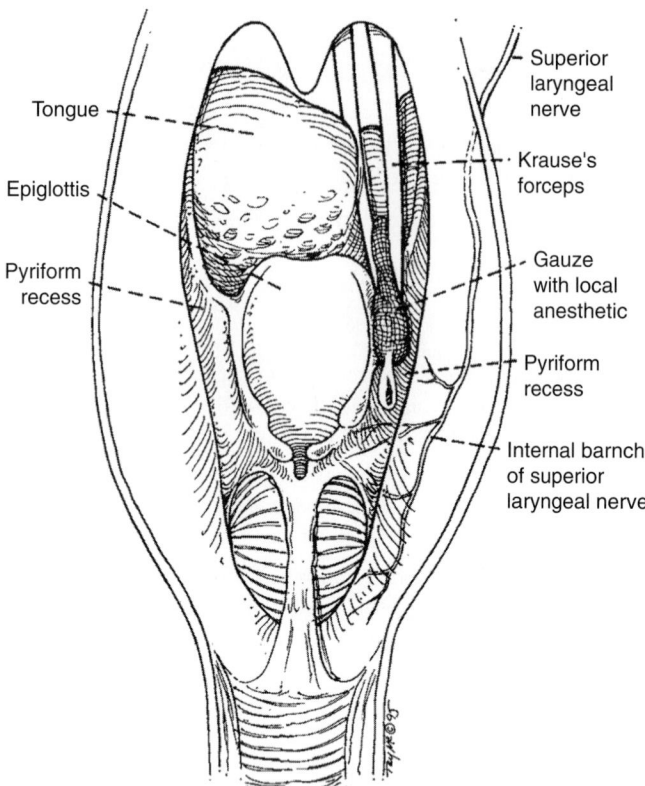

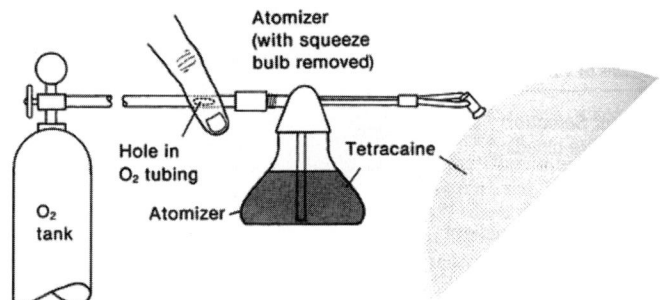

Figure 3.14 Continuous oxygen flow atomizer apparatus. Oxygen tubing is connected from an oxygen tank to the bulb attachment site of a DeVilbiss atomizer. A hole is cut in the oxygen tubing near the attachment site. Oxygen is allowed to flow into the tubing and out of the cut hole until a finger is applied covering the hole; then oxygen flows to the nebulizer and a fine mist of local anesthesia is emitted. The size and velocity of the spray is directly related to the flow of oxygen through the tubing.

Figure 3.13 Superior laryngeal nerve block by external approach ("topicalization"). Posterior view of the nasopharyngeal area showing the perforating branches of the superior laryngeal nerve. Krause's forceps are used with gauze soaked in local anesthetic fluid at the level of the pyriform sinus. (From University of California, Irvine, Department of Anesthesia D.A. teaching aids; with permission.)

Cocaine is topically applied to each nare by using Krause's forceps (Fig. 3.13) or a cotton-tipped applicator (Q-tip). Topicalization is initiated by painting the external nares and slowly working down the nasopharynx with the cocaine-impregnated Q-tip. By advancing the Q-tip into the pyriform fossa, the superior laryngeal nerve will also become blocked. The superior laryngeal nerve innervates the epiglottis, aryepiglottic folds, and mucus membranes of the laryngeal structures down to the false cords. When the Q-tip can be inserted into the deepest recesses of the nasal cavity without causing discomfort, a soft 34 Fr nasal airway can be inserted. If the patient is not inconvenienced by this, the topicalization of the nasopharynx is complete.

While the nasopharynx is being anesthetized, simultaneous topicalization of the oropharynx and larynx should occur by spraying a fine mist of 4% lidocaine via a DeVilbiss nebulizer. The DeVilbiss sprayer can be modified by connecting it to a low-flow O_2 source after removing the squeeze bulb, thus providing a continuous source of aerosolized lidocaine (Fig. 3.14). When utilizing the DeVilbiss sprayer in this way, the patient can entrain the aerosolized lidocaine well into the trachea and past the carina. The patient should be instructed to

"pant like a puppy dog" to facilitate the inhalation early in the process. Later, the patient will be able to inhale a full vital capacity breath of the aerosolized local anesthetic, indicating that the subglottic structures are anesthetized. Once the DeVilbiss sprayer can fully enter the oropharynx without the patient gagging, oropharyngeal and base of tongue topicalization is adequate for fiberoptic intubation. Provided the patient has breathed enough lidocaine mist into the airways, the trachea is usually adequately anesthetized at this point as well.

Some endoscopists prefer performing nerve blocks of the glossopharyngeal nerve at the palatoglossal arch (Fig. 3.15) and the superior laryngeal nerve externally, where it crosses the superior cornu of the hyoid, as well as administering transtracheal lidocaine (Fig. 3.16). These maneuvers are not necessary for FOB-aided or blind nasal intubation techniques in properly topicalized patients. However, if awake laryngoscopy is planned with either a conventional laryngoscope or another device utilizing a blade (e.g., Bullard laryngoscope, Wu Scope, or Airtraq), the deep mucosal pressure receptors require blockade to prevent gagging. When these pressure-inducing rigid laryngoscopic devices are used to intubate the tracheas of awake patients, supplemental glossopharyngeal nerve blocks should also be performed.

Technique of fiberoptic intubation
Awake nasal technique

The largest ETT that will fit the patient's nasal passage should be used, and most adults can accept an 8.0 ETT. Indeed, provided the patient's nares can be easily dilated with a 34 Fr soft nasal airway, an 8.0 ETT will almost always fit through the nares. This is possible because the external diameter of a 34 Fr soft nasal airway is approximately 11.0 mm, whereas the external diameter of an 8.0 ETT is approximately 10.5 mm. However, in emergency situations, and in cases of stridor, smaller ETTs are best.

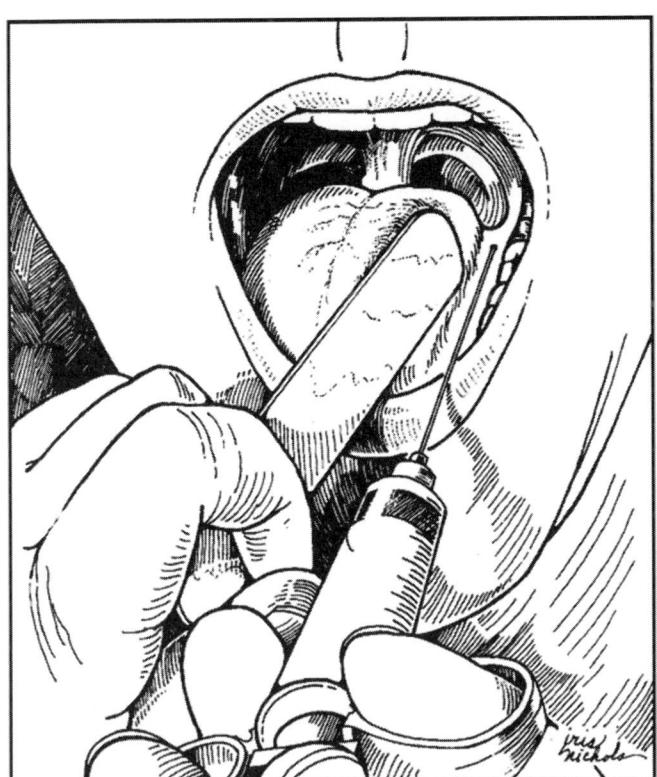

Figure 3.15 Glossopharyngeal nerve (lingual branch) block. The tongue is pushed medially with a tongue depressor, and a 3-inch spinal needle is inserted into the base of the anterior tonsillar pillar 0.5 cm lateral to the base of the tongue and advanced 0.5 cm deep. After negative aspiration, 2 mL of local anesthetic is injected. Both sides are injected for adequate block of the gag reflex. (From Mulroy MF. *Regional Anesthesia: an Illustrated Procedure Guide*, 3rd edition. Philadelphia, PA: Lippincott, Williams & Wilkins, 2002, p. 229; with permission.)

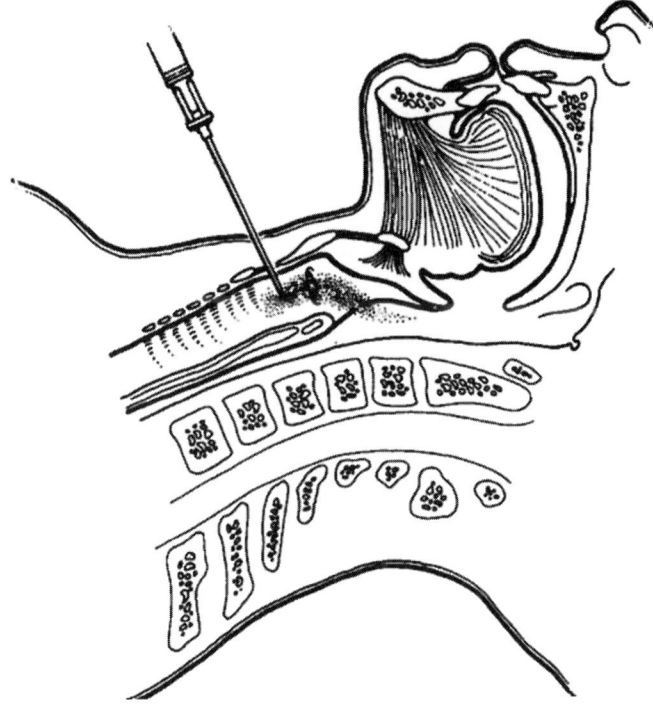

Figure 3.16 Transtracheal injection (topical subglottic anesthesia – recurrent laryngeal nerve distribution). A 20 gauge IV catheter is introduced through the cricoid membrane. Once tracheal entry is confirmed by air aspiration, 4 mL of topical anesthetic is injected as the patient inspires; the inward airflow carries the solution down the trachea, and the cough reflex will spread it up to the undersurface of the vocal cords. (From Mulroy MF. *Regional Anesthesia: an Illustrated Procedure Guide*, 3rd edition. Philadelphia, PA: Lippincott, Williams & Wilkins, 2002, p. 230; with permission.)

Following topicalization, the FOB, with preloaded ETT, is inserted into the patient's nares. Alternatively, an ETT can be placed in the nares to serve as an introducer and the FOB can then be placed through the ETT and into the nasal passage. The advantage of preloading the ETT over the FOB is elimination of the possibility that the FOB might exit the Murphy eye during intubation, which subsequently will not allow the ETT to enter the trachea. The advantage of the second technique is that the ETT serves as a dilating airway and a guide for the FOB. When the FOB exits the nasopharyngeally located ETT, it is frequently aiming directly into the laryngeal aperture.

When manipulating the FOB, it is useful to remember that small movements at the end of the FOB result in very large changes in the view that the endoscopist has. Regardless of the technique chosen for introducing the FOB into the nares, the endoscopist next advances the FOB under direct vision until the epiglottis or the laryngeal aperture is visualized. The FOB should never be advanced blindly, because structures that are not clearly identified can be damaged. Once the glottis or the epiglottis is in view, the FOB is maneuvered through the vocal cords and into the trachea. The FOB is then advanced further down the trachea to a position just above the carina. At this point, the ETT is threaded over the indwelling FOB, through the larynx, and into trachea.

If the ETT does not advance easily, it may be hung up at the arytenoids or at the laryngeal aperture. This can result from a large discrepancy between the internal diameter of the ETT and the outer diameter of the FOB, or because the ETT is simply too large for the glottis. Often rotating the ETT 90–180 degrees either clockwise or counterclockwise will facilitate passage of the ETT through the glottic aperture.

If the ETT will not pass despite the use of these maneuvers, then the ETT and FOB should be removed together as a unit and a smaller ETT utilized. If secretions become a problem during bronchoscopy, these can be managed by flushing saline down the working channel of the FOB and suctioning under direct vision. Alternatively, oxygen can be administered through the working channel and used to blow secretions out of the way. The additional benefit of the O_2 insufflation technique is the increased FiO_2 provided in spontaneously breathing patients. Switching back and forth between suction and O_2 insufflation is often useful.

Once the ETT is positioned approximately 3–4 cm above the carina, the FOB is removed. Difficulty in removing the FOB can result from a narrow nasal passage with crimping of the ETT, and also when the FOB is inadvertently passed through the Murphy eye of the ETT, trapping it in place. If this occurs, the FOB and the ETT may have to be removed as a unit and the procedure begun once again.

Oral technique

The FOB can be advanced through the oropharynx in both awake, spontaneously ventilating patients and those who are asleep and being ventilated with a mask or LMA. The sedation and local anesthesia preparation for an awake oral intubation is the same as that required for a nasal intubation.

With oral intubation in a spontaneously ventilating patient, the FOB is advanced into the airway through a rigid plastic Ovassapian oral airway intubator. Oral intubation can be more difficult in some patients, because the FOB must take a more acute bend at the oropharynx in order to be directed toward the larynx, compared with the more gentle curvature required for nasal intubation. Having an assistant perform a jaw-thrust or chin-lift maneuver may be helpful in this regard.

When FOB-assisted intubation is performed in patients under general anesthesia, concomitant ventilation can be achieved using an LMA, Intubating Fastrach LMA, or the Patil intubating mask with self-sealing diaphragm, along with the Ovassapian oral airway intubator, as described by Rogers and Benumof.[43] Entry into the glottis is generally easier with an LMA-FOB-assisted intubation than with an intubating mask-FOB-assisted technique.

Difficult airway algorithms
The ASA difficult airway algorithm

Practice guidelines for management of the difficult airway have been published by the ASA Task Force on Management of the Difficult Airway for 20 years. The original practice guidelines were developed by a task force of ASA members who expounded on the original ideas put forth in a medical intelligence article written by J. L. Benumof in 1991, entitled "Management of the difficult airway."[2]

In 1996, Benumof wrote another landmark article discussing the development and use of the LMA and its implications for the ASA algorithm.[10] This article contributed to the ASA's decision to revise the 1993 algorithm. The current version emerged after the ASA Task Force reviewed the literature published over the past 60 years and obtained expert opinions from other ASA members to build a consensus. The key points of the 2013 practice guidelines are summarized in Table 3.8.

Several critical decision-tree elements are present in the ASA difficult airway algorithm. These include recognition of the difficult airway, awake intubation techniques, and anesthetized intubation techniques. Fig. 3.17 shows the ASA algorithm as revised in 2003, along with modifications required for utilization in the trauma patient.

Table 3.8 Principles of the ASA difficult airway (DA) algorithm

Principles	Examples/comments
A. Airway history is useful	Ask patient, check chart/bracelet
B. Airway examination (11-step)	Should be conducted on all patients whenever feasible (Table 3.3)
C. Additional evaluation may be indicated in some patients	e.g., Rheumatoid arthritis patients may need flexion/extension C-spine x-rays
D. Basic preparation for a difficult airway, per 2013 ASA DA guidelines	Requires a portable DA storage unit with contents that include airway tools that can assist management of the difficult airway (Table 3.1).
E. When a patient is identified as having a DA several things should happen	1. Inform patient/family of risks, plans, and alternative management methods 2. Identify an experienced helper to assist in managing the DA 3. Preoxygenate 4. Pursue opportunities to administer O_2 to patient during DA management
F. The anesthesiologist should have a strategy for DA management – one such strategy is following the algorithm	1. Assess the likelihood of any one of the four basic problems: • Difficult ventilation • Difficult intubation • Difficulty with patient cooperation or consent • Difficult tracheostomy 2. Consider the merits of crossing the three basic bridges to airway access: • Awake vs. general anesthesia (RSI +/− modified with PPV) • Natural airway with ETT vs. surgical airway • Spontaneous ventilation vs. apnea 3. Identify the preferred primary approach (patient and condition specific) 4. Identify a back-up approach (i.e., Plan "B") 5. Exhaled CO_2 should be used for confirmation of tracheal intubation 6. Consideration of conducting surgery with regional/local technique. Significant judgment is required. Regional is seldom a wise choice for acute polytrauma patients (Table 3.6)

Table 3.8 (cont.)

Principles	Examples/comments
G. The anesthesiologist should also have a strategy for extubation or tube change of the DA patient. Every DA extubation strategy requires consideration of the following four elements:	1. Relative merits of awake extubation 2. Factors that may have an adverse impact on ventilation after extubation 3. Formulate an airway management plan that can be implemented if the patient is unable to maintain adequate ventilation after extubation 4. Consider use of an AEC for short-term use. An AEC can serve as a guide for expedited reintubation, or (via the hollow inner core) as a method to provide O_2 by insufflation (if patient breathing spontaneously) or via jet ventilation
H. Follow-up care and documentation	1. Inform patient/family of difficulty. Suggest patient get a card in wallet and a bracelet stating difficult airway 2. Document in chart specific problems with mask ventilation, LMA ventilation, or intubation. Also, document which tools were used successfully or unsuccessfully. Provide all guidance relevant for the next person managing the patient in the future

AEC, airway exchange catheter; ASA, American Society of Anesthesiologists; CO_2, carbon dioxide; DA, difficult airway; ETT, endotracheal tube; LMA, laryngeal mask airway; O_2, oxygen; PPV, positive-pressure ventilation; RSI, rapid sequence induction.

Recognition of the difficult airway

The ASA algorithm begins with recognition of airway difficulty. Penetrating trauma to the neck with stridor and cyanosis is easily recognized as a potentially difficult airway. However, more subtle anatomic or pathologic causes of airway difficulty can go unrecognized in the traumatized patient because of hasty preoperative evaluation or preoccupation with other aspects of care. Missed signs of a difficult airway can be minimized if one looks carefully for both pathologic and anatomic abnormalities. Whenever the patient is recognized to have a difficult airway, the clinician should consider securing the airway by using an awake technique, as long as the patient is cooperative, hemodynamically stable, and spontaneously ventilating.

Awake limb of the ASA difficult airway algorithm

After deciding to intubate the trachea by using an awake technique, the airway expert must select the most appropriate technique given the reason for airway difficulty and the clinical circumstances. The technique chosen is not as important as is the airway expert's experience and judgment as to suitability of a particular airway intubation technique given the patient's difficult airway circumstances.

Indeed, the ASA algorithm does not endorse any specific airway technique. However, it does emphasize that the patient must be properly prepared for an awake technique, and the physician must ensure that spontaneous ventilation continues and O_2 saturation is maintained throughout the procedure. In trauma scenarios, the patient must also be cooperative and stable.

The basic ASA algorithm recommends considering abandoning the airway attempt while maintaining spontaneous ventilation, and allowing the patient to recover from topicalization or sedative medications and resume management later with a better plan. However, stopping is rarely an option in emergency airway management situations. At any time during the awake intubation manipulation, if the patient is unable to ventilate by mask and intubation is not successful, then consideration should be given to use of emergency airway adjunct devices such as the LMA, Combitube, TTJV, or a surgical airway.

Uncooperative/unstable/anesthetized limb of the algorithm

The physician may be confronted with the need to intubate the trachea of an unconscious or anesthetized patient with a difficult airway. In the uncooperative patient, preinduction assessment should have identified factors that might make intubation of the trachea difficult, and the airway expert should consider using a technique that maintains spontaneous ventilation despite the need for anesthesia.

ASA difficult airway algorithm modified for trauma

Trauma patients who are hemodynamically stable without specific injuries to the head, neck, maxilla–face, or chest, can be managed as outlined by the ASA algorithm (Fig. 3.17). Isolated abdominal or extremity injuries in hemodynamically stable patients fall into this category. However, in this "uncomplicated" setting, the anesthesiologist must maintain a heightened vigilance for and undertake protective measures against aspiration (Table 3.9).

Trauma and associated conditions such as apprehension, opioid administration, alcohol ingestion, and gastrointestinal disorders are all associated with an increased volume of gastric contents. Pain, trauma, and apprehension decrease the gastric pH and further increase the risk that passive regurgitation will progress to aspiration syndrome. Therefore, all trauma patients are expected to have full stomachs, and RSI should always be considered (see Chapter 13).

However, many airway disasters have resulted from an inappropriate placement of gastric regurgitation and

(A)

DIFFICULT AIRWAY ALGORITHM (MODIFIED FOR TRAUMA)

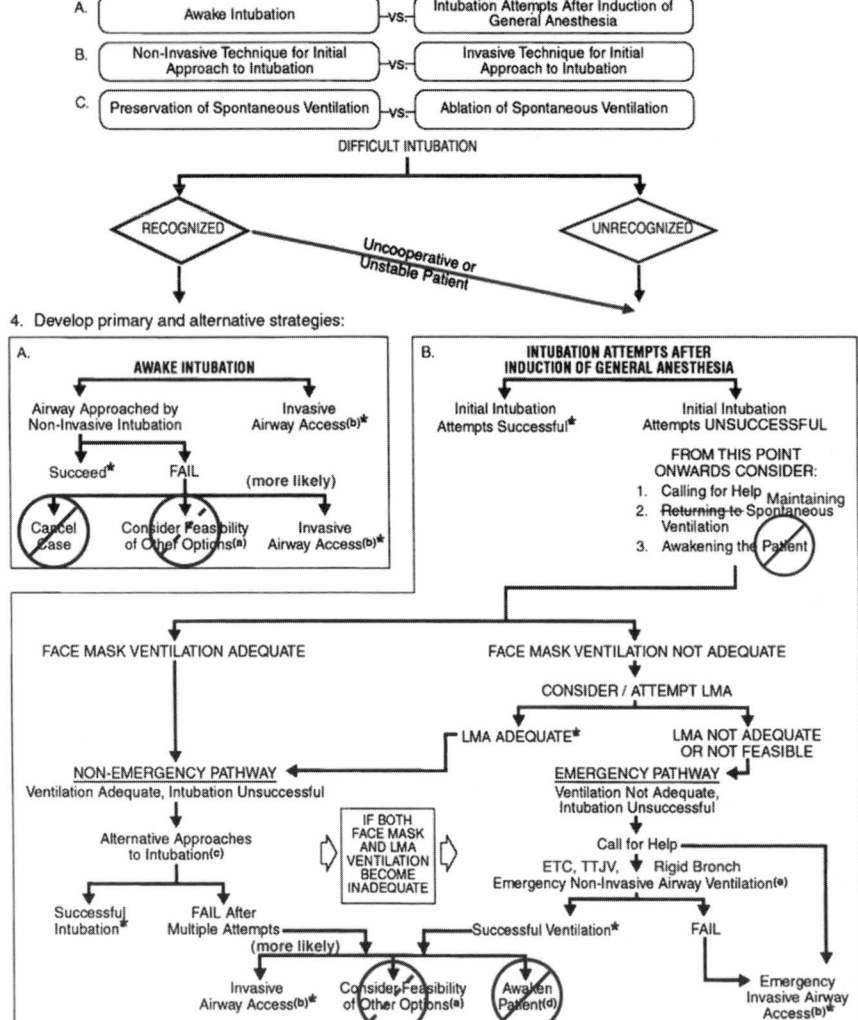

AMERICAN SOCIETY OF ANESTHESIOLOGISTS

2003 DIFFICULT AIRWAY ALGORITHM (MODIFIED FOR TRAUMA)

1. Assess the likelihood and clinical impact of basic management problems:
   A. Difficult Ventilation
   B. Difficult Intubation
   C. Difficulty with Patient Cooperation or Consent
   D. Difficult Tracheostomy

2. Actively pursue opportunities to deliver supplemental oxygen throughout the process of difficult airway management

3. Consider the relative merits and feasibility of basic management choices:

   A. Awake Intubation -vs- Intubation Attempts After Induction of General Anesthesia
   B. Non-Invasive Technique for Initial Approach to Intubation -vs- Invasive Technique for Initial Approach to Intubation
   C. Preservation of Spontaneous Ventilation -vs- Ablation of Spontaneous Ventilation

   DIFFICULT INTUBATION

   RECOGNIZED — Uncooperative or Unstable Patient — UNRECOGNIZED

4. Develop primary and alternative strategies:

   A. **AWAKE INTUBATION**
   Airway Approached by Non-Invasive Intubation / Invasive Airway Access(b)*
   Succeed* / FAIL / (more likely)
   Cancel Case / Consider Feasibility of Other Options(a) / Invasive Airway Access(b)*

   B. **INTUBATION ATTEMPTS AFTER INDUCTION OF GENERAL ANESTHESIA**
   Initial Intubation Attempts Successful* / Initial Intubation Attempts UNSUCCESSFUL
   FROM THIS POINT ONWARDS CONSIDER:
   1. Calling for Help
   2. Returning to Spontaneous Ventilation
   3. Awakening the Patient
   Maintaining Spontaneous Ventilation

   FACE MASK VENTILATION ADEQUATE / FACE MASK VENTILATION NOT ADEQUATE
   CONSIDER / ATTEMPT LMA
   LMA ADEQUATE* / LMA NOT ADEQUATE OR NOT FEASIBLE

   NON-EMERGENCY PATHWAY
   Ventilation Adequate, Intubation Unsuccessful

   Alternative Approaches to Intubation(c)

   IF BOTH FACE MASK AND LMA VENTILATION BECOME INADEQUATE

   EMERGENCY PATHWAY
   Ventilation Not Adequate, Intubation Unsuccessful
   Call for Help
   ETC, TTJV, Rigid Bronch Emergency Non-Invasive Airway Ventilation(e)

   Successful Intubation* / FAIL After Multiple Attempts / (more likely) / Successful Ventilation* / FAIL
   Invasive Airway Access(b)* / Consider Feasibility of Other Options(a) / Awaken Patient(d)
   Emergency Invasive Airway Access(b)*

   *Confirm ventilation, tracheal intubation, or LMA placement with exhaled CO_2

a. Other options include (but are not limited to): surgery utilizing face mask or IMA anesthesia, local anesthesia infiltration, or regional nerve blockade. Pursuit of these options usually implies that mask ventilation will not be problematic. Therefore, these options may be of limited value if this step in the algorithm has been reached via the Emergency Pathway. Judgement required. Rarely appropriate for trauma patients.

b. Invasive airway access includes surgical or percutaneous tracheostomy or cricothyrotomy.

c. Alternative non-invasive approaches to difficult intubation include (but are not limited to): use of different laryngoscope blades, LMA as an intubation conduit (with or without fiberoptic guidance), fiberoptic intubation (FOB), intubating stylet or tube changer (airway exchange catheter, AEC), light wand, retrograde intubation, and blind oral or nasal intubation.

d. Consider re-preparation of the patient for awake intubation or canceling surgery. Rarely applicable in the trauma patient.

e. Options for emergency non-invasive airway ventilation include (but are not limited to): rigid bronchoscope (Rigid Bronch), esophageal-tracheal combitube ventilation (ETC), or transtracheal jet ventilation (TTJV).

f. Extubation strategies include: evaluation of the airway with FOB and extubation over an airway exchange catheter (AEC).

Figure 3.17 ASA difficult airway algorithm, with modifications (in bold) required for trauma. The algorithm begins with recognition of the difficult airway. If the patient is recognized to have a difficult airway then the *awake* limb of the algorithm is followed. But if the patient is uncooperative or unstable, or was not recognized to have a difficult airway, the *anesthetized* limb is followed. Regardless of the technique used to secure a definitive airway, confirmation of mechanical ventilation with either end-tidal CO_2 or other test is mandatory. The original algorithm is from Caplan RA. Practice guidelines for management of the difficult airway. *Anesthesiology* 2003; **98**: 1273; with permission, along with modifications (in bold) as published in ASA Difficult Airway Algorithm modified for Trauma (Wilson WC. Trauma: airway management. ASA difficult airway algorithm modified for trauma – and five common trauma intubation scenarios. *ASA Newsletter* 2005; **69** (11): 10; with permission.)

(B)

Summary of the ASA Difficult Airway Algorithm Modifications for Trauma

A. Stopping to come back another day is seldom an option with trauma

B. A surgical airway may be the first/best choice in certain conditions

C. An awake ETT technique should be chosen in a DA patient providing the patient is cooperative, stable, and spontaneously ventilating.

D. If the patient becomes uncooperative/combative general anesthesia (GA) may need to be administered—but if the airway is difficult, spontaneous ventilation(SV)should be continued (if possible).

E. Awake limb of the ASA Algorithm—Trauma Notes. An awake intubation technique is recommended for all trauma patients with a recognized difficult airway…. Providing the patient is cooperative, stable, and maintains spontaneous ventilation and adequacy of O_2 saturation. The ASA DA Algorithm does not endorse any particular airway technique. However, it does emphasize that the patient must be properly prepared (mentally and physically) for an awake technique.

F. Anesthetized or uncooperative limb of ASA DA Algorithm—Trauma Notes. There are three common conditions when the need arises to intubate the trachea of an unconscious or anesthetized trauma patient with a DA:
1. Clinician fails to recognize a difficult airway in preoperative evaluation prior to the induction of anesthesia
2. The DA patient is already unconscious prior to being assessed by the trauma anesthesiologist
3. The patient obviously has a DA, but is hemodynamically unstable (e.g., following trauma) or absolutely refuses to cooperate with an awake intubation (e.g., child, mentally retarded, drugged, or head-injured adult).

Once the patient is anesthetized or is rendered apneic or presents comatose and the trachea cannot be intubated, O_2, enriched mask ventilation (MV) is attempted.

If MV adequate, a number of intubation techniques may be employed. Techniques allowing continuous ventilation during airwaymanipulations are favored over those requiring an interruption of MV (e.g., FOB, via an LMA or an airway intubating mask, with self-sealing diaphragm).

Alternatively, techniques requiring a cessation of ventilation (at least temporarily) can be employed.These techniques are relatively contraindicated for patients with large right-to-left transpulmonary shunt, or decreased FRC.

G. Confirmation of endotracheal tube (ETT) position. Immediately after the patient's trachea is intubated, one must confirm ETT position with end-tidal CO_2 measurement. If end-tidal CO_2 measurement is unavailable, Wee's esophageal detector device (EDD) is reasonably reliable (close to 100% sensitive and specific).

H. Extubation or ETT change of the DA. If the conditions that caused the airway to be difficult to intubate still exist at the time of extubation, or if new DA conditions exist (e.g., airway edema, halo), then the trachea should be extubated over an AEC and or with the assistance of a FOB.

Figure 3.17 (cont.)

pulmonary aspiration on a hierarchical level above airway difficulty. Thus, the clinician must always fully evaluate the airway. If the patient has an anticipated difficult airway, consideration should be given to using an awake technique. Awake techniques can be safely used provided the physician maintains close observation of the patient's mental status. If the patient is awake and following commands, then the patient's airway-protective mechanisms should be functional. Indeed, Ovassapian and colleagues intubated the tracheas of 123 patients considered to be at high risk for aspiration of gastric contents by using an awake technique.[44] Regurgitation occurred in only one patient, and no patients suffered aspiration. Therefore, the ASA algorithm can be followed without significant modification in patients with isolated extremity or abdominal injuries with documented absence of cervical spine, brain, neck, maxillofacial, or chest injury.

Previously, the traditional overriding goal in securing a difficult airway in patients with a full stomach was the

Table 3.9 Modification of the ASA difficult airway (DA) algorithm for trauma

Management choices	Standard ASA DA algorithm	Trauma ASA DA algorithm
Unsuccessful intubation after general anesthesia induced	Awakening the patient is always an option	Awakening/stopping is seldom an option
Surgical airway decision	Invasive surgical airway is performed for failed intubation/failed ventilation	Surgical airway may be the first/best choice
Management of recognized difficult airway	Awake intubation	Awake intubation technique only if cooperative, stable, and spontaneously ventilating
Failed awake intubation	Cancel is an option	Uncooperative/combative patient requires general anesthesia with or without spontaneous ventilation
Regional for anesthetic management	Regional anesthesia is usually an option	Regional anesthesia is occasionally an option

ASA DA, American Society of Anesthesiologists difficult airway algorithm

prevention of catastrophic aspiration. It is now more clearly understood that preventing hypoxia and brain injury is most important. The general principles of the ASA algorithm as they apply to the trauma airway are outlined in Fig. 3.17. The modifications of the algorithm for trauma as compared with the general algorithm are summarized in Table 3.9. First, stopping to come back another day is seldom an option with trauma. Second, an awake ETT technique should be chosen in a difficult-airway patient providing the patient is cooperative, stable, and spontaneously ventilating. Third, if the patient becomes uncooperative/combative or unstable, then sedative drugs may need to be administered to gain control. However, if the airway is deemed difficult, spontaneous ventilation should be maintained, if possible. Finally, a surgical airway may be the best choice in certain conditions.

Five common difficult intubation scenarios in trauma

Traumatic brain injury/intoxication

In the setting of traumatic brain injury (TBI), surgical decompression/evacuation is frequently the primary intervention required for resolution of increased intracranial pressure

(ICP). Tracheal intubation and subsequent modest hyperventilation constitute important temporizing modalities (Fig. 3.18). Hyperventilation serves to decrease cerebral blood flow by causing cerebral vasoconstriction via an increase in intracellular brain pH (see Chapter 21). Simultaneously, maintenance of mean arterial pressure (MAP) at a normal or slightly elevated level throughout these manipulations is important to maintain cerebral perfusion pressure (CPP = [MAP − ICP]). Patients with a CPP < 60 mmHg have a worse outcome for similar categories of head injury and Glasgow Coma Scale (GCS) than patients with normal CPP,[45] and a CPP > 70 mmHg is desirable if it can be accomplished.

Airway management considerations for the TBI patient begin with a determination of acuity followed by airway evaluation. If the patient has a GCS < 9, airway management begins at the anesthetized limb of the ASA difficult airway algorithm just as in any unstable uncooperative patient (see Chapter 35, Table 35.1 for GCS). If the patient has stable hemodynamics, a GCS ≥ 9, and an airway that appears difficult to intubate, then an awake intubation technique should be considered.

Cervical spine injury

C-spine injury should be suspected in all blunt trauma patients, especially those with a significant mechanism of injury (i.e., front-end motor vehicle collision > 35 miles per hour [56 km/h] without seatbelt), and in those patients admitted with altered mental status.[46,47] Because comatose patients cannot respond to a clinical examination, all head-injured and/or intoxicated patients, and others in whom a clinical exam cannot be performed, must initially be assumed to have cervical instability. Few well-controlled studies are available to guide airway management for these patients. However, several excellent reviews of C-spine injury and airway management exist.[48,49]

When confronted with the patient with suspected C-spine injury, six points should be considered. The C-spine airway management algorithm (Fig. 3.19) follows directly from concepts outlined in Table 3.10. First, intubation of the proved or suspected C-spine-injured patient is analogous to intubation of any other patient, except that there is an added handicap because the head and neck should not be moved. Second, the patient must have his or her airway evaluated for all the other factors that would predict a difficult airway. Third, outcome data indicate that there are no differences in terms of incidence of neurologic deficit between awake intubation and intubation under general anesthesia as long as the operator does not move the head on the neck.[50] Fourth, if the C-spine is known or suspected to be unstable, and the patient is awake, cooperative, and otherwise stable, an awake intubation, optimally with an FOB, should be pursued because this allows for neurologic evaluation after intubation. Fifth, if intubation is contemplated for neck surgery in a patient with known C-spine injury, both awake intubation and awake positioning should be pursued (see also Chapters 22 and 23). Finally, consideration must be

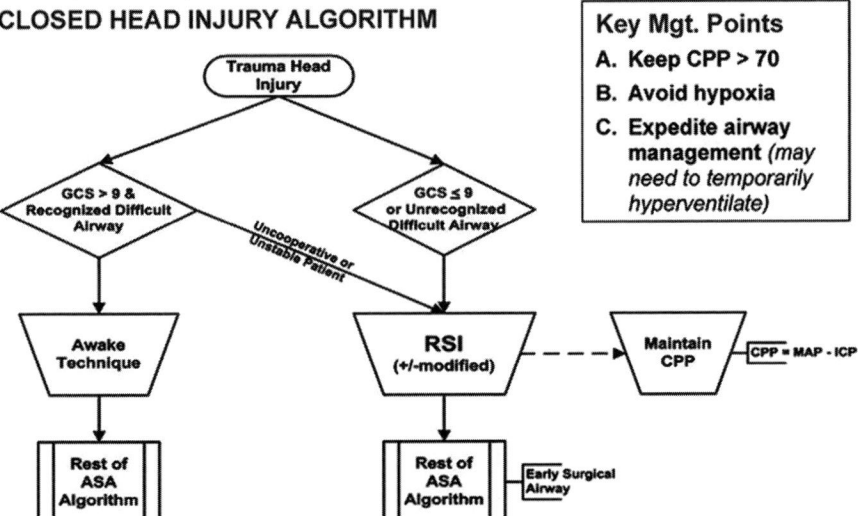

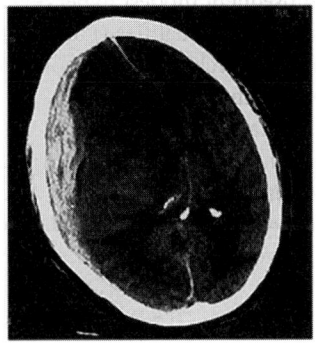

CLOSED HEAD INJURY / INTOXICATION

At left: CT of brain demonstrating severe closed head injury with right temporoparietal subdural hematoma.

General Considerations

IF Difficult Airway..... Do an awake intubation, provided the patient is cooperative, stable, maintains SV... ......and has a GCS > 9.

Key Questions........ Driving Algorithm Decision Making

A. How severe?
  1. GCS ≤ 9 = RSI (+/-modified–i.e., cricoid pressure, +/- PPV)
  2. GCS > 9 = Awake option
B. Cooperative? If yes, do awake technique

CLOSED HEAD INJURY ALGORITHM

Key Mgt. Points
A. Keep CPP > 70
B. Avoid hypoxia
C. Expedite airway management *(may need to temporarily hyperventilate)*

Figure 3.18 ASA difficult airway algorithm applied to closed-head injury/intoxication. ASA, American Society of Anesthesiologists; CPP, cerebral perfusion pressure; GCS, Glasgow coma scale; PPV, positive-pressure ventilation; RSI, rapid sequence intubation. (From Wilson WC. Trauma: airway management. ASA difficult airway algorithm modified for trauma – and five common trauma intubation scenarios. *ASA Newsletter* 2005; **69** (11): 12; with permission.)

given to using an intubation technique that does not require head extension or the sniffing position to optimally expose the glottis and intubate the trachea, especially when dealing with the uncooperative/unstable/anesthetized limb of the difficult airway algorithm. In a landmark review of C-spine injury and airway management, Hastings and Marks mention the occurrence of two cases of quadriplegia or death after laryngoscopy in patients with unrecognized C-spine injuries.[48]

The vast majority of cervical motion during glottic visualization and intubation with conventional laryngoscopy using a Macintosh blade is produced at the occipitoatlantal and atlantoaxial joints. The subaxial cervical segments are only minimally displaced. It is well known that immobilization of the C-spine results in a higher incidence of difficulty with visualization of the vocal cords when using conventional laryngoscopy. This is because optimal alignment of the airway axes requires a certain amount of cervical segmental and rotational motion, which is prevented by immobilization techniques. For example, Nolan and Wilson showed that immobilization of the

C-spine resulted in a 22% incidence of grade 3 views, and reduced the optimal view of the larynx in 45% of patients.[14] Use of a gum elastic bougie is invaluable whenever a grade 3 view of the glottis is encountered. While performing direct laryngoscopy, the operator maintains adequate force to keep the epiglottis in view. The bougie is then introduced by the operator and gently advanced anteriorly under the epiglottis and into the trachea. Often, tracheal clicks will be felt. With the operator still maintaining laryngoscopic force, the assistant threads the ETT over the bougie. The ETT may need to be rotated 90 degrees to facilitate its passage through the glottis. Intratracheal placement is confirmed with $P_{ET}CO_2$ detection.

As described above, video laryngoscopes have also been used successfully in patients with difficult airways and C-spine disorders, and they have high success rates in experienced hands. Rigid fiberoptic laryngoscopy with anatomically shaped blades such as the Bullard laryngoscope and Wuscope are reliable techniques to visualize the glottis and intubate the trachea in patients with known or suspected C-spine

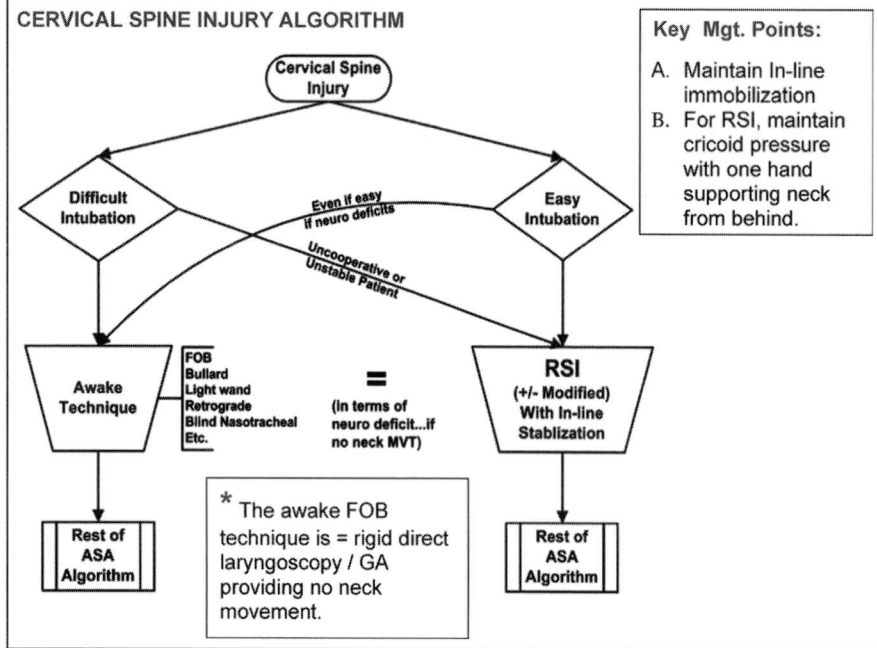

CERVICAL SPINE INJURY

At left: **A.** Lateral C-Spine X-Ray showing C5-6 bifacet dislocation.
B. Lateral C-Spine X-Ray showing atlanto-occipital dislocation

General Considerations

IF Difficult Airway..... Do an awake intubation, provided the patient is cooperative, stable, maintains SV... ...... Especially if the patient has neurological symptoms from SCI.

Key Questions

1. Does the rest of the airway exam (HMD < 6 cm, Mallampati Class IV, small mouth) predict a DA? If Yes, Do awake. 2. Does the patient have a neurological deficit? If Yes, Do Awake.

CERVICAL SPINE INJURY ALGORITHM

Key Mgt. Points:

A. Maintain In-line immobilization
B. For RSI, maintain cricoid pressure with one hand supporting neck from behind.

Figure 3.19 ASA difficult airway algorithm applied to cervical spine injury. ASA, American Society of Anesthesiologists; DA, difficult airway; FOB, fiberoptic bronchoscopy; GA, general anesthesia; RSI, rapid sequence intubation; SCI, spinal cord injury; SV, spontaneous ventilation. (From Wilson WC. Trauma: airway management. ASA difficult airway algorithm modified for trauma – and five common trauma intubation scenarios. *ASA Newsletter* 2005; **69** (11): 13; with permission.)

trauma.[51,52] Unlike conventional laryngoscopy, the Bullard and Wuscope devices do not require head and neck movement to obtain a grade 1 view of the vocal cords. Alternatively, the McCoy levering laryngoscope or Heine CL flex-tip blade can be used. This is a modified Macintosh laryngoscope that has a hinged tip controlled by a lever on the handle. The hinged tip allows the epiglottis to be elevated without requiring excessive lifting force. The McCoy levering laryngoscope has been shown to improve laryngeal visualization in patients whose necks cannot be extended.[53]

For patients with known or suspected C-spine injuries undergoing RSI, cricoid pressure can be maintained by an assistant utilizing a one- or a two-handed method. For the one-handed method, cricoid pressure is exerted by placing the thumb and middle finger on either side of the cricoid cartilage and the index finger above, thereby preventing lateral movement of the signet-shaped cricoid cartilage. With the two-handed method, the assistant uses one hand to support the back of the neck and the other hand to apply firm pressure on the cricoid cartilage (Sellick maneuver).

Airway disruption

Airway disruption is defined as any interruption of airway integrity due to either blunt or penetrating trauma. The literature provides little guidance for emergency airway management of patients with airway disruption because these injuries are relatively uncommon, occurring in only 14% of penetrating neck trauma cases. Thus, most studies are retrospective. The diversity of concomitant injuries and the hemodynamic status of the patient make universal recommendations difficult as well. Shearer and Giesecke reviewed their experience with

Table 3.10 Airway considerations for patients with known or suspected cervical spine injuries

Cervical spine injury considerations	Airway manipulation implications
Must not move the neck	Maintain in-line immobilization Consider use of intubation technique other than conventional laryngoscopy (e.g., video laryngoscope FOB, Bullard, Wuscope, McCoy blade) Routine use of gum-elastic bougie if rigid laryngoscopy technique chosen Other concerns similar to any other patient with no neck range of motion
Concomitant airway risks	Awake technique if otherwise high risk (HMD < 6 cm, Mallampati class IV) If otherwise low risk, awake or general anesthesia techniques are equal in terms of neurologic outcome, as long as the neck remains immobilized
Selection of awake technique	If awake technique chosen, the specific methodology does not appear to affect outcome, providing the anesthesiologist is proficient in using the instrumentation
Aspiration prophylaxis	If awake technique chosen, no increase in aspiration has been documented If RSI chosen, maintain cricoid pressure

FOB, fiberoptic bronchoscope; HMD, hyomental distance; RSI, rapid sequence induction/intubation.

107 patients with penetrating neck trauma requiring definitive airway management at Parkland Memorial Hospital and found that neither the zone of injury nor the mechanism correlated with degree of intubation difficulty or the primary choice of surgical airway.[54]

Despite the inherent complexity of managing airway disruptions, the ASA algorithm is useful (Fig. 3.20). If the airway injury is large or subglottic, an awake technique under direct vision is indicated (surgical airway or FOB intubation). If the disruption is very small or supraglottic, then the technique chosen is less critical. Importantly, whatever technique is selected, the clinician must avoid applying positive-pressure ventilation proximal to the injury, because this could convert a relatively small tear into a large or complete airway disruption and cause mediastinal air.

Awake intubation, with spontaneous ventilation, is indicated for a major airway tear because this avoids exposing the disruption to positive-pressure ventilation. Positive-pressure ventilation can cause further injury to the airway and increase the likelihood that air will dissect into the mediastinal tissues (i.e., mediastinal emphysema) with resultant obliteration of neck landmarks and impossibility of performing a surgical airway. Furthermore, the airway may be held together by muscle tone in the strap muscles along the airway, which is lost in an RSI technique with muscle paralysis. The FOB-assisted intubation is the awake technique of choice because it allows for visualization of airway disruption (diagnosis) as well as assured placement of the ETT cuff distal to the disruption (treatment). A double-lumen endobronchial tube can be placed using an awake technique under fiberoptic guidance in cases of a small distal unilateral bronchial disruption. Figure 3.20 shows the awake limb of the ASA algorithm applied to the problem of airway disruption.

In general, intubation by conventional laryngoscopy should not be the primary technique for a subglottic disruption, because the ETT could pass out through the disruption into the mediastinum, worsening or completing the disruption. Ideally, one would like to maintain a view of the airway (FOB, surgical airway). Use of an FOB may be problematic if the airway is grossly bloody. Finally, in addition, a complex distal tear may require cardiopulmonary support or bypass for resuscitation or definitive treatment if concomitant vascular injury is present.[55] Disruptions limited primarily to the airway can usually be repaired using a double-lumen tube (see Chapter 33).

The anesthetized limb of the ASA algorithm (Fig. 3.20) applies to the problem of airway disruption when the tear cannot be easily bypassed by conventional intubation or the patient has a major tear but refuses an awake intubation. In this case the neck should be prepped and landmarks identified, and the surgeon gloved and gowned prior to intubation so that the surgeon may quickly perform a surgical airway if difficulty is encountered following induction.

A patient with a small, easily bypassed tear can be intubated by conventional means, but a patient with a large tear, undergoing general anesthesia, should maintain spontaneous ventilation. Intubation options following the awake limb of the ASA algorithm should be utilized. If the cannot intubate–cannot ventilate situation arises, TTJV is contraindicated, as are supraglottic ventilatory techniques such as the LMA and Combitube. These methods will expose the disruption to positive-pressure ventilation, leading to possible complete disruption, mediastinal emphysema, tension pneumothorax, or massive subcutaneous emphysema. Thus, if a cannot intubate–cannot ventilate situation arises in a patient with a subglottic airway disruption, one should go immediately to a surgical airway and be prepared for cardiopulmonary bypass if the tear is distal. Finally, with open gaping neck wounds (e.g., knife, metal, glass) that transect the trachea, direct tracheal intubation via the wound is an appropriate first choice.

Maxillofacial trauma

Maxillofacial injuries are rarely life-threatening unless associated with airway obstruction or hemodynamic instability (see Chapters 24 and 25). Mask ventilation may be made more

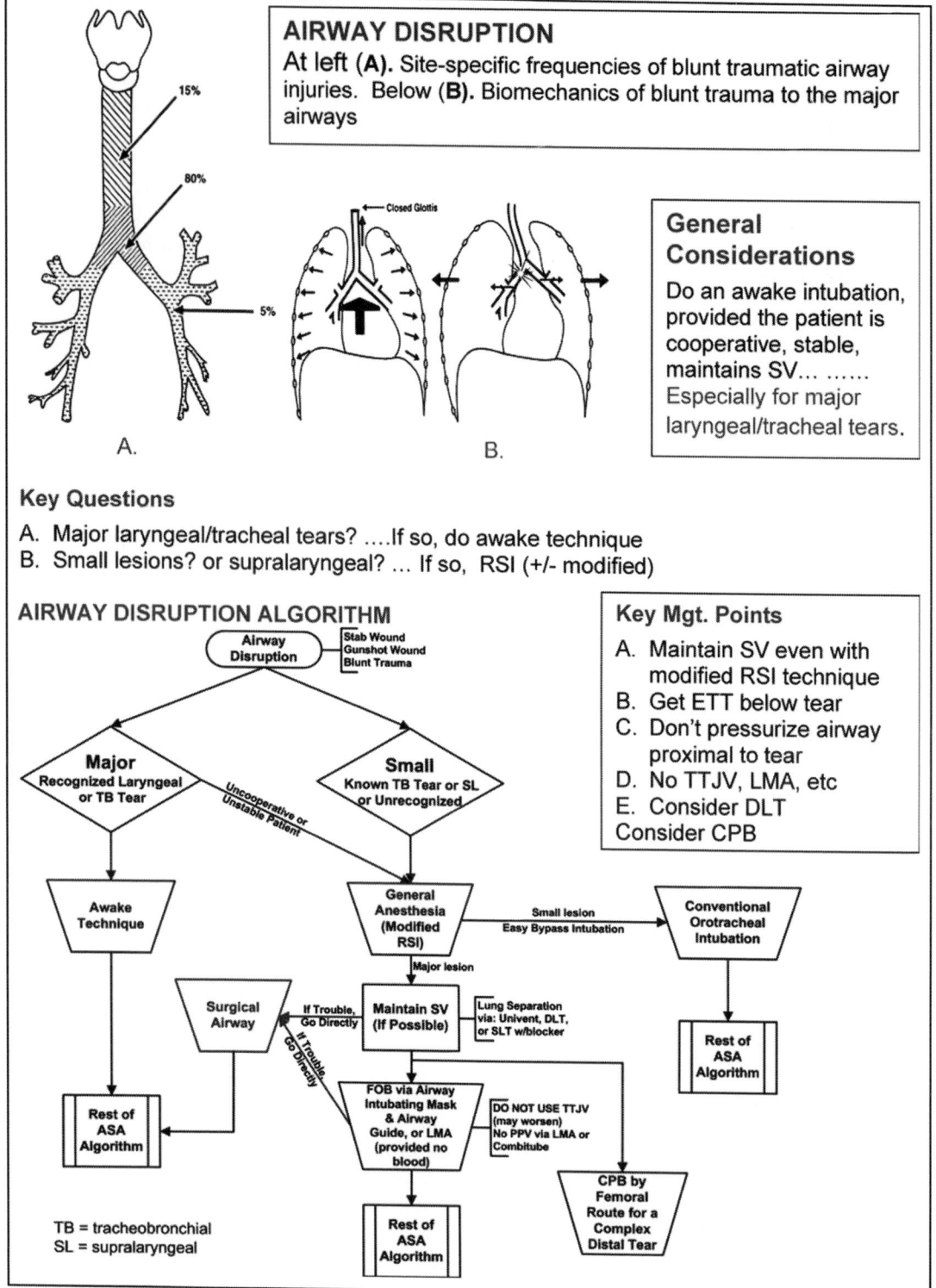

Figure 3.20 ASA difficult airway algorithm applied to airway disruption. ASA, American Society of Anesthesiologists; CPB, cardiopulmonary bypass; DLT, double-lumen endobronchial tube; ETT, endotracheal tube; LMA, laryngeal mask airway; RSI, rapid sequence intubation; SLT, single-lumen endotracheal tube; SV, spontaneous ventilation; TTJV, transtracheal jet ventilation. (From Wilson WC. Trauma: airway management. ASA difficult airway algorithm modified for trauma – and five common trauma intubation scenarios. *ASA Newsletter* 2005; **69** (11): 14; with permission.)

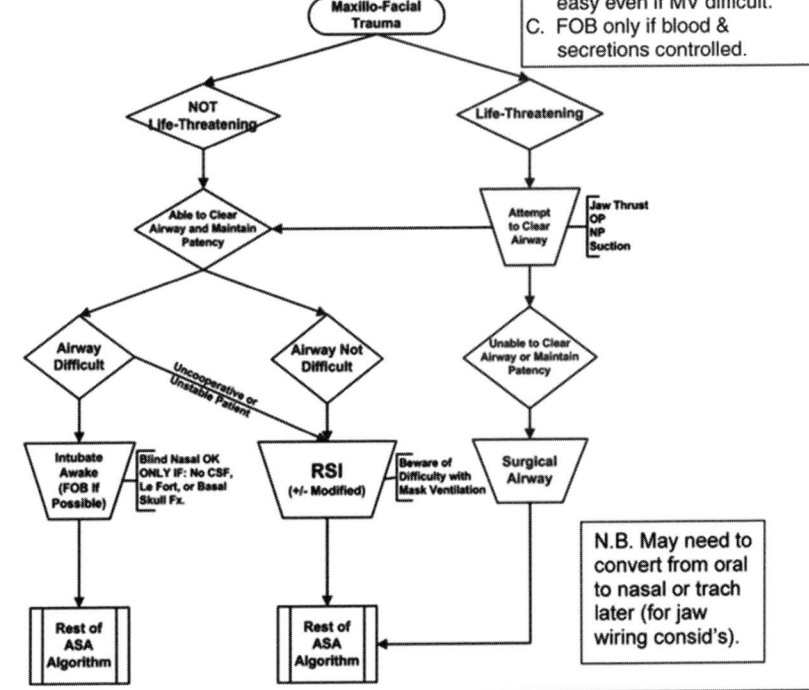

MAXILLARY-FACIAL TRAUMA

At left: Traumatic injury to face, maxilla, & mandible.

General Considerations

A. Do awake ETT, provided the pt. is cooperative, stable, maintains SV & O_2 sat., and..... able to clear airway of blood, foreign bodies, secretions, and maintain patency.
B. M.V. may be difficult even if ETT is easy.
C. Blind nasal technique is contraindicated if: .... CSF leak, Le Fort, or basal skull fracture.
D. Initial decision-making based upon A,B,C's...,later, must be practical with the need for future jaw wiring

(Figure courtesy of Pablo Pratesi, Hospital Universitario AUSTRAL, Argentina.)

Key Questions

A. Life-threatening obstruction? If yes, → surgical airway
B. Not life-threatening (i.e., able to clear airway)? Then, consider DA issues as well as need for jaw wiring.

Key Points

A. Early Surgical Airway if Life Threatening
B. Direct laryngoscopy often easy even if MV difficult.
C. FOB only if blood & secretions controlled.

MAX-FACIAL TRAUMA ALGORITHM

Figure 3.21 ASA difficult airway algorithm applied to maxillofacial trauma. ASA, American Society of Anesthesiologists; CSF, cerebrospinal fluid; DA, difficult airway; ETT, endotracheal tube; FOB, fiberoptic bronchoscopy; MV, mask ventilation; NP, nasopharyngeal airway;OP, oropharyngeal airway; SV, spontaneous ventilation. (From Wilson WC. Trauma: airway management. ASA difficult airway algorithm modified for trauma – and five common trauma intubation scenarios. *ASA Newsletter* 2005; **69** (11): 15; with permission.)

difficult by maxillofacial or mandibular injuries, even though intubation is typically achievable. Airway management priorities for maxillofacial trauma are shown in Figure 3.21. Airway obstruction can occur due to pharyngeal blood clots, vomitus, loose teeth, dentures, or posterior displacement of the tongue and periglottic soft tissue, especially with bilateral mandibular fractures. Zygoma or zygomatic arch fractures can impinge on the coronoid process of the mandibular ramus, limiting mouth opening.

Over a century ago, Le Fort described three facial fracture patterns that have some anesthetic significance today.[56] Le Fort II and III fractures are associated with disruption of the cribriform plate, and nasally placed tubes can enter the brain. Because disruption of the cribriform plate is very difficult to rule out in the acute setting, any evidence of a basal skull fracture or Le Fort II or III fracture, such as periorbital hematomas resembling "raccoon-eyes," hemotympanum, Battle's sign (ecchymosis overlying the mastoid process), or cerebrospinal fluid (CSF) rhinorrhea, should be presumed to involve cribriform plate disruption. The presence of CSF rhinorrhea or otorrhea should caution against prolonged positive-pressure ventilation by mask. Positive-pressure ventilation via a mask may force air across the site of the CSF leakage, resulting in a pneumocephalus. Because of the possibility of causing meningitis or further brain injury by blindly forcing a nasally placed object into the cranial vault, blind manipulations are contraindicated. However, nasal intubations under FOB guidance are acceptable provided that the fracture does not cross the midline or that the cribriform plate is intact on imaging studies. Indeed, Bahr and Stoll reported a series of 160 patients with frontobasilar fractures and documented CSF leak, and there was no difference in postoperative complications including meningitis regardless of the route of intubation (oral vs nasal).[57] Another potential consideration in patients suffering from Le Fort II and III fractures is airway obstruction. This can occur when a maxillary fragment becomes dislodged posteriorly, obstructing the airway.

The first decision that needs to be made is whether the injury is life-threatening (Fig. 3.21). If it is not, the condition can be treated in a nonemergent mode and time can be taken to plan appropriately. If the fracture is life-threatening, then first priorities are airway and breathing followed by intubation – logic that takes into consideration the need to wire the mandible to the maxilla. Oral intubation followed by elective changeover to a nasally placed ETT tube or a tracheostomy is appropriate.

For non-life-threatening maxillary/mandibular fractures, the intubation strategy outlined by the basic ASA algorithm works well. General anesthesia can be induced if the intubation is predictably easy; whereas, when intubation difficulty is expected, the trachea should be intubated awake as long as the patient is cooperative, stable, and spontaneously ventilating. Regardless of the specific intubation technique utilized, the need to wire the maxilla to the mandible (intermaxillary fixation) must be considered. Thus, a nasal technique should be performed in the absence of maxillary fractures. If significant bilateral nasal or maxillary injuries are present, the patient may undergo topicalized awake FOB-guided nasal intubation.

Airway compression

The airway can be externally compressed by an expanding hematoma, hemorrhage from a major vascular injury (blunt or penetrating trauma), or large abscess. As with maxillary/ mandibular fractures, the first determination is whether the condition is life-threatening. If the situation is life-threatening, then one should consider whether airway manipulation might dislodge a clot and further compromise the airway (Fig. 3.22). Oral tracheal intubation may be difficult and therefore unwise. A surgical airway is often the best choice.

If there is extrinsic airway compression from hematoma, swelling, or abscess, and it is not life-threatening, then the basic difficult airway algorithm applies. Regardless of the intubation technique performed, the anesthesiologist must avoid disturbing a mass compressing the airway, and the lesion must not be allowed to obscure the view of the airway. Thus, an FOB-guided technique is often the best choice. The trauma anesthesiologist must be willing to proceed to a surgical airway if the mass is obscuring the view of the airway.

Table 3.11 serves as a summary of the major points pertinent to the various trauma difficult airway clinical scenarios. The plan for securing the airway of the trauma patient must minimize the risks of airway loss, aspiration, and hemodynamic compromise. The priority list must be reorganized as the patient's condition changes. If there is any concern that the patient's airway will be difficult to mask ventilate or intubate, an awake technique with spontaneous ventilation should be considered. Alternative plans must have been thought out beforehand and be physically ready to go. In some cases, the best first choice is a surgical airway.

Emergency intubation complications

Complications of emergency trauma airway management are numerous. However, there are six life-threatening emergency airway complications that must be avoided when managing airways of critically ill patients: (1) failure to intubate/ventilate, (2) unrecognized esophageal intubation, (3) hemodynamic compromise, (4) aspiration of gastric contents, (5) creating or exacerbating a C-spine injury, and (6) causing a partial airway tear to become a complete transected airway.

Failure to intubate or ventilate

Failure to maintain a patent airway for more than a few minutes can lead to brain damage or death and is the single most common cause of anesthesia-related morbidity and mortality. Trauma patients in cardiorespiratory failure are at an even higher risk because they are starting out with a more compromised hemodynamic and respiratory status than elective patients in the operating room. Furthermore, difficulty can occur because proper equipment and help may be missing. The ASA algorithm was developed by a task force of academic clinicians with the goal of reducing airway-related catastrophes. Although not specifically created for emergency situations, the algorithm provides logical guidance for emergency airway management of the cannot intubate–cannot ventilate situation.

Unrecognized esophageal intubation

An esophageal intubation is not an error of commission; it is an error of omission – that is, failure to recognize it. Once the airway is secure, confirmation of placement and ventilation must occur immediately. Depending on the patient's underlying condition, confirmation of ETT position can be complicated and can lead to disastrous results, if not properly verified. ETT confirmation techniques can be characterized as direct and indirect methods.

Direct confirmation of intratracheal position

Direct vision of the ETT passing through the cords is considered the gold standard. The only foolproof techniques for confirming an endotracheal position are seeing the tube pass through the cords and looking through the ETT and visualizing the tracheal rings with an FOB, or in penetrating neck trauma the trachea may be exposed and the tube can be placed under direct vision.

Indirect confirmation of intratracheal position

Specific indirect methods for determining ETT position are utilized for all trauma intubations. These include $P_{ET}CO_2$ measurement (intact circulation) and the esophageal detector

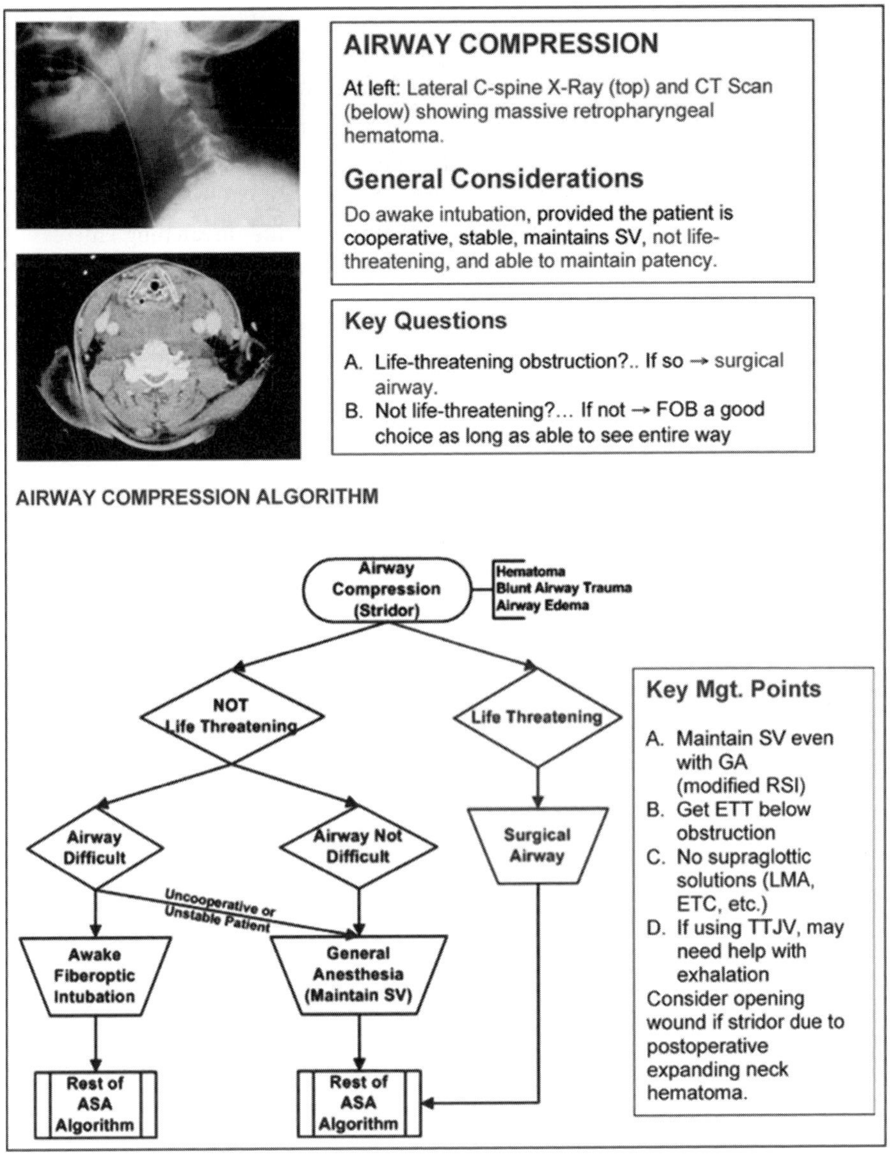

AIRWAY COMPRESSION

At left: Lateral C-spine X-Ray (top) and CT Scan (below) showing massive retropharyngeal hematoma.

General Considerations

Do awake intubation, provided the patient is cooperative, stable, maintains SV, not life-threatening, and able to maintain patency.

Key Questions

A. Life-threatening obstruction?.. If so → surgical airway.
B. Not life-threatening?... If not → FOB a good choice as long as able to see entire way

AIRWAY COMPRESSION ALGORITHM

Figure 3.22 ASA difficult airway algorithm applied to airway compression. ASA, American Society of Anesthesiologists; ETC, Combitube; ETT, endotracheal tube; FOB, fiberoptic bronchoscopy; GA, general anesthesia; LMA, laryngeal mask airway; RSI, rapid sequence intubation; SV, spontaneous ventilation; TTJV, transtracheal jet ventilation. (From Wilson WC. Trauma: airway management. ASA difficult airway algorithm modified for trauma – and five common trauma intubation scenarios. *ASA Newsletter* 2005; **69** (11): 16; with permission.)

device (cardiac arrest). All of the usual clinical endpoints are indirect methods and error-prone, including auscultating equal bilateral breath sounds, observing symmetrical chest rise, and fogging of the ETT.

End-tidal CO_2 measurement

$P_{ET}CO_2$ can be detected by capnography or capnometry. These devices are good predictors of esophageal intubation in patients with normal cardiovascular status. However, in code situations with little or no cardiac output, very little blood will traverse the pulmonary circulation and consequently very little CO_2 will be exhaled with each breath and be available to be detected. Indeed, $P_{ET}CO_2$ has been used to quantify the efficacy of CPR.[58]

Conversely, patients with high levels of CO_2 in their stomach (from sodium bicarbonate, $NaHCO_3$, or soft drinks) can give a false-positive test on the first few breaths. After six breaths, esophageal/gastric CO_2 levels drop. Barring these two relatively rare events, $P_{ET}CO_2$ measurement is a reliable indication of intratracheal placement of the ETT and should be used to confirm all intubations.

The Wee esophageal detector device, composed of an Ellicks evacuator applied to the supposed "tracheal" tube, has proved to be highly sensitive and specific for detection of esophageal intubation (Fig. 3.23). If the tube is in the esophagus, the deflated bulb fails to reexpand when released, because suction applied to the esophageal wall causes the mucosa to close in on and obstruct the ETT. In contrast, when the tube is in the trachea, air flows out of the lungs into the trachea and reinflates the bulb because the tracheal rings keep the airways from collapsing around the ETT. False negatives and false positives with the esophageal detector device have been

Table 3.11 Overview of airway considerations for five specific trauma scenarios

1. Closed head injury (GCS < 9)	Anesthetized limb of algorithm (Fig. 3.18) • Ventilate to normocarbia • Expeditiously secure definitive airway • Maintain CPP > 70 mmHg
2. Cervical spine injury	C-spine airway algorithm (Fig. 3.19) • Awake technique if otherwise high risk (HMD < 6 cm, Mallampati class IV) • IF otherwise low risk, awake or GA technique are the same in terms of neurologic outcome, as long as the neck remains immobilized
3. Airway disruption	Airway disruption algorithm (Fig. 3.20) • Goal is to get below the tear • Don't ventilate proximal to disruption • Surgical airway may be the first, best choice
4. Maxillary–mandibular fractures	Maxillary–mandibular fracture algorithm (Fig. 3.21) • IF emergency, RSI with laryngoscope or TTJV, LMA • IF nonurgent, nasal FOB acceptable providing the airways can be visualized in entirety. • Ultimate plan considers need for IMF • Surgical airway may be the first, best choice
5. Extrinsic airway compression	Extrinsic compression algorithm (Fig. 3.22) • Decide on urgency • Need to avoid, and get around, the mass • Surgical airway may be the first, best choice

CPP, cerebral perfusion pressure; FOB, fiberoptic bronchoscope; GA, general anesthesia; GCS, Glasgow Coma Scale; HMD, hyomental distance; IMF, intermaxillary fixation; LMA, laryngeal mask airway; RSI, rapid sequence induction/intubation; TTJV, transtracheal jet ventilation.

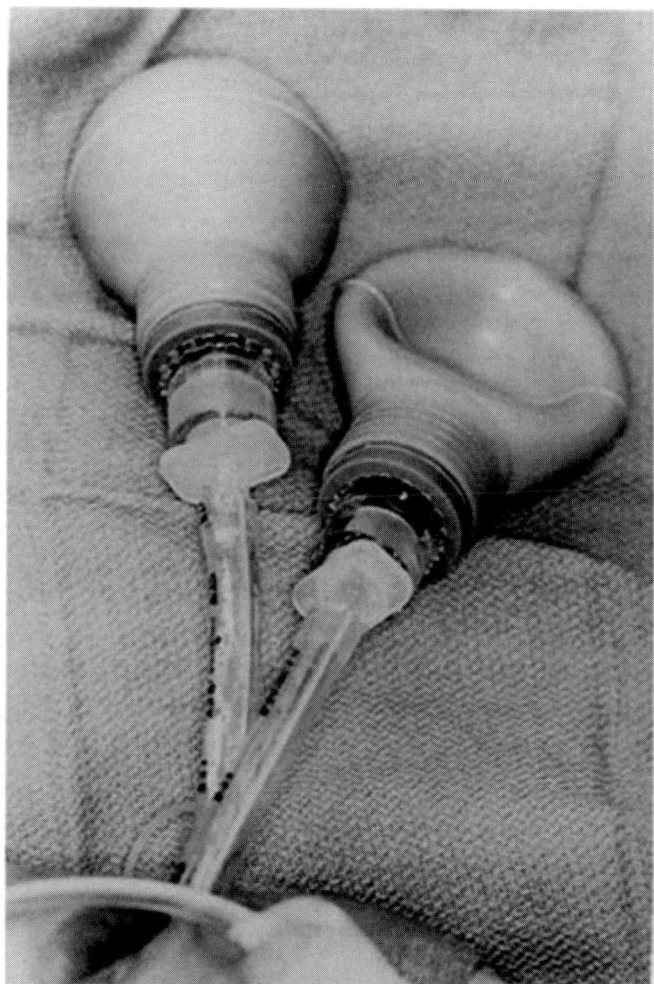

Figure 3.23 Collapsed self-inflating bulbs (SIBs) were connected simultaneously to tracheally and esophageally placed tubes. The SIB connected to the tube in the trachea instantaneously reinflated, while the SIB connected to the tube in the esophagus remained collapsed. (From Salem MR, Wafai Y, Joseph NJ, *et al.* Efficacy of the self-inflating bulb in detecting esophageal intubation. Does the presence of a nasogastric tube or cuff deflation make a difference? *Anesthesiology* 1994; **80**: 42–8; with permission.)

described in morbidly obese patients and those with severe asthma.[59]

Hemodynamic compromise

Trauma patients may be hovering on the edge of cardiopulmonary arrest from the primary process. Also, they may be at risk from the elevated circulating catecholamines that increase myocardial O_2 consumption and systemic vascular resistance (except in the rare circumstance of concomitant anaphylaxis, sepsis, or drug overdose). Furthermore, elevated catecholamines and $PaCO_2$ (if respiratory failure is present) sensitize the myocardium to ventricular ectopy.

More importantly, the elevated catecholamines tend to support the patient's blood pressure prior to intubation.

Therefore, the cardiovascular system of the critically ill patient frequently requires some exogenous catecholamine or vasopressor support during or after intubation. This support can come in the form of pharmacologic therapy or intravascular volume expansion. Hypotension following emergent intubation occurs secondary to loss of endogenous catecholamine output and due to the heart–lung interactions of positive-pressure ventilation, especially in hypovolemic patients.

Causes of preinduction increases of catecholamines

Prior to induction and intubation of a trauma patient, a hyperadrenergic state exists, serving to buoy the patient's blood pressure. Several factors promote this hyperadrenergic state through increased endogenous catecholamine elaboration: (1) stress and anxiety due to fear of dying and dyspnea, (2) pain, (3) elevated $PaCO_2$ (respiratory failure), (4) circulatory failure, and (5) hypovolemia and hemorrhage.

Causes of hypotension following induction and intubation

The hypotensive response can be attributed to four factors:

- **Loss of consciousness (decrease in sympathetic tone)** – All induction drugs such as etomidate, ketamine, propofol, and thiopental lead to a loss of consciousness and thereby a loss of preinduction stress-, fear-, and anxiety-mediated catecholamine production. Loss of this catecholamine elaboration can cause hypotension.

- **Direct myocardial depression and vasodilatation** – Thiopental and propofol cause direct myocardial depression and decreased systemic vascular resistance. Etomidate is associated with very little myocardial depression. Ketamine causes some myocardial depression but its sympathomimetic effect usually maintains or increases blood pressure, providing the patient is not already secreting the maximal amount of endogenous catecholamines.

- **Decreased right ventricular preload and increased right ventricular afterload** – Positive-pressure ventilation will decrease venous return to the right heart and thus decrease preload and increase right ventricular afterload when alveolar pressure is greater than pulmonary capillary pressure. These changes, in turn, decrease filling of the left heart, tending to decrease stroke volume. These effects are especially pronounced when the patient is intravascularly volume depleted or with cardiac tamponade.

- **Decreased $PaCO_2$** – Hyperventilation will blow off the previously elevated $PaCO_2$, resulting in a further decrement in the stimulus for catecholamine release. The combination of hypovolemia, decreased endogenous catecholamine elaboration, and mechanical factors inhibiting cardiac output such as positive-pressure ventilation can lead to catastrophic hypotension.

Techniques to limit hypotension following intubation

Avoid using an RSI technique when it is not necessary. A patient with an obvious difficult airway and full stomach can be intubated awake unless he or she is uncooperative or hemodynamically unstable. The use of smaller than usual doses of induction drugs may be helpful. Propofol and thiopental are best avoided in hypotensive unstable patients (see Chapter 7). If the airway is expected to be difficult to intubate, spontaneous ventilation with cricoid pressure can be done (e.g., debilitated patients, pericardial tamponade). Pretreatment with a fluid load may be helpful unless there is myocardial ischemia related to high preload. Vasopressors should be drawn up and immediately available for administration. Hyperventilation and large tidal volume ventilation after intubation is best avoided.

Aspiration of gastric contents

The severity of gastric aspiration is a function of the volume, pH, and nature of material aspirated. Patients at high risk for aspiration should either receive an RSI or have an awake, topicalized intubation technique.

The purpose of RSI with cricoid pressure is to seal the airway with a cuffed ETT as soon as possible after the loss of airway reflexes. Death can occur when the concern for a full stomach supersedes more important issues such as difficult airway, partial airway transection, and severe hypovolemia.

Creating a cervical spine injury in a patient with an unstable neck

The head and neck should remain neutral with in-line immobilization during trauma airway management unless the C-spine has been cleared. Radiographic C-spine clearance should be achieved prior to airway management whenever possible. Awake FOB-guided technique is recommended if the patient is awake, cooperative, and stable with a known C-spine injury.

An eye to the future

Preparation is the first step in management of the difficult trauma airway. Oxygen should be immediately applied for the duration of the assessment and treatment phase. The code bag should have all the necessary airway equipment for securing the airway of the most difficult patient. If possible, a complete history and 11-step airway evaluation is completed to elicit any predictors of difficult ventilation and intubation. In the absence of such an opportunity, an abbreviated exam of the upper incisors, mandibular space, thyromental distance, neck length, and neck thickness can briefly assess relative difficulty in the uncooperative patient. If the airway is deemed to be difficult, an awake intubation should be planned in the cooperative, stable, and spontaneously ventilated patient.

Regardless of technique, every intubation begins with the appropriate patient preparation and positioning. The optimal position is the sniffing position for RSI or the head elevated to 45 degrees for an awake topicalized FOB technique. However, in trauma patients with suspected cervical and lumbar spine injuries, in-line immobilization and full spine precautions dictate that the patient must remain flat and secure on the resuscitation table.

Ventilation is achieved with an appropriately sized mask and with the aid of oropharyngeal or nasopharyngeal airways and jaw thrust when indicated. In the cannot intubate–cannot ventilate situation, the use of LMA, Combitube, TTJV, rigid ventilating bronchoscope, or a surgical airway is indicated. Direct laryngoscopy and intubation is achieved with in-line cervical immobilization and cricoid pressure in a standard RSI or modified RSI technique with spontaneous or assisted ventilation.

With the introduction of the ASA difficult airway algorithm, the number of ASA closed claims for malpractice grievances has decreased dramatically and difficult airway management has improved significantly. In addition to institution of the trauma difficult airway algorithm, new modalities are necessary to improve the management of the difficult airway in trauma. The future promises new developments in airway management, including new tools with fiberoptic technology for better direct visualization of the airway when placing an ETT.

Technologic advances will work to improve patient safety in trauma airway management. Intubating imaging stylets and rigid fiberoptic and video laryngoscopes enable the practitioner to visualize the airway throughout the entire procedure. The LMA, an established conduit for an FOB-assisted endotracheal placement, is being used to place Aintree intubation catheters that serve as airway exchange catheters, facilitating placement of a large-sized ETT.[60] In most trauma airway scenarios, blind manipulation is not recommended.

The Cookgas intubating laryngeal airway, without the epiglottic elevating bar, is used to allow the FOB, preloaded with a standard-sized ETT, to pass through the intubating laryngeal airway's elliptically shaped aperture into the trachea. This obviates the need for an airway exchange catheter to place a larger sized tube. The Cookgas device has three major advantages over the regular LMA for use as an intubation conduit: (1) one can place a standard-size tube (i.e., 7.5–8.5) with adequate length, (2) it allows an ETT one size larger than the LMA (Table 3.5), and (3) the Cookgas device is easy to remove compared with the standard ETT.

One of the major factors in the appropriate management of the difficult airway is the need for appropriate skill and experience on the part of the airway manager. With the introduction of mannequins and simulators, there is ample opportunity to utilize and practice the different airway modalities discussed in the difficult airway algorithm. The development and widespread availability of mannequins with renewable cricothyroid membranes would provide much-needed training in cricothyroidotomy and TTJV.

Computerized simulators can be programmed for diverse scenarios, and they provide a safe, reproducible training environment. Simulators are being used to educate resident staff in addition to others who are involved in managing the airway to utilize all the appropriate tools and to follow the necessary steps in approaching the difficult airway. Practice with bag-mask ventilation, LMA placement, oropharyngeal/nasopharyngeal airways, and endotracheal intubation is easily obtained with simulators. Prospective studies have shown a decrement in management problems with the use of the simulator. However, further studies are needed to determine the utility of the simulator for trauma difficult airway.[61]

Questions

(1) Which of the following statements regarding O_2 administration is *false*?
   a. O_2 should be immediately applied as soon as the trauma patient is encountered by the anesthesia care team, either in the field or in the emergency department.
   b. O_2 should be administered throughout the trauma assessment and treatment phase.
   c. The administration of O_2 serves to increase the concentration of carboxyhemoglobin following inhalational smoke injury.
   d. Optimum preoxygenation requires that 100% O_2 be delivered by a tight-fitting mask during spontaneous ventilation for 3–5 minutes prior to administering drugs that cause apnea.

(2) Which of the following statements regarding cervical spine (C-spine) injuries and trauma is *false*?
   a. The "sniffing position" is contraindicated whenever C-spine injury is suspected. In these patients, in-line immobilization of the head and neck is maintained throughout airway manipulation.
   b. In-line traction is superior to in-line immobilization.
   c. When the C-spine is known or suspected to be unstable and the patient is awake, cooperative, and otherwise stable, an awake intubation (e.g., with a fiberoptic bronchoscope) should be pursued.
   d. When the patient requires a definitive airway and is uncooperative and/or hemodynamically unstable, tracheal intubation should proceed using general anesthesia even though the patient may be suspected of having a C-spine fracture or injury.

(3) Which of the following statements regarding trauma intubation is *false*?
   a. Rapid sequence induction/intubation (RSI) techniques were developed to minimize the likelihood of regurgitation and aspiration.
   b. The RSI technique can be modified to allow institution of bag-mask ventilation (with concomitant cricoid pressure) prior to placement of the ETT in patients at risk for arterial desaturation during apnea.
   c. Allowing spontaneous ventilation (SV) to be maintained (with concomitant cricoid pressure) during placement of the ETT is a suitable technique in patients with stridor, expanding airway hematomas, or partial airway tears.
   d. The RSI technique is required in all trauma patients, because they all should be considered to have a full stomach.

(4) True or false? Awake tracheal intubation, with spontaneous ventilation, is indicated for a major airway tear because this avoids exposing the disruption to positive-pressure ventilation.

(5) True or false? An awake intubation technique is recommended for trauma patients with known or anticipated difficult airways provided they are cooperative, stable, and spontaneously ventilating, and provided that time allows.

(6) True or false? When airway injuries involve a tear between the glottis and the distal tracheobronchial tree, TTJV is absolutely contraindicated because the positive-pressure ventilation can cause a pneumothorax

or pneumomediastinum, or even convert a partial airway tear into a complete airway separation.

(7) True or false? Mask ventilation can be made more difficult by maxillofacial or mandibular injuries, but tracheal intubation is typically achievable.

(8) True or false? The laryngeal mask airway (LMA) is an emergency aid used to establish ventilation in the cannot intubate–cannot ventilate situation, and can also serve as a conduit for tracheal intubation once ventilation has been established.

(9) True or false? Blind intubation techniques are contraindicated in the setting of stridor, known mass-expanding lesions, or known partial airway injuries, because blind manipulation can change a partial airway obstruction into a complete obstruction.

(10) True or false? Extreme caution is suggested when attempting to blindly pass an endotracheal tube

through a functioning LMA in trauma patients, because of the high blind passage failure rate and the risk of doing harm to a tenuous airway (especially when there is evidence of neck swelling or stridor).

Answers

(1) c
(2) b
(3) d
(4) True
(5) True
(6) True
(7) True
(8) True
(9) True
(10) True

References

1. Peterson GN, Domino KB, Caplan RA, *et al.* Management of the difficult airway: a closed claims analysis. *Anesthesiology* 2005; **103**: 33–9.

2. Benumof JL. Management of the difficult airway. *Anesthesiology* 1991; **75**: 1087–110.

3. American Society of Anesthesiologists. Practice Guidelines for Management of the Difficult Airway. An updated report by the American Society of Anesthesiologists Task Force on Management of the Difficult Airway. *Anesthesiology* 2013; **118**: 251–70.

4. Cormack RS, Lehane J. Difficult tracheal intubation in obstetrics. *Anaesthesia* 1984; **39**: 1105–11.

5. Wilson WC. Emergency airway management on the ward. In Hannowell LA, Waldron RJ, eds., *Airway Management*. Philadelphia, PA: Lippincott-Raven, 1996, pp. 443–51.

6. McIntyre JRW. The difficult intubation. *Can J Anaesth* 1987; **34**: 204.

7. Wilson ME, Spiegelhalter D, Robertson JA, *et al.* Predicting difficult intubation. *Br J Anaesth* 1988; **61**: 211.

8. Mallampati SR, Gatt SP, Gugino LD, *et al.* A clinical sign to predict difficult tracheal intubation: a prospective study. *Can Anaesth Soc J* 1985; **32**: 429–34.

9. Adnet F, Borron SW, Dumas JL, *et al.* Study of the "sniffing position" by magnetic resonance imaging. *Anesthesiology* 2001; **94**: 83–6.

10. Benumof JL. Laryngeal mask airway and the ASA difficult airway algorithm. *Anesthesiology* 1996; **84**: 686–99.

11. Pennet JH, White PF. The laryngeal mask airway. *Anesthesiology* 1993; **79**: 144–63.

12. Heath ML. Endotracheal intubation through the laryngeal mask – helpful when laryngoscopy is difficult or dangerous. *Eur J Anaesthesiol (Supp)* 1991; **4**: 41–5.

13. Ferson DZ, Rosenblatt WH, Johansen MJ, *et al.* Use of the intubating LMA-Fastrach in 254 patients with difficult-to-manage airways. *Anesthesiology* 2001; **95**: 1175–81.

14. Nolan JP, Wilson ME. Orotracheal intubation in patients with potential cervical spine injuries. An indication for the gum elastic bougie. *Anaesthesia* 1993; **48**: 630–3.

15. Wilson WC, Benumof JL. Pathophysiology, evaluation, and treatment of the difficult airway. *Anesthesiol Clin N Am* 1998; **16**: 29–75.

16. Wissler RN. The esophageal-tracheal combitube. *Anesthesiol Rev* 1993; **20**: 147–51.

17. Benumof JL, Scheller MS. The importance of transtracheal jet ventilation in the management of the difficult airway. *Anesthesiology* 1989; **71**: 769–78.

18. Inoue Y. Lightwand intubation can improve airway management. *Can J Anaesth* 2004; **51**: 1052–3.

19. Rose DK, Cohen MM. The airway: problems and predictions in 18, 500

patients. *Can J Anaesth* 1994; **41**: 372–83.

20. Healy DW, Maties O, Hovord D, Kheterpal A. A systematic review of the role of videolaryngoscopy in successful orotracheal intubation. *BMC Anesthesiology* 2012; **12**: 32.

21. Jungbauer A, Schumann A, Brunkhorst V, Borgers A, Groeben H. Expected difficult tracheal intubaton: a prospective comparison of direct laryngoscopy and video laryngoscopy in 200 patients. *Br J Anaesth* 2009; **102**: 546–50.

22. Ng I, Sim XLJ, Williams D, Segal R. A randomized controlled trial comparing the McGrath videolaryngoscope with the straight blade laryngoscope when used in adult patients with potential difficult airways. *Anaesthesia* 2011; **66**: 709–14.

23. Sun DA, Warrriner CB, Parsons DG, *et al.* The GlideScope Video Laryngoscope: randomized clinical trial in 200 patients. *Br J Anaesth* 2005; **94**: 381–4.

24. Andersen LH, Rovsing L, Olsen KS. GlideScope videolaryngoscope vs. Macintosh direct laryngoscope for intubation of morbidly obese patients: a randomized trial. *Acta Anaesthesiol Scand* 2011; **55**: 1090–7.

25. Aziz, MF, Dillman D, Rongwei F, Brambrink AM. Comparative Effectiveness of the C-MAC Video Laryngoscope versus Direct Laryngoscopy in the Setting of the Predicted Difficult Airway. *Anesthesiology* 2012; **116**: 629–36.

26. Enomoto Y, Asai T, Arai T, Kamishima K, Okuda Y. Pentax-AWS, a new videolaryngoscope, is more effective than the Macintosh laryngoscope for tracheal intubation in patients with restricted neck movements: a randomized comparative study. *Br J Anaesth* 2008; **100**: 544–8.

27. Griesdale DEG, Chau A, Isac G, *et al.* Video-laryngoscopy versus direct laryngoscopy in critically ill patients: a pilot randomized trial. *Can J Anaesth* 2012; **59**: 1032–9.

28. Noppens RR, Mobus S, Heid F, *et al.* Evaluation of the McGrath Series 5 videolaryngoscope after failed direct laryngoscopy. *Anaesthesia* 2010; **65**: 716–20.

29. Shippey B, Ray D, McKeown D. Case series: the McGrath videolaryngoscope – an initial clinical evaluation. *Can J Anaesth* 2007; **54**: 307–13.

30. Platts-Mills TF, Campagne D, Chinnock B, *et al.* A comparison of GlideScope video laryngoscopy versus direct laryngoscopy intubation in the emergency department. *Acad Emerg Med* 2009; **16**: 866–71.

31. Turkstra TP, Craen RA, Pelz DM, Gelb AW. Cervical spine motion: a flurorscopic comparison during intubation with lighted stylet, GlideScope, and Macintosh laryngoscope. *Anesth Analg* 2005; **101**: 910–15.

32. Kill C, Risse J, Wallot P, *et al.* Videolaryngoscopy with GlideScope reduces cervical spine movement in patients with unsecured cervical spine. *J Emerg Med* 2013; **44**: 750–6.

33. Robitaille A, Williams, SR, Tremblay M-H, *et al.* Cervical spine motion during trachael intubation with manual in-line stabilization: direct laryngoscopy versus glidescope videolaryngoscopy. *Anesth Analg* 2008; **106**: 935–41.

34. Dhonneur G, Abdi W, Ndoko S. *et al.* Assisted versus conventional tracheal intubation in morbidly obese patients. *Obes Surg* 2009; **19**: 1096–101.

35. Abdallah R, Galway U, You J, *et al.* A randomized comparison between the Pentax AWS video laryngoscope and the Macintosh laryngoscope in morbidly obese patients. *Anesth Analg* 2011; **113**: 1082–7.

36. Walker L, Brampton W, Halai M, *et al.* Randomized controlled trial of intubation with the McGrath Series 5 videolaryngoscope by inexperienced anaesthetists. *Br J Anaesth* 2009; **103**: 440–5.

37. Howard-Quijano KJ, Huang YM, Matevosian R, Kaplan MB, Steadman RH. Video-assisted instruction improves the success rate for tracheal intubation by novices. *Br J Anaesth* 2008; **101**: 568–72.

38. Doyle DJ. Glidescope-assisted fiberoptic intubation: a new airway teaching method. *Anesthesiology* 2004; **101**: 1252.

39. Walls RM. Did you miss the revolution? Presentation to ICEM, 2012. http://imgpublic.mci-group.com/ie/ICEM2012/Friday/track3/Ron_Walls.pdf (accessed July 2014).

40. Aziz MF, Healy D, Kheterpal, S, *et al.* Routine clinical practice effectiveness of the Glidescope in difficult airway management: an analysis of 2004 glidescope intubations, complications, and failures from two institutions. *Anesthesiology* 2011; **114**: 34–41.

41. Waters DJ. Guided blind endotracheal intubation. For patients with deformities of the upper airway. *Anesthesia* 1963; **18**: 158–62.

42. Powell WF, Ozdil TA. Translaryngeal guide for tracheal intubation. *Anesth Analg* 1967; **46**: 231–4.

43. Rogers SN, Benumof JL. New and easy techniques for fiberoptic endoscopy-aided tracheal intubation. *Anesthesiology* 1983; **59**: 569–72.

44. Ovassapian A, Krejcie TC, Yelich SJ, *et al.* Awake intubation in the patient at high risk of aspiration. *Br J Anaesth* 1989; **62**: 13–16.

45. Shields CB, McGraw CP. ICP and CPP as predictors of outcome following closed head injury. Presented at the Sixth International Symposium on Intracranial Pressure. Glasgow, Scotland, June 9–13, 1985.

46. Como JJ, Diaz JJ, Dunham CM, *et al.* Practice management guidelines for identification of cervical spine injuries following trauma: update from the Eastern Association for the Surgery of Trauma Practice Management Guidelines Committee. *J Trauma* 2009; **67**: 651–9.

47. Crosby ET, Lui A. The adult cervical spine: implications for airway management. *Can J Anaesth* 1990; **37**: 77–93.

48. Hastings RH, Marks JD. Airway management for trauma patients with potential cervical spine injuries. *Anesth Analg* 1991; **73**: 471–82.

49. Criswell JC, Parr MJA, Nolan JP. Emergency airway management in patients with cervical spine injuries. *Anaesthesia* 1994; **49**: 900–3.

50. Ghafoor AU, Martin TW, Viswamitra S, *et al.* Caring for the patients with cervical spine injuries: what have we learned? *J Clin Anesth* 2005; **17**: 640–9.

51. Smith CE, Sidhu TS, Lever J, Pinchak AB. The complexity of tracheal intubation using rigid fiberoptic laryngoscopy (Wuscope). *Anesth Analg* 1999; **89**: 236–9.

52. Smith CE. Cervical spine injury and tracheal intubation: a never-ending conflict. *Trauma Care* 2000; **10**: 20–6.

53. Uchida T, Hikawa Y, Saito Y, Yasuda K. The McCoy levering laryngoscope in patients with limited neck extension. *Can J Anaesth* 1997; **44**: 674–6.

54. Shearer VE, Giesecke AH. Airway management for patients with penetrating neck trauma: a retrospective study. *Anesth Analg* 1993; **77**: 1135–8.

55. Kawaguchi T, Kushibe K, Takahama M, *et al.* Bluntly traumatic tracheal transection: usefulness of percutaneous cardiopulmonary support for maintenance of gas exchange. *Eur J Cardiothorac Surg* 2005; **27**: 523–5.

56. Le Fort R. Etude experimentale sur les fractures de la machoire superieure. *Rev Chir* 1901; **23**: 360–70.

57. Bahr W, Stoll P. Nasal intubation in the presence of frontobasalar fractures: A retrospective study. *J Oral Maxillofac Surg* 1992; **50**: 445–7.

58. Levine RL, Wayne MA, Miller CC. End-tidal carbon dioxide and outcome of out-of-hospital cardiac arrest. *N Engl J Med* 1997; **337**: 301–6.

59. Wee M. The oesophageal detector device: assessment of a new method to distinguish oesophageal from tracheal intubation. *Anaesthesia* 1988; **43**: 27–9.

60. Zura A, Doyle DJ, Orlandi M. Use of the Aintree intubation catheter in a patient with an unexpected difficult airway. *Can J Anaesth* 2005; **25**: 646–9.

61. Barsuk D, Ziv A, Lin G, *et al.* Using advanced simulation for recognition and correction of gaps in airway and breathing management skills in prehospital trauma care. *Anesth Analg* 2005; **100**: 803–9.

Chapter

4

Shock management

Richard P. Dutton

Objectives

(1) Review the pathophysiology of traumatic shock.
(2) Describe the diagnosis and treatment of shock in trauma patients.

Introduction

Shock is a systemic disease caused by inadequate tissue oxygen delivery. Shock consists of primary cellular injury due to hypoperfusion and the secondary inflammatory response that follows. Shock is a complication of many traumatic conditions and is the cause of up to half of all deaths from trauma: 40% due to acute hemorrhage and up to 10% due to multiple organ system failure after the initial cause of shock has been controlled.[1] This chapter describes the mechanisms of injury that lead to shock, the pathophysiologic progression of shock, the way in which shock is diagnosed and monitored, and the ways in which shock is treated. The chapter concludes with specific recommendations for resuscitation and a brief review of active areas of research.

Pathophysiology

Shock may result from any traumatic or nontraumatic process that impairs the systemic delivery of oxygen or that prevents its normal uptake and utilization. Table 4.1 lists the causes of shock in trauma patients, and although hemorrhage is the most common of these, it is by no means the only one. It is not unusual for shock to result from the combination of multiple triggers. Hemorrhage, tension pneumothorax, and cardiac contusion can all coexist in the patient with chest trauma, with each contributing to systemic hypoperfusion. Underlying medical conditions can play a part, with decompensation of diseases such as diabetes and myocardial ischemia contributing to decreased oxygen delivery, especially in older trauma patients. The effects of alcohol, medications, and illicit drugs may also contribute to a state of hypoperfusion and may block normal compensatory mechanisms. Most of the discussion that follows assumes that shock is occurring as the result of hemorrhage, with systemic effects triggered by a lack of blood flow and oxygen delivery. Shock arising from sepsis,

Table 4.1 Causes of shock in the trauma patient

Cause	Pathophysiology
Lost airway or pulmonary injury	Inability of oxygen to reach the circulation
Tension pneumothorax	Diminished blood return to the heart
Cardiac tamponade	Diminished blood return to the heart
Hemorrhage	Inadequate oxygen-carrying capacity Inadequate intravascular volume
Cardiac injury	Inadequate pump function
Spinal cord injury	Inappropriate vasodilatation Inadequate pump function
Poisoning	Direct failure of cellular metabolism Inappropriate vasodilatation
Sepsis	Direct failure of cellular metabolism Inappropriate vasodilatation

poisoning, or chronic cardiac failure may manifest differently, although the fundamental pathology is the same and the final systemic pathways are similar.

By whatever means it arises, the hallmark of shock is cellular hypoperfusion. The cells of certain organ systems (e.g., skeletal muscle, the gut) have a generous anaerobic capacity and can tolerate periods of ischemia, whereas other organs (e.g., the central nervous system) must have a continuous flow of oxygen to survive. Shock must be defined, therefore, as a reduction of oxygen delivery below the threshold at which a cellular response occurs. Shock may be triggered in oxygen-dependent tissues such as the brain – due to the catastrophic failure of oxygen caused by an obstructed airway – even while skin and bone and muscle are functioning normally. Shock can result from prolonged absence of perfusion to skeletal muscle beds, due to subacute hemorrhage, even in the presence of continued cardiac and neurologic function. The "dose" of hypoperfusion necessary to trigger shock is a

Trauma Anesthesia, 2nd Edition, ed. Charles E. Smith. Published by Cambridge University Press. © Charles E. Smith, 2015.

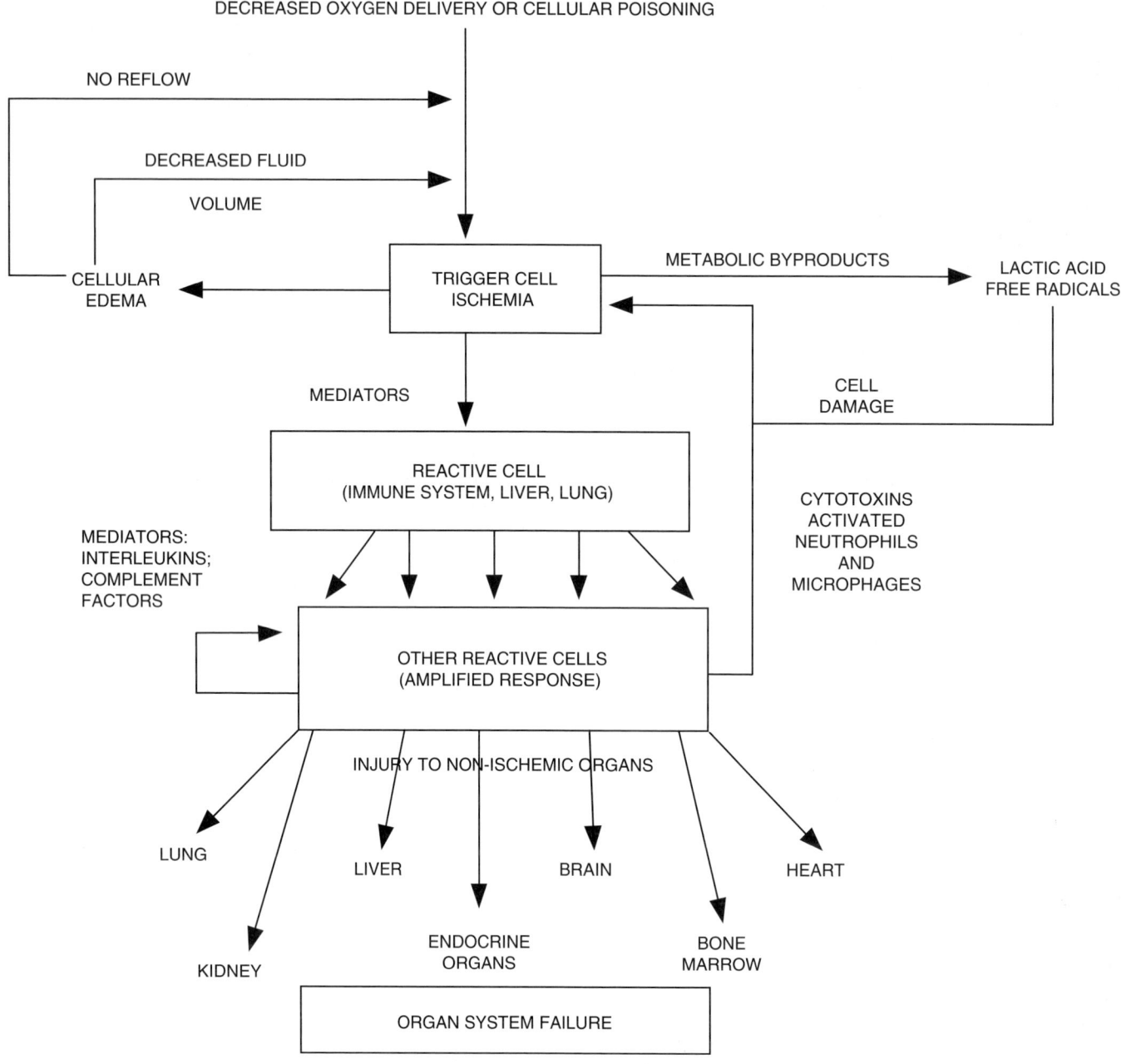

Figure 4.1 The inflammatory cascade triggered by an episode of shock can turn an episode of local hypoperfusion into a systemic disease. (Adapted from Dutton RP. Management of traumatic shock. In Prough DS, Fleisher L, eds., *Problems in Anesthesia: Trauma Care* **13** (3), London: Lippincott, Williams & Wilkins, 2002.[2])

function of both the depth of hypoperfusion – the number of cells experiencing a loss of oxygenation – and the duration. Whatever the trigger, and whatever the organ system that first becomes critically hypoperfused, the subsequent course of shock is driven by a cascade of humoral signaling and response that turns shock from a local condition into a systemic disease (Fig. 4.1).[2] It is important to recognize that shock continues even after the triggering event has been corrected.

The cellular response to critical ischemia can take many forms. Many cells (e.g., kidney, gut) can "hibernate" in the absence of adequate oxygenation by ceasing to function and

thus reducing metabolic demand.[3] Other cells (cardiac muscle, brainstem) do not have this option. Most cells take up free water as they become ischemic,[4] perhaps as a means of buffering accumulated intracellular toxins and perhaps due to a failure of energy-dependent membrane functions. This cellular edema can itself be problematic if it further limits perfusion of adjoining cells, and the "no-reflow" phenomenon has been identified as a cause of ongoing cellular hypoperfusion in the liver even after the restoration of adequate systemic blood flow.[5] As available oxygen drops even lower, cells become fatally injured and will die. This can occur chaotically, in the form of an infarction, or on a "programmed" basis known as apoptosis in which the cell engages in a specific series of chemical steps that result in its own death.[6] Apoptosis is primarily associated with brain tissue, and serves a functional role in brain development by "pruning" neural networks.[7] In response to ischemia, apoptosis may represent a planned triage process intended to preserve limited oxygen supplies for more critical cells at the expense of less critical ones.

Even before hypoperfusion has progressed to cellular ischemia, there will be local and systemic compensatory changes intended to mitigate damage. Injured blood vessels constrict to limit hemorrhage, while collateral vessels dilate to increase blood flow to ischemic tissue.[8] Perception of blood loss, augmented by pain, causes a reflex increase in sympathetic outflow from the central nervous system, leading to increased chronotropy and inotropy of the heart, and shunting of blood away from ischemia-tolerant vascular beds and into the central circulation. This redirection of blood flow allows for continued perfusion (and survival) of the brain and cardiac muscle even with loss of substantial intravascular blood volume. It is this central shunting that creates the potential for reperfusion injury. The sudden restoration of blood flow to vascular beds that have been intensely vasoconstricted may liberate large quantities of metabolic toxins, resulting in cardiac dysfunction and a systemic inflammatory response.[9]

Organ systems react differently to hypoperfusion, as listed briefly in Table 4.2.[10] The brain and spinal cord, which have limited capacity for anaerobic metabolism, will be permanently injured within minutes if deprived of oxygen. Some

degree of hibernation can occur as oxygen supplies drop and with it the cerebral metabolic rate; this may explain the change in level of consciousness seen in progressive hemorrhagic shock, from normal to agitated to lethargic to comatose.[11] Rapid cell death and infarction occur in areas of the brain completely lacking in blood flow, whereas apoptosis may occur in regions that are merely ischemic. Because the brain is the most oxygen-sensitive tissue of the body, and because systemic compensation functions to maintain brain perfusion for as long as possible, permanent neurologic injuries short of death are actually rare as a consequence of systemic shock, and usually occur only in the presence of stroke or traumatic brain injury.

Cardiac function in shock is initially augmented, as part of the systemic compensation for decreased oxygen delivery.[12] Heart rate and contractility increase, and coronary arterial flow increases accordingly. It is rare for the heart to be the sentinel organ for hypoperfusion unless the cessation of oxygen delivery is rapid and complete, as with a lost airway. Evidence of myocardial ischemia – elevated serum troponin levels, ST segment changes on electrocardiogram – usually occur only with direct myocardial injury (cardiac contusion) or underlying severe atherosclerotic disease. As shock progresses, however, cardiac dysfunction becomes more common. Increasing serum acidosis has a negative inotropic effect, as do the hypothermia, anemia, and hypocalcemia that result from rapid fluid resuscitation. Progressive ischemia leads eventually to vascular system failure, as vasoconstriction is an energy-dependent process.[13] Inappropriate vasodilatation with a lack of response to epinephrine is the hallmark of acute fatal shock and may occur despite the rapid infusion of resuscitative fluid. In the patient who achieves hemostasis and survives to reach the intensive care unit (ICU), cardiac dysfunction may be caused by the systemic inflammatory response syndrome (SIRS) or toxins released in association with septic episodes.

Although pulmonary tissue itself will always be exposed to oxygen, the capillary beds of the lung serve an important role as the downstream filter for the systemic circulation. The lungs are where acute shock affecting individual tissues and organs becomes a systemic disease. Much of the inflammatory upregulation that follows traumatic shock occurs in the lungs.[14] Simple blood loss, without the development of hypoperfusion, does not trigger the same amplified response as blood loss leading to hypoperfusion.[15] Accumulation of toxic byproducts leads to impairment of normal ventilation/perfusion (V/Q) matching, with subsequent arterial desaturation, while progression of the inflammatory cascade impairs normal membrane function and causes cellular edema and extracellular extravasation of fluid. The lungs are the sentinel organ for the development of multiple organ system failure, with the need for mechanical ventilation as the first clinical sign of this syndrome.[16]

The splanchnic circulation is more ischemia-tolerant than the brain or heart. Kidney and gut cells have the ability to conserve energy by limiting active membrane transport.[17] This

Table 4.2 Organ system response to ischemia

Organ system	Moderate ischemia	Severe ischemia
CNS	Anxiety, then lethargy	Coma, cellular apoptosis
Cardiovascular	Vasoconstriction Increased cardiac output and rate	Vascular failure Vasodilatation Myocardial ischemia Dysrhythmias
Pulmonary	Increased respiratory rate	V/Q mismatch ARDS
Renal	Hibernation	Acute tubular necrosis
Gastrointestinal	Ileus	Infarction Loss of barrier function
Hepatic	Increased glucose release	No reflow Reperfusion injury Loss of synthetic function
Hematopoietic	None	Decreased cell production Impaired immune function

CNS, central nervous system; ARDS, acute respiratory distress syndrome; V/Q, ventilation/perfusion.

leads to diminished urine output and an ileus in the short term, but both of these conditions are reversible without long-term consequences, if the dose of shock is small.[18] While the gut and kidney shut down in response to hypoperfusion, the liver and adrenals are part of the fight-or-flight response. Serum catechol levels increase with adrenal stimulation, leading to increased release of glucose from the liver.[19] If shock persists or deepens, these organs will become critically hypoperfused and will cease to function. Adrenal "exhaustion" is often apparent in established shock, such as that from sepsis or chronic cardiac failure.[20] Dysfunction of the liver is manifest first in loss of control over serum glucose levels, then in increased levels of liver proteins – indicating cell death – and finally in a loss of synthetic functions and persistent coagulopathy.[21] Liver cells are prone to the no-reflow phenomenon and may contribute to the perpetuation of shock from hemorrhage, even after restoration of systemic blood volume. With increasing ischemia, renal cells begin to fail, leading to the development of acute tubular necrosis, and gut cells will lose the ability to maintain a barrier between intraluminal contents and the circulation. Translocation of bacteria first to the liver and then to the lungs may play an important role in the development of systemic inflammation and multiple organ system failure.[22] Outright infarction of splanchnic organs is unusual in traumatic shock and is almost always the result of a direct arterial injury, but splanchnic dysfunction is common and problematic.

Skin, muscle, and bone are the most ischemia-tolerant tissues in the body, and therefore the organs that lose blood flow first in response to shock. Reduction of blood flow to the skin in response to hemorrhage causes the characteristic pallor of the trauma victim and is associated with peripheral cooling and diaphoresis.[23] Absorption of water from the vascular and extravascular space was first established in ischemic muscle cells, and it is this effect, occurring systemwide, that causes a severely shocked individual to become massively edematous (up to dozens of liters of positive fluid balance) in the first days following injury.[4] Muscle cells can remain dormant for extended periods in the resting individual, with only intermittent blood flow to support basic metabolic needs. Even complete ischemia, as with the use of a tourniquet during extremity surgery, is tolerated without consequence for periods as long as 2 hours.[24] It is this very ability to compensate, however, that makes the peripheral circulation the trigger for systemic shock in situations of sustained low-level hypoperfusion. Hemorrhage sufficient to trigger peripheral vasoconstriction but not severe enough to threaten the central circulation will leave the patient with normal mentation and vital signs, but a slowly accumulating metabolic debt. In time, the toxic byproducts and inflammatory mediators that accumulate in the periphery will make their way to the lung, triggering the systemic response.

The clinical outcome of traumatic shock from unchecked hemorrhage follows one of the four paths shown in Figure 4.2.[25] In early hemorrhage, reduced oxygen-carrying capacity is compensated by increased heart rate and contractility, leading to increased cardiac output. If hemorrhage is limited or rapidly controlled and fluid is provided to restore intravascular volume and compensate for extravascular losses, as in curve A, then there will be no long-term effect on the patient. A greater duration or severity of blood loss requires compensation by peripheral and splanchnic vasoconstriction. While effective at preserving core oxygen delivery, this mechanism is inherently unstable, as an "oxygen debt" is now accumulating in these tissues. This is a patient who requires rapid diagnosis and control of hemorrhage. If these efforts are unsuccessful, the clinical course will follow curve B, death from acute hemorrhagic shock. This is the patient who is said to exsanguinate, although with modern intravenous infusion technology, this is seldom strictly true. Rather, the state of systemic hypoperfusion becomes so severe that vascular system failure ensues, with inappropriate vasodilatation and loss of responsiveness to pressor agents. Elements of the "lethal triad" of acidosis, coagulopathy, and hypothermia will be apparent despite aggressive efforts to prevent them.[26] At this point shock is irreversibly severe and the patient will die of complete circulatory failure, usually after the decision that further transfusion therapy is futile.

Curves C and D in Figure 4.2 represent the subtle middle ground of shock progression, treatment, and long-term outcome. In both cases, control of hemorrhage occurs before the patient can "tip over" into acute irreversible shock. Once bleeding is controlled, fluid resuscitation can restore intravascular volume and macroperfusion to hypoperfused organs. However, the dose of shock sustained is large enough to trigger an inflammatory response in susceptible patients, with significant long-term consequences. The SIRS is characterized by fever and a hyperdynamic state in the first days following an episode of shock.[27] Organ system failure post resuscitation starts in the lungs, with increased need for supplemental oxygen and an inability to wean from the ventilator.[16] Renal failure is common and may be severe enough to require hemofiltration or dialysis. Gut function is impaired, with a protracted ileus and inability to tolerate enteral feeding. Instability of serum glucose levels and decreased clotting-factor activity indicate liver dysfunction, while persistent anemia and recurrent septic episodes may reflect failure or dysfunction of the immune system.[28] The development of SIRS and the degree of subsequent organ system failure is a complex interaction of age, the degree of injury, the nature and specificity of treatment, the patient's underlying genetic makeup, and the patient's premorbid medical condition (Table 4.3). In some patients (curve C) restoration of systemic perfusion is followed by an "overshoot" period of high cardiac output with limited and survivable organ system dysfunction. In other patients (curve D), organ failure is more severe, repeated episodes of sepsis occur, and the patient succumbs to a combination of respiratory failure and recurrent septic shock.

Table 4.3 Factors predisposing to the systemic inflammatory response syndrome (SIRS) and the development of the acute respiratory distress syndrome (ARDS)

Depth and duration of hypoperfusion ("dose" of shock)
- Predicted by maximum lactate level
- Predicted by rate of clearance of lactate to normal

Quantity of blood products transfused

Presenting injuries
- Long-bone fractures (fat/marrow embolus)
- Traumatic brain injury
- Aspiration prior to definitive airway
- Chest contusion/injury

Greater patient age

Underlying medical conditions
- Diabetes
- Coronary artery disease
- Chronic obstructive pulmonary disease
- Autoimmune disease

Patient genetics

Diagnosis

Given the potentially serious consequences of shock, rapid diagnosis leading to immediate treatment is critical to improving outcomes. The Advanced Trauma Life Support (ATLS) curriculum of the American College of Surgeons provides a common language for trauma practitioners and a framework for organizing diagnostic and resuscitative efforts.[29] The ATLS approach has become the standard for trauma centers and trauma training. The algorithm is organized to identify and eliminate the causes of shock in order of acuity, beginning with the mechanics of oxygen delivery to the bloodstream (A for airway and B for breathing). This is followed by an assessment of oxygen delivery to the tissue level (C for circulation), with search for any source of hemorrhage. Following the ABCs, a detailed secondary survey is undertaken to identify neurologic disability and specific injuries that require treatment.

Diagnosis of shock begins with suspicion based on the mechanism of injury. Any penetrating trauma and any high-energy event (a fall greater than 3 meters [10 feet], motor vehicle collision, pedestrian or bicyclist struck, gunshot wound, industrial explosion) has the potential to cause

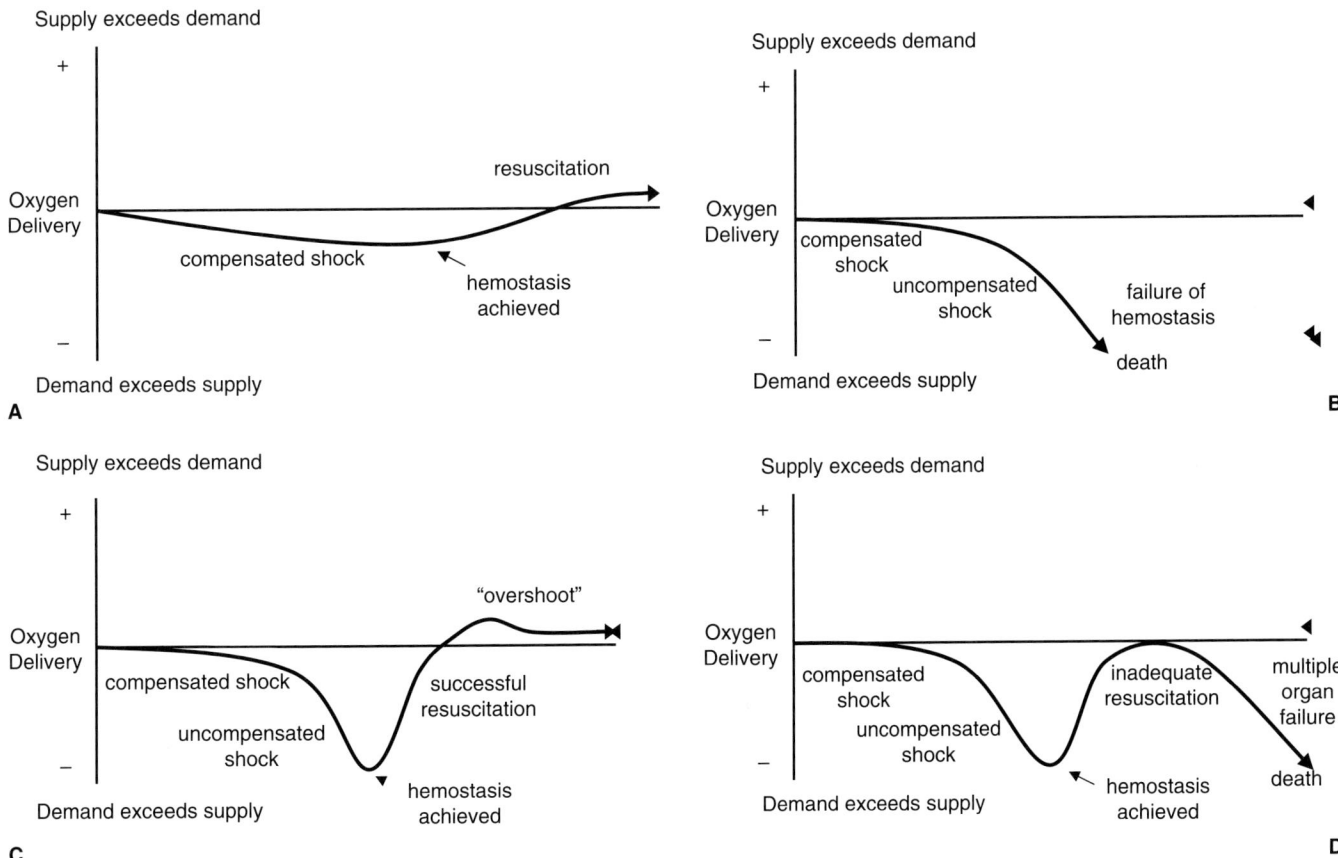

Figure 4.2 Outcomes from an episode of hemorrhagic shock, expressed as the ratio of tissue oxygen delivery to demand. Curve A shows hemorrhage within the range of compensation, with minimal tissue ischemia. Curve C shows a patient in whom hemorrhage is controlled short of death. Oxygen delivery is restored, and an "overshoot" occurs as the patient becomes hyperdynamic. Curve D shows a similar patient in whom the inflammatory response to hemorrhagic shock becomes overwhelming. Despite resolution of hemorrhage short of death, the patient dies of multiple organ system failure after days to weeks in the ICU. Curve B shows severe hemorrhage, with physiologic decompensation and total systemic ischemia. This is the patient who dies of acute hemorrhage in the emergency department or operating room.

Table 4.4 Early signs and symptoms of shock

Visible evidence of blood loss or long-bone fracture
Anxiety, progressing to lethargy and coma
Pallor, diaphoresis
Decreased skin turgor
Hypotension with narrowed pulse pressure
Tachycardia
Nonfunctioning pulse oximeter
Hypotension or unusual sensitivity to standard doses of analgesic or anesthetic medications
Decreased end-tidal CO_2 after tracheal intubation

bleeding, and should prompt transport to a trauma center and expert assessment. The first look at a trauma patient is often sufficient to make the diagnosis. A patient in shock will be pale, with cool and diaphoretic skin. Injuries associated with blood loss may be readily apparent: fractured long bones or deep lacerations. The patient's mental status is important, with patients in shock progressing from normal to anxious to agitated to lethargic to comatose.[11] Initial vital signs are helpful, but not pathognomonic. Classically, the shocked patient will be hypotensive, although young patients have enormous capacity to vasoconstrict and preserve normal blood pressure. The key to recognizing this phenomenon is often an abnormally narrow pulse pressure (such as 140/115), especially when seen on an automated noninvasive blood pressure system.[30] Based on one large retrospective analysis, two-thirds of hypotensive patients will be tachycardic.[31] An even more subtle indicator of peripheral hypoperfusion is failure of the pulse oximeter to function due to vasoconstriction of the fingers. Table 4.4 lists these early characteristics of shock. If any are present, then confirmatory laboratory testing should occur, along with an aggressive search for an inciting cause: mechanical obstruction of blood flow, hemorrhage, or spinal cord injury.

Laboratory tests are the most reliable indicators of tissue hypoperfusion in early shock. The instantaneous degree of shock is approximated by the base deficit measured on arterial blood gas, or by the pH when adjusted for respiratory function. Metabolic acidosis in a trauma patient is due to diminished perfusion. Serum lactate is another sensitive marker for shock; because lactate is cleared from the circulation more slowly than acidosis is corrected, the lactate level is a good approximation of the total dose of shock (i.e., the integral or "area under the curve" of the severity of shock and the amount of time it has persisted). Lactate level on admission is a sensitive predictor of outcome in severely injured trauma patients, and the rate at which lactate is cleared from the circulation correlates with the adequacy of resuscitation.[32] Because systemic compensation can produce normal vital signs even following substantial blood loss, metabolic acidosis

or elevated lactate may be the first and most sensitive indicator of hypoperfusion, especially in young trauma patients. A persistently elevated lactate level in an ICU patient with stable vital signs following initial surgery should raise the specter of the occult hypoperfusion syndrome (i.e., unrecognized shock) and should prompt a more aggressive fluid resuscitation strategy.[33]

Various devices have been developed to provide continuous monitoring of the depth of shock and the response to therapy. To date, none has achieved the ideal combination of sensitivity, rapid response, ease of use, and noninvasiveness that would make it a standard of care. Mixed venous oxygen saturation correlates closely with perfusion and is rapidly responsive to changing conditions, but requires placement of a central venous or pulmonary artery catheter. This monitor is of most use outside of initial resuscitation in patients who are hemodynamically stable.[34] Continuous measurement of gastric mucosal pH (gastric tonometry) is sensitive to the patient's state of perfusion.[35] However, because the monitor is cumbersome to use and requires careful calibration and time to achieve a steady-state equilibration, use of this device has been abandoned. A simpler version, based on rapid assessment of sublingual carbon dioxide concentration, was tested but not commercialized.[36] Near-infrared tissue oximetry of vulnerable muscle beds, typically the thenar eminence of the hand, has shown some promise. This is a noninvasive measure that is easy to use, and provides a value for muscle-bed tissue saturation that correlates with the mixed venous oxygen saturation.[37] This tissue oxygenation monitor has been used to guide the resuscitation of trauma patients in the ICU, with good results, but has not yet demonstrated value in the highly dynamic period of emergency department diagnosis and treatment. Other monitors in this category include minimally invasive cardiac output monitors based on esophageal Doppler technology,[38] lithium-ion dilution,[39] exhaled carbon dioxide,[40] or analysis of arterial pulse pressure variation.[41] All such monitors produce accurate data over time in relatively healthy patients, but show more variation during the rollercoaster of active hemorrhage and ongoing resuscitation that occurs during early hemorrhagic shock in trauma patients.

The value of simple continuous observation should not be underestimated. Trends in vital signs are more important than absolute values, especially considering the wide range of baseline physiologies seen in trauma patients. Even more important is close observation of the patient's response to therapeutic interventions, as illustrated in Figure 4.3. Decreased blood pressure in response to observed hemorrhage, in response to a switch from spontaneous to positive-pressure ventilation, or after administration of sedative or analgesic medications all indicate a state of critical hypovolemia and a patient who is close to the limits of compensation. Increased blood pressure in response to an intravenous fluid bolus is an indicator that the patient was hypovolemic to begin with. These effects are used by the ATLS curriculum to make the useful classification of hypotensive trauma patients as "responders," "transient

Table 4.5 Advanced Trauma Life Support (ATLS) classification of shock, based on the response of a hypotensive patient to an initial fluid bolus (500 mL of isotonic crystalloid)

Category	Response to fluid bolus	Clinical implications
Responder	Increased and sustained improvement in blood pressure	Not actively bleeding Unlikely to require transfusion
Transient responder	Increased blood pressure, followed by recurrent hypotension	Actively bleeding Should consider early transfusion
Nonresponder	No improvement	Must rule out other causes of shock • Tension pneumothorax • Cardiac tamponade • High spinal cord injury Likely active bleeding, with protracted or severe hypoperfusion Immediate transfusion, early use of plasma and platelets

Table 4.6 Sources of hemorrhage

Location	Cause	Diagnostic approach
Chest	Pulmonary injury	Physical examination (low yield)
	Intercostal arteries Great vessels	Chest radiograph CT scan Chest tube output
Abdomen	Solid organ injury Mesenteric bleeding	Ultrasound (FAST) CT scan Peritoneal lavage
Retroperitoneum	Posterior pelvic fracture (Rarely) renal, aortic, vena caval injury	Pelvic instability Pelvic radiograph CT scan
Thighs	Femur fracture	Physical examination Directed radiography
"The street"	Scalp lacerations Open fractures Massive soft tissue wounds	Physical examination

CT, computed tomography; FAST, focused assessment with sonography for trauma.

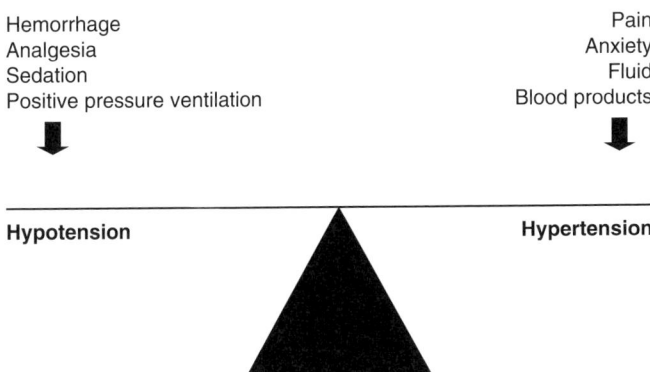

Figure 4.3 Hemodynamic "balance" in the hemorrhaging trauma patient. Observation of the response to therapy is an important clue to the presence of shock. Patients who become hypotensive in response to positive-pressure ventilation or analgesic medication should be presumed hypovolemic until proven otherwise.

responders," and "nonresponders," with clinical implications as illustrated in Table 4.5.[29]

Finally, determination of the presence of shock is only a portion of the diagnostic challenge. For therapy to be effective, the cause of shock must be identified and corrected. Shock as the result of airway obstruction or respiratory insufficiency will be rapidly corrected by tracheal intubation and mechanical ventilation. Mechanical obstruction of blood flow due to pneumothorax or tamponade will be identified by clinical suspicion, physical examination, ultrasound, chest radiography, or response to direct action (i.e., chest tube placement or emergency department thoracotomy). Spinal cord injury will become apparent on physical examination; hypoperfusion, due to decreased sympathetic outflow and inappropriate vasodilatation, will be associated with loss of motor and sensory function at a level of T6 or higher.[42] Traumatic brain injury (TBI) by itself should not produce a state of shock, but the presence of TBI will complicate diagnostic efforts and the course of resuscitation. Ongoing hemorrhage is left as the cause of shock that presents the greatest diagnostic challenge and is the subject of much of the ATLS curriculum.

Bleeding sufficient to produce life-threatening shock can occur in one of five regions, as listed in Table 4.6.[43] Each of these must be considered in the victim of high-energy trauma, and ongoing hemorrhage ruled out. Thoracic hemorrhage is identified by plain film or computed tomography (CT) imaging of the chest and quantified by placement of a tube thoracostomy. Peritoneal hemorrhage is diagnosed by the presence of free fluid on sonographic examination (FAST: focused assessment with sonography for trauma),[44] or by CT (in patients stable enough to undergo this test) or direct peritoneal lavage (in austere environments). Retroperitoneal bleeding is almost always the result of disruption of the pelvic ring; this diagnosis is suggested by gross instability of the pelvis on physical examination and confirmed by plain film and/or CT. Femoral compartment hemorrhage is almost always associated with femur fracture, and is readily apparent on physical examination. Bleeding outside the body should be easy to diagnose, but ongoing scalp hemorrhage can be easily overlooked during the primary survey, especially in patients with other injuries.

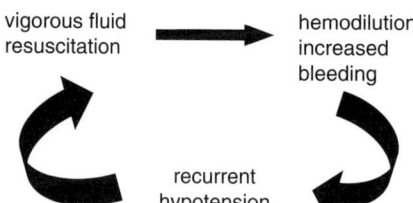

Figure 4.4 The vicious cycle of rapid crystalloid infusion in patients with active hemorrhage.

Fluid resuscitation

Resuscitation must begin as soon as shock is identified, to prevent deterioration of the patient beyond the point where salvage becomes impossible. Yet resuscitation cannot be successful unless the source of shock is corrected. As this invariably takes time – for diagnostic studies, for placement of intravenous access and invasive monitors, for transport to the operating room and induction of anesthesia – there is always a period of time in which resuscitation and primary therapy overlap. This time is analogous to pouring water into a bucket with a hole in the bottom, and is the most complex and critical portion of resuscitation. During this time the goal should be to support, but not necessarily normalize, the patient's physiology. Aggressive pursuit of "endpoints of resuscitation" in the patient who is still actively hemorrhaging may exacerbate the underlying pathology and make the ultimate treatment more difficult.

Table 4.6 lists the common sources of hemorrhage in trauma patients and the basic diagnostic approach for each. Shock is usually apparent at the time of admission to the trauma center, and the initial treatment steps are the ATLS "ABCs": airway control, mechanical ventilation, and circulatory support. Endotracheal intubation must be approached with caution, because administration of a normal induction dose of a sedative/hypnotic agent will cause profound hypotension in the patient with shock (see Chapter 7). Even cardiac-friendly agents such as etomidate or ketamine will cause hemodynamic distress in patients with high catecholamine levels at the time of induction.[45] Mechanical ventilation may exacerbate occult pneumothorax; chest tube placement based only on hypotension is appropriate in a patient with any chest injury who "crashes" immediately after intubation. Positive-pressure ventilation reduces venous return to the heart and may significantly lower blood pressure in hypovolemic patients or those patients with tamponade physiology. Low tidal volumes and a slow ventilatory rate are appropriate for patients in shock, with upward titration towards normal settings as tolerated by the patient's hemodynamic status.

While rapid administration of intravenous fluids has long been advocated by the ATLS curriculum, this therapy, more than any other, may be detrimental to the patient who is actively bleeding. Hypotension is a key contributor to early clotting.[46] Rapid crystalloid infusion to produce an increase in blood pressure may "pop the clot" and cause rebleeding and a subsequent further deterioration in vital signs, as illustrated by Figure 4.4.[47] Isotonic crystalloids, the most commonly

available fluid for early resuscitation, will further exacerbate hemorrhage by diluting the supply of clotting factors and platelets (already stressed by multiple sites of hemorrhage), by reducing the viscosity of the blood, and – unless administered with great care – by reducing body temperature. Numerous laboratory studies have demonstrated the value of deliberate hypotension in resuscitation of the actively bleeding animal,[48] and two large human trials have provided further evidence of the benefit of this approach.[49,50] Fluids should be administered in small boluses only, with the goal of maintaining a lower than normal systolic blood pressure (typically 80–90 mmHg), until definitive control of hemorrhage. The moment when active bleeding stops is usually readily apparent to clinicians, as the blood pressure will spontaneously rise toward the normal range ("autoresuscitation" caused by extravascular-to-intravascular fluid shifts) and the patient will become more tolerant of anesthetic agents.[50]

The quality of fluid administered is as important as the quantity. Each of the available intravenous volume expanders has its own risks and benefits (Table 4.7). The clinician must make an educated guess at the amount of fluid the patient is likely to require, and plan accordingly to achieve optimal blood composition at the conclusion of resuscitation. In general, patients will fall into one of the three broad categories shown in Table 4.5: (1) responders, (2) transient responders, and (3) nonresponders. Many patients in shock have already stopped bleeding at the time that treatment begins. This includes most patients with a single isolated femur fracture, for example. The patient may lose 1000–1500 mL of blood within the first minutes of injury, but the profound vasoconstrictive mechanisms of the peripheral circulation, tamponade within the surrounding muscle compartments, and a normal coagulation response will all contribute to spontaneous hemostasis while the patient is still in the prehospital phase. As long as fluid administration is not so aggressive as to wash off the existing clots or rapidly reverse local vasoconstriction, then this patient will remain hemodynamically stable throughout his or her course. Crystalloid fluids can be administered over time to replace losses to cellular edema and extravasation, and red blood cells (RBCs) and coagulation factors can be given as indicated by laboratory testing, and in precisely the quantities required.

Patients with ongoing active hemorrhage in the emergency department, such as those with high-grade splenic or hepatic trauma or with penetrating injuries to large arteries or veins, will emerge as transient responders to initial fluid

Table 4.7 Fluids available for resuscitation from hemorrhagic shock

Fluid	Benefits	Risks
Isotonic crystalloids		
0.9% saline	Inexpensive Compatible with blood	Dilutes blood composition Hyperchloremic metabolic acidosis
Lactated Ringer's	Inexpensive Physiologic electrolyte mix	Dilutes blood composition
Plasmalyte-A	Inexpensive Physiologic electrolyte mix	Dilutes blood composition
Colloids		
Albumin	Rapid volume expansion	Expensive No proven benefit Dilutes blood composition
Starch solutions	Rapid volume expansion	Coagulopathy with first-generation products No proven benefit Dilutes blood composition
Hypertonic saline	Rapid volume expansion Improved outcomes in TBI patients	Rapid increase in blood pressure may exacerbate bleeding Dilutes blood composition
Red blood cells	Rapid volume expansion Increased oxygen delivery	Expensive, limited resource Requires crossmatching TRALI Viral transmission
Plasma	Rapid volume expansion Clotting factor replacement	Expensive, limited resource Crossmatching required TRALI Viral transmission
Fresh whole blood	Rapid volume expansion Carries oxygen Includes clotting factors and platelets Ideal fluid for early resuscitation	Unavailable in civilian practice • Logistics (low demand) • Time required for viral testing

TBI, traumatic brain injury; TRALI, transfusion-related acute lung injury.

administration. It is critical to identify these patients, because of the strong correlation between speed of definitive hemostasis and ultimate patient outcome. Resuscitation is far more likely to be successful if hypothermia and coagulopathy can be avoided, and tissue perfusion preserved, while hemostatic efforts are under way. Transient responders are likely to hemorrhage at least a single blood volume (approximately 5000 mL), and will inevitably require transfusion. Patients who are actively bleeding but still somewhat compensated are those

most at risk from excessive crystalloid infusion. It is better to limit non-blood products from the outset – even below the ATLS recommended 2-liter threshold – and begin efforts to preserve blood composition as soon as the transient responder is identified. Uncrossmatched type O RBCs are safe and immediately available in most large hospitals and should be used aggressively to begin resuscitation.[51] Early use of plasma and platelets is indicated to preserve coagulation function and replace the losses inherent in massive or multiple injuries (see Chapter 6).[52] As Figure 4.5 illustrates, even a fluid resuscitation scheme consisting of nothing but equal quantities of RBCs, plasma, and platelets in a 1:1:1 ratio will barely suffice to maintain blood composition.[53] The only way in which this plan can be improved would be the use of fresh whole blood, thus avoiding the losses and dilution inherent in component production and storage, but this therapy is unavailable in US trauma centers (outside of the military).

Although early recognition of the actively bleeding patient and informed and organized steps to preserve blood composition will allow the clinician to keep up with the patient in compensated shock, this approach will be insufficient in the patient presenting in extremis. This patient has either been actively bleeding like the transient responder, but for long enough to exhaust compensatory mechanisms, or is so massively injured that profound shock is already present at the time of emergency department arrival. Markers for this condition include hypothermia, persistent hypotension despite fluid therapy, metabolic acidosis, decreased hematocrit on the first laboratory sample, and elevated prothrombin time.[54] This patient has a high prospective mortality even with prompt diagnosis and treatment. In addition to a hypotensive resuscitation scheme using RBCs and plasma in equal quantities, as outlined above, this patient needs a "jump start" to the coagulation system. Eight to ten units of cryoprecipitate and 1–2 pheresis packs of platelets (6–12 random donor packs) are administered as early as possible, to provide a substrate for clotting, and an "off-label" dose of recombinant human clotting factor VIIa (rFVIIa; 10–100 μg/kg) is administered to trigger coagulation at the sites of vascular injury.[55] Although not yet validated by prospective scientific study, this is the current approach of the US military and several large civilian trauma centers, and is justified by risk–benefit assessment in sufficiently desperate cases.

Adjuvant therapies

Successful resuscitation requires more than administration of the right quantity and quality of fluid. Obtaining intravenous access is an important first step, and many patients will require a central line. A single-lumen large-bore catheter (e.g., a 9 Fr introducer) will provide the best flow of resuscitative fluid, with specially designed shorter, large-bore double-lumen catheters a good second choice (see Chapter 5). Subclavian and femoral veins are more accessible in the trauma patient than the internal jugulars, because of the cervical collar. Femoral

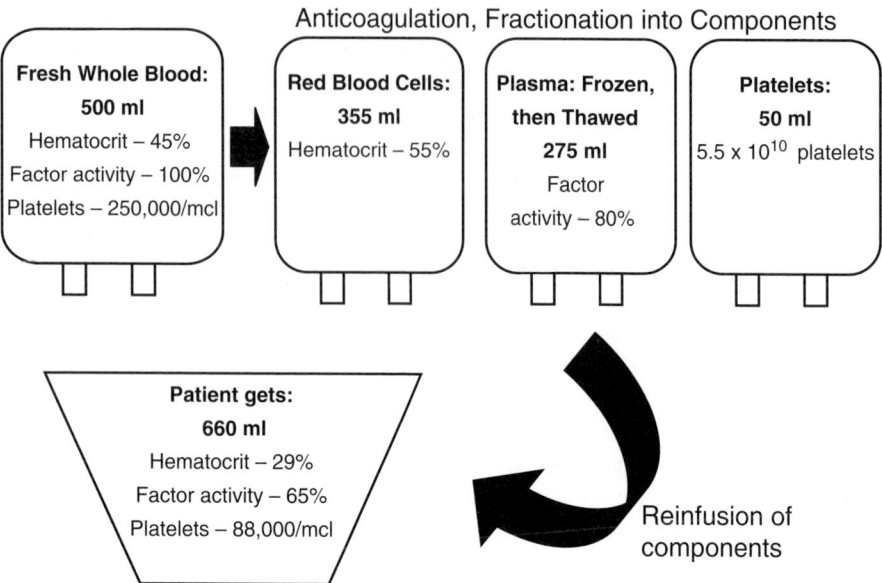

Figure 4.5 Fractionation and reconstruction of a unit of whole blood, illustrating the dilutional and storage-damage changes that occur between donation and transfusion.

lines and lines placed under less than fully sterile conditions have a high incidence of infection and should be removed or replaced at the conclusion of resuscitation.[56]

Preserving patient body temperature is a critical function of the anesthesiologist.[57] Hypothermia will exacerbate both acidosis and coagulopathy if allowed to persist. It is much easier to preserve body temperature than to restore it once the patient has become hypothermic, so attention to this issue throughout resuscitation is required. All infused fluids should be warmed, using a rapid infusion system if a large-volume transfusion is anticipated. The patient should be kept covered as much as possible, and the trauma bay and operating room should be warmed in advance of the patient's arrival, and kept warmer than normal for as long as the patient is exposed (see Chapter 14). Use of a forced-air heating blanket is strongly recommended, as is use of a passive humidity-capture device on the ventilator circuit. Irrigation and lavage fluids should be warmed, and the surgeon kept apprised of the patient's temperature; development of hypothermia is an indication for "damage control" maneuvers intended to minimize operative duration in unstable patients (see Chapter 18).[58]

Careful titration of mechanical ventilation is an important adjuvant to resuscitation. While respiratory acidosis should be avoided if possible, overventilation is also problematic because of impaired thoracic blood flow, inappropriate hypocapnia, oxygen toxicity, and the potential for barotrauma. Ventilator volumes, pressures, and rates should be as carefully titrated as all other aspects of resuscitation.[59]

Several recent studies have demonstrated the beneficial effect of tranexamic acid (TXA) administered early in resuscitation.[60,61] TXA is an inexpensive lysine analog that is known to have an antifibrinolytic effect. Prophylactic use in elective cardiac surgery patients has demonstrated a modest reduction in blood loss. The CRASH-2 trial, published in 2010, randomized 20,000 trauma patients to receive TXA or placebo early in the course of resuscitation.[60] This trial, one of the largest ever performed in trauma patients, demonstrated significant improvement in survival with TXA. Earlier administration was better than later. Of note, there was no difference in transfusion requirement between groups, raising a question regarding the beneficial mechanism of action. Regardless, other trials have confirmed the benefit to survival, and TXA has rapidly become standard for patients presenting with moderate or severe hemorrhagic shock.[61]

Recognition of the prognostic and therapeutic importance of the coagulation system during hemorrhage has led to experimental resuscitation strategies based around early whole-blood viscoelastic testing: thromboelastography or rotational thromboelastometry. These systems can rapidly identify specific defects in coagulation, and thus guide replacement strategies built around targeted administration of factor and platelet concentrates.[62] Several early case series have been published, and appear promising, but a large prospective randomized trial has not yet occurred.

In addition to preserving oxygen-carrying and clotting functions of blood, the anesthesiologist must carefully follow the chemical composition of the plasma. Hypocalcemia is common during massive resuscitation, due to both acidosis and "citrate intoxication," the binding of free calcium to the citrate solution used to keep banked blood from clotting.[45] While total body calcium stores are adequate to overcome this problem in the long run, any resuscitation more vigorous than 2 units of RBCs per hour runs the risk of causing hypocalcemia. Serum electrolytes should be assayed frequently during resuscitation, and calcium replaced (500–1000 mg IV over 3–5 minutes) if necessary. Hypotension unresponsive to a fluid bolus should raise the question of hypocalcemia, and empiric treatment should be given if this diagnosis is suspected.

Large quantities of 0.9% saline will produce a predictable hyperchloremic metabolic acidosis (see Chapter 8).[63] This fluid should be avoided in favor of lactated Ringer's solution or Plasmalyte-A. Hyperkalemia can occasionally result after transfusion of older RBC units, but is more commonly the result of hypoperfusion, acidosis, and failing resuscitation. Hyperkalemic cardiac dysrhythmias should be treated aggressively with insulin, dextrose, and calcium administration. Other electrolyte abnormalities are uncommon during massive resuscitation, especially if the majority of fluids used are blood products or an isotonic crystalloid.

Early treatment of hyperglycemia is an emerging standard for any patient undergoing major surgery.[64] Hyperglycemia is common after trauma, related to elevated serum catechol levels as part of the fight-or-flight response. Whereas formerly this condition was tolerated and allowed to correct itself over time, it is now recommended to treat hyperglycemia with intravenous regular insulin by intermittent "sliding-scale" dose or continuous infusion. A glucose level of 140–180 mg/dL is usually targeted. Close control of serum glucose has been associated with a reduced incidence of postoperative infections.[65]

Less clear at this time is the role of specific pro- or anti-inflammatory agents during early resuscitation. Activated protein C was shown to improve outcomes when given to patients with severe septic shock in one trial,[66] but has not had a consistently beneficial effect. Other inflammatory modulators are under study at this time. It seems sensible that pharmacotherapy directed at the inflammatory response will have its greatest impact when administered early after the inciting event. Unraveling the entire cascade of inflammation and learning how best to manipulate it will be a significant challenge, however, as the optimal inflammatory state for wound healing and recovery from trauma may vary with the patient's age, genetics, nutritional state, and the time since injury. This is an active and exciting area of trauma and critical care research at present, and it may bring significant change(s) to future clinical practice.

A final concern during resuscitation from shock is the interaction between hypotension, fluid resuscitation, and TBI (see Chapters 20 and 21). Many patients with hemorrhagic shock also have some degree of TBI, and the interaction between these conditions is known to be deadly.[67] This has led some authors to advocate higher blood pressure targets and more aggressive ventilation in patients with both shock and TBI. Exacerbation of hemorrhage and the need for a longer and more intense resuscitation would seem problematic, however, making it likely that rapid hemostasis is still the best course. At least one laboratory study of animals with both TBI and shock has confirmed the beneficial role of deliberate hypotension.[68]

Summary

With a clear understanding of the pathophysiology of shock in trauma patients, the anesthesiologist can titrate resuscitative therapy to produce the best possible clinical outcome. Rapid diagnosis of shock and treatment of hemorrhage are critical. Early fluid resuscitation should be titrated to a lower than normal blood pressure and should emphasize the preservation of normal blood composition and chemistry, using uncross-matched type O RBC and empiric plasma and platelet therapy in any patient who will require massive transfusion. For patients presenting with deep shock and evidence of physiologic decompensation an even more aggressive approach is indicated, with TXA, platelets and clotting factors given to rapidly restore an effective state of coagulation. Once the bleeding stops, laboratory markers of tissue perfusion are used to guide the completion of resuscitation. In the future, improved anesthetic and surgical techniques will lead to early survival of more severely injured patients, and enable exploration of the next frontier: direct manipulation of the systemic inflammatory response to provide recovery from severe trauma without organ system failure.

Questions

(1) Which of the following is *not* a possible site for exsanguinating blood loss in a trauma patient?
    a. Into the chest
    b. Into the abdomen
    c. Into the cranium
    d. Into the retroperitoneum
    e. Onto the "street"

(2) Which of the following is a negative effect of rapid crystalloid infusion in a hemorrhaging trauma patient?
    a. Increased cardiac output
    b. Increased hemorrhage
    c. Increased heart rate
    d. Increased hematocrit
    e. Increased urine output

(3) A 25-year-old man presents to the hospital following a motor vehicle collision. His initial blood pressure is 80/40, but it improves to 110/80 following 500 mL of intravenous fluid. Thirty minutes later, while the patient is in CT scan, his pressure falls again to 60/35. Which of the following pathologies is most likely to explain these findings?
    a. Traumatic brain injury
    b. Tension pneumothorax
    c. T12 spinal cord injury
    d. Myocardial ischemia
    e. Splenic laceration

(4) Which of the following laboratory abnormalities is most indicative of hemorrhagic shock?
    a. Hematocrit of 32%
    b. Arterial pH of 7.50
    c. Serum potassium of 2.5 mg/dL
    d. Serum glucose of 155 mg/dL
    e. Serum lactate of 10 mg/dL

(5) Which of the following best describes the patient with occult hypoperfusion syndrome in the ICU?

a. Normal vital signs, normal serum lactate
b. Normal vital signs, elevated serum lactate
c. Hypotension, normal serum lactate
d. Hypotension, elevated serum lactate
e. Hypotension, hypocapnia

(6) Which of the following best describes the sequence of vasoconstriction in a hemorrhaging patient?
a. Skin, then muscle, then gut
b. Muscle, then gut, then skin
c. Muscle, then skin, then gut
d. Gut, then skin, then muscle
e. Skin, then gut, then muscle

(7) Which of the following is the most appropriate initial fluid to administer to the hypotensive patient who presents with active hemorrhage and pH < 7.25?
a. Isotonic crystalloid
b. Uncrossmatched red blood cells
c. Plasma
d. Platelets
e. Hypertonic saline

(8) Which of the following electrolyte abnormalities is most common during massive transfusion therapy?
a. Hypocalcemia
b. Hypoglycemia
c. Hypernatremia
d. Hypokalemia
e. Hypermagnesemia

(9) Preservation of coagulation function in the actively hemorrhaging patient is best achieved with administration of which of the following?
a. Fresh whole blood

b. Equal numbers of units of RBC, plasma, and platelets
c. One liter of isotonic crystalloid for each unit of RBC
d. Three units of plasma for each unit of RBC
e. Hypertonic saline and platelets

(10) Factor VIIa as an off-label "rescue" therapy is most appropriate in which of the following clinical situations?
a. Urgent repair of an open femur fracture in a hemodynamically stable patient
b. Following emergent splenectomy in a patient who has not yet required transfusion
c. During exploratory laparotomy in a patient undergoing massive transfusion
d. For control of coagulopathic hemorrhage in a patient who has suffered a transcranial gunshot wound
e. Following return of spontaneous circulation in a patient who required cardiopulmonary resuscitation for a tension pneumothorax

Answers

(1) c
(2) b
(3) e
(4) e
(5) b
(6) a
(7) b
(8) a
(9) a
(10) c

References

1. Dutton RP, Stansbury LG, Leone S, et al. Trauma mortality in mature trauma systems: are we doing better? An analysis of trauma mortality patterns, 1997–2008. *J Trauma* 2010; **69**: 620–6.

2. Dutton RP. Management of traumatic shock. In Prough DS, Fleisher L, eds., *Problems in Anesthesia: Trauma Care.* London: Lippincott, Williams & Wilkins, 2002, Vol. **13** (3).

3. Peitzman AB. Hypovolemic shock. In Pinsky MR, Dhainaut JFA, eds., *Pathophysiologic Foundations of Critical Care.* Baltimore, MD: Lippincott, Williams & Wilkins, 1993, pp. 161–9.

4. Shires GT, Cunningham N, Baker CRF, et al. Alterations in cellular membrane function during hemorrhagic shock in primates. *Ann Surg* 1972; **176**: 288–95.

5. Peitzman AB, Billiar TR, Harbrecht BG, et al. Hemorrhagic shock. *Curr Probl Surg* 1995; **32**: 929–1002.

6. Honig LS, Rosenberg RN. Apoptosis and neurologic disease. *Am J Med* 2000; **108**: 317–30.

7. Hara MR, Snyder SH. Cell signaling and neuronal death. *Annu Rev PharmacolToxicol.* 2007; **47**: 117–41.

8. Collins JA, The pathophysiology of hemorrhagic shock. *Prog Clin Biol Res* 1982; **108**: 5–29.

9. Khalil AA, Aziz FA, Hall JC. Reperfusion injury. *Plast Reconstr Surg* 2006; **117**: 1024–33.

10. Runciman WB, Sjowronski GA. Pathophysiology of haemorrhagic shock. *Anaesth Intensive Care* 1984; **12**: 193–205.

11. Ba ZF, Wang P, Koo DJ, et al. Alterations in tissue oxygen consumption and extraction after trauma and hemorrhagic shock. *Crit Care Med* 2000; **28**: 2837–42.

12. Dark PM, Delooz HH, Hillier V, Hanson J, Little RA. Monitoring the circulatory responses of shocked patients during fluid resuscitation in the emergency department. *Intensive Care Med* 2000; **26**: 173–9.

13. Gann DS, Amaran JF. Endocrine and metabolic responses to injury. In Schwartz SI, Shires GT, Spencer FC, eds., *Principles of Surgery.* New York, NY: McGraw-Hill, 1989.

14. Thorne J, Blomquist S, Elmer O. Polymorphonuclear leukocyte sequestration in the lung and liver following soft tissue trauma: an in vivo study. *J Trauma* 1989; **29**: 451–6.

15. Fulton RL, Raynor AVS, Jones C. Analysis of factors leading to posttraumatic pulmonary insufficiency. *Ann ThoracSurg* 1978; **25**: 500–9.

16. Demling R, Lalonde C, Saldinger P, Knox J. Multiple organ dysfunction in the surgical patient: pathophysiology, prevention, and treatment. *Curr Probl Surg* 1993; **30**: 345–424.

17. Reilly PM, Bulkley GB. Vasoactive mediators and splanchnic perfusion. *Crit Care Med* 1993; **21**: S55–68.

18. Kutayli ZN, Domingo CB, Steinberg SM. Intestinal failure. *Curr Opin Anaesthesiol* 2005; **18**: 123–7.

19. Maitra SR, Geller ER, Pan W, Kennedy PR, Higgins LD. Altered cellular calcium regulation and hepatic glucose production during hemorrhagic shock. *Circ Shock* 1992; **38**: 14–21.

20. Marcu AC, Kielar ND, Paccione KE, *et al.* Androstenetriol improves survival in a rodent model of traumatic shock. *Resuscitation* 2006; **71**: 379–86.

21. Chun K, Zhang J, Biewer J, Ferguson D, Clemens MG. Microcirculatory failure determines lethal hepatocyte injury in ischemic-reperfused rat livers. *Shock* 1994; **1**: 3–9.

22. Redan JA, Rush BF, McCullogh JN, *et al.* Organ distribution of radiolabeled enteric *Escherichia coli* during and after hemorrhagic shock. *Ann Surg* 1990; **211**: 663–8.

23. Mullins RJ. Management of shock. In Mattox KL, Feliciano DV, Moore EE, eds., *Trauma*, 4th edition. New York, NY: McGraw-Hill, 2000.

24. Pedowitz RA, Gershuni DH, Schmidt AH, *et al.* Muscle injury induced beneath and distal to a pneumatic tourniquet: A quantitative animal study of effects of tourniquet pressure and duration. *J Hand Surg [Am]* 1991; **16**: 610–21.

25. Dutton RP. Pathophysiology of traumatic shock. *Semin Anesth Perioperative Med Pain* 2001; **20**: 7–10.

26. Moore EE. Staged laparotomy for the hypothermia, acidosis, coagulopathy syndrome. *Am J Surg* 1996; **72**: 405.

27. Ni Choileain N, Redmond HP. The immunological consequences of injury. *Surgeon* 2006; **4**: 23–31.

28. Hildebrand F, Pape HC, van Griensven M, *et al.* Genetic predisposition for a compromised immune system after multiple trauma. *Shock* 2005; **24**: 518–22.

29. Committee on Trauma, American College of Surgeons. *Advanced Trauma Life Support Program for Doctors.* Chicago, IL: ACS, 2008.

30. Davis JW, Davis IC, Bennink LD, *et al.* Automated blood pressure measurements accurate in trauma patients? *J Trauma* 2003; **55**: 860–3.

31. Demetriades D, Chan LS, Bhasin P. Relative bradycardia in patients with traumatic hypotension. *J Trauma* 1998; **45**: 534–9.

32. Abramson D, Scalea TM, Hitchcock, *et al.* Lactate clearance and survival following injury. *J Trauma* 1993; **35**: 584–8.

33. Blow O, Magliore L, Claridge JA, *et al.* The golden hour and the silver day: Detection and correction of occult hypoperfusion within 24 hours improves outcome from major trauma. *J Trauma* 1999; **47**: 964–9.

34. Scalea TM, Hartnett RW, Duncan AO, *et al.* Central venous oxygen saturation: A useful clinical tool in trauma patients. *J Trauma* 1990; **30**: 1539–43.

35. McKinley BA, Butler BD. Comparison of skeletal muscle PO_2, PCO_2, and pH with gastric tonometric $P(CO_2)$ and pH in hemorrhagic shock. *Crit Care Med* 1999; **27**: 1869–77.

36. Weil MH, Nadagawa Y, Tang W, *et al.* Sublingual capnometry: a new noninvasive measurement for diagnosis and quantification of severity of circulatory shock. *Crit Care Med* 1999; **27**: 1225–9.

37. Puyana JC, Soller BR, Zhang SB, Heard SO. Continuous measurement of gut pH with near-infrared spectroscopy during hemorrhagic shock. *J Trauma* 1999; **46**: 9–14.

38. Raghunathan K, Bloomstone JA, McGee WT. Cardiac output measured with both esophageal Doppler device and Vigileo-FloTrac device. *AnesthAnalg.* 2012; **114**: 1141–2

39. Ambrisko TD, Coppens P, Kabes R, Moens Y. Lithium dilution, pulse power analysis, and continuous thermodilutioncardiac output measurements compared with bolus thermodilution in anaesthetized ponies. *Br J Anaesth.* 2012; **109**: 864–9.

40. Young A, Marik PE, Sibole S, Grooms D, Levitov A. Changes in end-tidal carbon dioxide and volumetric carbon dioxide as predictors of volume responsiveness in hemodynamically unstable patients. *J Cardiothorac Vasc Anesth* 2012; **27**: 681–4.

41. Le Manach Y, Hofer CK, Lehot JJ, *et al.* Can changes in arterial pressure be used to detect changes in cardiac output during volume expansion in the perioperative period? *Anesthesiology* 2012; **117**: 1165–74.

42. Albin MS, White RJ. Epidemiology, physiopathology and experimental therapeutics of acute spinal injury. *Crit Care Clin* 1987; **3**: 441–52.

43. Scalea TM, Henry SM; Assessment and initial management in the trauma patient. *ProblAnesth* 2001; **13**: 271–8.

44. Rozycki GS. Abdominal ultrasonography in trauma. *Surg Clin N Am* 1995; **75**: 175–91.

45. Dutton RP, McCunn M. Anesthesia for trauma. In Miller RD, ed., *Miller's Anesthesia*, 6th edition. Philadelphia, PA: Elsevier, 2005, pp. 2451–95.

46. Shaftan GW, Chiu C, Dennis C, Harris B. Fundamentals of physiologic control of arterial hemorrhage. *Surgery* 1965; **58**: 851–6.

47. Stern A, Dronen SC, Birrer P, Wang X. Effect of blood pressure on haemorrhagic volume in a near-fatal haemorrhage model incorporating a vascular injury. *Ann Emerg Med* 1993; **22**: 155–63.

48. Shoemaker WC, Peitzman AB, Bellamy R, *et al.* Resuscitation from severe hemorrhage. *Crit Care Med* 1996; **24**: S12–23.

49. Bickell WH, Wall MJ, Pepe PE, *et al.* Immediate versus delayed fluid resuscitation for hypotensive patients with penetrating torso injuries. *N Engl J Med* 1994; **331**: 1105–9.

50. Dutton RP, Mackenzie CF, Scalea TM. Hypotensive resuscitation during active hemorrhage: Impact on in-hospital mortality. *J Trauma* 2002; **52**: 1141–6.

51. Dutton RP, Shih D, Edelman BB, Hess JR, Scalea TM. Safety of uncrossmatched Type-O red cells for resuscitation from hemorrhagic shock. *J Trauma* 2005; **59**: 1445–9.

52. Fries D, Innerhofer P, Schobersberger W. Coagulation management in trauma patients. *Curr Opin Anaesthesiol* 2002; **15**: 217–23.

53. Armand R, Hess JR. Treating coagulopathy in trauma patients. *Transfus Med Rev* 2003; **17**: 223–31.

54. Kauvar DS, Holcomb JB, Norris GC, Hess JR. Fresh whole blood transfusion: A controversial military practice. *J Trauma* 2006; **61**: 181–4.

55. Stein DM, Dutton RP. Uses of recombinant factor VIIa in trauma. *Curr Opin Crit Care* 2004; **10**: 520–8.

56. McGee DC, Gould MK. Preventing complications of central venous catheterization. *N Engl J Med* 2003; **348**: 1123–33.

57. Dutton RP. Hypothermia and hemorrhage. In Speiss B, Shander A, eds., *Perioperative Transfusion Medicine*. Philadelphia: Lippincott, Williams & Wilkins, 2006, pp. 481–6.

58. Moeng MS, Loveland JA, Boffard KD. Damage control: beyond the limits of the abdominal cavity. A review. *TraumaCare* 2005; **15**: 197–201.

59. McCunn M. Mechanical ventilation: weapon of mass destruction or tool for liberation? *Crit Care Med* 2003; **31**: 974–6.

60. CRASH-2 trial collaborators. Effects of tranexamic acid on death, vascular occlusive events, and blood transfusion in trauma patients with significant haemorrhage (CRASH-2): a randomised, placebo-controlled trial. *Lancet* 2010; **376**: 23–32.

61. Perel P, Ker K, Morales Uribe CH, Roberts I. Tranexamic acid for reducing mortality in emergency and urgent surgery. *Cochrane Database Syst Rev* 2013; (1): CD010245.

62. Schöchl H, Cotton B, Inaba K, *et al.* FIBTEM provides early prediction of massive transfusion in trauma. *Crit Care* 2011; **15**: R265.

63. DuBose TD. Hyperkalemic hyperchloremic metabolic acidosis: Pathophysiologic insights. *Kidney Int* 1997; **51**: 591–602.

64. Laird AM, Miller PR, Kilgo PD, Meredith JW, Chang MC. Relationship of early hyperglycemia to mortality in trauma patients. *J Trauma* 2004; **56**: 1058–62.

65. Sung J, Bochicchio GV, Joshi M, *et al.* Admission hyperglycemia is predictive of outcome in critically ill trauma patients. *J Trauma* 2005; **59**: 80–3.

66. Ely EW, Bernard GR, Vincent JL. Activated protein C for severe sepsis. *N Engl J Med* 2002; **347**: 1035–6.

67. Chestnut RM, Marshall LF, Klauber MR, *et al.* The role of secondary brain injury in determining outcome from severe head injury. *J Trauma* 1993; **134**: 216–22.

68. Novak L, Shackford SR, Bourguignon P, *et al.* Comparison of standard and alternative prehospital resuscitation in uncontrolled hemorrhagic shock and head injury. *J Trauma* 1999; **47**: 834–44.

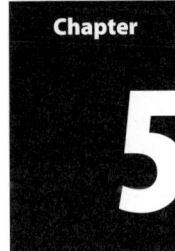

Establishing vascular access in the trauma patient

Matthew A. Joy, Donn Marciniak, and Kasia Petelenz Rubin

Objectives

(1) Describe in a structured approach the advantages and disadvantages of various types of intravascular access and infusion devices in the trauma patient.

(2) Present practical guidelines for the establishment of central venous access in the critically injured patient.

(3) Describe in detail the technique for insertion of various central access sites, with current standard of care recommendations in the trauma patient.

(4) Review peripheral arterial cannulation in the trauma setting.

(5) Discuss current recommendations regarding intraosseous access in the trauma patient.

Foreword

Since publication of the last edition of this textbook, the most recent change in establishing vascular access in the trauma patient has been the increased role and importance of ultrasound guidance. It is the authors' recommendation that real-time ultrasound be used for all elective internal jugular cannulations. However, real-time ultrasound guidance should also be used routinely for establishing internal jugular vein access in emergency situations, such as in trauma patients. In addition, ultrasound guidance can be instrumental in obtaining successful access for the femoral vein, for difficult peripheral vein cannulations, and for arterial line access. Indeed, several recommendations and guidelines have been released by professional societies since the last publication of this textbook, advocating the use of ultrasound for vascular access.[1-5] This chapter incorporates the use of ultrasound, but also provides the reader with a comprehensive landmark and surface-anatomy approach, which will aid in the success and appropriate integration of ultrasound guidance. The reader is also encouraged to review Chapter 12 on ultrasound-guided procedures for a more extensive discussion on this topic.

Introduction

Advanced Trauma Life Support (ATLS) guidelines recommend that in the initial management of hemorrhagic shock, prompt access must be obtained.[6] This is best accomplished by the insertion of two large-caliber (16 gauge angiocatheters or larger) peripheral intravenous catheters before consideration is given to central venous catheters or venous cutdowns.[6] Obviously the condition of the arriving trauma patient – e.g., massive extremity injury and extensive injury – may not allow for any reasonable peripheral venous access for IV insertion. This chapter reviews the management of intravascular access in the trauma patient in the hospital setting where definitive care is to be provided. The main areas to be covered include venous access, as well as arterial access, in critically injured patients. Clinical experience and evidence-based medicine is balanced to provide a framework for guiding the management of patients from a vascular access standpoint.

Peripheral intravenous catheters

Prior to arrival in the emergency department, peripheral intravenous (PIV) cannulation has usually been performed in the field by prehospital personnel.[6,7] Upon arrival, the in-situ access should be inspected for catheter size, flow dynamics, and insertion-site characteristics. Additional IV access may be required in the event that any of the prehospital IVs have poor flow quality, intermittent flow, or any apparent infiltration with extravasation.[7] Should the preexisting access be deemed inadequate, additional large-bore access should be placed. Ideally, either a 14 or 16 gauge angiocatheter may be inserted into any available upper extremity vein, preferably the antecubital or large forearm vein, if not previously cannulated.[6] According to the Hagen–Poiseuille law, the flow through a tube is directly proportional to the fourth power of the radius and inversely related to its length:

$$Q = \Delta P(\pi r^4 / 8 \eta L)$$

where Q = flow, P = pressure, r = radius of the catheter, η = viscosity, L = length of the catheter.

Trauma Anesthesia, 2nd Edition, ed. Charles E. Smith. Published by Cambridge University Press. © Charles E. Smith, 2015.

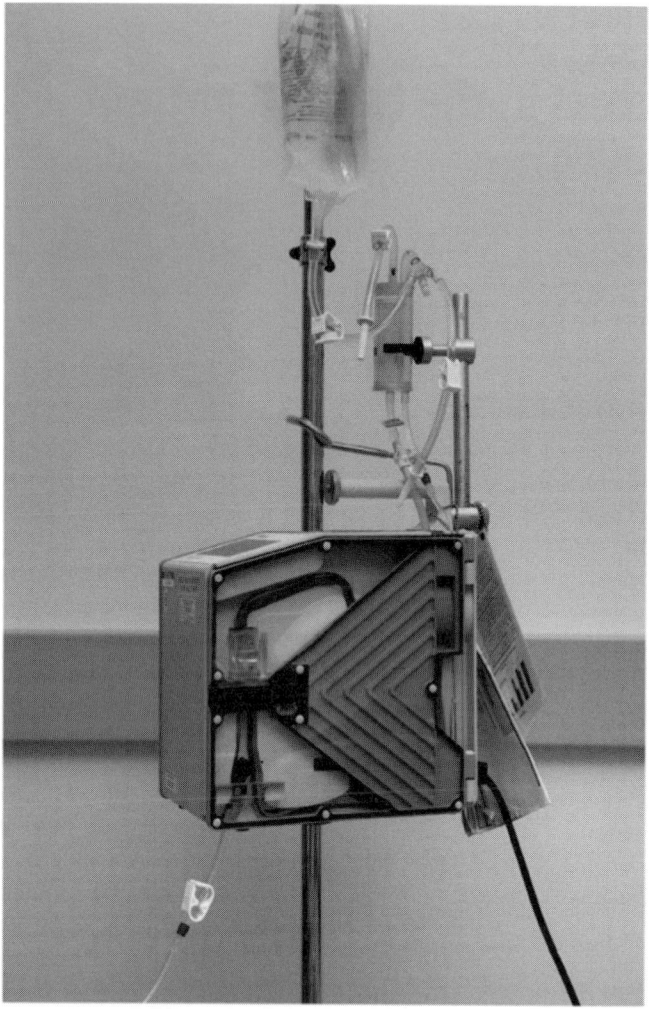

Figure 5.1 Belmont Instruments FMS 2000 rapid infusion device. Belmont Instrument Corp., Billerica, MA.

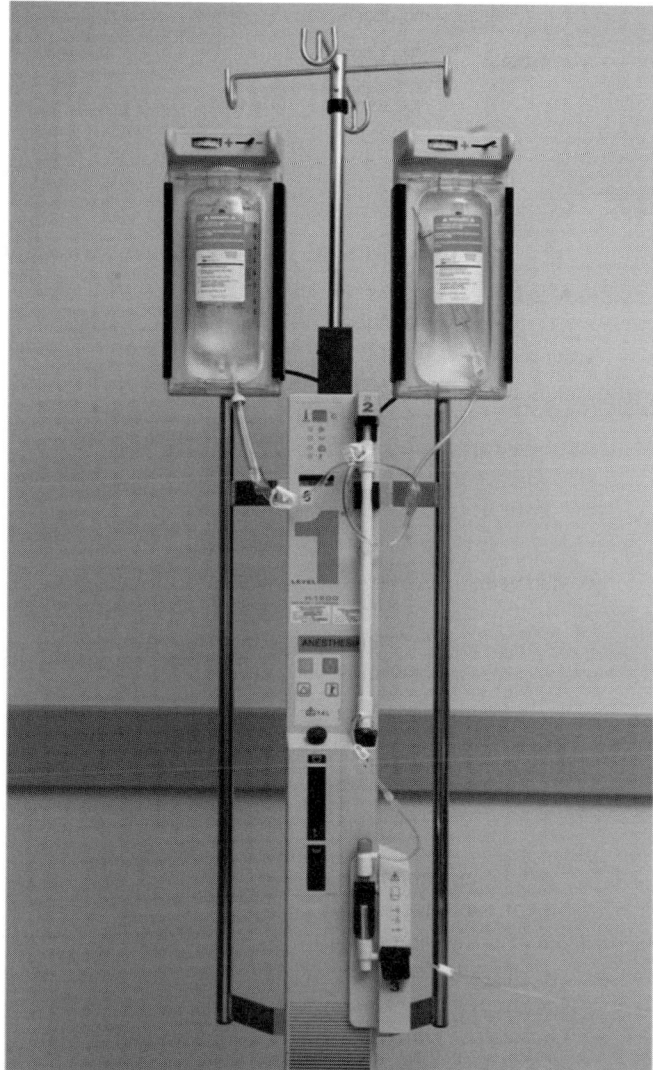

Figure 5.2 Level I rapid infusion device (H1025). SIMS Level 1, Inc., Rockland, MA.

Therefore, the primary variable for flow rate is the radius of the catheter. Equally important is the caliber of the IV fluid tubing sets. These should have large diameters at all points, including connectors and injection sites, to reduce turbulent flow. Once successfully cannulated, peripheral IV catheters should be connected to high-capacity fluid warmers or rapid infusion devices, depending on the patient's response to fluid therapy.[6,8–10] (Figs. 5.1, 5.2)

Repeated unsuccessful efforts at peripheral IV access should not be continued without considering the use of ultrasonography guidance[11–14] or concurrent attempts at central access. The initial site of choice for central venous access depends on the extent and location of injury.[8]

Central venous catheters

The use of central access in the trauma patient not only provides larger and more reliable vessels for administration of large volumes of fluid administration, but it also provides for the administration of medications that may not be suitable

for infusion via peripheral sites.[6] Additionally, central venous access allows for the monitoring of central venous pressures (see Chapter 9). Although conflicting reports exist regarding the safety of central venous access in trauma patients and the incidence of complications,[15,16] other evidence suggests that complication rates are no higher than in nonemergent settings.[16,17] This may be due in part to physicians with more experience placing the majority of central lines in trauma patients.

Femoral vein cannulation

First described by Duffy in 1949,[18] the common femoral vein, as a site for cannulation into the inferior vena cava, is probably the easiest and most accessible vessel for rapid central venous access in the trauma patient. There is no potential for pneumothorax, hemothorax, or arrhythmias (potentially preexisting conditions in a severely injured trauma patient). The vein is

Table 5.1 Advantages and disadvantages of central venous access sites

Mode of access	Advantages	Disadvantages	Contraindications
All	Access when peripheral veins unsuitable Larger fluid volumes may be delivered Monitoring of central venous pressure	Hematoma Infection Line misplacement Air embolism Arterial puncture Thrombosis of catheter	Coagulopathy Local infection or tumor at access site
Femoral vein	Accessible during CPR and airway management Compressible	Increased rate of thrombosis Femoral arterial injury	Extensive lower extremity injury – burns or trauma Abdominal trauma (possible IVC disruption)
Internal jugular vein	Provider familiarity PA catheter conversion	Pneumothorax Hemothorax Ventricular arrhythmia Myocardial injury Cardiac tamponade Carotid artery injury	Cervical spine injury Presence of cervical collar
Subclavian vein	Provider familiarity PA catheter conversion Remains patent in shock Stable catheter fixation Accessible during neck immobilization	Pneumothorax Hemothorax Ventricular arrhythmia Myocardial injury Cardiac tamponade Subclavian artery injury	Clavicular injury Kyphoscoliosis

CPR, cardiopulmonary resuscitation; IVC, inferior vena cava; PA, pulmonary artery.

easily accessible in patients with neck immobilization, and incidental hematoma formation is relatively easy to compress (Table 5.1). Femoral venous access can also be easily accomplished in patients receiving cardiopulmonary resuscitation.[17,19–22] The femoral vein may be unsuitable, however, in the trauma patient with extensive lower extremity injury, as well as in the patient with significant abdominal trauma injury, where inferior vena cava flow may be disrupted.[23,24]

Techniques for insertion first involve appropriate use of hand hygiene and cleansing the site with a sterile antiseptic solution, preferably chlorhexidine solution.[25–28] If necessary, topicalization is provided with subcutaneous administration of 1% lidocaine. The urgent need for intravascular access may supersede full Centers for Disease Control and Prevention (CDC) recommendations [6,25,26] and other guidelines for central line insertion [23,24] such as sterile scrub, gown, and full body drape. However, antiseptic solution, along with sterile gloves, mask, and cap can very quickly be obtained and used without adding any unnecessary time delays in achieving IV access. Once prepped and cleaned, the best approach to access the femoral vein is with the operator on the ipsilateral side facing the patient from below.[26,29]

Despite several reports documenting the safety of the femoral vein for central access, many clinicians still are hesitant to use this site, based upon a perceived increased risk of complications.[19,21,22,24] Although recent experience demonstrates relative safety with the femoral vein route for line access,[17,19] there are limited data establishing this as the preferred site for short-term access in the severely injured patient.[17,30]

In what is referred to as the femoral triangle (Fig. 5.3), the femoral vein lies medial to the femoral artery and lateral to the femoral canal in the middle compartment. Ultrasound to guide the procedure is recommended (see below, and Chapter 12).

A 20 gauge hypodermic needle attached to a 5 mL syringe is used as a "finder" or "scout" needle to locate the vein.[29] With the operator facing the patient from the ipsilateral side, and with the patient's leg in a slightly abducted and externally rotated position,[29,30] the needle is inserted 1 cm medial to the pulsating femoral artery, just below the inguinal ligament. Directing the needle cephalad, the femoral vein is typically entered approximately 2–4 cm below the skin. Utilizing negative pressure, blood is aspirated once the vein is entered (initially verified by color and lack of arterial pulsation). An 18 gauge angiocatheter is then placed immediately parallel to the needle and aspiration of the vein is once again obtained. The catheter is then advanced over the stylet until the catheter has completely entered the vessel.[29,31] With the hub transfixed at the skin level, the vessel can be transduced with sterile pressure extension tubing attached to the angiocatheter to verify venous flow. This step of mechanical transduction of the vein,[32,33] although rudimentary, can be completed in relatively little time, which is useful given the urgent nature of trauma line placement.

Once confirmed as a venous vessel, a trauma central line is placed. In our institution, the preferred central line is a 12 Fr

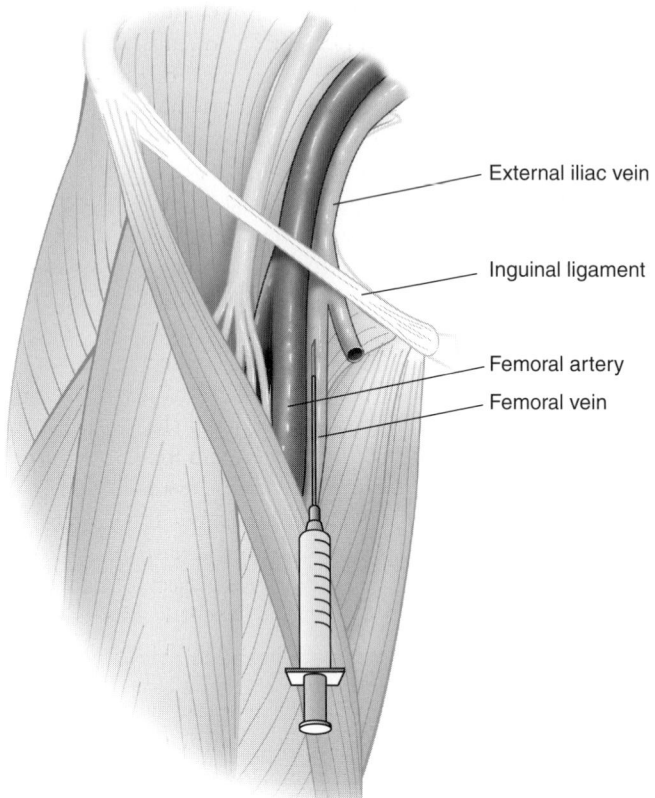

Figure 5.3 The femoral triangle, and **steps for insertion of femoral vein central catheters** (see text for additional detail on cannulation):
- The patient is prepped and draped in the usual fashion. Aseptic conditions are maintained throughout.
- The operator faces the patient from the ipsilateral side.
- The patient's legs are placed in a slightly abducted and externally rotated position.
- The needle is inserted 1 cm medial to the pulsating femoral artery and approximately 1 cm below the inguinal ligament.
- Directing the needle cephalad, the femoral vein is typically entered approximately 2–4 cm below the skin.
- Utilizing negative pressure, blood is aspirated once the vein is entered.

triple-lumen catheter (Arrow International, Figs. 5.4, 5.5). Utilizing the Seldinger technique[34] of guidewire placement, a thin flexible J-shaped wire is placed via the angiocatheter and advanced until at least half to two-thirds of the wire is entered into the vessel. Caution should be exercised with the advancement of the guidewire, and if any resistance is encountered the wire should be immediately removed and flow from the angiocatheter should be reconfirmed. Once the wire has been advanced to approximately half its length, the angiocatheter is removed and a dilator device is advanced over the wire.[30,31]

Care must be taken to avoid loss of the wire by embolization into the vessel. This can be prevented by allowing an adequate length of the wire to extend beyond skin, taking care not to remove the wire entirely from the intravascular lumen. In addition, when advancing any catheter over a wire, one end of the wire should always be visible, preferably within one's grasp. Once enough distance of catheter has been removed the

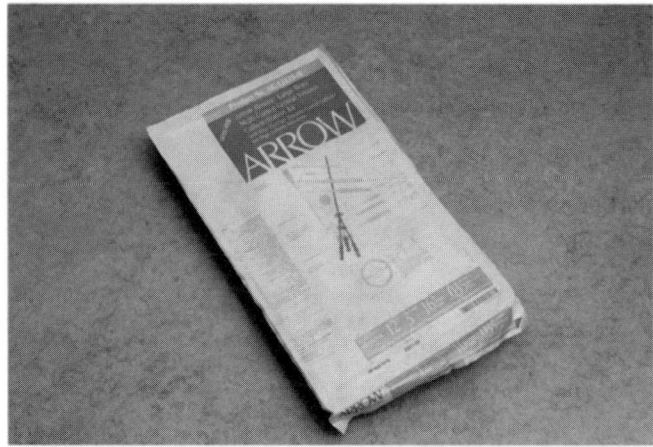

Figure 5.4 Arrow-Howes 12 Fr TLC (product AK-12123-H, Arrow International, Reading, PA).

dilator is advanced over the wire. Once again, the dilator should enter the vessel easily without resistance. Any hindrance to advancement should be immediately investigated. The skin incision around the wire may need to be enlarged, or the guidewire may be kinked. The dilator should never be inserted any further than necessary to achieve the maximum diameter, typically no further than the midpoint or beginning of the dilator taper. Any further advancement carries the potential risk of vessel injury from the rigid dilator.[35–37]

Once dilated, the catheter is placed over the wire utilizing the Seldinger technique. The wire is then removed and the catheter is sewn in place. Verification of placement is achieved once again by mechanical or pressure transduction,[33] and ease of flow of infusion fluids by gravity. The femoral vein site obviates the need for radiographic confirmation.

If at all possible, and if readily available, it is recommended to utilize real-time (dynamic) ultrasound guidance in the performance of femoral vein cannulation.[3–5] At the very least a static evaluation of the femoral vein course and its associated structures should be performed as a minimum prior to prepping the femoral vein for cannulation. For optimal success, it is the authors' recommendation to place the ultrasound machine on the contralateral side of the vein to be cannulated so as to obtain a direct alignment of view between the operator, the femoral vein, and the ultrasound machine screen. Again, strict adherence to aseptic conditions is recommended, and whenever possible a sterile probe cover should be utilized when placing the probe in the field.

Internal jugular vein cannulation

Many trauma patients present with limited accessibility to the neck due to cervical spine precautions with cervical collars. In general, it is not advisable to remove the collar for internal jugular venous access. However, if the patient's cervical spine has been cleared, such access may be attempted.

Utilizing the previously mentioned sterile technique and after placing the patient in a slight Trendelenburg position, the

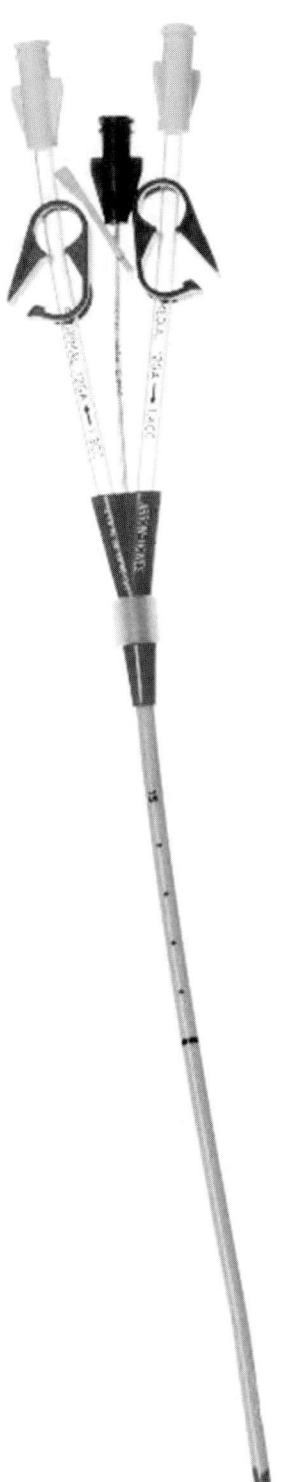

Figure 5.5 Arrow-Howes Large-Bore Multi-Lumen Central Venous Catheterization Kit with Blue FlexTip catheter for high-volume infusions (product AK-12123-F, Arrow International, Reading, PA, with permission).

thus potentially increasing the risk of pneumothorax on left-sided approaches. Ultrasound is valuable to guide the cannulation procedure (see Chapter 12). In the case of massive chest injury the site chosen should avoid the side of the unaffected lung, thereby avoiding the risk of contralateral lung injury. The central approach,[29,38] which is favored by the authors, is performed by identifying the clavicular and sternal heads of the sternocleidomastoid muscle at the base of the neck. These two heads join superiorly to form an apex of a triangle, at which point the needle is inserted. Depending on the circumstances and urgency of establishing access, a seeker needle may or may not be utilized. Either a 22 gauge × 3.8 cm seeker needle or 18 gauge × 6.35 cm angiocatheter is directed lateral to the pulsating carotid, which is best palpated and slightly retracted with the opposite hand, usually the left hand for right internal jugular cannulation. The needle is directed toward the ipsilateral nipple, at a 45 degree angle. The vein lies anterolateral to the carotid artery, and typically is entered at a depth of 1.3 cm (no greater than 3 cm) below the skin surface. Utilizing the Seldinger technique of guidewire placement as described in the femoral vein section, the trauma central line is placed into the internal jugular vein (Fig. 5.6).

Complication rates vary for the anatomic landmark technique of internal jugular vein catheter insertion, depending on the setting and classification of complications (i.e., mechanical vs. infectious vs. thrombotic). Complications have been reported to occur in the internal jugular route at a frequency of 6.3–11.8% in the general population,[28] and although there are limited data available regarding this approach in the emergency care setting, one study reports a rate of complications as low as 5.2%.[39] The most common major complications for the internal jugular route are pneumothorax, hemothorax, line misplacement, and hematoma formation (Table 5.1).[28,39,40] Other less common but serious complications include sustained ventricular arrhythmias, air embolism, and cardiac tamponade.[40] Rare but lethal complications occurring with this technique reported in the literature include vertebral artery and innominate pseudoaneurysms.[41,42] Preventive measures, including aseptic technique, verification of venous flow, use of ultrasound, and meticulous guidewire/dilator technique, serve to minimize the occurrence of potential complications. A postprocedural chest radiograph should be obtained after all internal jugular vein catheterizations if time permits.

Again it is highly recommended that ultrasound guidance be utilized in either a static or (preferably) a dynamic (real-time) fashion for cannulation of the internal jugular vein.[3,43–45] It is imperative, however, that the reader, especially the novice operator, appreciate that ultrasound guidance should not be used as a substitute for a thorough understanding of surface anatomy, landmarks, and structural relationships of the target vessel. If time allows, an initial surveillance of the vessel to be cannulated with an ultrasound probe permits identification of suitability for access. This "static" interrogation with the ultrasound probe is easily performed before prepping of the site and allows for proper identification of

internal jugular vein approach is preferred on the right side of the neck, because of the straighter course this vessel runs to the heart and for the avoidance of possible injury to the thoracic duct, which most typically is on the left side. Furthermore, the cupola of the left lung rises higher than that of the right lung,

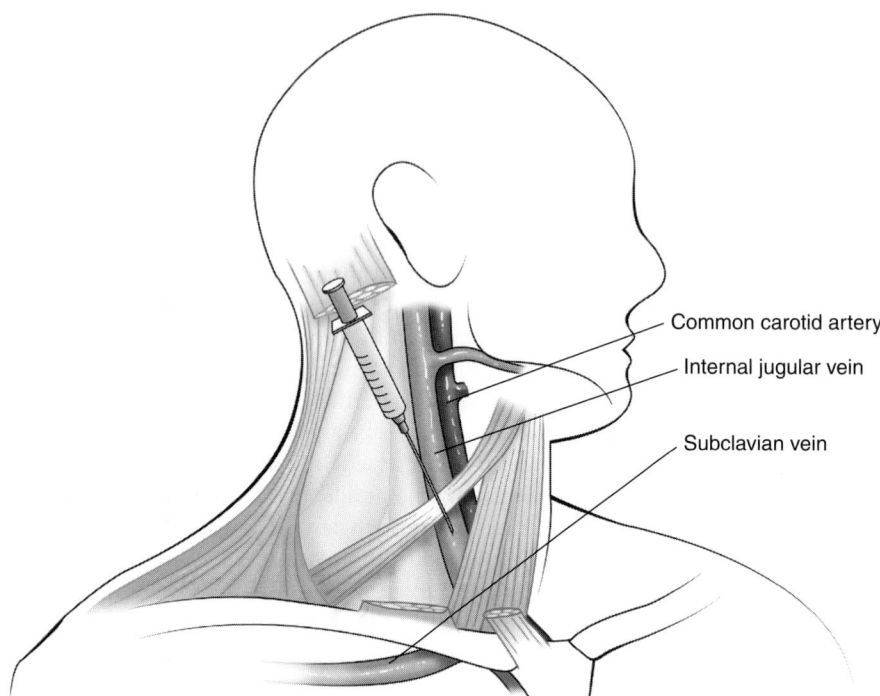

Figure 5.6 Internal jugular vein anatomy, and steps for insertion of internal jugular vein catheters, central approach (see text for additional detail on cannulation):

- The patient is prepped and draped in the usual fashion. Aseptic conditions are maintained throughout.
- The patient is placed in the Trendelenburg position.
- The needle is inserted lateral to the carotid artery, at the apex of the triangle formed by the two heads of the sternocleidomastoid muscle and the clavicle.
- At an angle of approximately 20 degrees to the skin surface, the internal jugular vein is typically entered at approximately 1.3 cm below the skin.

Common carotid artery

Internal jugular vein

Subclavian vein

possible anatomic variants, vessel disease states (e.g., thrombosed, atretic, or scarred vessels), enabling an alternative vessel to be chosen prior to prepping the site.[3–5,43] For vascular access in superficial percutaneoous procedures, such as internal jugular vein cannulation, a high-frequency linear-array 5–7 MHz transducer is usually an appropriate choice. It is the authors' practice to utilize the transverse view initially so as to visualize the adjacent structures, and once the vein is successfully cannulated a longitudinal view should be used to confirm either needle or guidewire position. As with femoral vein cannulation, proper orientation of the ultrasound machine is crucial for success in cannulation, and it is the authors' preference that the ultrasound machine be placed in an ergonomically favorable position so as to maintain a direct line of sight with the proceduralist, the vessel being cannulated, and the image screen (for instance, the ultrasound machine should be on the ipsilateral side of the internal jugular vein being cannulated). Again, for a more extensive review of ultrasound guidance for vascular cannulation, the reader should refer to Chapter 12.

Subclavian vein cannulation

Subclavian vein catheterization was first described by Aubaniac in 1952.[46] The procedure gained popularity as the practical use and high success rate of the procedure were substantiated.

Proponents of the subclavian technique in the trauma setting note that the anatomic properties of the vein lend themselves to expedient catheterization. There is a constant anatomic position, allowing for easy access; a low or negative intravascular pressure; a large diameter of 12 – 25 mm;[47] and

absence of valves. The walls are reinforced with a thick tunica fibrosa and adhere to the adjacent ligaments, fascia, and periosteum. The vein does not constrict, collapse, or displace. It remains patent in shock and death, allowing for central access even in situations of severe hypovolemia.[48] Other indications for placement of a subclavian catheter include: extremity burns or trauma; inaccessibility of the internal jugular vein (i.e., presence of cervical collar); and lack of adequate peripheral veins, as in drug abusers.[16] In abdominal or flank injuries, the subclavian vein is the recommended route of central venous access.[17]

Benefits of subclavian catheters exist in the posttrauma setting as well (Table 5.1). Indwelling subclavian catheters can be converted easily to pulmonary artery catheters. There is a decreased risk of catheter-related infections[24,49,50] compared with the internal jugular or femoral approaches in the emergency or high-risk setting.[51] Catheter fixation is more stable and more comfortable over the upper chest,[52] increasing patient satisfaction.

There is some opposition to the use of subclavian vein catheterization in trauma, which is derived from the concern regarding the potential for life-threatening complications in an already injured patient. The most common complications in both the elective and emergent settings include pneumothorax and hemothorax, with reported rates of 2–5%[53] and 0.4–5%,[16] respectively. In trauma, however, the complication rate increases significantly, with rates of serious complication attributable to the procedure of 14–15%.[15,54] Additional complications include: subclavian artery puncture; local hematoma formation; hydrothorax; hydromediastinum; myocardial penetration or perforation; thoracic duct laceration (left side);

venous stenosis; catheter-related thrombosis; damage to the phrenic nerve, recurrent laryngeal nerves, or brachial plexus; and local or systemic infection.

Relative contraindications specific to the placement of a subclavian catheter include kyphoscoliosis, clavicular deformity, and low toleration for pneumothorax (Table 5.1). Literature lore has suggested that mechanical ventilation is a contraindication to such line placement,[53] as the cupola of the lung may protrude into the neck and elevate the subclavian vein above its normal position, but clinicians may circumvent this by using lower tidal volumes. Coagulopathy is also considered a relative contraindication to the placement of any central line, and the subclavian vein is generally thought to be the least suitable approach in these patients. Hemorrhage from an inadvertent subclavian artery puncture is much more difficult to control by pressure alone, and may be missed, as the blood can track into the pleural cavity.[55]

Independent of patient characteristics, complication rates also increase in parallel with the level of operator experience.[12,56,57] Selection of the insertion site for a central venous catheter must therefore be based on both the ease of placement and the risks, taking into account both the individual patient and the practitioner performing the procedure.

An understanding of the relationship of the subclavian vein to the clavicle is necessary for successful subclavian vein cannulation, because, in this essentially blind procedure, the subclavian vein cannot be visualized or palpated. The subclavian vein enters the thorax as a continuation of the axillary vein of the arm, posterior to the clavicle. It passes over the first rib anterior to the scalene tubercle parallel to the subclavian artery, but is separated by the anterior scalene muscle. The subclavian vein is covered in its entire course by the clavicle, the costoclavicular ligament, and the subclavius muscle. It adheres to the adjacent ligaments, fascia, and periosteum through an extension of the fascia colli media. The cupola of the lung is mostly medial and posterior to the vein as it begins to course deeper into the thorax (Fig. 5.7).[45,47,58]

The infraclavicular route is widely used for access because of the ease with which the subclavian vein is located. The largest vein caliber is obtained with placement of the patient in moderate Trendelenburg position, with the head neutral and the shoulders flat.[59] Slight retraction of the shoulders may be used.[60] The Trendelenburg position is not always necessary, as the subclavian vein adheres firmly to the surrounding structures via the fascia colli media, and is well distended regardless of position. The initial puncture needle may be placed near the lateral border of the deltopectoral triangle, slightly lateral to the junction of the medial and distal thirds of the bone, below the midpoint of the clavicle, or at the medial and middle thirds of the clavicle.[61] The junction between the lateral concavity and the medial convexity of the clavicle creates a space (the superior margin of the deltopectoral triangle) in which a needle may be passed at a relatively superficial angle, preventing injury to deeper structures.[59] The needle is directed medially and cranially, toward the suprasternal notch, along the posterior surface of the clavicle, always in close proximity to the periosteum.[62,63]

Because of the consistent course of the subclavian vein at the clavicle, it is generally considered to be simple to access via this landmark-guided approach. Complications are certainly far less devastating than in failed internal jugular cannulations, in which the adjacent carotid artery may be injured, placing brain circulation in danger. In addition, as compared to ultrasound use for internal jugular cannulation, there are greater difficulties in utilizing ultrasound for subclavian vein access, as the ultrasound beam cannot penetrate bone, and proper alignment of the probe with the vessels is often cumbersome and difficult.[4] These issues have led to fewer studies documenting any benefits of ultrasound-guided venipuncture on the subclavian vein.[64] The data from a few large-scale studies indicate a generally improved success rate with fewer complications using an ultrasound-guided subclavian catheter placement method versus the landmark method,[4,44] but practice guidelines for ultrasound use in vascular access, published in 2012,

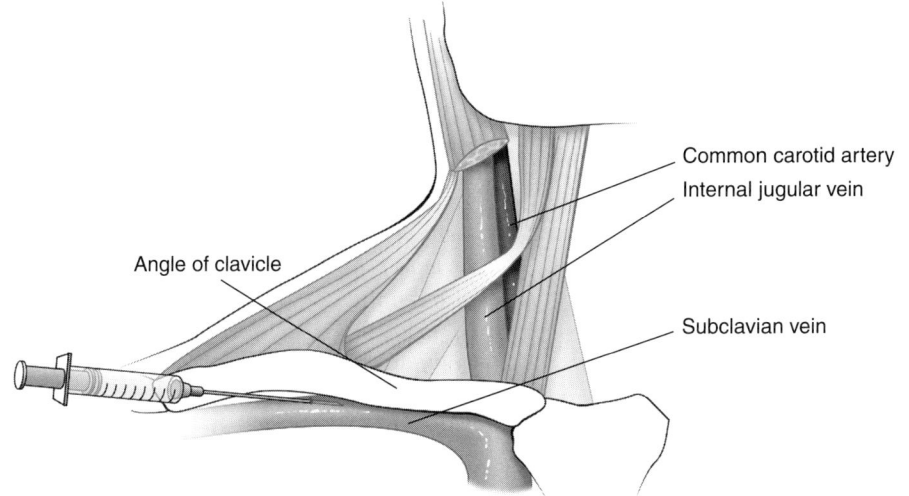

Angle of clavicle

Common carotid artery

Internal jugular vein

Subclavian vein

Figure 5.7 Subclavian vein anatomy, and **steps for insertion of subclavian vein catheters, infraclavicular approach** (see text for additional detail on cannulation):

- The patient is prepped and draped in the usual fashion. Aseptic conditions are maintained throughout.
- The patient is placed in moderate Trendelenburg position.
- An 18 gauge × 6.3 cm introducer needle is inserted at the lower border of the clavicle at the junction of the medial and middle thirds.
- The needle is directed medially and cranially beneath the inferior surface of the clavicle (in close proximity to the periosteum) toward the suprasternal notch while maintaining a slight negative pressure in the syringe.

state that at this time there is insufficient evidence to support the use of ultrasound for cannulation of the subclavian vein.[5] However, this standard is likely to change as large-scale studies continue to be published indicating that ultrasound-guided cannulation of the subclavian vein is superior to the landmark method, and it will likely become the method of choice for central venous access.[64,65]

Correct neutral positioning may be unattainable in the trauma bay, or in the presence of edema, bulky dressings, excessive fat distributed around the arms and upper chest, shoulder or joint pathologic conditions, or burns.[66] In clinical conditions that prevent shoulder retraction, a more medial approach to the vein is suggested, i.e., needle insertion at the junction between the middle and inner thirds of the lower border of the clavicle. This approach maintains a relatively constant course of the vein in relationship to the bone, but increased thickness of the bone mandates a steeper approach, increasing the possibility of damage to underlying structures.[52] Whenever possible, access should be attempted on the right side of the chest to avoid injury to the thoracic duct and more elevated pleural dome. In cases of thoracic injury, access should be via the ipsilateral subclavian vein, especially if an intercostal chest tube is already in place, rather than risking pneumothorax on the uninjured side. In mediastinal injury, access via the contralateral subclavian vein is recommended.[17]

Peripheral arterial cannulation

Direct blood pressure measurements were first performed in 1733 by an English scientist and clergyman, Stephen Hales, who inserted a brass pipe in the carotid artery of a horse and connected it to a glass manometer via the flexible trachea of a goose.[67] The practical application of perioperative arterial blood pressure measurements did not become a common practice until the middle to latter half of the twentieth century, however. A peripheral arterial catheter in a modern setting allows for continuous blood pressure monitoring, assessment of volume status if certain conditions are met, and a source for arterial blood sampling – all critical components in a trauma resuscitation.

Blood pressure and pulse are key monitoring parameters (see Chapter 9). Arterial blood pressure monitoring will provide immediate data to expedite the diagnosis of circulatory and electromechanical cardiac dysfunction. Trauma patients are susceptible to paroxysmal intraoperative hemodynamic disturbances owing to their presenting injury, subsequent resuscitation, exposure to vasoactive medications, and hemodynamic insults from surgical maneuvering. Rapid or profound blood loss is usually the culprit, but other conditions such as pneumothorax, hemothorax, cardiac tamponade, or primary cardiac or great vessel injury can also result in significant perfusion disturbances. An arterial line in these situations will allow for rapid diagnosis and intervention. If cardiopulmonary bypass is required, or if, in the era of circulatory

support devices, a patient presents with a left ventricular assist device (LVAD), an arterial line would be mandatory for monitoring blood pressure under nonpulsatile conditions. Additionally, pulse oximetry may be unreliable or unobtainable in hypotensive or hypothermic patients, and an invasive arterial catheter will provide definitive evidence of perfusion and determination of arterial oxygenation. There are some data to suggest that noninvasive blood pressure measurements may not be accurate in the shock state,[68,69] and in low flow states blood pressure may more accurately be monitored intraarterially. The practitioner should critically evaluate the potential for volume changes or loss of pulsatility and consider early arterial catheter placement before intraoperative changes make it an egregious challenge. If a discrete vessel injury is suspected, consideration should be given to the location of the arterial catheter, so that the measured value accurately represents aortic root pressure.

The radial artery is the most frequently chosen site for peripheral arterial cannulation, since it is readily accessible, often technically simple, and has favorable collateral circulation. In the typical adult, a 20 gauge peripheral angiocatheter is inserted in the radial artery supplying the nondominant hand, if available. After sterile preparation the catheter is often placed near the wrist crease, but it may be placed more proximally in the upper extremity. Depending on the practitioner's preferred technique, a radial arterial catheter set may be employed or a 20 gauge angiocatheter may be directly placed. If there is difficulty advancing the catheter, a guidewire may be passed. Many proprietary devices are available with a self-contained wire, which some find useful. Longer catheters are less likely to dislodge, and some evidence suggests that they decrease the incidence of post-decannulation arterial thrombosis.[70,71] Ultrasound guidance may increase the rate of first-pass success by up to 71% in the radial position,[72] and should strongly be considered in cases where the vessel is not palpable.[73] Furthermore, a micropuncture kit with a 20 gauge introducer needle and 0.025-inch (0.64 mm) diameter wire can often facilitate a challenging arterial cannulation when combined with ultrasound.

The safety and reliability of radial artery blood pressure monitoring has been proven in numerous studies,[74–76] yet it is not without risk. Recent data indicate a 0.09% risk of permanent ischemic injury,[67] similar to the femoral artery. The most common complication is transient arterial occlusion, with a reported range of 1.5–35%,[73,77,78] and a mean of 19.7%.[67] This is thought to typically resolve in 30 days for most patients.[79] Although there are reports describing digit or forearm amputation after radial artery cannulation, multiple emboli and prolonged circulatory failure with vasopressor support have typically been implicated as etiologies in such cases.[74,80] Retrograde cerebral air embolism is a theoretic concern, but it is unlikely unless very large amounts of air are introduced or the rate of flushing is above 4 mL/second.[81] Other complications include pseudoaneurysm (0.09%), hematoma (14.4%), and hemorrhage (0.53%).[70]

The Modified Allen test is often advocated as a tool to assess the risk of ischemia with radial artery compromise. The test is used to estimate the adequacy of the blood supply through the ulnar artery to the hand. Unfortunately, most studies examining this test or its several permutations have subjective endpoints and conflicting results. A common modification involves placing a pulse oximeter on a digit at risk for ischemia. Since pulse oximetry can be normal with as little as 5% of baseline flow, the correlation between a normal pulse oximetry value and tissue ischemia is not reliable. While it may be helpful for radial artery harvest, the Modified Allen test has not shown benefit in assessing candidacy for radial artery catheters.[82] A recent American Society of Anesthesiologists (ASA) closed claims analysis of peripheral vascular catheters showed 7 of 13 arterial line claims involved radial arterial lines, with only one case concerning ischemia.[83]

If the radial artery cannot be found or successfully cannulated, or if the nature of the injury prohibits placing a catheter in that location, other sites including the ulnar, brachial, axillary, femoral, or dorsalis pedis arteries are reasonable alternatives. Although highly debated and fraught with anecdote, data suggest that these sites offer overall minimal increased risk of complication over radial catheters.[68,74,84] The axillary and femoral arteries may have extra utility in the trauma setting, as they are more easily palpated in the hypothermic or hypotensive patient and demonstrate fairly regular anatomy. Clinical discretion based on scenario and vessel availability is the final determinant for the site of line placement.

The dorsalis pedis artery is considered a relatively safe site for cannulation. There is acceptable collateral blood flow provided by the posterior tibial and peroneal arteries. However, one must consider the presence of comorbid conditions such as diabetes or peripheral vascular disease when choosing this vessel, since a compromise of collateral flow could affect perfusion or healing. There is a lower rate of success in cannulating this vessel,[85] and it may be decreased even more in the setting of shock. There is some evidence that suggests there is a lower rate of thrombosis in this vessel compared to the radial artery,[78] and from this standpoint it may have some ancillary benefit. Overall, it is a safe alternative to the radial artery in a young and otherwise healthy patient.[86]

The ulnar artery is another alternative to radial artery cannulation. Some data indicate mild, transient paresthesias of the hand in a small number of patients at this site.[87] A concern exists that ischemia may be increased, since the ulnar artery is proximally the larger of the two vessels supplying the hand, but studies that evaluated complications of ulnar artery catheterization have not demonstrated this risk.[75,88,89] At the level of the wrist, the ulnar artery is often equal in size or smaller than the radial artery, as it provides several branches to form the interosseous supply in the forearm while the radial artery functions more as an arterial supply to the hand.[87] Ulnar artery catheters have been reported to be safely used in patients with known multiple ipsilateral radial artery punctures,[82] and even with chronic radial occlusion.[90]

A randomized study comparing radial versus ulnar cannulation for coronary angiography found both sites equally safe.[91] That being stated, long-term indwelling ulnar artery catheters should be used with caution and are best avoided if alternative sites are available, since most data series are small and institutional familiarity is usually lacking.

Many practitioners are hesitant to use the brachial artery for pressure monitoring, but it can be a valuable resource in trauma scenarios. There are concerns of an increased risk of ischemia owing to its lack of collateral flow, but this is not supported by data. One study evaluated 1000 patients with brachial artery catheters and revealed only one serious complication, an infected hematoma arising from a pseudoaneurysm.[92] In this same study, 157 minor complications including hematoma, evidence of microemboli, and transient median nerve paresthesias were described. Another large study of 6185 patients whose brachial arteries were employed for blood gas sampling had only a 0.2% complication rate, consisting mainly of paresthesias.[92] A large study of neonatal and pediatric patients with brachial artery complications also revealed no major complications. Anecdotal experience with the cardiac surgery population at the Cleveland Clinic and University Hospitals (Cleveland, OH) indicates that ischemic complications are rare and often accompanied by severe vasoplegia, sepsis, or embolic phenomena.

The axillary artery is another option for blood pressure monitoring in trauma patients. A recent review described the incidence of complication in the axillary artery catheter as follows: permanent ischemic damage 0.2%, temporary occlusion 1.18%, pseudoaneurysm 0.1%, hematoma 2.28%, and hemorrhage 1.14%.[75] Although the risk of bleeding and hematoma is low, there may be a concern for brachial plexopathy, but this is speculative. The axillary artery has been shown to be more difficult to cannulate,[93] but it is relatively safe given a lack of alternatives.[67,75,84,93]

The femoral artery may be chosen for reasons similar to the axillary artery. Ischemic complications are very rare, and other complications of femoral arterial lines include temporary vessel occlusion (1.45%), pseudoaneurysm (0.3%), hematoma (6.1%), and hemorrhage (1.58).[75] There is one report of death from retroperitoneal bleeding.[94] Femoral arterial lines should be placed below the inguinal ligament to avoid a retroperitoneal bleed. An iliac artery injury resulting in cardiac arrest from retroperitoneal bleeding was reported that resulted in an award in excess of $12,000,000.[83] While not without risk, the femoral artery is a safe choice and can be easily accessed in most patients in the trauma setting.

In a trauma patient, arterial lines are often placed under less than optimal conditions with a heightened sense of urgency. While sterile technique should always be followed, it can easily be breached in these situations. Considering that many trauma patients will have an extended stay in an intensive care unit, postoperative infectious risks should be of concern. Radial artery local infection has been estimated to be 0.43–0.72%, while catheter-related sepsis ranged from

0.13% to 0.14% in two very large reviews.[75,95] There is a concern that femoral arterial lines carry a higher rate of infection. Incidence of femoral local infection ranges from 0.78 to 1.17% and rates of catheter related sepsis of 0.34 to 0.44%.[75,95] Recent data point to a statistically significant increase in local and systemic infection rates of femoral arterial catheters compared to radial arterial catheters; there is no statistically significant increase in local or systemic infections for brachial or dorsalis pedis artery catheters.[95] Of note, axillary artery catheters may have an increased rate of local infection at 2.24% and a systemic infection rate of 0.51%.[70] While there is a definite risk of catheter-related local infection or sepsis, it is small in all cases. However, if alternative options are sought in sites other than the radial artery, the long-term effects of infection should be considered.

Intraosseous (IO) access

Intraosseous (IO) access has long been accepted as a means of vascular access in children (see Chapter 34). Adult use has been documented as safe and acceptable, but the recent advent of new access devices is permitting rapid, accurate access to the IO space.[76] Recent changes in the American Heart Association's resuscitation guidelines state that that the IO access should be established if the IV route is unavailable.[96]

It is likely that IO will be a rarity within the hospital, as ultrasound-guided vascular access is widely adopted in pediatric institutions as a technique that helps to save time and increase success in central venous access as well as peripheral vascular access.[97] The IO route will likely become limited to prehospital emergency situations, with the result that anesthesiologists may encounter these already in situ in the trauma bay or operating room. Anesthesiologists should understand the mechanisms and utility of these devices.

IO insertion sites include the sternum, tibia, humeral head, and even the pelvis.[98] IO cannulation accesses a noncollapsible venous plexus, enabling fluid and medication delivery similar to that achieved by central venous access.[96] Although adults have much less active bone marrow than children, the vascular sinusoids remain patent, and fluid injected into the bone marrow disperses via its venous drainage, which connects the marrow to the systemic circulation.[99] The IO device provides an effective, rapid alternative for the prehospital provider (see Chapter 2). Access time is reported to average 77 seconds. IO flow rates vary, with documentation of fluid delivery from 15 to 30 mL per minute via 1 meter gravity drip, or 125 mL per minute when a pressure cuff bag is used, or 150 mL per minute possible when infused with a syringe bolus.[98,100]

While IV access is the gold standard, there are situations where an IV cannot rapidly be placed, when the time required to place an IV may compromise patient care, or when other methods of IV access have failed,[101] especially as central venous catheter insertion is not an option in most prehospital settings. In hemodynamically unstable trauma patients, catheter placement may be extremely difficult secondary to collapse of veins. The IO vascular conduit remains open in the presence of shock.[102] Placement of an IO line may be a viable alternative to IV access in severely burned patients, in whom IV access may be extremely difficult, if not impossible. Other indications for IO line placement include combative patients, where precise access is not possible, and failed peripheral IV access in adult patients, where vascular access is critical.[99]

Contraindications to the placement of an intraosseous device include fractures or previous surgery at the bone of access; infection at the insertion site; local vascular compromise; burn injury at the IO cannulation site; severe osteoporosis; and obese patients in whom the IO needles may not be long enough to reach the bone marrow space. [76,98,100] Lack of fluid flow, or extravasation of fluid at the site, mandates discontinuation of the IO infusion.[103]

Conclusions

Venous access is initially accomplished using peripheral IV catheters. However, many patients will require central venous access and arterial line placement. Regardless of the site of central venous cannulation, the Seldinger technique is routinely performed using aseptic technique. The femoral vein is a large and relatively easy vessel to cannulate. In contrast to the internal jugular and subclavian veins, there is no risk of hemothorax or pneumothorax with the femoral vein. One major limitation of femoral vein cannulation, however, is abdominal trauma, where inferior vena cava flow may be disrupted. The internal jugular vein is often not easily accessible in trauma, because of a cervical collar. For this reason, the subclavian approach is usually preferred. Given its safety and reliability, radial artery cannulation is the preferred site for trauma. Arterial cannulation permits an accurate measure of blood pressure, including systolic and pulse pressure variability (see Chapter 9), and permits easy access for arterial blood gas measurements. Anesthesiologists should be familiar with the intraosseous (IO) route of access, especially IO catheters placed in the prehospital setting. Except in rare circumstances, however, ultrasound-guided vascular access has limited the need for establishing IO access in the hospital setting.

Questions

(1) **The flow rate through a catheter is primarily determined by which variable?**
   a. Change in pressure
   b. Radius of the catheter
   c. Density of the fluid
   d. Length of the catheter

(2) **Which of the following can provide the fastest possible infusion rate?**
   a. Packed red blood cells 2 m above the patient's chest, via a 12 Fr subclavian 16 cm length triple-lumen catheter

b. Lactated Ringer's via the rapid infusor (e.g., Belmont or level 1 infusion device) attached to a 14 gauge × 6.25 cm peripheral intravenous catheter

c. A hand-inflated pressure cuff bag set to 200 mmHg delivering lactated Ringer's via a sternal intraosseous cannula

d. Hetastarch via a hand-inflated pressure cuff bag set to 300 mmHg, connected to the 7 Fr internal jugular triple-lumen 20 cm length catheter

(3) Which of the following is *not* a characteristic of femoral venous catheterization?
   a. Ease of access
   b. Compressible location, should a hematoma occur
   c. Contraindicated in the presence of inferior vena cava disruption
   d. Decreased rate of infection

(4) Which one of the following sets of anatomic landmarks is correct?
   a. The femoral vein is located lateral to the femoral artery in the femoral triangle
   b. The central approach to the internal jugular vein requires the identification of the sternal and clavicular heads of the sternocleidomastoid muscle; the needle is inserted at the junction of these two heads, and is directed toward the contralateral nipple
   c. The internal jugular vein lies posteromedial to the carotid artery, at a depth no greater than 3 cm below the skin surface.
   d. The subclavian vein is an extension of the axillary vein of the arm, and courses parallel to the subclavian artery, separated by the anterior scalene muscle, posterior to the clavicle

(5) Internal jugular vein access should be obtained:
   a. Via the left side, to decrease risk of pneumothorax
   b. Preferentially via the right side because of the straighter course of the vein
   c. Ipsilateral to a preexisting mediastinal injury
   d. Contralateral to a preexisting pneumothorax

(6) Indications for invasive arterial blood pressure monitoring include:
   a. Significant hemodynamic changes in brief time periods
   b. Frequent blood sample measurements
   c. Improved blood pressure measurement, compared with noninvasive measurement
   d. Inability to assess oxygenation due to inaccurate pulse oximetry, secondary to hypotension or hypothermia
   e. All of the above

(7) Invasive arterial blood pressure monitoring:
   a. May be obtained at the axillary or femoral artery, as alternative sites, since these arteries may be easier to access in the hypotensive or hypothermic trauma patient

b. Should first be attempted at the dorsalis pedis artery in patients with severe diabetes or significant peripheral vascular disease
   c. Often leads to arterial occlusion that is thought to be permanent in most patients
   d. Is indicated in the American College of Surgeons shock classifications I and II

(8) Choose the true statement regarding intraosseous (IO) access in trauma patients:
   a. IO cannulation accesses an arterial vessel, enabling fluid and medication delivery similar to that achieved by central venous access
   b. The IO conduit tends to be a venous system that collapses quickly in states of hemodynamic compromise
   c. Placement of an IO line may be a viable alternative to IV access in severely burned patients, in whom IV access may be extremely difficult, if not impossible
   d. Lack of fluid flow, or extravasation of fluid at the site, mandate the application of a pressure cuff bag to improve flow

(9) Which of the following is appropriately paired with a recognized not-uncommon complication?
   a. Peripheral intravenous catheter – venous thrombosis
   b. Subclavian vein catheter – carotid artery puncture
   c. Internal jugular vein catheter – pneumothorax
   d. Femoral vein catheter – venous air embolism
   e. Subclavian vein catheter – pneumothorax

(10) Benefits of central venous catheters in the trauma patient include:
   a. Larger-caliber and more reliable vessels for the administration of large fluid volumes
   b. Monitoring of central venous pressures via the subclavian, femoral, and internal jugular routes
   c. Potential conversion of internal jugular and subclavian catheters to pulmonary artery catheters, should the need arise
   d. Ability to infuse medications that may not be compatible with peripheral intravenous administration
   e. All of the above

Answers

(1) b
(2) b
(3) d
(4) d
(5) b
(6) e
(7) a
(8) c
(9) e
(10) e

References

1. National Institute for Clinical Excellence. *Guidance on the Use of Ultrasound Locating Devices for Placing Central Venous Catheters.* Technology Appraisal 49. London: NICE, 2002. http://guidance.nice.org.uk/TA49 (accessed July 2014).

2. Agency for Healthcare Research and Quality. *Making Health Care Safer II: An Updated Critical Analysis of the Evidence for Patient Safety Practices.* http://www.ahrq.gov/research/findings/evidence-based-reports/ptsafetyuptp.html (accessed July 2014).

3. American Society of Anesthesiologists. Practice guidelines for central venous access: a report by the American Society of Anesthesiologists Task Force on Central Venous Access. *Anesthesiology* 2012; **116**; 539–73.

4. Weiner MM, Geldard P, Mittnacht A. Ultrasound-guided vascular access: a comprehensive review. *J Cardiothorac Vasc Anesth* 2013; **27**; 345–60.

5. Troianos C, Hartman G, Glas K, *et al.* Guidelines for performing ultrasound guided vascular cannulation: recommendations of the American Society of Echocardiography and the Society of Cardiovascular Anesthesiologists. *Anesth Analg* 2012; **114**; 46–72.

6. American College of Surgeons Committee on Trauma. *ATLS: Advanced Trauma Life Support For Doctors*, 7th edition. Chicago, IL: ACS, 2004.

7. Westfall MD, Price KR, Lambert M, *et al.* Intravenous access in the critically ill trauma patient: a multicentered, prospective, randomized trial of saphenous cutdown and percutaneous femoral access. *Ann Emerg Med* 1994; **23**; 541–5.

8. Revell M, Porter K, Greaves I. Fluid resuscitation in prehospital trauma care: a consensus view. *Emerg Med J* 2002; **19**; 494–8.

9. Comunale, M. A laboratory evaluation of the level 1 rapid infuser (H1025) and the Belmont instrument fluid management system (FMS 2000) for rapid transfusion. *Anesth Analg* 2003; **97**; 1064–9.

10. de la Roche M, Gauthier L; Rapid transfusion of packed red blood cells: effect of dilution, pressure and catheter size. *Ann Emerg Med* 1993; **22**; 1551–5.

11. Keyes L, Frazee B, Snoey E, Simon B, Christy D. Ultrasound-guided brachial and basilic vein cannulation in the emergency department patients with difficult intravenous access. *Ann Emerg Med* 1999; **34**; 711–14.

12. Brannam L, Blaivas M, Lyon M, Flake M. Emergency nurses' utilization of ultrasound guidance for placement of peripheral intravenous lines in difficult-access patients. *Acad Emerg Med* 2004; **11**; 1361–3.

13. Costantino TG, Fojtik JP. Success rate of peripheral IV catheter insertion by emergency physicians using ultrasound guidance. *Acad Emerg Med* 2003; **10**; 487a.

14. Joing S, Strote S, Caroon L, *et al.* Videos in clinical medicine. Ultrasound-guided peripheral IV placement. *N Engl J Med* 2012; **366** (25): e38. doi: 10.1056/NEJMvcm1005951.

15. Abraham E, Shapiro M, Podolsky S. Central venous catheterization in the emergency setting. *Crit Care Med* 1983; **11**; 515–17.

16. Pappas P., Brathwaite CE, Ross SE. Emergency central venous catheterization during resuscitation of trauma patients. *Am Surg* 1992; **58**; 108–11.

17. Scalea TM, Sinert R, Duncan AO, *et al.* Percutaneous central venous access for resuscitation in trauma. *Acad Emerg Med* 1994; **1**; 525–31.

18. Duffy BJ. The clinical use of polyethylene tubing for intravenous therapy. *Ann Surg* 1949; **130**: 929.

19. Mangiante EC, Hoots AV, Fabian TC. The percutaneous common femoral vein catheter for volume replacement in critically injured patients. *J Trauma* 1988; **28**; 1644–9.

20. Emerman CL, Bellon EM, Lukens TW, May TE, Effron D. A prospective study of femoral versus subclavian vein catheterization during cardiac arrest. *Annals Emerg Med* 1990; **19**; 26–30.

21. Swanson RS, Uhlig, PN, Gross PL, McCabe CJ. Emergency intravenous access through the femoral vein. *Ann Emerg Med* 1984; **13**; 244–7.

22. Durbec O, Viviand X, Potie F, *et al.* A prospective evaluation of the use of femoral venous catheters in critically ill adults. *Crit Care Med* 1997; **25**; 1986–9.

23. Joynt GM, Kew J, Gomersall CD, Leung VY, Liu EK. Deep venous thrombosis caused by femoral venous catheters in critically ill adult patients. *Chest* 2000; **117**; 178–83.

24. Merrer J, De Jonghe B, Golliot F, *et al.* Complications of femoral and subclavian venous catheterization in critically ill patients; *JAMA* 2001; **286**: 700–7.

25. Centers for Disease Control and Prevention. Guideline for Hand Hygiene in Health-Care Settings. Recommendations of the Healthcare Infection Control Practices Advisory Committee and the HICPAC/SHEA/APIC/IDSA Hand Hygiene Task Force. Society for Healthcare Epidemiology of America/Association for Professionals in Infection Control/Infectious Diseases Society of America. mm *WR Recomm Rep* 2002; **51** (RR-16): 1–45.

26. O'Grady NP, Alexander M, Dellinger EP, *et al.* Guidelines for the prevention of intravascular catheter-related infections. Centers for Disease Control and prevention. mm*WR Recomm Rep* 2002; **51** (RR-10): 1–29.

27. Berenholtz SM, Pronovost PJ, Lipsett PA, *et al.* Eliminating catheter-related bloodstream infections in the intensive care unit. *Crit Care Med* 2004; **32**; 2014–20.

28. McGee DC, Gould MK. Preventing complications of central venous catheterization. *N Engl J Med* 2003; **348**; 1123–33.

29. Latto IP, Ng WS, Jones PL, Jenkins BJ. *Percutaneous Central Venous and Arterial Catheterisation*, 3rd edition. Philadelphia, PA: Saunders, 2000. Chapter 9: The femoral vein; pp. 211–21.

30. Polderman KH, Girbes AJ. Central venous catheter use. Part 1: mechanical complications. *Intensive Care Med* 2002; **28**; 1–17.

31. Butterworth JF. *Atlas of Procedures in Anesthesia and Critical Care.* Philadelphia, PA: Saunders, 1992. Chapter 15: Central venous cannulation; pp. 95–9.

32. Jobes DR, Schwartz AJ, Greenhow DE, *et al.* Safer jugular vein cannulation: Recognition of arterial puncture and preferential use of the external jugular route. *Anesthesiology* 1983; **59**; 353–5.

33. Augoustides JG, Diaz D, Weiner J, Clarke C, Jobes DR. Current practice of

internal jugular venous cannulation in a university anesthesia department: influence of operator experience on success of cannulation and arterial injury. *J Cardiothorac Vasc Anesth* 2002; **16**; 567–71.

34. Seldinger SI. Catheter replacement of the needle in percutaneous arteriography: a new technique. *Acta Radiol* 1953; **39**; 368–76.

35. Scott WL, Collier P. The vessel dilator for central venous catheter placement: forerunner for success or vascular misadventure? *Intensive Care Med* 2001; **16**: 263–9.

36. Oropello JM, Leibowitz AB, Manasia A, Del Guidice R, Benjamin E. Dilator-associated complications of central vein catheter insertion: possible mechanisms of injury and suggestions for prevention; *J Cardiothorac Vasc Anesth* 1996; **10**: 634–7.

37. Lobato EB, Gravenstein N, Paige GB. Dilator-associated complications of central vein catheter insertion: possible mechanisms of injury and suggestions for prevention. *J Cardiothorac Vasc Anesth* 1997; **11**; 539–40.

38. Bailey PL, Whitaker EE, Palmer LS, Glance LG. The accuracy of the central landmark used for central venous catheterization of the internal jugular vein. *Anesth Analg* 2006; **102**; 1327–32.

39. Steele R, Irvin C. Central line mechanical complication rate in emergency medicine patients. *Acad Emerg Med* 2001; **8**; 204–7.

40. Eisen LA, Narasimhan M, Berger JS, et al. Mechanical complications of central venous catheters. *J Intensive Care Med* 2006; **21**; 40–6.

41. Aoki H, Mizobe T, Nozuchi S, Hatanaka T, Tanaka Y. Vertebral artery pseudoaneurysm: a rare complication of internal jugular vein catheterization. *Anesth Analg* 1992; **75**; 296–8.

42. Maddali MM, Badur RS, Rajakumar MC, Valliattu J. Pseudoaneurysm of the innominate artery: a delayed iatrogenic complication after internal jugular vein catheterization. *J Cardiothorac Vasc Anesth* 2006; **20**; 853–5.

43. Feller-Kopman D. Ultrasound-guided internal jugular access: a proposed standardized approach and implications for training and practice. *Chest* 2007; **132**; 302–9.

44. Balls A, Lovecchio F, Kroeger A, et al. Ultrasound guidance for central venous catheter placement: results from the central line emergency access registry database. *Am J Emerg Med* 2010; **28**; 561–7.

45. Fortune JB, Feustel P. Effect of patient position on size and location of the subclavian vein for percutaneous puncture. *Arch Surg* 2003; **138**; 996–1000.

46. Aubaniac R. L'injection intraveineuse sous-claviculaire: avantages et technique. *Presse Med* 1952; **60**; 1456.

47. Grant JP. Anatomy and physiology of venous system vascular access: implications. *JPEN J Parenter Enteral Nutr* 2006; **30**: S7–12.

48. Defalque RJ. Subclavian venipunture: a review. *Anesth Analg Curr Res* 1968; **47**; 677–82.

49. Ruesch S, Walder B, Tramer MR. Complications of central venous catheters: internal jugular versus subclavian access – a systematic review. *Crit Care Med* 2002; **30**; 454–9.

50. Lorente L, Henry C, Martin MM, Jimenez A, Mora ML. Central venous catheter-related infection in a prospective and observational study of 2595 catheters. *Crit Care* 2005; **9**: R631–5.

51. Nagashima G, Kikuchi T, Tsuyuzaki H, et al. To reduce catheter-related bloodstream infections: is the subclavian route better than the jugular route for central venous catheterization? *J Infect Chemother* 2006; **12**: 363–5.

52. Tan BK, Hong SW, Huang MH, Lee ST. Anatomic basis of safe percutaneous subclavian venous catheterization. *J Trauma* 1999: **48**: 82–6.

53. Agee KR, Balk RA. Central venous catheterization in the critically ill patient. *Crit Care Clin* 1992; **8**; 677–86.

54. Ferguson M, Max M, Marshall W. Emergency department infraclavicular sublavian vein catherization in patients with multiple injuries and burns. *South Med J* 1988; **81**; 433–5.

55. Timsit JF. Central venous access in intensive care unit patients: Is the subclavian vein the royal route? *Intensive Care Med* 2002; **28**: 1006–8.

56. Mansfield PF, Hohn DC, Fornage BD, Gregurich MA, Ota DM. Complications and failures of subclavian vein catheterization. *N Engl J Med* 1994; **331**; 1735–8.

57. Sznejder JI, Zveibel FR, Bitterman H, Weiner P, Bursztein S. Central vein catheterization: failure and complications by 3 percutaneous approaches. *Arch Intern Med* 1986; **146**; 259–61.

58. Thompson EC, Calver LE. Safe subclavian vein cannulation. *Am Surg* 2005; **71**; 180–3.

59. Moran SG, Peoples JB. The deltopectoral triangle as a landmark for percutaneous infraclavicular cannulation of the subclavian vein. *Angiology* 1993; **44**; 683–6.

60. von Goedecke A, Keller C, Moriggle B, et al. An anatomic landmark to simplify subclavian vein cannulation: the "deltoid tuberosity." *Anesth Analg* 2005; **100**: 623–8.

61. Porzionato A, Montisci M, Manani G. Brachial plexus injury following subclavian vein catheterization: a case report. *J Clin Anesth* 2003; **15**; 582–6.

62. Land RE. The relationship of the left subclavian vein to the clavicle. *J Thorac Cardiovasc Surg* 1972; **63**; 564–8.

63. Land RE. Anatomic relationships of the right subclavian vein. *Arch Surg* 1971; **102**; 178–80.

64. Lamperti M, Bodenham A, Pittiruti M, et al. International evidence-based recommendations on ultrasound-guided vascular access. *Intensive Care Med*, 2012; **38**: 1105–17.

65. Fragou M, Gravvanis A, Dimitriou V, et al. Real-time ultrasound-guided subclavian vein cannulation versus the landmark method in critical care patients: a prospective randomized study. *Crit Care Med* 2011; **39**; 1607–12.

66. Tan BK, Wong CH, Ng R, Huang M, Lee ST. A modified technique of percutaneous subclavian venous catheterization in the oedematous burned patient. *Burns* 2005; **31**; 505–9.

67. Gordon LH, Brown M, Brown OW, Brown EM. Alternative sites for continuous arterial monitoring. *South Med J* 1984; **77**; 1498–500.

68. Cohn JN. Blood pressure measurement in shock: mechanism of inaccuracy in ausculatory and palpatory methods. *JAMA* 1967; **199**; 118–22.

69. Gardner RM. Direct blood pressure measurement dynamic response

requirements. *Anesthesiology* 1981; **54**; 227–36.

70. Dahl MR, Smead WL, McSweeney TD. Radial artery cannulation: a comparision of 15.2- and 4.45cm catheters. *J Clin Monit* 1992; **8**; 193–7.

71. Kim JM, Arakawa K, Bliss J. Arterial cannulation: factors in the development of occlusion. *Anesth Analg* 1975; **54**; 836–41.

72. Shiloh AL, Savel RH, Paulin LM, Eisen LA. Ultrasound-guided catheterizationof the radial artery: a systematic review and meta-analysis of randomized controlled trials. *Chest* 2011; **139**; 524–9.

73. Gratrix AP, Atkinson JD, Bodenham AR. Cannulation of the impalpable section of radial artery: preliminary clinical and ultrasound observations. *Eur J Anaesthesiol* 2009; **26**; 887–9.

74. Slogoff S, Keats AS, Arlund C. On the safety of radial artery cannulation. *Anesthesiology* 1983; **59**; 42–7.

75. Scheer BV, Perel A, Pfeiffer UJ. Clinical review: complications and risk factors of peripheral arterial catheters used for haemodynamic monitoring in anaethesia and intensive care medicine. *Crit Care* 2002; **6**; 199–204.

76. Fowler R, Gallagher JV, Isaacs SM, *et al.* The role of intraosseous vascular access in the out-of-hospital environment (Resource document to NAEMSP position statement). *Prehosp Emerg Care* 2007; **11**; 63–6.

77. Soderstrom CA, Wasserman DH, Dunham CM, Caplan ES, Cowley RA. Superiority of the femoral artery for monitoring: a prospective study. *Am J Surg* 1982; **144**; 309–12.

78. Bedford RF. Wrist circumference predicts the risk of radial-arterial occlusion after cannulation. *Anesthesiology* 1978; **48**; 377–8.

79. Hoencamp R, Ulrich C, Verschuren AJ, van Baalan JM. Prospective comparative study on the hemodynamic and functional consequences of arterial monitoring catheters in intensive care patients on the short and long term. *J Crit Care* 2006; **21**; 193–6.

80. Green JA, Tonkin MA. Ischemia of the hand in infants following radial or ulnar artery catheterization. *Hand Surg* 1999; **4**; 151–7.

81. Murphy GS, Szokol JW, Marymont JH, Avram MJ, Vender JS. Retrograde air embolization during routine radial artery catheter flushing in adult cardiac surgical patients: an ultrasound study. *Anesthesiology* 2004; **101**; 614–19.

82. Brzezinski M, Luisetti T, London MJ. Radial artery cannulation: a comprehensive review of recent anatomic and physiologic investigations. *Anesth Analg* 2009; **109**; 1763–81.

83. Bhananker SM, Liau DW, Kooner PK, *et al.* Liability related to peripheral venous and arterial catheterization: a closed claims analysis. *Anesth Analg* 2009; **109**; 124–9.

84. Gurman GM, Kriemerman S. Cannulation of big arteries in critically ill patients. *Crit Care Med* 1985; **13**; 217–20.

85. Martin C, Saux P, Papazain L, Goutin F. Long-term arterial cannulation in ICU patients using the radial artery or dorsalis pedis artery. *Chest* 2001; **119**; 901–6.

86. Youngberg J, Miller ED. Evaluation of percutaneous cannulations of the dorsalis pedis artery. *Anesthesiology* 1976; **44**; 80–3.

87. Chopra PS, Kroncke GM, Dacumos GC, Young WP, Kahn DR. Use of the ulnar artery for monitoring arterial blood pressures and blood gases. *Ann Thorac Surg* 1973; **15**; 541–3.

88. Frezza EE, Mezghebe H. Indications and complications of arterial catheter use in surgical or medical intensive care units: analysis of 4932 patients. *Amer Surg* 1998; **64**; 127–31.

89. Kahler AC, Mirza FZ. Alternative arterial catheterization using the ulnar artery in critically ill pediatric patients. *Pediatr Crit Care Med* 2002; **3**; 370–4.

90. Lanspa TJ, Williams MA, Heirigs RL. Effectiveness of ulnar artery catheterization after failed attempt to cannulate a radial artery. *Am J Cardiol* 2005; **95**; 1529–30.

91. Aptecar E, Pernes JM, Chabane-Chaouch M, *et al.* Transulnar versus transradial artery approach for coronary angioplasty: the PCVI-CUBA study. *Catheter Cardiovasc Interv* 2006; **67**; 711–20.

92. Okeson GC, Wulbrecht PH. The safety of brachial artery puncture for arterial blood sampling. *Chest* 1998; **114**; 748–51.

93. Bryan-Brown CW, Kwun KB, Lumb PD, Pia RLG, Azer S. The axillary artery catheter. *Heart Lung* 1983; **12**; 492–7.

94. Muralidhar K. Complications of femoral artery pressure monitoring. *J Cardiothorac Vasc Anesth* 1998; **12**; 128–9.

95. Lanspa TJ, Reyes AP, Oldemeyer JB, Williams MA. Ulnar artery catheterization with occlusion of corresponding radial artery. *Catheter Cardiovasc Interv* 2004; **61**; 211–13.

96. Hazinski MF, Nadkarni VM, Hickey RW, *et al.* 2005 American Heart Association Guidelines for Cardiopulmonary Resuscitation and Emergency Cardiovascular Care. Part 7.2: Management of cardiac arrest. *Circulation* 2005; **112** (Suppl I): IV-58–66.

97. Schindler E, Schears G, Hall S, Yamamoto T. Ultrasound for vascular access in pediatric patients. *Paediatr Anesth* 2012; **22**; 1002–7.

98. Day MW. Using a sternal intraosseous device in adults. *Nursing* 1999; **29** (12): 22–3.

99. Waisman M, Waisman D. Bone marrow infusion in adults. *J Trauma* 1997; **42**; 288–93.

100. Frascone R, Kaye K, Dries D, Solem L. Successful placement of an adult sternal intraosseous line through burned skin. *J Burn Care Rehabil* 2003; **24**; 306–8.

101. Brown C, Wiklund L, Bar-Joseph G, *et al.* Future directions for resuscitation research. IV. Innovative advanced life support pharmacology. *Resuscitation* 1996; **33**; 163–77.

102. Calkins MD, Fitzgerald G, Bentley TB, Burris D. Intraosseous infusion devices: a comparison for potential use in special operations. *J Trauma* 2000; **48**; 1068–74.

103. Day MW. Act FASTwith intraosseous infusion. *Nursing* 2003; **33** (11): 50–2.

Chapter

6

Massive blood transfusion in trauma care

Joshua M. Tobin

Objectives

(1) Understand the definition of massive transfusion in the context of major traumatic injury.

(2) Appreciate the triggers for initiation of massive transfusion as well as the personnel involved in the implementation of a massive transfusion protocol (MTP).

(3) Review the current state of resuscitation and transfusion practices.

(4) Discuss adjunctive therapy, including tranexamic acid, vasopressin, and recombinant factor VIIa.

(5) Appreciate the role of inflammation and the immune response in trauma and resuscitation.

(6) Describe laboratory assays (including base excess, lactate, and point-of-care coagulation testing) available for monitoring the progress of massive transfusion.

Defining massive transfusion

The cornerstones of resuscitation in trauma are the transfusion of blood and blood products along with control of bleeding. An efficiently conducted resuscitation with appropriate transfusion practices is partnered with trauma surgery and interventional radiology to achieve source control of bleeding. In these cases, the need to transfuse large volumes of blood product in a short period of time is not uncommon. Establishing a massive transfusion protocol (MTP) can assist with making necessary blood products available in a timely fashion. In one study utilizing an historical control, mortality improved from 45% to 19% after institution of an MTP.[1] Interestingly, the ratio of fresh frozen plasma to packed red blood cells (FFP: RBC) was the same in both groups (1:1.8), but a decrease in mean time to administration of first blood product was noted. This illustrates the role that an MTP can play in timely and effective communication with the blood bank during a trauma emergency.

A massive transfusion is commonly defined as the administration of 10 units of RBCs in the first 24 hours of hospitalization (Table 6.1). Given the limited utility of a retrospective definition of massive transfusion in the acutely bleeding patient, other more practical definitions include loss of half a

Table 6.1 Definitions of massive transfusion

One blood volume loss in 24 hours (equivalent to 10 units of whole blood)
4 or more units replaced in 1 hour with continuing bleeding
50% blood volume loss in 3 hours (equivalent to 5 units of whole blood)
50 units lost in 48 hours
20 units lost in 24 hours
Blood loss exceeding 150 mL/min

Adapted from Repine TB, Perkins JG, Kauvar DS, Blackborne L. The use of fresh whole blood in massive transfusion. *J Trauma* 2006; **60** (6 Suppl): S59–69.

blood volume in 3 hours, or acute ongoing blood loss despite interventional radiologic or surgical management. The Assessment of Blood Consumption (ABC) score uses nonlaboratory parameters to identify patients who will require massive transfusion.[2] This tool assesses for penetrating trauma, a positive focused assessment with sonography for trauma (FAST), arrival systolic blood pressure less than 90 mmHg, and arrival heart rate greater than 120 bpm. An ABC score > 2 is 75% sensitive and 86% specific at predicting the need for massive transfusion.

An important component of massive transfusion is developing an agreed-upon MTP for use in emergencies. It is difficult to make the necessarily large volumes of blood and blood products available immediately from the blood bank without first designating what a massive transfusion will entail. Inputs from the blood bank, pathologists, surgeons, anesthesiologists, nursing, and operating room (OR) support staff are all vital to a well-organized MTP. There is considerable heterogeneity in the management of massive transfusion. One survey representing 25 countries found that 45% of respondents used an MTP regularly, 19% used MTPs inconsistently, and 34% did not use any protocol.[3] Furthermore, few MTPs addressed the need for adjuvant therapy such as the management of acidosis, hypothermia, and coagulopathy. Effective

---

Trauma Anesthesia, 2nd Edition, ed. Charles E. Smith. Published by Cambridge University Press. © Charles E. Smith, 2015.

Table 6.2 Sample criteria for massive transfusion protocol (MTP) initiation

5 units blood loss in one hour (50% blood volume) *or*

10 units blood loss anticipated in entire case, or within 12–24 hours of observation (one blood volume) *or*

Hypovolemic hypotension uncorrected by crystalloid and/or packed red blood cell resuscitation during ongoing hemorrhage *or*

Two or more of the following:
- penetrating mechanism
- positive focused assessment with sonography for trauma (FAST)
- systolic blood pressure < 90 mmHg
- heart rate > 120 beats per minute

communication can help provide consistency in the utilization of an MTP.

When an MTP is initiated, all members of the team must understand their role in the process, and must be prepared to act in that role immediately. The individual that enacts the MTP must clearly communicate with the blood bank, using predetermined triggers such as expected transfusion > one blood volume in 12 hours, significant ongoing blood loss, and/or more than 4 units of blood transfused in 1 hour (Table 6.2). Once the decision to enact the MTP has been made, appropriate support staff must be advised, including (and especially) the individual identified to physically go to the blood bank to pick up the blood. The blood bank staff must also understand that an MTP has been enacted, make the necessary assets available quickly, and work with the OR support staff who bring the blood to the OR. A standard "blood check" with the blood bank at the start of the day can save time when an MTP is enacted. This includes verification that the agreed-upon amounts of universal donor blood products are available (e.g., 6 units O negative RBCs, 6 units AB plasma, and 5–6 units of random donor platelets [1 standard adult dose]).

Once the MTP has been activated and the necessary blood products are available, then it is important to adhere to transfusion practices demonstrated to improve the care of the trauma patient.

Transfusion and resuscitation practices

As noted above, important concepts in trauma care are source control of hemorrhage and resuscitation with blood products. A thoughtful evaluation of the fluids and blood products needed to resuscitate the trauma patient is an important component of the anesthetic contribution to damage control resuscitation.[4,5]

A more thorough appreciation of transfusion practices, and a more refined definition of massive transfusion in the trauma patient, has led to improved resuscitation with blood products.[6] Improved understanding of trauma-induced coagulopathy has prompted early empiric treatment, rather than a more reactive response to documented coagulation abnormalities. This trend has led many trauma centers to revise their MTPs to include the use of 1:1 ratios of plasma to RBCs during massive transfusion.[7] Recent wartime studies on the ratio of plasma to RBCs have reported improved survival in the wounded combatant.[8] In 246 battle-wounded patients the FFP:RBC ratio was evaluated. It was found that mortality decreased from 65% with a 1:8 ratio to 19% with a 1:1.4 ratio. The civilian literature reported similar data, in which 467 massively transfused trauma patients were examined. Thirty-day survival improved in patients with FFP:RBC ratios greater than 1:2, as well as platelet:RBC ratios greater than 1:2.[9]

This apparent survival advantage associated with high FFP:RBC transfusion ratios could be explained by a "survival bias." Blood products are often not administered evenly and simultaneously in clinical practice, and many deaths occur early. This introduces the possibility that the survival benefit observed among patients receiving a higher FFP:RBC ratio merely reflects the fact that they live long enough to receive the higher ratio of products. Several investigations have reported that the association between higher FFP:RBC ratios and improved survival is not statistically significant when adjusted for survival bias.[10,11] One prospective observational study indicates that a 1:1 FFP:RBC ratio does not provide any additional benefit over ratios of 1:2 to 3:4, and that the hemostatic benefits of plasma therapy are limited to coagulopathic patients.[12] Some suggest that one of the reasons for these conflicting results is that the survival benefit of using 1:1 FFP to RBC is relatively small and only apparent within the first 3 hours of resuscitation.[13] The American Association of Blood Banks and the European task force recommend early intervention with FFP but stop short of endorsing a preset FFP:RBC ratio.

Recently, Ho and colleagues evaluated the presence of survivor bias in studies where 1:1 FFP:RBC ratios were used during massive transfusion of trauma patients.[14] Massive transfusion was defined as 10 units or more of RBCs transfused over the first 24 hours of hospitalization. Twenty-six studies were identified out of an initial pool of 216 abstracts selected from a MEDLINE search.

Studies in which cohorts were compared before and after a massive transfusion ratio of 1:1 was implemented (so-called "before and after" studies) were not considered to have a survivor bias, nor were studies in which the FFP:RBC ratio was considered a time-dependent covariate in the statistical analysis. Studies were considered "survivor bias-prone" if they included all patients from time of hospital admission (given that early deaths often received a lower FFP:RBC ratio). Studies in which patients were included only if they survived the first few hours of resuscitation or until intensive care unit admission were also considered to have a survivor bias. Overall, 21 of the 26 studies evaluated demonstrated an association between "1:1" and survival. Of those, only 10 did not have a survivor bias for or against "1:1" transfusion ratios.

A well-controlled randomized trial could answer the question of survivor bias more conclusively. The Pragmatic Randomized Optimum Platelet and Plasma Ratio (PROPPR) trial is an ongoing multicenter, prospective, randomized study that will evaluate different blood product ratios to be administered to trauma patients in need of more than 10 units of RBCs in the first 24 hours. This may offer an opportunity to prospectively evaluate the ideal ratio of blood products for use in trauma.

While massive transfusion is life-saving when indicated, there can be significant side effects.[15] A unit of red cells, mixed with a unit of platelets and a unit of plasma, has a hematocrit of 29% and a platelet count of approximately 85,000/μL. Transfusion of large volumes of these blood products can result in dilutional thrombocytopenia and coagulopathy. The cycle of hypothermia, acidosis and coagulopathy is well known in trauma and can be worsened by massive transfusion. In addition to the coagulopathic effect of hypothermia, the low temperatures commonly seen in trauma patients can decrease hepatic metabolism and drug clearance (see Chapter 14). Other complications of massive transfusion include transfusion-related lung injury and electrolyte abnormalities, including hypocalcemia and hyperkalemia.

Transfusion-related acute lung injury (TRALI) is defined as a partial pressure of oxygen in the arterial blood / fraction of inspired oxygen ratio (PaO_2/FiO_2 ratio) < 300 mmHg, bilateral pulmonary infiltrates, and absence of elevated pulmonary capillary wedge pressure or left atrial hypertension, all within 6 hours of blood transfusion. Even a small amount of transfused blood can lead to lung injury. A risk–benefit analysis of transfusion after control of bleeding must be undertaken to mitigate the increase in mortality seen in TRALI. Of course, patients who are actively bleeding must continue to be aggressively resuscitated. Treatment includes supportive therapy such as lung-protective ventilatory strategies (see Chapter 19) and limitation of unnecessary crystalloid administration.

Transfusion-associated circulatory overload (TACO) is a problem of pressure overload resulting in hydrostatic pulmonary edema, in contradistinction to TRALI, which is a problem of pulmonary vascular permeability. Assessment of diastolic dysfunction can help differentiate these two entities (see Chapter 10). Comparison of transmitral Doppler flow during early diastole and again during atrial contraction (E/A ratio) during cardiac echocardiography affords a quantitative and reproducible measure of diastolic function. Tissue Doppler (transmitral to mitral annular early diastolic velocity ratio, E/Ea or E/Em) and pulmonary venous flow velocities are routinely employed to assess diastolic function.

Transfusion of as few as 4 units of RBCs results in systemic inflammatory response syndrome (SIRS), compounding the hyperinflammatory response already seen with the initial traumatic insult. Transfusion-related immunomodulation is a poorly understood consequence of blood transfusion. In transfusion- associated micro-chimerism (TA-MC) a small population of donor hematopoietic stem cells engraft into the recipient, persisting sometimes for years. The clinical effect of this phenomenon is not clear, but it underscores the potent and enduring effects that transfusion can have on the immune system of a massively transfused trauma patient.

Immune response to trauma and resuscitation

The role that inflammation plays in trauma is the subject of great investigative interest. Perhaps a "Grand Unified Theory" of medicine will clarify the pathophysiology of acute illness as it pertains to the immune response. Conceivably, the inflammatory response of acute myocardial infarction, sepsis, and trauma may all be defined by one final common pathway. To better understand the role of inflammation in trauma, an appreciation of basic clinical immunology is necessary.

T cells are made up of two major subtypes, CD4+ and CD8+. CD4+ cells (helper T cells) are further divided into Th1 and Th2 subtypes. Th1 cells are responsible for cell-mediated response by activating macrophages and producing IL-2 and interferon gamma. Th2 cells are responsible for humoral response by assisting B cells with the production of antibodies. CD4+ cells (helper T cells) are activated when microbes are phagocytosed by antigen-presenting cells (e.g., macrophages, dendritic cells, B cells), whereupon the antigen is presented to the CD4+ receptor via the major histocompatibility complex II on the antigen-presenting cell. A second stimulatory signal is necessary for activation of the Th1 cell and production of cytokines. CD8+ cells (cytotoxic T cells) kill infected cells. Cytotoxic T cells are activated after proteins are presented to the CD8+ receptor via major histocompatibility complex I. Interleukin -2 (IL-2) from Th1 cells act as a second stimulator to activate the cytotoxic T cell to kill via induction of apoptosis.

B cells produce antibodies. Variable light- and heavy-chain portions of the antibody recognize antigens, while the Fc portion of the antibody fixes complement. Antibodies play important roles in preventing bacterial adherence to cell membranes, phagocytosis, and complement activation. Antibody production on B cells is assisted by CD4+ (helper T cell) activation. Production of IL-4, IL-5 and IL-10 from Th2 cells acts as a primary signal, followed by CD40 receptor stimulation on CD4+ (helper T cells).

The complement system involves a complex interaction of proteins that affect the inflammatory response and humoral immunity. Complement is activated via either the classic or the alternative pathway. Complement fulfills a number of functions including opsonization, viral neutralization, and cytolysis by membrane attack complex. Cytokines secreted by macrophages play important roles in the immune response. IL-1 is an important mediator of the inflammatory response, IL-8 serves as a chemotactic factor for neutrophils, and tumor necrosis factor alpha (TNF-α) has a role in endothelium activation and the resultant "vascular leak" that can accompany sepsis. Cytokines produced by Th1 cells include IL-2 and interferon gamma (IFN-γ). IL-2 stimulates helper and cytotoxic T cells.

IFN-γ inhibits Th2 cells and has an important antiviral function. Th2 cells secrete IL-4, IL-5 and IL-10. IL-10 inhibits Th1 cells and modulates the immune response.

Transfusion and inflammation

Blood transfusions can increase SIRS and mortality in trauma patients.[16] One study prospectively evaluated over 7000 trauma patients and found 954 had received blood transfusions in the first 24 hours of trauma center admission. Transfused patients were older, with higher Injury Severity Scores (ISS) and lower Glasgow Coma Scale (GCS) scores. Transfusion was found to be an independent predictor for intensive care unit (ICU) admission, mortality, and SIRS. Trauma patients who had received blood transfusions had a significantly increased risk of developing SIRS, with odds ratios ranging from 2.1 to 5.1. Association of blood transfusion with mortality had a similarly increased odds ratio (4.2), as did the association between transfusion and ICU admission (4.6).

Innate immune dysfunction in trauma involves complex interplay between a variety of immune-modulatory mechanisms (Fig. 6.1).[17] Much like microbial activation of pathogen-associated molecular patterns (PAMPs), the release of endogenous damage-associated molecular patterns (DAMPs) activates innate immunity.[18] Mitochondrial DAMPs, released after injury, activate polymorphonuclear neutrophils via a toll-like receptor 9 (TLR9) pathway. Mitochondrial DAMPs released after trauma bear an evolutionary similarity to bacterial PAMPs, providing a key link in the relationship between inflammation, trauma, and SIRS.

How exactly injury interacts with inflammation is not clearly understood. A variety of immune-regulatory pathways can counteract the deleterious effects of the innate immune response that characterizes SIRS.[19] Efforts to understand and manipulate the adaptive immune response of the compensatory anti-inflammatory response syndrome have demonstrated that injury induces an upregulation of Th2 phenotypic expression, with a suppression of Th1 immune function. The rapid expression of inflammatory cytokines such as TNF and IL-1, IL-6 and IL-10 suggest an innate immune cell source.

Factors related to injury (e.g., heat shock proteins and high-mobility group proteins) may induce an inflammatory response via toll-like receptor (TLR) pathways, thus providing a mechanistic link between injury and the inflammatory response. After injury the TLR4 response is augmented, whereas in sepsis the TLR4 response is not increased. This suggests an ability to upregulate the immune response to fight infection after injury, but to also attenuate that effect when TLR4-driven responses may be harmful. The balance between SIRS and compensatory anti-inflammatory response syndrome is fundamental to an overall understanding of the inflammatory response to injury.

Efforts to support immune function while avoiding unwanted inflammatory results have yielded improvements with immune-modulating diets rich in arginine, omega-3 fatty acids and antioxidants.[20] L-arginine can improve wound

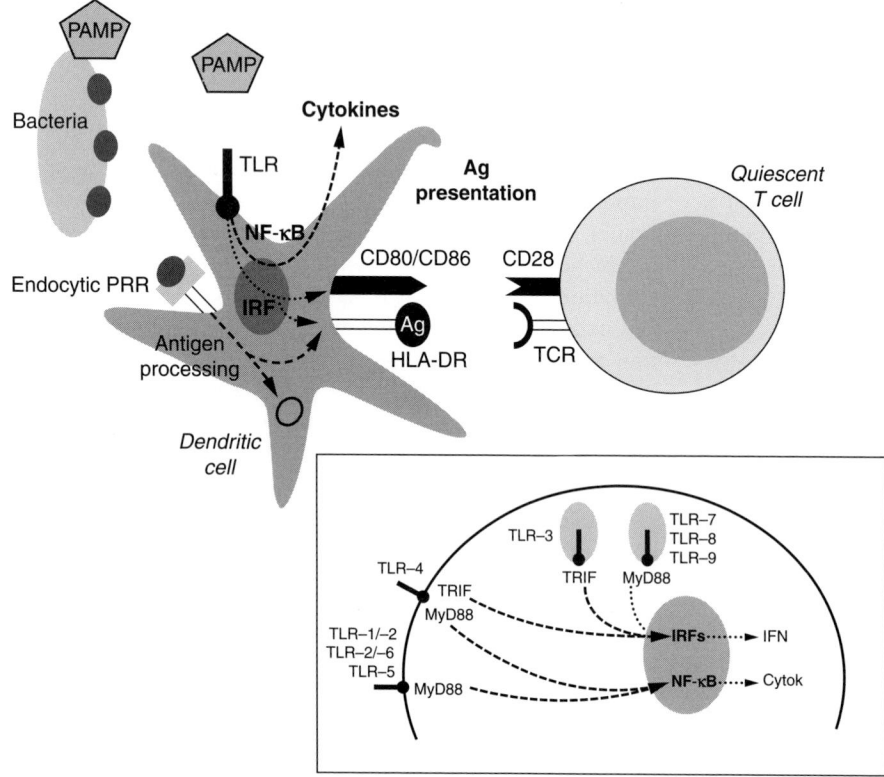

Figure 6.1 Innate immune function in trauma: functions of the dendritic cell. Pathogen-associated molecular patterns, expressed by bacteria, are recognized by toll-like receptors. Activation of the toll-like receptor signaling pathways induces expression of nuclear factor κ-dependent cytokines and interferon regulatory factor-dependent costimulatory molecules, CD80 and CD86. Pattern-recognition receptors mediate the phagocytosis of pathogens by dendritic cells. Proteins derived from the microorganisms are processed to generate antigens. The major-histocompatibility-complex class II molecules present antigens to the T-cell receptor, activating T cells. Recognition of the costimulatory molecules (CD80 and CD86) by CD28 on T cell membrane is required to fully activate T cells.

Ag, antigens; CD80, CD86, costimulatory molecules; DC, dendritic cell; HLA-DR, histocompatibility-complex class II molecules; IRF, interferon regulatory factor; NF-κB, nuclear factor κB; PAMP, pathogen-associated molecular patterns; PRR, pattern-recognition receptors; TCR, T-cell receptor; TLR, toll-like receptors. (Reproduced with permission from Asehnoune et al., 2012.[17])

A black and white version of this figure will appear in some formats. For the color version, please refer to the plate section.

healing and restore postoperative macrophage function and lymphocyte responsiveness. A shift in Th1/Th2 balance occurs following surgery and trauma, with a predominant Th2/anti-inflammatory response. Th2 cells secrete anti-inflammatory cytokines, as well as inhibiting macrophage activation and proinflammatory cytokines. Omega-3 fatty acids can shift the balance of Th1/Th2 in favor of a Th1 response.

In trauma, the inflammatory response is sufficient to block nuclear factor kappa-light-chain-enhancer of activated B cells (NF-κB) translocation from the first day post injury. This effect is seen for at least 10 days.[21] NF-κB is present in the enhancer and promoter regions of several important proinflammatory cytokines, and a decreased ability of leukocytes to mount an inflammatory response following trauma may lead to greater susceptibility to sepsis and higher mortality.

High-mobility group box 1 (HMGB1) is a DNA binding protein with potent proinflammatory properties. It is an important mediator of organ system dysfunction, such as acute lung injury (ALI), and increases mortality in animal models. It is also expressed in the lung after hemorrhage.[22] Anti-HMGB1 antibodies decrease the levels of proinflammatory cytokines and can improve survival. Blockade of HMGB1 via this mechanism can attenuate haemorrhage-induced increase in inflammatory cytokines, expression of NF-κB, and development of interstitial edema in the lung. The authors of this study speculate that trauma patients who are evaluated in trauma centers soon after injury and before ALI develops, may benefit from anti-HMGB1 therapy.

Vasopressors in resuscitation

Complications of massive transfusion, such as volume overload, respiratory failure, and TRALI, raise the question of the role vasopressors play in the management of resuscitation. An ICU database query at a Level I trauma center evaluated 1349 patients who were admitted to the ICU.[23] Patients were grouped according to exposure to dopamine, epinephrine, phenylephrine, norepinephrine, or vasopressin within the first 24 hours of ICU admission; or no exposure to any vasopressors. The patients were further grouped according to hypovolemia, as defined by a central venous pressure < 8 mmHg. Mortality in the vasopressor group was 43.6%, compared to mortality of 4.2% in the control group. In the vasopressor group, hypovolemia was not independently associated with higher mortality. The study offers important insights into the risks of vasopressor use in trauma. It is important to note, however, that this population had survived long enough to be admitted to the ICU, suggesting a possible survivor bias.

A prospective multicenter cohort study evaluated 921 blunt trauma patients in hemorrhagic shock who had survived 48 hours.[24] Those who survived and had received any vasopressor (including norepinephrine, vasopressin, dopamine, or phenylephrine) within 12 hours after injury had an 80% higher risk of mortality (hazard ratio = 1.8). Interestingly, the 95% confidence interval for the hazard ratio for mortality crossed unity

in patients who had received vasopressin, suggesting nonsignificance. The authors further compared early vasopressor use with "aggressive early crystalloid resuscitation" (defined as crystalloid resuscitation > 16 L at 12 hours and 20 L at 24 hours!). The authors noted a reduction in mortality associated with crystalloid use (hazard ratio = 0.59). Given the current trend toward transfusion of blood products and away from aggressive crystalloid resuscitation, the relevance of these data is difficult to determine.

Alternatives to transfusion

Adjunctive therapy includes pharmacologic agents that can maintain blood pressure, attenuate the systemic inflammatory response, and improve outcome in trauma. This approach is of increased significance in situations where the patient continues to deteriorate in spite of massive transfusion and surgery.

Tranexamic acid

Tranexamic acid (TXA) is a synthetic lysine derivative that competitively inhibits lysine binding sites on plasminogen, blocking the conversion of plasminogen to plasmin. This inhibits the proteolytic action of plasmin on fibrin clot and platelet receptors, and serves as an effective antifibrinolytic.

In a prospective multicenter trial (CRASH-2), 20,211 trauma patients were randomized to receive either TXA or placebo.[25] Mortality decreased from 16% in the placebo group to 14.5% in those treated with a 1 g bolus of TXA followed by an infusion of 1 g over 8 hours. The risk of death from bleeding was also reduced from 5.7% to 4.9%. There was no significant difference in death from vascular occlusive events (including myocardial infarction, stroke, and pulmonary embolus), multiorgan failure (MOF) or head injury. Inclusion in the study required a clinical assessment of hemorrhage. The clinical diagnosis of traumatic hemorrhage can be surprisingly difficult, and the authors acknowledged that some patients might have been included in the study who were not bleeding at the time of randomization. The large patient sample and numerous participating centers, however, can effectively exclude a large-scale inclusion bias. Although a decrease in the risk of death was conferred by TXA, the exact mechanism of action for this effect remains to be determined. Although it is presumably due to an antifibrinolytic effect, the authors did not document any measure of fibrinolytic activity.

Two hundred and seventy adult trauma patients at risk for extracranial bleeding, who also had a traumatic brain injury, were included in a subgroup analysis of the CRASH-2 trial.[26] Computed tomography (CT) was used to measure intracranial hemorrhage growth. There was no difference in mean total hemorrhage growth between the TXA arm and placebo. Also, new focal ischemic lesions were not significantly different in the two groups. It was thought that a decrease in the size of the intracranial hemorrhage would decrease local pressure on arteries and therefore decrease the risk of ischemia. This effect, however, was not demonstrated. A follow-up study, the CRASH-3 trial, will examine head injury more closely.

The Military Application of Tranexamic Acid in Trauma and Emergency Resuscitation (MATTERs) study evaluated the use of TXA in 293 wounded combatants suffering from hemorrhagic shock.[27] Despite more severe injuries, unadjusted mortality was lower in the TXA group. Patients who received massive transfusion (> 10 units of packed red blood cells [pRBCs] within 24 h) benefited the most from the administration of TXA, with improved survival and less coagulopathy.

In children undergoing craniosynostosis surgery, TXA decreases blood loss and transfusion requirements.[28] Forty-three children received either TXA (50 mg/kg bolus followed by an infusion of 5 mg/kg/h) or placebo. Compared to the placebo arm, the TXA group had significantly less blood loss, and significantly lower transfusion requirements. TXA plasma concentrations were maintained above in-vitro-derived thresholds for inhibition of fibrinolysis and plasmin-induced platelet activation. Interestingly, thromboelastograph (TEG) parameters (reaction time, coagulation time, maximum amplitude, alpha angle, and fibrinolysis) were no different in the two groups. This suggests a localized, rather than systemic, site of action and provides some insight into the mechanism of action for TXA. In an interesting cost analysis of TXA, 40 pediatric patients undergoing craniosynostosis surgery, who were pretreated with erythropoietin, were evaluated.[29] The volume of erythrocytes transfused was significantly reduced with administration of TXA, conferring significant savings (given a cost of US$0.70 per 500 mg TXA vs. US$240 per unit RBC).

Tranexamic acid can improve survival and reduce transfusion requirements, and it offers a lower-cost alternative in resuscitation of the trauma patient. Western European militaries (specifically the United Kingdom) use TXA as part of their resuscitation plan for the wounded combatant. A thoughtful evaluation of its use may also offer benefit to the severely injured trauma patient in the United States.

Vasopressin

Vasopressin is a potent vasoconstrictor that spares cerebral, pulmonary, and cardiac vascular beds. Although vasopressors in general are associated with increased mortality in trauma, vasopressin may prove to be an exception to the rule. Physiologically, vasopressin-mediated vasoconstriction decreases transmural pressure at the site of injury and facilitates clot formation. Pharmacologic amplification of the neuroendocrine stress response with vasopressin may provide further benefit.[30] Vasopressin also acts as a potent endogenous vasoconstrictor in low cardiac output states, with decreased vasopressin levels contributing to the shock state. Depletion of neurohypophyseal stores may contribute to this vasodilatory shock. Vasopressin blocks a number of vasodilatory pathways in shock, including potassium-ATP channels on vascular smooth muscle, and cGMP pathways via a nitric oxide/atrial naturetic peptide pathway.[31]

Of the several vasopressin subtypes (V1a, V1b and V2), V1a receptors are thought to mediate vasoconstriction on arterial smooth muscle via an increase in cytoplasmic calcium via the phosphatidyl–inositol–bisphosphonate pathway. Vasopressin is significantly more potent than norepinephrine and angiotensin II, and maintains its efficacy in hypoxia and severe acidosis, where catecholamines may not be as effective.[32]

A number of animal studies have demonstrated improved blood pressure and survival in subjects with profound hypovolemic shock treated with vasopressin. One porcine model utilizing liver injury to produce hemorrhagic shock demonstrated improved short-term survival with vasopressin.[33] Twenty-one pigs were injured, and then resuscitated with either vasopressin (0.4 U/kg), an equal volume of placebo, or 1 L each of lactated Ringer's and hetastarch. The vasopressin arm had higher mean arterial pressures and improved abdominal organ blood flow (as measured by ultrasound flowprobe) without further blood loss. All seven animals in the vasopressin arm survived until surgical control of hemorrhage, whereas all seven of the placebo and all seven of the fluid-resuscitation animals died. In another animal model, 21 pigs subjected to a standardized liver injury were resuscitated with either vasopressin (0.4 U/kg then 0.04 U/kg/min), epinephrine (45 μg/kg then 5 μg/kg/min), or saline placebo.[34] Mean arterial pressure was higher in the vasopressin arm at 2.5 and 10 minutes. Hepatic and renal artery blood flow was also significantly higher, with no increased bleeding. All seven animals in the vasopressin arm survived until surgical correction of bleeding (plus 60 minutes) without further vasopressor support, whereas all 14 animals in the epinephrine and placebo groups died.

In a canine hemorrhagic shock model, seven animals were resuscitated with blood and norepinephrine to maintain a mean arterial pressure of 40 mmHg.[35] Following an hour of aggressive resuscitation, vasopressin (1–4 mU/kg/min) was initiated, with improvement in the mean arterial pressure from 39 to 128 mmHg. Administration of angiotensin II only marginally increased the blood pressure. Plasma vasopressin levels, although elevated initially, were low immediately before vasopressin administration, suggesting the possibility of vasopressin depletion in late-stage hemorrhagic shock.

While animal studies have been encouraging, case reports form the bulk of the experience with humans. In one remarkable case report, a 41-year-old woman suffered a fall from a roof and was resuscitated with RBCs and coagulation factors prior to transport to a trauma center.[36] At the trauma center, an aggressive resuscitation was continued with fluids and norepinephrine, but the patient continued to be hemodynamically unstable. An infusion of high-dose vasopressin (10 U/min) was initiated, with sufficient stabilization of the blood pressure to emergently embolize bleeding pelvic blood vessels. Despite numerous orthopedic injuries, a liver injury, and a subdural hematoma, the patient was ultimately discharged from the ICU with no neurologic deficit.

Other case reports describe patients who suffered intraoperative or postoperative bleeding. In these cases low-dose vasopressin infusions (0.04 U/min) improved short-term survival.[37] In one case of a portal vein injury during surgery, a patient suffered systolic blood pressures in the 50s with a base deficit of –21 mEq/L. Following surgical correction of the injury, fluid resuscitation, and a norepinephrine infusion, the patient was admitted to the ICU, where a low-dose vasopressin infusion was part of the continued resuscitation. The authors speculate that in cases of advanced hemorrhagic shock, acidotic, vasodilated patients who are poorly responsive to volume and catecholamines may benefit from vasopressin. Other reports document cases of aortic and liver surgery in which patients suffered profound and prolonged hypotension secondary to hemorrhage.[38] Low-dose vasopressin infusions were part of an aggressive resuscitation in which patients survived.

While evidence of the utility of vasopressin in animal models and case reports is encouraging, there are few data from human trials. A multicenter European trial had hoped to evaluate prehospital administration of vasopressin versus 0.9% saline, but follow-up results have not been forthcoming.[39,40] Another project, the Arginine Vasopressin During the Early Resuscitation of Traumatic Shock (AVERT) study, is a phase 2 clinical trial that is recruiting patients to evaluate the use of vasopressin supplementation in the resuscitation of trauma patients, as well as the utility of using copeptin as a biomarker for vasopressin. Trauma patients who receive 6 or more units of blood product within 12 hours of arrival will receive either a 10-unit vasopressin bolus in addition to an infusion to maintain a mean arterial pressure $\geq$ 65 mmHg for 48 hours, or placebo. Data will be collected prospectively for 5 days post injury. The study will evaluate the need for blood and crystalloid resuscitation, as well as the incidence of transfusion related complications. It will be exciting to see what becomes of the results of these studies.

Recombinant factor VIIa

Recombinant factor VIIa (rFVIIa) accelerates formation of thrombin at the site of endothelial injury. It is thought to act locally at the site of tissue injury by binding to exposed tissue factor and generating a tight fibrin hemostatic plug through increased thrombin generation.

Initially used in hemophiliac patients, rFVIIa has also proven useful in the bleeding post-surgical patient. Initial case series in cardiac surgery reported favorable results with rFVIIa. In one assessment of five patients who underwent a variety of cardiac surgical procedures and received rFVIIa 30 µg/kg, "satisfactory haemostasis" was achieved with no adverse events.[41] A recent meta-analysis, however, found an increased risk of stroke with the use of rFVIIa in cardiac surgery with no significant reduction in the need for surgical re-exploration.[42] There was no difference in the rate of death.

In patients bleeding during prostate surgery, a 40 µg/kg bolus of rFVIIa produced a dose-dependent decrease in bleeding, as well as a decreased need for blood transfusion.[43] Patients were followed for 10 days postoperatively to screen for complications, including screening for venous thromboembolism via ultrasound examination of both legs. None of the patients suffered adverse events.

A group of 399 neurosurgical patients with intracerebral hemorrhage received either placebo or rFVIIa in doses of 40 µg/kg, 80 µg/kg, or 160 µg/kg.[44] The volume of intracerebral hemorrhage, as measured on CT scan, was decreased in all three groups treated with rFVIIa. Severe disability (as measured by modified Rankin Scale score) was higher in the control group. Ninety-day mortality was decreased in the rFVIIa groups. There was, however, a significant increase in arterial thromboembolic events in those treated with rFVIIa. A small case series of nine neurosurgical patients received rFVIIa in doses of 40–90 µg/kg prior to surgery.[45] Patients suffered from a variety of coagulation abnormalities including liver dysfunction, use of anticoagulation medication, and dilutional coagulopathy after trauma. Prothrombin time (PT), partial thromboplastin time (PTT) and international normalized ratio (INR) all normalized within 20 minutes of rFVIIa administration. No postoperative hemorrhagic or thromboembolic complications were noted in this observational study.

The use of rFVIIa in trauma was investigated in an audit of a multicenter trauma registry in which 380 patients received rFVIIa.[46] Death from hemorrhage was reported at a rate of 30%. rFVIIa nonresponders tended to have a pH < 7.1, platelet counts < 100,000/µL, and blood pressure $\leq$ 90 mmHg. A varied range of rFVIIa doses, as well as a broad range of "time to first dose of rFVIIa," make interpretation of these data difficult. In a case series of 81 heterogeneous trauma patients, rFVIIa reversed coagulopathy, as measured by decreased PT in 75% of patients.[47] While coagulation abnormalities were corrected, an outcome benefit was not demonstrated. Lower arterial pH, higher lactate, and worse base deficit were most predictive of rFVIIa nonresponders.

A retrospective database review evaluated the use of rFVIIa in combat casualties with high injury severity scores who had received massive transfusion.[48] Forty-nine of 124 patients received rFVIIa. Those patients who did not receive rFVIIa had lower temperature and lower admission systolic blood pressure. Twenty-four-hour and 30-day mortality were significantly decreased in the rFVIIa group. There was no statistically significant difference in death from hemorrhage between the two groups, nor was there an increase in the risk of severe thromboembolic events, such as pulmonary embolisms, deep venous thrombosis, or stroke. The efficacy of rFVIIa versus placebo at controlling bleeding in penetrating trauma and blunt trauma was evaluated in a randomized control trial.[49] RBC transfusions were significantly decreased with the use of rFVIIa in blunt trauma. Nonsignificant trends toward decreased RBC transfusion were observed in penetrating trauma. Thromboembolic complications in the placebo and rFVIIa groups were similar. This study is significant in that it represents one of the few efforts to subject rFVIIa use to a randomized, placebo-controlled trial.

While rFVIIa can reverse coagulation abnormalities and decrease blood loss, a well-defined outcome benefit is less clear. Use of rFVIIa merits consideration in trauma patients undergoing massive transfusion who continue to exsanguinate, with an understanding of the limitations of its effect.

Concentrated coagulation factors

Concentrated coagulation factors offer the advantage of targeting specific phases of the coagulation process with a minimal amount of volume. Fibrinogen concentrate is one such factor. Stinger and colleagues evaluated 252 patients to determine the effect of increased ratios of fibrinogen to RBC on mortality in patients who had received a massive transfusion at a military combat support hospital.[50] The typical amount of fibrinogen in each unit of blood product was used to calculate the fibrinogen-to-RBC ratio (F:R). High F:R was defined as 0.48 g fibrinogen/unit RBC and low F:R was defined as 0.1 g fibrinogen/unit RBC. Mortality in the high F:R group was 24%, compared to 52% in the low F:R group. Death from hemorrhage was also higher in the low F:R group. Logistic regression modeling demonstrated that F:R ratio was independently associated with mortality (odds ratio = 0.37). While the fibrinogen content of various blood products (e.g., fresh whole blood, fresh frozen plasma, cryoprecipitate) can be estimated, such estimations introduced an element of unreliability into the calculation of overall fibrinogen content. Ultimately, however, a mortality benefit was demonstrated, presumably due to improved clot firmness following fibrinogen administration.

Prothrombin complex concentrate (PCC) contains factor II, VII, IX, X and protein C. It has typically been used to treat hereditary coagulation disorders and to antagonize anticoagulation therapy. In a porcine model of uncontrolled hemorrhage and subsequent dilutional coagulopathy, fibrinogen and PCC together were able to restore impaired clot formation, reduce blood loss, and decrease mortality.[51] Twenty pigs were anesthetized and then had approximately 65% of their blood volume withdrawn and replaced with hydroxyethyl starch (HES). The animals were then randomized to receive either fibrinogen (200 mg/kg) and PCC (35 IU/kg) or placebo. Blood loss was significantly less in the fibrinogen + PCC group. Mortality was 80% in the control group, compared to zero in the treatment group. While this study offers insight into the role of fibrinogen and PCC in trauma, the large HES transfusion makes it difficult to translate this result into patients who have received massive blood transfusions.

Animal studies have been encouraging, but the efficacy of PCC has not been demonstrated in prospective human trials, and some investigators caution against its "uncritical" administration.[52] In one animal study fibrinogen and PCC decreased bleeding at the risk of fatal thromboembolism.[53] Following removal of approximately 60% of their blood volume,

50 anesthetized pigs were resuscitated with HES and randomized to receive fibrinogen, fibrinogen + PCC, fibrinogen + factor II, fibrinogen + factor II + factor VII + factor X, or saline. A standardized liver injury model was used to induce uncontrolled hemorrhage. Fibrinogen + factor II, as well as fibrinogen + PCC, improved survival. Additionally, all treatment groups saw a significant decrease in bleeding. One fatal thromboembolic event occurred in an animal that received fibrinogen + PCC.

Retrospective reports and animals studies on the use of fibrinogen in trauma are encouraging, but larger trials of prospective data are lacking. Ideally a large multicenter trial would produce a well-powered evaluation of the ideal "coagulation cocktail."

Hypotensive resuscitation

The concern that massive transfusion may worsen bleeding has led some investigators to advocate a plan of hypotensive resuscitation. The concept of hypotensive resuscitation dates back to World War I, when surgeons advocated limited fluid resuscitation of casualties out of concern for worsening blood loss prior to source control as a result of overcoming the hemostatic force of an established clot. A well-referenced study by Bickell et al. evaluated patients with penetrating torso trauma and a prehospital systolic blood pressure < 90 mmHg.[54] Patients received either standard crystalloid resuscitation or placement of intravenous access only. The investigators found that the delayed-resuscitation group had an improvement in mortality, acute respiratory distress syndrome (ARDS), sepsis, and other complications. Another study randomized trauma patients to be resuscitated either to a systolic blood pressure of 110 mmHg or to a systolic blood pressure of 70 mmHg.[55] There was no significant difference in mortality between the two groups. The authors speculated that this may be due to the heterogeneous nature of traumatic injury and the imprecision of systolic blood pressure as a marker for tissue perfusion.

The Resuscitation Outcomes Consortium has completed a study to prospectively evaluate hypotensive resuscitation strategies in penetrating and blunt trauma: the Field Trial of Hypotensive Resuscitation versus Standard Resuscitation in Patients with Hemorrhagic Shock after Trauma. Patients with a prehospital systolic blood pressure ≤ 90 mmHg were randomized to either the standard resuscitation group (2 L normal saline rapidly plus additional fluid to maintain a systolic blood pressure of 110 mmHg) or a hypotensive strategy (500 mL total of normal saline if the systolic blood pressure is < 70 mmHg or the radial pulse is absent). As the results of this interesting study are evaluated, they may help elucidate the optimal blood pressure trigger for transfusion in trauma patients.

It is possible, however, that systolic blood pressure is an imperfect measure of the efficacy of resuscitation and transfusion in trauma. Other more appropriate markers may include base excess/deficit, lactate, and/or viscoelastic testing such as TEG and rotational thromboelastometry (ROTEM).

Laboratory evaluation of transfusion and resuscitation

Oxygen serves as the final electron acceptor in the electron transport chain. When oxygen is no longer available, the cell switches to anaerobic metabolism. As lactate and other organic acids accumulate an acid excess, or base deficit, begins to build. Base deficit is the amount of base required to bring a sample of blood to a pH of 7.4 at body temperature (37 °C) with a carbon dioxide tension of 40 mmHg.[56] This calculation removes the respiratory component from the evaluation of the resuscitation. Actual base excess measures the acid load in an in-vitro sample, whereas the standard base excess calculates the acid load in a sample of extracellular fluid containing a hemoglobin (Hgb) of 5 g/dL, approximately one-third of the Hgb concentration in blood. Given that the base deficit is commonly evaluated with the arterial blood gas, and can sometimes be assayed in the OR, it may offer a more timely evaluation of the resuscitation than other laboratory studies.

A retrospective review of 2954 trauma patients found that transfusion requirement increased in patients with severe base deficit.[57] Seventy-two percent of patients with a base deficit worse than –6 required transfusion within 24 hours of admission, as opposed to 18% of patients with base deficit better than –6. A more severely deranged base deficit portended longer ICU and hospital length of stay, as well as higher frequency of ARDS, renal failure, coagulopathy, and MOF. In trauma, deranged base excess portends higher mortality. In one study 674 trauma patients with a base deficit worse than –6 within 1 hour of admission were evaluated.[58] Patients were categorized as having moderate (–6 to –9) or severe (worse than –10) base deficit. Survivors improved their base deficit and normalized their base deficit faster than nonsurvivors. Patients who did not improve their base deficit better than –6 had an increased incidence or ARDS, MOF, and death.

There are important considerations affecting the utility of base deficit evaluation in trauma. For instance, base deficit can be deranged by hyperchloremic metabolic acidosis, which often accompanies aggressive resuscitation with 0.9% saline solutions. Alcohol ingestion can also contribute to metabolic acidosis and affect the base deficit. The often coincident occurrence of alcohol intoxication and trauma serves as an important consideration when evaluating the patient's acid–base status. Patients with chronic renal failure and/or on renal replacement therapy in the ICU will have altered acid–base state at baseline, limiting the utility of base deficit in this population.

Elevated lactate levels suggest an imbalance between oxygen delivery and metabolic rate, with lactate levels higher than 4 mmol/L portending higher mortality. Other reasons for elevated lactate include microbial production of D-lactic acid, glycolysis stimulated by alkalosis, and impaired hepatic clearance of lactate. While liver failure can decrease clearance of lactate, it is unclear to what extent liver injury in the acute phase of trauma affects lactate levels. In a recent study of

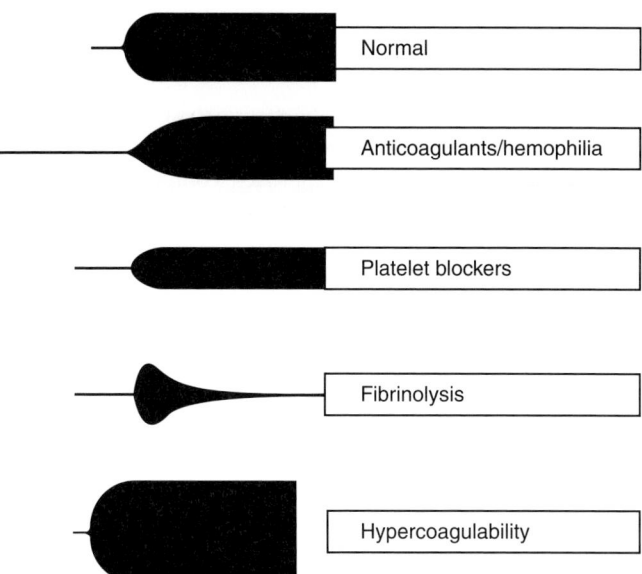

Figure 6.2 Examples of normal and abnormal tracings on TEG. (Reproduced with permission from da Luz LT, Nascimento B, Rizoli S. Thrombelastography (TEG(R)): practical considerations on its clinical use in trauma resuscitation. *Scand J Trauma Resus Emerg Med* 2013; **21**: 29.)

586 trauma patients, elevated lactate levels were associated with higher mortality. Early clearance of lactate (within 2 hours) provided a prognostic variable for decision making.[59] The authors suggested a "categorical approach" with a lactate clearance of 20% per hour or lower established as a threshold during resuscitation in trauma.

With thromboelastography (TEG) a sample of blood is placed under gentle rotational agitation in a cuvette. A torsion wire submerged in the blood sample transmits pressure changes to a graphic display where a characteristic waveform is generated (Fig. 6.2). The reaction time (R value), lasts from the start of the assay until the waveform amplitude reaches 2 mm. This is an enzymatic process that presents initial clot formation due to clotting factors. Prolonged R values can be treated with plasma. Clot kinetic time (K) lasts from R until the amplitude reaches 20 mm. This is an effect of clot kinetics and represents time to form clot, fibrinogen and the platelet plug. Maximal amplitude (MA) represents the clot strength and is a qualitative measure of platelet function. It measures the ultimate strength of the clot as it pertains to fibrin–platelet interactions via glycoprotein IIb/IIIa. Low MA can be treated with platelet transfusion. The alpha angle (α) measures the speed with which clot strengthening and crosslinking occurs; along with the MA, it is a measure of clot kinetics. Clot lysis at 30 minutes after the MA (LY30) defines the overall stability of the clot. An elevated LY30 is treated with antifibrinolytics.

TEG is a rapid and reliable method to assess coagulation in the trauma patient. In one study evaluating 272 trauma patients, activated clotting time (ACT), R value, and K time correlated with INR, PT, and PTT.[60] MA and alpha angle correlated with platelet count. The authors found that an ACT > 128 predicted the need for massive transfusion within

6 hours of arrival. The utility of TEG has prompted some investigators to advocate for the replacement of conventional coagulation tests with TEG.[61]

ROTEM (rotational thromboelastometry) offers a similar assessment of clot formation, kinetics, and strength via a slightly different mechanical approach compared with TEG. With ROTEM, an optical detector is suspended in a blood-containing cuvette and then the detector is rotated. Although both ROTEM and TEG assess similar elements of the clotting process, differences between the two methods have been noted.[62] It is important, therefore, to have an understanding of the advantages and limitations of both.

Future options for massive transfusion in trauma

Future options for the multisystem trauma patient requiring massive transfusion may involve blood component therapy with significantly longer shelf-life, such as freeze-dried plasma. Currently in use in the French military, PCSD is a pH-buffered, freeze-dried plasma pooled from 8–10 donors with a 2-year shelf life. There have been no adverse events reported in 8 years of use of PCSD. A German freeze-dried plasma named LyoPlas is drawn from a single donor and has a shelf life of 1.5 years. It is type-specific and must be reconstituted with buffering solution.

An exciting possible future approach to the trauma patient requiring massive transfusion may be administration of TXA and freeze-dried plasma in the field. Efficient transportation to the trauma center will extend the critical care continuum to the injured patient. At the trauma center a team of surgeons, anesthesiologists, intensivists, interventional radiologists, and other emergency personnel will initiate a practiced MTP while gaining source control of bleeding.

Questions

(1) Which of the following does *not* meet the definition of massive transfusion?
   a. One blood volume loss in 24 hours
   b. 4 units of blood replaced in 4 hours
   c. Ongoing blood loss exceeding 150 mL/minute
   d. 10% blood volume loss in 3 hours

(2) The Assessment of Blood Consumption (ABC) score to predict the need for a massive transfusion protocol (MTP) includes:
   a. Presence of penetrating trauma
   b. Systolic blood pressure < 90 mmHg
   c. Heart rate > 120 bpm
   d. Positive focused assessment with sonography for trauma (FAST)
   e. all of the above

(3) A sample "massive transfusion cooler" may contain all of the following, *except*:
   a. 6 units of RBCs
   b. 6 units of FFP
   c. Recombinant factor VIIa

(4) Triggers for initiation of an MTP include:
   a. ABC score = 1
   b. hypovolemic hypotension uncorrected by ongoing resuscitation
   c. chest tube output = 50 mL/h
   d. 10 units blood loss anticipated within 12 hours
   e. (b) and (d)

(5) Which of the following vasopressors is the subject of an ongoing prospective trial during the early resuscitation of traumatic shock?
   a. Epinephrine
   b. Vasopressin
   c. Norepinephrine
   d. Phenylephrine

(6) The initial bolus dose of tranexamic acid evaluated in the CRASH-2 trial is:
   a. 2 g over 10 minutes
   b. 1 g over 8 hours
   c. 2 g over 10 minutes
   d. 1 g over 10 minutes

(7) True or false? Thrombelastography (TEG) is used in some medical centers in lieu of conventional coagulation tests.

(8) A low maximal amplitude (MA) on a TEG suggests the need to transfuse:
   a. Platelets
   b. Fresh frozen plasma
   c. Antifibrinolytics
   d. Packed red blood cells

(9) True or false? Anti-high mobility group box 1 antibodies may benefit trauma patients with acute lung injury (ALI) if administered soon after injury.

(10) Th2 cells produce all of the following, *except*:
   a. IL-1
   b. IL-4
   c. IL-5
   d. IL-10

Answers

(1) d
(2) e
(3) c
(4) e
(5) b
(6) d
(7) True
(8) a
(9) True
(10) a

References

1. Riskin DJ, Tsai TC, Riskin L, *et al.* Massive transfusion protocols: the role of aggressive resuscitation versus product ratio in mortality reduction. *J Am Coll Surg* 2009; **209**: 198–205.

2. Nunez TC, Voskresensky IV, Dossett LA, *et al.* Early prediction of massive transfusion in trauma: simple as ABC (assessment of blood consumption)? *J Trauma Acute Care Surg* 2009; **66**: 346–52.

3. Hoyt DB, Dutton RP, Hauser CJ, *et al.* Management of coagulopathy in the patients with multiple injuries: results from an international survey of clinical practice. *J Trauma Acute Care Surg* 2008; **65**: 755–64.

4. Hess JR, Holcomb JB, Hoyt DB. Damage control resuscitation: the need for specific blood products to treat the coagulopathy of trauma. *Transfusion* 2006; **46**: 685–6.

5. Gunter OL, Au BK, Isbell JM, *et al.* Optimizing outcomes in damage control resuscitation: identifying blood product ratios associated with improved survival. *J Trauma Acute Care Surg* 2008; **65**: 527–34.

6. Como JJ, Dutton RP, Scalea TM, Edelman BB, Hess JR. Blood transfusion rates in the care of acute trauma. *Transfusion* 2004; **44**: 809–13.

7. Malone DL, Hess JR, Fingerhut A. Massive transfusion practices around the globe and a suggestion for a common massive transfusion protocol. *J Trauma Acute Care Surg* 2006; **60** (6 Suppl): S91–6.

8. Borgman MA, Spinella PC, Perkins JG, *et al.* The ratio of blood products transfused affects mortality in patients receiving massive transfusions at a combat support hospital. *J Trauma Acute Care Surg* 2007; **63**: 805–13.

9. Holcomb JB, Wade CE, Michalek JE, *et al.* Increased plasma and platelet to red blood cell ratios improves outcome in 466 massively transfused civilian trauma patients. *Ann Surg* 2008; **248**: 447–58.

10. Snyder CW, Weinberg JA, McGwin G, *et al.* The relationship of blood product ratio to mortality: survival benefit or survival bias? *J Trauma Acute Care Surg* 2009; **66**: 358–62.

11. Magnotti LJ, Zarzaur BL, Fischer PE, *et al.* Improved survival after hemostatic resuscitation: does the emperor have no clothes? *J Trauma Acute Care Surg* 2011; **70**: 97–102.

12. Davenport R, Curry N, Manson J, *et al.* Hemostatic effects of fresh frozen plasma may be maximal at red cell ratios of 1: 2. *J Trauma Acute Care Surg* 2011; **70**: 90–5.

13. de Biasi AR, Stansbury LG, Dutton RP, *et al.* Blood product use in trauma resuscitation: plasma deficit versus plasma ratio as predictors of mortality in trauma. *Transfusion* 2011; **51**: 1925–32.

14. Ho AM, Dion PW, Yeung JH, *et al.* Prevalence of survivor bias in observational studies on fresh frozen plasma: erythrocyte ratios in trauma requiring massive transfusion. *Anesthesiology* 2012; **116**: 716–28.

15. Sihler KC, Napolitano LM. Complications of massive transfusion. *Chest* 2010; **137**: 209–20.

16. Dunne JR, Malone DL, Tracy JK, Napolitano LM. Allogenic blood transfusion in the first 24 hours after trauma is associated with increased systemic inflammatory response syndrome (SIRS) and death. *Surg Infect (Larchmt)* 2004; **5**: 395–404.

17. Asehnoune K, Roquilly A, Abraham E. Innate immune dysfunction in trauma patients: from pathophysiology to treatment. *Anesthesiology* 2012; **117**: 411–16.

18. Zhang Q, Raoof M, Chen Y, *et al.* Circulating mitochondrial DAMPs cause inflammatory responses to injury. *Nature* 2010; **464**: 104–7.

19. Murphy TJ, Paterson HM, Mannick JA, Lederer JA. Injury, sepsis, and the regulation of Toll-like receptor responses. *J Leukoc Biol* 2004; **75**: 400–7.

20. Marik PE, Flemmer M. The immune response to surgery and trauma: Implications for treatment. *J Trauma Acute Care Surg* 2012; **73**: 801–8.

21. Adib-Conquy M, Asehnoune K, Moine P, Cavaillon JM. Long-term-impaired expression of nuclear factor-kappa B and I kappa B alpha in peripheral blood mononuclear cells of trauma patients. *J Leukoc Biol* 2001; **70**: 30–8.

22. Kim JY, Park JS, Strassheim D, *et al.* HMGB1 contributes to the development of acute lung injury after hemorrhage. *Am J Physiol Lung Cell Mol Physiol* 2005; **288**: L958–65.

23. Plurad DS, Talving P, Lam L, *et al.* Early vasopressor use in critical injury is associated with mortality independent from volume status. *J Trauma Acute Care Surg* 2011; **71**: 565–70.

24. Sperry JL, Minei JP, Frankel HL, *et al.* Early use of vasopressors after injury: caution before constriction. *J Trauma Acute Care Surg* 2008; **64**: 9–14.

25. Shakur H, Roberts I, Bautista R, *et al.* Effects of tranexamic acid on death, vascular occlusive events, and blood transfusion in trauma patients with significant haemorrhage (CRASH-2): a randomised, placebo-controlled trial. *Lancet* 2010; **376**: 23–32.

26. CRASH-2 Intracranial Bleeding Study. Effect of tranexamic acid in traumatic brain injury: a nested randomised, placebo controlled trial. *BMJ* 2011; **343**: d3795.

27. Morrison JJ, Dubose JJ, Rasmussen TE, Midwinter MJ. Military Application of Tranexamic Acid in Trauma Emergency Resuscitation (MATTERs) Study. *Arch Surg* 2012; **147**: 113–19.

28. Goobie SM, Meier PM, Pereira LM, *et al.* Efficacy of tranexamic acid in pediatric craniosynostosis surgery: a double-blind, placebo-controlled trial. *Anesthesiology* 2011; **114**: 862–71.

29. Dadure C, Sauter M, Bringuier S, *et al.* Intraoperative tranexamic acid reduces blood transfusion in children undergoing craniosynostosis surgery: a randomized double-blind study. *Anesthesiology* 2011; **114**: 856–61.

30. Raab H, Lindner KH, Wenzel V. Preventing cardiac arrest during hemorrhagic shock with vasopressin. *Crit Care Med* 2008; **36** (11 Suppl): S474–80.

31. Robin JK, Oliver JA, Landry DW. Vasopressin deficiency in the syndrome of irreversible shock. *J Trauma Acute Care Surg* 2003; **54** (5 Suppl): S149–54.

32. Krismer AC, Dunser MW, Lindner KH, *et al.* Vasopressin during cardiopulmonary resuscitation and different shock states: a review of the literature. *Am J Cardiovasc Drugs* 2006; **6**: 51–68.

33. Raedler C, Voelckel WG, Wenzel V, *et al.* Treatment of uncontrolled hemorrhagic shock after liver trauma: fatal effects of fluid resuscitation versus

improved outcome after vasopressin. *Anesth Analg* 2004; **98**: 1759–66.

34. Voelckel WG, Raedler C, Wenzel V, *et al.* Arginine vasopressin, but not epinephrine, improves survival in uncontrolled hemorrhagic shock after liver trauma in pigs. *Crit Care Med* 2003; **31**: 1160–5.

35. Morales D, Madigan J, Cullinane S, *et al.* Reversal by vasopressin of intractable hypotension in the late phase of hemorrhagic shock. *Circulation* 1999; **100**: 226–9.

36. Krismer AC, Wenzel V, Voelckel WG, *et al.* Employing vasopressin as an adjunct vasopressor in uncontrolled traumatic hemorrhagic shock. Three cases and a brief analysis of the literature. *Anaesthesist* 2005; **54**: 220–4.

37. Sharma RM, Setlur R. Vasopressin in hemorrhagic shock. *Anesth Analg* 2005; **101**: 833–4.

38. Tsuneyoshi I, Onomoto M, Yonetani A, Kanmura Y. Low-dose vasopressin infusion in patients with severe vasodilatory hypotension after prolonged hemorrhage during general anesthesia. *J Anesth* 2005; **19**: 170–3.

39. Lienhart HG, Wenzel V, Braun J, *et al.* [Vasopressin for therapy of persistent traumatic hemorrhagic shock: The VITRIS.at study]. *Anaesthesist* 2007; **56**: 145–8.

40. Lienhart HG, Lindner KH, Wenzel V. Developing alternative strategies for the treatment of traumatic haemorrhagic shock. *Curr Opin Crit Care* 2008; **14**: 247–53.

41. Al Douri M, Shafi T, Al Khudairi D, *et al.* Effect of the administration of recombinant activated factor VII (rFVIIa; NovoSeven) in the management of severe uncontrolled bleeding in patients undergoing heart valve replacement surgery. *Blood Coagul Fibrinolysis* 2000; **11** (Suppl 1): S121–7.

42. Ponschab M, Landoni G, Biondi-Zoccai G, *et al.* Recombinant activated factor VII increases stroke in cardiac surgery: a meta-analysis. *J Cardiothorac Vasc Anesth* 2011; **25**: 804–10.

43. Friederich PW, Henny CP, Messelink EJ, *et al.* Effect of recombinant activated factor VII on perioperative blood loss in patients undergoing retropubic prostatectomy: a double-blind placebo-controlled randomised trial. *Lancet* 2003; **361**: 201–5.

44. Mayer SA, Brun NC, Begtrup K, *et al.* Recombinant activated factor VII for acute intracerebral hemorrhage. *N Engl J Med* 2005; **352**: 777–85.

45. Park P, Fewel ME, Garton HJ, Thompson BG, Hoff JT. Recombinant activated factor VII for the rapid correction of coagulopathy in nonhemophilic neurosurgical patients. *Neurosurgery* 2003; **53**: 34–8.

46. Knudson MM, Cohen MJ, Reidy R, *et al.* Trauma, transfusions, and use of recombinant factor VIIa: A multicenter case registry report of 380 patients from the Western Trauma Association. *J Am Coll Surg* 2011; **212**: 87–95.

47. Dutton RP, McCunn M, Hyder M, *et al.* Factor VIIa for correction of traumatic coagulopathy. *J Trauma Acute Care Surg* 2004; **57**: 709–18; discussion 18–19.

48. Spinella PC, Perkins JG, McLaughlin DF, *et al.* The effect of recombinant activated factor VII on mortality in combat-related casualties with severe trauma and massive transfusion. *J Trauma Acute Care Surg* 2008; **64**: 286–93.

49. Boffard KD, Riou B, Warren B, *et al.* Recombinant factor VIIa as adjunctive therapy for bleeding control in severely injured trauma patients: two parallel randomized, placebo-controlled, double-blind clinical trials. *J Trauma Acute Care Surg* 2005; **59**: 8–15.

50. Stinger HK, Spinella PC, Perkins JG, *et al.* The ratio of fibrinogen to red cells transfused affects survival in casualties receiving massive transfusions at an army combat support hospital. *J Trauma Acute Care Surg* 2008; **64** (2 Suppl): S79–85.

51. Fries D, Haas T, Klingler A, *et al.* Efficacy of fibrinogen and prothrombin complex concentrate used to reverse dilutional coagulopathy–a porcine model. *Br J Anaesth* 2006; **97**: 460–7.

52. Fries D. The early use of fibrinogen, prothrombin complex concentrate, and recombinant-activated factor VIIa in massive bleeding. *Transfusion* 2013; **53** (Suppl 1): 91S–5S.

53. Mitterlechner T, Innerhofer P, Streif W, *et al.* Prothrombin complex concentrate and recombinant prothrombin alone or in combination with recombinant factor X and FVIIa in dilutional coagulopathy: a porcine model. *J Thromb Haemost* 2011; **9**: 729–37.

54. Bickell WH, Wall MJ, Pepe PE, *et al.* Immediate versus delayed fluid resuscitation for hypotensive patients with penetrating torso injuries. *N Engl J Med* 1994; **331**: 1105–9.

55. Dutton RP, Mackenzie CF, Scalea TM. Hypotensive resuscitation during active hemorrhage: impact on in-hospital mortality. *J Trauma Acute Care Surg* 2002; **52**: 1141–6.

56. Juern J, Khatri V, Weigelt J. Base excess: a review. *J Trauma Acute Care Surg* 2012; **73**: 27–32.

57. Davis JW, Parks SN, Kaups KL, Gladen HE, O'Donnell-Nicol S. Admission base deficit predicts transfusion requirements and risk of complications. *J Trauma Acute Care Surg* 1996; **41**: 769–74.

58. Davis JW, Kaups KL, Parks SN. Base deficit is superior to pH in evaluating clearance of acidosis after traumatic shock. *J Trauma* 1998; **44**: 114–18.

59. Regnier MA, Raux M, Le Manach Y, Asencio Y, Gaillard J, Devilliers C, *et al.* Prognostic significance of blood lactate and lactate clearance in trauma patients. *Anesthesiology* 2012; **117**: 1276–88.

60. Cotton BA, Faz G, Hatch QM, *et al.* Rapid thrombelastography delivers real-time results that predict transfusion within 1 hour of admission. *J Trauma Acute Care Surg* 2011; **71**: 407–14.

61. Holcomb JB, Minei KM, Scerbo ML, *et al.* Admission rapid thrombelastography can replace conventional coagulation tests in the emergency department: experience with 1974 consecutive trauma patients. *Ann Surg* 2012; **256**: 476–86.

62. Sankarankutty A, Nascimento B, Teodoro da Luz L, Rizoli S. TEG(R) and ROTEM(R) in trauma: similar test but different results? *World J Emerg Surg* 2012; **7** (Suppl 1): S3.

Chapter

7

Blood loss: does it change my intravenous anesthetic?

Ken Johnson and Talmage D. Egan

Objectives

(1) Review emerging data on the influence of blood loss and resuscitation on the behavior of commonly used intravenous sedative hypnotics and opioids.

(2) Discuss the rational selection and dosing of sedative hypnotics and opioids in settings of intravascular volume depletion.

Introduction

Anesthesiologists have long recognized the need to moderate doses of intravenous anesthetics in settings of significant blood loss. The scientific rationale for this practice, however, has not been well established. This chapter reviews recent investigations that have quantified how blood loss influences intravenous anesthetic behavior and synthesizes these findings into a set of clinical "take-home messages" targeted at improving patient safety.

Influence of blood loss on intravenous anesthetics

Dr. Halford, a surgeon, wrote a letter to the editor of *Anesthesiology* after caring for several trauma victims after the attack on Pearl Harbor in 1941. He noticed that anesthetists had started using the intravenous (IV) anesthetic sodium pentothal (thiopental). His comments were:

> Then let it be said that intravenous anesthesia is also an ideal form of euthanasia ... With this heterogeneous mass of emergency anesthetists, it is necessary to choose an anesthetic involving the *WIDEST MARGIN OF SAFETY* for the patient ... Stick with *ETHER*.[1]

Anesthesiologists recognize the need to select certain IV anesthetics over others, to incrementally dose these anesthetics, and to moderate the overall dose for patients who have significant blood loss before or during surgery. Through experience, they have learned that a full dose of certain IV anesthetics can lead to pronounced and often unwanted side effects with potentially disastrous consequences. To that end, researchers have

quantified how the extent of blood loss influences the behavior of selected IV anesthetics.

The purpose of this chapter is to synthesize their findings into a set of clinical "take-home messages" targeted at improving patient safety. This chapter will (1) review what is known about the impact of **blood loss** and **resuscitation** on the pharmacologic behavior of commonly used sedative hypnotics and opioids and (2) discuss the rational selection and dosing of these anesthetics when used for induction and/or maintenance of anesthesia using mathematical descriptions of drug pharmacokinetics and pharmacodynamics.

Pharmacokinetics

Prior work has investigated how blood loss influences the behavior of opioids,[2-5] sedative hypnotics,[6-12] benzodiazepines,[11,13] and local anesthetics.[14] This body of work has been primarily done in animal models, given the ethical limitations of studying blood loss in human volunteers and patients. The most important finding consistent throughout is that equivalent dosing leads to higher drug concentrations with severe blood loss when compared with unbled controls. A decrease in blood volume and cardiac output,[15,16] along with compensatory changes in regional blood flow, are the likely physiologic mechanisms explaining these pharmacokinetic changes.

As an example, consider prior work exploring the impact of moderate hemorrhage on the pharmacokinetic profile of propofol.[8] In this study, a series of pilot studies in swine determined (1) the extent of blood loss (milliliters per kilogram) required to reach and maintain a selected target mean arterial blood pressure (MAP) and (2) the propofol infusion rate (in micrograms per kilogram per minute) that would achieve near-maximal drug effect (i.e., Bispectral Index scale [BIS] near 0) but allow animal subjects to survive the study period.

Based on prior work with remifentanil,[4] a hemorrhage protocol removed a large volume of blood (48 mL/kg) to maintain a MAP of 40 mmHg. Subsequently, a large dose of remifentanil 10 μg/kg/min was administered for 10 minutes. This dose is approximately 50–100 times greater than a typical dose of 0.1–0.2 μg/kg/min. Of note, all animals survived severe hemorrhage followed by a high-dose remifentanil infusion.[4]

In unbled animals, a propofol infusion of 750 µg/kg/min for 10 minutes was required to reach maximal effect (i.e., BIS near 0). With hemorrhage, a propofol dose of 750 µg/kg/min for 10 minutes was lethal. So were doses of 500, 250, and 125 µg/kg/min. What quickly became clear was that the cardiovascular depressant properties of propofol were dangerous with severe blood loss.

Unlike remifentanil, doses required to achieve maximal effect under normal unbled conditions would in no way be tolerated after a 50% loss in blood volume. Important take-home messages from these pilot studies were: (1) In comparison with opioids, selected sedative hypnotics known to have cardiovascular depressant properties, such as propofol and sodium pentothal, are poorly tolerated following blood loss. (2) Conventional doses in this setting can lead to cardiovascular collapse and death. If these drugs are to be used, doses should be markedly reduced to achieve desired clinical endpoints in sedation and hypnosis.

Following the pilot studies, a comparison of plasma propofol concentrations between an unbled control group and a hemorrhagic shock group were made. Bled animals (30 mL/kg) developed a hemodynamic and metabolic profile consistent with hemorrhage shock (i.e., tachycardia, low central venous pressure, low cardiac index, and lactic acidemia). The cardiac index was 5.0 and 2.6 L/min/m² for the control and shock groups, respectively. Following hemorrhage, each animal subject received a 10-minute propofol infusion at 200 µg/kg/min. Plasma propofol levels during and 3 hours following a brief 10-minute infusion were approximately twofold higher in the shock group.

As part of the pharmacokinetic analysis, the propofol plasma concentration profile over time was described using a three-compartment model. A comparison between groups revealed that compartmental clearances were decreased and compartment volumes were smaller in the shock group.

In terms of drug effect, BIS was used as a surrogate measure of effect. The propofol infusion produced a large decrease in the BIS that returned to baseline within 30 minutes of the infusion, but had minimal effect on the BIS in the control group. In order to achieve a similar change in the BIS in unbled animals, the dose had to be increased to 500 µg/kg/min. The magnitude of the propofol-induced decrease in BIS was similar between the control (500 µg/kg/min µg) and shock (200 µg/kg/min) groups.

Although these compartment volumes and clearances do not reflect true organ drug distribution and clearance, these analyses indicate that during severe blood loss blood flow to peripheral tissues is markedly decreased. Hence, anesthetics delivered intravenously are pumped straight to the brain in higher concentrations, producing a more pronounced anesthetic effect.[17]

In more recent work, Kurita et al. studied the pharmacokinetic profile of simultaneous continuous infusions of propofol (100 µg/kg/min) and remifentanil (0.5 µg/kg/min) during compensated and uncompensated hemorrhagic shock in a swine model.[5] They found that plasma propofol and remifentanil concentrations increased during compensated and uncompensated hemorrhagic shock, but that the increase in drug concentrations were substantially larger during uncompensated hemorrhagic shock.

They defined uncompensated hemorrhagic shock as the transition from increasing to decreasing systemic vascular resistance. Their hemorrhage protocol consisted of 10% of estimated blood volume removed every 30 minutes for 90 minutes followed by 5% of estimated blood volume removed every 20 minutes until circulatory collapse. The transition from compensated to uncompensated hemorrhagic shock required approximately 3–4 hours. This corresponded to removal of 35–40% of the estimated blood volume.

Important findings from this study were that the rise in remifentanil and propofol concentrations as a percentage change from baseline concentrations prior to hemorrhage were different between drugs during compensated hemorrhagic shock. As a function of blood loss, remifentanil plasma concentrations rose three times faster than propofol. For example, remifentanil concentrations increased by 95% over baseline within 30 minutes of the hemorrhage protocol, while propofol concentrations required 50 minutes into the hemorrhage protocol to achieve the same endpoint. After decompensation, plasma concentrations of the drug rose at an even faster rate with remifentanil, once again outpacing propofol until cardiovascular collapse.

Proposed mechanisms to describe these observations were that propofol concentrations were relatively insensitive to changes in cardiac output during compensated hemorrhagic shock, but became very sensitive during the uncompensated phase associated with a large decrease in cardiac output. Remifentanil was somewhat less sensitive to cardiac output changes. The authors suggest that remifentanil metabolism by nonspecific esterases occurs primarily in peripheral tissues and not in blood. This would explain the marked increase in remifentanil plasma concentrations once perfusion to peripheral tissues was decreased during hemorrhagic shock.[5]

Pharmacodynamics

Pharmacodynamics describes the concentration–effect relationship for a given drug. This is pictorially represented by how a measure of drug effect (i.e., the BIS) changes with effect-site concentrations. These curves are sigmoid in nature. Terms used to describe the sigmoid curve include the C_{50} (the effect site concentration that produces 50% of the maximal effect), gamma (a measure of curve steepness), and E_{max} (a measure of the maximal effect). Changes in drug potency can be illustrated with this relationship. For example, an increase in end-organ sensitivity would result in a leftward shift in the sigmoid curve.

Comparison of pharmacodynamic parameters between the shock and control groups for propofol revealed that the C_{50} was 2.7-fold less in the shock group (4.6 µg/mL vs. 1.7 µg/mL for the control and shock groups, respectively). The most interesting finding is that hemorrhagic shock *increased* the potency of propofol in swine. This has also been reported in a rat hemorrhage model.[6]

The mechanism of *how* hemorrhagic shock increases the potency of propofol is not clear. A potential mechanism may be a rise in circulating endorphins that act in a synergistic fashion with propofol. Propofol's potency is well known to increase in the presence of opioids.[18,19] With this synergistic relationship in mind, it interesting to point out that blood loss leads to a rise in circulating beta-endorphins.[20–22] During blood loss, high levels of beta-endorphins may act synergistically with propofol to increase its potency. Work by DePaepe *et al.*, however, has revealed that endorphin antagonism with naloxone does not influence end-organ sensitivity to propofol during hemorrhagic shock in rats.[6]

Other potential sources of increased end-organ sensitivity to propofol include (1) an alteration in the end-organ response to propofol as a consequence of the lactic acidemia, hyperkalemia, tissue hypoxia, or other metabolic disturbances associated with severe hemorrhagic shock, and (2) an undetected increase in the fraction of unbound propofol as a consequence of decreased lipophilic binding sites within whole blood.[23]

Clinical implications

One of the more dangerous uses of IV anesthetics is during the induction of anesthesia. Here, bolus doses are used to rapidly render a patient analgesic or unconscious. After a bolus of propofol, the concentration almost instantaneously rises and then slowly decays. Effect-site concentrations lag behind changes in plasma concentrations. This lag time represents the time required for a drug to diffuse from the plasma to the site of action and to exert its pharmacologic effect.

Prior work has explored the propofol effect-site concentration thresholds associated with important clinical endpoints, such as loss of responsiveness to various stimuli (e.g., verbal or noxious). By using these thresholds, plots of the effect-site concentration over time that result from commonly used dosing regimens allow us to visualize key clinical points of interest, such as the time to onset of effect and the duration of effect.

From Figure 7.1, the time to loss of response to verbal prompting occurs in approximately 1 minute followed by the loss of response to a noxious stimulus in 90 seconds. The duration of effect for loss of response to verbal stimuli and noxious stimuli are 5 and 3 minutes, respectively. These times are for a propofol bolus only and perhaps do not reflect the routine practice of using an opioid and a sedative hypnotic during the induction of anesthesia.

Figure 7.2 represents a simulation of the propofol effect-site concentration following a propofol bolus dose in a patient with an estimated blood loss of 35% of his/her blood volume. This simulation illustrates how both pharmacokinetic and pharmacodynamic changes influence the duration of effect. This simulation accounts for the kinetic changes as manifest by a roughly 2.5-fold increase in the peak plasma propofol concentration and also the dynamic changes as manifest by a 2.7-fold decrease in the effect-site concentration required for loss of response to verbal and noxious stimuli. The onset of effect is accelerated by approximately 60–90 seconds, and the duration of effect for both stimuli is more than doubled (from 6 to 28 minutes for verbal stimuli, and from 3 to 18 minutes for noxious stimuli).

Perhaps the most important consequence of blood loss for propofol behavior is the exaggerated hemodynamic response following a bolus dose. Propofol is a peripheral vasodilator and suppresses contractility.[25–28] As observed in the simulations, a

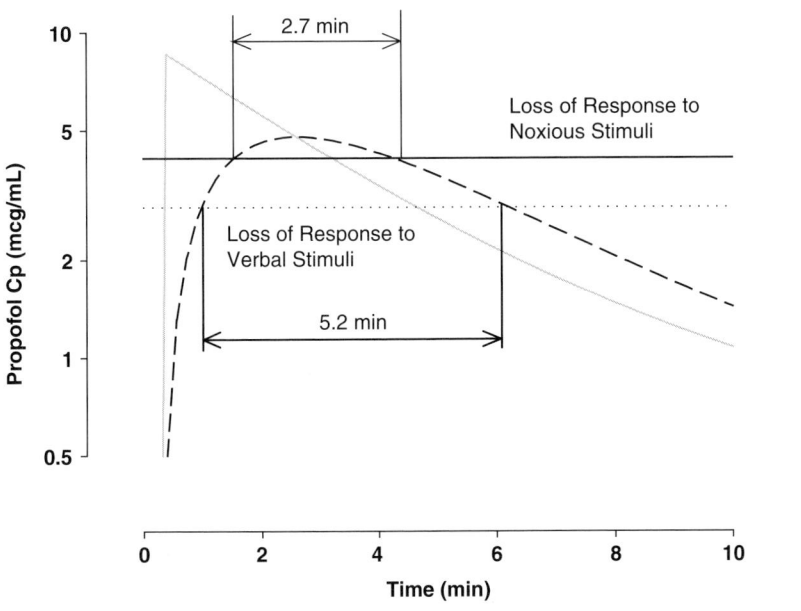

Figure 7.1 Simulation of a bolus dose of propofol 2 mg/kg. The solid gray line represents the plasma concentration. The dashed black line represents the effect-site concentration. The solid black line represents the propofol effect-site concentration (4.1 µg/mL) required for a loss of response to noxious stimuli, and the dotted black line represents the propofol effect-site concentration (2.9 µg/mL) at which there is a loss of response to verbal stimuli.[24]

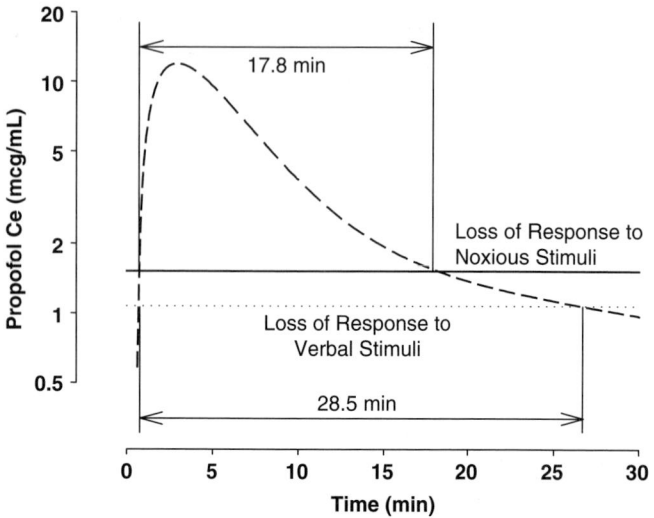

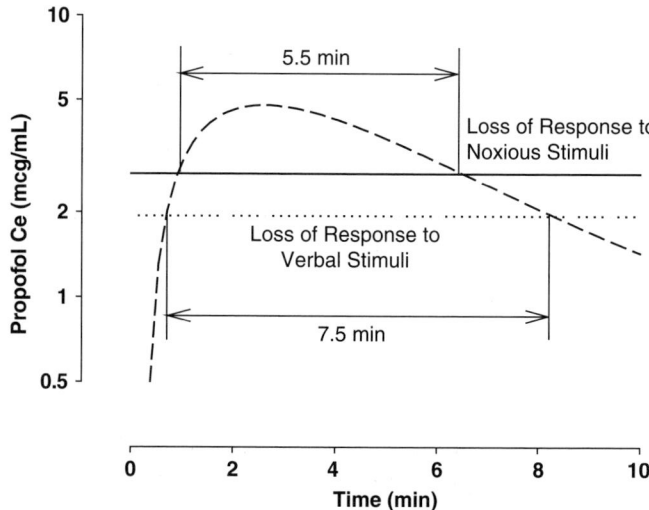

Figure 7.2 Combined pharmacokinetic and pharmacodynamic simulation of a propofol bolus dose of 2 mg/kg following severe blood loss. The dashed black line represents the effect-site concentration. The solid black line represents the propofol effect-site concentration (1.5 µg/mL) required for a loss of response to noxious stimuli and the dotted black line represents the propofol effect-site concentration (1.1 µg/mL) at which there is a loss of response to verbal stimuli.

Figure 7.3 Combined pharmacokinetic and pharmacodynamic simulation of a propofol bolus dose of 2 mg/kg after severe blood loss followed by resuscitation. The dashed black line represents the effect-site concentration. The solid black line represents the propofol effect-site concentration (2.7 µg/mL) required for a loss of response to noxious stimuli, and the dotted black line represents the propofol effect site concentration (1.9 µg/mL) at which there is a loss of response to verbal stimuli.

propofol bolus dose yields higher effect-site concentrations that remain elevated for a prolonged period, amplifying propofol's cardiovascular suppression. This phenomenon is most likely why Dr. Halford was so adamant about the dangers of IV anesthetic induction agents in victims of trauma at Pearl Harbor. With large blood loss, propofol should be used, if at all, with extreme caution. From these simulations, if we were to work backward and determine the appropriate dose for a person suffering from severe blood loss that would be equivalent to a person with normal cardiovascular physiology, the dose of propofol would be reduced fivefold (e.g., 0.4 mg/kg).

Resuscitation

Although interesting, the impact of severe blood loss on propofol behavior does not reflect the clinical practice of providing some degree of resuscitation prior to the administration of an anesthetic. Based on the premise that resuscitation will restore cardiac output and systemic blood flow, the shock-induced kinetic and dynamic changes may be reversed.

In a similar set of experiments, a comparison was made between unbled controls and bled and then resuscitated swine.[29] Blood loss was severe (42 mL/kg). Following hemorrhage, 59 mL/kg of lactated Ringer's solution was infused over an hour to keep the MAP at 70 mmHg. The propofol plasma concentrations were nearly identical. Resuscitation restored the shock-induced changes in propofol pharmacokinetics to near-baseline values. Distribution volumes and compartment clearances were nearly identical between groups.

The shock-induced increase in end-organ sensitivity to propofol after blood loss, however, was reduced but still persisted with resuscitation. Although the propofol C_{50} increased

from 2.7-fold following hemorrhage, it was still 1.5-fold higher following hemorrhage and resuscitation. Although the mechanism for this phenomenon is not well understood, increased end-organ sensitivity associated with severe blood loss persisted after resuscitation despite near normalization of the pharmacokinetics.

In this study, the hemorrhage protocol produced an estimated 60% decrease in blood volume. The resuscitation protocol replaced approximately 140% of the shed blood volume with lactated Ringer's solution to maintain a near-normotensive MAP. The near-normal blood pressure was deceiving. The resuscitative effort was incomplete. Although the hemodynamic function appeared near-normal, as manifest by a return of central venous pressure and cardiac index to baseline levels, the cardiovascular response to propofol remained exaggerated. During the propofol infusion, the cardiac index dropped 1.7 L/min/m² in the shock-resuscitation group but only dropped 0.2 L/min/m² in the control group. The large hemodynamic changes in the shock-resuscitation group illustrate how propofol can lead to large cardiovascular changes despite a near-normal hemodynamic profile following partial resuscitation.

Figure 7.3 represents a simulation of the propofol effect-site concentration following a propofol bolus dose in a patient suffering from severe blood loss followed by partial resuscitation with crystalloid (1.5 mL of crystalloid per mL of estimated blood loss). This simulation accounts for the pharmacodynamic changes as manifest by a 1.5-fold decrease in the effect-site concentration required for loss of response to verbal and noxious stimuli. The onset of effect is accelerated by approximately 30–60 seconds, and the duration of effect for both stimuli is increased (from 6 to 8 minutes for verbal stimuli and from 3 to 6 minutes for noxious stimuli).

Table 7.1 Clinical implications of blood loss and resuscitation on a 2 mg/kg bolus of propofol: a summary of simulations exploring how pharmacokinetic and pharmacodynamic changes influence the pharmacologic behavior of propofol

	Normal	Blood loss	Resuscitation following blood loss
	Euvolemia Normotensive	Hypovolemia Hypotensive	Mild hypovolemia Normotensive
Propofol C_e for LOR to verbal stimuli	2.9 µg/mL	1.1 µg/mL	1.9 µg/mL
Time to LOR to verbal stimuli	1 min	< 1 min	1 min
Duration of LOR to verbal stimuli	5 min	28 min	7 min
Propofol C_e for LOR to noxious stimuli	4.1 µg/mL	1.5 µg/mL	2.7 µg/mL
Time to LOR to noxious stimuli	1 min	< 1 min	1 min
Duration of LOR to noxious stimuli	3 min	18 min	5 min

C_e, effect-site concentration; LOR, loss of responsiveness.
Simulations were performed using drug infusion simulation software (STANPUMP, Stanford University, Palo Alto, CA). Pharmacokinetic and pharmacodynamic parameters were adapted for simulation from Johnson et al.[8,29] Thresholds for LOR to verbal and noxious stimuli were adapted from work by Struys et al.[24]

Three take-home messages are evident here. With partial crystalloid resuscitation, (1) the exaggerated hemodynamic response to propofol is diminished but persists and may produce potentially dangerous cardiovascular depression, (2) shock-induced changes in propofol kinetics previously observed after hemorrhagic shock are restored to near baseline, and (3) shock-induced changes in pharmacodynamics are diminished yet persist to a degree such that conventional dosing can lead to a more pronounced drug effect. A summary of the propofol bolus simulation (normal conditions, blood loss, and resuscitation following resuscitation) is presented in Table 7.1.

Opioids in hemorrhagic shock

Similar to propofol, opioids have an altered pharmacologic profile following severe blood loss. In experiments similar to those described for propofol, brief high-dose infusions led to plasma concentrations of opioid that were up to twofold higher in bled animals than in unbled controls.[3,4] Both fentanyl and remifentanil exhibited pharmacokinetic changes to include a reduced volume of distribution and a decrease in drug clearance that were consistent with what has been observed with propofol[6,8] following blood loss. These pharmacokinetic changes suggest that in the presence of moderate to severe blood loss, opioid dosing can be reduced by 50% to achieve a desired analgesic effect.

There are, however, some important differences between the pharmacologic profiles of opioids and propofol following hemorrhagic shock. When compared with propofol, the doses of opioid delivered following moderate to severe hemorrhage were much higher. For example, following a 30 mL/kg hemorrhage, swine would only tolerate a propofol dose of 200 µg/kg/min for 10 minutes. This dose is notable for three reasons: (1) It was adequate to achieve the desired effect (near-maximal effect in the BIS) and higher doses were found to lead to *irreversible* cardiovascular collapse. (2) It was 2.5-fold less than the dose required to achieve near-maximal effect in the unbled controls. (3) This dose represents only a modest increase in what is typically administered to achieve sedation during a general anesthetic. By contrast, following a 25 mL/kg hemorrhage, swine tolerated a brief fentanyl infusion of 10 µg/kg/min for 5 minutes.[3] This infusion rate represents a dose that is nearly 5–10 times what is required to produce analgesia. The infusion was tolerated in both bled and unbled animal subjects. The cardiovascular depression from high-dose fentanyl in the presence of moderate blood loss was minimal. An important take-home message is that higher doses of fentanyl are better tolerated, with less cardiovascular depression, during hemorrhagic shock and demonstrate the wider therapeutic range of opioids when compared with propofol.

With regard to the influence of hemorrhagic shock on the pharmacodynamic profile of opioids, prior work has reported that the dynamics of remifentanil is relatively immune to the consequences of severe blood loss. This is again in stark contrast to what has been observed with propofol.

The impact of blood loss on etomidate and ketamine

By comparison with propofol, both ketamine and etomidate have a higher degree of acceptance among clinicians caring for patients with significant blood loss. This is largely because the cardiovascular depression known to be exaggerated with propofol and sodium pentothal is not as apparent with etomidate, and even to a lesser extent with ketamine. For example, although etomidate is known to produce mild cardiovascular depression, prior work surprisingly has revealed minimal cardiovascular change following a high-dose, brief continuous etomidate infusion during moderate hemorrhagic shock (30 mL/kg).[9] As well, the kinetic and dynamic profile of etomidate following blood loss has also been found to be minimally influenced by blood loss.

Table 7.2 Summary of studies investigating the influence of blood loss and resuscitation on intravenous drug behavior

Drug	Pharmacokinetic changes with BL	Pharmacodynamic changes with BL	Pharmacokinetic changes with BL & R	Pharmacodynamic changes with BL & R	Reference
Sedative hypnotics					
Propofol	+++	+++	+	+	DePaepe et al.[6] Johnson et al.[8] Johnson et al.[28]
Sodium thiopental	+++	—	—	—	Halford[1] Weiskopf et al.[12]
Etomidate	+	0	—	—	DePaepe et al.[7] Johnson et al.[9]
Ketamine	+	—	—	—	Black et al.[29] Weiskopf et al.[12]
Midazolam	++	—	—	—	Adams et al.[13]
Opioids					
Morphine	++	—	—	—	DePaepe et al.[2]
Fentanyl	+++	—	—	—	Egan et al.[3]
Remifentanil	+++	0	—	—	Johnson et al.[4]

BL, blood loss; R, resuscitation.
+++, ++, +, 0 indicate large, moderate, small, and no change in parameters that lead to more pronounced and/or prolonged drug effect.
— indicates that no data are available.

Similar to etomidate, preliminary work has suggested that severe blood loss minimally influences the pharmacokinetic behavior of ketamine.[30] Ketamine is known to increase sympathetic tone, serve as a potent analgesic, and perform favorably in patients with poor cardiovascular function. During severe hemorrhage (39 mL/kg) in swine, equivalent dosing surprisingly led to near-equivalent plasma levels during and after a brief high-dose infusion. One disadvantage to studying ketamine is that it is difficult to characterize the influence of blood loss on the pharmacodynamic behavior. This is because it is difficult to identify and measure a surrogate of ketamine's sedative or analgesic effect (i.e., BIS is not a reliable measure of ketamine's sedative effect).

Nevertheless, these preliminary results suggest that dosing requirements for ketamine and etomidate require minimal adjustment following moderate to severe blood loss, and that these are important drugs to maintain in our pharmacologic armamentarium when caring for patients suffering from life-threatening blood loss.

Summary

As anesthesiologists navigate patients suffering from blood loss through often perilous anesthetics, hemorrhage – and even hemorrhage followed by resuscitation that appears to restore hemodynamic function to near normal – can lead to dramatic alterations in the pharmacologic behavior of commonly used sedative hypnotics and opioids. Duration of effect, peak effect-site concentrations, and extent of cardiovascular depression should all be considered when selecting an intravenous anesthetic and formulating an appropriate dose. The hemodynamically compromised patient is especially susceptible to the cardiovascular suppression of some sedative hypnotics, whereas others appear to be much safer. Propofol appears to be an especially poor choice even after some degree of resuscitation. Ketamine or etomidate are better suited in patients suffering from hemorrhagic shock. In contrast to propofol, opioids enjoy a wide therapeutic margin in the presence of blood loss. A summary of how blood loss and resuscitation influence intravenous drug behavior is presented in Table 7.2.

What remains unexplored is the influence of blood loss on drug behavior when sedatives and opioids are administered simultaneously, as is often done when providing a general anesthetic. It is well established that sedative hypnotics and opioids have a synergistic relationship, but how that interaction behaves in the presence of intravascular volume depletion has not been described.

Questions

(1) Likely mechanisms to explain pharmacokinetic changes in intravenous drug behavior following severe blood loss include all of the following, *except*:
   a. Decreased cardiac output
   b. Decreased protein binding of active drug
   c. A rightward shift in the concentration–effect relationship
   d. Decreased blood flow to essential organs
   e. Decreased volume of distribution

(2) An exaggerated response in processed EEG measures of sedation (i.e., the Bispectral Index scale) to intravenous propofol administration following severe hemorrhage is most likely a function of:
   a. Changes in propofol pharmacokinetics
   b. Changes in propofol pharmacodynamics
   c. A leftward shift in propofol's concentration effect curve
   d. Elevated effect site concentrations
   e. All of the above

(3) Similarities in opioid and propofol behavior following severe blood loss include all of the following, *except*:
   a. Blood loss leads to a decrease in the volume of distribution
   b. Administration causes severe cardiovascular depression
   c. Blood loss leads to a decrease in clearance
   d. Administration yields elevated effect-site concentrations in response to conventional dosing
   e. None of the above

(4) Extreme caution should be used when administering all of the following sedative hypnotic dosing regimens in the setting of moderate to severe blood loss, *except*:
   a. Propofol 2 mg/kg
   b. Propofol 150 µg/kg/min
   c. Thiopental 4 mg/kg
   d. Etomidate 0.1 mg/kg
   e. Propofol 2 mg/kg + fentanyl 3 µg/kg

(5) Following a 2 mg/kg induction dose of propofol, moderate blood loss would be expected to lead to the following changes in propofol's behavior, *except*:
   a. A rightward shift in the concentration–effect curve
   b. Higher effect-site concentrations
   c. A lower effect-site concentration threshold for loss of responsiveness
   d. Prolonged duration of effect
   e. Higher plasma concentrations

(6) Preliminary research exploring the influence of partial resuscitation following severe blood loss on propofol behavior has revealed all of the following, *except*:
   a. Pharmacokinetic changes seen in blood loss are reversed
   b. Pharmacodynamic changes in blood loss are reversed
   c. The potentially dangerous cardiovascular depressant effect of propofol is not fully reversed with partial resuscitation
   d. Presence of a leftward shift in the concentration–effect curve of smaller magnitude than observed with moderate to severe blood loss
   e. Persistence of a lower effect-site concentration threshold for loss of responsiveness as observed with blood loss when compared with euvolemic normotensive conditions

(7) Features that make administration of opioids attractive to administer during severe blood loss when compared with propofol include:
   a. Decrease in the volume of distribution
   b. Conventional dosing leads to higher than expected plasma concentrations
   c. Minimal cardiovascular depressant effects even at high doses
   d. Conventional dosing leads to lower than expected effect site concentrations
   e. A lower effect-site concentration threshold for loss or responsiveness to painful stimuli

(8) Comparing ketamine and propofol behavior following severe blood loss, which of the following is *not* true?
   a. Ketamine increases sympathetic tone, whereas propofol is a cardiovascular depressant
   b. Propofol and to a lesser extent, ketamine, have a decreased volume of distribution
   c. Both require a significant reduction in dose to minimize the risk of cardiovascular collapse
   d. Ketamine has a significant analgesic component, whereas propofol does not
   e. None of the above

(9) During hemorrhagic shock, pronounced drug effect may be due to:
   a. Decreased cardiac output
   b. Redistribution of blood flow to essential organs, the brain and heart
   c. Possible decreased protein binding of active drug yielding more drug per dose available to exert an effect
   d. Decreased clearance
   e. All of the above

(10) Recent investigations have shown that the C_{50}, a pharmacodynamic parameter used to characterize the drug–effect relationship, is shifted to the left in severe blood loss for which of the following drug(s)?
   a. Remifentanil
   b. Remifentanil and fentanyl
   c. Remifentanil, fentanyl, and propofol
   d. Propofol
   e. Propofol and etomidate

Answers

(1) c
(2) e
(3) b
(4) d
(5) a
(6) b
(7) c
(8) c
(9) e
(10) d

References

1. Halford F. A critique of intravenous anesthesia in war surgery. *Anesthesiology* 1943; **4**: 67–9.

2. De Paepe P, Belpaire FM, Rosseel MT, Buylaert WA. The influence of hemorrhagic shock on the pharmacokinetics and the analgesic effect of morphine in the rat. *Fundam Clin Pharmacol* 1998; **12**: 624–30.

3. Egan TD, Kuramkote S, Gong G, *et al*. Fentanyl pharmacokinetics in hemorrhagic shock: a porcine model. *Anesthesiology* 1999; **91**: 156–66.

4. Johnson KB, Kern SE, Hamber EA, *et al*. Influence of hemorrhagic shock on remifentanil; a pharmacokinetic and pharmacodynamic analysis. *Anesthesiology* 2001; **94**: 322–32.

5. Kurita T, Uraoka M, Morita K, *et al*. Influence of haemorrhage on the pseudo-steady-state remifentanil concentration in a swine model: a comparison with propofol and the effect of haemorrhagic shock stage. *Br J Anaesth* 2011; **107**: 719–25.

6. De Paepe P, Belpaire FM, Rosseel MT, *et al*. Influence of hypovolemia on the pharmacokinetics and the electroencephalographic effect of propofol in the rat. *Anesthesiology* 2000; **93**: 1482–90.

7. De Paepe P, Belpaire FM, Van Hoey G, Boon PA, Buylaert WA. Influence of hypovolemia on the pharmacokinetics and the electroencephalographic effect of etomidate in the rat. *J Pharmacol Exp Ther* 1999; **290**: 1048–53.

8. Johnson KB, Egan TD, Kern SE, *et al*. The influence of hemorrhagic shock on propofol: a pharmacokinetic and pharmacodynamic analysis. *Anesthesiology* 2003; **99**: 409–20.

9. Johnson KB, Egan TD, Layman J, *et al*. The influence of hemorrhagic shock on etomidate: a pharmacokinetic and pharmacodynamic analysis. *Anesth Analg* 2003; **96**: 1360–8.

10. Kazama T, Kurita T, Morita K, Nakata J, Sato S. Influence of hemorrhage on propofol pseudo-steady state concentration. *Anesthesiology* 2002; **97**: 1156–61.

11. Klockowski P, Levy G. Kinetics of drug action in disease states. XXV. Effect of experimental hypovolemia on the pharmacodynamics and pharmacokinetics of desmethyldiazepam. *J Pharmacol Exp Ther* 1988; **245**: 508–12.

12. Weiskopf RB, Bogertz MS, Roizen MF, Reid IA. Cardiovascular and metabolic sequelae of inducing anesthesia with ketamine or thiopental in hypovolemic swine. *Anesthesiology* 1984; **60**: 214–19.

13. Adams P, Gelman S, Reves JG, *et al*. Midazolam pharmacodynamics and pharmacokinetics during acute hypovolemia. *Anesthesiology* 1985; **63**: 140–6.

14. Benowitz N, Forsyth RP, Melmon KL, Rowland M. Lidocaine disposition kinetics in monkey and man II. Effect of hemorrhage and sympathomimetic drug administration. *Clin Pharmacol Ther* 1973; **16**: 99–109.

15. Kurita T, Morita K, Kazama T, Sato S. Influence of cardiac output on plasma propofol concentrations during constant infusion in swine. *Anesthesiology* 2002; **96**: 1498–503.

16. Upton RN, Ludbrook GL, Grant C, Martinez AM. Cardiac output is a determinant of the initial concentrations of propofol after short-infusion administration. *Anesth Analg* 1999; **89**: 545–52.

17. Shafer S. Shock Values. *Anesthesiology* 2004; **101**: 568–70.

18. Kazama T, Ikeda K, Morita K. The pharmacodynamic interaction between propofol and fentanyl with respect to the supression of somatic or hemodynamic responses to skin incision, peritoneum incision, and wall retraction. *Anesthesiology* 1998; **89**: 894–906.

19. Pavlin DJ, Arends RH, Gunn HC, *et al*. Optimal propofol-alfentanil combinations for supplementing nitrous oxide for outpatient surgery. *Anesthesiology* 1999; **91**: 97–108.

20. McIntosh TK, Palter M, Grasberger R, *et al*. Endorphins in primate hemorrhagic shock: beneficial action of opiate antagonists. *J Surg Res* 1986; **40**: 265–75.

21. Molina P. Opiate modulation of hemodynamic, hormonal, and cytokine response to hemorrhage. *Shock* 2001; **15**: 471–8.

22. Tuggle D, Horton J. beta-Endorphin in canine hemorrhagic shock. *Surg Gynecol Obstet* 1986; **163**: 137–44.

23. Dutta S, Matsumoto Y, Ebling WF. Propofol pharmacokinetics and pharmacodynamics assessed from a cremophor EL formulation. *J Pharmaceutical Sci* 1997; **86**: 967–9.

24. Struys MM, Vereecke H, Moerman A, *et al*. Ability of the bispectral index, autoregressive modelling with exogenous input-derived auditory evoked potentials, and predicted propofol concentrations to measure patient responsiveness during anesthesia with propofol and remifentanil. *Anesthesiology* 2003; **99**: 802–12.

25. Brussel T, Theissen JL, Vigfusson G, *et al*. Hemodynamic and cardiodynamic effects of propofol and etomidate: negative inotropic properties of propofol. *Anesth Analg* 1989; **69**: 35–40.

26. Goodchild C, Serrao J. Cardiovascular effects of propofol in the anaesthetized dog. *Br J Anaesth* 1989; **63**: 87–92.

27. Graham M, Thiessen D, Mutch W. Left ventricular systolic and diastolic function is unaltered during propofol infusion in newborn swine. *Anesth Analg* 1998; **86**: 717–23.

28. Pagel PS, Warltier DC. Negative inotropic effects of propofol as evaluated by the regional preload recruitable stroke work relationship in chronically instrumented dogs. *Anesthesiology* 1993; **78**: 100–8.

29. Johnson K, Egan T, Kern S, *et al*. Influence of hemorrhagic shock followed by crystalloid resuscitation on propofol: a pharmacokinetic and pharmacodynamic analysis. *Anesthesiology* 2004; **101**: 647–59.

30. Black I, Grathwohl K, IB T, Martini W, Johnson K. The influence of hemorrhagic shock on ketamine: a pharmacokinetic analysis. *Anesthesiology* 2006; ASA Annual Meeting Abstracts: A203.

8

Fluid and blood therapy in trauma

Maxim Novikov and Charles E. Smith

Objectives

(1) Understand the timing, extent, and immediate goals for initial fluid resuscitation in trauma victims, individualized to specific patients, including the concept of delayed fluid resuscitation (hypotensive resuscitation).

(2) Review the factors influencing the choice of fluid for the initial and ongoing resuscitation.

(3) Discuss factors influencing the decision for initiating transfusion therapy, the choice of blood products, and the risks and benefits of transfusion therapy.

(4) Become familiar with the current state of therapies intended for the most severely injured patients, including factor concentrates and massive blood transfusion protocols.

Introduction

Initial evaluation of an acutely volume-depleted trauma patient will include a primary and secondary survey according to Advanced Trauma Life Support (ATLS) principles (see Chapter 2), estimates of blood volume deficit (Table 8.1) and the rate of ongoing blood loss, and an evaluation of cardiopulmonary reserve and coexisting hepatic or renal dysfunction. The major goal in resuscitation is to stop the bleeding, replete intravascular volume, and restore tissue oxygenation. Perfusion pressure and oxygenated blood flow to vital organs are important determinants of outcome. Hypotensive resuscitation, where the rate of fluid infusion is carefully titrated to a predetermined level of lower than normal blood pressure (BP) until the bleeding is controlled, is currently advocated in patients who are not pregnant and do not have traumatic head injury. The early use of tranexamic acid (TXA) appears to be a life saving, safe, and inexpensive treatment and is discussed in detail in Chapter 6.

Management priorities in an acutely bleeding trauma patient include control of bleeding, ventilation and oxygenation (see Chapter 3), establishment or verification of adequate intravenous (IV) access (see Chapter 5), measurement of BP, placement of electrocardiogram (ECG), pulse oximeter, and capnograph, and laboratory studies. Placement of an arterial

Table 8.1 Estimation of blood volume deficit in trauma

Unilateral hemothorax	3000 mL
Hemoperitoneum with abdominal distension	2000–5000 mL
Full-thickness soft tissue defect 5 cm^3	500 mL
Pelvic fracture	1500–2000 mL
Femur fracture	800–1200 mL
Tibia fracture	350–650 mL
Smaller fracture sites	100–500 mL

line and close monitoring of systolic pressure and pulse pressure variability (see Chapter 9), temperature, urine output, arterial blood gases, hemoglobin, hematocrit, electrolytes, and parameters of coagulation are routine in severely injured trauma patients. Consideration is given to the use of additional monitors (e.g., central venous pressure, transesophageal echocardiography) and provision of anesthesia as needed.

Timing and aggressiveness of fluid resuscitation

Early aggressive crystalloid fluid resuscitation aimed at restoration of "normal" hemodynamics, once the mainstay of trauma management, is no longer recommended in hemorrhagic shock. In animal models of uncontrolled hemorrhage, this strategy leads to increased duration and volume of bleeding and decreased survival. The proposed mechanisms include dilution of clotting factors, decreased blood viscosity, and blow-out of hemostatic plugs with increasing blood pressure (Table 8.2). Delayed fluid resuscitation, also known as permissive hypotension, is preferred, together with source control of bleeding. The question of immediate versus delayed fluid resuscitation for hypotensive trauma patients was first addressed two decades ago in a landmark randomized clinical trial which demonstrated improved survival, shorter hospital stay, and fewer postoperative complications in patients who did not receive fluid resuscitation until arrival to operating room.[1] Patients receiving fluids on the way to the hospital had

Table 8.2 Disadvantages of immediate crystalloid fluid resuscitation

Decreased blood viscosity
Blow-out of hemostatic plug
Dilution of coagulation factors
Increased blood loss
Delayed transport to definitive care

higher BP on arrival, but were more tachycardic and acidotic; BP was similar between the two groups on arrival to the operating room (OR), whereas coagulopathy and acidosis persisted in the immediate-fluid group. The study was limited to isolated penetrating torso injuries and the receiving trauma center had a rapid response time such that most patients were in the OR within 1 hour of injury. Benefits of delayed fluid resuscitation in the prehospital setting include minimal delay in transfer and surgical intervention, and avoidance of increased BP or hemodilution, which could disrupt the clot or alter resistance to flow around a partially formed thrombus.

Prehospital crystalloid fluid administration was associated with higher mortality in the National Trauma Data Bank analysis of 766,734 patients.[2] In the analysis, approximately half the patients received prehospital IV fluids. After adjustment for other relevant factors, prehospital fluid increased mortality by 11% overall, by 25% in penetrating trauma, by 44% in hypotensive patients, by 35% in patients requiring immediate surgery, and by 34% in patients with severe head injury. Emergency department crystalloid resuscitation was associated with increased mortality after trauma.[3] In the chart review study, 1.5 L (or more) of crystalloid fluids doubled mortality in younger patients (age < 70), and nearly tripled mortality in the elderly (age ≥ 70). At 3 liters, risk of death was 8.6 times higher in the elderly and 2.7 times higher in younger patients.

The concept of limited crystalloid fluid resuscitation applies to in-hospital and intraoperative management as well. In a pilot project (first 90 patients recruited for a larger study), trauma patients who had at least one in-hospital BP < 90 mmHg and required an emergent laparotomy or thoracotomy were randomized to either maintaining an intraoperative mean BP of at least 65 mmHg, or to allowing mean BP to decrease to 50 mmHg.[4] The lower BP group had less blood loss (2 vs. 3 L), required less blood products (1.6 vs. 3 L), and had better 24-hour survival (6 vs. 10 deaths) with the difference maintained at 30 days (10 vs. 13 deaths).

Consequently, in uncontrolled hemorrhagic shock, resuscitation is aimed at restoring radial artery pulse, improved mental status, and systolic BP of 70–80 mmHg, until the bleeding is surgically controlled. The concept of damage control resuscitation (also known as hemostatic resuscitation) is routinely practiced at many trauma centers.[5] Damage control resuscitation consists of early measures to stop bleeding,

limiting crystalloid fluids, accepting lower than normal systolic BP, giving thawed plasma and blood early and in higher ratios (e.g., 1:1:1 ratios of plasma to red cells to platelets; see Chapter 6), and aggressively maintaining normothermia (heat conservation measures, including using fluid warmers for each IV line, warming the OR; see Chapter 14). Damage control resuscitation has been associated with decreased mortality, especially related to attenuating the bloody vicious cycle of coagulopathy, acidosis, and hypothermia.[5] However, higher BP (systolic > 100 mmHg, mean arterial pressure [MAP] > 70 mmHg) is generally sought in head-injured and in pregnant patients (see Chapters 21 and 37). Guidelines from the American Association of Neurological Surgeons published in 2007 call for maintaining systolic BP at or above 90 mmHg and cerebral perfusion pressure (MAP – intracranial pressure) in the 50–70 mmHg range, including after the dura is opened. The European guidelines on management of bleeding and coagulopathy after major trauma recommend "a target systolic BP of 80 to 90 mmHg until major bleeding has been stopped in the initial phase following trauma without brain injury" and "a MAP ≥ 80 mmHg in patients with combined hemorrhagic shock and severe traumatic brain injury (TBI)."[6]

Fluid options
Crystalloids

There is controversy concerning which IV solutions should be used for resuscitation, or if any asanguinous fluid should be used at all. Studies quoted above suggest that administration of crystalloid fluids in the prehospital setting increases mortality. Certainly, a patient with uncontrolled bleeding requires rapid source control of bleeding, and resuscitation with crystalloids may negatively impact outcome.

During hemorrhage, a compensatory increase in reabsorption of fluid into capillaries partially restores the intravascular compartment, but depletes the interstitial space. To replete the intravascular and interstitial compartments, crystalloid solutions such as isotonic normal saline (0.9% saline) or lactated Ringer's (LR) solution are traditionally used. LR is mildly hypotonic with respect to plasma and may be detrimental if given in large volumes to patients with head injury (Table 8.3). European task force guidelines suggest that "hypotonic solutions, such as Ringer's lactate, be avoided in patients with severe head trauma."[6] Since LR contains 3 mEq/L of calcium, it has been traditionally contraindicated for co-infusion with or dilution of RBCs. This view has been challenged, because dilution of RBCs with LR in a ratio up to 2:1 (RBC:LR) with subsequent incubation at 37 °C for up to 2 hours does not lead to clot formation, and dilution of RBCs to a hematocrit of 35% does not slow down the passage of blood through the standard 170 micron filter.[7]

Plasmalyte is also an option. One liter of Plasmalyte has an ionic concentration of 140 mEq sodium, 5 mEq potassium, 3 mEq magnesium, 98 mEq chloride, 27 mEq acetate, and

Table 8.3 Asanguinous fluid options for trauma

Crystalloids (lactated Ringer's, Plasmalyte, normosol, normal saline)	Early aggressive crystalloid fluid resuscitation aimed at restoration of "normal" hemodynamics is not recommended.
Lactated Ringer's (LR)	Isotonic crystalloid solution for many trauma resuscitations. Physiologic Na:Cl ratio. Mildly hypotonic and avoided in patients with severe head trauma. Contains calcium (theoretical risk of blood clot if used to dilute RBCs or in blood lines).
Plasmalyte	Isotonic crystalloid with higher osmolarity than LR. Physiologic Na:Cl ratio. Does not contain calcium and may be co-administered with RBCs or used as a diluent for RBCs.
Normosol	Isotonic crystalloid with higher osmolarity than LR. Physiologic Na:Cl ratio. Does not contain calcium and may be co-administered with RBCs or used as a diluent for RBCs.
Normal saline (0.9%)	Isotonic crystalloid solution for head trauma. Can be used in blood transfusion lines and to dilute pRBCs. Associated with hyperchloremic metabolic acidosis, renal failure and increased mortality due to excess chloride.
Hyperoncotic starches (Hespan, Hextend, and others)	Not recommended because of adverse effects on hemostasis and renal function and increased mortality.
Albumin (5%)	Not recommended. Increased mortality after head trauma in SAFE study (vs. 0.9% saline). May pass into interstitial compartment if impaired vascular integrity with resultant endothelial swelling and impaired microcirculatory perfusion. Little effect on coagulation.
Dextrans and gelatins	These colloid solutions have been largely abandoned in the US because of negative effects on coagulation and potential for anaphylaxis and hypersensitivity reactions.
Hypertonic saline	Variety of solutions/concentrations. May be combined with colloid to prolong duration of action. Efficiently restores intravascular volume and decreases extravascular volume and tissue edema. Decreases ICP and increases CPP. Advantageous in prehospital situations and in head trauma with refractory increased ICP. Not associated with improved outcomes in trauma.

CPP, cerebral perfusion pressure; ICP, intracranial pressure; MW, molecular weight; pRBC, packed red blood cells; SAFE, Saline versus Albumin Fluid Evaluation.

23 mEq gluconate. The osmolarity is 294 mOsm/L. Plasmalyte does not contain calcium and may be co-administered with RBCs or used as a diluent for RBCs. Normosol is another isotonic crystalloid fluid option. The electrolyte concentration of Normosol is isotonic in relation to the extracellular fluid (approximately 280 mOsm/L) and provides a physiologic sodium-to-chloride ratio, normal plasma concentrations of potassium and magnesium and two bicarbonate alternates, acetate and gluconate (sodium 140 mEq; potassium 5 mEq; magnesium 3 mEq; chloride 98 mEq; acetate 27 mEq; gluconate 23 mEq). Like Plasmalyte, Normosol does not contain calcium.

Normal saline has a chloride concentration of 154 mmol/L, well above the normal serum chloride concentration of 100 mmol/L, and is a well-known cause of hyperchloremic metabolic acidosis. Unlike patients with lactic acidosis, those with hyperchloremic metabolic acidosis have a normal anion gap and elevated serum chloride. In patients undergoing noncardiac and nontransplant surgery, hyperchloremia has been associated with postoperative renal dysfunction and increased 30-day mortality.[8] Other adverse effects of hyperchloremia and acidosis include altered splanchnic and renal blood flow, altered hemoglobin oxygen binding, impaired coagulation, and amplification of the inflammatory response in sepsis.

The effects of crystalloid solutions on the coagulation system are complex. With hemodilution up to 20–40%, crystalloids produce a hypercoagulable state due to dilution of anticoagulant factors such as antithrombin, and by platelet activation.[9–11] After 60% hemodilution, both crystalloids and colloids produce a hypocoagulable state. However, animal studies point to attenuation of hypercoagulability and increased blood loss in uncontrolled hemorrhagic shock treated with 0.9% saline as opposed to LR. A head-to-head comparison of these two crystalloid solutions in patients undergoing abdominal aortic aneurysm repair found an increased need for bicarbonate, platelets, and blood products in patients receiving 0.9% saline compared with LR.

Glucose-containing solutions are avoided because hyperglycemia is associated with increased mortality rate, hospital length of stay, ICU length of stay, and incidence of nosocomial infection. Hyperglycemia is also associated with worse neurologic outcomes in patients with TBI. Intensive insulin therapy guided by specific target glucose levels was shown to improve in-hospital survival, with the benefit preserved over a 4-year follow-up, to prevent critical illness neuropathy, to decrease the need for long-term ventilation, and to shorten ICU stay. Paradoxically, the effect was most prominent in nondiabetic patients. The effect is seemingly dependent more on strict glucose control than on the dose of insulin, even though nonhypoglycemic effects of insulin are generally well recognized and might play a role. It should be noted that in observational studies, patients with more severe TBI have higher blood glucose levels, i.e., hyperglycemia might be a marker of injury severity and a predictor of the outcome rather than the causative agent. Improved outcome with strict glucose control might then be due to effects of insulin infusion rather than lowering the glucose level. Some animal studies have suggested that hyperglycemia induced by rapid glucose infusion does not worsen different markers of neurologic injury, survival, and neurologic sequelae of head trauma. Based on the NICE-SUGAR trial (Normoglycemia in Intensive Care Evaluation Survival Using Glucose Algorithm Regulation), a glucose level of 140–180 mg/dL is generally targeted after trauma. Insulin is often required.[12] Tight glucose control (80–110 mg/dL) is undesirable after trauma because of the increased incidence of severe hypoglycemia. In any case, the routine use of glucose-containing solutions is not justified.

Colloids

Although colloid solutions such as albumin and various hydroxyethyl starch (HES) solutions are more effective plasma expanders than crystalloids, these solutions are not recommended for trauma patients, as discussed below. An intact endovascular glycocalyx is critical to prevent extravasation of these colloids into extravascular compartments.[13] Classic teaching postulates that oncotic pressure serves to retain the intravascular volume. As long as the endovascular glycocalyx remains intact, the large molecules do not migrate into the extravascular space; therefore, the same increase in intravascular volume and preload can be achieved with a smaller volume, less peripheral edema, less endothelial swelling, improved tissue perfusion, improved wound and anastomotic healing, and decreased risk of pulmonary complications and brain swelling. Despite the differences between colloid solutions, a Cochrane review of 86 studies did not find a significant difference in mortality between albumin, starches, dextran, and gelatin.[14]

In relatively stable patients, there is evidence that limited use of colloids is beneficial. For example, intraoperative use of colloid solutions has been associated with improved outcome and decreased hospital stay, possibly due to decreased tissue edema, nausea, vomiting, and pain in elective surgery patients with moderate blood loss. In critically ill patients (e.g., sepsis, shock, endotoxemia, hypoxia, ischemia), however, the glycocalyx is degraded; this decreases the ability of the colloid to expand the plasma volume and may result in accumulation of the colloid in the extravascular space with resultant adverse effects.

The European Society of Intensive Care Medicine (ESICM) task force on colloid volume therapy in critically ill patients reviewed the data available as of May 2011. The consensus statement issued in Feb 2012 stated:

> We recommend not to use HES with molecular weight ≥ 200 kDa and/or degree of substitution > 0.4 in patients with severe sepsis or risk of acute kidney injury and suggest not to use 6% HES 130/0.4 or gelatin in these populations. We recommend not to use colloids in patients with head injury and not to administer gelatins and HES in organ donors. We suggest not using hyperoncotic solutions for fluid resuscitation. We conclude and recommend

that any new colloid should be introduced into clinical practice only after its patient-important safety parameters are established.[15]

Since then, another large study in sepsis patients has shown an increased risk of kidney failure and of the duration of ventilator support with HES and gelatin as opposed to crystalloids, with minimal, if any, benefit in normalizing the volume status.[16] HES-based fluid therapy has also resulted in significantly higher need for platelets and plasma transfusion. The US Food and Drug Administration (FDA) has issued a black box warning against using HES. In Great Britain, all starches have been withdrawn from market.

HES solutions are now avoided in trauma, as they increase the risk of acute kidney injury, the need for renal replacement therapy, and mortality. Dextrans have been largely abandoned for fluid resuscitation due to the negative effects on coagulation and high anaphylactic potential. Similarly, gelatins were abandoned in the USA due to the high incidence of hypersensitivity reactions.

Albumin

Albumin is derived from pooled human plasma, does not affect kidney function nor coagulation, and does not disrupt glycocalyx. Albumin is generally accepted to be safe in terms of transmission of infectious diseases. It saves lives in some situations. For example, a meta-analysis on fluid therapy in spontaneous bacterial peritonitis has shown that use of albumin reduced mortality by a factor of three and risk of kidney damage by a factor of five.[17] In CABG patients, use of albumin instead of hetastarch and/or dextran reduced mortality.[18]

Aside from its volume-replacing properties, albumin may have some additional specific effects such as transport function for various drugs and endogenous substances or effects on membrane permeability secondary to free-radical scavenging. Of note, in patients with impaired vascular endothelial integrity, albumin may pass into the interstitial compartment with resultant endothelial swelling and impaired microcirculatory perfusion.

However, in trauma and in the general critical care population, albumin confers no benefits or is outright detrimental. The lack of benefit has been known since the publication of the first Cochrane review on the subject in 1998.[19] In subgroup analysis, albumin has actually increased mortality. A recent Cochrane review has found no difference in outcomes between patients treated with albumin and crystalloids.[20]

The single largest trial to date is the Saline versus Albumin Fluid Evaluation (SAFE) study, in which there was no difference in 28-day mortality, length of stay, ventilation days, and new organ failure.[21] With albumin, there were trends for an improved survival in severe sepsis patients and for increased mortality in trauma patients. Mortality for head trauma patients was 25% if treated with albumin versus 15% if treated with normal saline. In a post-hoc analysis of patients with TBI, the 24-month mortality was significantly worse with albumin (relative risk [RR] = 1.63, $p = 0.003$) and even more so in patients with severe brain injury (RR = 1.88, $p < 0.001$).[22]

Hypertonic fluids

Use of hypertonic solutions for different populations of critically ill patients has been investigated for more than two decades. The obvious rationale is that a minimal volume of hypertonic saline will draw intracellular water into the extracellular space. Volume expansion with hypertonic saline is more efficient and better sustained than with normosmolar fluids. In comparison of the peak hemodilution in healthy volunteers, 7.5% saline and 7.5% saline in 6% dextran were 4.4 and 6.2 times more effective than similar volumes of 0.9% saline, respectively. The area under the hemodilution–time curve was seven times larger for 7.5% saline in dextran and 3.8 times larger for 7.5% saline than for 0.9% saline. As expected, addition of colloid to hypertonic saline increased the magnitude and markedly prolonged the duration of volume expansion.[4] When a 30-minute infusion of 4 mL/kg of 7.5% saline in 6% dextran was compared to 25 mL/kg of LR, the peak volume expansion was similar – about 7 mL/kg. However, 30 minutes later, the volume expansion with hypertonic saline–dextran was three times higher than with LR (5.1 ± 0.9 vs 1.7 ± 0.6 mL/kg). At 2 hours, for each mL of the fluid infused, the remaining intravascular volume expansion was 0.07 mL for LR and 0.7 mL for hypertonic saline–dextran. Hypertonic fluids are especially advantageous in military trauma and other situations (e.g., prehospital, helicopter) when the weight/benefit ratio is crucial.

In hemorrhagic shock or local ischemia, cells swell, absorb water, chloride, and sodium, and lose their resting membrane potential. They return to normal volume, electrolyte balance, and resting potential with hypertonic saline better than with isotonic resuscitation. Capillary lumens narrow as a result of this swelling, and return to normal diameter with hypertonic resuscitation but not with LR. Further, hypertonic saline restores intravascular volume and hemodynamics while decreasing extravascular volume and tissue edema. With LR, extravascular volume increased by 60% of the infused volume at the end of the infusion and by 43% at 2 hours, while with hypertonic saline–dextran extravascular water decreased by 170% and 430%, respectively. In brain injury associated with pulmonary edema, hypertonic saline depletes tissue water content better than mannitol. This feature may be crucial in situations such as head trauma (see Chapter 35).

Prehospital infusion of 250 mL of 7.5% saline, with or without dextran, followed by usual fluid resuscitation, to hypotensive trauma patients was compared to LR.[23] The bolus of hypertonic fluid resulted in improved blood pressure, decreased fluid requirements, and increased survival to discharge, especially in patients with Glasgow Coma Scale < 8. The rise in the circulating blood volume and cardiac output is immediate, although a transient decrease in blood pressure due to vasodilatation may occur. Hypertonic solutions increase cardiac contractility, venous return, and coronary blood flow. Moreover, hypertonic saline–dextran solution is effective in treating dehydration and massive hemorrhage in animals with preexisting dehydration.

Hypertonic solutions used in clinical studies vary. The most common regimen is 100–250 mL or 1.5–2 mL/kg of 7.2–7.5% saline with or without colloid. The US military recommends 7.5% saline; in Europe, 7.5% saline in 6% dextran-70 is used. Other regimens include single boluses of 30 mL of 23.4% saline, 75 mL of 10% saline, or continuous infusions of 3% saline. For most studies in head trauma, regardless of concentration used, the dose of sodium chloride infused with a single fluid bolus in adult patients ranges approximately from 7 to 15 g, or 120 to 300 mEq. Accordingly, results are fairly uniform. A single infusion of hypertonic saline will decrease intracranial pressure by around 70% or 10–25 mmHg and increase the cerebral perfusion pressure by 10–30 mmHg, both effects evident in a matter of minutes, reaching maximum effect by 20–60 minutes, and lasting for 1.5–4 hours, sometimes longer. Similar effects have been observed in patients with stroke and subarachnoid hemorrhage. Effects of hypertonic saline on intracranial and cerebral perfusion pressure were more rapid and more profound than a comparable or double volume of 20% mannitol, and lasted longer.

In a study on trauma patients whose elevated intracranial pressure was refractory to all other modalities, 2 mL/kg of hypertonic saline was compared to a similar volume of 20% mannitol.[24] In the hypertonic saline group, the number of episodes of elevated intracranial pressure was reduced by almost a half and their cumulative duration by about a third as compared to patients treated with mannitol. Similarly, patients in the hypertonic saline group required 50% less volume of cerebrospinal fluid drainage to maintain target intracranial and cerebral perfusion pressure, and the success rate in achieving these targets was 90% in the hypertonic saline group versus only 30% in the mannitol group. The clinical outcome at 90 days was, however, similar in both groups.

In a study of pediatric head-injured patients whose elevated intracranial pressure had been refractory to all other modalities including mannitol and barbiturate coma, continuous infusion of 3% saline for the mean of 7.6 days (range 4–18 days) led to a rapid and sustained improvement in intracranial and cerebral perfusion pressure.[25] The treatment was surprisingly well tolerated, even though on average the serum sodium was 171 mEq/L (range 157–187 mEq/L) and serum osmolarity was 365 mOsm/L (range 330–431 mOsm/L).

A cohort study in patients with TBI and hypotension compared 7.5% saline/6% dextran-70 with conventional crystalloid fluid treatment.[26] With the hypertonic fluid, there was a trend for improved survival to discharge in all the subgroups (odds ratio = 1.6–1.8). For patients with initial Glasgow Coma Scale < 8, the odds ratio for survival until discharge was 2.12 with hypertonic saline–dextran versus conventional treatment. On the other hand, in a randomized controlled trial of patients with TBI who were comatose (Glasgow Coma Scale < 9) and hypotensive (systolic blood pressure < 100 mmHg), at 6 months after injury the patients who received prehospital resuscitation with 250 mL of 7.5% saline had almost identical neurological function to the ones resuscitated with conventional fluid.[23] There was no significant difference between the groups in terms of favorable outcomes or in any other measure of post-injury neurological function.

Hypertonic saline has some immune-modulating effects. For example, hypertonic saline resuscitation in traumatic hemorrhagic shock in humans blunts the usual response in distribution of monocyte receptors, decreases tumor necrosis factor alpha (TNF-α), and increases anti-inflammatory interleukins (IL-1ra and IL-10). In a meta-analysis of studies of hypertonic saline in patients with trauma, burns, or those undergoing surgery, the pooled relative risk (RR) for death in trauma patients was 0.84 (95% confidence interval [CI] 0.69–1.04); in patients with burns 1.49 (95% CI 0.56–3.95); and in patients undergoing surgery 0.51 (95% CI 0.09–2.73).[27] In the one trial that gave data on disability using the Glasgow outcome scale, the relative risk for a poor outcome was 1.00 (95% CI 0.82–1.22).

Two important multicenter studies designed to provide the definitive answers were stopped early, having satisfied the predetermined criteria for futility. Both were three-arm studies, randomizing patients to 250 mL of normal saline, hypertonic saline, or hypertonic saline in dextran, given as early as possible and after not more than 2 L of total IV fluids, followed by the usual fluid resuscitation. One enrolled patients with severe TBI who were not in hypovolemic shock.[28] The other included trauma patients presenting with hypovolemic shock.[29] In both, there was no difference in outcomes and it was judged, by a predetermined interim analysis, that continuing enrollment was unlikely to produce significant results. There was a trend to worse outcomes in patients who received hypertonic saline and did not require transfusion later.

The European guidelines suggest that hypertonic solutions during initial treatment may be used, but demonstrate no advantage compared to crystalloids or colloids in blunt trauma and TBI. They recommend that "hypertonic solutions be used in hemodynamically unstable patients with penetrating torso trauma."[6]

Red blood cell transfusions (RBCs)
General considerations

In a hemodynamically stable nonbleeding patient, the safest transfusion is no transfusion and the best transfusion is the transfusion not given.[30] The fact that a certain level of anemia is dangerous does not necessarily mean that correcting it with allogeneic RBCs is going to benefit the patient. In many cases, transfusion causes more harm than treating the anemia conservatively. However, we should also keep in mind that despite the limited ability of RBCs to restore tissue oxygenation, and despite all the harmful effects of transfusion, we routinely treat patients who exsanguinate, receive massive transfusion of several blood volumes, recuperate from their injuries, and survive (see Chapter 6).

The lower limit of anemia is not established in humans. Observational studies on surgical patients refusing transfusion for religious reasons suggest that the risk of mortality and/or morbidity is increased with hemoglobin levels below 5–6 g/dL.[31] After adjusting for age, cardiovascular disease, and Acute Physiology and Chronic Health Evaluation II (APACHE II) score, the odds of death in patients with a postoperative hemoglobin level ≤ 8 g/dL increase by a factor of 2.5 for each 1 g decrease in hemoglobin level. A retrospective cohort study of patients who declined RBCs for religious reasons demonstrated that in patients with a postoperative hemoglobin level of 7.1–8.0 g/dL, none died and 9% had a morbid event such as myocardial infarction, arrhythmia, or congestive heart failure. In patients with a postoperative hemoglobin level of 4.1–5.0 g/dL, 34% died and 58% had a morbid event or died. Of note, age, systolic BP at admission, Glasgow Coma Scale score, and type of trauma were more important predictors of mortality than religious objection to blood.

Normally, oxygen delivery exceeds oxygen consumption three- to fourfold. Consumption is thus independent of delivery over a wide range of hemoglobin concentrations. The "critical hematocrit" (or hemoglobin) is defined as the threshold below which the body oxygen consumption becomes dependent on oxygen delivery.

Several factors help maintain tissue oxygenation in acutely anemic patients. Sympathetic stimulation increases heart rate and contractility. Decreased blood viscosity increases venous return and lowers systemic vascular resistance (SVR), thus increasing the stroke volume. Indeed, the observed increase in stroke volume closely parallels the calculated one produced by the decreased blood viscosity. Importantly, the increase in cardiac output occurs without an increase in cardiac workload and without detectable cardiac ischemia. Redistribution of blood flow to vital organs may protect them even if whole-body perfusion/oxygen delivery is falling. Oxygen extraction ratio by most organs, including the brain, increases. Mobilization of capillary flow increases the oxygen extraction, since only about one-third of capillaries are usually perfused. In the setting of shock and severe hypoperfusion, oxygen extraction will increase as a result of the expected rightward shift in oxygen dissociation due to tissue acidosis and/or hypercarbia. Later, the oxyhemoglobin dissociation curve shifts to the right as a result of increased production of 2,3-diphosphoglyceric acid (2,3-DPG, also known as 2,3-bisphosphoglycerate or 2,3-BPG). The heart, as opposed to other organs, does not have a large oxygen extraction reserve, and compensates for anemia by increasing coronary blood flow. This mechanism might be impaired by coronary artery disease. In a series of experiments on dogs, presence of a critical coronary stenosis significantly impaired the heart's tolerance to acute anemia. In CABG patients, hemodilution to hematocrit of 30% combined with increased heart rate resulted in decreased myocardial contractility.

BP decreases in the setting of decreased blood viscosity and SVR. Both are beneficial, and the resulting hypotension is not an indication for transfusion. Conversely, transfusion of RBCs impedes peripheral perfusion (see below) and increases blood viscosity, thus increasing SVR, which in turn will raise the measured BP; this in itself, however, cannot be considered a beneficial change.

In a series of human experiments with acute normovolemic hemodilution to hemoglobin 5 g/dL, subcutaneous tissue perfusion increased and oxygen tension remained stable, even in the subjects who were mildly hypoperfused at baseline. Transient and asymptomatic ECG changes were observed in only 3 out of 55 volunteers, all at hemoglobin of less than 7 g/dL, in conjunction with movement or tachycardia. Subtle cognitive function impairment only appeared at or below hemoglobin 6 g/dL and was readily reversible with administration of 100% oxygen.[32] The same authors used invasive monitoring to investigate the effects of acute normovolemic hemodilution in awake volunteers and in patients without cardiovascular comorbidities (mean age 50; range 35–69 years) undergoing major surgery with general anesthesia. Gradual hemodilution resulted in increased cardiac index and stable oxygen delivery down to hemoglobin of approximately 7.5–8 g/dL in males, and 5.5–6 g/dL in females. Below this level, and down to 4.5–5.4 g/dL, oxygen delivery decreased in parallel to the fall in oxygen-carrying capacity. Tissue oxygen extraction ratio increased from 23% to 30%, and oxygen consumption actually increased by approximately 12%. pH increased, base excess was more positive, and there was a trend to a lower lactate level.[33]

The cardiovascular and metabolic response to acute, severe isovolemic anemia was studied in elderly patients (76 ± 2 years, range 66–88), many of them with diabetes and other significant risk factors, undergoing major abdominal surgery.[33] Patients were hemodiluted from hemoglobin of 11.6 to 8.8 g/dL before surgery. Hemoglobin further decreased on average to 7.7 g/dL due to surgical blood loss. Oxygen consumption was stable throughout surgery, and signs of myocardial ischemia such as ST segment changes, arrhythmias, and hypotension were absent. In patients separating from cardiopulmonary bypass, hemodilution to a hematocrit of 15% resulted in decreased MAP and oxygen delivery, increased cardiac output and oxygen extraction ratio, and stable oxygen consumption across the tested range.

The physiologic changes described above have been repeatedly demonstrated in studies on acute hemodilution, with oxygen consumption remaining stable and without signs of myocardial ischemia in the range of 7.5–8 g/dL in moribund elderly patients, 4.5–5.5 g/dL in healthy awake volunteers and healthy surgical patients and in CABG patients, and at 3 g/dL in children undergoing major spine surgery.

Of note, in awake normovolemic patients, heart rate increases linearly with normovolemic anemia. In patients under general anesthesia, however, anemia does not induce tachycardia. The increased cardiac output is due to increased stroke volume alone. An increase in the heart rate should raise suspicion for hypovolemia.

A literature review published in 1994 reported on Jehovah's Witnesses with hemoglobin < 8 g/dL or hematocrit < 24%.[34] With the exception of three patients who died after cardiac surgery, all of the deaths attributed to anemia occurred when hemoglobin was lower than 5 g/dL, adding to the anecdotal evidence of human tolerance to anemia.

In surgical patients without cardiovascular comorbidities, there are anecdotal reports of survival without major complications despite extreme levels of normovolemic anemia. Fewer data are available in patients with coronary artery or valvular heart disease. In observational studies, any level of anemia has been associated with increased perioperative mortality, and more so in patients with preexisting cardiovascular disease. However, anemia might be a result of and a marker for ill health rather than a cause for the adverse outcome. For example, in patients undergoing cardiopulmonary bypass, after correction for comorbidities, only a nadir hematocrit of lower than 14% (17% for high-risk patients) was an independent risk factor of adverse outcome.[35]

Under normal conditions, oxygen dissolved in the blood accounts for only about 2% of the blood oxygen content. With hemodilution and thus a relatively larger plasma volume, and especially if high inspired oxygen concentrations are used, dissolved O_2 becomes clinically relevant. Switching from room air to pure oxygen is equivalent to increasing hemoglobin by at least 3 g/dL. In a series of experiments on pigs, hyperoxia improved tolerance of extreme anemia and decreased critical hemoglobin levels from 2.4 when breathing room air to 1.5 g/dL at $FiO_2 = 0.6$, and to 1.2 g/dL at $FiO_2 = 1.0$. There was 100% mortality at critical hemoglobin and $FiO_2 = 0.21$, whereas switching to 100% oxygen increased oxygen delivery and resulted in 100% survival at 6 hours.[36] In healthy human volunteers breathing room air, acute normovolemic hemodilution from 12.7 to 5.7 g/dL resulted in hypotension, tachycardia, and cognitive changes.[37] Oxygen administration decreased heart rate and restored cognitive function even though BP did not change.

More relevant is the question of whether correcting anemia with stored RBCs will improve the oxygen consumption, and how will it affect outcome. First, despite the immediate improvement in the oxygen-carrying capacity of the blood and oxygen delivery, transfusion may not improve the target tissue oxygen utilization, unless the patient has already reached the critical hemoglobin concentration. Second, older RBC units have low levels of 2,3-DPG. Their ability to release transported oxygen into the peripheral tissues is compromised; it takes 6–24 hours to restore the normal levels of 2,3-DPG. Third, older RBCs lack normal deformability and thus impair the capillary flow. These effects are clinically significant. For example, in cardiac patients with hemoglobin 7.5–8.5 g/dL, transfusion of 1–2 red cell units increased the calculated oxygen delivery but did not increase oxygen consumption or tissue oxygenation.[38] In an ICU study on critically ill septic patients, transfusion of 3 red cell units failed to improve the tissue oxygenation for up to 6 hours.[39] More importantly, there was an inverse correlation between age of blood units and tissue pH. Transfusion of red cell units older than 15 days consistently worsened the tissue acidosis.

Two main approaches factor into the decision to transfuse. First is the so-called transfusion trigger – the level of anemia at which there is a favorable risk–benefit ratio for the transfusion, usually determined by patient factors, clinical experience, practice setting, and judgment. Second are real-time physiologic data such as hemodynamic instability despite normovolemia, decreased mixed venous oxygen saturation, evidence of target-organ ischemia, and direct or indirect measurement of brain oxygenation. Threshold-based transfusion is not appropriate for trauma patients with uncontrolled hemorrhage, because it requires waiting for hemoglobin levels to be reported, and the result might not reflect the magnitude of the ongoing or recent blood loss.

Jehovah's Witness (JW) patients undergoing coronary bypass surgery were compared to the regular patients chosen from almost 90,000 patients, allowing for a very precise propensity score matching.[40] Compared to their transfused counterparts, JW patients experienced fewer myocardial infarctions (0.31% vs. 2.8%), had fewer reoperations for bleeding (3.7% vs. 7.1%), less need for prolonged ventilation (6% vs. 16%), had a day shorter length of stay in the hospital and in the ICU, had a better survival at 1 year (95% vs. 89%) and similar survival at 20-year follow-up (34% vs. 32%). Outcomes in the nontransfused non-JW patients were similar to those in JW patients.[40] In another study on open heart surgery, transfusion increased infection by 238%, ischemic outcomes by 235% and the cost of admission by 42%, decreased the chance of discharge alive by 37%, increased the risk of 30-day mortality more than 6-fold, and the one-year mortality by 32%.[41] Chance of stroke after CABG is increased with transfusion in a dose-dependent manner. In carotid endarterectomy, transfusion of 1–2 units increases the chance of stroke fivefold.

Since burn patients die from sepsis and transfusion increases infection risk, it is plausible that transfusion would increase mortality in thermal injury. Surprisingly, we could not find many data on these patients. In one large study, transfusion increased mortality by a factor of five.[42] In a trial of burn patients randomized to hemoglobin < 10 g/dL versus > 10 g/dL, there was no difference in skin graft take between groups.[43] The authors concluded that mild to moderate anemia does not cause any deleterious effect on wound healing.

For perioperative vision loss, in multivariate models built for different clinical scenarios, anemia either is not an independent risk factor or enters the models together with transfusion – i.e., for a given level of anemia, allogeneic transfusion further increases the risk of blindness.[44] Exclusions are cardiac surgery, where transfusion is an independent risk factor while the anemia is not, and spine fusion, where the opposite is true. In a landmark trial (the TRICC study), critically ill euvolemic patients with hemoglobin < 9 g/dL were randomized to transfusion trigger of hemoglobin 7 g/dL or 10 g/dL.[45] Patients in both the restrictive and liberal arms of the study had an average of 2 or more units of blood transfused prior to randomization. Patients in the restrictive arm received 54% fewer transfusions, and their chance to receive any transfusion after randomization was diminished by 33%. As expected, shock was diagnosed more often in the restrictive group. However, the patients in the restrictive arm had a one-third lower incidence of acute respiratory distress syndrome (ARDS) and 35% fewer cardiac complications such as myocardial infarction (MI) or pulmonary edema. Adjusted multiple-organ failure scores were lower with the restrictive protocol. Mortality was lower with the restrictive strategy in patients younger than 55 years and with APACHE II score of ≤ 20, and similar or nonsignificantly lower for all other subgroups, including separate analyses for patients with trauma and cardiovascular disease.[46,47] Surprisingly, the association of decreased incidence of infections and bacteremia in the restrictive group did not reach statistical significance, possibly because of transfusion before randomization, which would blunt the difference between the groups. The rate of pneumonia was about 20% in both groups. Rates of all other individual complications (aside from shock) were nonsignificantly lower in the restrictive compared with the liberal transfusion group. Overall, the rate of complications was about 10% lower in the restrictive than in the liberal transfusion group, but this was not a statistically significant difference.

In critically ill children randomized to RBC transfusion at the trigger of 7 versus 9.5 g/dL, there was no difference in either mortality or multiorgan dysfunction. Patients in the restrictive-strategy group received 44% fewer transfusions; no significant differences were found in other outcomes, including adverse events, although the length of stay in the ICU was prolonged from 7.7 to 11.6 days by the liberal transfusion.[48] The authors concluded that a restrictive transfusion strategy can decrease transfusion requirements without increasing adverse outcomes.

In the Transfusion After Cardiac Surgery (TRACS) study, patients undergoing cardiac surgery with cardiopulmonary bypass were randomized to a liberal strategy of blood transfusion (to maintain a hematocrit ≥ 30%) or to a restrictive strategy (hematocrit ≥ 24%).[49] As per routine hospital policy, only new (< 14 days old) units were used. A liberal transfusion strategy led to increased RBC transfusions. Independent of transfusion strategy, the number of transfused RBC units was an independent risk factor for clinical complications or death at 30 days.

In the CRIT Pilot study anemic patients with acute MI were randomized to a liberal (hematocrit > 30%) or restrictive (target hematocrit 24–27%) transfusions.[50] Liberal transfusion increased in-hospital death, recurrent MI, or new or worsening congestive heart failure from 13% to 38%.

Finally, a 2012 Cochrane review of 19 studies on the transfusion threshold, enrolling a total of 6264 patients, demonstrated an overall decrease of 23% in in-hospital mortality with a restrictive transfusion threshold.[51]

Regarding the effect of anemia and transfusions on mortality in cardiac patients, a post-hoc analysis of 24,112 patients with acute coronary syndrome pooled from three large

Table 8.4 Approach to transfusing red blood cells (RBCs) in bleeding trauma patients, based on the American Society of Anesthesiologists Practice Guidelines and review of the literature.

Transfuse RBCs if hemoglobin < 6 g/dL
Do not transfuse RBCs if hemoglobin > 10 g/dL
Decision to transfuse RBCs should be individualized based on: (1) presence of organ ischemia (e.g., altered mental status, myocardial ischemia, acidosis, low mixed venous oxygen saturation) (2) rate of bleeding (3) magnitude of bleeding (4) ability of physicians to stop the bleeding (5) intravascular volume status (6) cardiopulmonary reserve

Table 8.5 American Association of Blood Banks (AABB) red blood cell transfusion guidelines for hemodynamically stable patients without active bleeding

Hemoglobin concentration	Recommendation
< 6 g/dL	Transfusion recommended except in exceptional circumstances
6–7 g/dL	Transfusion likely to be indicated
7–8 g/dL	Transfusion should be considered in postoperative surgical patients, including those with stable cardiovascular disease, after evaluating the patient's clinical status
8–10 g/dL	Transfusion generally not indicated, but should be considered for some populations (e.g., those with symptomatic anemia, ongoing bleeding, acute coronary syndrome with ischemia)
> 10 g/dL	Transfusion not indicated except in exceptional circumstances

Note that the decision to transfuse should incorporate individual patient characteristics and symptoms. Clinical judgment is critical in the decision to transfuse. Similarly, the decision not to transfuse RBCs to a patient is also a matter of clinical judgment. Adapted from Carson JL, Grossman BJ, Kleinman S, et al. Red blood cell transfusion: a clinical practice guideline from the AABB. *Ann Intern Med* 2012; **157**: 49.

cardiology trials revealed a fourfold increase in 30-day mortality with transfusion at a hematocrit higher than 25%, and a trend to increased mortality below this level.[52,53] In a meta-analysis of 10 observational studies on transfusion in acute MI involving a total of 203,665 patients, transfusion tripled the all-cause 30-day mortality, and doubled the risk of recurrent myocardial infarction.[54] There was an additional death for every eight patients transfused.

Recommendations for RBC transfusion

The American Society of Anesthesiologists (ASA) practice guidelines, last updated in 2006, recommend transfusion if hemoglobin concentration is below 6 g/dL and do not recommend transfusion with hemoglobin concentration above 10 g/dL.[55] The decision to transfuse in the 6–10 g/dL hemoglobin concentration range should be individualized according to presence of organ ischemia, rate and magnitude of potential or actual bleeding, intravascular volume status, and risk factors for complications of inadequate oxygenation, such as low cardiopulmonary reserve and high oxygen consumption (Table 8.4). The decision not to transfuse RBCs to an anemic patient is a matter of clinical judgment (Table 8.5). Although some authorities recommend using mixed venous oxygen saturation (SvO_2) < 50% or mixed venous oxygen tension (PvO_2) < 32 mmHg as a trigger for transfusion, clinical and laboratory evidence are more frequently used. Use of factor concentrates, more effective use of blood salvage devices, and possibly other means of bleeding control may significantly decrease the need for allogeneic transfusion in the future.

The European task force notes that the use of a single hematocrit measurement may be misleading and may not accurately reflect blood loss due to the confounding influence of resuscitative measures on the hematocrit. Decreasing serial hematocrit measurements, however, typically reflect continued bleeding. The European task force recommends a target hemoglobin of 7–9 g/dL.[6]

One unit of RBCs will usually increase the hematocrit by approximately 3% or the hemoglobin by 1 g/dL in a 70 kg nonbleeding adult. Available options are type O negative, type-specific, typed and screened, or typed and crossmatched packed RBCs. Type O negative red cells have no major antigens and can be given reasonably safely to patients with any blood type. Unfortunately, only 8% of the population has O negative blood, and blood bank reserves of O negative, low-antibody-titer blood are usually very low. For this reason, O positive red cells are frequently used. This is a reasonable approach in males but may be a problem in females of child-bearing age. If 50–75% of the patient's blood volume has been replaced with type O blood (e.g., approximately 10 units of red cells in an average-size adult patient), one should continue to administer type O red cells, unless directed otherwise by the blood bank. The concern is that the patient may have received enough anti-A or anti-B antibodies to precipitate hemolysis if A, B, or AB units are subsequently given.

Obtaining type-specific red cells requires 5–10 minutes in most institutions, and "temporizing" measures can sometimes be employed to gain the necessary time. Switching to a type-specific blood transfusion as soon as possible would spare the scarce supply of O-type blood, reduce the risk of hemolytic transfusion reaction and allow to continue with a type-specific and crossmatched blood transfusion once it becomes available. If one can wait 15 minutes, typed and screened blood should be available. A full crossmatch generally requires about 45 minutes and involves mixing donor cells with recipient serum to rule out any unexpected antigen/antibody reactions.

Coagulation factors and platelets

The primary cause of bleeding after trauma is surgical, while other major causes are hypothermia, acidemia, dilutional coagulopathy, and trauma-induced coagulopathy (TIC, also known as posttraumatic coagulopathy, acute coagulopathy of trauma, and acute traumatic coagulopathy). TIC develops rapidly after injury, and is associated with shock, inflammation, tissue hypoperfusion, and activation of protein C (inhibiting thrombin formation) and tissue plasminogen activator (resulting in hyperfibrinolysis).[56,57]

There is a lack of evidence to identify a critical international normalized ratio (INR), prothrombin time (PT), partial thromboplastin time (PTT), fibrinogen level, or platelet count to trigger a blood component transfusion in patients with critical bleeding requiring massive transfusion. This is likely due to the dynamic and complex interactions of thrombin, fibrinogen, tissue factor, platelets, other clotting factors, and endothelium in the bleeding patient, which is modified by shock, resuscitation, hypothermia, and acidosis.[58] Current European guidelines recommend early, repeated, and combined measurement of PT, PTT, fibrinogen, and platelets. The guidelines also recommend that viscoelastic coagulation testing be performed to assist in characterizing the coagulopathy and in guiding hemostatic therapy (Fig. 8.1). Platelet function tests may also be required (e.g., whole blood impedance aggregometry). Point-of-care coagulation testing (e.g., thromboelastography [TEG], thromboelastometry) provides real-time information on the coagulation system and can help guide hemostatic therapy (Fig. 8.2).[59] In the absence of point-of-care coagulation testing, traditional tests such as PT, INR, PTT, fibrinogen, and fibrinogen degradation products are measured. Rapid TEG seems to correlate better with the relevant clinical outcomes and provide faster results at a comparable cost. Murray *et al.* have showed microvascular bleeding and clinical evidence of coagulopathy occurred in the setting of massive transfusion and was associated with decreased coagulation factor levels, decreased fibrinogen, and elevated prothrombin times.[60] Microvascular bleeding in this instance was treated with fresh frozen plasma (FFP).

Two units of thawed plasma (10–15 mL/kg) will achieve 30% factor activity in most adults. Liquid plasma, approved by the FDA to be stored for up to 26 days at 1–6 °C without being ever frozen, might have a better hemostatic profile than the thawed frozen plasma.

Coagulation factor deficiencies may be present due to other causes such as preexisting defects, disseminated intravascular coagulopathy (DIC), and TIC. Cryoprecipitate and factor concentrates may be indicated to correct specific factor deficiencies. Cryoprecipitate is a highly concentrated source of fibrinogen: one unit of cryo contains approximately 200–400 mg of fibrinogen in a volume of 10–15 mL. Additionally, cryoprecipitate contains high concentrations of factor VIII and von Willebrand factor, which further enhance platelet adhesion and coagulation. In Europe, factor concentrates are routinely used instead of cryoprecipitate or thawed plasma.

Dilutional thrombocytopenia and microvascular bleeding is likely after 1.5–2.0 blood volumes have been transfused. For example, Leslie and Toy showed that platelet count was reduced to < 50,000/μL after administration of 20 units of red cells.[61] Platelet transfusions are usually indicated in the presence of clinical bleeding and a platelet count of less than 75,000–100,000/μL. Platelet concentrates are stored at room temperature (thus a higher risk of bacterial contamination) and contain about 70% of the platelets in a unit of blood. One unit of platelets, equivalent to 50 mL, increases the platelet count in an average adult by 5,000–10,000/μL. Transfusion of single-donor pooled platelet units, equivalent each to 6 units of random donor platelet units, has become routine at many institutions. Since platelets are suspended in plasma, 1 unit of single-donor apheresis platelets or 4–5 multiple donor platelet units will provide factor levels similar to 1 unit of thawed plasma.

Factor concentrates

Fibrinogen

Fibrinogen, or factor 1, is a key component in the coagulation cascade and facilitates effective coagulation and platelet function. During massive transfusion, fibrinogen is the first

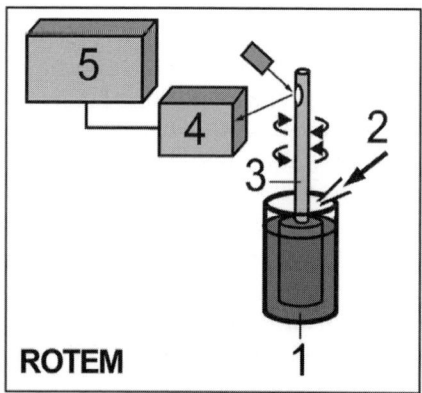

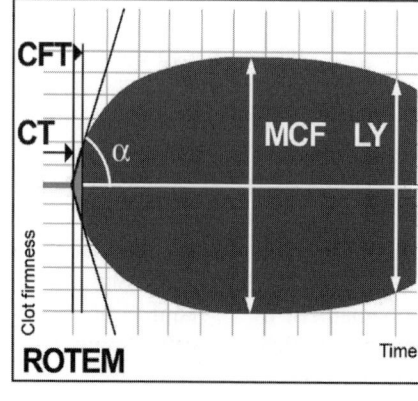

Figure 8.1 Viscoelastic point-of-care coagulation monitoring with rotational thromboelastometry (ROTEM). (**A**) Working principle: (1) stationary cuvette with blood, (2) coagulation activator added by automated pipette, (3) rotating pin stabilized by a high-precision ball-bearing system, (4) electromechanical signal detection via light source and mirror mounted on the shaft of the pin, (5) data processing unit. (**B**) ROTEM tracing: CT, clotting time; CFT, clot formation time; α, slope of tangent at 2 mm amplitude; MCF, maximal clot firmness; LY, lysis. (Courtesy of Michael Ganter, MD.)

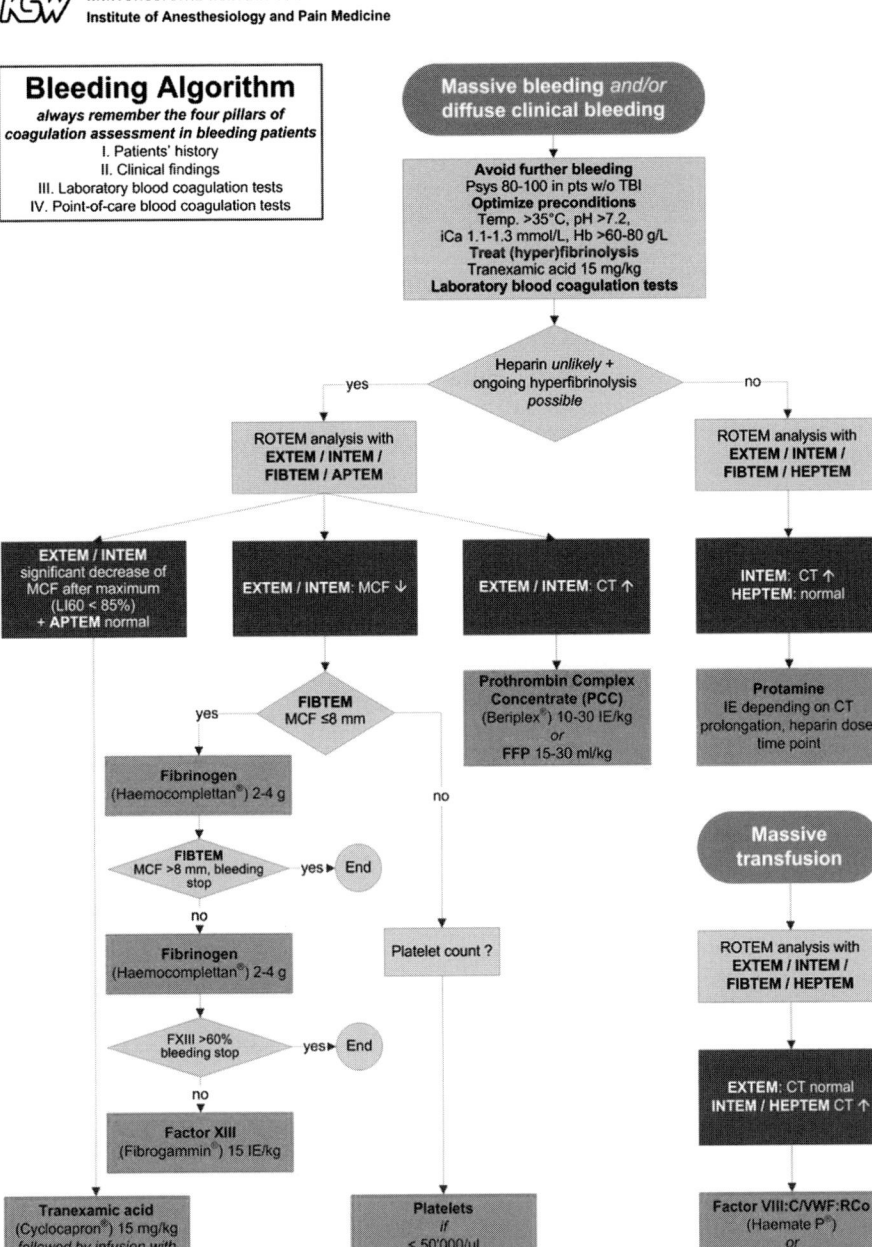

KSW KANTONSSPITAL WINTERTHUR
Institute of Anesthesiology and Pain Medicine

Bleeding Algorithm
always remember the four pillars of
coagulation assessment in bleeding patients
I. Patients' history
II. Clinical findings
III. Laboratory blood coagulation tests
IV. Point-of-care blood coagulation tests

Massive bleeding *and/or* diffuse clinical bleeding

Avoid further bleeding
Psys 80-100 in pts w/o TBI
Optimize preconditions
Temp. >35°C, pH >7.2,
iCa 1.1-1.3 mmol/L, Hb >60-80 g/L
Treat (hyper)fibrinolysis
Tranexamic acid 15 mg/kg
Laboratory blood coagulation tests

Heparin *unlikely* + ongoing hyperfibrinolysis *possible*

yes — no

ROTEM analysis with **EXTEM / INTEM / FIBTEM / APTEM**

ROTEM analysis with **EXTEM / INTEM / FIBTEM / HEPTEM**

EXTEM / INTEM significant decrease of MCF after maximum (LI60 < 85%) + APTEM normal

EXTEM / INTEM: MCF ↓

EXTEM / INTEM: CT ↑

INTEM: CT ↑
HEPTEM: normal

FIBTEM MCF ≤8 mm

yes

no

Prothrombin Complex Concentrate (PCC) (Beriplex®) 10-30 IE/kg *or* FFP 15-30 ml/kg

Protamine IE depending on CT prolongation, heparin dose, time point

Fibrinogen (Haemocomplettan®) 2-4 g

FIBTEM MCF >8 mm, bleeding stop — yes ▶ End

no

Platelet count ?

Fibrinogen (Haemocomplettan®) 2-4 g

FXIII >60% bleeding stop — yes ▶ End

no

Massive transfusion

ROTEM analysis with **EXTEM / INTEM / FIBTEM / HEPTEM**

Factor XIII (Fibrogammin®) 15 IE/kg

EXTEM: CT normal
INTEM / HEPTEM CT ↑

Tranexamic acid (Cyclocapron®) 15 mg/kg *followed by infusion with* 1 mg/kgxh

Platelets *if* < 50'000/µl (TBI < 100'000/µl)

Factor VIII:C/VWF:RCo (Haemate P®) *or* FFP 15-30 ml/kg

Figure 8.2 Bleeding algorithm. This bleeding algorithm has been developed for the Level I trauma center at the Kantonsspital Winterthur, Switzerland. The basis of the algorithm is the four pillars of coagulation diagnostics and the frequent reassessment of the patient. After initial steps to avoid further bleeding (controlled hypotension, damage control surgery), preconditions of coagulation are being optimized (maintaining homeostasis) and tranexamic acid administered. Thereafter, laboratory and point-of-care blood coagulation tests are being performed to treat the underlying coagulopathy in an individual and goal-directed way. (Courtesy of Michael Ganter, MD.)

coagulation factor to decrease below critical values. Fibrinogen is now available as a lyophilized product, can be stored at room temperature, and may be rapidly constituted and administered IV.[62] It does not require thawing or blood type matching. The fibrinogen content is standardized in each vial: 900–1300 mg per vial. Target fibrinogen levels after major trauma are higher (1.5–2 g/L) than with congenital fibrinogen deficiency (0.8–1 g/L). Fibrinogen administration using point-of-care coagulation testing (e.g., thromboelastometry FIBTEM component) or fibrinogen levels can be done. Risks of fibrinogen concentrate consist of anaphylaxis, deep venous thrombosis,

pulmonary embolus, and myocardial infarction. The European task force "recommend[s] treatment with fibrinogen concentrate or cryoprecipitate in the continuing management of the patient if significant bleeding is accompanied by thromboelastometric signs of a functional fibrinogen deficit or a plasma fibrinogen level of less than 1.5–2.0 g/l." The task force "suggest[s] an initial fibrinogen concentrate dose of 3–4 g or ... cryoprecipitate, ... approximately ... 15 to 20 single donor units in a 70 kg adult. Repeat doses may be guided by viscoelastic monitoring and laboratory assessment of fibrinogen levels."[6]

Prothrombin complex concentrate

Prothrombin complex concentrates (PCCs) are now available for the rapid reversal of warfarin in the case of bleeding. The hemostatic efficacy of PCCs depends on the available commercial product – e.g., three-factor (adequate levels of factor II, IX, and X) versus four-factor (adequate levels of factors II, IX, VII, and X). The four-factor PCC is preferred. Normalization of vitamin K-dependent factors occurs within 30 minutes using four-factor PCC, much more quickly and with less risk compared with plasma transfusion. PCCs have a half-life of 40–72 hours. Adverse reactions to PCCs consist mainly of thromboembolic complications. The European task force recommends "early use of PCCs for the emergency reversal of vitamin K-dependent oral anticoagulants." PCCs can also be used for bleeding patients with point-of-care evidence of delayed coagulation initiation.[6]

Factor VIIa

Recombinant factor VIIa (rFVIIa) was developed initially for use in hemophiliacs who developed inhibitors to factor VIII, and it is licensed only for this use. rFVIIa combines with tissue factor at the site of endothelial damage to activate factor X, which promotes conversion of prothrombin to thrombin and to trigger platelet activation. This "thrombin burst" is dependent on adequate levels of fibrinogen and mainly occurs at the site of injury, thus limiting the risk of thrombotic events. rFVIIa can also bind to activated platelet membranes, where it activates factor X directly, which leads to a massive rise in thrombin generation at the platelet surface. The dose currently recommended for bleeding episodes in patients with hemophilia is 90 µg/kg. Pharmacokinetics of rFVIIa based on a two-compartment model is compatible with an initial half-life of 0.6 hours and a terminal half-life of 2.4 hours. The use of rFVIIa for reversal of coagulopathy and/or treatment of bleeding in nonhemophilic patients is off-label.

rFVIIa can reverse coagulation abnormalities and decrease blood loss. However, a well-defined outcome benefit is less clear. The first case report on rFVIIa use in a trauma patient complicated with coagulopathy was reported in Israel in 1999. Initial anecdotal reports and small series suggested a striking effectiveness of the intervention. Two randomized, double blinded, placebo-controlled trials with 143 blunt and 134 penetrating trauma patients have been carried out.[63] The initial dose of rFVIIa was given after the eighth RBC unit and then 1 and 3 hours after (200, 100, 100 µg/kg). RBC transfusion was significantly reduced in blunt trauma patients, as was the need for massive transfusion (14% vs. 33%). There was a trend towards similar results in penetrating trauma which did not reach statistical significance. Subgroup analysis of coagulopathic patients from both trials showed reduced blood component per patient, fewer massive transfusions (6% vs. 29%) and less multiorgan failure and ARDS (3% vs. 20%) in the rFVIIa group. Thromboembolic complications were similar to the placebo group. In a study of early versus late administration of rFVIIa (before vs. after 8 RBC units) in combat casualties, the early group required less blood (20.6 vs. 25.7 units).[64] Mortality, ARDS, infection and thrombotic events were similar between groups. In the CONTROL trial, rFVIIa decreased RBC, FFP, and total allogeneic blood product use but did not affect mortality.[65] The study was terminated early because of low mortality and there was no difference in arterial and venous thrombotic events in the rFVIIa vs the placebo group.

In a review of 35 randomized clinical trials involving 4468 subjects, the rate of venous thromboembolic events was similar between rFVIIa and placebo-treated subjects (approximately 5.3–5.7%).[66] However, arterial thromboembolic events were higher in patients who received rFVIIa versus placebo (2.9% vs 1.1%). The rate of arterial events was highest in patients > 65 years receiving rFVIIa (9.0%).

The initial great enthusiasm for using rFVIIa has diminished after several trials, the subsequent meta-analyses and a Cochrane review failed to demonstrate a consistent decrease in mortality.[66,67] The transfusion requirements, both the average volume of transfusion and the percentage of patients in need of ongoing massive transfusion, were consistently decreased. ARDS rates were also consistently lower. However, the drug is almost prohibitively expensive, with the cost estimate being in excess of $100,000 per year of life saved for most patients. The drug is less efficient in acidosis and loses about 90% of its efficacy at pH = 7.0. Clinically, it has been shown that patients with pH of 6.9–7.02 do not benefit from rFVIIa. The efficiency of the drug is also affected, although to a lesser degree, by hypothermia. Other coagulation factors should be replaced in order for the drug to work. The usual dose of rFVIIa is in the 100–200 µg/kg range. Possible caveats in the trials include the late use of the drug, which might affect its efficacy, and the use of the drug in patients with known injury to major arteries, which might have increased the rate of thrombosis.

European guidelines suggest that the use of rFVIIa "be considered if major bleeding and traumatic coagulopathy persist despite standard attempts to control bleeding and best-practice use of conventional hemostatic measures" and that rFVIIa should not be used in patients with intracerebral hemorrhage caused by isolated head trauma. Because of the risk of serious adverse effects, treatment with rFVIIa must be individualized based on a risk-benefit analysis.[6]

Massive blood transfusion

Massive transfusion protocols (MTPs) are employed in order to provide the large quantities of blood products required for the resuscitation of rapidly exsanguinating trauma patients (see Chapter 6).[68] These protocols are designed to stabilize blood volume, support tissue, and prevent or correct coagulation deficits often associated with hemorrhagic shock. Different definitions of massive transfusion threshold exist (Table 8.6), such as one total blood volume loss (and replacement) in 24 hours, roughly equivalent to 10 units of whole

Table 8.6 Definitions of massive transfusion

One blood volume loss in 24 hours (equivalent to 10 units of whole blood)

4 or more units replaced in 1 hour with continuing bleeding

50% blood volume loss in 3 hours (equivalent to 5 units of whole blood)

50 units lost in 48 hours

20 units lost in 24 hours

Blood loss exceeding 150 mL/min

Adapted from Repine TB, Perkins JG, Kauvar DS, Blackborne L. The use of fresh whole blood in massive transfusion. *J Trauma* 2006; **60** (6 Suppl): S59–69.

blood, or 4 or more units replaced in 1 hour with continuing bleeding, 50% blood volume loss in 3 hours (equivalent to 5 units of whole blood), 50 units lost in 48 hours, 20 units lost in 24 hours or blood loss exceeding 150 mL/min. MTPs have been modified and now generally consist of administering RBCs and thawed plasma initially, then adding platelet units and cryoprecipitate depending on local preference and point-of-care and standard coagulation tests. An example of the MTP used at the authors' institution is shown in Table 8.7. An algorithmic approach to massive transfusion (Fig. 8.2) is commonly used in some European countries based on point-of-care testing and availability of factor concentrates such as PCCs and fibrinogen. The reason behind designing MTPs is to prevent coagulopathy rather than wait for coagulopathy to develop. One rule of thumb (personal communication with

Table 8.7 Massive transfusion protocol (MTP) at MetroHealth Medical Center.

Massive transfusion – adult/pediatric	POLICY No: NEW
Originated by: Surgery: Division of Trauma	Original date: 9/12/2013
Last review date:	Policy owner(s): Division of Trauma; Blood Bank
Last Revised Date:	Approval: Signatures on file

I. POLICY: The MetroHealth System has established a process for use when massive transfusions are necessary to achieve intravascular volume support, increase oxygen-carrying capacity, and stabilize the coagulation process for the adult and pediatric population

II. PURPOSE: To provide optimal patient safety while rapidly restoring blood volume during resuscitation from traumatic and/or hemorrhagic shock in emergent situations.

III. SCOPE: The MetroHealth System

IV. DEFINITION:
I. **Adult patients** – All patients age 15 years of age and above or greater than 50 kg.
    Adult massive transfusion is defined as the transfusion of 10 or more red blood cell (RBC) units in a 24-hour period.
II. **Pediatric patients** – pediatric patients weighing less than 50 kg and/or less than 15 years of age.
    Pediatric massive transfusion is defined as the transfusion of packed red cells in the amount > 40mL/kg in the first 4 hours and/or > 80mL/kg pRBC in the first 24 hours.

V. PROCEDURE:

A. Initiating massive transfusion process: adult/pediatrics
(1) The attending physician determines that the patient requires massive transfusion.
(2) The physician, or his designee, contacts the Blood Bank by calling the distinct-ring Massive Transfusion Protocol (MTP) Hot line phone (x89000) and gives a verbal order to begin the MTP.
(3) The lab technician completes a pink verbal Phone Order form. The lab technician will record two patient identifiers, date, location, physician's name/PIN #, and the person calling to initiate the MTP.
(4) Submit a properly labeled blood sample to the Blood Bank as soon as possible.
(5) Consider tranexamic acid (TXA).

B. Retrieving blood products from blood bank: adult/pediatrics
(1) Transporting blood products
    a. A runner will be provided by the area in which the patient is residing to obtain the products from the Blood Bank. On the off–shifts and weekends, a call should be placed by the Trauma team, or their designee in the trauma bay, to the nursing supervisor for assistance with runner resource identification. If a runner cannot be provided, the Blood Bank will tube the blood to the appropriate area providing the area is approved to receive tubed blood products.
    b. The runner is to be provided with the swipe card that provides access to the Operating Room when they pick up the cooler. The swipe card will be kept near the MTP hot-line phone located in the Blood Bank. Record the runner's name on the Insulated Cooler Sign-Out sheet.

Table 8.7 (cont.)

Massive transfusion – adult/pediatric	POLICY No: NEW

C. Issuing blood products from blood bank: adult

(1) FIRST MTP PACK:
   a. Four (4) O negative red blood cells (RBCs) and two (2) AB plasma units will be packed in a Blood Bank Insulated Cooler.
   b. The pink ALERT label for the insulated cooler, the Insulated Cooler – Blood Storage Tracking Sheet, and the Insulated Cooler Signout Sheet must all be completed. (Refer to Massive Transfusion Protocol BB1 43.5)
   c. As soon as the 1st MTP pack is issued, begin preparing the 2nd MTP pack.
   d. If a sample has not yet been submitted, contact the Blood Bank Medical Director and inquire as to whether the patient should be switched to O Rh Positive.
(2) SECOND AND ALL SUBSEQUENT MTP PACKS:
   a. Six (6) units of RBCs: O Neg/Pos, or type specific, if sample has been submitted
   b. Four (4) units of Plasma: AB, or type specific, if sample has been submitted
   c. Six (6) random A/AB platelets, (or one five day pool, or one apheresis platelet product)
   d. Second insulated cooler; do NOT place platelets in cooler; for RBCs/Plasma only
   e. Necessary emergency release/insulated cooler paperwork
   f. Consider fibrinogen at this time (10 units cryoprecipitate or 3–4 g fibrinogen concentrate in setting of thrombelastometric signs of a functional fibrinogen deficit or a plasma fibrinogen level of less than 150 mg/dL to 200 mg/dL)
(4) As soon as the second MTP pack is issued, begin preparing the third MTP pack.
(5) Third and subsequent packs should have the RBCs crossmatched using the BB1 43.0-Massive Transfusion Abbreviated Crossmatch Procedure since 10 RBCs will at that point be issued in less than a 24-hour period.

D. Issuing blood products from blood bank: pediatrics

1. Anticipate replacement of one blood volume within 24 hours or 4 units of packed red blood cells:

Age	Blood volume
Neonates: less than 30 days	85–90 mL/kg
Infants: 30 days to 1 year	75–80 mL/kg
Children: 1 to 14 years	70–75 mL/kg

* To estimate weight of patient use the parent's estimated weight of child or use the Broselow Pediatric Emergency Tape.

Neonates 0–4 kg

MTP Pack 1	MTP Pack 2	MTP Pack 3	MTP Pack 4
1 unit of pRBCs	1 unit of pRBCs	1 unit of pRBCs	1 unit of pRBCs
1 unit of FFP	1 unit of FFP	1 unit of FFP	1 unit of FFP
	(½) 6 pack plts	(½) 6 pack plts	(½) 6 pack plts
		1 unit cryo	1 unit cryo

Infants 5–10 kg

MTP Pack 1	MTP Pack 2	MTP Pack 3	MTP Pack 4
1 unit of pRBCs	1 unit of pRBCs	1 unit of pRBCs	1 unit of pRBCs
1 unit of FFP	1 unit of FFP	1 unit of FFP	1 unit of FFP
	(½) 6 pack plts	(½) 6 pack plts	(½) 6 pack plts
		1 unit cryo	1 unit cryo

Small children 11–30 kg

MTP Pack 1	MTP Pack 2	MTP Pack 3	MTP Pack 4
2 units of pRBCs	2 units of pRBCs	2 units of pRBCs	2 units of pRBCs
2 units of FFP	2 units of FFP	2 units of FFP	2 units of FFP
	(½) 6 pack plts	(½) 6 pack plts	(½) 6 pack plts
		6 units cryo	6 units cryo

Table 8.7 (cont.)

Massive transfusion – adult/pediatric		POLICY No: NEW	
Large children 30–50 kg			
MTP Pack 1	**MTP Pack 2**	**MTP Pack 3**	**MPT Pack 4**
4 units of pRBCs	4 units of pRBCs	4 units of pRBCs	4 units of pRBCs
2 units of FFP	4 units of FFP	4 units of FFP	4 units of FFP
	(1) 6 pack ptls	(1) 6 pack ptls	(1) 6 pack ptls
		6 units cryo	6 units cryo

* Platelets will be used as available.
(1) If additional products are required for each or any of the Packs, for clinical reasons or for patient weight requirements, the attending physician or their designee caring for the patient will notify the Blood Bank.
(2) The pink ALERT label for the insulated cooler, the Insulated Cooler – Blood Storage Tracking Sheet, and the Insulated Cooler Sign-out Sheet must be completed.
(3) If a blood bank sample has not yet been submitted, contact the Blood Bank Medical Director and inquire as to whether the patient should be switched to O Rh positive.

E. Terminating MTP process: adult/pediatrics

Continue with preparing an MTP PACK until the Blood Bank has been notified by a clinician to discontinue the MTP. The lab technician will record on a verbal Phone Order the two patient identifiers, the date, location, the physician's name/PIN #, and the person calling to inactivate the MTP order.

VI. Cross references
a. Massive Transfusion Protocol BB1 43.5
b. Transportation of Blood in an Insulated Cooler BB1 65.0
c. Massive Transfusion Abbreviated Crossmatch Procedure BB1 43.0
d. Massive Transfusion – Adult Policy III-54

Dr. Cotton) is that if the trauma team leader reaches for the O negative blood in the emergency department, the MTP is activated. In a more formal study of early predictors of massive transfusion, a massive transfusion score included a point assigned to each one of the following being abnormal: INR, systolic BP, hemoglobin, base deficit, positive result for focused assessment for sonography with trauma (FAST) examination, and temperature.[69] Penetrating injury mechanism and heart rate were not good predictors of the need for massive transfusion. With a score of two or higher, the chance of getting massively transfused was 33%, as opposed to 11% for the patients with fewer than two predictive factors. More importantly, the sensitivity was 85%, meaning that in patients with fewer than two positive factors the chance of needing a massive transfusion was low. An even simpler and still highly efficient Assessment of Blood Consumption (ABC) score assigns one point to each of heart rate > 120 bpm, systolic BP < 90 mmHg, positive FAST, and penetrating injury mechanism; a score of two or more was highly predictive for the need for massive transfusion.[70]

Mathematical modeling has shown that initial resuscitation with > 5 units of red cells together with crystalloid inevitably leads to dilutional coagulopathy. Ongoing resuscitation with plasma, platelets, and RBCs in a 1:1:1 ratio just barely keeps up. A mix of 1 unit of RBC, an apheresis unit of platelets, and a unit of thawed plasma together has an approximate hematocrit of 29%, about 65% of initial coagulation factor activity, and a platelet count of about 88,000/μL. Despite the primarily retrospective military and civilian data, lack of prospective randomized trials, survival bias of many studies, blood component resuscitation is often driven by MTPs trending towards 1:1:1 plasma:platelet:RBC ratios together with a reduction in crystalloid use. Current prospective national observational studies are being done to help assess both benefit and potential unintended consequences of ratio-guided massive transfusion (e.g., PROPPR study, Pragmatic Randomized Optimal Platelet and Plasma Ratios to investigate different ratios of blood products given to trauma patients who are predicted to require massive transfusions, http://cetir-tmc.org/research/proppr).

Some authors make a strong case that most trauma patients have enough oxygen-carrying capacity reserve, but are severely coagulopathic on their arrival to the hospital or before surgery. Trauma-induced coagulopathy is common, especially in the setting of hypoperfusion and acidosis, and is strongly associated with mortality. For the trauma patient in hemorrhagic shock with ongoing bleeding, the benefits of administering blood products in the absence of confirmatory laboratory tests often outweigh the risks of transfusion. High plasma-to-RBC transfusion ratios benefit patients regardless of the initial INR. The logistics of such protocols to treat hemorrhagic shock need to involve several departments, including anesthesia, surgery, and blood bank (transfusion medicine). In military trauma, it is possible to transfuse fresh warm whole blood collected in real time from the "walking blood bank" (see Chapter 38). The practice is dictated mainly by specific logistic limitations in the war environment, but seems to be safe and possibly even more effective than transfusion of stored blood components.

Complications of transfusions

In several high-quality retrospective trauma studies, transfusion was a strong predictor of mortality even after meticulous adjustment for age and severity of trauma and shock.[71] In a study of 15,534 trauma patients by Malone *et al.* in 2003, after adjustment for severity of trauma, demographics and physiologic data, transfusion almost tripled the mortality and more than tripled the need for admission to the ICU.[72] Anemia on admission did not increase mortality. In patients with blunt liver and spleen injury, transfusion independently increased risk of death in all patients (OR = 4.75), and especially in the patients treated nonoperatively (OR = 8.45). Mortality increased by 16% for every unit transfused. Length of stay was increased as well. Similarly, transfusion increased (more than quadrupled) mortality in patients with grade IV and V liver injury.[73] In head trauma patients, transfusion was associated with more than double the mortality and more than triple the rate of complications and led to worse neurologic outcomes.[74]

At the beginning of the last decade, two similar multicenter analyses of thousands of ICU patients were performed, one in Europe in 2002 and one in the US in 2004.[75,76] In both, the average transfusion trigger was about 8.5 g/dL. Hematocrit on admission was not a risk factor for either death or ICU length of stay (LOS); transfusion tripled the average LOS in the European study and increased it in a dose-dependent manner in the American one, and increased mortality by an average of 37% and 65%, respectively, in a dose-dependent manner.

Analysis of almost 1 million surgeries performed in 2005–2009 in the US has identified 15,186 patients who received exactly 1 unit of RBC.[77] Transfusion of this one single unit increased LOS by 1.5 days, and also increased mortality by 17%, wound problems by 18%, pulmonary complications by 31%, renal problems by 24%, cardiac complications by 20%, sepsis by 29%, with numbers needed to treat (NNT) of 110, 58, 28, 77, 250 and 42, respectively. There was one additional, unnecessary death for every 110 surgical patients given a single unit of blood. The article was accompanied by a very expressive invited comment by Dr. Holcomb stressing the "all or nothing approach: in the setting of exsanguination, transfuse early and aggressively; in a more or less stable one, disregard the temptation to treat the number."

Several strategies might be used to decrease the rate of complications, such as lower transfusion triggers (almost uniformly adopted), cell salvage, preoperative erythropoietin, and oxygen-carrying RBC substitutes (not commercially available to date) (Table 8.8). Immunomodulation by allogeneic blood transfusion has long been recognized. In cadaveric kidney recipients, transfusion of RBCs increased graft survival and the effect persisted after 5 years.[78] Decreased natural killer cytotoxicity and various T-cell subpopulations could be demonstrated two decades after blood transfusion.

Infection risk may increase 10-fold, and immunologic effects are still evident 1 month after transfusion. Transfusions, especially of non-leukodepleted blood, have been associated with poor wound healing, failure of bowel anastomosis, sepsis, multiple organ failure, and death. These effects are more significant with transfusions of older RBCs. Donor leukocytes survive in significant numbers in the recipient blood flow for decades after transfusion – described by the term "microchimerism" – and this is not affected by leukodepletion. In a meta-analysis enrolling a total of 13,152 patients, transfusion was associated with increased risk of infection in 17 out of 20 studies, with a total risk ratio of 3.45 and, for trauma patients specifically, RR = 5.23.[79] Transfusion has been associated with a poor wound healing, failure of bowel anastomosis, sepsis, multiple organ failure, ARDS, ventilator-associated pneumonia, and death.

Blood banks discard RBC units after 42 days of storage, but cells older than 14 days have been associated with an increased rate of the complications. The red cell membrane undergoes changes with storage, cells become stiffer and their aggregability increases, interfering with the passage of blood through the capillaries, although all these effects can be attenuated by leukodepletion. 2,3-DPG is undetectable after 2 weeks of storage and takes time to return to normal levels. Finally, transfusion of stored erythrocytes, especially the old ones, can deplete nitric oxide (NO) and cause vasoconstriction. RBC units also accumulate cytokines and inflammatory mediators, although these are most prominent in the units stored with leukocytes and are greatly reduced by leukodepletion, which is now universally performed immediately after donation.

Observational studies report a several-fold increase in infection, pulmonary complications, ARDS, ventilator-associated pneumonia, multiorgan failure, and mortality with older blood. For example, in 4993 patients admitted with acute cardiovascular conditions, 535 of whom died, there was a 2% increase in the risk of death for every 1 day increase in the age of the oldest blood unit transfused to a patient, and a 48% difference in mortality between the lowest and the highest quartile of the age.[80] In another study of 6002 cardiac surgery patients, transfusion of blood older than 14 days, as compared with newer units, was associated with increased risk of: in-hospital mortality, by 64% (2.8% vs. 1.7%, $p = 0.004$); intubation beyond 72 hours, by 73% (9.7% vs. 5.6%, $p < 0.001$); renal failure, by 69% (2.7% vs. 1.6%, $p = 0.003$); sepsis or septicemia, by 43% (4.0% vs. 2.8%, $p = 0.01$); multiorgan failure, 3-fold (0.2% vs. 0.7%, $p = 0.007$); limb ischemia, by 136% (0.2% vs 0.6%, $p = 0.05$); and 1-year mortality by 49% (7.4% vs. 11.0%, $p < 0.001$).[81] In a study of trauma patients

Table 8.8 Clinical strategies to reduce complications of transfusion therapy

Complication	Clinical strategies to reduce complication
Impaired oxygen release from hemoglobin	Warm all IV fluids and blood. Avoid alkalosis. Maintain normothermia (core temperature 36–37 °C).
Dilutional coagulopathy	Thawed plasma, cryoprecipitate, PCCs, and/or fibrinogen for clinically excessive bleeding, signs of functional fibrinogen deficit, plasma fibrinogen level < 1.5 g/L, prothrombin > 1.5 x normal. Platelets for thrombocytopenia (< 100,000/µL if TBI; < 75,000/µL without TBI) and clinically excessive bleeding.
Hypothermia	Warm all IV fluids and blood. Warm room > 28 °C. Convective warming. Gel pad warming (see also Chapter 14).
Decreased ionized calcium	Treat with calcium chloride, 20 mg/kg, in setting of massive transfusion and hypotension.
Hyperkalemia	Monitor ECG and treat with calcium chloride, 20 mg/kg, if hemodynamically significant. Otherwise, monitor and treat with glucose and insulin and/or bicarbonate.
Hemolytic transfusion reaction	Check and recheck every donor unit. Once occurred, stop transfusion and maintain systemic perfusion and renal blood flow. Alkalinize urine. Watch for DIC. Send suspected unit to blood bank for crossmatch.
Infection	Lower transfusion trigger. Red cell salvage. Avoid indiscriminate blood product transfusions. Increased use of PCCs and fibrinogen concentrates instead of thawed plasma.
Transfusion-induced immunosuppression/ immunomodulation	Lower transfusion trigger. Red cell salvage. Leukodepletion. Avoid indiscriminate blood product transfusions. Increased use of PCCs and fibrinogen concentrates instead of thawed plasma.
Transfusion-related acute lung injury (TRALI)	Increased use of PCC and fibrinogen concentrates instead of thawed plasma. Blood bank strategies to mitigate risk. Red cell salvage. Avoid indiscriminate blood product transfusions.
Transfusion-associated circulatory overload (TACO)	Increased use of PCC, especially for reversal of warfarin in elderly trauma patients with cardiac disease. Lower transfusion trigger. Red cell salvage. Avoid indiscriminate blood product transfusions.

DIC, disseminated intravascular coagulation; PCCs, prothrombin complex concentrate; TBI, traumatic brain injury.

transfused in ICU with mean pre-transfusion hematocrit of 22%, units older than 21 days were associated with a significant decrease in tissue oxygenation, roughly from 87% to 81%, over 2–3 hours after the transfusion, while the younger ones did not affect the oxygenation – although they did not improve it either.[82] However, a recent analysis of nearly 7000 non-cardiac-surgery patients did not confirm the effect of RBC age (in this case, the median age of the units) on mortality. Further, 3-week-old autologous RBCs were as efficient as fresh RBCs in restoring the mental capacity of volunteers undergoing acute isovolemic hemodilution[83] and caused a similar reduction in the gas exchange pulmonary function.[84]

Figures 8.3 and 8.4 illustrate the age of RBC units issued by the blood bank to consecutive trauma patients in our hospital, a tertiary care Level I trauma center. To date, there are no completed prospective randomized controlled studies examining the effect of storage duration of transfused red cells on morbidity and mortality.

According to Kleinman, "available studies do not present compelling enough evidence to alter transfusion practice toward the selective use of fresher RBCs or to answer the paired questions of whether 'fresh blood is better' and 'older blood is potentially harmful.'"[85] The ongoing Red Cell Storage Duration Study (RECESS) will compare young versus older RBC units in cardiac surgery (young = stored ≤ 10 days; old = stored ≥ 21 days).

Immunomodulation is dose-dependent, regarding both the number of units transfused (the usual threshold being 3–4 units of RBCs) and the degree of leukodepletion. For the last several years the blood provided to US hospitals by the American Red Cross is leukodepleted unless requested otherwise. In most other developed countries, universal leukodepletion was adopted years ago. Thus old findings might not apply to the current practice. One has to recognize that "leukodepleted" does not mean free from leukocytes. Buffy-coat reduction removes about 70% of white blood cells (WBCs), while filtering the blood removes more than 99.9%, leaving several million leukocytes per unit of RBC. The incidence of microchimerism (long-term survival of the donor WBCs in the recipient body) is approximately 30% and not diminished by leukodepletion. Storage of blood with leukocytes allows them to release significant amounts of cytokines. Thus, early leukodepletion should reduce the inflammatory impact of the transfused blood. Bedside leukodepletion has also been associated with a reduction in the risk of perioperative infection associated with blood transfusion. Current American Red Cross standards require that RBC units be leukodepleted no later than 5 days after donation, and contain no more than 5×10^6 WBCs per unit. Leukodepletion seems to decrease the rate of febrile reactions and postoperative infections. Cell salvage is an important way to reduce allogeneic blood consumption. It reduces the postoperative infections and mortality in some studies, but others do not confirm the results.

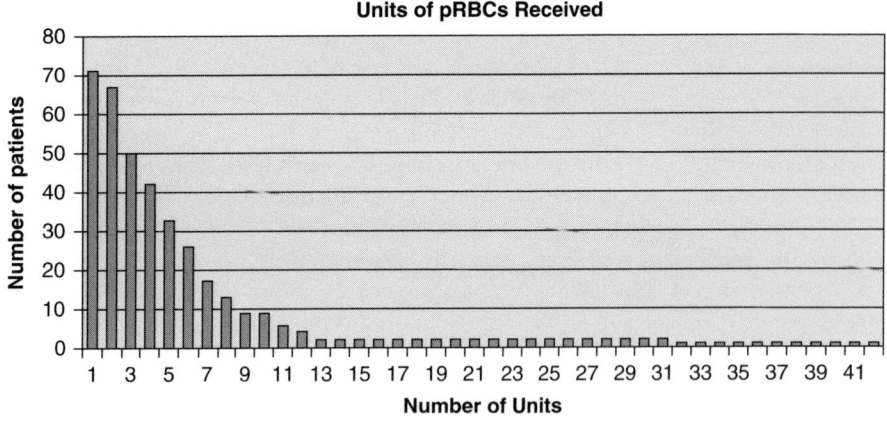

Figure 8.3 Number of packed red blood cell (pRBCs) units transfused per patient. Data are from 115 trauma patients requiring emergency surgery at MetroHealth Medical Center between June 2003 and June 2004. A total of 2595 units was transfused.

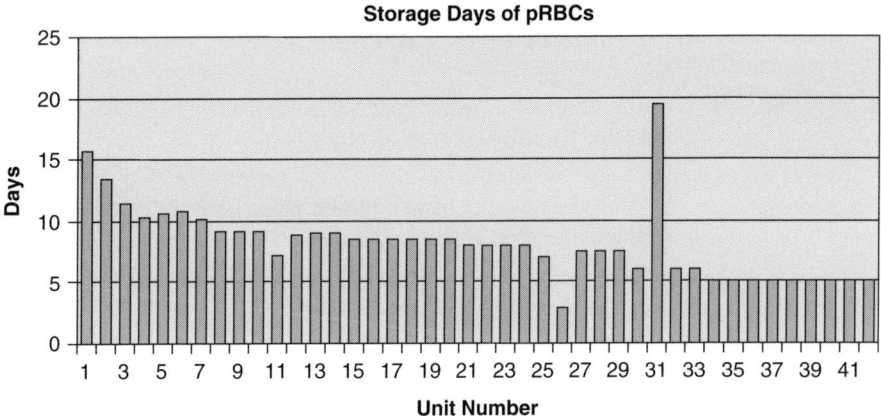

Figure 8.4 Number of storage days for packed red blood cell (pRBCs) units prior to transfusion in 115 trauma patients requiring emergency surgery at MetroHealth Medical Center between June 2003 and June 2004. A total of 2595 units was transfused.

Transfusion-related acute lung injury (TRALI) is defined as new acute lung injury (ALI)/ARDS occurring during or within 6 hours after blood product administration. According to Kleinman and Kor, TRALI likely occurs via a two-hit mechanism: (1) neutrophil sequestration and priming in the lung microvasculature, due to recipient factors such as endothelial injury (endothelial cells may be responsible for both the neutrophil sequestration [through adhesion molecules] and priming [through cytokine release]), and (2) neutrophil activation by a factor in the blood product with damage to the pulmonary capillary endothelium and an inflammatory (nonhydrostatic) pulmonary edema.[86] The severity of TRALI depends upon the susceptibility of the patient to develop a more clinically significant reaction as a result of an underlying disease process, and upon the nature of triggers in the transfused blood components. Other causes of ALI should be excluded in order to definitively diagnose TRALI. The incidence of TRALI has decreased following the institution of TRALI mitigation strategies for transfused plasma and platelet components (e.g., deferral of multiparous female donors for plasma donation, and testing of parous apheresis donors of platelets or plasma for anti-HLA antibodies).

Transfusion-associated circulatory overload (TACO) is another obvious danger, especially in the elderly, small children, and those with heart failure and compromised cardiac function.

Hypothermia

The adverse effects of hypothermia in the trauma patient include major coagulation derangements, peripheral vasoconstriction, metabolic acidosis, compensatory increased oxygen requirements during rewarming, and impaired immune response (see Chapter 14). Standard coagulation tests are temperature-corrected to 37 °C and may not reflect hypothermia-induced coagulopathy. Hypothermia impairs coagulation because of slowing of enzymatic rates and reduced platelet function. Even worse, different coagulation cascade steps are affected to different degrees, disrupting synchronization of the cascade. Hypothermia can cause cardiac dysrhythmias and even cardiac arrest due to electromechanical dissociation, standstill, or fibrillation, especially with core temperatures below 30 °C. Hypothermia also impairs citrate, lactate, and drug metabolism; increases blood viscosity; impairs RBC deformability; increases intracellular potassium release; and causes a leftward shift of the oxyhemoglobin dissociation curve. A mortality of 100% has been reported in trauma patients whose body temperature fell below 32 °C, regardless of severity of injury, degree of hypotension, or fluid replacement. In our own study of 880 acute trauma victims, hypothermia, and especially hypothermia towards the end of the surgery, was an independent predictor of mortality.

In isolated moderate to severe head trauma, hypothermia on admission and in severe brain injury hypothermia on admission to ICU have been independently associated with increased mortality.

Selective therapeutic hypothermia prevents secondary injury to the brain, prevents inflammatory response, and lowers intracranial pressure, but the net effect on survival and long-term outcomes remains controversial. Hypothermia is not currently recommended as a routine but can be used at the discretion of the neurosurgeon (see Chapter 14). Hyperthermia is universally recognized as being detrimental, and should be prevented.

The importance of fluid warming cannot be overestimated in the trauma patient. It requires 16 kCal of energy to raise the temperature of 1 L of crystalloid infused at room temperature (21 °C) to body temperature (37 °C), and 30 kCal to raise the temperature of cold (4 °C) blood to 37 °C. Infusion of 4.3 L of crystalloid at room temperature to an anesthetized adult trauma patient who cannot increase heat production can result in a decrease of 1.5 °C in core temperature. Similarly, infusion of 2.3 L of red cells could result in a core temperature decrease of between 1 and 1.5 °C. Since the thermal stress of infusing fluids at normothermia is essentially zero, it follows that use of fluid warming devices effective at delivering normothermic fluids to the patient at clinically relevant flow rates permits more efficient rewarming of hypothermic trauma patients than using other methods such as the patient's own metabolically generated heat, or externally provided heat such as convective warming. Several models of fluid warmers with set points of 42 °C are now commonly used for trauma (see Chapter 14). Countercurrent water and other fluid warmers using 42 °C set points will not damage red cells, will result in consistently warmer fluid delivery, and will allow the clinician to maintain thermal neutrality with respect to fluid management over a wide range of flow rates.

Citrate intoxication, hyperkalemia, and acid–base abnormalities

Blood is stored in citrate phosphate dextrose with adenine or Adsol at 4 °C. Citrate binds calcium, which is why it is added to the RBCs in the first place, and citrate intoxication decreases serum levels of ionized calcium. Administration of calcium is warranted during massive transfusion if the patient is hypotensive and measured serum ionized serum calcium is low, or if large amounts of blood are infused rapidly (50–100 mL/min). Ionized serum calcium levels will usually return to normal when hemodynamic status is improved.

The potassium level in stored blood rises with length of storage and can be as high as 78 mmol/L after 35 days. The potential for clinically important hyperkalemia still exists in patients receiving blood administered at rates > 120 mL/min and in patients with severe acidosis. Monitoring the ECG for signs of hyperkalemia is always warranted, and treatment of hyperkalemia with calcium chloride, bicarbonate, glucose, and insulin may be life-saving.

The pH of bank blood decreases to about 6.9 after 21 days of storage because of accumulation of CO_2, lactic acid, and pyruvic acid by RBC metabolism. Thus, the acidosis seen in stored blood is partly respiratory and partly metabolic. The respiratory component is of little consequence with adequate patient ventilation. The metabolic component is not usually clinically significant. It is unwise to administer sodium bicarbonate on an empiric basis, because there is already a pool of bicarbonate generated from the metabolism of citrate, which is present in large quantities in stored blood.

Hemolytic transfusion reactions

Immediate reactions occur from error involving ABO incompatibility. More than half of these errors happen after the blood has been issued by the blood bank, which highlights the importance of verifying and identifying each and every donor unit for recipient compatibility. Intravascular hemolysis occurs when recipient antibody coats and immediately destroys the transfused red cells. Classic signs of hemolytic transfusion reaction are masked by general anesthesia. The only evidence may be hemoglobinuria, hypotension, and a bleeding diathesis. Treatment is supportive and involves stopping the transfusion and maintaining systemic and renal perfusion.

Microaggregates

Microaggregates begin forming after approximately 2 days of blood storage. During the first 7 days, microaggregates are mostly platelets or platelet debris. After the first week, the larger fibrin–WBC–platelet aggregates begin to accumulate. Whether these microaggregates contribute to lung dysfunction during blood transfusion and whether they need to be removed by micropore filters is controversial.

Infection

The risk of infection after transfusion of a single unit of blood product in developed countries was approximately 1 in 2–3 million for hepatitis C, 1 in 30,000–200,000 for hepatitis B, 1 in 1.5–4.7 million for HIV, 1 in 2000–8000 for bacterial contamination with platelet units, and 1 in 28,000–143,000 for pRBC.[87] In addition, several cases of possible transfusion-transmitted variant Creutzfeldt–Jakob disease (vCJD) have been described. The risk per unit for *Yersinia*, malaria, babesiosis, and Chagas is estimated at < 1 in 1,000,000. Other types of infectious diseases such as toxoplasmosis and cytomegalovirus, Epstein–Barr virus, and bacterial infections may also be transmitted by transfused blood and blood products. Each unit of FFP or platelets has the same risk of infection as a unit of pRBCs.

Table 8.9 Resuscitation endpoints within the first 24 hours after trauma

Parameter	Value
Mixed venous oxygen tension	> 35 mmHg
Mixed venous oxygen saturation (central venous or pulmonary artery)	> 65%
Base deficit	> –3 mmol/L
Lactate	< 2.5 mmol/L

Adapted from Ivatury RR, Simon RJ. Assessment of tissue oxygenation (evaluation of the adequacy of resuscitation). In Ivatury RR, Cayten CGC, eds. *The Textbook of Penetrating Trauma.* Baltimore, MD: Williams & Wilkins, 1996, pp. 927–38.

Endpoints of resuscitation

Blood and fluid resuscitation is continued until perfusion has been improved and organ function has been restored. Manifestations of improved perfusion include improved mental status, increased pulse pressure, decreased heart rate, increased urine output, resolution of lactic acidosis and base deficit, brisk capillary refill, and improvement in oxygen delivery, oxygen consumption, and mixed venous oxygen saturation (Table 8.9).

Summary

Fluid management is a challenging task in trauma patients undergoing urgent and emergent surgery. The major goal is to stop the bleeding, and after this to replete the intravascular volume to optimize tissue oxygen delivery. Choice, volume, and timing of intraoperative fluid resuscitation are based on correlates of hypoperfusion such as tachycardia, hypotension, low pH, base deficit, and lactate. Blood transfusion is currently the most effective therapy for hemorrhagic shock. Large volumes of crystalloids used to maintain or restore blood pressure in general cause fluid overload resulting in dilution of hemostatic and other beneficial mediators. It is strongly suggested that synthetic colloids not be used in critically ill patients; albumin is contraindicated in head trauma patients.

The bleeding trauma patient requires rapid evaluation and treatment to ensure adequate tissue perfusion and successful outcome. Resources such as thermally efficient warmers, effective transfusion services, rapid and timely availability of blood products (red blood cells, thawed plasma, platelets, cryoprecipitate), point-of-care coagulation testing, factor concentrates (fibrinogen, prothrombin complex concentrate), and tranexamic acid (see also Chapter 6) are practical aspects of trauma resuscitation. Preventing hypothermia (see Chapter 14) and recognizing other complications of massive transfusion, as well as following trends in vital signs, systolic and pulse pressure variability, urinary output, central venous pressures, and arterial and central venous blood gas analysis, are of vital importance in managing trauma patients with hemorrhagic shock.

Questions

(1) Delayed or hypotensive fluid resuscitation:
   a. Increases survival in patients with ruptured aortic aneurysm and in military trauma patients
   b. Is superior in animal studies
   c. Is aimed at restoration of systolic blood pressure to more than 80 mmHg in pregnant patients and head trauma patients, and to restore mental status in all others
   d. Is detrimental in some human studies

(2) **When comparing different crystalloid solutions:**
   a. 0.9% saline and lactated Ringer's solution have similar effect on intravascular volume, acid–base balance, and coagulation profile
   b. Lactated Ringer's solution cannot be co-infused with blood products or used to dilute packed red blood cells
   c. Hemodilution leads to coagulopathy
   d. Volume expansion with lactated Ringer's solution is approximately a third of the infused volume immediately after the infusion, and drops to about 7% of the infused volume half an hour later

(3) **When comparing different iso-osmolar crystalloid solutions:**
   a. Lactated Ringer's solution is a standard choice for head trauma due to better coagulation and acid–base profile compared with 0.9% saline
   b. Infusion of more than 30 mL/kg of 0.9% saline leads to hyperchloremic acidosis
   c. Infusion of more than 30–40 mL/kg of lactated Ringer's solution leads to lactic acidosis and/or severe respiratory acidosis
   d. Hyperglycemia is associated with improved neurologic outcomes in patients with traumatic brain injury

(4) **Regarding colloid- and crystalloid-based volume replacement regimens, which of the following is true?**
   a. In relatively stable patients, use of colloid solutions has been associated with worsened outcome and increased tissue edema in elective surgery patients
   b. Most hetastarch solutions improve coagulation and platelet function in a dose-dependent manner
   c. Hetastarch solutions increase the risk of acute kidney injury, the need for renal replacement therapy, and mortality in critically ill patients
   d. Hetastarch solutions and other colloids improve survival in patients with massive blood loss

(5) Hypertonic saline (HS):
   a. Is rarely used in head trauma patients, as it is often associated with rapidly developing dose-dependent hypernatremia and hyperosmolarity which might lead to seizures and central pontine myelolysis (CPM)
   b. In head trauma patients is at least as effective as mannitol in decreasing intracranial pressure
   c. Improves short- and long-term outcomes in head trauma patients

d. Is not effective for volume replacement in dehydrated patients

(6) **Regarding anemia:**
   a. Oxygen-carrying capacity is not affected by anemia until hemoglobin falls below a certain level
   b. Tissue oxygenation is independent of the oxygen-carrying capacity
   c. Oxygen delivery in euvolemic anemic patients is maintained over a wide range of hematocrits as a result of decreased peripheral vascular resistance, decreased blood viscosity, tachycardia, and increased stroke volume.
   d. In a healthy adult, tissue oxygenation decreases when hemoglobin falls below 7–8 g/dL; vital organs (brain, heart, kidneys, gut) compensate by increasing the oxygen extraction ratio

(7) **Regarding blood transfusions, which of the following is true?**
   a. In the TRICC study, patients in the liberal transfusion arm had significantly higher rate of pulmonary and cardiac complications
   b. In the TRICC study, patients with coronary artery disease did worse with the restrictive transfusion strategy
   c. Current American Society of Anesthesiologists guidelines recommend transfusion at hemoglobin below 10 g/dL
   d. Transfusion improves tissue oxygenation parallel to the increase in oxygen carrying capacity

(8) **Transfusion in trauma:**
   a. Should be done with O negative blood only
   b. Should be done without the use of a blood warmer
   c. Should be delayed until surgical control of bleeding is achieved
   d. In case of massive ongoing blood loss, should combine transfusion of packed red blood cells, coagulation factors, and platelets

(9) **Match the following:**
   (i) Fibrinogen or factor 1
   (ii) Prothrombin complex concentrates (PCCs)
   (iii) Recombinant factor VIIa
   a. Available for the rapid reversal of warfarin in the case of bleeding
   b. First coagulation factor to decrease below critical values during massive transfusion
   c. Developed for use in hemophiliacs with inhibitors to factor VIII, and licensed only for this use; not enough data available so far to make definite recommendations about patient selection, timing, and dosage in trauma patients

Answers

(1) b
(2) d
(3) b
(4) c
(5) b
(6) c
(7) a
(8) d
(9) (i) b; (ii) a; (iii) c

References

For a complete list of references please email Dr. Smith: csmith@metrohealth.org.

1. Bickell, WH, Wall MJ, Pepe PE *et al.* Immediate versus delayed fluid resuscitation for hypotensive patients with penetrating torso injuries. *N Engl J Med* 1994; **331**: 1105–9.

2. Haut ER, Kalish BT, Cotton BA, *et al.* Prehospital intravenous fluid administration is associated with higher mortality in trauma patients: a National Trauma Data Bank analysis. *Ann Surg* 2011; **253**: 371–7.

3. Ley EJ, Clond MA, Srour MK, *et al.* Emergency department crystalloid resuscitation of 1.5 L or more is associated with increased mortality in elderly and nonelderly trauma patients. *J Trauma* 2011; **70**: 398–400.

4. Morrison CA, Carrick MM, Norman MA, *et al.* Hypotensive resuscitation strategy reduces transfusion requirements and severe postoperative coagulopathy in trauma patients with hemorrhagic shock: preliminary results of a randomized controlled trial. *J Trauma* 2011; **70**: 652–63.

5. Cotton BA, Reddy N, Hatch QM, *et al.* Damage control resuscitation is associated with a reduction in resuscitation volumes and improvement in survival in 390 damage control laparotomy patients. *Ann Surg* 2011; **254**: 598–605.

6. Spahn DR, Bouillon B, Cerny V. Management of bleeding and coagulopathy following major trauma: an updated European guideline. *Critical Care* 2013; **17**: R76. http://ccforum.com/content/17/2/R76 (accessed July 2014).

7. Cull DL, Lally KP, Murphy KD. Compatibility of packed erythrocytes and Ringer's lactate solution. *Surg Gynecol Obstet* 1991; **173**: 9–12.

8. McCluskey SA, Karkouti K, Wijeysundera D, *et al.* Hyperchloremia after noncardiac surgery is independently associated with increased morbidity and mortality: a propensity-matched cohort tudy. *Anesth Analg* 2013; **117**: 412–21.

9. Ruttmann TG, Jamest MF, Lombard EH. Haemodilution-induced enhancement of coagulation is attenuated in vitro by restoring antithrombin III to pre-dilution concentrations. *Anaesth Intensive Care* 2001; **29**): 489–93.

10. Ruttmann TG, James MFM, Aronson I, *In vivo* investigation into the effects of haemodilution with hydroxyetil starch (200/0.5) and normal saline on coagulation. *Br J Anaesth* 1998; **80**: 612–16.

11. Ruttmann TG, James MFM, Finlayson J. Effects on coagulation of intravenous crystalloid or colloid in patients

undergoing peripheral vascular surgery. *Br J Anaesth* 2002; **89**: 226–30.

12. The NICE-SUGAR Study Investigators. Intensive versus Conventional Glucose Control in Critically Ill Patients. *N Engl J Med* 2009; **360**: 1283–97.

13. Weiskopf R. Equivalent Efficacy of Hydroxyethyl Starch 130/0.4 and Human Serum Albumin: If Nothing Is the Same, Is Everything Different? The Importance of Context in Clinical Trials and Statistics. *Anesthesiology* 2013; **119**: 1249–54.

14. Mandel J, Palevsky PM. Treatment of severe hypovolemia or hypovolemic shock in adults. http://www.uptodate.com/contents/treatment-of-severe-hypovolemia-or-hypovolemic-shock-in-adults?source=search_result&search=colloids&selectedTitle=1~26 (accessed July 2014).

15. Reinhart K, Perner A, Sprung CL, *et al.*; European Society of Intensive Care Medicine. Consensus statement of the ESICM task force on colloid volume therapy in critically ill patients. *Intensive Care Med* 2012; **38**: 368–83.

16. Bayer O, Reinhart K, Kohl M, *et al.* Effects of fluid resuscitation with synthetic colloids or crystalloids alone on shock reversal, fluid balance, and patient outcomes in patients with severe sepsis: a prospective sequential analysis. *Crit Care Med* 2012; **40**: 2543–51.

17. Salerno F, Navickis RJ, Wilkes MM. Albumin infusion improves outcomes of patients with spontaneous bacterial peritonitis: a meta-analysis of randomized trials. *Clin Gastroenterol Hepatol* 2013; **11**: 123–30

18. Sedrakyan A, Gondek K, Paltiel D, Elefteriades JA. Volume expansion with albumin decreases mortality after coronary artery bypass graft surgery. *Chest* 2003; **123**: 1853–7.

19. Bunn F, Lefebvre C, Li Wan Po A, *et al.* Human albumin administration in critically ill patients: systematic review of randomized controlled trials. Cochrane Injuries Group Albumin Reviewers. *BMJ* 1998; **317**: 235–40.

20. Perel P, Roberts I. Colloids versus crystalloids for fluid resuscitation in critically ill patients. *Cochrane Database Syst Rev* 2012; (6): CD000567.

21. Finfer S, Bellomo R, Boyce N, *et al.* A comparison of albumin and saline for fluid resuscitation in the intensive care unit. *N Engl J Med* 2004; **350**: 2247–56.

22. SAFE Study Investigators, Australian and New Zealand Intensive Care Society Clinical Trials Group, Australian Red Cross Blood Service, *et al.* Saline or albumin for fluid resuscitation in patients with traumatic brain injury. *N Engl J Med* 2007; **357**: 874–84.

23. Cooper DJ, Myles PS, McDermott FT, *et al.*; HTS Study Investigators. Prehospital hypertonic saline resuscitation of patients with hypotension and severe traumatic brain injury: a randomized controlled trial. *JAMA* 2004; **291**: 1350–7.

24. Vialet R, Albanese J, Thomachot L, *et al.* Isovolume hypertonic solutes (sodium chloride or mannitol) in the treatment of refractory posttraumatic intracranial hypertension: 2 mL/kg 7.5% saline is more effective than 2 mL/kg 20% mannitol. *Crit Care Med* 2003; **31**: 1683–7.

25. Khanna S, Davis D, Peterson B, *et al.* Use of hypertonic saline in the treatment of severe refractory posttraumatic intracranial hypertension in pediatric traumatic brain injury. *Crit Care Med* 2000; **28**: 1144–51.

26. Wade CE, Grady JJ, Kramer GC, *et al.* Individual patient cohort analysis of the efficacy of hypertonic saline/dextran in patients with traumatic brain injury and hypotension. *J Trauma* 1997; **42** (Supplement): 61S–65S.

27. Bunn F, Roberts I, Tasker R, Akpa E. Hypertonic versus near isotonic crystalloid for fluid resuscitation in critically ill patients. *Cochrane Database Syst Rev* 2004; (3): CD002045.

28. Bulger EM, May S, Brasel KJ, *et al.* Out-of-hospital hypertonic resuscitation following severe traumatic brain injury: a randomized controlled trial *JAMA*. 2010; **304**: 1455–64.

29. Bulger EM, May S, Kerby JD, *et al.* Out-of-hospital hypertonic resuscitation after traumatic hypovolemic shock: a randomized, placebo controlled trial. *Ann Surg* 2011; **253**: 431–41.

30. Fergusson DA. Evidence-based transfusion medicine: TRICC & BART revisited. Blood Day, Winnipeg, November 4th, 2009.

31. Carson JL, Noveck H, Berlin JA, Gould SA. Mortality and morbidity in patients with very low postoperative Hb levels who decline blood transfusion. *Transfusion* 2002; **42**: 812–18.

32. Weiskopf RB, Toy P, Hopf HW *et al.* Acute isovolemic anemia impairs central processing as determined by P300 latency. *Clin Neurophysiol* 2005; **116**: 1028–32.

33. Weiskopf RB, Viele MK, Feiner J, *et al.* Human cardiovascular and metabolic response to acute, severe isovolemic anemia. *JAMA* 1998; **279**: 217–21.

34. Viele MK, Weiskopf RB. What can we learn about the need for transfusion from patients who refuse blood? The experience with Jehovah's Witnesses. *Transfusion* 1994; **34**: 396–401

35. Fang WC, Helm RE, Krieger KH, *et al.* Impact of minimum hematocrit during cardiopulmonary bypass on mortality in patients undergoing coronary artery surgery. *Circulation* 1997; **96** (9 Suppl): II-194–9.

36. Meier J, Kemming GI, Kisch-Wedel H, *et al.* Hyperoxic ventilation reduces 6-hour mortality at the critical hemoglobin concentration. *Anesthesiology* 2004; **100**: 70–6.

37. Weiskopf RB, Feiner J, Hopf HW, *et al.* Oxygen reverses deficits of cognitive function and memory and increased heart rate induced by acute severe isovolemic anemia. *Anesthesiology* 2002; **96**: 871–7.

38. Suttner S, Piper SN, Kumle B, *et al.* The influence of allogenic red blood cell transfusion compared with 100% oxygen ventilation on systemic oxygen transport and skeletal muscle oxygen tension after cardiac surgery. *Anesth Analg* 2004; **40**: 457–60.

39. Marik PE, Sibbald WJ. Effect of stored-blood transfusion on oxygen delivery in patients with sepsis. *JAMA* 1993; **269**: 3024–9.

40. Pattakos G, Koch CG, Brizzio ME, *et al.* Outcome of patients who refuse transfusion after cardiac surgery: a natural experiment with severe blood conservation. *Arch Intern Med* 2012; **172**: 1154–60.

41. Murphy GJ, Reeves BC, Rogers CA, *et al.* Increased mortality, postoperative morbidity, and cost after red blood cell transfusion in patients having cardiac surgery. *Circulation* 2007; **116**: 2544–52.

42. Boral L, Kowal-Vern A, Yogore M, Patel H, Latenser BA. Transfusions in

burn patients with/without comorbidities. *J Burn Care Res* 2009; **30**: 268–73.

43. Agarwal P, Prajapati B, Sharma D. Evaluation of skin graft take following post-burn raw area in normovolaemic anaemia. *Indian J Plast Surg* 2009; **42**: 195–8.

44. Shen Y, Drum M, Roth S. The prevalence of perioperative visual loss in the United States: a 10-year study from 1996 to 2005 of spinal, orthopedic, cardiac, and general surgery. *Anesth Analg* 2009; **109**: 1534–45.

45. Hebert PC, Wells G, Blajchman MA, *et al.* A multicenter, randomized, controlled clinical trial of transfusion requirements in critical care. Transfusion Requirements in Critical Care Investigators, Canadian Critical Care Trials Group. *N Engl J Med* 1999; **340**: 409–17.

46. McIntyre L, Hebert PC, Wells G, *et al.* Is a restrictive transfusion strategy safe for resuscitated and critically ill trauma patients? *J Trauma* 2004; **57**: 563–8.

47. Hebert PC, Yetisir E, Martin C, *et al.* Is a low transfusion threshold safe in critically ill patients with cardiovascular diseases? *Crit Care Med* 2001; **29**: 227–34.

48. Lacroix J, Hébert PC, Hutchison JS, *et al.* Transfusion strategies for patients in pediatric intensive care units. *N Engl J Med* 2007; **356**: 1609–19.

49. Hajjar LA, Vincent JL, Galas FR, *et al.* Transfusion requirements after cardiac surgery: the TRACS randomized controlled trial. *JAMA* 2010; **304**: 1559–67.

50. Cooper HA, Rao SV, Greenberg MD, *et al.* Conservative versus liberal red cell transfusion in acute myocardial infarction (the CRIT Randomized Pilot Study). *Am J Cardiol* 2011; **108**: 1108–11.

51. Carson JL, Carless PA, Hebert PC. Transfusion thresholds and other strategies for guiding allogeneic red blood cell transfusion. *Cochrane Database Syst Rev* 2012; (4): CD002042.

52. Rao SV, Jollis JG, Harrington RA, *et al.* Relationship of blood transfusion and clinical outcomes in patients with acute coronary syndromes. *JAMA* 2004; **292**: 1555–62.

53. Al-Sarraf A, Fowler RA. Is blood transfusion harmful in patients with acute coronary syndromes? *CMAJ* 2005; **172**: 182.

54. Chatterjee S, Wetterslev J, Sharma A, Lichstein E, Mukherjee D. Association of blood transfusion with increased mortality in myocardial infarction: a meta-analysis and diversity-adjusted study sequential analysis. *JAMA Intern Med* 2013; **173**: 132–9.

55. American Society of Anesthesiologists. Practice guidelines for perioperative blood transfusion and adjuvant therapies. An updated report by the American Society of Anesthesiologists Task Force on Perioperative Blood Transfusion and Adjuvant Therapies. *Anesthesiology* 2006; **105**: 198–208.

56. Hess JR, Brohi K, Dutton RP, *et al.* The coagulopathy of trauma: a review of mechanisms. *J Trauma* 2008; **65**: 748–54.

57. Kashuk JL, Moore EE, Sawyer M, *et al.* Postinjury coagulopathy management: goal directed resuscitation via POC thrombelastography. *Ann Surg* 2010; **251**: 604–14.

58. Smith CE, Bauer AM, Pivalizza EG, *et al.* Massive transfusion protocol (MTP) for hemorrhagic shock. ASA Committee on Blood Management. http://www.asahq.org/for-members/about-asa/asa-committees/committee-on-blood-management.aspx (accessed July 2014).

59. Schochl H, Maegele M, Solomon C, Gorlinger K, Voelckel W. Early and individualized goal-directed therapy for trauma-induced coagulopathy. *Scand J Trauma Resus Emerg Med* 2012; **20**: 15.

60. Murray OJ, Pennell BJ, Weinstein SL, Olson JD. Packed red cells in acute blood loss: dilutional coagulopathy as a cause of surgical bleeding. *Anesth Analg* 1995; **80**: 336.

61. Leslie SO, Toy PT. Laboratory hemostatic abnormalities in massively transfused patients given red blood cells and crystalloid. *Am J Clin Pathol* 1991; **96**: 770.

62. Tanaka KA, Esper S, Bolliger D. Perioperative factor concentrate therapy. *Br J Anaesth* 2013; **11**: i35–49.

63. Boffard KD, Riou B, Warren B, *et al.* Recombinant factor VIIa as adjunctive therapy for bleeding control in severely injured trauma patients: two parallel randomized, placebo-controlled, double-blind clinical trials. *J Trauma* 2005; **59**: 8–15.

64. Perkins JG, Schreiber MA, Wade CE, Holcomb JB. Early versus late recombinant factor VIIa in combat trauma patients requiring massive transfusion. *J Trauma* 2007; **62**: 1095–9

65. Hauser CJ, Boffard K, Dutton R, *et al.* Results of the CONTROL trial: efficacy and safety of recombinant activated Factor VII in the management of refractory traumatic hemorrhage *J Trauma* 2010; **69**: 489–500.

66. Levi M, Levy JH, Andersen HF, Truloff D. Safety of recombinant activated factor VII in randomized clinical trials. *N Engl J Med* 2010; **363**: 1791–800.

67. Simpson E, Lin Y, Stanworth S, *et al.* Recombinant factor VIIa for the prevention and treatment of bleeding in patients without haemophilia. *Cochrane Database Syst Rev* 2012; (3): CD005011.

68. Young PP, Cotton BA, Goodnough LT. Massive transfusion protocols for patients with substantial hemorrhage. *Transfus Med Rev* 2011; **25**: 293–303.

69. Callcut RA, Cotton BA, Muskat P, *et al.* Defining when to initiate massive transfusion: a validation study of individual massive transfusion triggers in PROMMTT patients. *J Trauma Acute Care Surg* 2013; **74**: 59–65, 67–8.

70. Krumrei NJ, Park MS, Cotton BA, Zielinski MD. Comparison of massive blood transfusion predictive models in the rural setting. *J Trauma Acute Care Surg* 2012; **72**: 211–15.

71. Malone DL, Dunne J, Tracy JK, *et al.* Blood transfusion, independent of shock severity, is associated with worse outcome in trauma. *J Trauma* 2003; **54**: 898–905.

72. Robinson WP 3rd, Ahn J, Stiffler A, *et al.* Blood transfusion is an independent predictor of increased mortality in nonoperatively managed blunt hepatic and splenic injuries. *J Trauma* 2005; **58**: 437–44.

73. Di Saverio S, Catena F, Filicori F, *et al.* Predictive factors of morbidity and mortality in grade IV and V liver trauma undergoing perihepatic packing: single institution 14 years experience at European trauma centre. *Injury* 2012; **43**: 1347–54.

74. Salim A, Hadjizacharia P, DuBose J, *et al.* Role of anemia in traumatic brain

injury. *J Am Coll Surg* 2008; **207**: 398–406.

75. Vincent JL, Baron JF, Reinhart K, *et al.*; ABC (Anemia and Blood Transfusion in Critical Care) Investigators. Anemia and blood transfusion in critically ill patients. *JAMA* 2002; **288**: 1499–507.

76. Corwin HL, Gettinger A, Pearl RG, *et al.* The CRIT Study. Anemia and blood transfusion in the critically ill: current clinical practice in the United States. *Crit Care Med* 2004; **32**: 39–52.

77. Ferraris VA, Davenport DL, Saha SP, *et al.* Surgical outcomes and transfusion of minimal amounts of blood in the operating room. *Arch Surg* 2012; **147**: 49–55.

78. Opelz G, Vanrenterghem Y, Kirste G, *et al.* Prospective evaluation of pretransplant blood transfusions in cadaver kidney recipients. *Transplantation* 1997; **63**: 964–7.

79. Hill GE, Frawley WH, Griffith KE, Forestner JE, Minei JP. Allogeneic blood transfusion increases the risk of postoperative bacterial infection: a meta-analysis. *J Trauma* 2003; **54**: 908–14.

80. Eikelboom JW, Cook RJ, Liu Y, Heddle NM. Duration of red cell storage before transfusion and in-hospital mortality. *Am Heart J* 2010; **159**: 737–43.

81. Koch CG, Li L, Sessler DI, *et al.* Duration of red-cell storage and complications after cardiac surgery. *N Engl J Med* 2008; **358**: 1229–39.

82. Saager L, Turan A, Dalton JE, *et al.* Erythrocyte storage duration is not associated with increased mortality in noncardiac surgical patients: a retrospective analysis of 6,994 patients. *Anesthesiology* 2013; **118**: 51–8.

83. Weiskopf RB, Feiner J, Hopf H, *et al.* Fresh blood and aged stored blood are equally efficacious in immediately reversing anemia-induced brain oxygenation deficits in humans. *Anesthesiology* 2006; **104**: 911–20.

84. Weiskopf RB, Feiner J, Toy P, *et al.* Fresh and stored red blood cell transfusion equivalently induce subclinical pulmonary gas exchange deficit in normal humans. *Anesth Analg* 2012; **114**: 511–19.

85. Kleinman S. Red blood cell transfusion in adults: storage, specialized modifications, and infusion parameters. http://www.uptodate.com/contents/red-blood-cell-transfusion-in-adults-storage-specialized-modifications-and-infusion-parameters?source=search_result&search=older+blood+and+risks&selectedTitle=2~150 (accessed July 2014).

86. Kleinman S, Kor DJ. Transfusion-related acute lung injury (TRALI). http://www.uptodate.com/contents/transfusion-related-acute-lung-injury-trali?source=see_link (accessed July 2014).

87. Marcucci C, Madjdpour C, Spahn DR. Allogeneic blood transfusions: benefit, risks and clinical indications in countries with a low or high human development index. *Br Med Bull* 2004; **70**: 15–28.

Chapter

9

Monitoring the trauma patient

Elizabeth A. Steele, P. David Soran, Donn Marciniak, and Charles E. Smith

Objectives

(1) List the basic guidelines for monitoring of patients receiving anesthesia.

(2) Evaluate options, functions, use, and problems associated with monitoring devices, particularly in the trauma setting.

(3) Interpret the information provided by monitoring devices.

Introduction

In 1986, the American Society of Anesthesiologists (ASA) prepared and approved *Standards for Basic Anesthetic Monitoring*.[1] This document outlines the responsibilities of the anesthesiologist in assessing patients' vital signs throughout the anesthetic period. Similar guidelines have been published by the Australian and New Zealand College of Anaesthetists (ANZCA) and the Royal College of Anaesthetists.[2,3] Both the Royal College and the ASA note that, in extreme circumstances, provision of life-saving measures takes precedence over application of monitors. Nonetheless, monitoring is intended to improve the quality of care and outcome for patients, and every attempt should be made to appropriately monitor the trauma patient.

All anesthesia providers have an obligation to carefully assess their patients receiving any form of anesthetic. Basic principles include monitoring the physiologic variables of oxygenation, ventilation, circulation, and temperature. Oxygenation can be assessed with pulse oximetry, inhaled and exhaled gas analysis, and blood gas analysis. Ventilation is assured by end-tidal carbon dioxide (CO_2) measurement, listening to the patient's breath sounds, and monitoring the ventilator. Circulation is assessed by electrocardiogram (ECG) and blood pressure (BP) measurements, whether noninvasively by a cuff or invasively by an intraarterial catheter. Circulation can also be monitored minimally invasively through echocardiography and invasively with pulmonary artery (PA) catheter measurements. Urine output provides a rough estimate of tissue perfusion and thus is another monitor for circulation. Temperature measurement can take place at any number of sites, esophageal, tympanic, and rectal being three options. Neurologic monitoring is frequently employed for the trauma patient. A good outcome is often synonymous with a good neurologic outcome. Regardless of the type of technologic monitoring methods employed, anesthesia providers are never relieved of their obligations of vigilance and utilization of clinical skills.

Basic standards

Monitoring standards as outlined by the three major professional organizations are remarkably similar. The ASA standards are helpfully organized into physiologic variables that must be assessed on a regular basis: (1) oxygenation, (2) ventilation, (3) circulation, and (4) temperature (Table 9.1). The Royal College adds "general principles" such as patient identification and availability of support services. Additional requirements include keeping adequate medical records, equipment with functioning alarm systems, and personnel.

Intuitively, we believe that improvements in monitoring improve patient safety and outcomes. However, few randomized prospective studies exist that validate the use of intraoperative monitors and these standards. Most analyses have been pre and post adoption of new monitoring devices. The closed-claims studies by the ASA Committee of Professional Liability noted a decrease in claims for severely injured patients secondary to esophageal intubation and inadequate ventilation in the 1990s as compared with the prior decade. They theorized that this was due to the widespread adoption of pulse oximetry and end-tidal CO_2 monitoring.[4] The Australian Incident Monitoring Study (AIMS) analyzed the role of monitors in detecting critical events in patients undergoing general anesthesia. In more than 50% of cases, a monitor detected the incident prior to clinical observations. The authors concluded that the analysis of events support monitoring standards.[5]

Table 9.2 shows examples of the monitoring technology that is used for various organ systems.

Trauma Anesthesia, 2nd Edition, ed. Charles E. Smith. Published by Cambridge University Press. © Charles E. Smith, 2015.

Table 9.1 American Society of Anesthesiologists (ASA) monitoring standards

Standard I				
Qualified personnel in the room at all times				
Standard II				
Oxygenation	Inspired gas	Oxygen concentration in breathing circuit Low oxygen concentration alarm		
	Blood oxygenation	Quantitative measurement	Pulse oximetry	Variable pitch pulse tone Low-threshold audible alarm
		Observation	Patient color	Adequate exposure and illumination
Ventilation	Observation	Clinical signs: chest excursion; reservoir bag movement; auscultation of breath sounds		
	Quantitative	Volume of expired gas		
	Monitoring	End-tidal CO_2 analysis	Audible alarm	
	Ventilator alarm	Mechanical ventilator disconnect audible alarm		
Circulation	ECG	Continuous monitoring		
	Arterial BP	At least every 5 minutes		
	Heart rate	At least every 5 minutes		
	One additional modality	Pulse palpation, auscultation of heart sounds, intraarterial pressure tracing, ultrasound peripheral pulse monitoring, or pulse plethysmography or oximetry		
Temperature	When clinically significant changes are intended, anticipated, or suspected			

Oxygenation

Pulse oximetry

The first commercially viable pulse oximeter was introduced into clinical practice in 1974 and by the late 1980s was commonly used.[6] It quickly became the standard of care for its ease of use, no need for special training, and freedom from deleterious side effects and risks for the patient.

Pulse oximeters use two wavelengths of light: red (660 nm) and infrared (940 nm). The light is transmitted through tissue (usually a finger) from one side of the sensor to a photodetector on the opposite side. The lights rapidly cycle on and off, with background light being detected during the "off" phase and subtracted from the equation. The lights cycle frequently enough to detect changes in absorbance secondary to arterial pulsations when larger amounts of oxyhemoglobin are flowing through the tissues.

Oxyhemoglobin and deoxyhemoglobin vary in light absorption at different wavelengths. By comparing the absorption at two wavelengths for oxy- and deoxyhemoglobin, a ratio is calculated by using both pulsatile (AC) and static (DC) absorption. This wavelength absorption ratio is converted to percent oxygen saturation.

$$R = \frac{AC_{660}/DC_{660}}{AC_{940}/DC_{940}}$$

One of the few randomized trials for commonly used intraoperative monitors involved more than 20,000 patients. Patients were randomly assigned to the pulse oximetry group except for neurosurgical and cardiac procedures.[7] Patients monitored with pulse oximetry had significantly more respiratory events

noted in the operating room (OR) and post-anesthesia care unit (PACU). Those without oximetry monitoring had more myocardial ischemia, defined by angina and/or ST changes. Overall, however, reductions in postoperative complications were not realized.[8] In a pediatric study, anesthesia providers were blinded to pulse oximeter data. More than twice as many patients with concealed oxygen saturation (SpO_2) data suffered a major desaturation event ($SpO_2 \le 85\%$ for at least 30 seconds) compared with those with available SpO_2 data.[9]

Delivery of oxygen to the tissues is accomplished by adequate cardiac output and the oxygen-carrying capacity of blood. Hemoglobin is the main transport system for oxygen in the body, with a smaller amount of oxygen dissolved in blood. Several other hemoglobin species are commonly seen in clinical practice that are not quantifiable by the standard pulse oximeter but can interfere with oxyhemoglobin measurement. In the trauma patient with inhalational injury or poisoning, methemoglobin (MetHgb) and/or carboxyhemoglobin (COHgb) may be present in significant amounts. The patient with COHgb may have a high saturation on pulse oximetry but truly have a low oxyhemoglobin, because much of the hemoglobin is bound with CO (see Chapters 39 and 40). Similarly, the patient with MetHgb has unreliable pulse oximetry values, commonly reading about 85% regardless of their true oxyhemoglobin value. Arterial blood gas co-oximetry must be sent in these cases or a pulse co-oximeter must be used. A pulse co-oximeter is commercially available in which multiple wavelengths of light are used to measure COHgb, MetHgb, and SpO_2.[10] Use of this pulse oximeter may be of benefit in patients suspected of having COHgb and MetHgb.

Pulse oximetry provides several useful pieces of information. Besides oxygen saturation, pulse oximetry gives a heart

Table 9.2 Monitoring technology for various organ systems

Organ monitored	Technology
Lungs	Arterial blood gas (ABG) Pulse oximeter Mixed venous oxygen saturation* Capnography
Brain	Intracranial pressure monitor Transcranial Doppler Electroencephalogram (EEG) Bispectral Index Cerebral oximetry Jugular venous saturation
Brain and spinal cord	Somatosensory evoked potentials (SSEP) Motor evoked potentials (MEP)
Heart	Electrocardiogram (ECG) Pulse contour analysis of arterial line Echocardiography Central venous pressure Pulmonary artery catheter
Liver and gut	Lactate Gastric tonometry
Kidneys	Urine output Blood urea nitrogen (BUN) Creatinine Creatinine clearance Urinary excretion of Na and Cr
Hematological	Hemoglobin Hematocrit Coagulation tests (PT, PTT, INR) Platelet count and function Thromboelastography Thromboelastometry Fibrinogen

* Mixed venous oxygen saturation is a monitor of global oxygen delivery and consumption.
INR, international normalized ratio; PT, prothrombin time; PTT, partial thromboplastin time.
Modified from Wilson WC, Shapiro B. Perioperative hypoxia. *Anesthiol Clin N Am* 2001; **19**: 769–812.

rate and a plethysmographic tracing of the pulse. The heart rate tone is pitched to vary with saturation so that the anesthesia provider can watch the patient while simultaneously listening for heart rate and saturation. In a trauma case with multiple interventions occurring simultaneously, the volume of the pulse oximeter should be loud enough to hear over the activities in the OR.

In the healthy patient, saturation should be greater than 95%, particularly when receiving supplemental oxygen. A decrease in SpO_2 should prompt an investigation into the cause of desaturation (e.g., hypoventilation, dead-space ventilation, low cardiac output states). The display of a pulse oximetry tracing also gives information about tissue perfusion. Poorly perfused tissue may have a flattened tracing. The amplitude of the wave tracing and the dicrotic notch position can vary with vascular tone.[11] Sensors are usually placed on fingers, but toes and earlobes are also commonly used. Sensors have also been developed for noses and foreheads. Motion artifact may interfere with pulse oximetry readings. Other confounders may be dark fingernail polish, intravenous dyes, COHgb, MetHgb, and deeply pigmented skin.[12]

Blood gas analysis

Pulse oximetry provides near-instantaneous information regarding patient oxygenation, but it has limitations. Moller noted a 2.5% failure rate of oximetry overall, which increased to 7.2% in ASA physical status IV patients. Sicker patients, including trauma patients, are more likely to suffer from low-perfusion states, which may hamper pulse oximetry readings. Trauma patients may also have dyshemoglobinemias, which give inaccurate pulse oximetry readings. Blood gas analysis is a more sensitive measurement of oxygenation. Lysed red blood cells are suspended in a cuvette. By using Beer's law, absorption of light at different wavelengths is calculated to provide concentrations of the various hemoglobin species. It provides dissolved oxygen content (PaO_2) as well as oxyhemoglobin, MetHgb, and COHgb measurements. Using the PaO_2 value as compared with the alveolar oxygen (P_AO_2), one can calculate the A–a gradient ($P_AO_2 - PaO_2$) to provide diagnosis of relative hypoxemia. The alveolar gas equation is used to calculate P_AO_2:

$$P_AO_2 = FiO_2(PB - PH_2O) - (PCO_2/0.8)$$

where FiO_2 = inspired O_2 concentration; PB = barometric pressure at sea level, 760 mmHg; PH_2O = saturated water vapor pressure, 47 mmHg; PCO_2 = arterial CO_2; 0.8 = respiratory quotient.

Additionally, the PaO_2/FiO_2 ratio can be used for classification of lung injury:

$$PaO_2/FiO_2 < 300 \text{ mmHg} = \text{acute lung injury (ALI)}$$

$$PaO_2/FiO_2 < 200 \text{ mmHg}$$
$$= \text{acute respiratory distress syndrome (ARDS)}$$

Blood gas analysis also provides information regarding ventilation ($PaCO_2$), perfusion (pH, lactate), cellular metabolism (cyanide or propofol toxicity), resuscitation (hemoglobin/hematocrit), and electrolyte balance (Na, Cl, HCO_3, K, glucose). Mixed venous and central venous blood oxygenation analysis can also be followed for resuscitation (Table 9.2). Blood is sampled from the PA catheter or cental venous line, which is covered later in this chapter.

Continuous intraarterial blood gas monitoring is a method for measuring arterial pH, PCO_2, PO_2, and temperature in real time. These devices are composed of a series of fiberoptics as well as sensing electrodes that provide continual measurements of pH, PCO_2, PO_2, and temperature.[13–15] The major advantage is availability of immediate data without having to wait for an offline laboratory to analyze the sample. This allows for more timely clinical intervention to correct abnormalities.

Inhaled/exhaled gas analysis/monitor alarms

Monitoring standards have long recognized the importance of verifying the concentration of oxygen in breathing circuits.[16] Alarms, both audio and visual, alerting anesthesia providers to low oxygen concentration must be active when anesthesia machines are used to provide general anesthesia. The Australian Incident Monitoring Study noted that 5 of 1256 incidents were not detected by the oxygen analyzer because the alarm had been disabled. The incidents that were detected included ventilator-driving-gas leaks, hypoxic mixtures, gas leaks, and partial and total ventilation failures.[17] Most anesthetic delivery systems analyze inspired concentrations of oxygen via electrochemical analyzers or paramagnetic analysis. Electrochemical analyzers (polarographic or galvanic) are used in many anesthesia machines. A gas-permeable membrane allows gas to access a metal cathode in an electrolyte solution. The solution reduces oxygen and generates a charge. The current flow is proportional to the amount of oxygen in the sample.[18] Oxygen analyzers are on the inspiratory limb of the anesthesia circuit, so they do not detect disconnects as gas continues to flow past the sensor. However, they are below the flow control valves and thus can detect distal failures as a last line of defense against a hypoxic gas mixtures.

Paramagnetic oxygen analysis is used in parallel with infrared analysis of polar molecules such as nitrous oxide, CO_2, and the halogenated anesthetic agents. This allows the sample taken for agent analysis to be used for oxygen concentration levels as well. The sample gas is compared to a reference gas via a differential transducer exposed to a magnetic field that is rapidly switched on and off. The magnetic field causes the oxygen molecules to become agitated, and the pressure increases. The transducer pressure is converted to an electrical signal, which, in turn, is converted to a partial pressure or FiO_2.

Redundant safety measures such as gas-sampling measurements in addition to an oxygen analyzer on the anesthesia machine, proportioning systems for oxygen and nitrous oxide, minimum oxygen flow rates on ventilators, low oxygen pressure alarms, and backup oxygen tanks help to minimize the potentially catastrophic delivery of hypoxic gas mixtures.

Ventilation
End-tidal CO_2 analysis

CO_2 is in low concentrations in atmospheric air (about 0.03%), but several times this amount is present in exhaled air.[19] CO_2, a byproduct of metabolism, is commonly monitored to assess the ventilatory status of a patient. The efficacy of ventilation, that is, the elimination of CO_2, can be assessed by both $P_{ET}CO_2$ values and capnogram analysis. There is a pressure gradient, typically 3–5 mmHg, from arterial ($PaCO_2$) to alveolar (P_ACO_2) to end-tidal CO_2 ($P_{ET}CO_2$) that is attributable to physiologic shunting and ventilation/perfusion (V/Q) mismatch.[20] During general anesthesia, this pressure gradient increases to 5–10 mmHg.[21]

CO_2 concentration is measured using infrared spectroscopy. The absorbance of light at 4.28 μm is proportional to the amount of CO_2 in a sample.[22] The infrared radiation that passes through the sample is measured by a photodetector and converted to an electric signal and graph. Gas may be sampled by removing air (about 150 mL/min) from the circuit in sidestream analysis, or a monitor can be inserted into the circuit in main-stream analysis, measuring CO_2 concentrations as air moves past a sampling window. For the ventilated patient, the sample is taken from the anesthesia circuit just proximal to the endotracheal tube. Exhaled CO_2 should also be measured from the spontaneously breathing patient via an attachment to the nasal cannula or tubing secured to the upper lip and nares. This method has been validated even in small children.[23]

$P_{ET}CO_2$ monitoring comes in many forms. A capnograph is an instrument that measures CO_2 throughout the respiratory cycle. The graphical display of a capnograph is called a capnogram ($P_{ET}CO_2$ concentration over time) (Fig. 9.1). Although capnometry displays only numerical values for CO_2, capnography is preferred for the OR, as it gives valuable information regarding a patient's cardiopulmonary function.

Measurement of exhaled CO_2 is used throughout hospitals, not just in ORs, to verify endotracheal tube placement. In the OR, exhaled CO_2 measurement is used for the duration of the case. Members of Eichhorn's group in Boston were among the first to advocate monitoring standards.[16] A few years later Eichhorn analyzed severe intraoperative events attributable solely to anesthetic management. In 7 of 11 cases, unrecognized hypoventilation was the cause. Capnography presumably would have prevented these cases.[24]

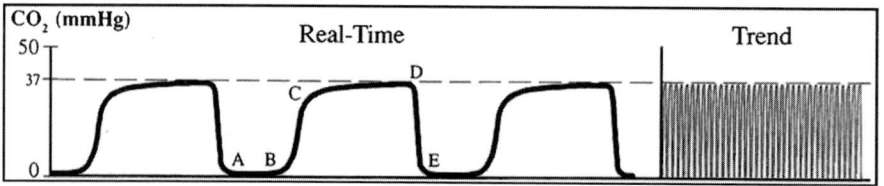

Figure 9.1 Normal capnogram. Line A–B represents the baseline of 0. Line B–C is the ascending limb of the expiratory gas with a mixture of dead space and alveolar air. Line C–D is the alveolar plateau where end-tidal CO_2 is measured. Line D–E is the descending limb with decreasing concentration of CO_2. (From Idris AH. End-tidal carbon dioxide physiology and monitoring during resuscitation. *Anesthesiol Clin N Am* 1995; **13**: 790. Used with permission.)

Table 9.3 Causes of increased or decreased end-tidal CO_2

High CO_2		Low CO_2	
Increased production	**Decreased elimination**	**Decreased production**	**Increased elimination**
Hyperthermia	Asthma	Anesthesia	Hyperventilation
Malignant hyperthermia	COPD	Paralysis	Anxiety Ventilation strategy
Cancer	Inadequate ventilation	Hypothermia	
Burn	(Ventilator settings, drugs, patient fatigue)	Coma	
Sepsis			
Tourniquet and aortic crossclamp release, IV bicarbonate administration, and CO_2 insufflation for laparoscopy may all increase $P_{ET}CO_2$ transiently. Rebreathing and exhausted soda lime may give elevated CO_2 levels that are unrelated to patient conditions and attributable to ventilator errors.		Esophageal intubation, airway obstruction, partial or complete disconnection of ventilator can present as low $P_{ET}CO_2$ (or absent $P_{ET}CO_2$). Arterial CO_2 may be normal or high in actuality. Hypotension, shock, and pulmonary embolus (PE) may give low $P_{ET}CO_2$ values due to decreased blood flow through the lungs.	

COPD, chronic obstructive pulmonary disease; $P_{ET}CO_2$, end-tidal CO_2.

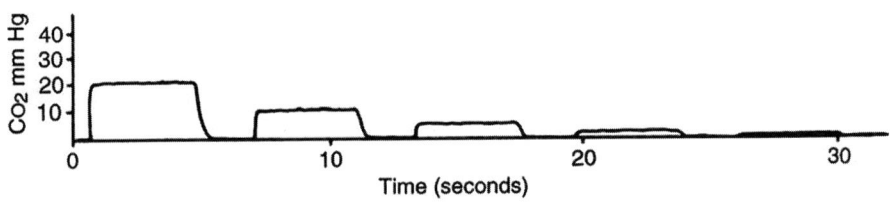

Figure 9.2 Capnogram showing esophageal intubation. Initially there may be some end-tidal CO_2 from the stomach. However, the end-tidal CO_2 will then rapidly decline to zero over the next five breaths. For this reason, capnometry should be verified after five breaths. (From Idris AH. End-tidal carbon dioxide physiology and monitoring during resuscitation. *Anesthesiol Clin N Am* 1995; **13**: 792. Used with permission.)

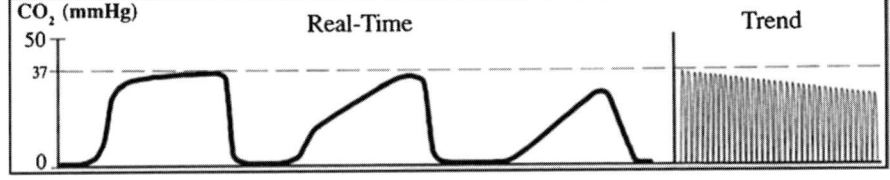

Figure 9.3 Capnogram in a patient with chronic obstructive pulmonary disease (COPD) or acute asthma. Obstruction in the expiratory gas flow is seen as a change in the slope of the ascending limb. The expiratory portion may decrease without a plateau. (From Idris AH. End-tidal carbon dioxide physiology and monitoring during resuscitation. *Anesthesiol Clin N Am* 1995; **13**: 790. Used with permission.)

Pulse oximetry alone will not detect hypoventilation/hypercapnia in the patient receiving supplemental oxygen. In a sample of pediatric patients undergoing dental procedures with sedation and supplemental nasal cannula oxygen, two anesthesia providers simultaneously monitored patients. One used "traditional" methods of assessment – precordial stethoscope and observation of chest movement and skin color. The second observer added pulse oximetry and a capnograph. Ten of 39 sedated patients had airway compromise. All 10 incidences were detected by capnography, three by traditional methods, and none by pulse oximetry.[25]

CO_2 monitoring ensures that ventilation is taking place and is adequate, either keeping the patient in a physiologic range or in a therapeutic range, such as decreased $P_{ET}CO_2$ for the patient with increased intracranial pressure. Coté and colleagues studied 331 children and found 35 events with exhaled CO_2 monitoring, of which 20 were potentially critical, including malignant hyperthermia, accidental extubation, and endobronchial intubation.[26] In another series, 11 of 153 patients had major capnographic events, including esophageal intubation, accidental extubation, disconnection or endotracheal tube obstruction (Fig. 9.2). Of these 11, eight went on to desaturate.[27]

CO_2 production can vary between patients, as can elimination (Table 9.3). Patients with chronic obstructive pulmonary disease (COPD) may have a sloped plateau on their capnogram indicating CO_2 trapping (Fig. 9.3). A patient with normal CO_2 production may have a low $P_{ET}CO_2$ if there are large amounts of dead-space ventilation (pulmonary embolism) or if blood flow through the lungs is decreased (profound hypotension, shock). In fact, a sudden decrease in $P_{ET}CO_2$ can be a first warning of impending circulatory collapse. Capnography also

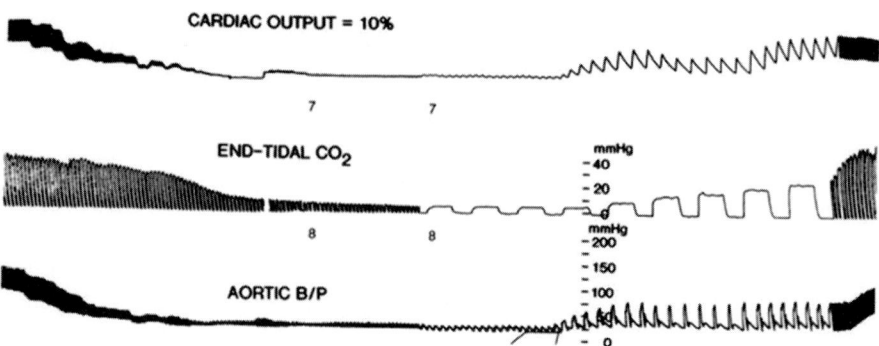

Figure 9.4 During steady state, end-tidal CO_2 reflects cardiac output and blood flow. In this calf experiment (125 kg), blood flow was reduced to 10% of baseline and then back to baseline. The second half of the tracing is at higher speed. B/P, blood pressure. (From Idris AH. End-tidal carbon dioxide physiology and monitoring during resuscitation. *Anesthesiol Clin N Am* 1995; **13**: 793. Used with permission.)

gives an easy visualization for respiratory rate, in particular if the patient is covered with surgical drapes, as with eye surgery. Alarms are linked to the capnogram for high and low CO_2 values as well as respiratory rate.

End-tidal CO_2 monitoring has been used to predict cardiac output after weaning from cardiopulmonary bypass and to predict outcome after resuscitation from cardiac arrest.[28] $P_{ET}CO_2$ concentrations appear to correlate with cardiac output (Fig. 9.4). There is a rapid increase in $P_{ET}CO_2$ with restoration of spontaneous circulation. Thus, if alveolar ventilation and CO_2 production are constant, $P_{ET}CO_2$ can be used to monitor lung perfusion and cardiac output. The relationship between cardiac output and $P_{ET}CO_2$ is not linear. Decreased presentation of CO_2 to the lungs is the major, rate-limiting determinant of the $P_{ET}CO_2$ during low-flow hemorrhagic shock states. As the cardiac output increases during resuscitation from shock or cardiac arrest, respiration becomes the rate-limiting controller of the $P_{ET}CO_2$ after tissue washout of CO_2 has occurred. Under such conditions, the $P_{ET}CO_2$ provides useful information about the adequacy of ventilation, provided that there is little V/Q mismatch.[28]

Precordial/esophageal stethoscope

As the capnogram provides valuable information about the ventilation of the patient, precordial and esophageal stethoscopes can also be used to monitor ventilation. A precordial stethoscope is placed on the chest wall with tubing connected to an ear piece. This allows the anesthesia provider to listen to breath sounds and the heart rate during a case, in particular if the patient is covered with surgical drapes. Left-chest placement, for example, will allow one to detect a main-stem intubation if breath sounds markedly diminish. Others prefer a sternal notch placement over the trachea. An esophageal stethoscope is a small tube placed into the distal portion of the esophagus at a depth of 28–32 cm in the adult. This places the stethoscope behind the heart, making this site advantageous for heart sounds and breath sounds.[29] The tubing connected to the ear piece should be long enough to comfortably reach the anesthesia provider and not interfere with the surgical field. Most esophageal stethoscopes currently in clinical use have a sensor at the distal end used to monitor patient temperature.

In an analysis by the Australian Incident Monitoring Study, only 5% of reported cases used continuous stethoscope monitoring. The authors theorize that slightly over half of the 1256 incidents could have been detected with stethoscope alone if the event had been allowed to evolve.[30] Almost a decade later, pediatric anesthesiologists in Great Britain and Ireland responded to a survey that one-third never used stethoscopes and two-thirds used them occasionally. Nonetheless, one-third admitted to having critical incidents detected through stethoscope use.[31] Meanwhile, at an academic institution in the United States more than half of 520 cases used an esophageal stethoscope.[32]

Once ubiquitous, continuous monitoring by stethoscope has fallen out of favor. Stethoscopes are unlikely to cause complications, unlikely to have device failure, and are inexpensive and easy to replace. Their use has been superseded by more complex monitors such as end-tidal gas analysis and pulse oximetry, but they should not be omitted.

Ventilator settings/alarms

Anesthesia ventilators are sophisticated pieces of equipment. With each case, settings should be checked and adjusted to suit the patient and case needs. Some alarms provide information about the patient and others about the function of the machine. Examples include a low limit on oxygen concentration and low minute ventilation and pressure alarms. Pressure alarms are set for both high and low pressure. Low pressure may indicate a leak in the machine or breathing circuit such as a disconnect. High-pressure alarms are likely due to patient conditions such as reduced lung compliance, secretions in the endotracheal tube, and dyssynchronous ventilation. An important safety feature of the anesthesia machine is a low-gas-pressure alarm alerting the anesthesia provider to a failing gas supply. All ventilators are equipped with alarms, which should be activated for optimum patient safety.

Circulation

Electrocardiogram

The ASA monitoring standards mandate the placement of surface electrocardiograms (ECGs). ECG leads should be placed on all trauma patients in the OR. Ideally, ECG data

Table 9.4 Etiologies of pulseless electrical activity (PEA): 5 H and 5 T

Hypovolemia
Hypothermia
Hyper- and hypokalemia
Hydrogen ion acidosis
Hypoxemia
Tension pneumothorax
Tamponade
Thrombosis: pulmonary embolus
Thrombosis: coronary artery thrombosis
Tablets: drug overdose

obtained in the OR should be compared with the preoperative ECG. This enables the anesthesia provider to determine whether abnormalities seen during surgery are the result of new pathology or a reflection of baseline preoperative status.

Most surface ECG systems employ five electrodes (one on each limb plus one placed in the precordium). This enables simultaneous recording of the six standard frontal-limb leads and one precordial lead. The precordial lead is traditionally placed in the V_5 position in the fifth intercostal space in the anterior axillary line. One of the advantages of this system is that leads II and V_5 can both be monitored simultaneously. This allows for detection of 90% of ischemic episodes. Lead II is also extremely useful in detecting atrial and ventricular arrhythmias. ECG electrodes are traditionally placed by using adhesive gel buttons. These pads improve the conduction of electrical signals from the heart through the skin. In the setting of severe skin burns, the electrodes can be placed on the patient by using small-gauge needles placed subdermally.

There are multiple ECG changes that can be seen in the trauma patient. These can be due to metabolic derangements as a result of hemorrhage and resuscitation, structural injury to the heart itself, or central nervous system injury. The presence of an ECG signal, however, does not guarantee perfusion, such as with pulseless electrical activity.

Pulseless electrical activity, or PEA, occurs when there is electrical activity in the heart but no appreciable cardiac output. PEA can be from multiple causes pertinent to the trauma patient, including cardiac tamponade, tension pneumothorax, hypovolemia, hyperkalemia, and hypothermia, among others (Table 9.4).

Patients are at risk for ischemia in the setting of hemorrhage, high circulating catecholamines, and/or the presence of baseline coronary disease. Patients are also prone to ECG changes related to electrolyte abnormalities. Trauma patients are resuscitated with intravenous crystalloid and blood products. Blood products contain citrate, which chelates calcium. As a result, blood-product volume resuscitation often leads to hypocalcemia. ECG changes associated with this include prolonged QT and ST changes. Potassium abnormalities are also common in trauma patients. Hyperkalemic patients have peaked T waves, shortened QT, diminished P waves, and bundle branch block. Hypokalemic patients can have widened QRS, ST depression, T wave flattening, and U waves. Trauma patients are frequently hypothermic, and they may have ECG changes consistent with this such as sinus bradycardia, Osborn waves, and prolonged QT intervals.[33]

Cardiac contusion from trauma can also cause ECG changes. Rhythm disturbances such as SA nodal abnormalities, AV junctional dysfunction, and intraventricular conduction delay have all been described. More commonly, nonspecific ST and T wave changes may be present.[34,35] Low-voltage ECG and electrical alternans can be seen in pericardial effusion (Fig. 9.5).

ECG changes are often seen in patients with cerebral trauma. Multiple changes have been described in subarachnoid hemorrhage, including ST and T wave changes, rhythm disturbances, and, more commonly, QT prolongation with giant negative T waves.[36]

The correct diagnosis of ECG changes is essential in the safe management of the trauma patient.

Blood pressure

ASA monitoring standards mandate that BP be checked at least every 5 minutes. BP can be measured noninvasively with a BP cuff or invasively with an intraarterial catheter.

Three measurements of arterial BP are commonly recorded on anesthetic records: systolic and diastolic BP (SBP and DBP) and mean arterial pressure (MAP). With the forceful expulsion of blood from the left ventricle, a pressure wave and a flow wave are generated. The pulse pressure wave moves at a rate of 10 m/s and is transmitted throughout the arterial vascular tree. This wave is measured by invasive or noninvasive means to determine arterial BP. The further one moves from the aorta, SBP as measured in peripheral arteries is greater; similarly, the lower the MAP and DBP, the narrower the wave form.[37] Arterial BP can be calculated as the product of vascular resistance and cardiac output. Multiple factors influence both resistance and cardiac output, including heart rate, stroke volume, blood volume, compliance of the vascular system, and sympathetic stimulation.

Noninvasive monitoring is accomplished by an inflatable cuff that is placed around an extremity and inflated to a pressure greater than systolic BP. As the cuff is deflated, BP is determined either by auscultation of Korotkoff sounds or by oscillations of air pressure in the cuff from arterial pulsations. The automated BP cuffs most frequently employed in ORs use oscillometric measurements.

Continuous noninvasive arterial pressure (CNAP) measures BP continuously in real time like an invasive arterial catheter system but is noninvasive. The major advantage of this technology is that invasive catheter placement is not required, meaning that the anesthesia provider is not potentially exposed to needle injuries and blood contamination

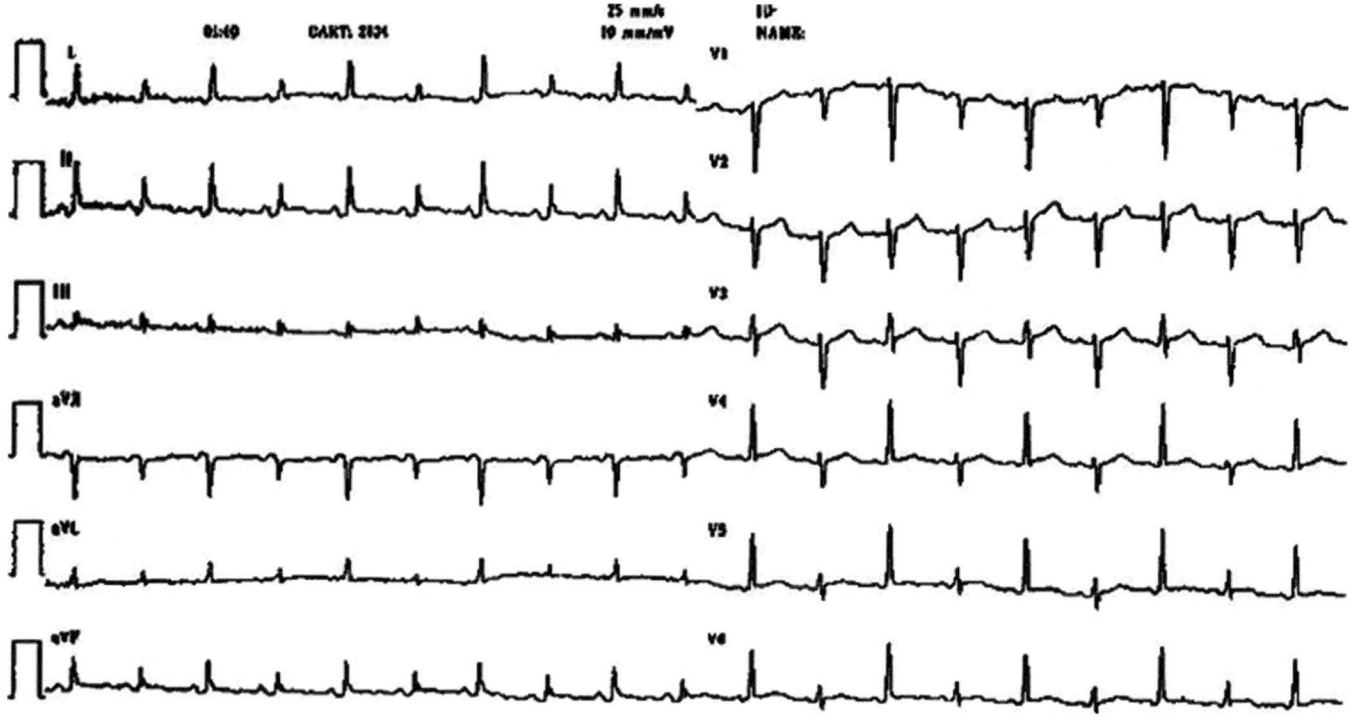

Figure 9.5 Electrical alternans is the beat-to-beat variation in the direction and amplitude of the QRS complex, which represents "swinging" of the heart in the pericardial fluid. Low-voltage QRS complexes are also seen with large effusions and tamponade. (Image courtesy of Kara Quan, MD, MetroHealth Medical Center, Cleveland, OH.)

associated with invasive catheter placement. Also, there is no risk of vascular injury and ischemic complications for the patient. Mathematical analysis of noninvasive pulse waves allows noninvasive estimation of stroke volume and cardiac output using arterial pulse contour algorithms (see *Arterial pulse contour analysis*, below). Disadvantages of continuous noninvasive BP measures are related to changes in vascular tone due to the sympathetic nervous system, anesthetic agents, and vasoactive drugs such as inotropes, vasopressors, and vasodilators. Patient movement makes measurement inaccurate, proper placement is required, and blood samples cannot be obtained. Noninvasive continuous arterial BP monitoring has been shown to correlate with invasive data.[38] However, in the trauma setting, with hemodynamic instability and shock, an arterial line is generally preferred.

To measure BP invasively, a catheter is inserted in a peripheral artery, commonly the radial or femoral (see Chapter 5), and attached to fluid-filled stiff tubing with a sampling port, flushing device, and pressurized fluid bag. The pressure wave of ventricular ejection is transmitted through the fluid to a sensor. Deformation of the sensor changes electric current and resistance through a transducer that converts it to a wave form. The transducer pressure is "zeroed" to atmosphere at the level of the right atrium in most cases but can be placed at the level of the circle of Willis for estimation of brain perfusion. Arterial pressure information can also be obtained by an intraaortic balloon pump. The balloon pump inflates and deflates in time with the cardiac cycle as detected by ECG

and pressure wave. The intraaortic balloon pump is used to "off-load" the failing heart and is not a primary monitoring device for anesthetic care.

Intraarterial monitoring is most commonly used for the trauma patient for multiple reasons: rapid fluctuations in BP may accompany the resuscitation as patients lose large amounts of blood, and cardiothoracic and cranial injuries require close monitoring of physiologic variables and frequent lab draws to assess ventilation, oxygenation, and resuscitation parameters (see Chapter 4).

Arterial pulse contour analysis

Assessing the volume status in trauma patients is a critical and often difficult task, as many patients will have hypotension from various causes (Tables 9.5 and 9.6).[39]

The literature suggests that, overall, only about 50% of hypotensive patients respond to volume administration.[40] Underresuscitation ultimately results in decreased tissue perfusion, while hypervolemia results in interstitial and pulmonary edema with subsequent tissue hypoxia. As an arterial line is commonly placed in the trauma setting, arterial pulse waveform analysis provides useful information in the form of pulse pressure and systolic pressure variation.

The Frank–Starling curve (Fig. 9.6) describes the curvilinear relationship between stroke volume and preload. In the condition of preload dependence, reflected on the ascending portion of the curve, an increase in preload will induce an increase in

Table 9.5 Differential diagnosis of hypotension in trauma

Undetected or underestimated blood loss

Other causes of hypovolemia
- Insensible losses
- Redistribution to extravascular space
- Gastrointestinal loss
- Renal loss
- Excessive venodilatation

Obstructive shock
- Tension pneumothorax
- Pericardial tamponade
- Massive pleural effusion
- Hemothorax
- Abdominal compartment syndrome
- Venous occlusion: air embolism, thrombus, tumor,
- Pregnancy: aortocaval compression
- Atrial occlusion: air embolism, tumor, thrombus

Cardiogenic shock
- Blunt cardiac injury with myocardial contusion and ventricular dysfunction
- Preexisting medical disease (e.g., cardiomyopathy, valvular heart disease)
- Myocardial infarction

Vasodilated shock
- Spinal cord injury
- Anaphylaxis (see Table 9.6)
- Adrenal insufficiency
- Arteriovenous fistula
- Sepsis
- Systemic inflammatory response syndrome (SIRS)
- Hepatic failure

Miscellaneous
- Acidosis
- Hypothermia
- Hypocalcemia

Modified From Duan Y, Smith CE, Como JJ. Cardiothoracic trauma. In Wilson WC, Grande CM, Hoyt DB, eds., *Trauma: Emergency Resuscitation, Perioperative Anesthesia, Surgical Management.* New York, NY: Informa Healthcare, 2007, pp. 469–99; and Palter MD, Cortes V. Secondary triage of the trauma patient. In Civetta JM, Taylor RW, Kirby RR, eds., *Critical Care*, 3rd edition. Philadelphia, PA: Lippincott-Raven, 1997, pp. 1045–63.

Table 9.6 Monitoring for anaphylaxis during anesthesia

System	Symptoms and signs
Pulmonary	Dyspnea, tachypnea, stridor (laryngeal edema), wheezing (bronchospasm), decreased compliance, increased airway pressures, hypoxia
Cardiovascular	Hypotension, shock, tachycardia, arrhythmias
Skin	Hives, edema, itching, burning, edema, diaphoresis, increased skin temperature
Neurologic	Altered level of consciousness

Modified from Levy JH, Yegin A. Anaphylaxis. What is monitored to make a diagnosis? *Anesthesiol Clin N Am* 2001; **19**: 705–15.

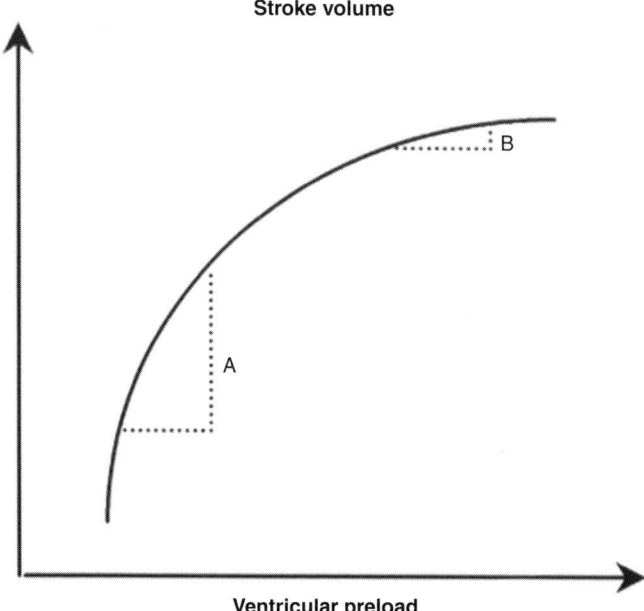

Stroke volume

Ventricular preload

Figure 9.6 Frank–Starling relationship between ventricular preload and stroke volume. A given change in preload results in a larger change in stroke volume on the steep portion (A) compared with the flat portion (B) of the curve. (From Michard F, Teboul JL. Using heart–lung interactions to assess fluid responsiveness during mechanical ventilation. *Crit Care* 2000; **4**: 283. Used with permission.)

stroke volume. These patients are considered volume responders. If the left ventricle (LV) is operating on the flat portion of the curve, an increase in preload will not induce the same change in stroke volume. These patients are considered volume nonresponders. Interpretation of arterial waveform analysis can aid in determining in which portion of the curve the patient is operating and guide volume resuscitation.

Arterial waveform changes stem largely from fluctuations in preload during the respiratory cycle. The patient must be mechanically ventilated and in sinus rhythm to derive meaningful data when analyzing these changes. This is because right heart filling will be irregular with variations in tidal volume or cardiac rhythm. Tidal volumes should be at least 8 mL/kg for data to be most accurate.[41] When pleural and transpulmonary pressures are increased during mechanical ventilation of the lung, systemic venous return is impaired, causing a decrease in right ventricular (RV) filling [42] and an increase in RV afterload, and thus a transient decrease in RV ejection.[43] Left heart filling is subsequently impaired. The reverse process occurs during expiration. This respiratory variation in LV stroke volume can be observed in arterial pressure throughout the respiratory cycle.[44] When the LV is functioning on the steep portion of the Frank–Starling curve and small changes in preload can produce significant changes in cardiac output, these

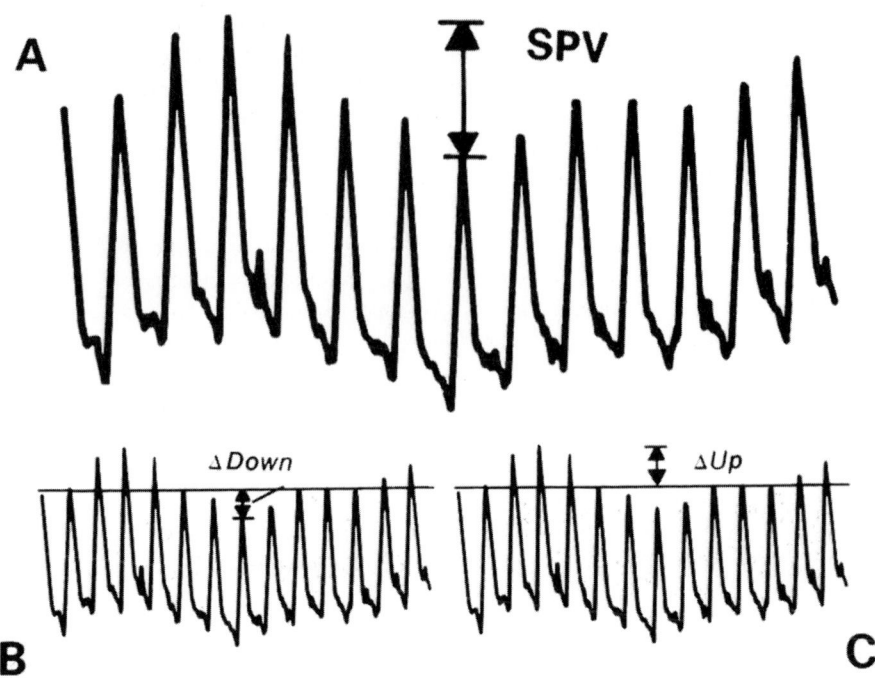

Figure 9.7 Respiratory changes during mechanical ventilation. The difference between maximal and minimal values of systolic BP over a single respiratory cycle is the systolic pressure variation (SPV). (From Michard F, Teboul JL. Using heart–lung interactions to assess fluid responsiveness during mechanical ventilation. *Crit Care* 2000; **4**: 286. Used with permission.)

changes are exaggerated. During periods of volume loading, it is hypothesized that there is a decrease is West's zone 2 of the lung resulting in a decrease in RV afterload, so that the changes seen in the arterial waveform are probably not due entirely to preload factors.

Systolic pressure variation (SPV) is the difference between minimum and maximum systolic BP (SBP) over one respiratory cycle (Fig. 9.7A). SPV occurs via changes in aortic transmural pressure and extramural changes, such as effects of pleural pressure. It can be calculated with the following equation:

$$SPV(\%) = 100 \times (SPBmax - SBPmin)/[(SBPmax + SBPmin)/2]$$

SPV is divided into two components, Δup and Δdown (Fig. 9.7B, C) These values represent the maximum and minimum variation in systolic BP during one respiratory cycle compared to a reference value. These changes represent fluctuations in LV stroke volume by a combination of changes in LV preload and afterload, or extramural aortic pressure. SPV $\geq$ 12 mmHg is considered a threshold value for volume responders versus nonresponders.[45] Δdown may be a more significant predictor of fluid responsiveness than SPV as a whole, with 5 mmHg being the threshold.[46]

Pulse pressure variation (PPV) is the difference between the systolic and diastolic arterial pressures, with a peak and a trough over a single respiratory cycle. It can be calculated with the following equation:

$$PPV(\%) = 100 \times (PPmax - PPmin)/[(PPmax + PPmin)/2]$$

PPV depends on changes in aortic transmural pressure, since the effects of positive-pressure ventilation will influence both systolic and diastolic pressures. In patients undergoing coronary artery bypass grafting, a PPV $\geq$ 11% was found to have a

sensitivity of 100% and a specificity of 93% for an increase in cardiac output after volume administration.[45] A meta-analysis determined that PPV is a more a reliable determinant of volume responsiveness than SPV, with sensitivity, specificity, and diagnostic odds ratio of 0.89, 0.88, and 59.9 versus 0.84, 0.82, and 27.3.[47] Thresholds for significant PPV range from 11% to 13%.

SPV and PPV can be valuable tools in assessing volume status in trauma patients. Much research has been done in septic patients showing the predictive value of PPV, but those findings have been validated in hemorrhagic shock as well. SPV has been evaluated in assessing the effects of hemorrhage on pulse contour in human and animal subjects[48–50] and has been compared to PPV in conditions of severe hemorrhage in an animal study.[51] Data support using these measures as assessors of intravascular depletion. However, there is some evidence that PPV may overestimate the severity of hemorrhage by up to 10% when blood loss approaches 40–50%, although the clinical relevance of this is not clear.[51] A particular advantage of PPV and SPV in the trauma setting is that it is a dynamic estimate of volume status. Blood loss can occur quickly and profoundly in this population, and central venous pressure (CVP), a more "static" measure of volume, will take longer to reflect such change, and in reality lacks any predictive value to volume responsiveness in any patient population.[40] A practical advantage to using arterial waveform analysis as a guide to fluid resuscitation in trauma is that it is relatively safe, is less prone to complications, and is typically much faster than placing a central venous line or a PA catheter.

PPV is most often determined with three techniques: direct calculation, use of a proprietary device, or most commonly the "eyeball" method. The "eyeball" method is considered reasonably accurate[52,53] and can be improved with sweep speeds adjusted to 6.25 mm/s. In a hectic trauma setting when time to get advanced monitoring equipment may not be available, visual interpretation of the arterial waveform is an acceptable method to determine volume responsiveness. Regardless of the method used, the information obtained from the arterial waveform should be used cautiously in the setting of RV dysfunction or elevated PA pressures. Under these conditions, significant PPV can give a false indication of volume responsiveness,[52] and echocardiography (see Chapter 10) is likely a superior indicator.[54] However, PPV appears to be an accurate predictor of volume responsiveness in patients with LV dysfunction.[55]

The emergent thoracotomy patient poses many challenges to anesthesiologists, most notable being fluid management. Resuscitating these patients is often a challenge, because of the hemorrhage that typically precedes the procedure, surgical maneuvering and traction to control the bleeding, and the large insensible losses that occur perioperatively. Typical monitors such as CVP are of questionable reliability because altered intrathoracic pressure clouds their meaning. Since SPV is derived in part from intrapleural pressure effects, it too should be used cautiously. An abundance of data does not exist for monitoring volume status in this subset of patients. However, it appears that PPV is a reliable, dynamic indicator to guide volume administration when the chest is open.[56,57]

Volume management is often a difficult task for the trauma anesthesiologist. Starting points may be unclear, and volume changes are rapid and occasionally harrowing. In patients in normal sinus rhythm receiving mechanical ventilation, PPV is probably the best indicator of fluid responsiveness because of its ease of implementation, use of a preexisting monitor (arterial line), and dynamic and continuous nature.

Central venous pressure

For the anesthesiologist, central venous access most commonly is obtained in the internal jugular vein. Other options include the subclavian and femoral veins (see Chapter 5). The internal jugular and subclavian approaches provide pressures for the superior vena cava, as the tip of the catheter sits at the superior vena cava/right atrial junction. Traditional thinking maintains that CVP is an indicator of preload. Right atrial pressure is a major determinant of right ventricular volume, which in turn supplies the left side of the heart. By monitoring trends in CVP, one can assess fluid status. CVP should be measured at end-expiration as intrathoracic pressures are transmitted to the venous system. The preferred position for the CVP transducer is at the top of the right atrium, approximately 5 cm below the sternal border at the fourth intercostal space.[58] Cardiac events are reflected in the CVP waveform. A wide variety of hemodynamic abnormalities can be identified by analyzing the components of the CVP. For example, in atrial fibrillation, the a wave disappears and the c wave becomes more prominent. With pericardial tamponade, there is elevation and equalization of diastolic filling pressures. The x descent is preserved and the y descent is dampened because of restricted early right ventricular filling.[59] Tricuspid regurgitation produces abnormal systolic filling of the right atrium through the incompetent valve, which results in a ventricularized pressure trace. During a premature ventricular contraction, cannon a waves can be seen on the CVP tracing. This is caused by the right atrium contracting against a closed tricuspid valve.[33] Absence of normal atrioventricular synchrony (AV dissociation or junctional rhythm) can also result in cannon a waves. With pulmonary contusion, CVP was found to be a better estimate of cardiac preload than pulmonary capillary wedge pressure,[60] likely due to increased pulmonary vascular resistance, airway resistance, and dead-space ventilation.

Clinical use of central venous access in the trauma patient is mostly for resuscitation and monitoring (Table 9.7). For the

Table 9.7 Conditions in which invasive monitoring is recommended

Condition	Examples/comments
General	Shock unresponsive to perceived adequate fluid resuscitation Oliguria unresponsive to perceived adequate fluid resuscitation Assessment of intravascular volume and cardiac function Evaluation of cardiovascular contribution to multiple organ system dysfunction
Surgical	Perioperative management of high-risk patients undergoing extensive surgery Cardiac or major vascular surgery Postoperative cardiac complications Multisystem trauma with hemodynamic instability despite fluid resuscitation Severe burns
Pulmonary	Respiratory failure Evaluate effects of ventilatory support on cardiovascular status
Cardiac	Blunt cardiac injury with cardiac dysfunction Complicated myocardial infarction Unstable angina unresponsive to conventional treatment Congestive heart failure unresponsive to conventional treatment Pulmonary hypertension during acute drug therapy

Note: Since the advent of echocardiography (see Chapter 10), pulmonary artery catheters are rarely used in trauma unless the patient requires cardiac surgery.

Modified from Duan Y, Smith CE, Como JJ. Cardiothoracic trauma. In Wilson WC, Grande CM, Hoyt DB, eds, *Trauma: Emergency Resuscitation, Perioperative Anesthesia, Surgical Management*. New York: Informa Healthcare, 2007, pp. 469–99; and Varon AJ. Arterial, central venous, and pulmonary artery catheters. In Civetta JM, Taylor RW, Kirby RR, eds. *Critical Care*, 3rd edition. Philadelphia: Lippincott-Raven, 1997, pp. 847–65.

patient facing a prolonged hospitalization and recovery period, central access is used for frequent blood sampling, infusion of caustic substances such as vasoactive pharmaceuticals, and hyperalimentation. Central venous access has utility in trauma patients long after they have left the OR.

Goal-directed therapy for resuscitating septic patients gives target CVPs between 8 and 12 mmHg to optimize tissue perfusion.[61] But using central pressures to guide therapy has been called into question, because the outcomes are not necessarily better. In addition, multiple studies have shown that measured hemodynamic pressures do not correlate with volume changes. Even healthy subjects do not show a "predictable relationship" between pressure and volume preload indices and cardiac performance variables.[62] Nonetheless, trends in CVP are commonly used to guide fluid therapy. Other methods for assessing volume status are often employed, such as arterial pulse contour analysis, PA occlusion pressure, urine output, capillary refill, and direct visualization with echocardiography.

Central venous oxygen saturation can also be measured to assess tissue perfusion in the critically ill patient. As perfusion decreases, more oxygen is extracted from the blood, resulting in lower saturations as blood returns to the heart. Mixed venous saturation is obtained from the PA catheter, whereas central venous saturation is measured from the CVP.

Pulmonary artery catheter

PA catheters have been used in the United States for more than four decades in the management of critically ill patients. The PA catheter allows the clinician to measure RV pressure or PA pressure, PA occlusion pressure, and cardiac output, and it allows for sampling of mixed venous blood. Although all of these measurements can be helpful in managing the trauma patient, it is generally accepted that echocardiography has supplanted the PA catheter as the preferred method for assessing the patient with cardiac dysfunction and for evaluating the hemodynamic state (see Chapter 10).

The PA catheter is placed through an introducer located in a central vein. The most common sites for placement are the right internal jugular vein, which allows for the shortest, straightest route, and the left subclavian vein. The catheter has a balloon tip that allows for flow-directed placement into the PA. The catheter tip must be in the PA for accurate measurements, both pressure and blood oxygen levels, to take place.

Right atrial or CVP and RV pressure waveforms may be a clue to potentially life-threatening cardiac pathology in the trauma patient. Patients in hypovolemic shock have low systemic and intracardiac pressures and often a dampened PA waveform. Patients with cardiac tamponade, RV contusion, and/or severe tricuspid regurgitation will have a high CVP.

As little as 50 mL of blood in the pericardium can significantly limit ventricular filling, resulting in low cardiac output, hypotension, and elevated CVP (see Chapters 29 and 30). In tamponade, the patient is normally tachycardic and

hypotensive with an elevated CVP. The ventricles are unable to fill during diastole, which causes equalization of diastolic pressures. Because the RV cannot fill in diastole, the CVP tracing is altered. Passive flow of blood from the right atrium to the ventricle is impaired because of compression from pericardial fluid. This results in a blunted y descent and a prominent x descent.[63]

PA occlusion pressure (PAOP), or pulmonary capillary wedge pressure (PCWP) can be measured from the PA catheter. When the balloon is inflated, the branch of the PA in which the catheter is sitting becomes occluded. No blood is flowing past the catheter tip. There are no valves between the PA and the left atrium, so the pressure transducer measures the pressure in the left atrium when the occlusion balloon is inflated. This pressure corresponds to the left ventricular end-diastolic pressure, as the mitral valve is open in diastole. This pressure measurement has been used as a surrogate for left ventricular end-diastolic volume (LVEDV) and thus as a tool for guiding fluid resuscitation. For example, a PAOP of 10 mmHg would tend to indicate a low LVEDV, and therefore fluid administration would be warranted, whereas a PAOP of more than 18 mmHg would tend to indicate volume overload. Some clinicians use the PAOP to guide fluid therapy in an effort to maximize cardiac output and organ perfusion. The major pitfall to using the PAOP as a measure of LVEDV is that, as the compliance of the LV changes, the pressure required to fill it also changes. For example, a patient with severe LV hypertrophy and diastolic dysfunction will require a much higher pressure to fill during diastole. PAOP of more than 18 mmHg may be needed to generate adequate ventricular filling and cardiac output in the stiffened ventricle.

The PA catheter can also be used to measure cardiac output. Most PA catheters use thermodilution measurements to calculate RV cardiac output. Barring any intracardiac shunts, right-sided cardiac output approximates left-sided output. Thermodilution methods to assess cardiac output measure changes in blood temperature from either an injected solution or a thermal filament in the catheter. The computer makes a temperature versus time curve from the data. The change in blood temperature is inversely proportional to the cardiac output. The cardiac output should then be divided by the patient's body surface area to generate a cardiac index. For the injectate method, a discrete quantity of saline at a known temperature is injected through the CVP port of the PA line. A thermistor located near the catheter tip measures the change in blood temperature due to the addition of the saline. Injections should be made at end-expiration to minimize respiratory variations in venous return. There are numerous possible errors inherent in bolus or intermittent cardiac output measurement. Using too little or too much injectate and injecting too rapidly or slowly will result in spurious data. Tricuspid or pulmonic regurgitation will also yield poor data. Continuous cardiac output removes variability in the measurement due to user characteristics but has the same limitations due to patient characteristics as bolus measurements.

Mixed venous saturation (SvO$_2$) can be measured by blood gas analysis from the tip of the PA catheter (Table 9.2). Alternatively, a continuous oxygen saturation catheter with wavelength oximetry may be used. Mixed venous saturation is related to oxygen delivery and thus cardiac output by the following equation, known as the Fick equation:[35]

$$SvO_2 = SaO_2 - VO_2/(13.9 \times CO \times Hgb)$$

where SaO$_2$ = oxygen saturation of the arterial blood, VO$_2$ = oxygen consumption, CO = cardiac output, and Hgb = hemoglobin.

The mixed venous saturation is a reflection of oxygen delivery and consumption by the tissues. For example, in a hypovolemic trauma patient with low cardiac output and anemia from traumatic bleeding, SvO$_2$ will be decreased. Therapy can be guided with the goal of improving SvO$_2$ as a marker for overall improved oxygen delivery. Many factors can interfere with accurate SvO$_2$ measurements. If the catheter is wedged or the patient has significant mitral regurgitation, the blood at the distal tip will contain oxygenated blood from the lungs. This will raise the saturation of the sample and result in false assessment of cardiac output and organ perfusion. Intracardiac or peripheral left-to-right shunts such as an arteriovenous fistula, as well as conditions of systemic shunt such as sepsis, will also result in falsely elevated SvO$_2$. In a multicenter trial, mortality in septic patients treated with early goal-directed therapy was highest in patients with low central venous oxygen saturation, followed by patients with high central venous oxygen saturation, and lowest in patients with normoxia.[63] Most complications of PA catheters are a result of obtaining central venous access. Those more specific to the PA line itself include arrhythmias due to iatrogenic right bundle branch block from PA line placement, PA rupture from overinflation of the flow balloon, and pulmonary infarction from leaving the occlusion balloon inflated for a period of time.

Numerous studies have evaluated the usefulness of PA catheters in treating patients. Many studies have shown little or no improvement in outcome in terms of mortality or hospital stay.[64,65] Data have shown improved outcomes when trauma patients were resuscitated to certain endpoints available from a PA line, such as cardiac index and mixed venous saturation.[66] One study suggested that the use of PA catheters in severely injured patients reduced mortality, in particular in older patients and those presenting to medical attention in severe shock.[67]

PA catheter monitoring in and of itself cannot be expected to improve outcome. Rather, the monitoring system must provide accurate numbers; pathologic causes must be identified; the need for therapy must be recognized; and a specific therapy must be selected and appropriately administered.[59] Although it is reasonable to assume that more precise knowledge of cardiovascular parameters will permit more appropriate treatment and improved outcome, there is little clinical evidence that PA catheter monitoring benefits patients.

Echocardiography

Echocardiography is an excellent monitor of ventricular performance and volume (see Chapter 10). In patients with injury, blood volume and fluid loading should be measured, because ventricular preload is critical for BP stability. Echocardiography assesses ventricular preload more accurately than PA catheterization. Other clinical applications of echocardiography in trauma include assessment of ventricular function, wall motion abnormalities, valvular disease, pericardial effusion, cardiac tamponade, aortic injury, interatrial shunt, and pulmonary embolism.[68] Because of the possibility of exacerbating an esophageal rupture, patients with known or suspected esophageal injury should not have a transesophageal echo probe placed. Esophagoscopy and gastroscopy can be used to rule out significant esophageal pathology prior to placing the probe.

Over the past few years, transthoracic echocardiography (TTE) has been implemented more frequently in the management of hemodynamically unstable patients. A TTE can be rapidly performed in the ED or the OR to evaluate the cause of hypotension without risk of further injury to the patient. A specific protocol (FATE protocol) has been developed to rapidly assess wall thickness, chamber sizes, biventricular function, and pleural pathology in order to determine cause of hypotension in an unstable patient. The protocol involves four scanning views: (1) subcostal four-chamber, (2) apical four-chamber, (3) parasternal, (4) pleural scanning (Fig. 9.8). In experienced hands, this can be performed in less than 70 seconds and provide critical information in the management of the trauma patient.[68]

Urine output

Traditional resuscitation guidelines use urine output as an endpoint. In the perioperative period, approximately 0.5 mL/kg/h is desired for urine production. While not all patients arriving in the OR will be catheterized, major trauma patients should be, making the measurement of urine output a routinely assessed parameter. Urine production in the perioperative period can be influenced by antidiuretic hormone (vasopressin) production during hypovolemia prior to resuscitation, catecholamines, medications, and third-spacing of crystalloids.

Urine output is used as a surrogate measure of organ perfusion. Presumably, with adequate urine output, one is providing oxygen delivery to the metabolically sensitive renal parenchyma. Unfortunately, urine output is a rough approximation and does not guarantee renal protection. Use of more sophisticated measurements of perfusion such as hemodynamic measurements and acid–base status, while not showing clear improvements in outcome, is recommended.[69] Differentiating the various causes of oliguria is critical (Table 9.8). Measurement of blood urea nitrogen (BUN), creatinine, urinary specific gravity, and fractional excretion of sodium can be done to uncover the cause of oliguria.

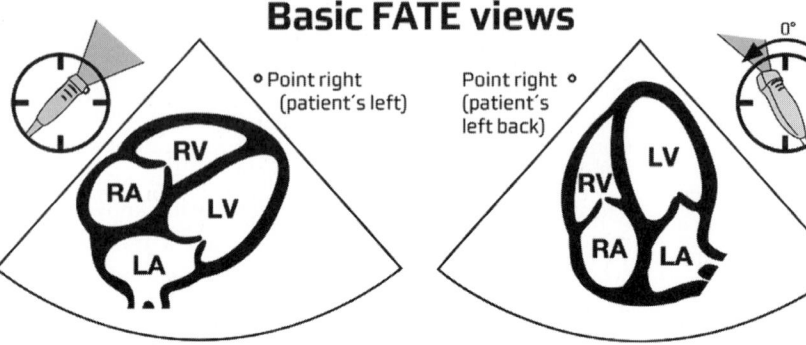

Figure 9.8 The FATE protocol is used to evaluate circulatory problems in five steps, as follows: (1) look for obvious pathology (e.g., left ventricular failure, severe pulmonary embolism, pericardial effusion); (2) assess wall thickness and chamber dimensions; (3) assess biventricular function; (4) visualize pleura on both sides; (5) relate the information to the clinical context.[69] (Figure used with permission from Erik Sloth.)

regionmidtjylland **mıdt**

Focus Assessed Transthoracic Echo (FATE)

Scanning through position 1-4 in the most favourable sequence

Basic FATE views

Pos 1: Subcostal 4-chamber

Pos 2: Apical 4-chamber

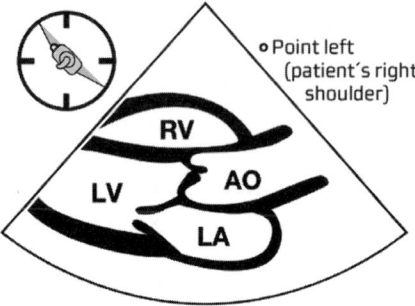

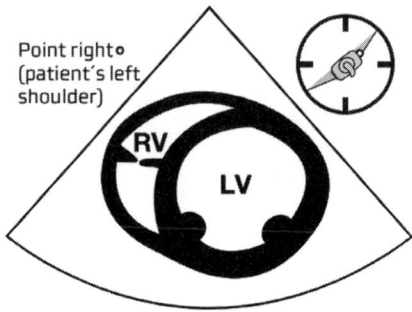

Pos 3: Parasternal long axis

Pos 3: Parasternal LV short axis

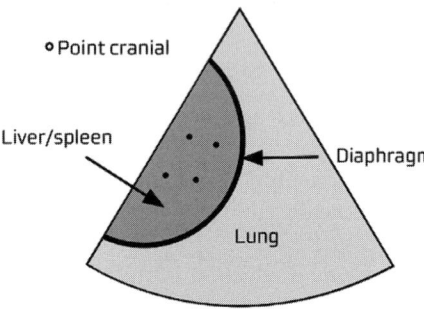

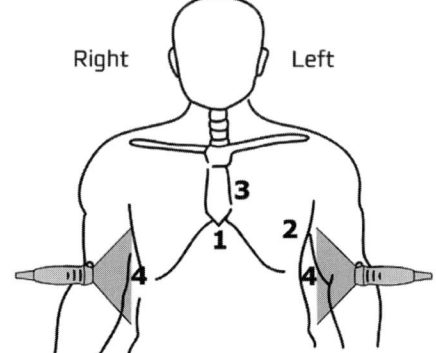

Pos 4: Pleural scanning

Temperature

Maintaining normothermia is a particular challenge in trauma (see Chapter 14). With large-volume resuscitations and much of the patient exposed, hypothermia quickly sets in. In most trauma cases, hypothermia should be avoided because it causes coagulation disturbances, cardiac arrhythmias, and inappropriate diuresis, it delays the metabolism of drugs, and it increases the risk of infections.[70] Hypothermia is selectively used for neurologic trauma (e.g., intracranial hypertension and pediatric brain injury: see Chapter 35) and cardiothoracic repairs under cardiac bypass.

The first assessment of temperature is not of the patient but of the temperature control for the OR. The room should be heated (> 24 °C) to prevent further hypothermia. In cases of damage control resuscitation, OR temperature can be increased to > 28 °C to minimize the risk of the bloody vicious cycle of hypothermia, coagulopathy, and acidosis (see Chapter 18). Esophageal stethoscopes are helpful for listening to heart and breath sounds but also contain a temperature sensor. Of note, gastric suctioning will artifactually lower esophageal temperatures.[71] The distal esophagus is considered a core temperature measuring site, as are the tympanic membrane, PA catheter sensor, and nasopharynx. Tympanic temperatures

Table 9.8 Perioperative conditions causing decreased urine output in trauma

Prerenal	Hypotension, multiple causes (see Table 9.5) Renal arterial obstruction: • Thrombosis • Embolus • Aortic crossclamp • Aortic dissection/transsection
Renal	Acute tubular necrosis: • Nephrotoxins • Radiographic contrast • Myoglobinuria • Rhabdomyolysis Vasculitis or glomerulonephritis Interstitial nephritis Trauma to urinary system
Postrenal	Obstructed urinary catheter Urinary calculi Injury to ureters or bladder

reflect brain temperature and are commonly employed with total circulation arrest for repair of the aorta. Intermediately accurate sites for temperature measurement are the bladder, rectum, mouth, and axilla. Skin temperatures are less helpful, as they may reflect ambient temperatures and superficial vaso-constriction of the skin.[72]

Neurologic monitoring

Traumatic brain injury (TBI) is unfortunately frequent, and frequently catastrophic (see Chapters 20, 21, and 35). A good outcome from a trauma includes an excellent neurologic prognosis. However, in the trauma setting, sophisticated neurologic monitoring, beyond intracranial pressure monitoring, is not commonly utilized. Systemic monitoring can improve outcome by limiting secondary brain injury from hypotension and hypoxemia.

Intracranial pressure (ICP)

The skull contains brain tissue, blood, and cerebrospinal fluid (CSF). Autoregulation provides for a relatively stable flow of blood to the brain over a range of BP (typically MAPs of 60–160 mmHg). For the brain-injured patient, autoregulation is disrupted and cerebral blood flow can change dramatically. This contributes to secondary brain injury. In addition, systemic hypotension and hypoxemia associated with the trauma can cause cytotoxic and vasogenic edema. Systemic monitors can assist in limiting hypotension and hypoxemia.

By measuring ICP, the anesthesiologist can track cerebral perfusion pressure (CPP = MAP – ICP) and optimize brain perfusion (see Chapters 20 and 21). Maneuvers such as raising BP, decreasing CSF volume (drainage, decreased production via pharmacologic agents), decreasing brain swelling (osmotic diuresis, steroids), and upright positioning may be used to increase CPP. Treatment of intracranial hypertension should begin with pressure levels above 20 mmHg,[73] though some would suggest above 15 mmHg.[74] The CPP goal should be approximately 60 mmHg. Levels below 50 mmHg are associated with poor outcome, and aggressively treating a patient to raise CPP above 70 mmHg with pressors and fluids is associated with systemic morbidity such as acute respiratory distress syndrome (ARDS).[75]

ICP is most commonly measured supratentorially through a ventriculostomy or an intracranial "bolt." A ventriculostomy is a catheter placed in the lateral ventricle, which is attached to a fluid-filled column and a pressure sensor. Through the catheter, CSF may be drained, medications injected, and ICP measured. Thus, the ventriculostomy acts as a monitor and a therapeutic device. The bolt or screw is a hollow device placed in the subarachnoid space and attached to a pressure transducer or fiberoptic cable. ICP can be measured but CSF cannot be withdrawn. The bolt has a lower infection rate and is easier to place than the ventriculostomy. The Brain Trauma Foundation considers the ventricular catheter "the most accurate, low-cost and reliable method of monitoring ICP."[76]

Electroencephalogram (EEG)

EEG monitoring records spontaneous electrical activity in the cerebral cortex. Electrodes are placed on the scalp in a standardized fashion. Waveforms are characterized by varying frequency and amplitude and the location in which the signal was obtained. Four basic frequencies are described: delta (0–4 Hz), theta (4–8 Hz), alpha (8–13 Hz), and beta (> 13 Hz). Delta waves, which are slow, synchronized waves, are seen with deep anesthesia or sleep, but may also occur with ischemia or severe metabolic disturbances. An awake patient will usually have disorganized, more complex waveforms such as beta waves.[77]

EEG monitoring is most commonly used for detecting seizure foci. Intraoperatively, EEG is frequently used to monitor cerebral ischemia during carotid surgery when one carotid artery is occluded. EEG has been used in the neurointensive care setting for patients with TBI. It is used to detect subclinical seizure activity and to aid in prognosticating outcomes in TBI patients. Studies of EEG in TBI have shown that TBI patients have a high risk of developing seizure activity, particularly older patients and those with baseline seizure disorders.[78]

Bispectral Index (BIS)

Interpreting raw EEG data in the OR is cumbersome and a highly technical skill. Several monitors are available that convert selected EEG signals into a single number that reflects the patient's level of consciousness. The algorithm used to convert the raw EEG is guarded. This number is used to guide pharmacologic therapy and depth of anesthesia. The BIS Monitor by Aspect is the most commonly used model.

Specialized gel pads are placed on the patient's forehead and attached to the corresponding monitor. The gel pad must be firmly attached to the patient, as impedance will reduce

151

signal quality. Patients may require muscle relaxation to obtain reliable processed EEG information, because muscle activity can interfere with the interpretation of EEG signals.

In trauma patients, depth of anesthesia monitors would be predicted to behave normally. The brain-injured patient potentially presents a special case. Several studies have tried to correlate the Glasgow Coma Scale (GCS) score and observational sedation scales with BIS levels in the brain-injured patient. A correlation exists between GCS and BIS such that the higher the GCS score, the higher the BIS. This relationship was maintained both with and without sedation, validating the use of anesthetic depth monitors in brain-injured patients.[79,80] Of note, use of a processed EEG monitor does not guarantee lack of awareness, as numerous case reports show.[81,82]

Evoked potentials

Evoked potentials measure nervous-system electrical activity that has been elicited by a stimulus. Evoked potentials are described in terms of amplitude, latency, and morphology (see also Chapter 23). The most common evoked potentials used in the OR are sensory and motor. Evoked potentials are not commonly employed during the initial trauma surgery. However, patients often return for definitive stabilization of injuries, which is are appropriate for evoked potential monitoring. As anesthetic agents can affect evoked potentials, protocols have been developed to provide optimal signal strength and interpretation. Sample guidelines from MetroHealth Medical Center in Cleveland, Ohio, are shown in Table 9.9 (J. Lovich-Sapola, personal communication, 2013).

Table 9.9 Somatosensory evoked potential (SSEP) and motor evoked potential (MEP) protocols at MetroHealth Medical Center

Protocol

1. The type of neuromonitoring should be placed on the surgical schedule (i.e., SSEP, MEP, or SSEP + MEP) to allow for appropriate planning and preparation by the anesthesia team.
2. Communication between the anesthesia team, neuromonitoring clinician, and surgeon is critical. Inform the neuromonitoring clinician prior to any significant changes in the administration of anesthesia during the case (i.e., any **bolus** of medication, volatile anesthetic change). The goal should be to make no major anesthetic changes after the induction of anesthesia and baseline measurements.
3. In the management of patient hemodynamics, **boluses of medications should be avoided.** Adjusting the infusion rates of the intravenous mediations is preferred. Boluses of β-blockers, hydralazine, phenylephrine, and ephedrine are preferred if a bolus is required. (Remember that the goal is hemodynamic stability throughout the case.)
4. Compatibility of a given anesthetic protocol with SSEP or MEP monitoring is not all-or-nothing; it is a continuum. It depends on multiple factors, and the same anesthetic protocol will not work with all patients. Each patient should have baseline measurements once anesthesia is induced and the patient is positioned.
5. Changes in levels of inhaled anesthetics, temperature, CO_2, and blood pressure affect interpretations of SSEP/MEP monitoring. Therefore, these levels should be kept as constant as possible during the case.
6. **The anesthesia and surgical teams must provide full disclosure of the risks and benefits of the above neuromonitoring and anesthesia, including but not limited to the possibility of intraoperative awareness and movement, tongue injury, and vision changes.**

SSEP monitoring anesthesia protocol

- 1–2 mg of midazolam preoperative (do not repeat)
- Induction: etomidate, propofol, thiopental, or ketamine
- Muscle relaxant (rocuronium or vecuronium) for induction and as needed throughout the case.
- ≤ 0.5 MAC of isoflurane, sevoflurane, or desflurane
- No N_2O
- Continuous infusion of propofol (75–300 µg/kg/min)
- Continuous infusion of fentanyl or remifentanil
- MAP should be maintained around the 90s (modify based on patient's medical history)

MEP monitoring anesthesia protocol

- 1–2 mg midazolam preoperative (do not repeat)
- Induction: etomidate, propofol, thiopental, or ketamine
- A single dose of muscle relaxant for intubation (do not repeat)
- ≤ 0.5 MAC of isoflurane, sevoflurane, or desflurane
- No N_2O
- Continuous infusion of propofol (75–300 µg/kg/min)
- Continuous infusion of fentanyl or remifentanil
- MAP should be maintained around the 90s (modify based on patient's medical history)
- A bite block must be placed prior to turning the patient prone to decrease the risk of tongue and lip lacerations (consider checking its placement if possible during long cases)

Somatosensory evoked potentials (SSEPs)

The somatosensory system relays vibration, proprioception, and light touch information from the periphery to the central nervous system. Electrical stimuli are applied to peripheral nerves (most commonly median, ulnar, common peroneal, and posterior tibial) and signals are assessed along the path of the nerve to the cortex. Typically, electrical potentials are assessed at the level of the cortex by scalp electrodes. Many signals are averaged from repeated stimulation to obtain a clinically useful waveform.[77] SSEP signals are carried mostly in the posterior spinal column; thus, anterior damage may not be recorded by the SSEP. SSEPs are most commonly used during spinal surgery and thoracic aneurysm repair. Anesthetic agents have variable effects on the signal.

Motor evoked potentials (MEPs)

Transcranial or spinal cord electrical stimulation produces a descending signal that can be recorded over the spinal cord, peripheral nerve, or muscle. Damage to anterior spinal tracts (motor tracts) not identified by SSEPs might be recognized by MEPs. MEPs are sensitive to inhaled anesthetic agents, and a total intravenous anesthetic approach is commonly employed with muscle relaxant to prevent gross motor movement.[83]

Cerebral oximetry

Cerebral oximetry can be measured either noninvasively with near-infrared spectroscopy, or invasively with a catheter placed in the jugular bulb to measure jugular bulb oxygen saturation ($SjvO_2$).

Venous blood from the brain drains into the jugular bulb located at the base of the skull. A catheter, placed through a 4 Fr sheath and into the jugular bulb, measures the saturation of cerebral venous blood in real time. In head trauma patients, the catheter is typically placed either on the side of the injury or bilaterally.[84,85] Treatment can thus be tailored toward optimizing cerebral saturation. This can be done by therapeutic maneuvers geared toward improving cerebral blood flow, such as treating elevated ICP with mannitol or hyperventilation, or by using volume or vasoactive drugs to improve perfusion pressure (see also Chapters 20, 21, and 35). Risks of jugular bulb monitoring include procedural when placing the catheter, complications of the intravascular device (e.g., infection, thrombosis), and incorrect placement leading to spurious oximetric values.[86] A study published in 2001 found that jugular bulb monitoring did not significantly influence the management of head trauma patients.[87] Most centers now use noninvasive near-infrared spectroscopy in place of jugular bulb catheters to evaluate cerebral oximetry.

Regional cerebral saturation monitors use near-infrared spectroscopy (NIRS), similar to pulse oximetry, to measure tissue saturation (rSO_2). Regional cerebral saturation is measured noninvasively by using cutaneous patches placed on the forehead. The alteration of regional cerebral perfusion and thus rSO_2 can be detected by the sensors. Cerebral oximetry is frequently used in cardiac and carotid surgery. Multiple studies have shown improvements in stroke rates and major organ morbidity and mortality when cerebral saturation is measured and interventions performed to keep the saturation within 75% of baseline.[88] Cerebral oxygen saturation can be improved by increasing cardiac output, FiO_2, hematocrit, or PCO_2.

Cerebral oximetry is also useful in trauma patients. Cerebral blood flow depends on CPP. Therapy in head trauma patients is guided toward improving CPP and thus cerebral perfusion in the setting of elevated ICP. In the past, many patients needed to have invasive ICP monitors placed in order to determine CPP. A study in 2002 showed, not surprisingly, a correlation of CPP to cerebral saturation. An rSO_2 greater than 75% suggested CPP was adequate to meet metabolic demands, whereas rSO_2 less than 55% suggested inadequate CPP.[89] A follow-up study showed a correlation of cerebral hypoxia (rSO_2) less than 60% with lower GCS scores, lower CPP, more severe head computed tomography (CT) score, and decreased survival.[90]

Cerebral oximetry monitoring can be useful in managing the trauma patient, offering a noninvasive measure of cerebral perfusion. Anesthetic interventions can be made in an effort to improve cerebral perfusion in the head trauma patient by using the rSO_2 as an objective measure of the efficacy of intervention. Limitations of cerebral oximetry include the effect of temperature on near-infrared absorption spectrum, contamination of the signal by chromophores in the skin, and differences between the various manufacturers' devices. There is also a large amount of variation from patient to patient in the "normal range." As a result, the current recommendation is to use cerebral oximetry more as a trend monitor than as an absolute one.[91]

Conclusions

Standard monitoring, including auscultation of breath and heart sounds and secure venous access, is the cornerstone of any anesthetic technique for patients with trauma. Standard monitoring includes ECG, noninvasive BP, pulse oximetry, $P_{ET}CO_2$, precordial or esophageal stethoscope, and core temperature. A peripheral nerve stimulator is used to assess the degree of neuromuscular blockade. Invasive monitoring, including arterial line and CVP, is routine in seriously ill trauma patients. Arterial pulse contour analysis is useful to assess fluid responsiveness. Consideration should also be given to monitoring for awareness in trauma patients, as many patients have hemodynamic instability that limits their ability to tolerate sufficient anesthetic agents to blunt awareness and recall.

Anesthetic outcomes have improved dramatically over the past few decades, in large part due to technological advances. Technology developed for primary use in other fields has found its way into perioperative use. While not all anesthesiologists will be well versed in every modality, a familiarity with options for monitoring and assessing patients is encouraged. Echocardiography is a rapid mode of assessing cardiac function and volume status (see Chapter 10). Doppler ultrasound, useful in locating blood vessels and assessing cerebral blood flow, is another technology that has a place in the trauma OR. Pulse wave analysis for cardiac output without a PA catheter is a technology that is in clinical use and gaining acceptance as a viable monitor. Monitors should improve outcome, not just add to the amount of information that must be interpreted and integrated by the anesthesia provider. In the increasingly mechanized OR, the potential for distraction, false negatives, and equipment malfunction exists. According to ASA closed claims analysis, however, most anesthesia machine malfunctions were user errors.[92] Electronic monitoring adds another dimension to the care we provide in the OR. Although research may not validate improvement in patient outcomes, we believe clinical monitoring helps avoid medical mismanagement.

Having a wide array of monitors within easy reach does not absolve the clinician from utilizing clinical skills. The power of the physical exam – watching, listening, and laying hands on our patients – has not yet been replaced.

Questions

(1) Which of the following does *not* interfere with pulse oximetry readings?
   a. Patient movement
   b. Dark nail polish
   c. Carboxyhemoglobin
   d. Deoxyhemoglobin
   e. Deeply pigmented skin

(2) The CO_2 pressure gradient from arterial to end-tidal increases under general anesthesia to what level?
   a. 1–3 mmHg
   b. 5–10 mmHg
   c. 15–20 mmHg
   d. 40–50 mmHg
   e. 95–100 mmHg

(3) Elevated CO_2 levels caused by increased production of CO_2 can be attributed to all of the following, *except*:
   a. Malignant hyperthermia
   b. Cancer
   c. Coma
   d. Fever
   e. Burn

(4) Low-pressure alarms are caused by which factor?
   a. Breathing circuit disconnect
   b. Dyssynchronous ventilation
   c. Disconnection from wall oxygen
   d. Reduced lung compliance
   e. Endotracheal tube obstruction

(5) Information obtained from a PA catheter includes all of the following, *except*:
   a. Cardiac output
   b. Central venous pressure
   c. Pulmonary artery pressure
   d. Left ventricular volume
   e. Pulmonary artery wedge pressure

(6) A falsely low mixed venous oxygen measurement will occur in which condition?
   a. Sample taken in "wedged" position
   b. Mitral regurgitation
   c. Left-to-right intracardiac shunt
   d. AV fistula
   e. Sample taken in the cardiac sinus

(7) Blood gas analysis provides information about all of the following, *except*:
   a. Oxygenation
   b. Cardiac function
   c. Ventilation
   d. Cellular metabolism
   e. Electrolytes

(8) Interference with processed EEG signals (BIS) may occur by all of the following, *except*:
   a. Electromyography (EMG) activity
   b. Traumatic brain injury
   c. Dry gel
   d. High impedance
   e. Forehead surgery

(9) Neurologic monitoring does *not* include:
   a. Doppler
   b. Processed EEG
   c. ICP measurements
   d. End-tidal gas analysis
   e. Peripheral nerve stimulator

(10) Most anesthesia machine malfunctions are due to:
   a. User error
   b. Gas pressure failure
   c. False negatives
   d. Obstruction of oxygen flow meter
   e. Failure of proportioning system

Answers

(1) d
(2) b
(3) c
(4) a
(5) d
(6) e
(7) b
(8) b
(9) d
(10) a

References

1. American Society of Anesthesiologists. Standards for Basic Anesthetic Monitoring, Approved by the ASA House of Delegates on October 21, 1986, and last amended on October20, 2010. www.asahq.org.

2. Australian and New Zealand College of Anaesthetists. Recommendations on monitoring during anesthesia. ANZCA Professional Document PS18, 2008. www.anzca.edu.au.

3. Royal College of Anaesthetists. Guidelines for the provision of anaesthetic services, 2009. www.rcoa.ac.uk.

4. Cheney FW. Changing trends in anesthesia-related death and permanent brain damage. *ASA Newsletter* 2002; **66**: 6–8.

5. Webb RK, van der Walt JH, Runciman WB, *et al*. The Australian Incident Monitoring Study. Which monitor? An analysis of 2000 incident reports. *Anesth Intensive Care* 1993; **21**: 529–42.

6. Tremper K, Barker S. Monitoring of oxygen. In Lake CL, Hines RL, Blitt CD, eds., *Clinical Monitoring: Practical Applications for Anesthesia and Critical Care*. Philadelphia, PA: Saunders, 2001, p. 324.

7. Moller JT, Pedersen T, Rasmussen LS, *et al*. Randomized evaluation of pulse oximetry in 20,802 patients: I. Design, demography, pulse oximetry failure rate, and overall complication rate. *Anesthesiology* 1993; **78**: 436–44.

8. Moller JT, Johannessen NW, Espersen K, *et al*. Randomized evaluation of pulse oximetry in 20,802 patients: II. Perioperative events and postoperative complications. *Anesthesiology* 1993; **78**: 445–53.

9. Cote CJ, Rolf N, Liu LM, *et al*. A single-blind study of combined pulse oximetry and capnography in children. *Anesthesiology* 1991; **74**: 980–7.

10. Barker SJ. Recent developments in oxygen monitoring. *ASA Annual Meeting Refresher Course Lectures* 2006; **320**: 1–6.

11. Shelley K, Shelley S. Pulse oximeter waveform: photoelectric plethysmography. In Lake CL, Hines RL, Blitt CD, eds., *Clinical Monitoring: Practical Applications for Anesthesia and Critical Care*. Philadelphia, PA: Saunders, 2001, p. 427.

12. Al-Shaikh B, Stacey S. *Essentials of Anaesthetic Equipment*, 2nd edition. London: Churchill Livingstone, 2002, p. 117.

13. Venkatesh B, Clutton Brock TH, Hendry SP. A multiparameter sensor for continuous intra-arterial blood gas monitoring: a prospective evaluation. *Crit Care Med* 1994; **22**: 588–94.

14. Coule LW, Truemper EJ, Steinhart CM, Lutin WA. Accuracy and utility of a continuous intra-arterial blood gas monitoring system in pediatric patients. *Crit Care Med* 2001; **29**: 420–6.

15. Myles PS, Buckland MR, Weeks AM, Bujor M, Moloney J. Continuous arterial blood gas monitoring during bilateral sequential lung transplantation. *J Cardiothorac Vasc Anesth* 1999; **13**: 253–7.

16. Eichhorn JH, Cooper JB, Cullen DJ, *et al*. Standards for patient monitoring during anesthesia at Harvard Medical School. *JAMA* 1986: **256**: 1017–20.

17. Barker L, Webb RK, Runciman WB, Van der Walt JH. The Australian Incident Monitoring Study. The oxygen analyzer: applications and limitations – an analysis of 200 incident reports. *Anaesth Intensive Care* 1993; **21**: 570–4.

18. Tremper K, Barker S. Monitoring of oxygen. In Lake CL, Hines RL, Blitt CD, eds., *Clinical Monitoring: Practical Applications for Anesthesia and Critical Care*. Philadelphia, PA: Saunders, 2001, pp. 315–16.

19. Keeling CD, Whorf TP. *Atmospheric CO2 records from sites in the SIO air sampling network. Trends: a Compendium of Data on Global Change*. Oak Ridge, TN: Carbon Dioxide Information Analysis Center, Oak Ridge National Laboratory, U.S. Department of Energy, 2005.

20. Gravenstein J, Paulus D, Hayes T. *Capnometric Methods: Gas Monitoring in Clinical Practice*, 2nd edition. Boston, MA: Butterworth-Heinemann, 1995, p. 17.

21. Barash P, Cullen B, Stoelting, R. *Clinical Anesthesia*, 5th edition. Philadelphia, PA: Lippincott, Williams & Wilkins, 2006, p. 670.

22. Davis P, Kenny G. *Basic Physics and Measurement in Anaesthesia*, 5th edition. New York, NY: Butterworth Heinemann, 2003, p. 214.

23. Campbell FA, McLeod ME, Bissonnette B, Swartz JS. End tidal carbon dioxide measurement in infants and children during and after general anesthesia. *Can J Anaesth* 1994; **41**: 107–10.

24. Eichhorn JH. Prevention of intraoperative anesthesia accidents and related severe injury through safety monitoring. *Anesthesiology* 1989; **70**: 572–7.

25. Croswell RJ, Dilley DC, Lucas WJ, Vann WF. A comparison of conventional versus electronic monitoring of sedated pediatric dental patients. *Pediatr Dent* 1995; **17**: 332–9.

26. Coté CJ, Liu LM, Szyfelbein SK, *et al*. Intraoperative events diagnosed by expired carbon dioxide monitoring in children. *Can Anaesth Soc J*. 1986; **33**: 315–20.

27. Baraka AS, Aouad MT, Jalbout MI, *et al*. End-tidal CO_2 for prediction of cardiac output following weaning from cardiopulmonary bypass. *J Extra Corpor Technol* 2004; **36**: 255–7.

28. Ornato JP, Garnett AR, Glauser FL. Relationship between cardiac output and the end-tidal carbon dioxide tension. *Ann Emerg Med* 1990; **19**: 1104–6.

29. Manecke GR Jr, Popper PJ. Esophageal stethoscope placement depth: Its effect on heart and lung sound monitoring during general anesthesia. *Anesth Analg* 1998; **86**: 1276–9.

30. Klepper ID, Webb RK, Van der Walt JH, Ludbrook GL, Cockings J. The Australian Incident Monitoring Study. The stethoscope: applications and limitations – an analysis of 2000 incident reports. *Anaesth Intensive Care* 1993; **21**: 575–8.

31. Watson A, Visram A. Survey of the use of oesophageal and precordial stethoscopes in current paediatric anaesthetic practice. *Paediatr Anaesth* 2001; **11**: 437–42.

32. Prielipp RC, Kelly JS, Roy RC. Use of esophageal or precordial stethoscopes by anesthesia providers: are we listening to our patients? *J Clin Anesth* 1995; **7**: 367–72.

33. Barash PG, Cullen BF, Stoelting RK. *Clinical Anesthesia*, 3rd edition. Philadelphia, PA: Lippincott-Raven Publishers, 1997, pp. 194–200.

34. Kaye P, O'Sullivan, I. Myocardial contusion: emergency investigation and diagnosis. *Emerg Med J* 2002; **19**: 8–10.

35. Potkin RT, Werner JA, Trobaugh GB, *et al.* Evaluation of noninvasive tests of cardiac damage in suspected cardiac contusion. *Circulation* 1983; **66**: 627–33.

36. Wittebole X, Hantson P. Electrocardiographic changes after head trauma. *J Electrocardiol* 2005; **38**: 77–81.

37. Shah N, Bedford RF. Invasive and noninvasive blood pressure monitoring. In Lake C, Hines R, Blitt C, eds., *Clinical Monitoring: Practical Applications for Anesthesia and Critical Care*. Philadelphia, PA: Saunders, 2001, pp. 181–203.

38. Janelle GM, Gravenstein N. An accuracy evaluation of the T-Line Tensymeter versus conventional invasive radial artery monitoring in surgical patients. *Anesth Analg* 2006; **102**: 484–90.

39. Duan Y, Smith CE, Como JJ. Cardiothoracic trauma. In Wilson WC, Grande CM, Hoyt DB, eds., *Trauma: Emergency Resuscitation, Perioperative Anesthesia, Surgical Management*. New York, NY: Informa Healthcare, 2007, pp. 469–99.

40. Marik PE, Baram M, Vahid B. Does central venous pressure predict fluid responsiveness? A systematic review of the literature and the tale of seven mares. *Chest* 2008; **134**: 172–8.

41. De Backer D, Heenen S, Piagnerelli M, Koch M, Vincent JL. Pulse pressure variations to predict fluid responsiveness: influence of tidal volume. *Intensive Care Med* 2005; **31**: 517–23.

42. Morgan BC, Martin WE, Hornbein TF, Crawford EW, Guntheroth WG. Hemodynamic effects of positive pressure ventilation. *Anesthesiology* 1966; **27**: 584–90.

43. Jardin F, Delorme G, Hardy A, *et al.* Reevaluation of hemodynamic consequences of positive pressure ventilation: emphasis on cyclic right ventricular afterloading by mechanical lung inflation. *Anesthesiology* 1990; **72**: 966–70.

44. Jardin F, Farcot JC, Gueret P, *et al.* Cyclical changes in arterial pulse pressure during respiratory support. *Circulation* 1983; **68**: 266–74.

45. Tavernier B, Makhotine O, Lebuffe G, Dupont J, Scherpereel P. Systolic pressure variation as a guide to fluid therapy in patients with sepsis-induced hypotension. *Anesthesiology* 1998; **89**: 1313–21.

46. Coriat P, Vrillon M, Perel A, *et al.* A comparison of systolic pressure variations and echocardiographic measurements of end-diastolic left ventricular size in patients after aortic surgery. *Anesth Analg* 1994: **78**; 46–53.

47. Marik PE, Cavallazzi R, Vasu T, Hirani A. Dynamic changes in arterial waveform derived variables and fluid responsiveness in mechanically ventilated patients: a systematic review of the literature. *Crit Care Med* 2009; **37**: 2642–7.

48. Perel A, Pizov R, Cotev S. The systolic pressure variation is a sensitive indicator of hypovolemia in ventilated dogs subjected to graded hemorrhage. *Anesthesiology* 1987; **67**: 498–502.

49. Rooke GA, Schwid HA, Shapira Y. The effects of graded hemorrhage and intravascular volume replacement on systolic pressure variation in humans during spontaneous mechanical variation. *Anesth Analg* 1995; **80**: 925–32.

50. Preisman S, DiSegni E, Vered Z, Perel A. Left ventricular preload and function during graded hemorrhage and retransfusion in pigs: analysis of arterial pressure waveform and correlation with echocardiography. *Br J Anaesth* 2002; **88**: 716–18.

51. Berkenstadt H, Friedman Z, Preisman S, *et al.* Pulse pressure and stroke volume variations during severe haemorrhage in ventilated dogs. *Br J Anesth* 2005; **94**: 721–6.

52. Kramer A, Zygun D, Hawes H, Easton P, Ferland A. Pulse pressure variation predicts fluid responsivness following coronary artery bypass surgery. *Chest* 2004; **126**: 1563–8.

53. Thiele RH, Colquhoun DA, Blum FE, Durieux ME. The ability of anesthesia providers to visually estimate systolic pressure variability using the "eyeball" technique. *Anesth Analg* 2012; **115**: 176–81.

54. Wyler von Ballmoos M, Takala J, Roeck M, *et al.* Pulse-pressure variation and hemodynamic response in patients with elevated pulmonary artery pressure: a clinical study. *Crit Care* 2010; **14**: R111.

55. Preisman S, Kogan S, Berkenstadt H, Perel A. Predicting fluid responsiveness in patients undergoing cardiac surgery: functional haemodynamic parameters including the Respiratory Systolic Variation Test and static preload indicators. *Br J Anaesth* 2005; **95**: 746–55.

56. Ornstein E, Eidelman L, Drenger B, Elami A, Pizov R. Systolic pressure variation predicts the response to acute blood loss. *J Clin Anesth* 1998; **10**: 137–40.

57. Reuter DA, Goepfert MSG, Goresch T, *et al.* Assessing fluid responsiveness during open chest conditions. *Br J Anaesth* 2005; **94**: 318–23.

58. Mark JB. Monitoring with CVP and PAC. *ASA Annual Meeting Refresher Course Lectures* 2006; **322**; 1–6.

59. Varon AJ. Arterial, central venous, and pulmonary artery catheters. In Civetta JM, Taylor RW, Kirby RR, ed., *Critical Care*, 3rd edition. Philadelphia: Lippincott-Raven, 1997. pp. 847–65.

60. Moomey CB, Fabia TC, Croce MA, *et al.* Determinants of myocardial performance after blunt chest trauma. *J Trauma* 1998; **45**: 988–96.

61. Rhodes A, Bennett ED. Early goal directed therapy: an evidence-based review. *Crit Care Med* 2004; **32**: S448–50.

62. Kumar A, Anel R, Bunnell E, *et al.* Pulmonary artery occlusion pressure and central venous pressure fail to predict ventricular filling volume, cardiac performance, or the response to volume infusion in normal subjects. *Crit Care Med* 2004; **32**: 691–9.

63. Pope JV, Jones AE, Gaieski DF, *et al.* Multi-center study of central venous oxygen saturation ($ScvO_2$) as a predictor of mortality in patients with sepsis. *Ann Emerg Med* 2010; **55**: 40–6.

64. Sandham JD, Hull RD, Brant RF. A randomized controlled trial of the use of pulmonary artery catheters in high risk surgical patients. *N Engl J Med* 2003; **348**: 5–14.

65. Shah MR, Hasselblad V, Stevenson LW. Impact of pulmonary artery catheters in critically ill patients: meta-analysis of randomized controlled trials. *JAMA* 2005; **294**: 1664–70.

66. Bishop MH, Shoemaker WC, Appel PL, *et al.* Prospective randomized trial of survivor values of cardiac index, oxygen delivery, and oxygen consumption as resuscitation endpoints

in severe trauma. *J Trauma* 1995; **38**: 780–7.

67. Friese RS, Shafi S, Gentilello LM. Pulmonary artery catheter use is associated with reduced mortality in severely injured patients. *Crit Care Med* 2006; **34**: 1597–601.

68. Holm JH, Frederiksen CA, Juhl-Olsen P, Sloth E: Perioperative use of focus assessed transthoracic echocardiography (FATE). *Anesth Analg* 2012: **115**: 1029–32.

69. Tisherman SA, Eastern Association for the Surgery of Trauma. Clinical practice guideline: endpoints of resuscitation. www.east.org.

70. Sessler D. Mild perioperative hypothermia. *N Engl J Med* 1997; **336**: 1730–7.

71. Nelson EJ, Grissom TE. Continuous gastric suctioning decreased measured esophageal temperature during general anesthesia. *J Clin Monit* 1996; **12**: 429–32.

72. Cork RC, Vaughan RW, Humphrey LS. Precision and accuracy of intraoperative temperature monitoring. *Anesth Analg* 1983; **62**: 211–14.

73. Brain Trauma Foundation, American Association of Neurological Surgeons, Congress of Neurological Surgeons. Guidelines for the management of severe traumatic brain injury. VIII. Intracranial pressure thresholds. *J Neurotrauma* 2007; **24** (Suppl 1): S55–8.

74. Saul TG, Ducker TB. Effects of intracranial pressure monitoring and aggressive treatment on mortality in severe head injury. *J Neurosurg* 1982; **56**: 498–503.

75. Brain Trauma Foundation, American Association of Neurological Surgeons, Congress of Neurological Surgeons. Guidelines for the management of severe traumatic brain injury. IX. Cerebral perfusion thresholds. *J Neurotrauma* 2007; **24** (Suppl 1): S59–64.

76. Intracranial Pressure Monitoring Technology. *J Neurotrauma* 2007 ; **24** (Suppl 1): S45–54.

77. Mahla M. Neurologic monitoring. In Cucchiara RF, ed., *Clinical Neuroanesthesia*. New York, NY: Churchill Livingstone, 1998, pp. 125–76.

78. Ronne-Engstrom E, Winkler T. Continuous EEG monitoring in patients with traumatic brain injury reveals a high incidence of epileptiform activity. *Acta Neurol Scand* 2006; **114**: 47–53.

79. Deogaonkar A, Gupta R, DeGeorgia M, *et al.* Bispectral Index monitoring correlates with sedation scales in brain-injured patients. *Crit Care Med* 2004; **32**: 2545–6.

80. Paul DB, Umamaheswara Rao GS. Correlation of bispectral index with Glasgow coma score in mild and moderate head injuries. *J Clin Monit Comput* 2006; **20**: 399–404.

81. Bevacqua B, Kazdan D. Is more information better? Intraoperative recall with a Bispectral Index Monitor in place. *Anesthesiology* 2003; **99**: 507–8.

82. Mychaskiw G, Horowitz M, Sachdev V, Heath BJ. Explicit intraoperative recall at a bispectral index of 47. *Anesth Analg* 2001; **92**: 808–9.

83. Mahla M, Black S, Cucchiara RF. Neurologic monitoring. In Miller RD, ed., *Miller's Anesthesia*. Philadelphia, PA: Elsevier, 2005, pp. 1511–50.

84. Coplin WM, O'Keefe GE, Grady MS, *et al.* Thrombotic, infectious, and procedural complications of the jugular bulb catheter in the intensive care unit. *Neurosurgery* 1997; **41**: 101–9.

85. Andrews PJD, Dearden NM, Miller JD. Jugular bulb cannulation: description of a cannulation technique and validation of a new continuous monitor. *Br J Anaesth* 1991; **67**: 553–8.

86. Edmonds HL. Pro: all cardiac surgical patients should have intraoperative cerebral oxygenation monitoring. *J Cardiothorac Vasc Anesth* 2006; **20**: 445–9.

87. Latronico N, Beindorf AE, Rasulo FA, *et al.* Limits of intermittent jugular bulb oxygen saturation monitoring in the management of severe head trauma patients. *Neurosurgery* 2001; **48**: 454–6.

88. Murkin JM, Adams SJ, Novick RJ, *et al.* Monitoring brain oxygen saturation during coronary bypass surgery: a randomized, prospective study. *Anesth Analg* 2007; **104**: 51–8.

89. Dunham CM, Sosnowski C, Porter JM, Siegal J, Kohli C. Correlation of noninvasive cerebral oximetry with cerebral perfusion in the severe head injured patient: a pilot study. *J Trauma* 2002; **52**: 40–6.

90. Dunham CM, Ransom KJ, Flowers LL, *et al.* Cerebral hypoxia in severely brain injured patients is associated with admission Glasgow Coma score, CT severity, cerebral perfusion pressure, and survival. *J Trauma* 2004; **56**: 482–91.

91. Chosh A, Elwell C, Smith M. Cerebral near-infrared spectroscopy in adults: a work in progress. *Anesth Analg* 2012: **115**: 1373–83.

92. Caplan RA, Vistica MF, Posner KL, Cheney FW. Adverse anesthetic outcomes arising from gas delivery equipment: a closed claims analysis. *Anesthesiology* 1997; **87**: 741–8.

Chapter

10

Use of echocardiography and ultrasound in trauma

Colin Royse and Alistair Royse

Objectives

(1) Identify the wide range of uses of ultrasound in trauma.
(2) Understand the concept of hemodynamic state assessment.
(3) Understand how echocardiography interpretation can guide clinical management.
(4) Understand the basics of focused abdominal sonography in trauma (FAST) and other surface ultrasound diagnostic studies.
(5) Understand how to get started using ultrasound.

Introduction

The use of ultrasound in trauma anesthesia is increasing rapidly, including transesophageal echocardiography (TEE), transthoracic echocardiography (TTE), and a multitude of surface ultrasound applications including the focused abdominal sonography in trauma (FAST) scan, and assessment for pneumothorax, pleural effusion, and deep venous thrombosis. It is being used as a guide for a number of procedures including vascular access, nerve blocks, pleural drainage, and percutaneous tracheostomy. This chapter will focus on hemodynamic assessment with echocardiography, as well as surface ultrasound diagnostic skills, while ultrasound-guided procedures are considered further in Chapter 12.

How many ways can ultrasound be used during trauma anesthesia?

The key to successful use of ultrasound during trauma anesthesia is to understand that it provides rapid diagnostic information to assist patient management. The FAST scan is well established in the emergency department for the assessment of abdominal trauma. Although this is a useful test, it is just one of many uses of ultrasound that are available in trauma. Hemodynamic state evaluation is a process of categorizing the underlying hemodynamic conditions by using echocardiography as an adjunct to our conventional clinical monitors. This is the single most useful application of ultrasound in trauma. Better diagnostic information will translate into

improved management. Although transesophageal echocardiography has been commonly used by anesthesiologists, the use of transthoracic echocardiography should be encouraged because it is rapid to perform and noninvasive. Once practitioners understand how to use ultrasound equipment, then it is a small step to check for pneumothorax or pleural effusion, to perform ultrasound-guided vascular access, and to use ultrasound to help place nerve blocks for anesthesia or pain relief, to assess blood flow in compromised limbs, or even to check for deep venous thrombosis.

In recent years, the concept of goal-focused echocardiography has become very popular in anesthesia, perioperative medicine, intensive care, and emergency medicine.[1] The concept is to perform a limited ultrasound examination to answer clinically relevant questions when treating the patient. In more general terms, it can be considered *ultrasound-assisted examination*, and it can apply to any form of surface ultrasound. For example, goal-focused echocardiography is ultrasound-assisted examination of the cardiovascular system, and lung ultrasound is ultrasound-assisted examination of the respiratory system. Defining limited studies and naming them with easy-to-remember acronyms such as iHEARTscan,[2] FATE (focus assessed transthoracic echocardiography), BLEEP (bedside limited echocardiography), and FOCUS (focused cardiac ultrasound) has popularized this. The studies vary in the amount of imaging performed, from simple two-dimensional imaging and assessment of ventricular function, to the incorporation of color flow Doppler imaging to assess valve function. However, they are all variants of a system designed to incorporate ultrasound examination into clinical decision making in real time. This is a different paradigm to conventional cardiology or radiology-based ultrasound services, where a technologist conducts a comprehensive study, an imaging specialist reports the study, and at some distant time the clinician treating the patient receives the information. The ability of the treating clinician to use ultrasound in real time dramatically improves the diagnosis, allowing more rational therapy to be instituted.

Clinical examination is well known to be quite unreliable in diagnosing cardiac pathology. Even with experienced clinicians, the addition of goal-focused echocardiography will

Trauma Anesthesia, 2nd Edition, ed. Charles E. Smith. Published by Cambridge University Press. © Charles E. Smith, 2015.

change the clinical diagnosis in 30–50% of patients.[3–6] In the trauma setting, hemodynamic state is often the first diagnosis made with echocardiography, upon which changes in management are based. However, there will be many occasions when significant ventricular or valvular pathology is identified, and this will further alter management. For example, an elderly patient presenting after a motor vehicle accident may have significant aortic stenosis contributing to the hypotension. Identification of the aortic stenosis allows the clinician to proactively manage the patient so as to minimize the effect of the stenotic valve.

Understanding ultrasound equipment

Ultrasound machines of the current generation are typically suitable for multiple examination types, including abdominal, vascular, cardiac, and musculoskeletal studies. Furthermore, advances in computer technology have allowed miniaturization of ultrasound machines, with portable and robust machines no bigger than a laptop computer. There are now handheld systems that fit in one's palm which are capable of two-dimensional and color flow Doppler transthoracic imaging. The same probe can be used for some abdominal imaging as well. These systems are the forerunners of what is likely to be the personal ultrasound machine, and a likely replacement for the stethoscope. What is more important, however, is the type of probe available for the particular application. The typical trauma anesthesia "setup" would include:

- console
- 2.5–3.5 MHz phased-array transducer for TTE
- 5–7 MHz TEE probe
- 10–15 MHz linear-array transducer for vascular access, musculoskeletal examination, and nerve block insertion
- 3–6 MHz curved linear abdominal probe for FAST and abdominal aortic examination.

The reason for the range of probes is the trade-off between depth of ultrasound penetration and image quality. The higher the frequency, the better the image, but the lower the depth of penetration. For example, a 15 MHz probe provides excellent resolution for assessment of nerves and vessels, but it is of no use beyond about 3–4 cm. For TTE, or abdominal ultrasound, depths of 10–20 cm are commonly required. Conversely, the resolution provided by a lower-frequency transducer would not be adequate for musculoskeletal examination or for identifying vessels and nerves.

Hemodynamic state assessment

When managing patients, we broadly determine whether their cardiovascular parameters represent normal or abnormal values. Typically, we will identify a problem when there is a change in blood pressure or heart rate, or some evidence of poor tissue perfusion (such as cold, blue periphery, reduced urine output, or metabolic acidosis). When using pressure-based monitoring, it is difficult to determine whether the cause of the hemodynamic abnormality is due to volume or ventricular function. Even with advanced monitoring systems such as the thermodilution pulmonary artery catheter, there is still a large element of guesswork in determining the underlying hemodynamic abnormality. The problem with pressure-based assessment of myocardial function is that it does not provide an accurate assessment of ventricular volume. A high pulmonary capillary wedge pressure in the setting of low cardiac output and hypotension could be caused by left ventricular systolic failure, right ventricular failure, or left ventricular diastolic failure. Echocardiography gives us a unique insight because we can directly assess volume and function, estimate ventricular filling pressure, and therefore estimate ventricular compliance.

The hemodynamic state can be categorized into a number of broad entities.[7] The following example describes the problem. An elderly patient undergoing hip surgery starts with a blood pressure of 140/90 mmHg, but this falls to 85/50 mmHg after 10 minutes of anesthesia. His heart rate is unaltered. Although the blood pressure is temporarily increased by the administration of a vasopressor, it soon falls to 80/50 mmHg again. After some time the anesthesiologist is able to insert a central venous catheter, and the right atrial pressure is 17 mmHg. Clearly, there is an abnormal hemodynamic state. The blood pressure information tells us only that there is abnormality, but we are unable to determine which of the hemodynamic states is the cause. The addition of right atrial pressure estimation probably rules out hypovolemia as the cause, but cannot identify further whether there is systolic or diastolic failure, vasodilatation, or right ventricular failure. The anesthesiologist then inserts a pulmonary artery catheter and determines that the cardiac index is 1.8 L/min/m^2, and the pulmonary capillary wedge pressure is 18 mmHg. At this stage, vasodilatation is unlikely, but we still cannot further differentiate between primary diastolic failure or systolic failure, or indeed right ventricular failure. The anesthesiologist remains uncertain as to the cause of problem, and what the best course of therapy is. Fortunately, his colleague has just arrived in the operating room with the TEE probe.

There are seven basic hemodynamic states, and four basic steps to work it out:

(1) normal
(2) empty (hypovolemic)
(3) primary diastolic failure
(4) primary systolic failure
(5) systolic and diastolic failure
(6) vasodilatation
(7) right ventricular failure

The four steps to determining the basic hemodynamic assessment are:

(1) estimate volume
(2) estimate systolic function
(3) estimate filling pressure
(4) final assessment (putting it all together)

Step 1. Estimate left ventricular end-diastolic volume (preload)

Echocardiography gives us the direct assessment of ventricular volume. This can be performed using TEE or TTE. Classically, the transgastric mid-short-axis view is used for repeated assessment of volume for TEE, and the parasternal long-axis view is used for TTE examinations. Much of the assessment, however, is frequently visual, and estimates of ventricular size can be performed from any view where there is adequate imaging. One tip is to set the depth of the image to the same value at the commencement of all studies, so that relative ventricular size is easily appreciated. In this step, one only needs to categorize the ventricle as hypovolemic (empty), normal, or dilated. Table 10.1 gives approximate estimates of ventricular size, though one should be aware that the range of normal values will vary between populations and will be dependent on body surface area (see also Fig. 10.1).

Step 2. Estimate systolic function

Estimates of ejection fraction can be used to determine systolic function. For TEE, this is based on the fractional area change (FAC) derived from the transgastric mid short-axis view; for TTE, fractional shortening (FS) is used. Volumetric methods can also be used to estimate ejection fraction (EF). Because the end-diastolic volume has already been estimated, the next step is to measure the smallest area or dimension, which occurs at the end of the T wave (end-systole). Fractional area change is calculated using the formula:

$$FAC = (EDA - ESA)/EDA$$

where EDA = end-diastolic area, ESA = end-systolic area; while fractional shortening is calculated as:

$$FS = (LVEDD - LVESD)/LVEDD$$

where LVEDD = left ventricular end-diastolic diameter, LVESD = left ventricular end-systolic diameter.

Figure 10.2 illustrates three grades of systolic function based on the FAC and FS. Ejection fraction estimates have the same numerical values as FAC. Systolic function may be categorized as increased, normal, or reduced, using Table 10.2 as a guideline.

Table 10.1 Assessment of ventricular dimensions: end-diastolic volume

Measurement	Hypovolemia	Normal	Dilated
M-mode PLAX (TTE)	< 2.3 cm	2.3–5.4 cm	> 5.4 cm
TG mid SAX (TEE)	< 8 cm^2	8–14 cm^2	> 14 cm^2

M-mode is a one-dimensional estimate of left ventricular volume. It is measured at the tips of the mitral leaflets during diastole. PLAX is the parasternal long-axis view, and an example is shown in Figure 10.1.
TG mid SAX is the transesophageal view used to estimate volume. It is at the midpapillary level and is identified by a continuum of the papillary muscle with the pericardium.
PLAX, parasternal long-axis; SAX, short-axis; TG, transgastric; TTE, transesophageal echocardiography; TTE, transthoracic echocardiography.

Transesophageal Echocardiogram Transgastric mid short axis view

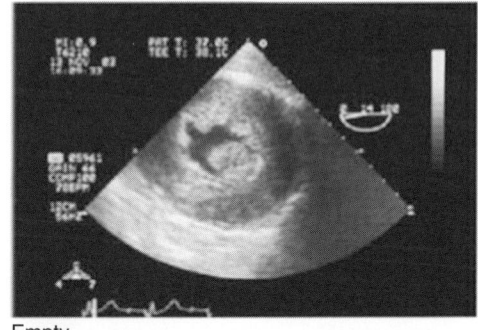 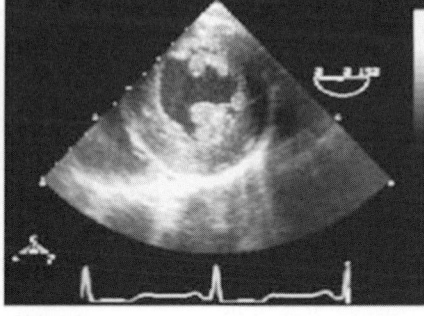 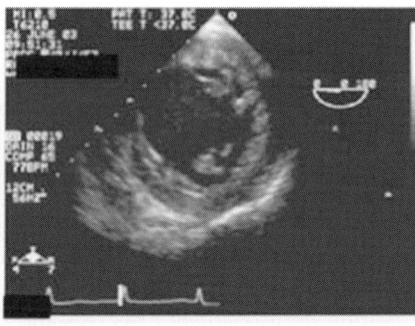

Empty   Normal   Dilated

Transthoracic Echocardiogram Parasternal long axis view

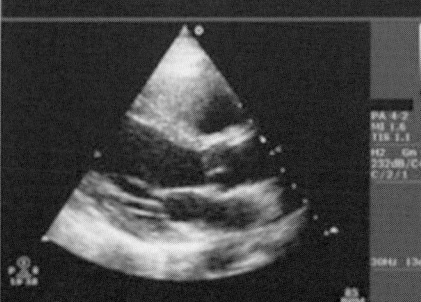 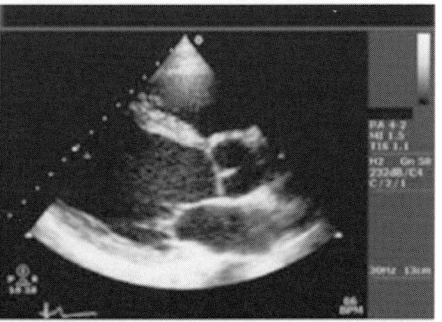

Empty   Normal   Dilated

Figure 10.1 Assessment of ventricular dimension.

Step 3. Estimate left atrial pressure

In this step, we aim to simply categorize left atrial pressure as "high" or "normal." It is of some additional use to determine when the left atrial pressure might be "low," as this can help to identify a hypovolemic state. Much work has been done on echocardiographic estimation of left atrial pressure, and while qualitative assessment is reasonable, quantitative assessment is poor. This does not really matter too much for basic hemodynamic state assessment, because we are primarily interested in identifying whether it is abnormal (high) or normal. The definition of "high" left atrial pressure state is somewhat arbitrary and is based on years of experience with invasive pressure monitoring such as a pulmonary artery catheter. It is probably reasonable, however, to define a "high" left atrial pressure as > 15 mmHg.

Table 10.2 Assessment of systolic function: fractional shortening (FS), fractional area change (FAC), ejection fraction (EF)

Measurement	Increased (%)	Normal (%)	Reduced (%)
M-mode PLAX (TTE) FS	> 44	28–44	< 28
TG mid SAX (TEE) FAC/EF	> 65	50–65	< 50

PLAX, parasternal long-axis; SAX, short-axis; TG, transgastric; TTE, transesophageal echocardiography; TTE, transthoracic echocardiography.

The following two methods are examples of estimating left atrial pressure state, arranged in the order of our personal preference. Other methods have been described, but they are beyond the scope of this chapter.

The shape and movement of the interatrial septum

The normal direction of the interatrial septum is moving from left to right for most of the cardiac cycle. During midsystole, however, there is transient reversal so that it bows from right to left. As the left atrial pressure rises, this directional change is reduced, and in the elevated left atrial pressure state the interatrial septum remains bowed from left to right throughout the cardiac cycle. These changes are accentuated by ventilation such that there is increased movement of the interatrial septum. The transition between normal and high pressure is quite easily seen when the septum does not move during inhalation, but is seen to move right to left with exhalation (if the patient is mechanically ventilated). When the interatrial septum remains fixed left to right with ventilation, this is a sign of raised left atrial pressure.[8,9] When the atrium is empty, the movement of the interatrial septum is increased such that there is marked movement in both directions through the cardiac cycle. The interatrial septum may appear concertinaed or buckled upon itself, and this shape reflects a low left atrial pressure state.

Transthoracic echocardiogram LV M-mode

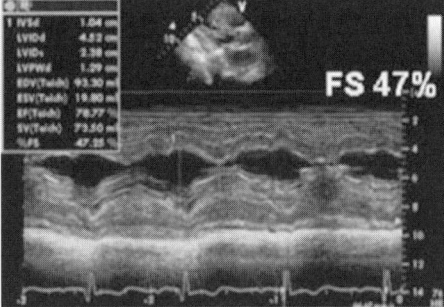
Increased

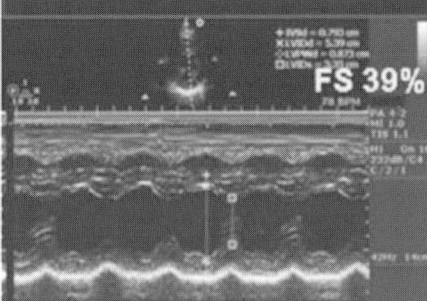
Normal

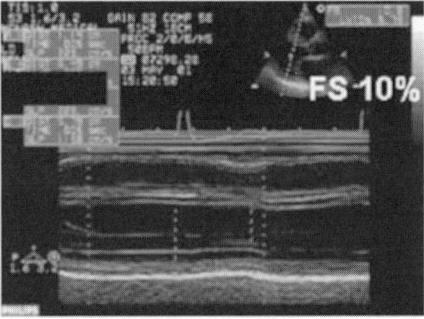
Reduced

Transesophageal echocardiogram

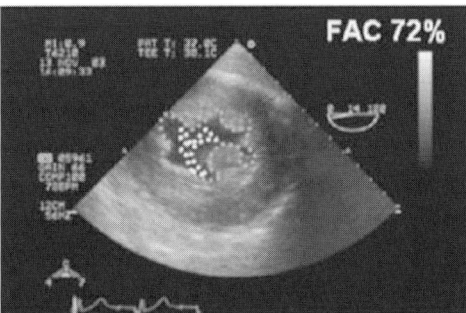
Increased   Normal   Reduced

Figure 10.2 Assessment of systolic function.

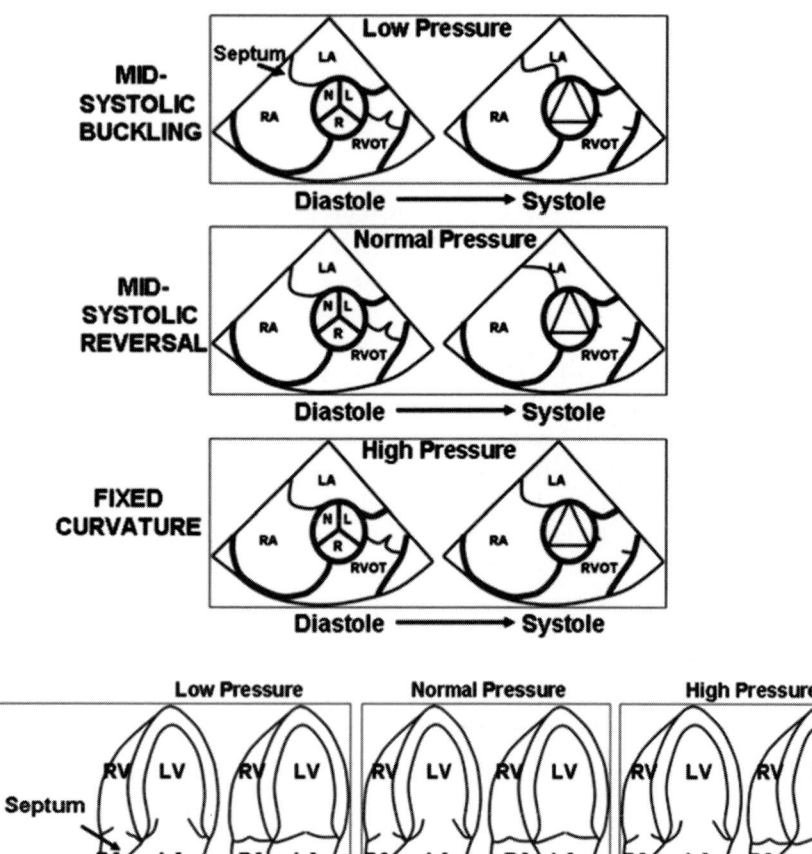

Figure 10.3 Estimation of left atrial pressure: interatrial septum trend for TEE (top) and TTE (bottom).

The best analogy to help conceptualize the movement is to think of the left atrium as a water-filled balloon. When the balloon is full of water and pressure is high, the balloon is circular in shape and if you were to cut a slice across the balloon, it would appear as a semicircle going outward. This is analogous to the "fixed curvature" seen in the high left atrial pressure state. If a little water is let out, a tap on the edge with your hand would move the wall inwards briefly before it springs out, which is analogous to the "systolic reversal" seen with normal left atrial pressure. Finally, if the balloon is relatively empty, the walls of the balloon will concertina or shrink down and appear to overlap, and a small tap of the hand will produce excessive motion: this is analogous to the "systolic buckling" pattern of the interatrial septum. This is illustrated in Figure 10.3.

The systolic versus diastolic components of the pulmonary vein flow

With normal left atrial pressure, the proportion of flow in systole exceeds that in diastole. As the left atrial pressure rises, this proportion changes such that the diastolic proportion predominates (Fig. 10.4).

Step 4. Putting it all together

The key difference between echocardiography and invasive pressure monitoring when used to diagnose hemodynamic state is that echocardiography allows direct assessment of volume, systolic function, and filling pressure. This combination of knowledge allows us to estimate preload, ventricular function, and, importantly, ventricular compliance. Only when we can estimate compliance and volume together can we differentiate diastolic heart failure from other hemodynamic states. Use Table 10.3 as a guide to interpretation. The hardest hemodynamic state to understand is primary diastolic failure. This is because the left ventricle appears empty, yet appears to have normal systolic function. This gives the appearance of hypovolemia, but the difference between primary diastolic failure and hypovolemia is that in hypovolemia the left atrial pressure is low, whereas in primary diastolic failure it is high. It is only by integrating pressure and volume that we can infer compliance.

Table 10.3 is a guide to interpretation, but the process is quite simple. For example, if preload is normal, function is normal, and filling pressure is normal, then we have defined the first hemodynamic state – that is, "normal."

Table 10.3 Ultrasound-guided hemodynamic state assessment

LV volume	N	↓	N/↓	↑	↑	N	RV↑
LV systolic function	N	N/↑	N	↓	↓	↑	RV↓
LV filling pressure	N	↓	↑	N	↑	N	↑
Basic state	Normal	Empty	Primary diastolic failure	Systolic failure	Systolic and diastolic failure	Vasodilatation	Right ventricular failure

LV, left ventricle; RV, right ventricle; N, normal; arrows show increased or decreased.

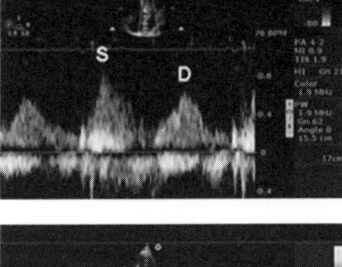
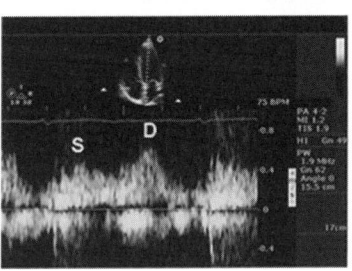
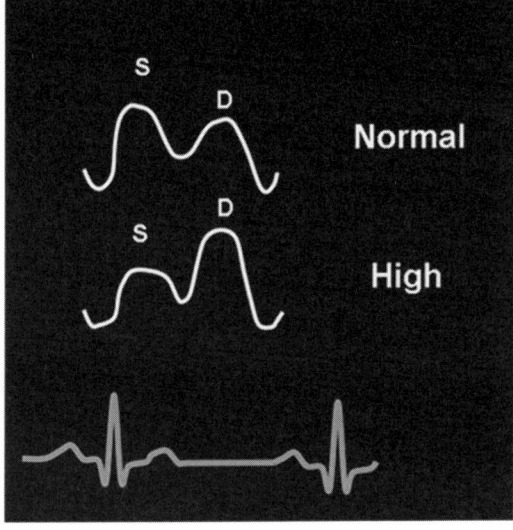

Figure 10.4 Estimation of left atrial pressure: pulmonary vein Doppler.

(1) **Normal hemodynamic state**. This is characterized by normal volume, normal systolic function, and normal left atrial pressure (LAP).

(2) **Empty (hypovolemic)**. This is characterized by reduced volume, normal or increased systolic function, and low LAP.

(3) **Primary diastolic failure**. The ventricle will appear hypovolemic (reduced volume), and will have normal systolic function but high LAP. This hemodynamic state is very difficult to appreciate because it looks normal. It is a *conceptual leap* to believe that the normal-looking ventricle constitutes heart failure. The key to identifying the state is to see a normal-looking ventricle operating at a high filling pressure.

(4) **Primary systolic failure**. This is characterized by increased volume (dilated ventricle), reduced systolic function, and normal LAP. Essentially, the compliance of this ventricle is normal or increased. It is important to differentiate dilated cardiomyopathy that is associated with normal filling pressure from that associated with increased filling pressure, because the hemodynamic performance may be quite different.

(5) **Systolic and diastolic failure**. In this hemodynamic state, the volume is increased, the systolic function is reduced, and the LAP is increased. These patients may represent the worst end of the heart failure spectrum, and may be associated with right ventricular failure as well. The diastolic failure is evident because of the raised filling pressure.

(6) **Right ventricular failure**. This is characterized by a dilated right ventricle, with reduced inward excursion, and elevated LAP state. Although isolated right ventricular failure can occur, it is frequently associated with left ventricle failure as well. The right ventricle will compress the left ventricle, causing left ventricular diastolic dysfunction (and the raised LAP state).

Using the basic hemodynamic state to influence management

The premise is that good diagnosis leads to good management. The treatment of each hemodynamic state can be very different, even though the signs and symptoms presenting to the practitioner may appear the same. Although the management of systolic failure appears straightforward, the management of diastolic failure is very different. For example, the use of an inodilator such as dobutamine or milrinone is reasonably standard therapy for patients with dilated cardiomyopathy. It appears logical that increasing systolic function and at the same time facilitating ejection will improve global myocardial

163

Table 10.4 Possible therapeutic interventions for hemodynamic state abnormalities

Hemodynamic state	Possible therapeutic interventions
Normal	No need for therapy
Empty	Infuse volume
Primary diastolic failure	Maintain preload Control heart rate Treat concomitant vasodilatation with a vasopressor Consider low-dose inotropes to support right ventricular function
Primary systolic failure	Inodilators/inotropes
Systolic and diastolic failure	Improve systolic performance at a reduced preload Inodilators Increase heart rate (e.g., pacing if available)
Vasodilatation	Vasoconstrictors
Right ventricular failure	Inodilators Treat excessive vasodilatation with vasoconstrictors in order to maintain normotension Consider pulmonary artery dilators, e.g., nitric oxide

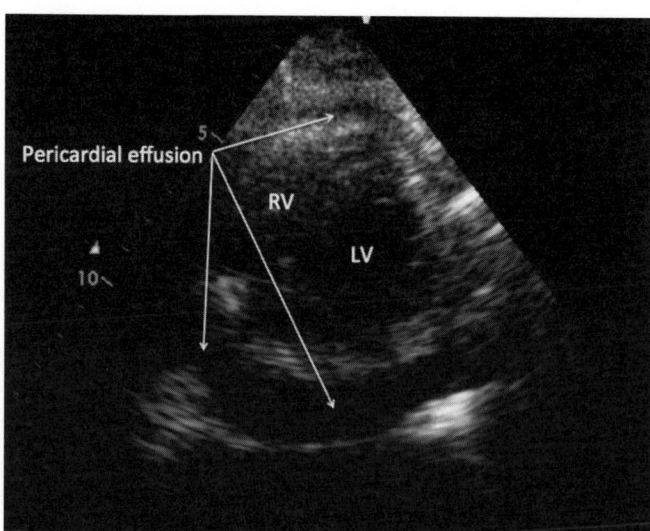

Figure 10.5 Example 1. Parasternal short-axis view showing a moderate-sized anterior pericardial effusion.

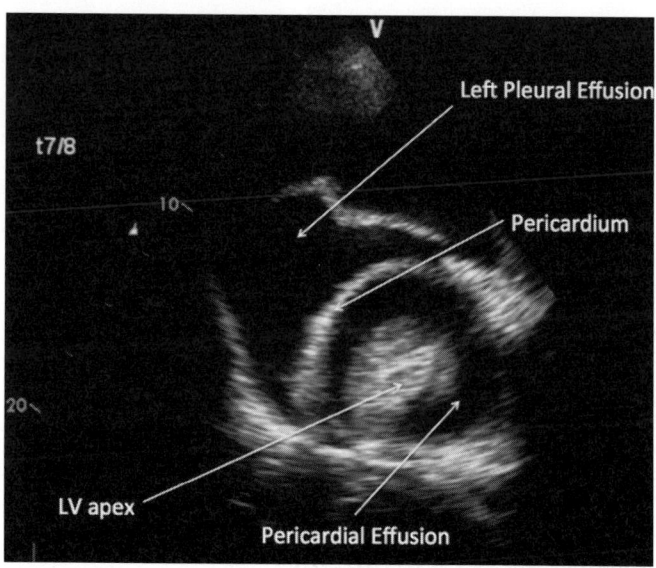

Figure 10.6 Example 1. Lateral view of the left chest showing a large left pleural effusion, and pericardial fluid surrounding the apex of the left ventricle.

performance. The primary limitation in diastolic heart failure, however, is that stroke volume is reduced because of reduced end-diastolic volume rather than because of poor systolic function. The use of an inodilator may reduce preload even further because of tachycardia (reduced filling time) and increased ejection fraction. The aim of this section is not to outline detailed therapeutic options, but rather to highlight that accurate diagnosis will lead to a logical choice of therapy. The exact choice of what type of volume to infuse, or which inotrope combination is best for each condition, is largely a matter of experience and familiarity. Table 10.4 suggests possible therapeutic approaches for each hemodynamic state.

Clinical examples

The following examples illustrate the value of echocardiography in the trauma setting.

Example 1

A 39-year-old previously healthy male presents to the emergency department after being stabbed by a kitchen knife in the left chest. He is hypotensive and has a week and thready pulse. You are concerned about trauma to the lung and heart, and conduct a focused transthoracic examination (Figs. 10.5, 10.6).

Comment: There is always a risk of trauma to the lung or heart from a left-sided stabbing. Severe hypotension could be associated with blood loss, or pericardial tamponade if the

ventricle is punctured. In this example, there is a small to moderate-sized pericardial effusion, and though the still images do not display this well, there was no chamber collapse consistent with tamponade. The presence of fluid in the pericardial space confirms that ventricular puncture has occurred, but the degree of effusion is unlikely to be the major contributor to hypotension. The large left pleural effusion is certainly a contributor to hypotension from blood loss as well as from external compression of the heart, which along with the pericardial effusion would restrict ventricular filling. The patient was resuscitated and underwent thoracotomy to repair the lacerated lung and to oversew a small right ventricular puncture.

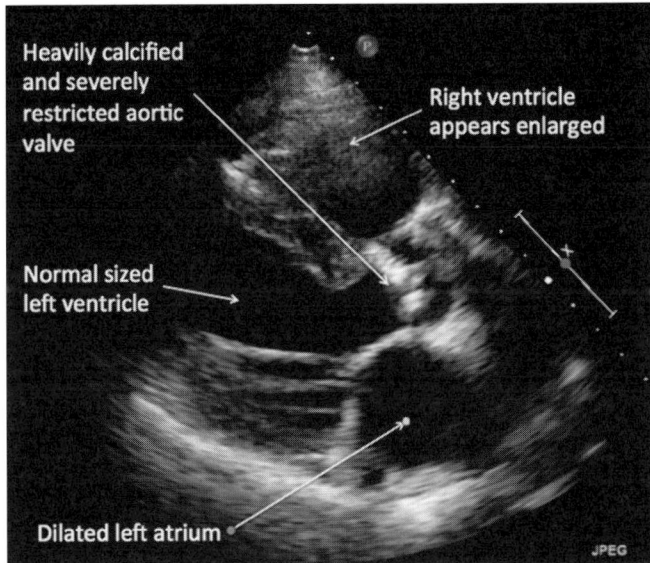

Figure 10.7 Example 2. A parasternal long-axis image showing severe aortic stenosis, as well as an enlarged right ventricle and left atrium. The left ventricular end-diastolic dimension is normal.

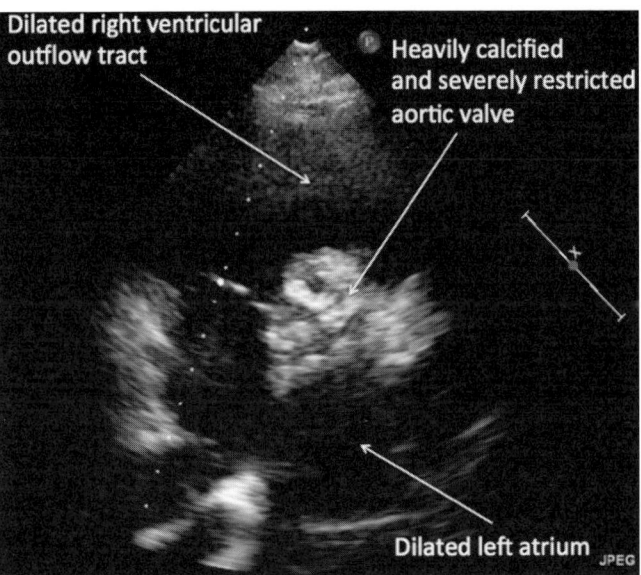

Figure 10.8 Example 2. A parasternal short-axis image showing the heavily calcified and severely restricted aortic valve. There is also right ventricular dilatation and left atrial dilatation.

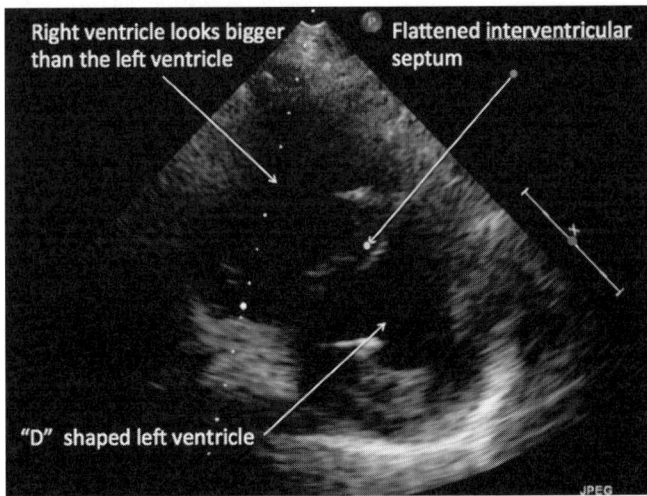

Figure 10.9 Example 2. A parasternal short-axis view of the left and right ventricles. The right ventricle appears larger than the left, there is flattening of the interventricular septum, and the left ventricle has a "D" shape, which is consistent with the right ventricular failure.

Example 2

An 85-year-old female presents to your emergency surgery session with a fractured neck of femur, following a fall at home. She denies any history of cardiac disease, but is relatively immobile due to advanced arthritis and mild dementia. She has been a long-term heavy smoker and does get short of breath doing household activities. On auscultation you detect a very soft ejection systolic murmur, and perform a goal-focused TTE examination (Figs. 10.7–10.9).

Comment: This patient has suffered relatively mild trauma but has severe underlying cardiac disease. She has obvious severe aortic stenosis, which alone will increase her mortality substantially, though recognition of it will alter the anesthetic and perioperative management. The left ventricle is normal size, and, though not shown, has a low-normal systolic function. The left atrium is dilated, and this pattern is consistent with diastolic heart failure, which is common in patients with aortic stenosis. But there is more. The right ventricle is dilated and is physically squashing the left ventricle. This pattern of enlarged right ventricle, interventricular septal flattening, and a D-shaped left ventricle is consistent with right ventricular failure. The most likely cause will be pulmonary hypertension secondary to her diastolic heart failure and aortic stenosis, and probably her long-term smoking. This combination of pathologies places her at extreme risk for surgery.

Example 3

A 75-year-old female is involved in a motor vehicle accident and has sustained fractures to her left tibia, right humerus, and right ribs. She also has a history of ischemic heart disease and received a drug eluting stent 4 months previously, and stopped antiplatelet therapy 1 month ago. She is hypotensive and tachycardiac, and has nonspecific changes on her ECG. Focused imaging is performed (Figs. 10.10–10.12).

Comment: The degree of trauma is potentially substantial, as there are fractures on both sides of the body and in both upper and lower limbs. Fractured ribs indicate significant chest trauma. However, the history of cardiac disease, a stent implantation, and relatively recent cessation of antiplatelet therapy raises the possibility of myocardial infarction as a major contributor to her hypotension. However, it is important not to have a focus error and consider myocardial

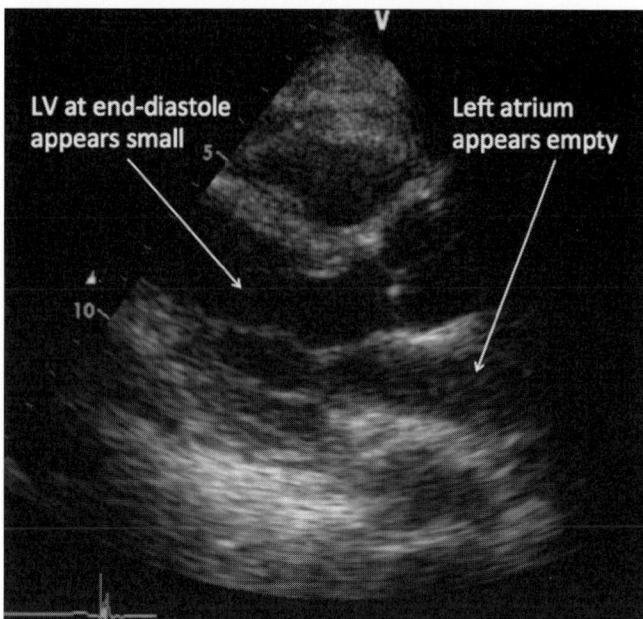

Figure 10.10 Example 3. A parasternal long-axis view showing a small left ventricle and empty left atrium.

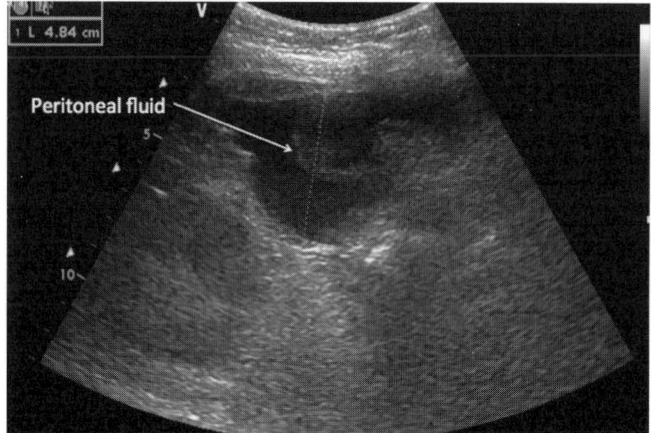

Figure 10.12 Example 3. An abdominal scan showing a large peritoneal fluid collection.

Table 10.5 Divisions of the abdomen

Division	Structures
Intrathoracic	The part of the upper abdomen that lies beneath the rib cage and contains the diaphragm, liver, spleen, and stomach
Pelvic	Defined by the bony pelvis and contains the urinary bladder, urethra, rectum, small intestine (and in females the ovaries, fallopian tubes, and uterus)
Retroperitoneal abdomen	Contains kidneys, uterus, pancreas, abdominal aorta, and inferior vena cava
True abdomen	Contains the small and large intestines, gravid uterus, or distended bladder

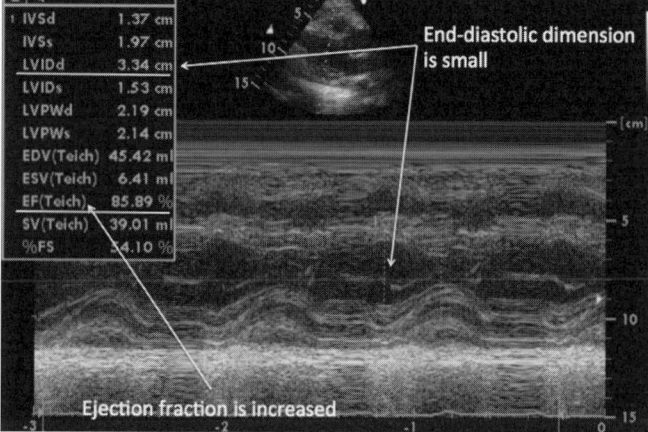

Figure 10.11 Example 3. An M-mode image of the left ventricle showing a small end-diastolic dimension and increased ejection fraction.

infarction as the most important pathology, as the nature of the injuries does suggest the potential for major organ damage. In this example, the TTE study showed a relatively empty heart with normal function, making acute myocardial ischemia an unlikely possibility. However, the empty heart and tachycardia points to blood loss, which in this case was from a ruptured abdominal viscus leading to a large intraperitoneal collection.

The basics of the FAST examination

The primary use of the focused abdominal scanning in trauma (FAST) examination is to identify whether there is a free fluid within the peritoneum, which could indicate organ rupture and internal bleeding. It has become an important tool in the decision-making algorithm during the early management of trauma. FAST has the advantage of being a rapid and easy scan to perform and, importantly, a bedside investigation. While its primary role is to assess abdominal pathology, the user can estimate ventricular filling and function from the subcostal view.

It is important to understand where major organs lie and how the peritoneum is structured. The abdomen can be arbitrarily divided into four areas (Table 10.5). There are four scanning windows for the FAST examination (Table 10.6). These windows are shown diagrammatically in Figure 10.13.

Conducting the study

Use an ultrasound machine with a live two-dimensional mode (rapid B-mode), transducer frequencies between 3 and 6 MHz, and a depth of 8–15 cm. Use lots of gel to ensure good ultrasound probe contact with the abdomen. The scan is performed with the patient in the supine position. For the perihepatic position, the probe is placed in the right mid-to-posterior axillary line at the level of the eleventh and twelfth

Table 10.6 Scanning windows for the FAST examination

Window	Structures identified
Perihepatic	Right upper quadrant structures including right lobe of liver, kidney, and the hepatorenal space
Perisplenic	Structures in the left upper quadrant, including spleen, kidney, and perisplenic area
Pelvic	Structures in the pelvis are identified including the pouch of Douglas (in females) or the retrovesical pouch (in males)
Pericardial	A subcostal view of the heart to identify pericardial effusions and to observe ventricular filling and function

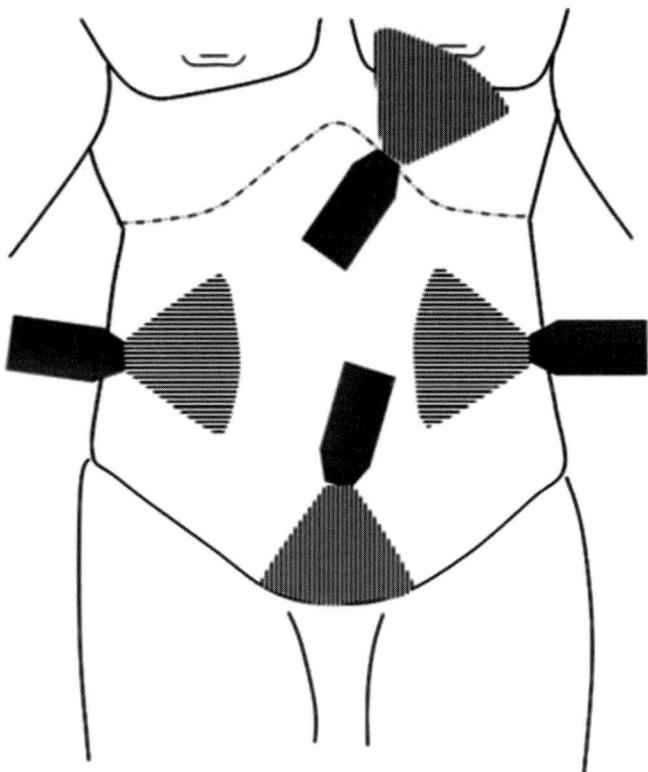

Figure 10.13 The four scanning windows of the FAST examination. Clockwise from top: pericardial, perisplenic, pelvic, and perihepatic.

ribs. Identify the hepatorenal space and look for fluid, which will appear as a black or dark stripe between liver and kidney. The perisplenic scan is conducted in a similar manner but on the left-hand side of the patient. Look for fluid between spleen and kidney. For the pelvic examination, place the transducer in the midline just above the symphysis pubis, and angle it to identify the bladder and look for fluid between the bladder and the uterus or rectum. The pericardial scan is essentially a subcostal view of the heart. The probe needs to be firmly placed beneath the xiphisternum and angled toward the heart. Views can be made in either the short or long axis. The primary aim of this view is to identify fluid in the pericardial space; however, it is a very useful view for identifying left ventricular filling and function of the heart as an aid to resuscitation during trauma. Line diagrams and ultrasound images are presented for each of the four views in Figure 10.14.

Detection of pneumothorax

Using ultrasound to identify the pneumothorax is remarkably simple. It is difficult to appreciate from still images, but is easy to identify when seen during real-time imaging. The key is to identify movement of the visceral pleura over the parietal pleura. The pleura–lung interface is a strong echo reflector, and so the surface of the lung is seen as a bright white line moving with respiration (called the "sliding sign"). It is also common to see white streaks perpendicular to the line of the pleura, which are "comet-tail" artifacts. These also move with respiration. When there is a pneumothorax, these signs disappear and neutral gray reflections appear beneath the ribs, which do not move. As the lung is relatively superficial to the chest wall, a variety of probes can be used for this diagnosis, including high-frequency transducers. Figure 10.15 shows line drawings and still images to illustrate normal versus pneumothorax.

Detection of pleural effusion

The key to identifying a pleural effusion using surface ultrasound is to understand that the fluid will collect in the dependent position. For supine patients, this means that the effusions will collect in the paraaortic gutters and may be difficult to identify from the lateral or anterior approaches. Conversely, if the patient is sitting, a black or gray space will easily be seen with ultrasound placed between the lower ribs posteriorly. The texture of the fluid will give different echo densities: clear fluid appears almost black, whereas hematoma is gray and gives an appearance similar to liver. It is not uncommon to see a clot floating within free fluid. TEE is very sensitive for detecting pleural effusion, with effusion seen with as little as 100 mL of fluid. By rotating the probe toward the aorta, the left pleural space is identified; and by rotating a long way to the right, the right pleural space can be identified if there is fluid within it. When using TEE, pleural effusions have the appearance of a "tiger claw." Figure 10.16 shows left and right pleural effusions using TEE.

Use of TEE in trauma anesthesia

Provided that the patient is intubated, and that there are no contraindications to insertion of the TEE probe, TEE provides the most reliable and rapid assessment of ventricular function and filling and can be used throughout the anesthetic to guide management. Because the images are usually of excellent quality, it is easier to conduct a full diagnostic study to identify potential damage to the heart or major vessels. The presence of a pericardial effusion, severe valvular dysfunction (especially tricuspid valve regurgitation), or evidence of major vessel

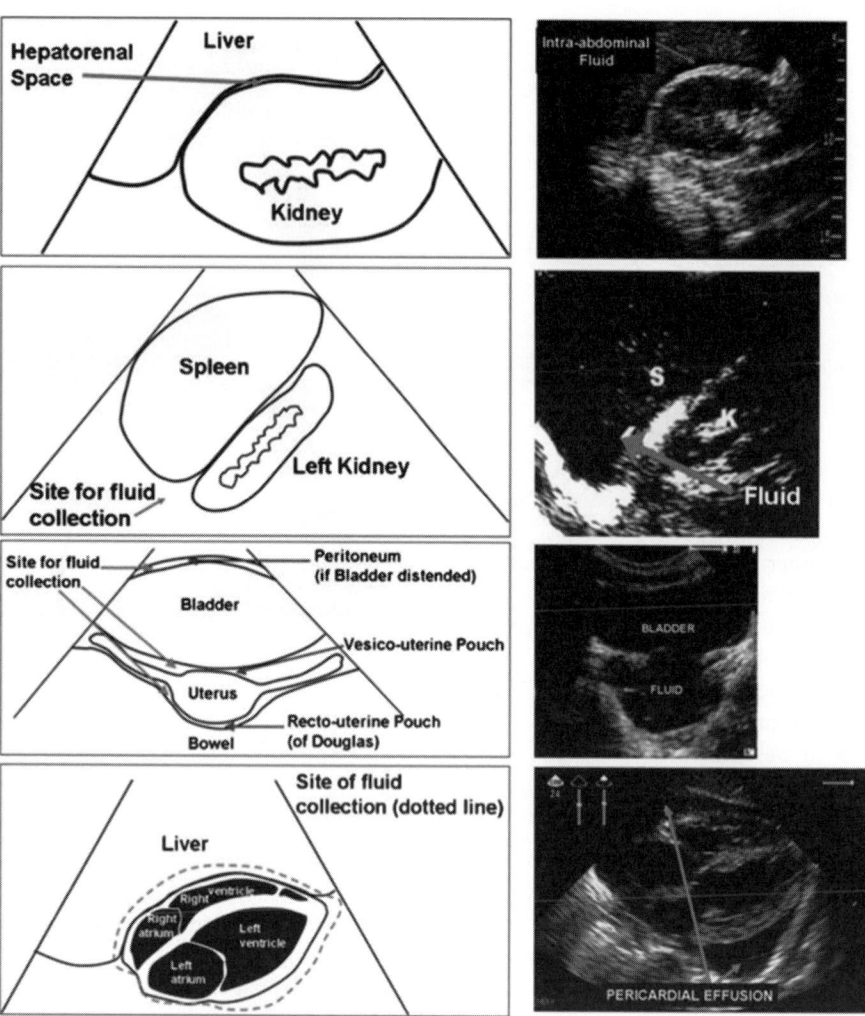

Figure 10.14 FAST examination, positive scans. Top to bottom: perihepatic, perisplenic, pelvic, and pericardial windows.

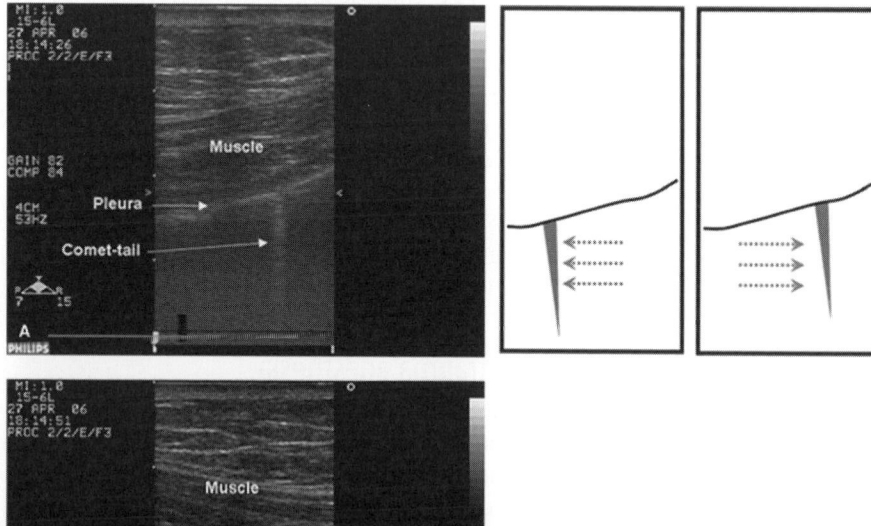

Figure 10.15 Detection of pneumothorax. (Top) Normal: moving comet-tail artifact. (Bottom) Pneumothorax: no comet-tail artifact.

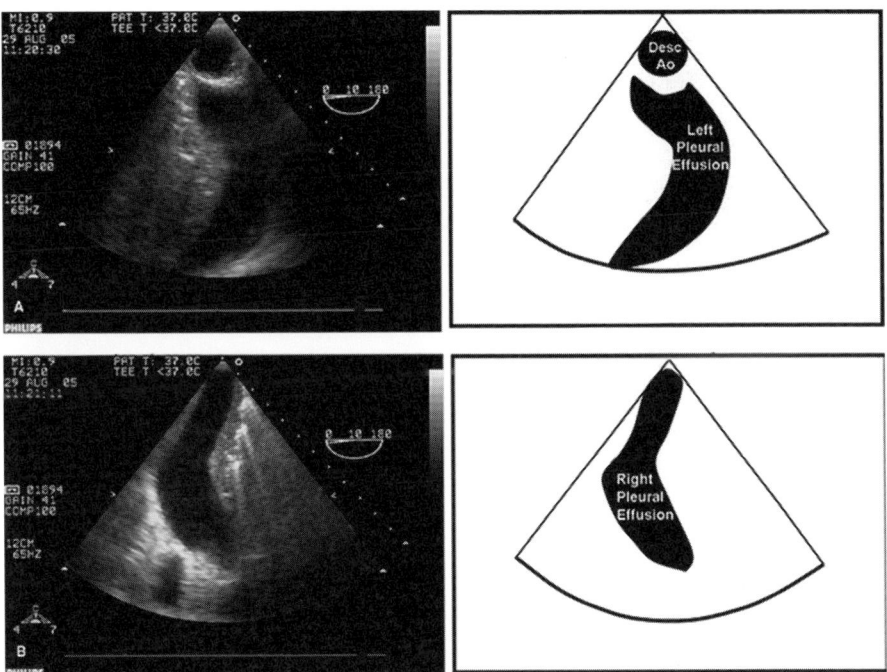

Figure 10.16 Detection of pleural effusion. (Top) Transesophageal echocardiogram of left pleural effusion. Desc Ao, descending aorta. (Bottom) Transesophageal echocardiogram of right pleural effusion.

disruption are diagnoses that are often detected during intra-operative echocardiography, rather than prior to the onset of surgery. A dilated and poorly contracting right heart may be indicative of myocardial contusion or, alternatively, could be caused by a pulmonary embolism such as fat emboli from long-bone fractures. A particularly difficult diagnosis is that of aortic transection. The most common place for transection to occur is just distal to the left subclavian artery. The key to diagnosis is to understand that imaging of the descending thoracic aorta is normally excellent, but when disrupted and surrounded by hematoma, there is echocardiography "drop-out" leading to poor imaging. Furthermore, the aorta decreases in size as it travels distally. If the aortic diameter increases in size from the arch to the descending aorta, then transection should be suspected. Finally, severe aortic atheroma is very uncommon in people younger than 50 years of age. Disruption to the intima can appear like severe aortic atheroma, and, in the setting of a young person with a deceleration injury, this points to aortic transection. Also look for associated features such as pleural effusion that could indicate hemothorax. Figure 10.17 shows the normal descending thoracic aorta and an example of transection.

Blunt injury to the abdominal aorta

Although the classic mechanism for thoracic aortic disruption is a deceleration injury, blunt trauma can injure the major abdominal vessels as well. Acute rupture is associated with high immediate mortality, and survival depends on incomplete rupture or containment of hematoma in the retroperitoneal space. The principles of ultrasound diagnosis are similar for the abdominal and for the thoracic aorta. First, in the young

patient the aorta should be 2 cm or less in diameter, and diminished in size as it courses more distally. The intima should be free of thickening (it is uncommon to have severe atheroma in young people), and there should not be a large space evident between the aorta and the posterior vertebral body. If there is significant hematoma, then the aorta will be poorly visualized due to attenuation of the ultrasound signal; this serves as an indirect clue that there may be pathology. It is not possible to see the abdominal aorta with TEE, and the image quality is variable with TTE because it is a posteriorly located structure. In older patients, there may be preexisting pathology such as aortic aneurysm or significant atheroma. It is important to consider the mechanism of injury when deciding whether the aortic pathology is acute or chronic. However, abdominal scanning with an abdominal probe will identify the abdominal aorta, which should be < 2 cm in diameter.

Myocardial contusion and blunt cardiac injury

Blunt cardiac injury may occur from a direct force or secondary to deceleration injury when the chest wall comes in contact with the steering wheel or seatbelt. Because the right ventricle lies immediately beneath the sternum, it is the ventricle most likely to show evidence of contusion. Valve rupture can also occur with blunt injury, with the tricuspid valve being most commonly affected. The echocardiographic features of contusion are those of acute segmental dysfunction and possibly ventricular dilatation (Fig. 10.18). It is important to consider the mechanism of injury and the patient's premorbid health to better gauge whether these findings are acute or chronic. Right ventricular dilatation can occur from wall contusion and dysfunction, or from severe tricuspid valve regurgitation

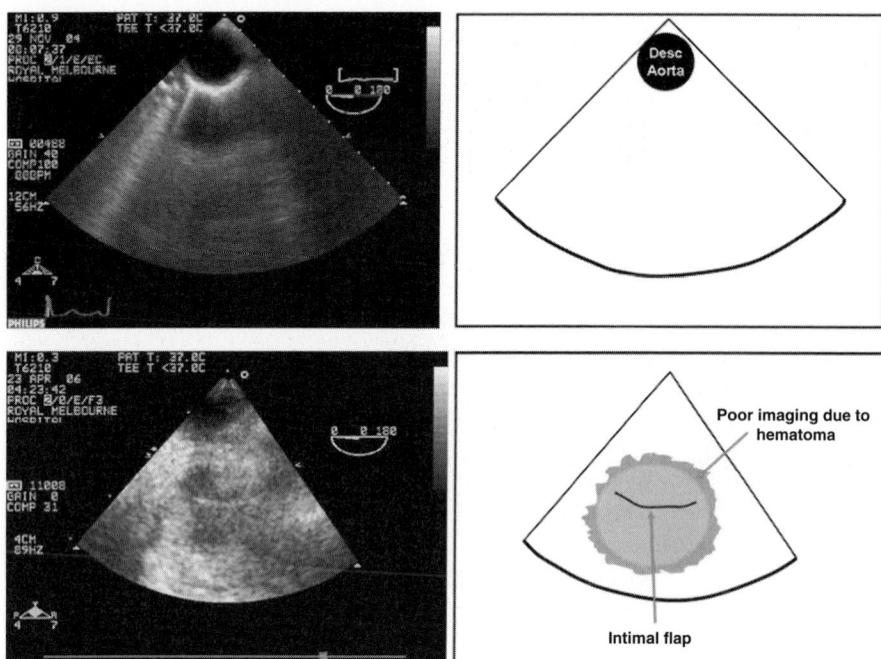

Figure 10.17 Detection of aortic transection. (Top) Normal descending aorta in short axis. (Bottom) Transected descending aorta in short axis.

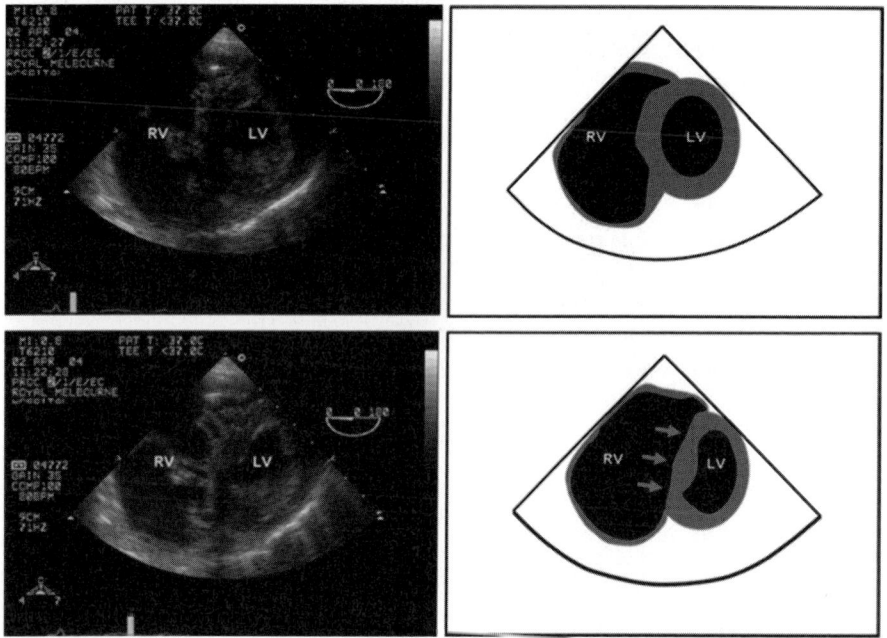

Figure 10.18 Transesophageal echocardiogram: dilated right ventricle (RV) with reduced systolic function and "D-shaped" left ventricle (LV)/septal flattening (arrows) consistent with myocardial contusion.

following rupture. Other valves can be affected. These patients may require inotrope or other circulatory support until the myocardial dysfunction resolves. Valve rupture usually requires corrective surgery.

Pericardial tamponade

In the trauma setting, pericardial tamponade is suggestive of ascending aortic rupture with blood escaping into the pericardial sac, or blunt or penetrating myocardial injury. It should be detected as part of the FAST scan, but may be initially detected during hemodynamic assessment using either TTE or TEE. For TEE, the transgastric views are best, and for TTE, the subcostal view is the first view to use to look for pericardial tamponade. You must decide two things: first, is the effusion causing compression of the heart; and second, is the compression leading to hemodynamic compromise? This should fit in with the clinical scenario and signs of a raised jugular venous pressure, hypotension, and evidence of poor tissue perfusion. Because pericardial tamponade is physiologically "severe acute

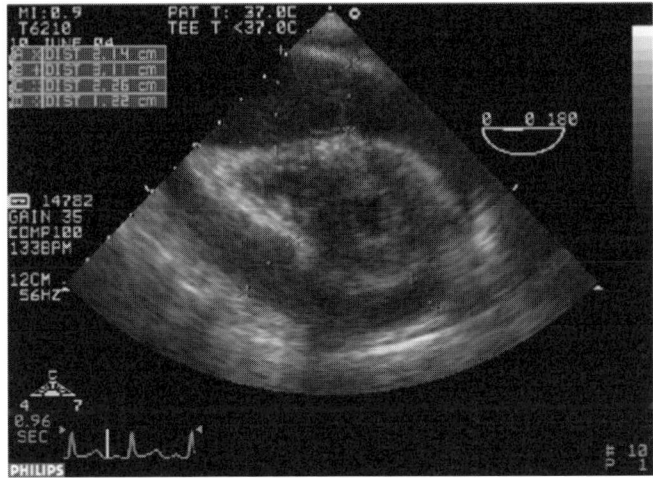

Figure 10.19 Transesophageal echocardiogram image showing a pericardial effusion causing tamponade.

diastolic dysfunction," there may be a prominent pulsus paradoxus, or marked respiratory variation in the arterial blood pressure waveform.

Because the right atrium and right ventricle are thin-walled, they are the chambers most commonly affected, leading to diastolic collapse. In Figure 10.19, the ventricle is seen as a small structure within a "sea of black," which is the effusion. This sort of picture demonstrates physical compression of the heart leading to tamponade.

Effusions are graded according to size (small, < 0.5 cm; moderate, 0.5–2.0 cm; large, > 2.0 cm). In the supine patient, small effusions tend to be localized behind the posterior LV wall, expanding laterally, apically, and anteriorly as the effusion increases. Large effusions are often circumferential. Size alone, however, does not dictate whether the effusion will cause compression or not.

In the trauma setting, a two-dimensional appearance of a large effusion is enough to give you the diagnosis, but analysis of the tricuspid or mitral inflow Doppler can then be used to help quantify tamponade. If the respiratory variation in peak tricuspid inflow velocity exceeds 40%, or the mitral inflow exceeds 25%, then this is highly suggestive of tamponade, as shown in Figure 10.20.

Some cautionary tips: tamponade occurs when the heart is physically compressed. Though this classically occurs as a result of blood in the pericardium, it can occur from a large pleural effusion, and also from lung inflation from gas trapping. In the setting of hypovolemia, the effect will be pronounced. Finally, if blood in the pericardium has clotted, then it can have the same appearance as liver and may be misdiagnosed as such.

Getting started in ultrasound

The two major hurdles for anesthesia and ultrasound are education and the availability of equipment. Ultrasound equipment is becoming smaller, more portable, and importantly

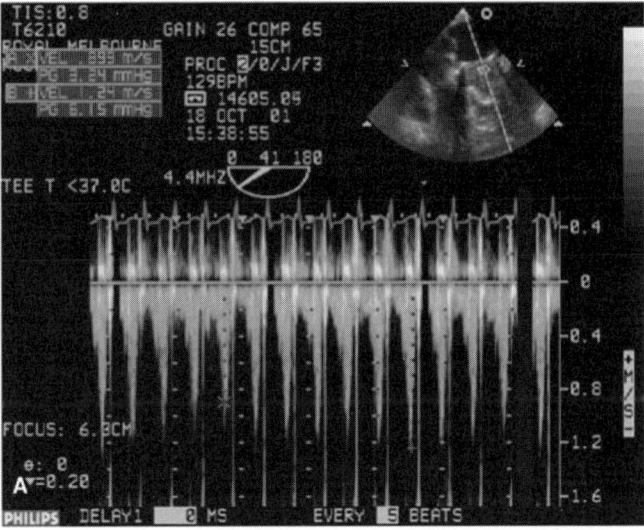

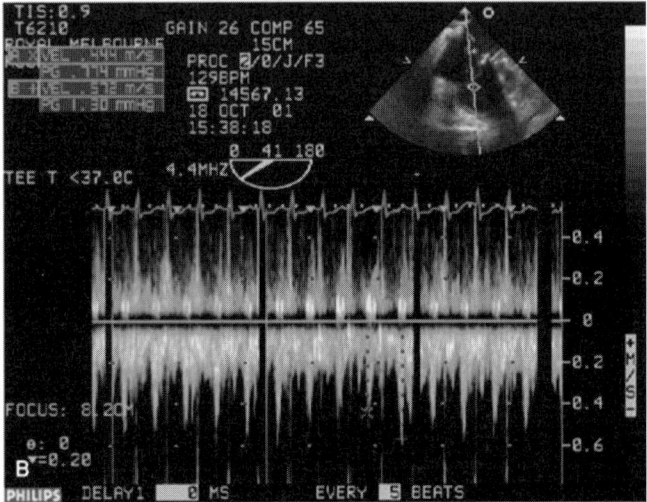

Figure 10.20 Transesophageal echocardiogram mitral inflow pulsed-wave Doppler. (Top) Transmitral inflow. (Bottom) Tricuspid inflow showing respiratory variation is consistent with tamponade.

more affordable, with a range of ultrasound machines now available. These range from surface ultrasound scanning machines all the way to comprehensive echocardiography and general imaging platforms. Laptop-sized machines are available that have the capability of full transthoracic, transesophageal, and abdominal imaging, and there are now palm-sized TTE machines. The cost of these ultrasound machines has decreased considerably, increasing the availability of ultrasound to more practitioners.

For many anesthesiologists, embarking on ultrasound means learning a new skill set and knowledge base. Simple surface ultrasound techniques and ultrasound-guided procedures require minimal instruction and limited practice prior to using them in clinical practice.[2] Short hands-on workshops are an ideal way to get started, especially for ultrasound-guided procedures or limited transthoracic echocardiography studies such as iHEARTscan (haemodynamic echocardiography assessment in real time – see www.heartweb.com.au). Diagnostic echocardiography, however, requires considerably greater knowledge and practice to achieve a level of confidence that important diagnoses will not be missed. Either TTE or TEE can be used for hemodynamic state assessment with relatively little training, but to move on and assess pathology, valve function, or aortic conditions requires a much greater knowledge base. Traditionally, fellowships in echocardiography have been the method to gain such knowledge and experience, but this is very restrictive for people who are already qualified and in established practice. Distance education providers can satisfy the knowledge-based requirements with a shorter period than required to acquire hands-on skills. An example of a distance education program is the Online Clinical Ultrasound and Echocardiography Courses conducted through the University of Melbourne. These courses are now available as the Society of Cardiovascular Anesthesiologists Online Clinical Ultrasound and Echocardiography (On-CUE) program (see www.heartweb.com). In the authors' experience, acquiring the manual skills is relatively simple, and the real hurdle to becoming an advanced practitioner in echocardiography is acquiring the knowledge base.

Acknowledgments

We thank Danielle Nicholas for her help with image acquisition, drawings, and content review.

Questions

(1) Assessing the abdominal aorta:
   a. Can accurately detect a ruptured abdominal aortic aneurysm
   b. Can accurately assess the size of the aneurysm
   c. Can accurately detect the presence of a retroperitoneal hematoma
   d. Can always assess all parts of the abdominal aorta

(2) When assessing the size of a pneumothorax using ultrasound:
   a. The size can be quantified in percentage terms as for an x-ray
   b. The pneumothorax will not normally be present anteriorly in a supine patient
   c. The presence of a pneumothorax can be distinguished based on the absence of both the movement at the pleural surface and the comet-tail artifacts
   d. A pneumothorax can be reliably determined in patients with bullae from chronic airways disease

(3) An elderly patient is involved in a motor vehicle accident. After induction of anesthesia, the blood pressure is 80/40 mmHg. A central venous catheter is inserted and the right atrial pressure is 5 mmHg. TEE examination reveals systolic buckling of the interatrial septum, LVEDA 6 cm^2, and LVESA 1 cm^2. The basic hemodynamic state is:
   a. Hypovolemia
   b. Primary diastolic failure
   c. Normal
   d. Right ventricular failure

(4) Which one of the following is consistent with primary diastolic failure?
   a. LVEDA = 6.5 cm^2
   b. LVESA = 13 cm^2
   c. Pulmonary vein systolic/diastolic velocity time integral (VTI) ratio of 1.2
   d. LVEDA = 12 cm^2 and LVESA 4 cm^2

(5) A patient with a recent myocardial infarct presents for surgery. He has a long history of severe asthma. He is breathless and hypotensive. A transthoracic echocardiograph is ordered prior to anesthesia. The left ventricular end-diastolic diameter is 3.2 cm, and there are no left ventricular wall motion abnormalities. The pulmonary vein Doppler shows diastolic flow predominance. The right ventricle is dilated with poor systolic function. The most likely hemodynamic state is:
   a. Primary systolic failure
   b. Systolic and diastolic failure
   c. Right ventricular failure
   d. Normal

(6) FAST can be technically difficult in:
   a. Obese patients
   b. Subcutaneous emphysema
   c. Uncooperative patients
   d. All of the above

(7) Which statement is correct? Ejection fraction (EF) calculated from M-mode measurements:
   a. Gives an accurate assessment of global ventricular contraction
   b. Identifies regional wall motion abnormalities
   c. Provides an assessment based on the contraction in a single plane
   d. Is only accurate in the setting of normal systolic contraction

(8) Overall ventricular systolic contraction is best evaluated by:
   a. M-mode echocardiography
   b. Two-dimensional imaging in all cardiac imaging views
   c. Two-dimensional imaging of the parasternal views
   d. Pulsed-wave Doppler assessment of left ventricular outflow tract velocity time integral (VTI)

(9) In the FAST examination, four sonographic views are used because:
   a. Sensitivity is maximized
   b. Specificity is maximized
   c. Speed of the examination is maximized
   d. It is a compromise between speed and sensitivity of the examination

(10) In the perihepatic window of FAST:
    a. The liver is normally not seen
    b. The kidney is surrounded by an echogenic fascia
    c. Free fluid is brightly echogenic
    d. The liver has the same echodensity as fluid

Answers

(1) b
(2) c
(3) a
(4) a
(5) c
(6) d
(7) c
(8) b
(9) d
(10) b

References

1. Royse CF, Canty DJ, Faris J, *et al.* Core review. Physician-performed ultrasound: the time has come for routine use in acute care medicine. *Anesth Analg* 2012; **115**: 1007–28.

2. Royse CF, Haji DL, Faris JG, *et al.* Evaluation of the interpretative skills of participants of a limited transthoracic echocardiography training course (H.A.R.T. scan course). *Anaesth Intensive Care* 2012; **40**: 498–504.

3. Faris JG, Hartley K, Fuller CM, *et al.* Audit of cardiac pathology detection using a criteria-based perioperative echocardiography service. *Anaesth Intensive Care* 2012; **40**: 702–9.

4. Canty DJ, Royse CF, Kilpatrick D, Williams DL, Royse AG. The impact of pre-operative focused transthoracic echocardiography in emergency non-cardiac surgery patients with known or risk of cardiac disease. *Anaesthesia* 2012; **67**: 714–20.

5. Canty DJ, Royse CF, Kilpatrick D, Bowyer A, Royse AG. The impact on cardiac diagnosis and mortality of focused transthoracic echocardiography in hip fracture surgery patients with increased risk of cardiac disease: a retrospective cohort study. *Anaesthesia* 2012; **67**: 1202–9.

6. Canty DJ, Royse CF, Kilpatrick D, Bowman L, Royse AG. The impact of focused transthoracic echocardiography in the pre-operative clinic. *Anaesthesia* 2012; **67**: 618–25.

7. Royse CF. Ultrasound-guided haemodynamic state assessment. *Best Pract Res Clin Anaesthesiol* 2009; **23**: 273–83.

8. Kusumoto FM, Muhiudeen IA, Kuecherer HF, Cahalan MK, Schiller NB. Response of the interatrial septum to transatrial pressure gradients and its potential for predicting pulmonary capillary wedge pressure: an intraoperative study using transesophageal echocardiography in patients during mechanical ventilation. *J Am Coll Cardiol* 1993; **21**: 721–8.

9. Royse CF, Royse AG, Soeding PF, Blake DW. Shape and movement of the interatrial septum predicts change in pulmonary capillary wedge pressure. *Ann Thorac Cardiovasc Surg* 2001; **7**: 79–83.

Imaging in trauma

Claire Sandstrom

Objectives

(1) Be familiar with imaging that may supplement the primary survey of Advanced Trauma Life Support for hemodynamically unstable victims of blunt and penetrating trauma.

(2) Review the indications and technique for CT obtained in evaluation of hemodynamically stable victims of blunt trauma.

(3) Identify differences in traditional trauma workup for special patient populations, including pregnant patients and children.

(4) Review the indications for emergent angiography by interventional radiology in the setting of trauma.

Diagnostic radiology in trauma

Emergent imaging of the unstable trauma patient

The imaging algorithm in the setting of blunt trauma depends on the patient's clinical stability. In unstable patients, the role of radiology is secondary and complementary to clinical stabilization of airway, breathing, and circulation. In this setting, imaging should be directed toward diagnoses directly related to these clinical endpoints: for example, tension pneumothorax, craniocervical dissociation, endotracheal tube malposition, severe pelvic fractures, or massive hemoperitoneum may contribute to ongoing cardiopulmonary instability and may be identified with emergent imaging.

Ultrasound assessment

Focused assessment with sonography for trauma (FAST) can demonstrate hemoperitoneum (see Chapter 10). Free fluid in a hemodynamically unstable blunt trauma patient can expedite laparotomy (Fig. 11.1).[1] It is not sensitive enough, however, to exclude intraperitoneal injury.[2] If the FAST is negative, therefore, some trauma centers will perform diagnostic peritoneal lavage on hemodynamically unstable trauma patients, although the role for this is diminishing. If this too is negative, other causes of hypotension are considered, including retroperitoneal/pelvic hemorrhage, hemorrhage

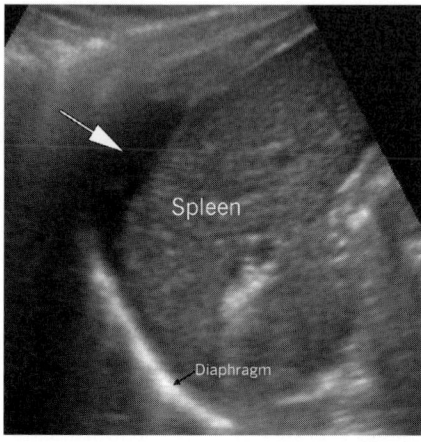

Figure 11.1 Left upper quadrant longitudinal gray-scale sonographic image from FAST in a hemodynamically unstable man hit by a truck demonstrates perisplenic free fluid (white arrow). Subsequent emergency laparotomy confirmed grade V splenic rupture.

Spleen

Diaphragm

into the pleural space or mediastinum, myocardial contusion, and neurogenic shock.[1]

Radiographic assessment

Frontal chest and pelvic radiographs can be obtained as adjuncts to the ATLS (Advanced Trauma Life Support) primary survey and may be called the "radiographic trauma series."[3] These images can be obtained and interpreted quickly and may prompt immediate interventions that are potentially life-saving. Some institutions routinely acquire these exams, or some combination, while others do not. These radiographs are often limited by patient positioning, overlying trauma backboard artifact, and exclusion of anatomy, and should not be relied upon to exclude subtle but significant injuries.

Chest radiography in the setting of blunt trauma is obtained in anteroposterior (AP) projection and in supine position. The location of endotracheal tube, chest tubes, or central venous catheter can be readily determined. Malpositioning of the endotracheal tube in a bronchus or the esophagus may contribute to hemodynamic instability and should be evident on radiograph (Fig. 11.2). In addition, signs of large pneumothorax, potentially under tension, extensive rib fractures with possible flail chest, and mediastinal contours suggesting traumatic aortic injury may also be detected in the acutely unstable patient (Fig. 11.3).[4]

Trauma Anesthesia, 2nd Edition, ed. Charles E. Smith. Published by Cambridge University Press. © Charles E. Smith, 2015.

However, supine radiography is limited in its sensitivity for pneumothorax, with a sensitivity of 75%, compared to 98% with beside ultrasound.[5] Moreover, despite historical teaching, a "widened mediastinum" on a supine chest radiograph is neither sensitive nor specific enough to exclude or diagnose acute aortic injury.[6]

Pelvic radiography can confirm the presence of pelvic ring disruption, which may prompt pelvic angiography and embolization for control of pelvic hemorrhage (Fig. 11.4).[7,8] Closed reduction of an open-book pelvic fracture reduces pelvic volume and may help tamponade bleeding temporarily until more definitive treatment is possible (Fig. 11.4b; see Chapter 27).[7]

A lateral radiograph of the cervical spine can be obtained when neurogenic shock is suspected as the cause of cardiovascular instability, looking for evidence of craniocervical dissociation or high cervical spine injury (Fig. 11.5). This radiograph is often suboptimal for visualization of the lower cervical spine due to positioning of the shoulders, and thus should not be relied upon to exclude significant cervical spine injury.

Resuscitation room CT

Multidetector computed tomography (MDCT) has a proven role in the diagnosis of acute traumatic injuries in stable patients and is now finding increasing use in the primary survey in semi-stable patients.[9,10] Historically, CT was not recommended in unstable patients because image acquisition required removal of the patient from the resuscitation room, separating the patient from close clinical monitoring and from easy access to appropriate interventional equipment. Transfer of the patient from resuscitation bed to CT table takes time and risks dislodging tenuous and life-sustaining vascular access and airway devices. Furthermore, acute decompensation of the patient on the CT table may have delayed recognition and response because of distance of the patient from clinicians. Thus, CT evaluation was historically deferred to the secondary survey of ATLS and was targeted to specific body parts based on findings from the primary survey and radiographs.

Recognizing that CT is far superior to radiographs for the diagnosis of traumatic injuries, and that rapid diagnosis can result in more prompt and definitive treatment, early whole-body CT protocols are gaining acceptance.[9,10] To facilitate their use in unstable patients, some trauma centers have redesigned resuscitation suites to include a portable or integrated CT scanner that can be used as part of the primary trauma survey without the risks of transferring the patient. However, resuscitation room-based CT scanning may be difficult to implement in some centers because of cost, operational, and infrastructural limitations.

Radiology in the stable trauma patient

Imaging evaluation of the stable blunt trauma patient begins with radiographic assessment of chest and pelvis and possibly cervical spine. Ultrasound can also be performed, understanding that FAST is not reliable for excluding hemoperitoneum (particularly less than 200 mL of fluid), solid organ injuries without hemoperitoneum, or hollow visceral injuries.[1]

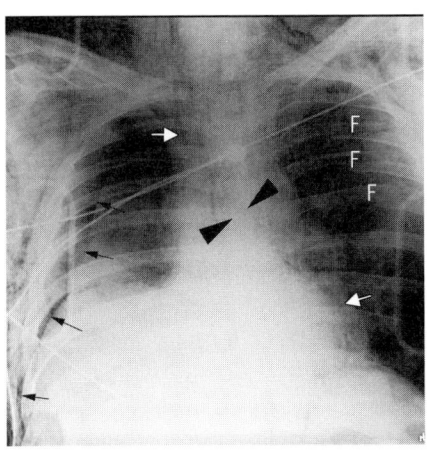

Figure 11.2 Frontal chest radiograph in a 51-year-old man after a motor vehicle crash shows left mainstem bronchus intubation (black arrowheads). Subcutaneous emphysema accompanies right pneumothorax (black arrows), pneumomediastinum (white arrows), and multiple left posterior rib fractures (F).

(A)

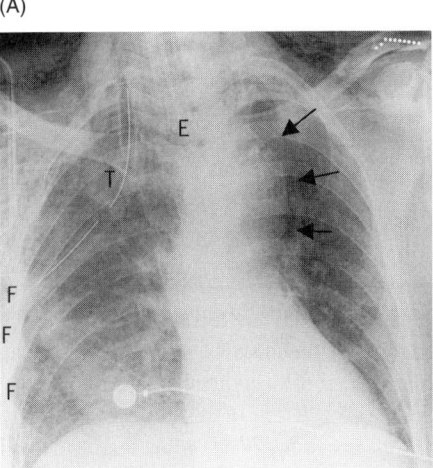

(B)

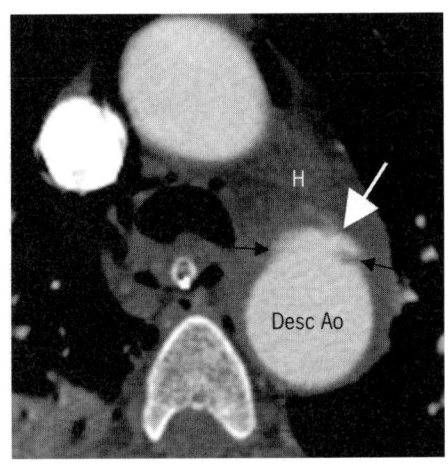

Figure 11.3 (A) Frontal chest radiograph in a 55-year-old man after a 90-foot (27 m) fall. Good position of endotracheal tube (E) and right chest tube (T), with multiple right rib fractures (F). Aorta is indistinct with abnormal contour (black arrows). (B) Axial chest CT angiography image through the aortic isthmus (Desc Ao) shows intimal flaps (small black arrows) and small aortic pseudoaneurysm (white arrow), surrounded by mediastinal hematoma (H), diagnostic of acute aortic injury.

(A)

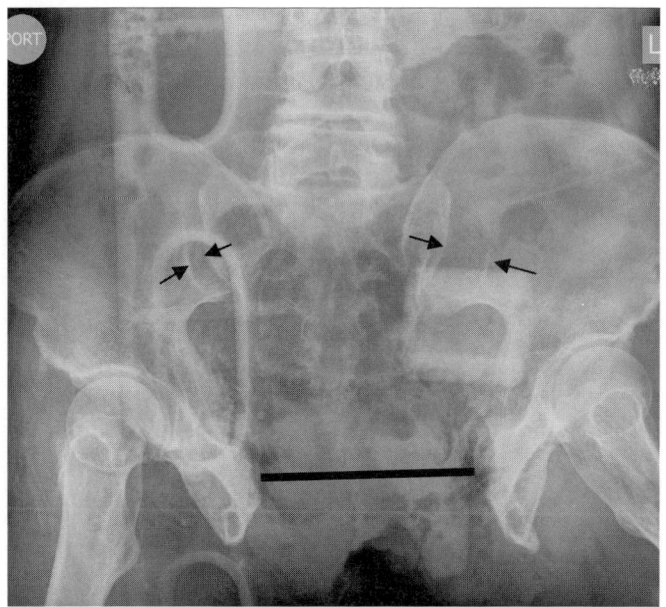

(B)

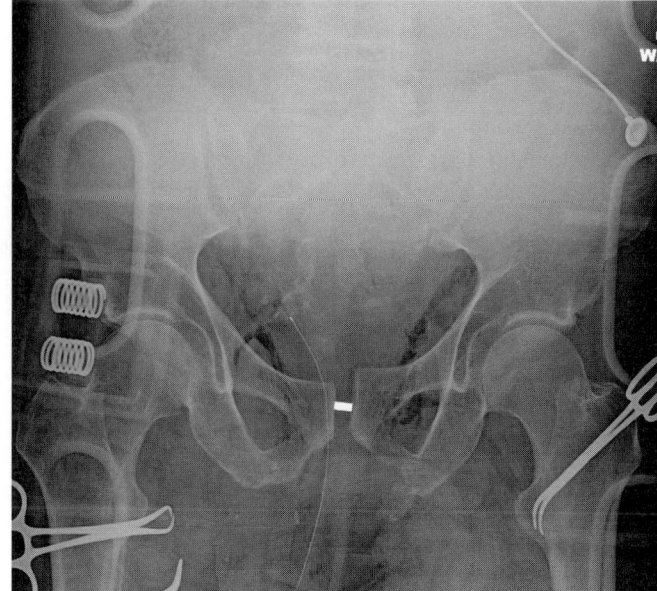

(C)

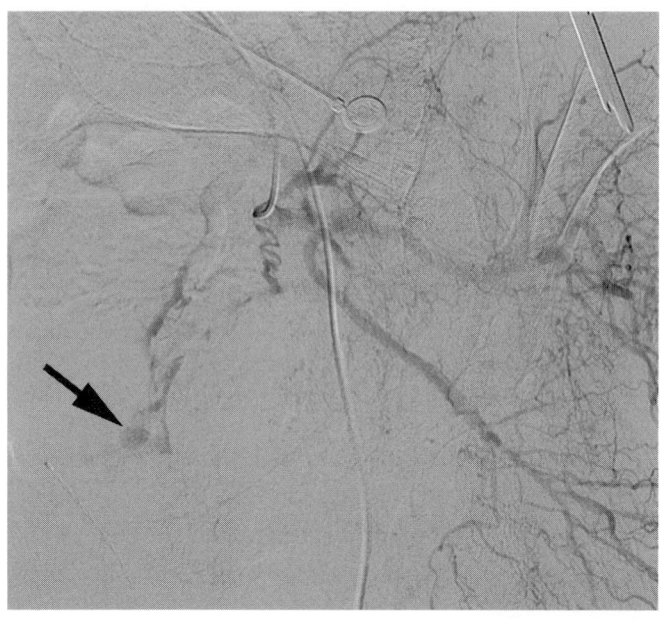

Figure 11.4 (**A**) Frontal pelvic radiograph in a 67-year-old man with an open perineal wound from a farm equipment accident. Marked pubic symphysis diastasis (black line) and bilateral sacroiliac joint disruption (black arrows) reflect anterior–posterior compression-type mechanism, the "open-book pelvis." (**B**) After pelvic sheeting, pubic symphyseal diastasis is improved (short white line). (**C**) Selective left internal iliac artery injection during digital-subtraction pelvic angiogram shows contrast extravasation (large black arrow) from the anterior division, which was successfully embolized.

Traditionally, the findings on these screening exams affect which segments of the body are imaged during subsequent targeted CT evaluation. Alternatively, many trauma centers now use a standard whole-body CT approach for all trauma patients,[9,11] lessening the benefit of radiographs for triage. Use of whole-body CT has been shown to decrease overall time in the emergency room (ER), but effects on outcome and overall radiation dose have not yet been adequately studied.[9,10] Results of a prospective, randomized controlled trial (REACT-2) of immediate whole-body CT are pending at the time of this publication.[12]

CT in stable trauma patients

Head

No intravenous contrast is administered for routine posttraumatic head CT, as both intravenous contrast and acute intracranial hemorrhage are hyperdense relative to normal brain tissue (Fig. 11.6). CT also helps with the characterization of calvarial, skull base, and facial fractures. In most centers, patients who have symptoms or risk factors for blunt cerebrovascular injury (Table 11.1) undergo CT angiogram (CTA) of the neck and head after the noncontrast CT of the brain (Fig. 11.7).[13]

(A)

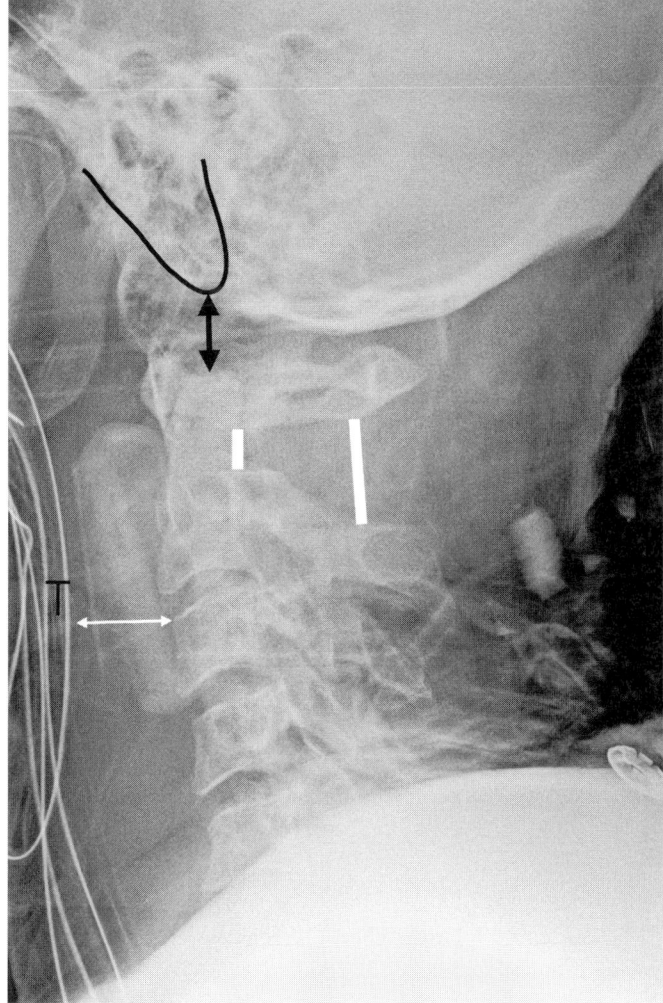

(B)

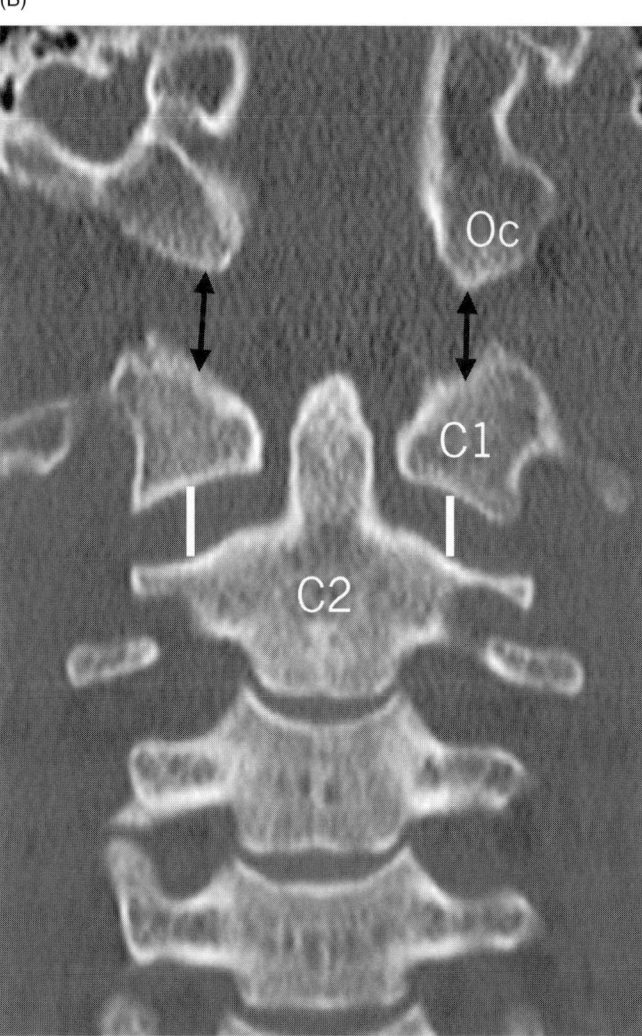

Figure 11.5 (**A**) Lateral cervical radiograph in a 37-year-old man who arrived at the emergency department in extremis after a motor vehicle collision. Marked prevertebral soft tissue swelling (white double arrow) displaces forward the endotracheal and orogastric tubes (T). Abnormal widening between the posterior elements and lateral masses of C1 and C2 (white lines) and increased distance between the clivus (black outline) and odontoid tip (black double arrow) were consistent with atlantoaxial and atlantooccipital dissociation, respectively. (**B**) Coronal cervical spine CT image through the craniocervical junction confirms bilateral widening of Oc–C1 and C1–C2 facet joints (Oc, occipital condyle; C1, lateral mass of axis; C2, vertebral body of C2). The patient expired shortly thereafter.

Chest

Chest CTA has replaced catheter aortography for diagnosis of blunt aortic injury. Depending on institutional policies, screening chest radiography may be used to determine if the aortic contour appears abnormal or indeterminate. Contingent upon clinical factors and/or chest radiographic appearance, chest CTA may be obtained to evaluate the thoracic aorta (Fig. 11.3b). Alternatively, the chest CT may be included as part of routine whole-body CT for trauma patients. Axial images with sagittal oblique reformations along the long axis of the aortic arch are particularly useful for this purpose (Fig. 11.8). A pseudoaneurysm of the aortic isthmus is the most typical finding of acute aortic injury.[4] Mediastinal hematoma usually accompanies acute aortic injury (Fig. 11.3b) but also occurs in the absence of aortic injury from sternal fractures, branch vessel injury, or venous

hemorrhage. Minimal aortic injuries can also be diagnosed on chest CTA (Fig. 11.9).[4]

Even when traumatic aortic injury is excluded, chest CT is useful for evaluating injuries to the lung parenchyma, mediastinum, and chest wall. Pulmonary contusion, laceration, and aspiration can be overlooked or indistinguishable on radiographs but are usually readily apparent on CT (Fig. 11.10). Radiographically occult pneumothorax or hemothorax may be detected even when small or inconspicuously located (Fig. 11.10). The number of rib fractures and the severity of underlying cardiopulmonary disease predict mortality from blunt chest trauma in the elderly,[14] and minimally or nondisplaced rib fractures may only be identified by CT. CT may identify pneumomediastinum and may differentiate aerodigestive tract origin from alveolar rupture origin (with dissection along bronchovascular sheaths into the mediastinum: the

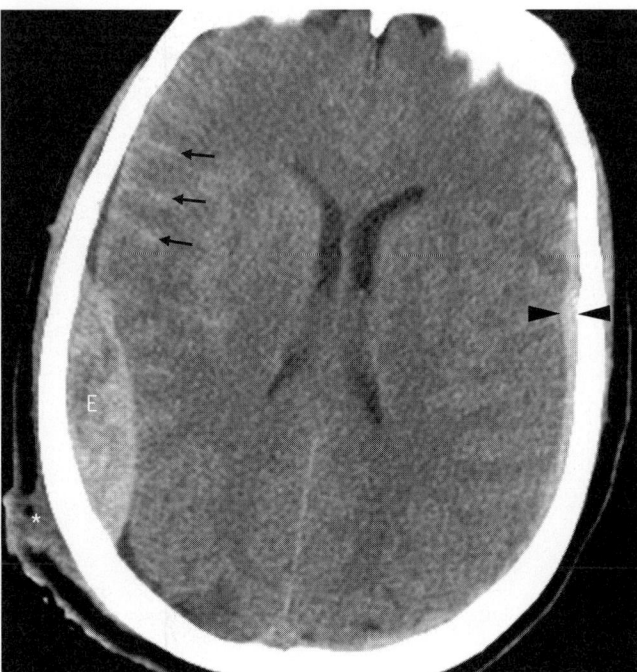

Figure 11.6 Axial noncontrast head CT image shows multifocal intracranial hemorrhage. Adjacent to the right parietal scalp laceration (asterisk), a lentiform hemorrhage reflects epidural hematoma (E). On the left is a thin subdural hematoma (bracketed by black arrowheads). Subarachnoid blood layers within right frontal sulci (black arrows).

Table 11.1 Presence of any of the following signs/symptoms or risk factors for blunt cerebrovascular injury should prompt CT angiography of the neck

Signs/symptoms	Risk factors
Arterial hemorrhage from neck, nose, or mouth Expanding cervical hematoma Cervical bruit < 50 years of age Focal neurologic deficit: • TIA • Hemiparesis • Vertebrobasilar symptoms • Horner's syndrome	High-energy mechanism resulting in: • Le Fort II or III fractures • Mandible fracture • Complex skull fracture • Petrous bone fracture • Basilar skull fracture • Occipital condyle fracture
Neurologic deficit inconsistent with head CT Stroke by CT or MRI	Closed head injury consistent with diffuse axonal injury and GCS < 6 Cervical subluxation or ligamentous injury Fracture of cervical transverse foramen Cervical vertebral body fracture Any fracture of C1–C3 Scalp degloving Near-hanging with anoxic brain injury Seatbelt sign or clothesline type injury with significant swelling, pain, or altered mental status Traumatic brain injury and thoracic injuries Thoracic vascular injuries Blunt cardiac rupture

CT, computed tomography; GCS, Glasgow Coma Scale; MRI, magnetic resonance imaging; TIA, transient ischemic attack.
Reproduced with permission from Burlew et al., 2012.[13]

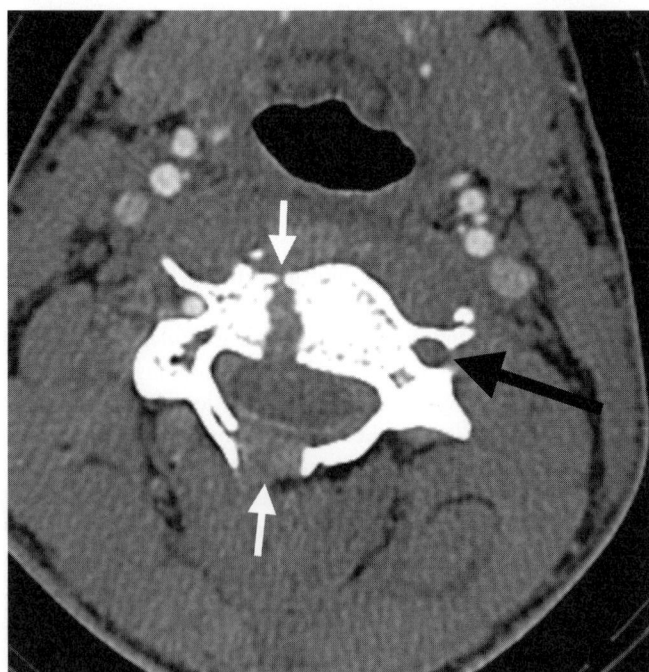

Figure 11.7 Axial image from contrast-enhanced neck CT angiography shows a sagittal-split fracture of C3 (white arrows) and complete occlusion of the left vertebral artery at the same level (black arrow).

"Macklin effect"). Lastly, chest CT enables reliable evaluation of the thoracic spine.

Abdomen and pelvis

Abdominopelvic CT in the setting of blunt trauma should almost invariably be performed with intravenous contrast to allow evaluation of parenchyma of solid abdominal organs and to detect and differentiate signs of direct arterial injury, namely active contrast extravasation and pseudoanuerysm. Imaging in the portal venous phase is most sensitive for solid organ injury, while arterial-phase imaging may be more sensitive for arterial injuries.[15] Regardless of phases of contrast opacification, biphasic imaging may improve specificity.[15] Ideally, the radiologist reviews abdominal images while the patient is still on the CT table, to facilitate rapid diagnosis and communication of findings, and to recommend and target delayed images to characterize positive CT findings. Noncontrast examination of these patients is severely limited and should be reserved for patients with significant renal impairment (acute renal impairment or stages 3, 4, or 5 chronic kidney disease) or prior life-threatening contrast reaction. Oral and rectal contrast is usually unnecessary in blunt trauma but may be used in the setting of penetrating flank or abdominal injuries when subtle bowel perforation is possible.[16]

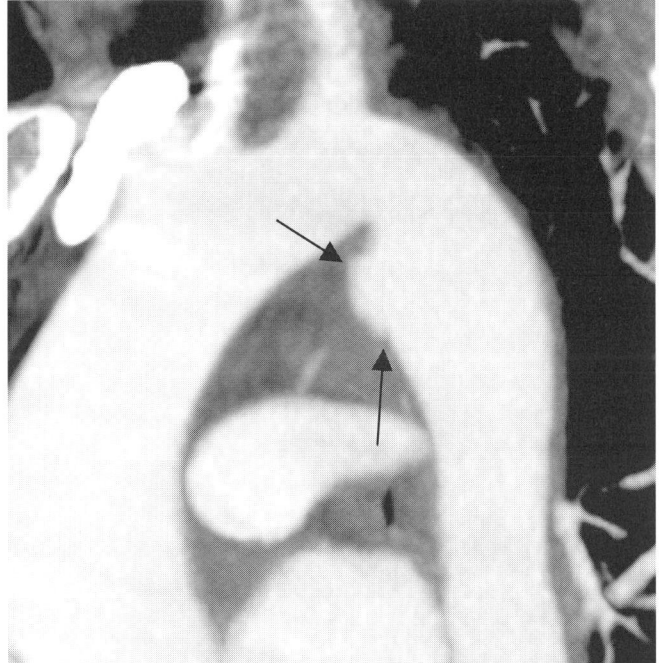

Figure 11.8 Sagittal oblique maximum intensity projection reconstructed from the chest CTA shown in Figure 11.3, showing pseudoaneurysm at the aortic isthmus (black arrows). This reconstruction often allows improved visualization of acute aortic injuries.

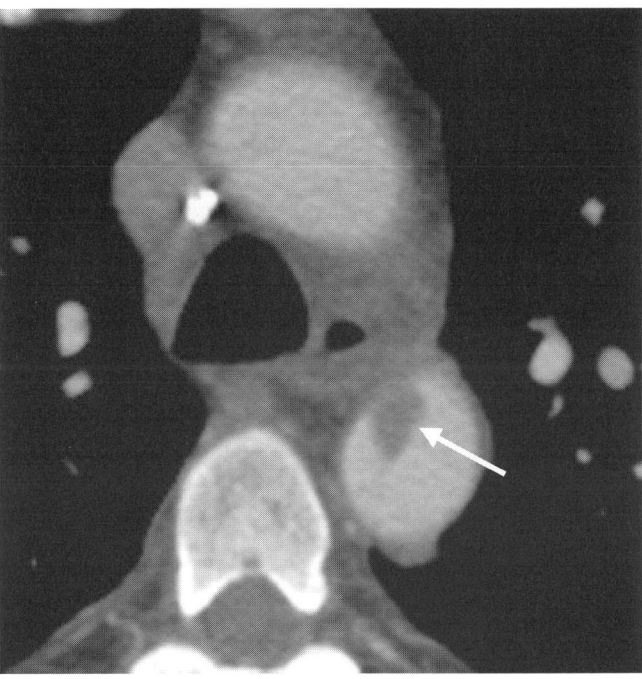

Figure 11.9 Axial image from contrast-enhanced chest CTA shows a thrombus (white arrow) within the lumen of the proximal descending aorta, compatible with minimal aortic injury. This was managed conservatively with blood pressure control and anticoagulation.

(A) (B) (C)

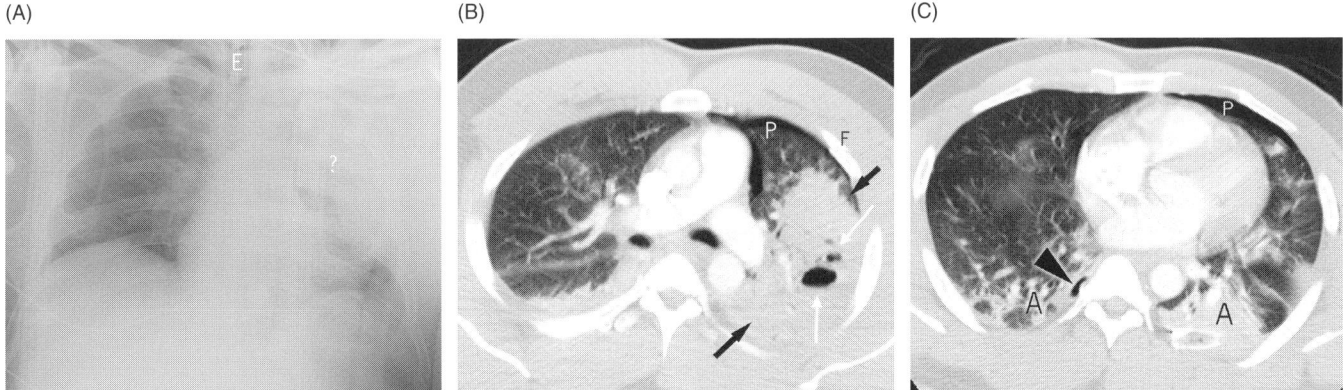

Figure 11.10 (A) Frontal chest radiograph from radiographic trauma series, 42-year-old man after high-speed motor vehicle crash. The endotracheal tube (E) is appropriately positioned. Left hemithorax opacity (?) is nonspecific, potentially contusion, aspiration, and hemothorax. No pneumothorax was detected radiographically. Select axial images from subsequent chest CTA in lung windows through the (B) mid and (c) lower thorax show multiple left lung lacerations (white arrows) within much larger contusion (black arrows). Radiographically occult left pneumothorax (P) is demonstrated anteriorly, adjacent to fracture (F) of the left third rib. A small right paraspinal lung laceration (black arrowhead) and bilateral lower lobe atelectasis (A) were also occult.

Contrast-enhanced abdominal CT in the venous phase is the preferred modality for detection of solid organ injury, with reported sensitivity of 92–97.6%, specificity of 98.7%, and negative predictive value of 99.63%.[1] Hepatic, splenic, adrenal, renal, and pancreatic lacerations or hematomas are usually readily appreciated (Figs. 11.11–11.13). Without intravenous contrast, organ injury severity is difficult to assess, and subtle parenchymal injuries may be invisible, particularly if there is no or minimal adjacent hemorrhage. Hollow visceral injuries and mesenteric injuries can be difficult to detect on CT, and

diagnostic peritoneal lavage (DPL) may be performed on patients with high likelihood of bowel and mesenteric injuries based on exam, history, or CT.[1] Intraperitoneal and retroperitoneal hematoma can be readily quantified by CT, and active vascular contrast extravasation can be localized if present at the time of imaging. The densest clot formation, known as the "sentinel clot sign,"[17] often occurs adjacent to the site of active bleeding (Fig. 11.14). Active bleeding can be differentiated from pseudoaneurysm using biphasic contrast-enhanced CT (Figs. 11.14, 11.15).

Venous-phase CT can identify renal parenchymal injuries, and delayed images, performed 5–15 minutes after contrast injection, can diagnose urine extravasation from the renal collecting system or ureter (Fig. 11.12). In patients with gross hematuria in the setting of pelvic fractures or fluid adjacent to the bladder without other explanation, a CT cystogram (with retrograde contrast injection into the urinary bladder via Foley catheter) can be performed to exclude or localize intraperitoneal and extraperitoneal bladder rupture (Fig. 11.16).

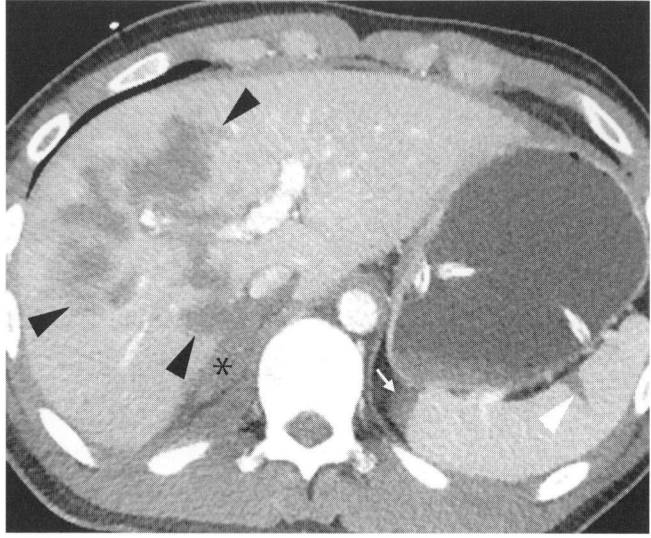

Figure 11.11 Axial contrast-enhanced CT of the upper abdomen in venous phase shows high-grade hepatic laceration (black arrowheads), right adrenal hematoma (asterisk), and small splenic laceration (white arrowhead) with small perisplenic hematoma (white arrow).

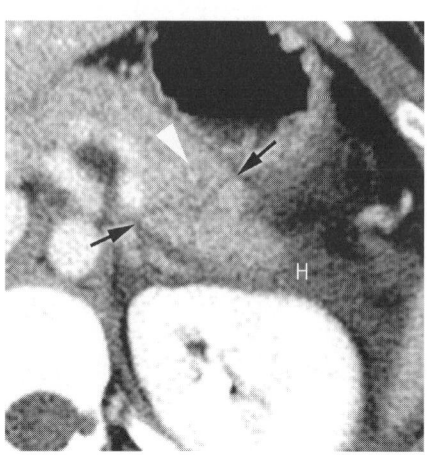

Figure 11.13 Axial contrast-enhanced CT image of the abdomen shows a laceration (black arrows) across the body–tail junction of the pancreas, surrounded by subtle, ill-defined contusion (white arrowhead). Retroperitoneal hematoma (H) is secondary to pancreatic injury and a splenic laceration (not shown). Injury to the pancreatic duct was suspected, based on the extent of the laceration. In the setting of increasing epigastric abdominal pain and serum amylase levels, the patient underwent laparotomy with splenectomy and distal pancreatectomy, which confirmed the CT findings.

(A)

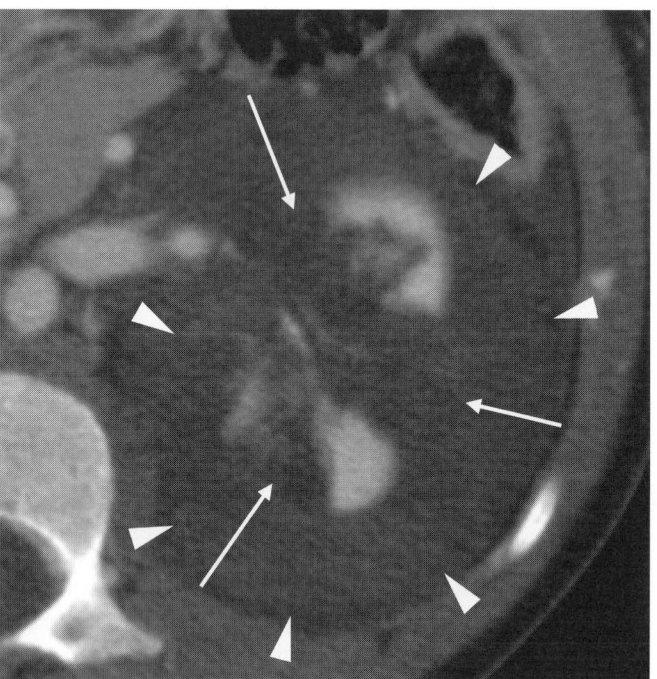

(B)

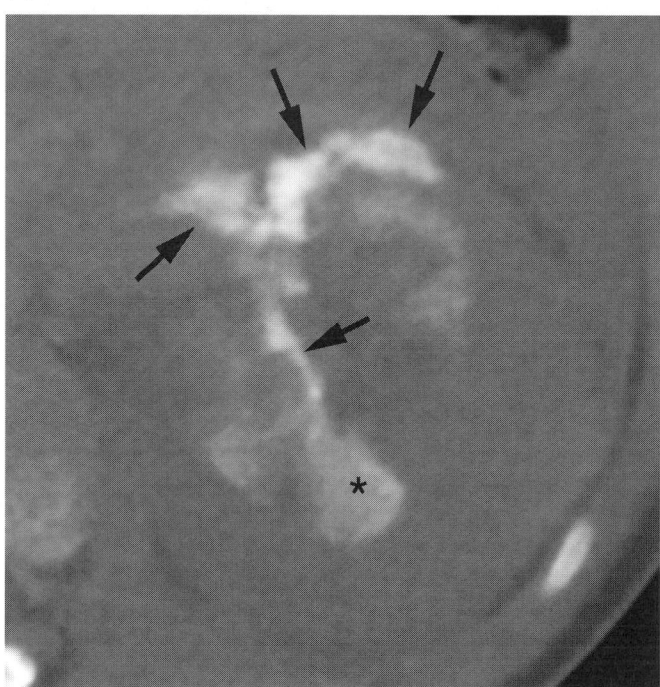

Figure 11.12 (**A**) Axial image from venous phase of contrast-enhanced CT of the kidneys in a 6-year-old girl after a fall shows multiple lacerations of the upper pole of the left kidney (white arrows), extending full-thickness from renal cortex to renal pelvic fat, and large perinephric hematoma (white arrowheads). (**B**) Corresponding axial image after 10-minute delay shows extravasation of contrast-opacified urine (black arrows) from the injured urinary collecting system, upgrading the Organ Injury Scale (OIS) grade from III to IV. Residual contrast staining of enhancing renal parenchyma (asterisk) indicates contrast retained within dysfunctional renal tubules, often as a result of renal contusion or parenchymal swelling.

(A)

(B)

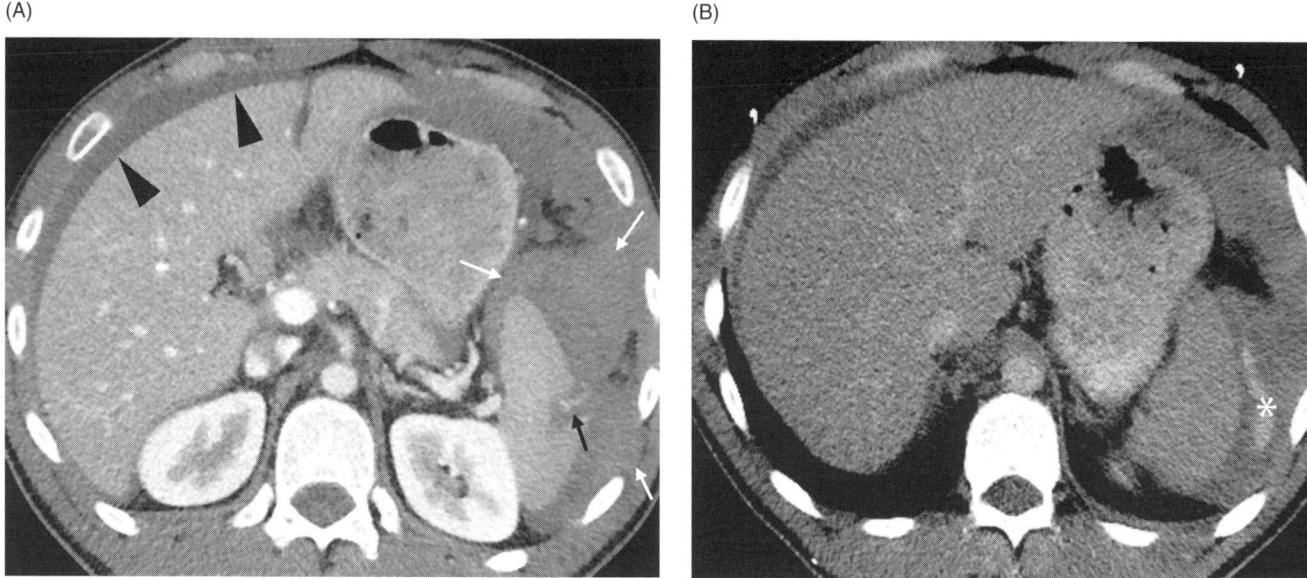

Figure 11.14 (**A**) Axial contrast-enhanced abdominal CT image in a 32-year-old man stabbed multiple times shows increased density of intraperitoneal hemorrhage in the left upper quadrant (white arrows) compared with the right upper quadrant (black arrowheads). This "sentinel clot sign" suggests hemorrhage most recently occurred in the left upper quadrant. The culprit is 17 mm deep splenic laceration with active contrast extravasation (black arrow). (**B**) Delayed axial image obtained 5 minutes later shows increased volume and redistribution of extravasated vascular contrast, now extending superiorly along the lateral aspect of the spleen (asterisk).

(A)

(B)

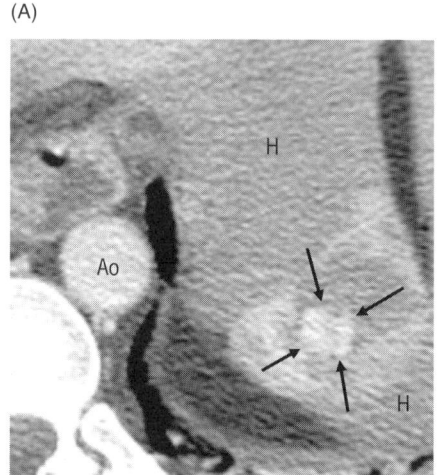

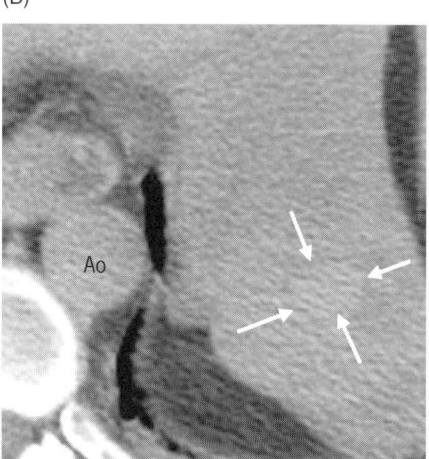

Figure 11.15 (**A**) Axial contrast-enhanced abdominal CT image in a 43-year-old man following a motor vehicle crash shows a complex splenic laceration and large parasplenic hematoma (H). Within the center of the laceration, a focal contrast collection (black arrows) is similar in density to the abdominal aorta (Ao). On this single phase, this could represent active contrast extravasation or pseudoaneurysm. (**B**) Delayed axial image obtained 12 minutes later shows a focal contrast collection (white arrows) of similar size and location, density again mirroring that of the abdominal aorta (Ao). This favors pseudoaneurysm with ongoing flow, rather than free contrast extravasation, though both indicate arterial vascular injury.

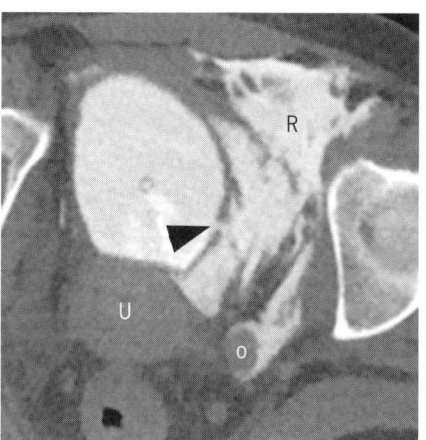

Figure 11.16 Axial image from CT cystogram shows extraperitoneal extravasation of contrast through a small defect (large black arrowhead) in the left lateral wall of the urinary bladder. No intraperitoneal contrast was detected. R, space of Retzius; O, left ovary; U, uterus.

Spine

Most patients sustaining blunt trauma qualify for some type of cervical spine imaging, whether by radiographs or by CT. Two clinical prediction rules exist to guide cervical spine radiography in low-risk patients after blunt trauma – the Canadian C-spine Rule (CCR) and the National Emergency X-radiography Utilization Study (NEXUS) low-risk criteria.[18] CT has superior sensitivity compared to plain radiographs for cervical spine injuries, particularly in older patients, and has been shown to be cost-effective, but has a higher radiation dose.[18]

Modern CT scanners are able to acquire images with near-isotropic voxels (equal resolution in three planes), allowing multiplanar reformations (MPR) in coronal and sagittal planes

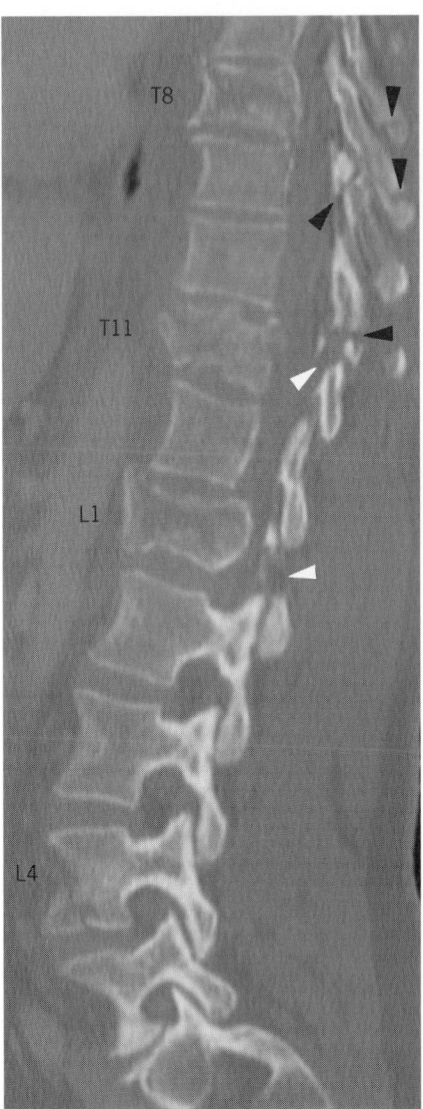

Figure 11.17 Reconstructed lumbar CT image in sagittal plane is shown in bone windows. Multilevel burst fractures resulting from motor vehicle crash are demonstrated at T8, T11, L1, and L4 (labeled), including laminar fractures at L1 and T11 (white arrowheads). Spinous process fractures are also seen at T7 through T10 (black arrowheads).

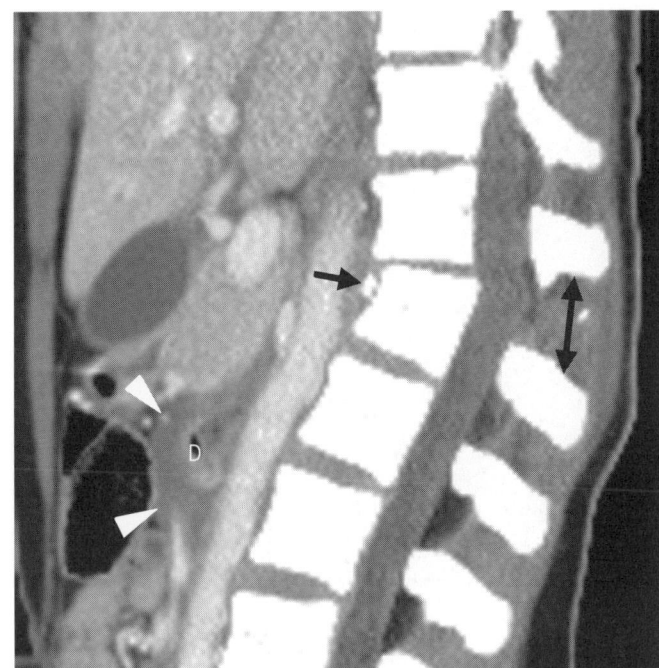

Figure 11.18 Sagittal image from abdominopelvic CT performed on a 14-year-old girl after a motor vehicle crash is shown in soft tissue windows. At L1 is a three-column flexion–distraction seatbelt-type injury, including focal kyphosis at T12–L1, widening of the T12–L1 interspinous space (double black arrow), and a small avulsion from the anterior superior endplate of L1 (black arrow). Hematoma (white arrowheads) encircling the third portion of the duodenum (D) reflects duodenal injury from compression between lapbelt and spine.

with image quality almost comparable to the axial images. This allows reformations of the spine in three dimensions from the body images without rescanning the patient, saving both time and radiation dose.[19]

Whole-spine imaging, whether by CT or by radiography, is important for almost all high-energy blunt trauma patients, with few exceptions. Spinal fractures can coexist at multiple levels and are often noncontiguous (Fig. 11.17). Even relatively mild-appearing fractures at the time of trauma may have progressive deformity and/or neurologic symptoms if not promptly recognized and appropriately treated (see Chapter 22). Axial-loading type injuries, such as resulting from falls, include anterior compression fractures and burst fractures, the latter of which are not infrequently associated with neurologic deficits. Seatbelt-type flexion–distraction injuries, including bony Chance fractures, are typically diagnosed after high-speed motor vehicle crashes and may have coexistent bowel, pancreatic, and aortic injuries detected on abdominal CT

(Fig. 11.18). Fracture–dislocations can follow any significant high-energy trauma and are highly unstable.

Certain patient populations benefit from primary CT assessment of the spine rather than radiographs. Anterior compression fractures, particularly prevalent in osteoporotic patients, may be difficult to age accurately by radiographs, often prompting a follow-up CT.[20] Morbidly obese patients often have suboptimal radiographic evaluation because of overlying soft tissue, contributing to poor photon penetration, excessive image noise, and higher radiation dose. Another special population of trauma patients includes those with ankylosing spondylitis, diffuse idiopathic spinal hyperostosis (DISH), or extensive surgical fusion or degenerative ankylosis. The relative rigidity of these spines predisposes to potentially devastating hyperextension-type fracture–dislocations with even minimal trauma (Fig. 11.19).[21] Radiographs in particular, but also CT, may underestimate or miss injuries in these patients, who may require a combination of CT and magnetic resonance imaging (MRI) for comprehensive spine evaluation.

Special considerations in specific trauma populations
Imaging the pregnant trauma patient

Following trauma, a fetus' best chance of survival depends on the survival of the mother, and thus appropriate radiography, CT, and angiography should not be delayed or avoided due to

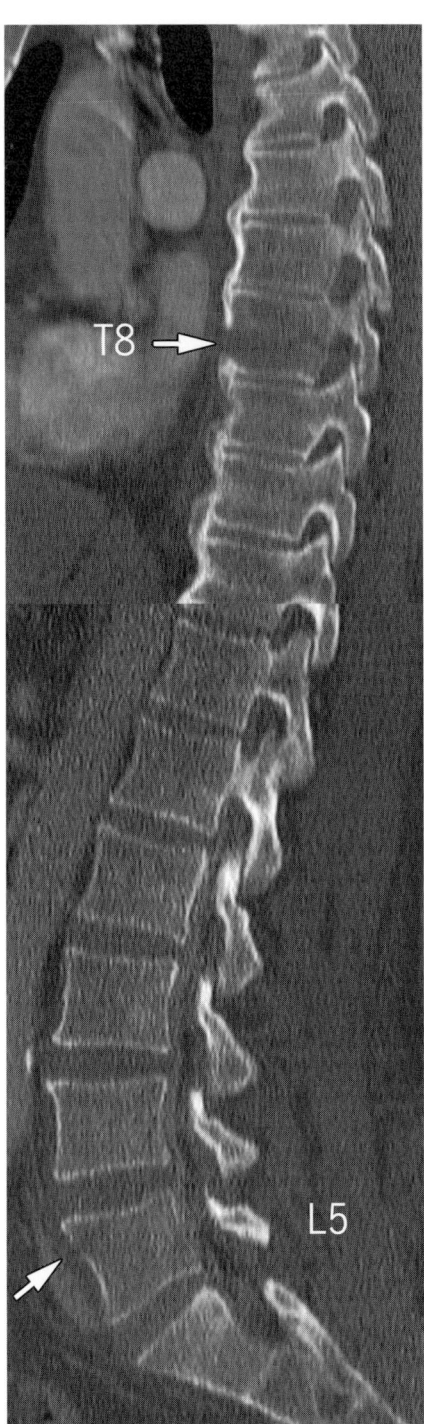

Figure 11.19
Composite sagittal image from thoracolumbar spine CT on a 58-year-old man with DISH hit by a car. Hyperextension fractures are present at T8 and L5 (white arrows). The T8 fracture predominantly involves bone, while the L5 fracture extended through the L5 superior endplate and propagated posteriorly through the disk space and ligamentous structures.

malformations, although any exposure to ionizing radiation likely increases the risk of childhood malignancy. For example, reported ranges for estimated fetal absorbed doses for abdominopelvic CT are 13–25 mgy. However, in severely traumatized women who undergo multiple CTs as well as catheter angiography, angioembolization, and orthopedic surgery, cumulative radiation doses can quickly exceed this acceptable threshold. In all cases, fetal dose can be calculated by a medical physicist, even retrospectively if pregnancy is not discovered until after image acquisition, such that the patient can be appropriately counseled.[23] MRI and ultrasound alternatives may be considered when appropriate, and informed consent is recommended when performing CT on stable pregnant patients.[23] CT should be performed with intravenous contrast, if indicated, while gadolinium should not be administered to pregnant patients during MRI.

When imaging is obtained in the pregnant trauma patient, close attention should be directed to evaluation of the uterus, placenta, and fetus, though these structures can be difficult to assess on CT. External fetal monitoring is essential, and is more sensitive than imaging, for diagnosis of placental abruption and other traumatic injuries resulting in fetal distress.[22]

Pediatric trauma patients

Blunt trauma in young children differs significantly from that in adults, and familiarity with the particular injury patterns and mechanisms commonly encountered in children is important to appropriate imaging and diagnosis. Given the higher radiation sensitivity of children, use of ionizing radiation should be limited to those exams that are absolutely necessary and should utilize appropriate radiation dose-reducing techniques.

Differences in pediatric anatomy, biomechanics, and mechanisms of trauma result in unique patterns of injury in children. The most common posttraumatic injuries in pediatric populations are upper and lower extremity fractures and intracranial injuries,[24] for which extremity radiographs and noncontrast head CT, respectively, are diagnostic. Types and location of spine and torso injuries also differ from those in adults, and diagnostic imaging may thus be tailored. For example, large cranial proportions, shape and articulation of partially ossified vertebral bodies, and relatively weak neck muscles predispose children younger than 9 years to upper cervical spine injuries (craniocervical junction to C2), while older children have mid and lower cervical spine injuries more typical of adult populations.[25] The focus of pediatric cervical spine imaging in young children should be primarily directed toward the upper cervical spine. If the child is undergoing head CT for exclusion or evaluation of intracranial injuries, the CT can be extended to the C3 midbody to include the upper cervical spine. If not performing head CT, radiographs can be obtained, but the odontoid process may be difficult to clear radiographically due to difficulty obtaining the open-mouth odontoid view. Imaging of the lower cervical spine in young children can usually be performed adequately with frontal and

pregnancy in a critically injured woman (see Chapter 37).[22,23] Imaging decisions for stable pregnant patients after trauma should be made on a case-by-case basis, weighing the risks of missing maternal injury with risks to the fetus of ionizing radiation.[23] Fetal risks of ionizing radiation depend both on gestational age and on dose magnitude, and include childhood cancer, cognitive impairment, organ malformation, and spontaneous abortion.[22] Most single diagnostic exams have fetal doses below 50 mgy, a level that likely confers no risk of fetal lateral radiographs without the need for CT. Spinal cord injury without radiologic abnormality (SWICORA) occurs more commonly in children than in adults. By definition, radiographs and CT are negative, and MRI is used to determine location and extent of spinal cord abnormalities.

Abdominopelvic CT is still the modality of choice for the evaluation of pediatric abdominal trauma, despite the use of ionizing radiation, though FAST exams may have some utility when used appropriately.[26] The relative paucity of intraabdominal fat in most children, and image noise from appropriately low-dose technique, may make characterization of subtle or low-grade intraabdominal injuries difficult even by CT. Chest CT is less frequently obtained in the pediatric population because of the low incidence of thoracic vascular injuries compared with adults.[27] Nevertheless, venous-phase CT may be appropriate to characterize lung and other thoracic injuries in a child with a high level of clinical suspicion or abnormalities detected on chest radiography.[27]

Emergent preoperative imaging in suspected brain herniation

Some victims of blunt trauma are identified in the field or early in their emergency department course as having severe head trauma with clinical signs indicating evolving brain herniation. In these otherwise hemodynamically stable patients, expedient craniotomy may avert this otherwise devastating event. Recognizing that even minutes' delay in surgery could be fatal, imaging in these patients is targeted to (1) confirming the presence of intracranial pathology, and if possible identifying its cause (e.g., epidural hemorrhage, intraparenchymal bleed), and (2) excluding other injuries that may become life-threatening while the patient is in the operating room. To this end, some facilities may adopt a CT protocol for rapidly screening these patients from head to thigh, without or with contrast. Image acquisition with modern scanners takes a matter of seconds, and the patient can then be transported quickly to surgery while the radiologist reviews axial images, alerting the surgeons and anesthesiologists to any significant findings within minutes. Of particular emphasis should be signs of active hemorrhage within the torso or abdomen, or of large pneumothorax, as these could shortly become clinically significant, and may manifest to the anesthesiologist as worsening patient instability in the operating room. Time can then be spent creating optimized reformations for detailed radiologist review and reporting, or the patient can be rescanned at a later time after stabilization by the emergent craniotomy.

Radiographs in stable trauma patients

As described, CT provides the bulk of diagnostic imaging of the torso and cranial soft tissues in the blunt trauma patient. Radiographs are particularly helpful in the timely assessment of the extremities for evidence of osseous injury when soft tissue swelling, laceration, deformity, or focal tenderness are elicited on clinical survey. Standard long-bone radiographs include frontal and lateral views, while joint imaging usually

entails a standard set of three to four images, aiding assessment of complex overlapping bony structures. Radiographic assessment of the bone and joints above and below a level of injury is usually advised. If complex intraarticular fractures or fracture-dislocation are detected, CT of the affected joint may be obtained to aid in orthopedic surgical planning and to detect additional radiographically occult injuries. Evidence of concomitant vascular injury on physical exam, such as asymmetric reduction in the ankle–brachial index (< 0.9) in the setting of a knee dislocation or diminished upper extremity pulses with concern for scapulothoracic dissociation, can be further assessed with CTA through the affected extremity.

MRI in acute trauma

Magnetic resonance imaging (MRI) is an imaging technique that allows better soft tissue characterization than CT without the use of ionizing radiation. Its utility is limited in the setting of trauma, however, for several reasons. First, the use of high magnetic fields for image acquisition requires meticulous pre-MRI screening to exclude ferromagnetic foreign material in the body and removal of certain equipment from the patient, all of which may be difficult in acute trauma. Secondly, most MRI exams routinely take 30–60 minutes to perform, compared with mere seconds for CT, and during this time the patient is isolated in the exam room without direct supervision or close monitoring. Furthermore, to obtain optimal MR images, patient cooperation must be maintained throughout the exam, which may be difficult for confused or injured patients. Lastly, in most cases, the soft tissue differentiating capacity of MRI is simply not needed for evaluation of acute injuries to solid organs. The primary exception to this, and thus the most likely reason a trauma patient will be referred for MRI, is for evaluation of spinal cord and ligamentous spinal injuries.[28] MRI may detect more extensive ligamentous injuries in a patient with relatively minimal displacement at the time of supine CT or radiographic assessment. In a patient with acute neurologic symptoms following trauma, with or without associated radiographic abnormalities, MRI is capable of differentiating spinal cord contusion from cord hemorrhage, an important prognostic indicator.[28] MRI is also useful in completion spine evaluation for patients with ankylosing spondylitis or DISH,[29] when bone marrow edema or fluid within an otherwise subtle fracture through bone or disk space may be detected.

Radiology in penetrating trauma

In penetrating trauma, the affected body regions are localized and usually readily identified on physical exam, while blunt trauma more often risks injury to the whole body and imaging must be more extensive. Hemodynamically unstable penetrating trauma patients usually undergo emergent surgical exploration with minimal initial imaging. This may include a complete FAST or limited sonographic assessment of the heart for evidence of pericardial effusion and possible tamponade.

For gunshot wounds, radiography (usually two views) is valuable to assess the final location of the bullet and to predict the bullet tract and likelihood of specific organ injuries. Preoperative chest radiography may be also obtained to identify the location of tubes and lines, and to exclude or characterize injuries to the thoracic cavity prior to laparotomy and/or thoracotomy.

Hemodynamically stable patients can have diagnostic imaging targeted to the region of penetrating injury. For penetrating injuries of the torso, imaging will often depend on the estimated depth of the wound based on direct exploration. Gunshot wounds suspected to penetrate the peritoneal cavity will often proceed directly to surgery without imaging. Conversely, low-velocity penetrating trauma such as stab wounds, and some gunshot wounds, may be evaluated with CT. If the penetrating wound is at a location where bowel injury may have occurred, triple-contrast CT using rectal, oral, and intravenous contrast should be considered,[16] along with delayed-phase CT if the trajectory is near the kidneys or ureters. If the penetrating trauma is localized to the extremities, radiographs, and extremity CTA if indicated, are usually sufficient for workup.

Interventional radiology in trauma

Twenty-four-hour access to interventional radiology (IR) is essential for Level I and Level II Trauma Center designation by the American College of Surgeons.[30] In coordination with trauma surgical services, IR plays a vital role in the control of hemorrhage and other traumatic vascular injuries. Triage of patients to surgery or to IR should be individualized based on availability and patient characteristics including hemodynamic stability, mechanism and injury types, and preexisting conditions.

Angiography and embolization of pelvic hemorrhage

Hemorrhage due to pelvic fractures from blunt trauma is associated with significant morbidity and mortality. Hemorrhage may occur from venous or arterial sources or from exposed bone edges.[8] The location of hemorrhage deep within the closed pelvic ring makes open surgical access difficult and time-consuming, increasing the risk of significant, potentially fatal, hemorrhage before obtaining surgical control. Angiography and transcatheter embolization, combined with open surgical and orthopedic stabilization, has therefore become the standard of care for control of pelvic hemorrhage.

Fracture pattern is not predictive of the presence of arterial hemorrhage.[7] Indications for angiography therefore include other clinical and imaging factors, as listed in Table 11.2.[7]

Only arterial sources of bleeding, which are found in 3–10% of patients, can be evaluated by angiography; however, embolization is highly successful in such cases.[31] An

Table 11.2 Indications for angiography in the setting of pelvic trauma[7]

Major pelvic fracture with signs of bleeding and ongoing transfusion requirements after nonpelvic bleeding sources are excluded
Pelvic fractures with hemodynamic instability after exclusion of nonpelvic sources of bleeding, even without evidence of active extravasation on CT
Pelvic fractures with active contrast extravasation at CT, regardless of hemodynamic status
Major pelvic fracture, with or without other associated injury, when pelvic bleeding cannot be surgically controlled

CT, computed tomography.

aortogram is usually obtained initially, followed by dedicated injections of the internal, and possibly external, iliac artery on each side. More selective catheterization can be performed if warranted. The arterial sheath can be left in short-term, after appropriately securing the device, if adequate hemostasis is expected to be difficult due to coagulopathy, if early repeat angiography is expected, or if the patient is going emergently to surgery. When feasible, the sheath is then removed and manual compression is applied until hemostasis is achieved at the femoral access site.

Signs of acute arterial injury on digital subtraction angiography, both in the pelvis and elsewhere, include active extravasation of contrast (Figs.11.4c and 11.20) or contrast "blush," pseudoaneurysm, sharp vessel cutoff, or slow flow.[8] Nonselective embolization is generally preferred in the anterior internal iliac artery distribution, while external iliac artery branch vessel injury (Fig. 11.20) requires more delicate selective angiography to prevent reflux of embolic material into the common femoral artery. Current embolic materials include permanent devices such as coils or an Amplatzer plug, or temporary materials such as gelatin sponge or slurry. The advantage of temporary embolic materials is that vascular recanalization occurs naturally within several weeks while promoting local thrombus formation for immediate vascular control.

Repeat angiography may sometimes be necessary. This may be particularly true in patients in whom initial embolization was selective, and in those with two or more injured vessels at initial embolization, recurrent hypotension, absence of intraabdominal injury, or persistent base deficit, or in those requiring pre-embolization blood transfusions.[7]

Complications can occur at the femoral access site or secondary to embolization. Most common is a self-limiting groin hematoma at the access site.[8] Femoral artery pseudoaneurysm or arteriovenous fistula are other potential complications that require intervention. Male erectile dysfunction has been attributed to the pelvic injury itself as opposed to bilateral internal iliac artery embolization.[32] Thus, pelvic trauma angioembolization is considered safe and effective.

(A)

(B)

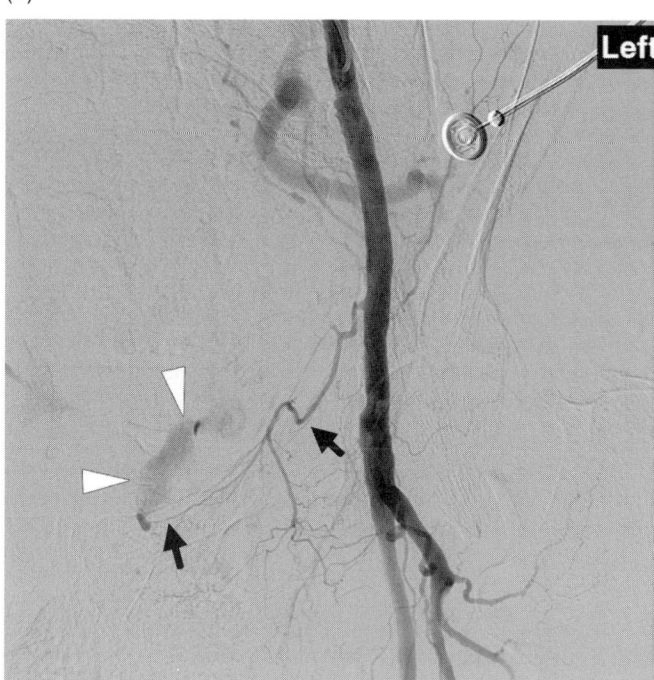

Figure 11.20 (**A**) Coronal reformation of contrast-enhanced abdominopelvic CT in an 86-year-old hypotensive woman after a motor vehicle crash shows active arterial contrast extravasation (white arrows) into a large pelvic hematoma (H), adjacent to minimally displaced fracture of the left superior pubic ramus (arrowheads). (**B**) Subsequent digital-subtraction angiogram of the left external iliac artery shows active extravasation (white arrowheads) arising from the replaced left obturator artery (black arrows). The patient's blood pressure stabilized after microcatheter embolization of this artery.

Visceral angiography and embolization for trauma

Endovascular treatment for intraperitoneal and retroperitoneal injuries is an alternative to surgical control. On occasion, an unstable patient sent to angiography because of concern for pelvic hematoma will instead have intraabdominal hemorrhage with active visceral contrast extravasation discovered at aortic angiogram. Temporary balloon occlusion of the feeding vessel may be performed, allowing transfer of the patient to the operating room for definitive open repair. Occasionally, emergent endovascular treatment might be preferred.

Preemptive endovascular treatment can be considered for stable patients with injuries with a high likelihood of hemorrhage or other complications. Actively bleeding or potentially hemorrhagic lesions that cannot be easily surgically controlled are an indication for angioembolization; these include intraparenchymal vascular injuries, such as are encountered in the spleen or kidneys, and posterior liver lacerations.[31] Remaining controversy regarding endovascular treatment of visceral lesions is primarily due to uncertainty in the natural history of these vascular injuries.

Splenic angioembolization

In recent decades, the trend toward nonoperative management of splenic injuries in stable patients has been highly successful. In some cases, embolization of traumatic splenic vascular lesions can avoid the need for splenectomy (Fig. 11.21a).[33] CT findings of active contrast extravasation,

pseudoaneurysm, high grade splenic laceration (Organ Injury Scaling, OIS grades 3–5), or large hemoperitoneum are associated with increased rate of failure of conservative management and therefore may benefit from early angiography and preemptive embolization if nonsurgical management is being considered.[33]

Hepatic angioembolization

Hepatic injuries detected by CT in stable patients will often be successfully managed by conservative observation regardless of grade. If CT evidence of active contrast extravasation or high-grade liver injury is found in a marginally stable patient responsive to initial resuscitation, angioembolization can be attempted, with a reported high rate of success (Fig. 11.21b).[34] Temporary embolization material is preferred, and embolization should be as selective as achievable to minimize tissue necrosis. IR can also assist with the management of delayed posttraumatic hepatic complications, including bile leak, infection, and delayed hemorrhage.[34]

Renal interventions

Traumatic renal lesions may involve the main renal artery or the renal parenchyma. Traumatic main renal artery injuries include intimal flaps, dissections, or transections, and can progress to renal artery thrombosis. Untreated, potential risks include retroperitoneal hemorrhage, renal infarct, or healing with residual renal artery stenosis and secondary hypertension.[35]

(A)

(B)

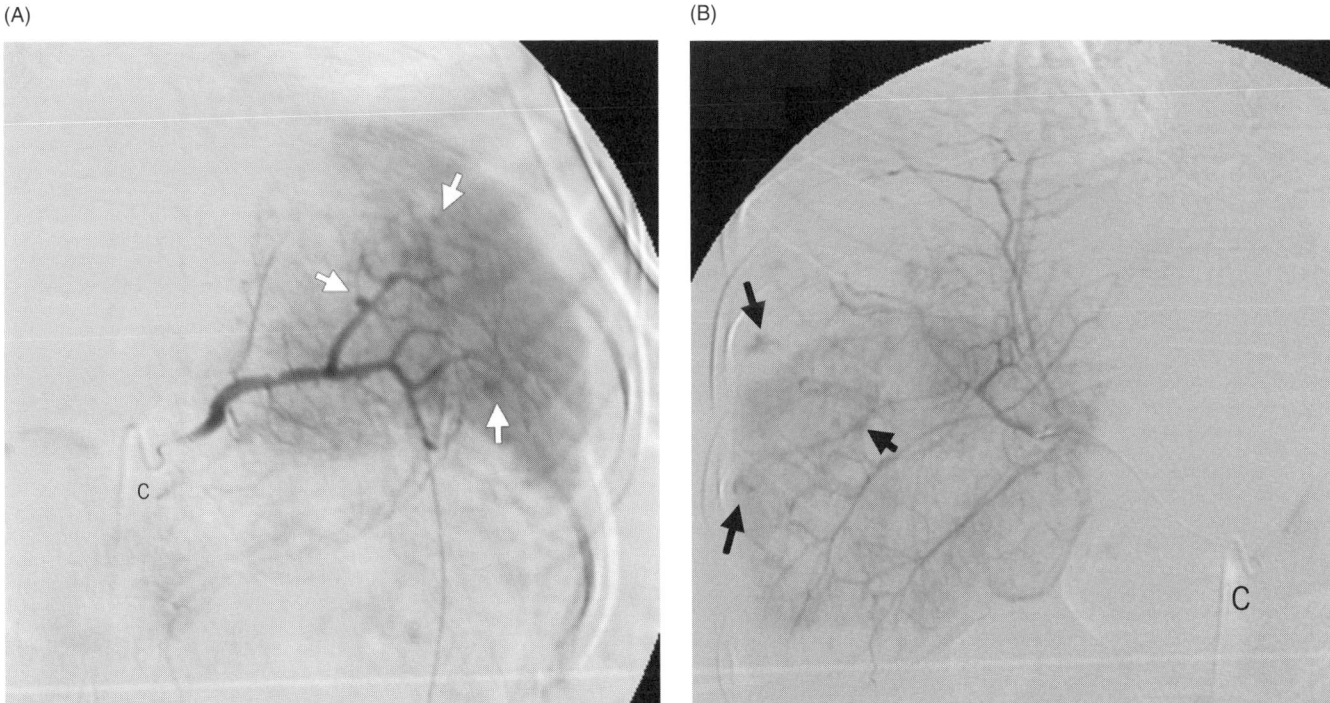

Figure 11.21 Spot images from digital-subtraction celiac angiogram in a 26-year-old woman with hepatic and splenic lacerations after a motor vehicle crash. (**A**) With a catheter (C) in the celiac axis, selective injection of the splenic artery shows multiple foci of contrast extravasation (white arrows), which were successfully embolized with gelatin slurry. (**B**) With the catheter (C) still in the celiac axis and a microcatheter advanced into the right hepatic artery, contrast injection shows multiple foci of contrast extravasation (black arrows) in the right hepatic lobe, which were successfully embolized with gelatin slurry and particles.

Endovascular treatment with main renal artery stenting has found some success compared with the poor outcomes generally achieved by surgical revascularization.[35]

Renal parenchymal lacerations, from either blunt or penetrating trauma, may result in pseudoaneurysm (Fig. 11.22) or arteriovenous fistula, both of which can result in pain, hematuria, or bleeding.[36] Intraparenchymal vascular lesions are usually treated with selective embolization by coils or gelatin slurry.[36] In selected patients, percutaneous ultrasound-guided embolization can be performed. The goal is to stop bleeding while preserving renal function. Repeat embolization may be needed if evidence suggests ongoing hemorrhage.[31]

Thoracic endovascular treatment

Arch aortography has been replaced by CTA for the detection of acute aortic injuries following blunt and penetrating trauma.[37] Endovascular treatment of traumatic thoracic aorta pseudoaneurysms (Fig. 11.23) is successful, with lower procedural mortality and morbidity rates compared to open repair (see Chapters 29 and 30).[38] Procedure success requires appropriate pre-procedural injury localization, graft choice, sizing, and anatomical characterization. Limitations to endovascular treatment include aortic arch diameter too large or too small for appropriate endograft sizing, and iliac arterial narrowing or stenosis precluding retrograde placement of the necessary large-caliber sheath.[39] Short-term complications include endoleak and access-related injuries, as well as those common to

open aortic repair, most importantly death, paraplegia, and stroke.[38] Long-term outcomes are still unknown, particularly in young patients with a narrow aortic diameter at the time of repair but who may develop luminal dilatation with age.

Cerebrovascular angiography in neurologic trauma

Catheter angiography for the diagnosis of acute blunt cerebrovascular trauma has been replaced in many centers by CTA.[40] Many patients with blunt cerebrovascular trauma can be managed conservatively with antithrombotics or anticoagulation. For patients with contraindications to anticoagulation, or pseudoaneurysm enlargement, progressive dissection, or neurologic deterioration while on conservative management, endovascular stenting can be considered as an alternative to surgery.[40] Endovascular techniques may also be considered for distal carotid artery injuries, where surgery entails extensive and difficult dissection at the mandibular angle.[40] Procedural success is related to operator experience. Controversy remains regarding type and duration of post-stent anticoagulation and imaging follow-up intervals.

Summary

Radiology plays an important role in the triage, diagnosis, and treatment of patients following blunt and penetrating trauma. Preliminary imaging workup can be performed in parallel to the primary trauma survey, particularly in hemodynamically

(A)

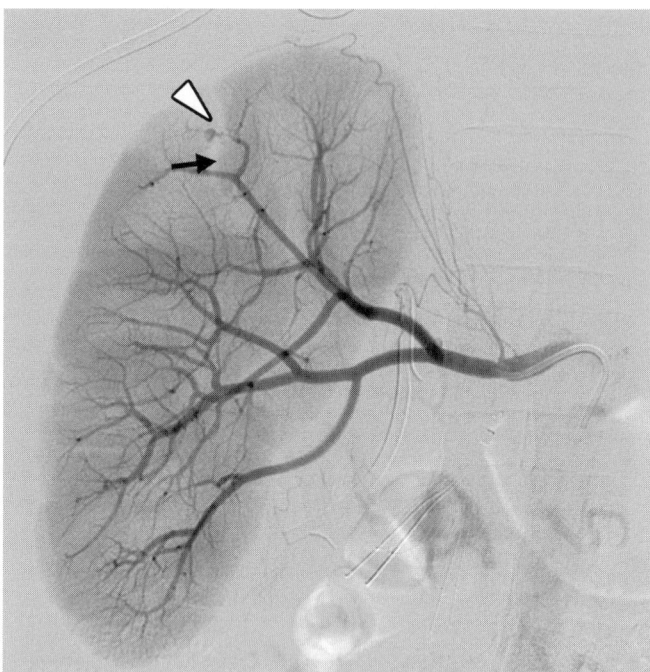

(B)

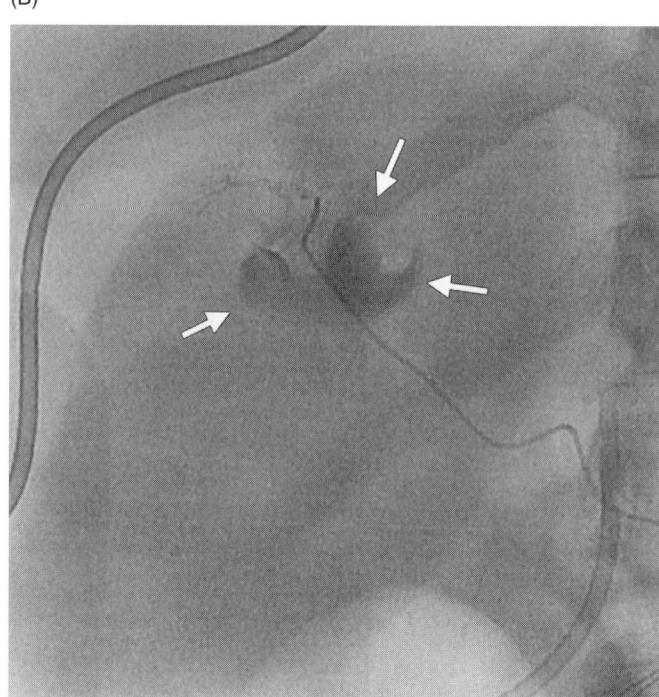

Figure 11.22 (**A**) Right renal artery digital-subtraction angiogram in a 45-year-old woman with intractable hematuria following right flank stab wound. Defect in enhancing right upper pole parenchyma (arrowhead) corresponds to known renal laceration. Within the laceration is a small pseudoaneurysm (black arrow). (**B**) Microcatheterization of the culprit upper pole branch shows extravasation of contrast from the pseudoaneurysm into the upper pole renal collecting system (white arrows). This was successfully controlled with a straight coil, with resolution of hematuria.

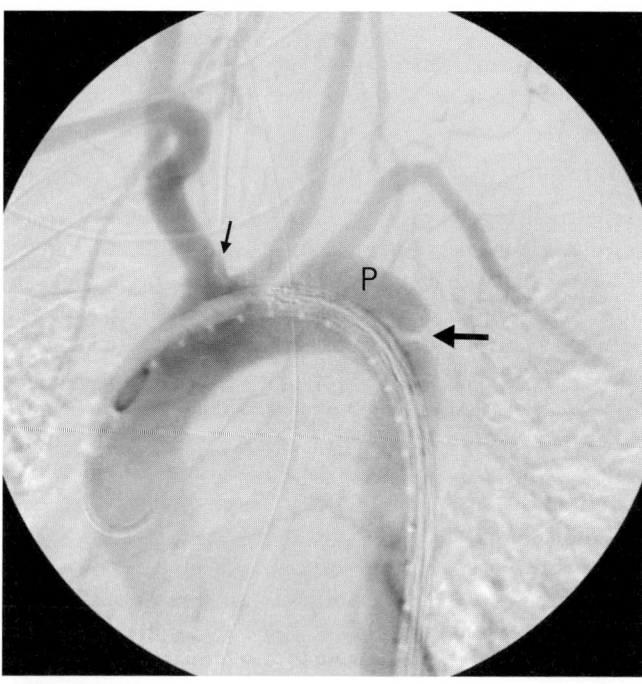

Figure 11.23 Spot image from intraprocedural digital-subtraction aortogram during endovascular repair of a traumatic aortic arch pseudoaneurysm. The pseudoaneurysm (P) and intimal flap (large black arrow) are most apparent at the superolateral wall of the aortic arch, as well as a small intimal flap at the origin of the brachiocephalic artery (small black arrow). Contrast is injected via a pigtail catheter with radiopaque markers, while the collapsed stent graft is positioned within the arch over a guidewire before deployment.

unstable patients. CT is the preferred modality for evaluation of the head and torso in stable patients.

Questions

(1) **Complementary to the primary trauma survey, initial imaging evaluation of an unstable blunt polytrauma patient may include:**
   a. Upright chest radiograph
   b. Frontal cervical spine radiograph
   c. Decubitus abdominal radiograph
   d. Frontal pelvic radiograph

(2) **Which of the following causes of acute hemodynamic instability cannot be suspected based on radiographs?**
   a. Saddle pulmonary embolism
   b. Tension pneumothorax
   c. Displaced pelvic ring disruption
   d. Traumatic aortic pseudoaneurysm
   e. Craniocervical dissociation

(3) **Of the following, mediastinal hematoma on chest CT is *least* likely attributed to:**
   a. Traumatic aortic pseudoaneurysm
   b. Tracheal laceration
   c. Mediastinal venous hemorrhage
   d. Sternal fracture
   e. Brachiocephalic artery injury

(4) Which of the following may be missed if abdominopelvic CT is performed only in the venous phase in the setting of trauma?
a. Splenic branch vessel injury with active contrast extravasation
b. Grade 1 hepatic laceration
c. Vena caval transection
d. Organ injury severity (OIS) grade 4 renal laceration
e. Full-thickness bowel wall laceration

(5) Noncontrast CT of the abdomen and pelvis would be the most valid emergent alternative to contrast-enhanced CT in which of the following trauma patients?
a. Stable 70-year-old woman without recent creatinine but history of mild renal insufficiency
b. Stable 17-year-old football player with mild left upper quadrant pain and concern for splenic laceration
c. Marginally stable 3-year-old boy with severe abdominal trauma and distended abdomen
d. 35-year-old type 1 diabetic on chronic hemodialysis with history of anaphylactic reaction during prior fistulogram

(6) Of the following spine injury types, which is most frequently associated with additional intraabdominal injuries, including aortic, duodenal, and pancreatic injuries?
a. Three-column burst fracture
b. Hyperextension fracture–dislocation
c. Flexion–distraction injury
d. Anterior compression fractures at three or more levels

(7) MRI is used in the setting of trauma for which of the following?
a. Characterization of bony Chance fracture extent
b. Noncontrast evaluation of the aorta for acute aortic injury
c. Differentiation of spinal cord hemorrhage from cord contusion
d. Alternative to CT for evaluation of extraaxial intracranial hemorrhage

(8) Regarding imaging of penetrating trauma, which of the following is *false*?
a. Primary survey imaging may include chest radiograph, complete FAST or even more focused

sonographic assessment, and if applicable radiograph of the body region through which a bullet has passed
b. Imaging can be limited to specific body regions based on the external exam
c. Because of potential ricochet and blast effect, all patients with gunshot wounds should have whole-body imaging
d. Abdominopelvic CT may be performed with rectal, oral, and intravenous contrast (triple contrast)

(9) Which of the following is among the indications for pelvic angiography?
a. Hemodynamically stable patient with open-book pelvic fracture
b. Hemodynamically stable patient with several foci of active contrast extravasation on pelvis CT
c. Patient with pelvic fractures and positive DPL (diagnostic peritoneal lavage), requiring ongoing blood transfusions
d. Vertical shear pelvic ring disruption
e. Hemodynamically unstable patient with pelvic fracture and positive FAST

(10) Conservative (nonsurgical) management of traumatic injuries may include endovascular treatment of which of the following injury types?
a. Intraparenchymal splenic artery pseudoaneurysm
b. Inferior vena cava transection
c. Minimal aortic injury without distal embolization
d. Mesenteric injury with devascularized segment of small bowel
e. Intracranial epidural hematoma

Answers

(1) d
(2) a
(3) b
(4) d
(5) d
(6) c
(7) c
(8) c
(9) b
(10) c

References

1. Hoff WS, Holevar M, Nagy KK, *et al.* Practice management guidelines for the evaluation of blunt abdominal trauma: the East practice management guidelines work group. *J Trauma* 2002; 53: 602–15.

2. Friese RS, Malekzadeh S, Shafi S, Gentilello LM, Starr A. Abdominal ultrasound is an unreliable modality for the detection of hemoperitoneum in patients with pelvic fracture. *J Trauma* 2007;63:97–102.

3. Kool DR, Blickman JG. Advanced Trauma Life Support. ABCDE from a radiological point of view. *Emerg Radiol* 2007; 14: 135–41.

4. Gunn ML. Imaging of aortic and branch vessel trauma. *Radiol Clin N Am* 2012; 50: 85–103.

5. Blaivas M, Lyon M, Duggal S. A prospective comparison of supine chest radiography and bedside ultrasound for the diagnosis of traumatic pneumothorax. *Acad Emerg Med* 2005; 12: 844–9.

6. Ekeh AP, Peterson W, Woods RJ, *et al.* Is chest x-ray an adequate screening tool for the diagnosis of blunt thoracic aortic injury? *J Trauma* 2008; 65: 1088–92.

7. Cullinane DC, Schiller HJ, Zielinski MD, *et al.* Eastern Association for the Surgery of Trauma practice management guidelines for hemorrhage in pelvic fracture: update and systematic review. *J Trauma* 2011; **71**: 1850–68.

8. Frevert S, Dahl B, Lonn L. Update on the roles of angiography and embolisation in pelvic fracture. *Injury* 2008; **39**: 1290–4.

9. Yeguiayan JM, Yap A, Freysz M, *et al.* Impact of whole-body computed tomography on mortality and surgical management of severe blunt trauma. *Crit Care* 2012; **16**: R101.

10. Sierink JC, Saltzherr TP, Reitsma JB, *et al.* Systematic review and meta-analysis of immediate total-body computed tomography compared with selective radiological imaging of injured patients. *Br J Surg* 2012; **99** (Suppl 1): 52–8.

11. Huber-Wagner S, Lefering R, Qvick LM, *et al.* Effect of whole-body CT during trauma resuscitation on survival: a retrospective, multicentre study. *Lancet* 2009; **373**: 1455–61.

12. Sierink JC, Saltzherr TP, Beenen LF, *et al.* A multicenter, randomized controlled trial of immediate total-body CT scanning in trauma patients (REACT-2). *BMC Emerg Med* 2012; **12**: 4.

13. Burlew CC, Biffl WL, Moore EE, *et al.* Blunt cerebrovascular injuries: redefining screening criteria in the era of noninvasive diagnosis. *J Trauma Acute Care Surg* 2012; **72**: 330–5.

14. Battle CE, Hutchings H, Evans PA. Risk factors that predict mortality in patients with blunt chest wall trauma: a systematic review and meta-analysis. *Injury* 2012; **43**: 8–17.

15. Dreizin D, Munera F. Blunt polytrauma: evaluation with 64-section whole-body CT angiography. *Radiographics* 2012; **32**: 609–31.

16. Chiu WC, Shanmuganathan K, Mirvis SE, Scalea TM. Determining the need for laparatomy in penetrating torso trauma: a prospective study using triple-contrast enhanced abdominopelvic computed tomography. *J Trauma* 2001; **51**: 860–8.

17. Orwig D, Federle MP. Localized clotted blood as evidence of visceral trauma on CT: The sentinel clot sign. *AJR Am J Roentgenol* 1989; **153**: 747–9.

18. Anderson PA, Gugala Z, Lindsey RW, Schoenfeld AJ, Harris MB. Clearing the cervical spine in the blunt trauma patient. *J Am Acad Orthop Surg* 2010; **18**: 149–59.

19. Sheridan R, Peralta R, Rhea J, Ptak T, Novelline R. Reformatted visceral protocol helical computed tomographic scanning allows conventional radiographs of the thoracic and lumbar spine to be eliminated in the evaluation of blunt trauma patients. *J Trauma* 2003; **55**: 665–9.

20. Lenchik L, Rogers LF, Delmas PD, Genant HK. Diagnosis of osteoporotic vertebral fractures: importance of recognition and description by radiologists. *AJR Am J Roentgenol* 2004; **183**: 949–58.

21. Westerveld LA, Verlaan JJ, Oner FC. Spinal fractures in patients with ankylosing spinal disorders: a systematic review of the literature on treatment, neurological status and complications. *Eur Spine J* 2009; **18**: 145–56.

22. Puri A, Khadem P, Ahmed S, Yadav P, Al-Dulaimy K. Imaging of trauma in a pregnant patient. *Semin Ultrasound CT MR* 2012; **33**: 37–45.

23. Sadro C, Bernstein MP, Kanal KM. Imaging of trauma. Part 2, abdominal trauma and pregnancy: a radiologist's guide to doing what is best for the mother and baby. *AJR Am J Roentgenol* 2012; **199**: 1207–19.

24. Guice KS, Cassidy LD, Oldham KT. Traumatic injury and children: a national assessment. *J Trauma* 2007; **63**: S68–80.

25. Mohseni S, Talving P, Branco BC, *et al.* Effect of age on cervical spine injury in pediatric population: a National Trauma Data Bank review. *J Pediatr Surg* 2011; **46**: 1771–6.

26. Schonfeld D, Lee LK. Blunt abdominal trauma in children. *Curr Opin Pediatr* 2012; **24**: 314–18.

27. Hammer MR, Dillman JR, Chong ST, Strouse PJ. Imaging of pediatric thoracic trauma. *Semin Roentgenol* 2012; **47**: 135–46.

28. Lammertse D, Dungan D, Dreisbach J, *et al.* Neuroimaging in traumatic spinal cord injury: an evidence-based review for clinical practice and research. Report of the National Institute on Disability and Rehabilitation Research Spinal Cord Injury Measures Meeting. *J Spinal Cord Med* 2007; **30**: 205–14.

29. Campagna R, Pessis E, Feydy A, *et al.* Fractures of the ankylosed spine: MDCT and MRI with emphasis on individual anatomic spinal structures. *AJR Am J Roentgenol* 2009; **192**: 987–95.

30. Amcrican College of Surgeons. Consultation/verification program: reference guide of suggested classification. VRC criteria type I and type II for level I trauma centers. 2006. http://www.facs.org/trauma/vrc1.pdf (accessed July 2014).

31. Velmahos GC, Toutouzas KG, Vassiliu P, *et al.* A prospective study on the safety and efficacy of angiographic embolization for pelvic and visceral injuries. *J Trauma* 2002; **53**: 303–8.

32. Ramirez JI, Velmahos GC, Best CR, Chan LS, Demetriades D. Male sexual function after bilateral internal iliac artery embolization for pelvic fracture. *J Trauma* 2004; **56**: 734–41.

33. van der Vlies CH, van Delden OM, Punt BJ, *et al.* Literature review of the role of ultrasound, computed tomography, and transcatheter arterial embolization for the treatment of traumatic splenic injuries. *Cardiovasc Intervent Radiol* 2010; **33**: 1079–87.

34. Taourel P, Vernhet H, Suau A, *et al.* Vascular emergencies in liver trauma. *Eur J Radiol* 2007; **64**: 73–82.

35. Lopera JE, Suri R, Kroma G, Gadani S, Dolmatch B. Traumatic occlusion and dissection of the main renal artery: endovascular treatment. *J Vasc Interv Radiol* 2011; **22**: 1570–4.

36. Ngo TC, Lee JJ, Gonzalgo ML. Renal pseudoaneurysm: an overview. *Nat Rev Urol* 2010; **7**: 619–25.

37. Demetriades D, Velmahos GC, Scalea TM, *et al.* Diagnosis and treatment of blunt thoracic aortic injuries: Changing perspectives. *J Trauma* 2008; **64**: 1415–19.

38. Kwolek CJ, Blazick E. Current management of traumatic thoracic aortic injury. *Semin Vasc Surg* 2010; **23**: 215–20.

39. Adams JD, Garcia LM, Kern JA. Endovascular repair of the thoracic aorta. *Surg Clin North Am* 2009; **89**: 895–912, ix.

40. Moulakakis KG, Mylonas S, Avgerinos E, Kotsis T, Liapis CD. An update of the role of endovascular repair in blunt carotid artery trauma. *Eur J Vasc Endovasc Surg* 2010; **40**: 312–19.

Chapter

12

Ultrasound procedures in trauma

Paul Soeding and Peter Hebbard

Objectives

(1) Identify the role of ultrasound in trauma.
(2) Understand the technique of neurovascular and pleural/lung examination.
(3) Identify normal neurovascular appearance and injury.
(4) Understand ultrasound-guided regional anesthesia.
(5) Understand ultrasound-guided vascular cannulation.
(6) Identify ultrasound features of both normal pleura and lung in addition to abnormalities following trauma.

Introduction

Ultrasound examination plays an increasingly important role in trauma management and anesthesia. Sonographic examination of peripheral nerves and vasculature can not only assess injury, but also guide needles for vascular access and regional anesthesia. Ultrasound-guided cannulation of arteries and veins allows invasive hemodynamic monitoring and fluid resuscitation in the trauma patient. Regional anesthesia provides immediate analgesia of injured limbs and enables specific surgical intervention. This chapter will focus on neurovascular anatomy and its recognition by ultrasound. The examination and identification of individual sonoanatomy is the basis for all ultrasound-guided procedures.

The recent development of portable high-frequency ultrasound units has made ultrasound examination an important component in the assessment of the trauma patient. Trauma management requires both resuscitation and careful systematic assessment of individual wounds, both evident and suspected. Injury, however, can often be difficult to evaluate, especially when it is concealed, such as in the case of blunt abdominal trauma or neurovascular injury associated with limb fracture. Sonography can be applied first as a diagnostic tool in the individual patient (see Chapter 10), and second as a guide in therapeutic procedures.[1]

A focused sonographic examination of the chest and abdomen can identify internal organ injury and hemorrhage and diagnose life-threatening injury such as cardiac tamponade and tension pneumothorax. Ultrasound-guided pericardiocentesis and thoracic chest-tube placement are valuable procedures in resuscitation. Clinical neurologic assessment is limited in the unconscious patient, and ultrasonic examination of limbs can provide assessment of neurovascular injury associated with fractured bones. High-resolution sonography can be used to support clinical and electrophysiologic testing in the detection of nerve abnormalities, including entrapment neuropathies, traumas, infectious disorders, and tumors. The advantages of bedside ultrasound examination are the immediate visualization of anatomical injury and the support of clinical examination and diagnosis.

In addition to their diagnostic role, ultrasound-guided procedures enable regional anesthesia and vascular cannulation to be performed under direct imaging (Table 12.1). Neural blockade may be performed to provide immediate analgesia or anesthesia for definitive surgical management (see Chapter 16). The use of ultrasound in the combat trauma patient illustrates this point perfectly.[2] Wounded soldiers with multiple injuries can have regional anesthesia performed in the field under ultrasound guidance, for immediate analgesia and management. For example, ultrasound can guide regional blockade of the brachial plexus in upper limb fracture or amputation, the femoral nerve in femoral fracture, the posterior tibial nerve in ankle fracture, or the intercostal nerves in rib fracture. In limb trauma, ultrasound can guide injection for regional anesthesia and has the advantage of targeting nerves without the need to elicit painful motor responses with neurostimulation. Regional anesthesia may also bring the benefits of preemptive analgesia and improvement of microcirculatory flow in the injured limb.

Vascular cannulation is an important component of resuscitation, and is necessary for invasive hemodynamic monitoring (see Chapter 5). The reflex vasoconstriction and reduced circulating blood volume resulting from hemorrhage can make palpation of the vasculature difficult. Ultrasound can be used to identify vascular structures, both arterial and venous, and accurately guide needles for cannulation using the Seldinger

---

Table 12.1 Advantages and disadvantages of ultrasound for nerve blocks and vascular procedures

	Advantages	Disadvantages
Nerve blocks	Improved reliability • Surface landmarks not required • Individual anatomy identified • New approaches possible • Accurate deposition of local anesthetic Reduced complications • Avoidance of neural, vascular, pleural contact • Monitoring of injectate spread and adjustment of needle Lower doses Improved patient comfort	More complex procedure • May require assistant • Increased set-up time • New skill to learn • Training and credentialing • Sterility Technical variations in image quality • Resolution poorer at greater depths/low frequencies • Difficulty visualizing needle at acute angles to beam • Inter-individual variation in visibility • Overconfidence if needle tip not clearly visualized May become reliant on new technology
Vascular access	Reduced complications • Arterial puncture • Pleural puncture Faster procedure • Ability to avoid unfavorable anatomy, e.g., small veins • Fewer needle passes • Improved patient comfort Detection of pathology • Thrombosis • Low flow states/ischemia	More complex procedure • May require assistant • Increased set up time • New skill to learn • Training and credentialing • Sterility Overconfidence if needle tip not clearly visualized

technique. Cannulation of the radial or femoral arteries allows transduction of systemic blood pressure. Cannulation of central veins enables rapid fluid and drug administration during resuscitation.

Ultrasound-guided regional anesthesia

Since the first report of supraclavicular brachial plexus block using Doppler ultrasound in 1978, ultrasound-assisted nerve block has been described for localization of the brachial plexus, lumbar plexus, and sciatic and femoral nerves. Outcome studies have shown ultrasound-guided techniques to provide greater accuracy, quicker onset, and less morbidity than conventional techniques. Conventional techniques rely on surface anatomical landmarks that define the probable location of nerves, and in trauma these may be distorted or even inaccessible from bandaging and splinting. With ultrasound, neural structures can be individually identified, and percutaneous injection can be directed under direct vision toward a target nerve. Successful regional anesthesia requires an accurate knowledge of nerves and their pathways, and relationship to vascular and anatomical structures.

In contrast, neurostimulation requires the tip to be in close proximity to the nerve in order to elicit a motor or sensory response. As with all landmark techniques, neurostimulation essentially remains a blind technique. The use of techniques that cause the limb to move may be painful, particularly in trauma. The risk of needle contact with vascular and neural structures remains, and in some patients, despite an elicited motor response, unexplained failure of anesthesia can occur. Ultrasound studies have shown that, even when a stimulating needle is in direct contact with a nerve, stimulation may not occur. Mechanical contact with nerves, intraneural injection, or local anesthetic toxicity can all result in neurapraxia. The use of ultrasound-guided regional anesthesia can, in experienced hands, reduce the complications of nerve contact and vascular puncture, reducing morbidity.[3,4]

Ultrasonography of nerve probes

Modern ultrasound probes comprise an array of piezoelectric elements that transmit and receive ultrasound waves. As sound waves travel through tissue, they are reflected at interfaces of altered acoustic impedance. These reflected waves form a real-time sonographic image of neural anatomy. Linear-array probes have multiple channels that emit parallel beams for enhancement of resolution, whereas sector probes with divergent beams provide less resolution. The wavelength of transmission determines penetration depth, with shorter wavelengths having less tissue penetration but higher image resolution. As frequency decreases, tissue penetration is increased, but image resolution is diminished. Probes with a frequency range between 5 and 15 MHz enable greater flexibility when examining different anatomical regions for neural elements.

Modern ultrasound systems enable high-resolution imaging of nerves by using appropriate software to enhance tissue contrast (Fig. 12.1). Subcutaneous tissues reflect sound waves at varying degrees, depending on acoustic impedance. The manner in which the dynamic range of this input signal is processed determines the image quality on screen. High-level gray-scale contrast results in precisely defined sonographic images. In general, a high-frequency, linear-array probe should be used for nerve, musculoskeletal, or vascular imaging.

Sonographic appearance of nerves

The appearance of a peripheral nerve depends on its size and the angle of insonation. Connective tissue surrounding nerve fascicles is often strongly reflected, producing a bright (hyperechogenic) circular or oval rim on transverse scanning (Table 12.2, Fig. 12.2). The interior of the nerve often appears dark (hypoechoic) and can have a granular appearance, depending on its fascicular architecture. Individual fascicles are surrounded by perineurium, and larger nerves with several fascicles may be invested within a capsule called the epineurium. In the long axis, nerves appear as a band of strongly

reflective interrupted parallel lines, distinguished from tendons, which have a continuous linear-patterned appearance (Fig. 12.3). This linear fascicular pattern is a feature of larger nerves and is absent in small nerves.

The sonographic appearance of neural structures may be altered if the angle of insonation is oblique, and reflection is

Table 12.2 Ultrasound characteristics of different body tissues

Tissue	Deformability	Texture	Anisotropy
Fat	Deformable	Hypoechoic with fine lines	No
Muscle	Deformable Slides in fascial planes	Coarse texture generally hypoechoic	No
Bone	No	Fine bright line, shadowing behind	No
Proximal nerve	Slides	Hypoechoic center, bright outside rim	Yes, only outer rim
Distal nerve	Slides	Fascicular, showing as parallel lines in long axis	Yes
Tendon	Slides	Fine-textured fascicular, more distinct than nerves	Yes
Vein	Compresses easily, sometimes pulsatile if large	Anechoic	No
Artery	Compresses with firm pressure, often not completely; pulsatile	Anechoic	No

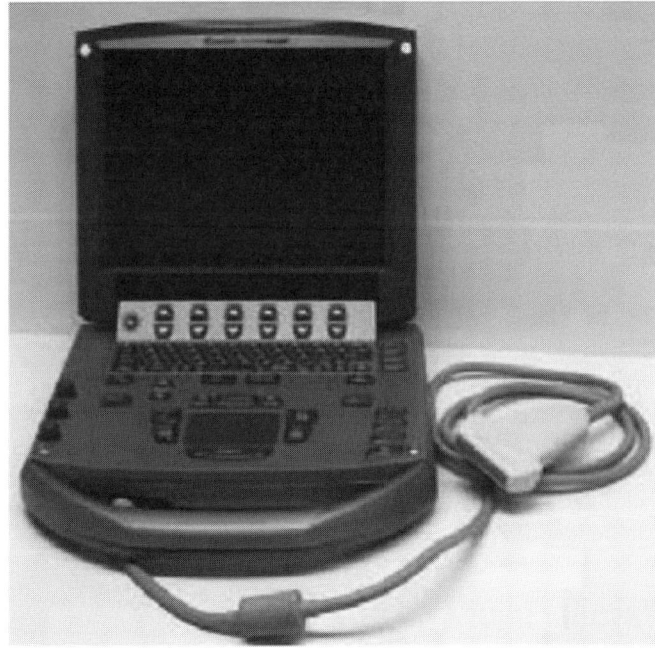

Figure 12.1 Portable ultrasound system: SonoSite MicroMaxx with linear-array transducer.

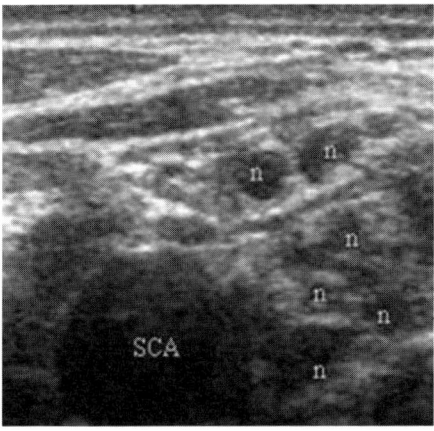

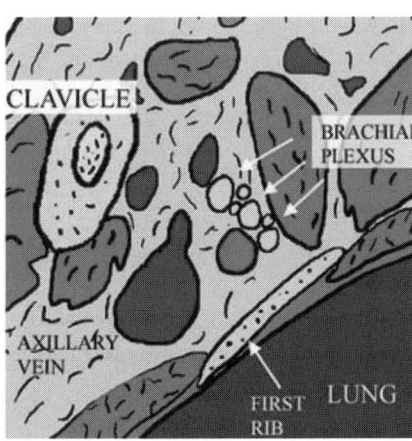

Figure 12.2 Supraclavicular sonogram of neural elements (n) adjacent to subclavian artery (SCA). *A black and white version of this figure will appear in some formats. For the color version, please refer to the plate section.*

193

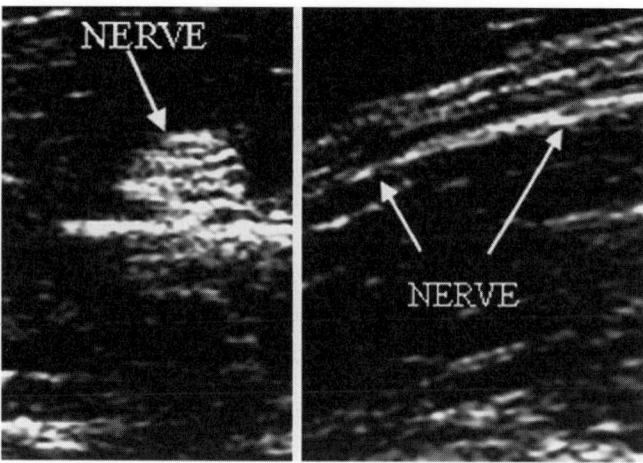

Figure 12.3 Long- and short-axis view of a typical peripheral nerve, the median nerve in the forearm.

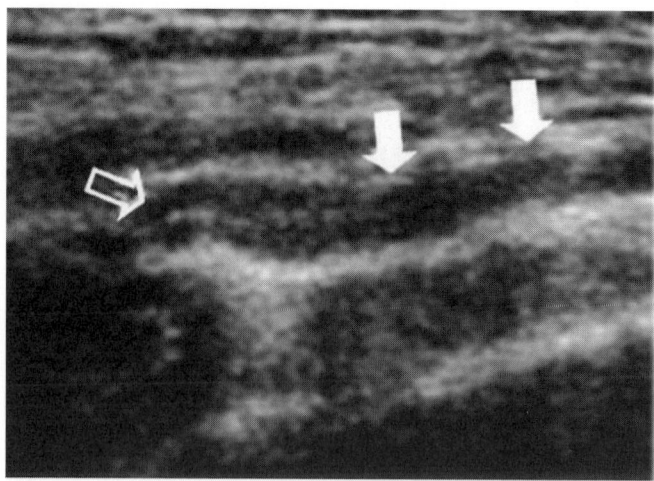

Figure 12.4 Longitudinal view of hypoechoic and enlarged radial nerve (solid arrows) with disrupted proximal end (open arrow) in spiral fracture of the humerus.

returned tangentially to the transducer. In such situations nerve rims may appear hypoechoic rather than hyperechoic in relation to surrounding tissues. This appearance due to oblique reflection is known as anisotropy, and it is dependent on examination technique. Anisotropy is useful when identifying distal nerves, as they characteristically "light up" on the ultrasound image when the beam is perpendicular. Surrounding vascular structures are poorly reflective and appear anechoic, though arterial vessels often appear pulsatile. Veins are nonpulsatile in the periphery (although the central veins may show a pulse with a dominant inwards movement) and are easily compressed by surface pressure. Arteries pulsate outwards, particularly if partly compressed, whereas large veins pulse inwards. Fat and muscle (except perimysium) appear hypoechoic, tendons hyperechoic with pronounced anisotropy, and bone strongly hyperechoic.

Peripheral nerve injury

Sonographic neural mapping requires a sound knowledge of anatomy as well as acquisition of skills in ultrasound technique. Examination of a peripheral nerve for injury requires identification of its proximal position or origin and tracing of its course distally down a limb. Neurovascular and muscular relationships need to be identified, and neural echotexture needs to be evaluated for the appearance of injury. The sciatic nerve, for example, can be mapped with ultrasound as it exits the greater sciatic foramen, travels beneath the gluteal muscles into the thigh, and extends distally to become the posterior tibial nerve at the popliteal fossa. Similarly the brachial plexus can be examined sonographically above and below the clavicle and followed to the axilla where it branches into its terminal branches: the radial, ulnar, median, and musculocutaneous nerves.

The mechanism of traumatic nerve injury can involve laceration, contusion, compression, or stretching of a nerve.[5] This may be associated with surrounding soft tissue injury, hematoma formation, or displacement of bone fractures. Radial nerve injuries associated with fractures of the humerus are the most common nerve injury seen in traumatic long-

bone fractures. The radial nerve is particularly susceptible to injury because of its close relationship to the humerus and its relative immobility as it pierces the lateral intermuscular septum of the arm. Injury is more likely to occur with fractures of the middle and distal thirds of the humerus. Direct contact with bony fragments can result in laceration, while entrapment of the nerve within hematoma can also occur. Ultrasound examination can identify altered nerve size and shape,[6] with enlargement and loss of normal fascicular pattern being a diagnostic feature of diffuse nerve swelling (Fig. 12.4). In other cases, complete rupture of nerve continuity, partial laceration, formation of traumatic neuroma, or entrapment within hematoma or callus may be seen. Once the technique of sonographic examination is mastered, the site and extent of neural injury can be identified and correlated to clinical findings.

Vascular injury

Similarly, traumatic arterial injury can present clinically as active bleeding, rapidly growing and pulsatile hematoma, pale and cold extremities, absent or very weak distal pulses, associated neurologic deficits, and associated injuries to bony and soft tissues. Traumatic brachial artery injuries constitute a relatively large proportion of peripheral arterial injury. Doppler ultrasonography of the upper extremity has been shown to be as specific and sensitive as arteriography in detecting brachial artery injuries.[7] Doppler ultrasonography can detect reduced arterial systolic pressures and flow, which is diagnostic for arterial injury.

Technique of ultrasound-guided regional anesthesia
Terminology

Because ultrasound is essentially a two-dimensional medium, a terminology has grown to describe the orientation between the beam and structures imaged. Images that are transverse to a

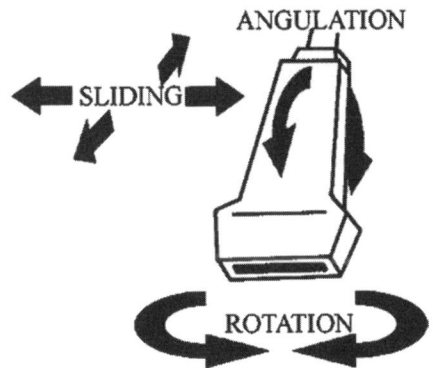

Figure 12.5
Movements of the ultrasound probe.

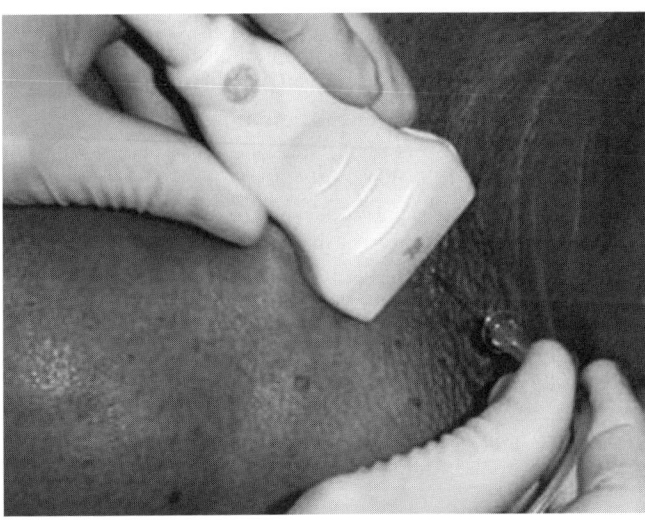

Figure 12.6 Regional anesthesia using an ultrasound probe (across-plane approach).

given structure are said to be "short axis," whereas images that are longitudinal are called "long axis."

Movements of the probe

The most common movement of a linear probe involves angulation. With angulation, deep structures will move far more than those near the surface, as the beam is angled from a fixed line on the surface. Probe rotation is used to align structures either in the short axis or the long axis. Only in the axis of rotation is the image constant. The probe may also be slid along the skin either in the plane of the beam or transversely; if the probe remains in the same orientation, all structures are moved equally within the beam (Fig. 12.5).

Angulation

The initial preparation involves an appropriate choice of settings for frequency and gain. The image gain should be adjusted to obtain an even brightness from top to bottom. For color Doppler, scale settings should have a low-velocity limit (about 15 cm/second) and the gain adjusted to the maximum that does not produce color on solid tissues. A sterile sheath should be used for ultrasound-guided procedures. Sterile gel, water, saline, or antiseptic may be used on the skin as an ultrasonic coupling medium. Removal of air from the injectate syringe, tubing, and regional needle is mandatory, since injected air grossly obscures sonographic anatomy. The technique of ultrasound examination involves the use of gentle pressure on the skin to avoid anatomical distortion. Fine movements of the probe are used to visualize target nerves and surrounding anatomy. By using a gentle sweeping pattern of the probe, individual sonography can be better visualized initially. The use of pressure from the probe may help define anatomical structures as they move relative to one another. Rotating the probe from short- to long-axis planes also defines relational anatomy. Color flow Doppler can help identify vascular structures, and gentle pressure can compress venous structures, distinguishing them from arterial vessels. Once a target nerve is identified sonographically, the image is centered and a direct route for needle advancement is chosen.

The probe is held either transversely or longitudinally with respect to the nerve (Fig. 12.6), and local anesthetic infiltration is applied to the skin adjacent to the probe. The regional needle

is initially advanced through the skin only a few millimeters. The needle tip position is monitored on the screen and, if not readily seen, can be identified by a gentle oscillatory movement of the needle shaft, which causes surrounding tissue movement. Transverse positioning of the probe with respect to the needle (out of plane) enables imaging of only part of the needle, with the rest of the needle shaft remaining out of the visual plane. Movements of the probe, angulation, or sliding (translation) are used to identify the needle tip. Longitudinal positioning (in plane) enables visualization of the whole needle shaft and tip, and this is a preferred alignment for some practitioners. Rotation from transverse to longitudinal axes is determined by the size of the probe footprint and the anatomical area under investigation.

Needle imaging

The major factors determining the visibility of a needle under ultrasound are the angle of the needle to the ultrasound beam, the reflecting characteristics of the needle, and the ultrasound texture of the surrounding tissue.[8] All needles reflect ultrasound best when positioned so that the ultrasound waves are traveling at close to perpendicular to the needle. When angled acutely to the beam smaller needles become difficult to see, particularly at depth. Larger needles are generally easier to see, and some needles are available with coatings to improve visibility. Fluid injected via the needle is seen as an expanding hypoechoic (black) area on the image; this may help to locate the position of the tip. In general, if the needle tip has a machined cutting edge it is more brightly reflecting than the shaft. Needle placement with respect to the ultrasound beam is either out of plane or in plane. If the needle is introduced some distance from the probe to subsequently come into the beam at the same depth as the target (from around a curved body surface), it is then introduced in an in-plane perpendicular orientation (Fig. 12.7).

The needle tip is advanced under direct vision, avoiding contact with vascular or neural structures. Regardless of orientation, keeping the tip in vision requires careful technique and repeated small angulation movements of the probe to ensure that the tip is seen. Once the tip is placed adjacent to a target nerve, local anesthetic solution is injected and monitored as it invests the nerve. Local anesthetic may be seen depositing in the wrong plane, in which case the needle can be repositioned after only a small amount of injectate. Sometimes injectate may start in an apparently ideal position but stream away from the nerve, often up the needle track. The injection should be stopped and the needle repositioned. Intravascular injection is evident by the lack of injectate seen distending tissues. Careful aspiration is still required before injection; however, the visualization of injectate spreading in the tissue is reassuring and further evidence for the correct deposition of local anesthetic. For each target nerve the needle tip can be repositioned and local anesthetic injected separately. Often the injection itself may move the nerve, and the needle can be repositioned to achieve full paraneural infiltration. Since injectate can be accurately placed, less total volume is often required. Local anesthetic completely surrounding the nerve appears to be optimal for rapid block onset. Most large nerves are known to have a paraneural sheath, outside the anatomical epineurium, which may be the optimal site for injection.[9] In this position the local anesthetic both curves around the nerve in the short-axis view and passes along the nerve.

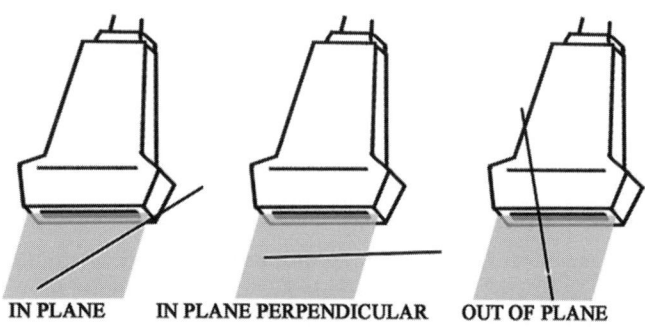

IN PLANE **IN PLANE PERPENDICULAR** **OUT OF PLANE**

Figure 12.7 Orientation of the needle with respect to the ultrasound probe.

Placement of catheters is also facilitated by ultrasound, with ultrasound imaging ensuring that the catheter lies adjacent to the nerve as it is railroaded into place. Studies have shown high success with catheter placement using ultrasound guidance.[10]

Brachial plexus examination

The brachial plexus originates from cervical (C5–C8) and thoracic (T1) nerve roots that form the superior, middle, and inferior trunks. The plexus travels to the base of the posterior triangle of the neck, where the trunks divide into anterior and posterior divisions, at the lateral edge of the first rib. These pass infraclavicularly to form cords around the axillary artery before entering the axilla.[11]

Interscalene block

Ultrasound examination begins by placing the ultrasound probe on the neck, adjacent to the cricoid cartilage, then moving it laterally over the sternocleidomastoid muscle. Identification of the carotid artery, internal jugular vein, and adjacent thyroid tissue provides reference landmarks. With further movement of the probe, the trunks of the plexus are located within the interscalene groove formed by anterior and medial scalene muscles (Fig. 12.8). Deep and medial to these trunks, the acoustic shadow of the C6 transverse process may be seen. The vertebral artery and vein may also be identified anterior to the posterior bony process of the C7 transverse process, with proximal nerve roots posterior to the vertebral vessels. Important anatomical variations seen at this level include slips of muscle dividing the interscalene groove into two, intramuscular location of nerves, and the presence of a large transverse cervical artery crossing the interscalene groove. Pre-procedural scanning is necessary to identify the plexus and branches such as the phrenic nerve, which typically arises from C4–C5 to travel on the anterior surface of the anterior scalene muscle. Similarly, the dorsal scapular nerve leaves the upper interscalene plexus posteriorly and travels through the scalenus medius muscle to supply the rhomboid muscle. Both these nerves should be identified before needle insertion, to avoid contact.

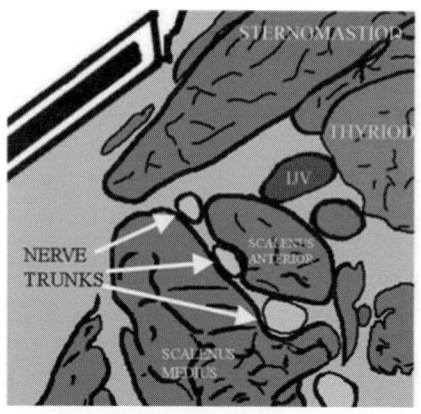
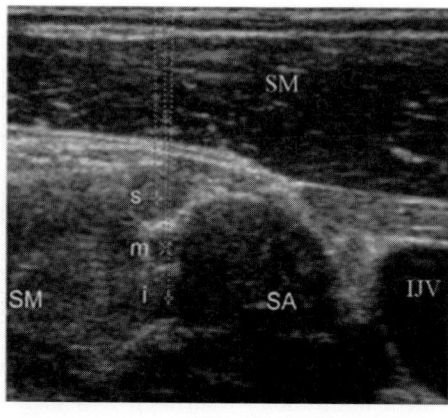

Figure 12.8 Sonographic anatomy of the brachial plexus in the interscalene region: scalenus medius (SM), scalenus anterior (SA), and sternomastoid muscle (SM); superior (s), middle (m), and inferior (i) trunks. IJV, internal jugular vein. *A black and white version of this figure will appear in some formats. For the color version, please refer to the plate section.*

If the plexus is not clearly imaged the nerves may also be followed upwards from the supraclavicular area.

Supraclavicular block

Ultrasonography of the supraclavicular region involves placement of the transducer above the midpoint of the clavicle. Alternatively, the imaged interscalene brachial plexus can be followed downward and laterally to reach the supraclavicular region. The key structure for orientation is the subclavian artery, which is located between the scalene muscles. Color flow Doppler will readily identify this vessel as well as distinguish neural elements from arterial and venous branches (in particular, the suprascapular and transverse cervical branches).

The primary trunks divide into their anterior and posterior branches, which appear as a cluster of nodules adjacent to the subclavian artery, usually in a cephaloposterior relation (Fig. 12.9). Distribution can vary, with elements of the inferior trunk occasionally positioned inferior to the artery, which may lead to ulnar sparing after blockade. The omohyoid muscle is seen overlying the plexus superficially, and the strong reflective signal of the first rib is noted inferiorly. The cervical pleura lies behind the rib and is an important landmark to define, in order to prevent inadvertent pleural puncture with injection. The dorsal scapular artery, if present, may be seen passing through the supraclavicular brachial plexus. The suprascapular nerve may be imaged leaving the plexus in a superficial and posterior position immediately deep to the omohyoid.

Infraclavicular block

Infraclavicular examination requires placement of the probe below the midpoint of the clavicle. The plexus and axillary vessels are located deep to the overlying pectoralis major and minor muscles as well as to the clavipectoral fascia. A lower ultrasound frequency is often required for adequate penetration. Deep to these structures, the ribs appear highly reflective and the pleura is easily identified.

Color flow Doppler is helpful in identifying the axillary artery and its thoracoacromial branch in this area. More distal branches of the axillary artery include the long thoracic, subscapular, and humeral circumflex arteries. The axillary vein is located inferomedial to the artery and receives the cephalic vein at this level of the clavipectoral triangle. The plexus divisions are initially located cranial to the axillary artery and, as they travel over the first rib, they group to form medial, lateral, and posterior cords around the artery. The medial cord is often positioned between the artery and vein (Fig. 12.10). Identification of individual cords using ultrasound is only possible in optimally imaged subjects. The block can be successfully performed by periarterial deposition of local anesthetic. It is important to place local anesthetic deep to the artery for successful blockade.

Axillary block

The axillary artery enters the axilla and lies within the internal bicipital groove formed by biceps and coracobrachialis superiorly and triceps inferiorly. A transverse view of the axillary artery is obtained by placing the probe 90 degrees over the sulcus, adjacent to the pectoral fold. The nerves are positioned around the artery and, in general, the median nerve lies anterior, ulnar nerve inferior, and radial nerve posterior to the artery. The nerves are easily identified using a technique to

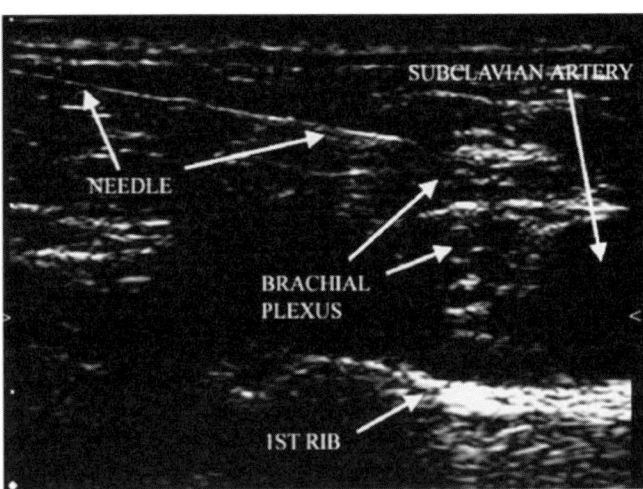

Figure 12.9 Sonogram of supraclavicular block.

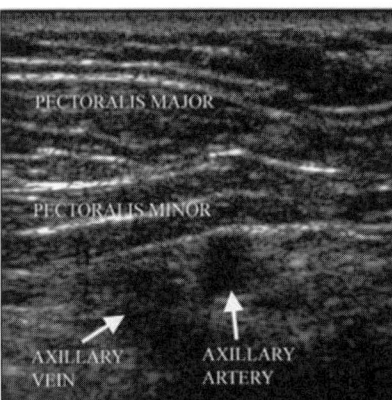

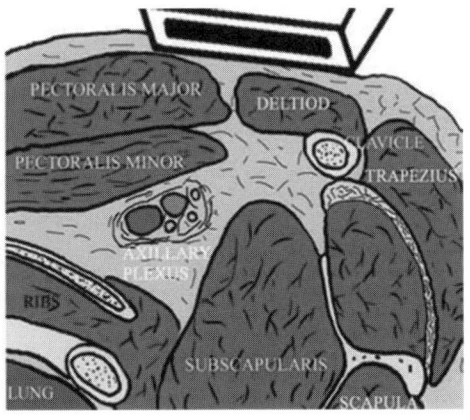

Figure 12.10 Sonographic anatomy of the brachial plexus in the infraclavicular region, medial to the coracoid. *A black and white version of this figure will appear in some formats. For the color version, please refer to the plate section.*

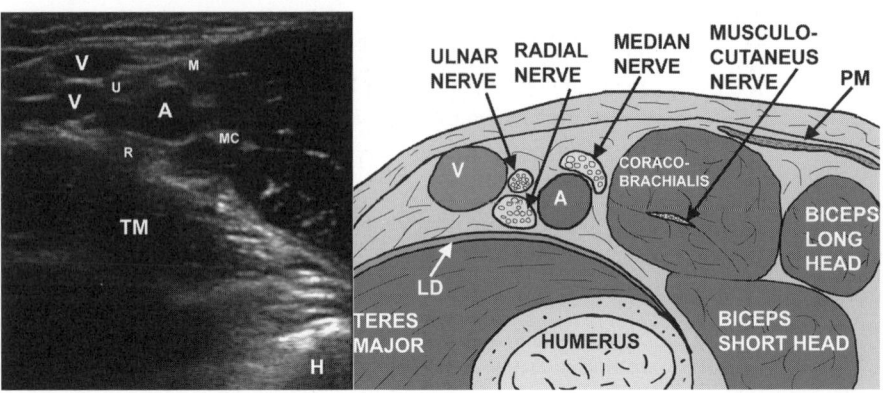

Figure 12.11 Sonographic anatomy of the brachial plexus in the axillary region: median nerve (M) ulnar nerve (U), radial nerve (R), musculo-cutaneous nerve (MC), axillary artery (A), axillary vein (V), humerus (H), teres major muscle (TM), pectoralis major tendon (PM), latissimus dorsi tendon (LD). *A black and white version of this figure will appear in some formats. For the color version, please refer to the plate section.*

trace the nerves down the arm. The median nerve stays in association with the brachial artery, the ulnar nerve courses posteriorly just deep to the deep fascia and towards the medial epicondyle, and the radial nerve passes deep and into the radial groove of the humerus in association with a prominent artery. Because the radial nerve passes away deeply from the ultra-sound probe, angulation towards the posterior axilla is required to highlight the nerve by anisotropy as the probe slides down the arm. The musculocutaneous nerve originates high in the axilla and travels on the aponeurotic surface or within the body of coracobrachialis. This accounts for its sparing during axillary brachial plexus anesthesia. The distri-bution of nerve positions can vary, as shown in Figure 12.11. Multiple venous structures are usually present, increasing the risk of intravascular injection with blind percutaneous tech-niques. Axillary block can be performed as a fascial sheath block using a large volume of local anesthetic or as four individual nerve blocks using a small volume for each nerve.[12] Provided circumferential spread of local anesthetic is achieved by needle manipulation, successful axillary block has been described with as little as 4 mL of local anesthetic in total. This may therefore be the block of choice for the upper limb if performing multiple limb blocks or needing to minimize the dose of local anesthetic.

The distal nerves in the forearm

The terminal branches of the brachial plexus can be mapped individually as they travel from the axilla down the arm. A nerve block of these branches at the elbow produces effective analgesia and anesthesia in their respective distributions (Fig. 12.12). Targeted injection in the lower forearm is an effective approach for hand surgery.

The radial nerve travels from the axilla between the medial and lateral heads of triceps obliquely along the spiral groove of the humerus, and pierces the intermuscular septum to enter the posterior compartment of the arm. Above the elbow it then travels anteriorly to lie between brachialis and brachioradialis muscles. The nerve enters the lateral part of the cubital fossa, dividing into the superficial radial and posterior interosseous branches. In the cubital fossa it is well identified in the short

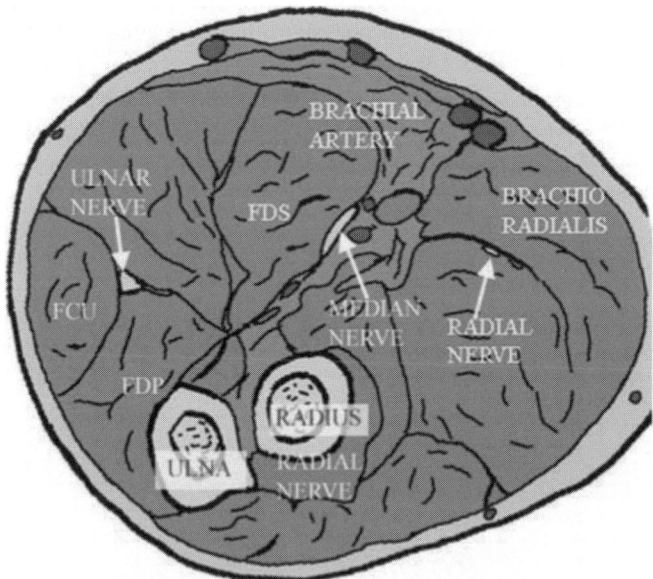

Figure 12.12 Diagram of cross-section at the cubital fossa, showing relations of radial, median, and ulnar nerves. *A black and white version of this figure will appear in some formats. For the color version, please refer to the plate section.*

axis by ultrasound in the fascial plane beneath brachioradialis, often accompanied by an artery. The nerve is typically flat-tened in cross-section. Local anesthetic is injected perineurally into the plane in which the nerve lies, spreads widely, and produces effective block (Fig. 12.13).

The median nerve travels down the arm in close proximity to the brachial artery, entering the forearm at the cubital fossa between the two heads of pronator teres muscle (pronator teres tunnel) and over the ulnar artery. It travels down the forearm between flexor digitorum superficialis (FDS) and profundus (FDP) muscles to enter the wrist between flexor retinaculum and flexor digitorum tendons. The nerve is most easily blocked in the cubital fossa, where it is identified proximally by its relation to the brachial artery. Further distally it leaves the artery to pass deep to FDS. It is often at this level flattened in short axis, although as it passes distally it becomes rounded.

The ulnar nerve travels down the arm, medial to the brachial artery, and at mid-humerus passes posteriorly to pierce the

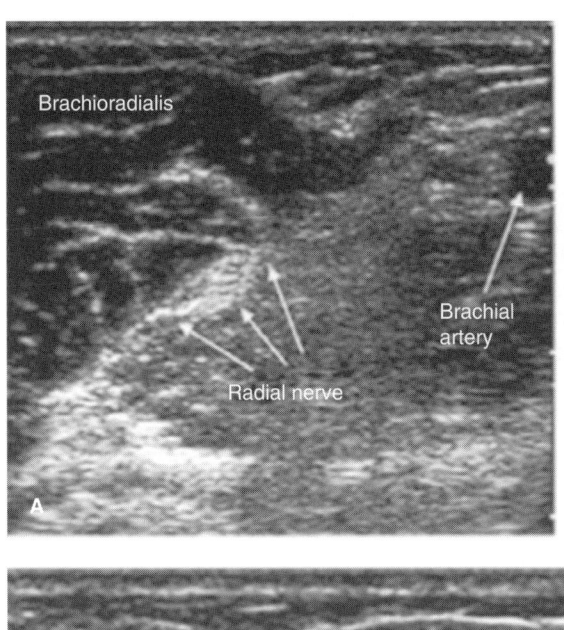
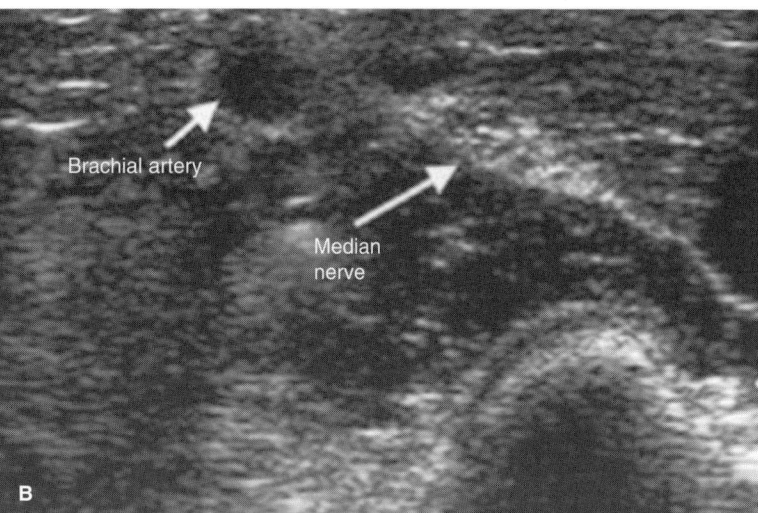
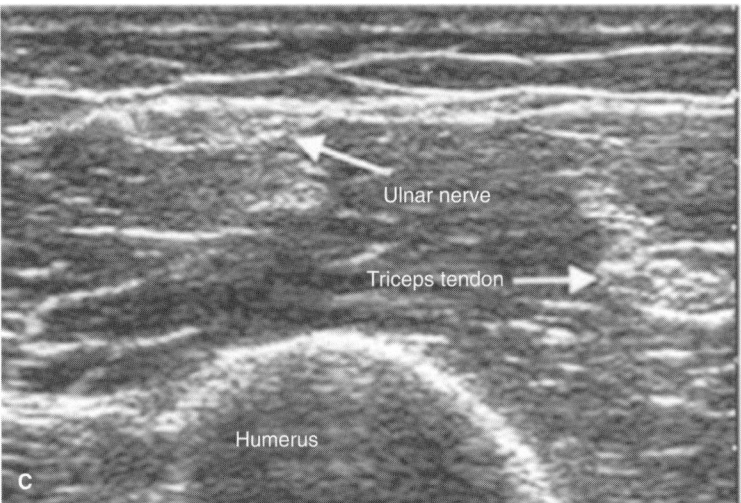
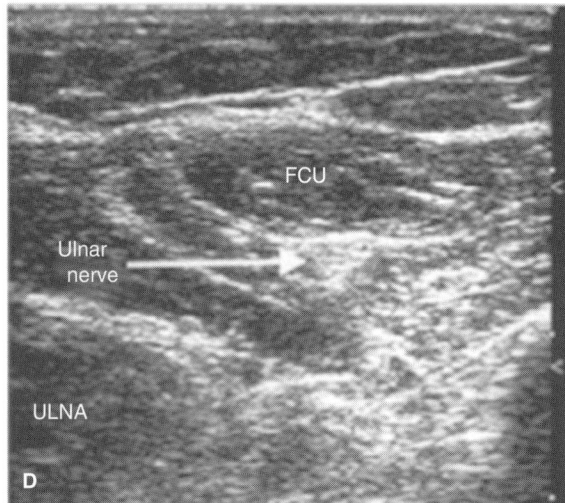

Figure 12.13 (**A**) Sonogram of radial nerve at the cubital fossa. (**B**) Sonogram of the median nerve in the cubital fossa at the point where it leaves the brachial artery to pass deep to flexor digitorum superficialis (FDS). (**C**) Ulnar nerve above the elbow. Note the similarity to the tendon of triceps; the ulnar nerve is more superficial. (**D**) Ulnar nerve in the proximal forearm in the Y beneath flexor carpi ulnaris (FCU).

medial intermuscular septum. It travels to the elbow on the anterior face of the medial head of triceps, and then turns behind the medial condyle of the humerus, over the elbow capsule, to enter the forearm between the humeral and ulnar heads of flexor carpi ulnaris (FCU). In the forearm the ulnar nerve descends on the FDP and is covered by the FCU, the tendon of which lies medial to the nerve at the wrist. It crosses the flexor retinaculum lateral to the pisiform. Blockade of the ulnar nerve may occur easily both proximal and distal to the elbow. Proximal to the ulnar groove of the humerus it may be identified lying on the distal belly of triceps on the medial side of the arm. There is a tendon within the substance of triceps at this level with which it may be confused; the nerve may be followed proximally to confirm its identity, as the tendon is short.

The ulnar nerve may also be approached below the elbow. The nerve runs in a constant course in a Y beneath the belly of FCU. It is easily identified and blocked in this position on the

medial forearm. More distally the nerve is joined by the ulnar artery, which may aid identification.

Lumbosacral plexus examination

The lumbar plexus (T12, L1–L4) is located deep within the psoas muscle and lies anterior to the transverse processes of each lumbar vertebra. The sacral plexus (L3–L4, S1–S4) passes through the greater and lesser sciatic foramina. The lumbosacral plexus supplies the motor and sensory innervation of the leg predominately via the femoral nerve anteriorly and the sciatic nerve posteriorly.

The femoral nerve

The femoral nerve (L2–L4) is the largest branch of the lumbar plexus; it passes beneath the inguinal ligament in a groove between the psoas and iliacus muscles. It is both a sensory

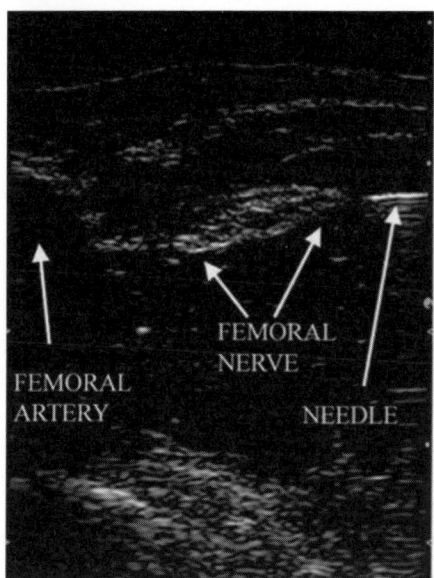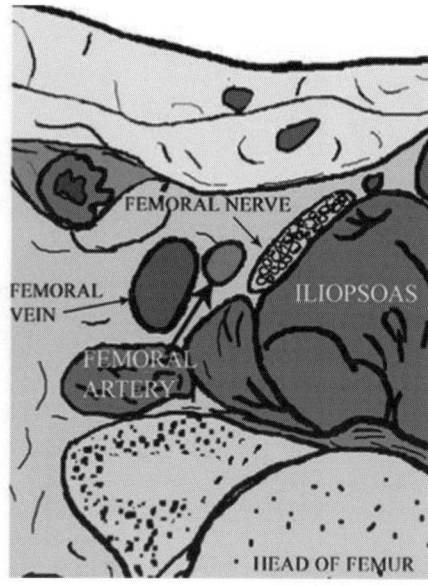

Figure 12.14 Sonographic anatomy of the femoral nerve below the inguinal ligament. *A black and white version of this figure will appear in some formats. For the color version, please refer to the plate section.*

and a motor nerve, with blockade producing both sensory anesthesia of the anterior upper thigh and the medial calf and inability to abduct the leg or extend the lower leg. It lies on iliopsoas muscle immediately lateral (one finger-breadth) to the femoral artery and is covered by fascia lata and fascia iliaca. The femoral nerve gives off an anterior and posterior division, of which a cutaneous branch continues to the lower leg as the saphenous nerve.

Since the femoral nerve is relatively superficial, a high-frequency probe placed just distal to the inguinal ligament will identify the nerve lateral to the artery, with a portion of psoas separating the two structures (Fig. 12.14). The femoral vessels and lymphatics lie in a separate fascial plane medial to the nerve. This fascial plane is, however, difficult to appreciate on ultrasound. The femoral nerve may be blocked in isolation or, as many believe, in conjunction with the obturator and lateral cutaneous nerves (3-in-l block) when larger injectate volumes spread perivascularly to reach the proximal lumbar plexus. The efficacy of this approach is questioned, and targeting of individual femoral, lateral cutaneous, and obturator nerves is recommended. Ultrasound guidance in performing a femoral nerve 3-in-1 block, however, is well described and has been shown to have increased accuracy and low morbidity.[13]

The sciatic nerve

The sciatic nerve (L3–L4, S1–S3) exits the pelvis through the greater sciatic foramen to enter the leg between the greater trochanter and ischial tuberosity. It is a large flattened nerve, over 1 cm in width, which travels inferior to piriformis and deep to gluteus maximus and medius muscles. The superior gluteal artery is superomedial to the sciatic nerve at this proximal point; in a small percentage of patients, the nerve may have a high bifurcation, dividing into tibial and peroneal branches as it emerges from the sciatic foramen. At this level

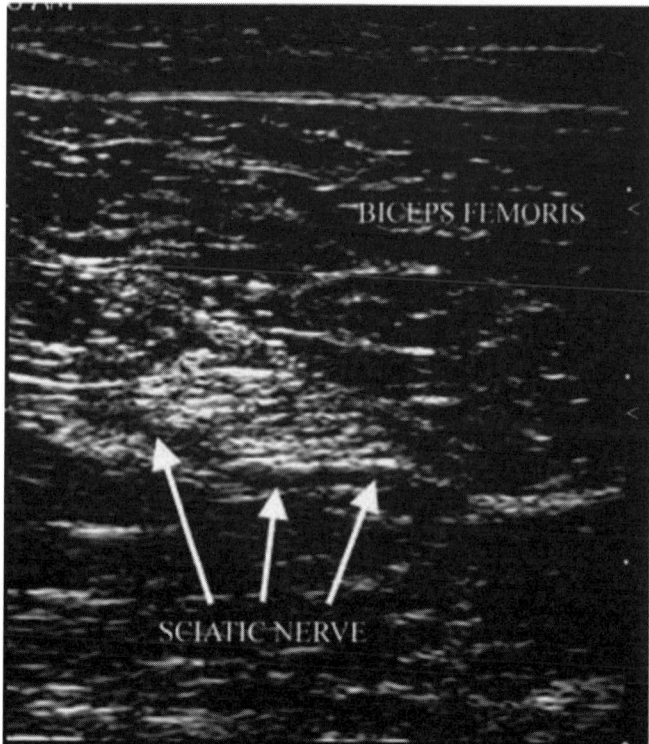

Figure 12.15 Sonographic anatomy of the sciatic nerve in the infragluteal region.

the posterior femoral cutaneous nerve also emerges. Ultrasonic examination requires the use of a lower-frequency probe, since insonation may need a penetration depth of 3–5 cm. It travels into the thigh posterior to the lesser trochanter of the femur, and distally along the posterior border of the adductor magnus muscle beneath biceps femoris (Fig. 12.15). The popliteal artery and vein, a continuation of the femoral vessels, enter the popliteal fossa via the adductor canal to lie anteromedial to the sciatic nerve. The sciatic nerve divides into posterior tibial and peroneal branches. The tibial nerve travels to the ankle, passes beneath the flexor retinaculum, and gives off the medial and lateral plantar nerves. The peroneal nerve leaves the popliteal fossa laterally by crossing the head of gastrocnemius to wind subcutaneously around the fibula head. It gives rise to the deep peroneal nerve that enters the foot between the extensor hallucis longus and tibialis anterior muscles and lateral to the dorsalis pedis artery. The second branch, the superficial peroneal nerve, travels down the leg in the lateral compartment to innervate the lower leg and foot.

Blockade of the sciatic nerve will provide anesthesia to the foot and the lower extremity distal to the knee. Ultrasound can scan the buttock and thigh posteriorly, to identify the sciatic nerve as it travels down to the popliteal fossa. Ultrasonic mapping of sciatic nerve size, depth, and position has been accurately described with reference to the ischial spine, ischial tuberosity, and lesser trochanter level.[14] It is most superficial in the subgluteal region, and is suitable for block at this point. Imaging can be difficult if beam angulation is not perpendicular to the nerve and poor muscle penetration occurs. In the thigh the sciatic nerve is quite varied in shape, from round to ribbon-like in short axis. Imaging in the popliteal fossa also identifies the sciatic nerve, the point at which it divides, and the relationship between peroneal and tibial nerves (Fig. 12.16). The nerve is often easy to identify in the popliteal fossa, because of its superficial location and high connective tissue content. This may provide a convenient starting point to

follow the nerve more proximally to be blocked in the thigh. Alternatively, the nerve may be blocked in the popliteal fossa, as a block distal to the division of the nerve leads to faster block onset.

Blocks below the knee

The common peroneal nerve may be identified as it passes around the fibula; this is not a recommended site for blockade because of the risk of neurapraxia. Distal to this, the deep peroneal branch accompanies the anterior tibial artery, where it may be blocked. The superficial peroneal nerve has no similarly convenient vascular landmark, although it lies deep to peroneus longus in the proximal leg; it may be imaged emerging from the deep fascia about halfway down the leg, and it often divides rapidly into multiple branches. The posterior tibial nerve lies deep in the calf until it emerges on the medial side of the distal leg above the ankle. It is readily identified at this level in conjunction with the posterior tibial artery and may be blocked at this level.

Epidural anesthesia

In adults, ultrasound imaging of the epidural space is poor even with the use of a low-frequency probe. The epidural space is deeply situated and is surrounded by bone of the vertebral column. Ultrasound has been used to identify vertebral landmarks in obese gravid patients and to reduce the number of puncture attempts for epidural catheter placement. In infants and children, however, the incomplete ossification of vertebrae enables ultrasound to accurately visualize the epidural space, assisting in puncture of the ligamentum flavum and placement of the catheter.

Intercostal and paravertebral blocks

Ultrasound scanning in the longitudinal plane shows the ribs in short-axis with their adjacent neurovascular bundle, intercostal muscles, and parietal pleura. Needles can be visually placed beneath the inferior rib border for intercostal block or advanced to the paravertebral region. An advantage is immediate screening for post-block pneumothorax and the identification of ribs when extensive tissue swelling is present. However, the presence of subcutaneous emphysema may make ultrasound imaging difficult. Paravertebral block is an advanced technique, and ultrasound guidance techniques have been described including in-plane along the line of the ribs, and in-plane and out-of-plane techniques from posterior to the transverse processes.

Abdominal wall blocks

Compared with neuraxial blocks, peripheral abdominal blocks are an attractive option for analgesia in abdominal trauma as there are fewer of the management problems of neuraxial blocks, such as hypotension, as well as decreased concerns regarding anticoagulation. Although abdominal wall blocks

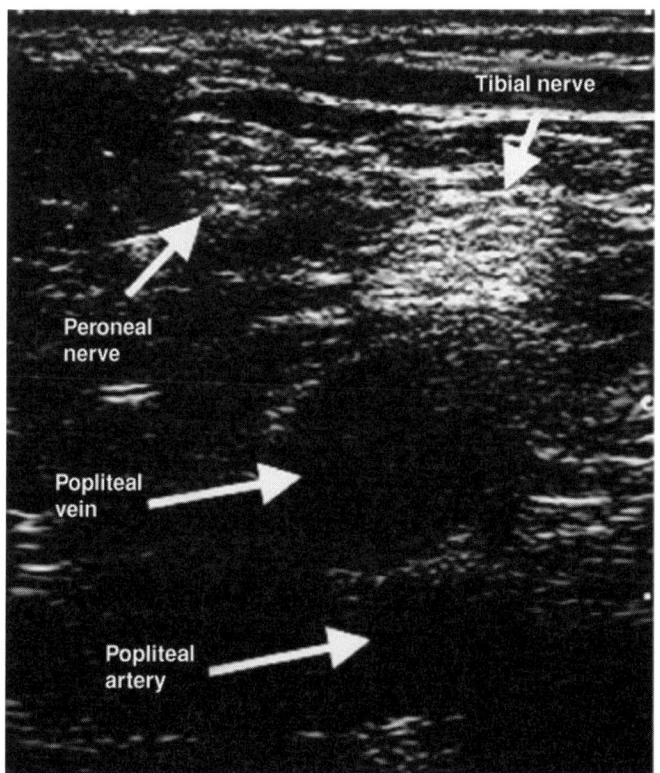

Figure 12.16 Sonogram of the bifurcated sciatic nerve in the popliteal fossa.

are well described, the evidence base is incomplete, partially due to a substantial decrease in open elective abdominal surgery and consequent limited clinical trials.[15] In particular, trials are lacking for upper abdominal midline incisional surgery. Spread of local anaesthetic in the transversus abdominis plane (TAP) has been shown to be dependent on the site of injection, and, as with other nerve block techniques, the nerves involved in the incision should be targeted for optimal analgesia. A thorough knowledge of the anatomy of the abdominal wall nerves will allow placement of optimal blocks.

The anatomy of the abdominal wall nerves follows a segmental pattern, passing from T6 at the xiphoid to L1 at the pubis. Each nerve gives off a lateral branch that supplies the external oblique muscle and the lateral skin to around the midclavicular line. This branch comes off in a posterior position as a branch of the intercostal section of the nerve and is not accessible to local anesthetic in the abdominal wall. The upper nerves (T6–T8) pass into the TAP by passing deep to the costal cartilages, emerge deep to the rectus sheath, and then penetrate the rectus sheath to supply the rectus and the overlying skin. The optimal place to target these nerves is deep to the rectus sheath superficial to transversus abdominis and as close as possible to the costal margin, as the nerves may penetrate into the rectus muscle close to the costal margin. Lateral to the rectus muscle (T9–T12) the nerves emerge directly into the TAP superficial to the transversus muscle. They may be targeted within this plane lateral to the rectus muscle. After passing into the rectus sheath they lie posterior to the rectus muscle, where they may also be blocked. Injection below the umbilicus may result in incomplete anesthesia, since nerves can have a short or absent passage deep to the rectus. The L1 nerves show more variation, passing into the transversus plane more anteriorly, near the anterior superior iliac spine (ASIS) and then passing superficially through external oblique without passing into the rectus muscle. The optimal anatomical position to block L1 is in the transversus plane just lateral to the ASIS.

Several approaches to the TAP block have been described, some of which likely have anatomical limitations. Individual injections may be placed anywhere along the oblique subcostal line between the xiphoid and the ASIS. A posterior injection is well described midway between the costal margin and the iliac crest in the midclavicular line; this is anatomically more likely to miss L1 and unlikely to spread much above the umbilicus. Approaches to make a more extensive block include a dual injection technique, medial and lateral to the rectus muscle along the oblique subcostal line; and a hydrodissection approach, passing a long needle along the oblique subcostal line, which allows one catheter on each side to maintain the block.[16,17] Both techniques can spread the block extensively in the abdomen and are suitable for catheter placement. Published experience of TAP techniques in trauma are limited to case studies with reported benefits of early extubation and improved analgesia.[18]

Ultrasound of the lung and pericardium

"Lung" ultrasound is now an established technique in emergency medicine and critical care for detection of pleural fluid, pneumothorax, interstitial lung disease, and consolidation (see Chapters 2 and 10). It may also be useful for the detection of endobronchial intubation and inadvertent one-lung ventilation.

The normal appearance of the lung with ultrasound imaging is essentially the reflection of the highly echogenic pleura and artifact resulting from the pleural surface, seen projecting deeper into the ultrasound image (Figs. 12.17, 12.18). There are two normal movements at the lung–pleural interface, lung sliding and the lung pulse. Lung sliding is caused by ventilation of the lung with subsequent movement

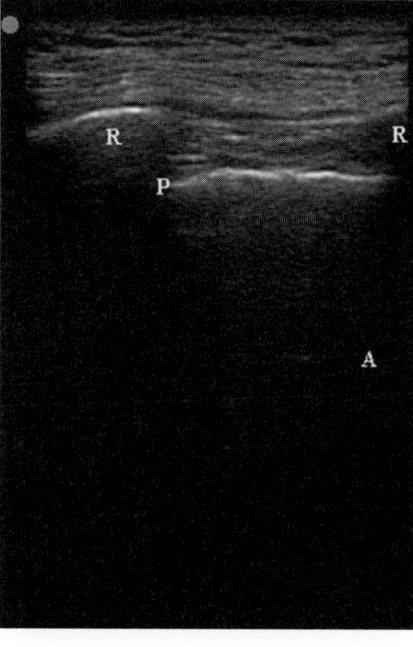

Figure 12.18 Normal lung. The pleura (P) is not visible but shadowed deep to the ribs (R). A faint reflected pleural line (A line) is visible.

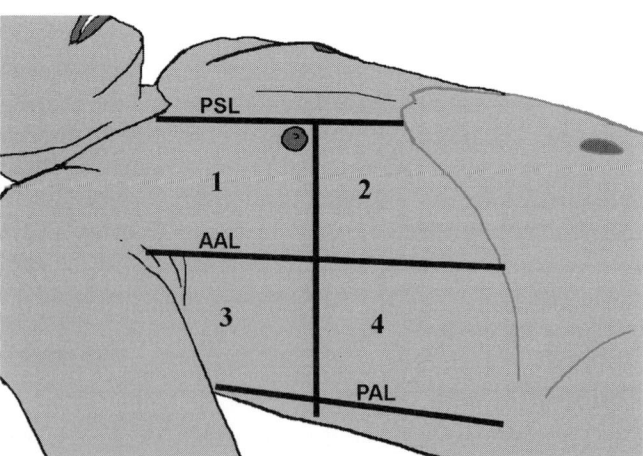

Figure 12.17 Recommended four chest areas per side for eight-zone lung examination in the supine patient. Upper and lower anterior zones and upper and basal lateral zones. AAL, anterior axillary line; PAL, posterior axillary line; PSL, parasternal line.

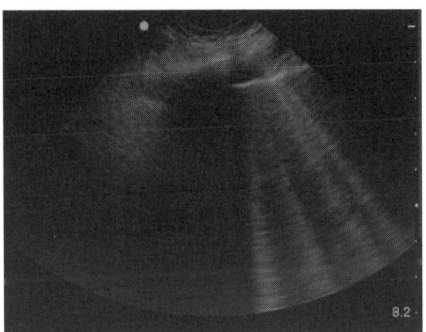

Figure 12.19 Interstitial syndrome. Multiple B lines are present in the transverse scan between ribs.

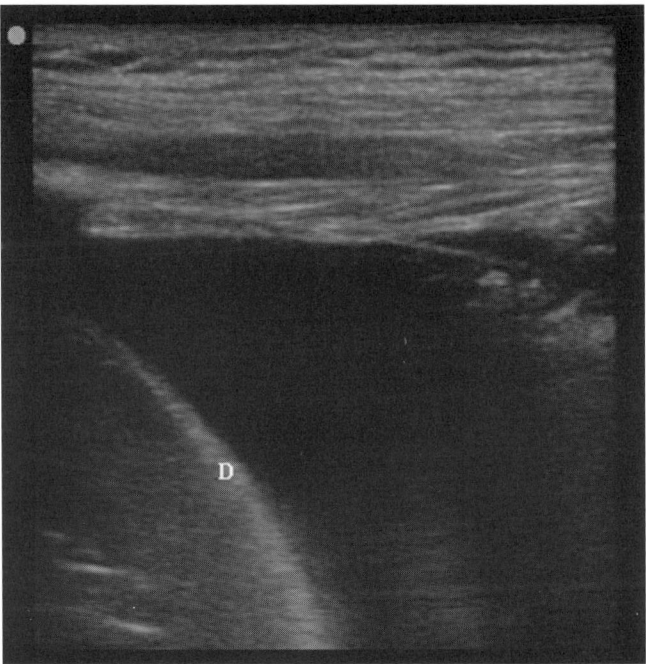

Figure 12.20 Pleural effusion. The diaphragm (D) is visible deep to a dark sonolucent effusion.

of the visceral and parietal pleura. It appears as a cyclical "shimmering" movement, and is most pronounced at the diaphragmatic base of the chest and least obvious at the apex. The lung pulse is a similar pleural movement secondary to the transmitted cardiac impulse. The air–fluid interface of lung tissue causes reverberation artifact when examined with ultrasound. A lines represent horizontal artifacts arising from the pleural line, and in the presence of a sliding sign usually indicate aerated lung. M-mode examination can further differentiate the presence of a sliding sign, with normal lung producing a granular "seashore" pattern, while the presence of a pneumothorax has absent lung sliding due to subpleural air, and exaggeration of the linear reverberation A lines, producing a "stratosphere" pattern. B lines, also termed "comet-tail" artifact, reflect the subpleural fluid–air interface of alveoli. In the examination of normal lung fewer than three B lines are present in the ultrasound scan plane transversely across an intercostal space (Fig. 12.18). Parenchymal changes to the lung such as increased interstitial fluid can increase the size and number of B-line artifacts, then termed lung rockets or B+ lines (Fig. 12.19). Large numbers of these are diagnostic of interstitial lung disease, including pulmonary edema.

Different zones of the lung show characteristic changes because of the gravitational distribution of pleural fluid and the tendency of lower zones to experience more atelectasis, interstitial fluid, and consolidation, whereas pleural air is confined initially to the uppermost parts of the chest, anteriorly in the supine patient. Supine examination of the lung requires placement of the ultrasound probe over four zones bilaterally, defining upper and lower anterior zones (anterior to the anterior axillary line) and upper and basal lateral zones (Fig. 12.17). A pneumothorax can be excluded if lung sliding, B lines, or lung pulse is present. A pneumothorax is strongly suspected with absence of lung sliding and presence of A lines. However, sliding absence can also occur with consolidation, endobronchial intubation, and apnea. Confirmation of pneumothorax is made by examining for the lung point, a transition point between normal and deflated lung, where air separates the partly deflated lung from the pleura with loss of lung sliding. If a lung point cannot be found and lung sliding, lung pulse, and B lines are not present, a pneumothorax may still be diagnosed.

Apart from pneumothorax, pleural fluid including hemothorax can be readily detected by pleural sonography (Figs. 12.20, 12.21), and drainage may be planned either by marking the optimal point or by real-time needle guidance under imaging. Further consolidation and atelectasis also have specific sonographic appearance, and evidence-based recommendations exist for point-of-care lung examination and diagnosis.[19]

Ultrasound-guided tube thoracoscopy

A high-frequency linear probe can define the shallow outer chest wall and pleura, though convex-array or phased-array probes (2–5 MHz) are also suitable for thoracic procedures. Chest tubes are typically inserted into the fourth or fifth intercostal space, at the level of the mid-axillary line, for immediate management of large pneumothoraces. However, with a smaller pneumothorax the entry site may be determined by the ultrasound findings. In cases of hemopneumothorax, insertion nearer to the diaphragm may be indicated to facilitate fluid drainage. Upright positioning is ideal to define fluid collections, but this is often not possible in the acutely injured patient. Once a diagnosis of pneumothorax is made, it is necessary to scan the hemithorax and to identify the presence of a collection and the position of the diaphragm, liver, and adjacent kidney. A pitfall is misinterpretation of Morrison's pouch (on the right) or the left-sided splenic–renal recess as the diaphragm, with subsequent risk of inadvertent tube placement into these organs. The technique of insertion requires identification of the intercostal space, noting the rib and inferiorly positioned intercostal nerves and vessels, and the measurement of the depth between the pleura and adjacent organs. A trochar is then inserted into the chest, over the top of the rib, with or without ultrasound in real time. Once the tube is

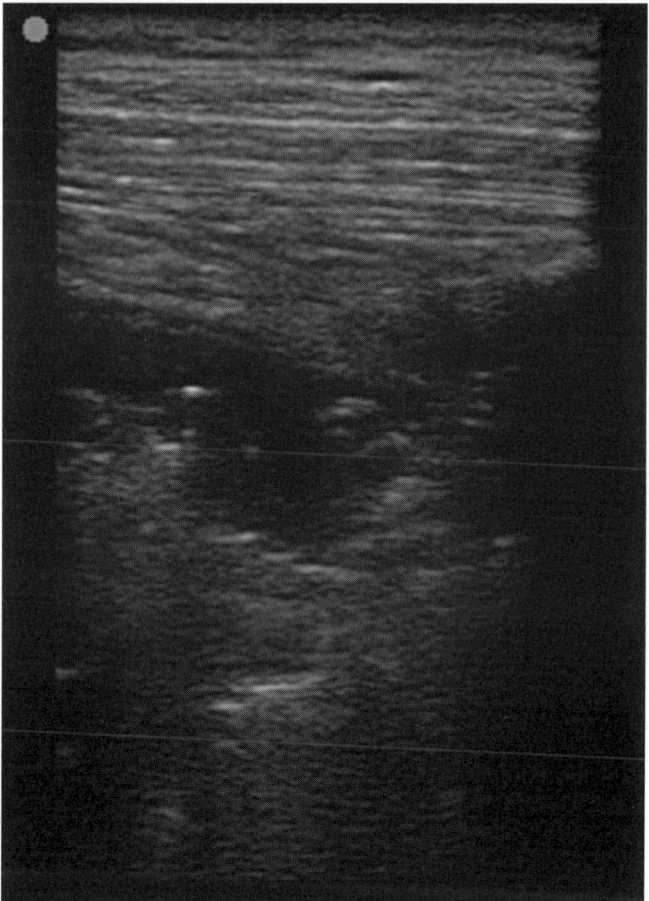

Figure 12.21 Pleural effusion and partial consolidation. Partly aerated lung is imaged deep to a small pleural effusion.

connected to an underwater-seal drain, re-expansion of the lung should occur, and repeat examination should show the return of lung sliding.

Ultrasound-guided pericardiocentesis

An acute bleed into the pericardium is potentially life-threatening and requires immediate diagnosis and treatment. Echocardiography is an important component of a focused ultrasound examination since it can identify the presence of a pericardial effusion and its size, distribution, and effect on cardiac filling (see Chapter 10). Chamber inversion and marked respiratory variation in filling are cardinal signs of tamponade physiology. The technique of ultrasound-guided pericardiocentesis is well established but requires experience and expertise.[20] A phased-array probe is commonly used, and the patient is positioned semi-laterally if appropriate. The needle entry point for pericardiocentesis is ideally adjacent to where the pericardial expansion is greatest, and closest to the chest wall. Injection here will reduce the risk of lung or liver penetration during needle advancement, and cardiac laceration on entering the pericardial space. The left chest wall is commonly used, though subcostal approaches are described. Subcostal entry has a longer trajectory and is more likely to involve

the liver. Injection can be performed blindly following the initial scan and measurement of the skin to pericardial distance, or alternatively needle advancement can be viewed with real-time imaging. Once puncture of the pericardium is achieved, the needle is quickly withdrawn and the sheath left within the pericardium to enable catheter insertion. Catheter position within the pericardium can be confirmed by injection of agitated saline.[20]

Ultrasound-guided vascular access

Ultrasound guidance for central venous catheter (CVC) placement has been shown to reduce the risk of inadvertent arterial puncture, pneumothorax, and failed line placement (see Chapter 5). Ultrasound is particularly useful for CVC placement via the internal jugular and femoral veins; it may also be used for placement of subclavian and peripheral CVCs, peripherally inserted central catheters (PICC), and arterial cannulas.

The UK National Institute of Clinical Excellence (NICE) guidelines in 2002 recommended the use of ultrasound for the placement of adult and pediatric CVCs via the internal jugular vein (IJV).[21] The US Agency for Healthcare Research and Quality (AHRQ) in 2001 recommended the use of real-time ultrasound guidance during central line insertion.[22]

For many CVC insertions, ultrasound-guided and landmark techniques are essentially the same in terms of needle insertion, point, and depth. Use of routine ultrasound identifies patients with difficult or variant anatomy and pathology before the insertion is commenced, and skills in ultrasound anatomy and eye–hand coordination are improved by regular use. Time to establish venous access from first needle insertion is generally improved by ultrasound, but setting up the equipment may sometimes result in slower insertion. Equipment availability and experience will minimize this.

As with all ultrasound-guided needle techniques, continuous identification of the needle tip is the key to safe practice. Short-axis out-of-plane techniques are generally preferred for vascular access, and the NICE and AHRQ recommendations are based on this approach.

Veins may be distinguished from arteries, using ultrasound, by their more irregular outline, less obvious pulsatility, and easier occlusion under pressure. Color Doppler characteristics of veins include lower-velocity flow, sometimes varying with respiration and augmented by squeezing the distal limb. Arteries are usually rounder with more distinct calcified walls, visibly pulsatile, and with strongly pulsatile flow in color Doppler imaging.

Jugular venous puncture

The ultrasound transducer is placed in short axis displaying a cross-section of the IJV and the carotid artery. The first view establishes the size of the vein and its position relative to the carotid artery. Unlike the carotid artery, the vein is easily occluded by pressure from the ultrasound transducer. If the vein is small, the other IJV should be examined, because there is occasionally a large difference in size. Venous distension is

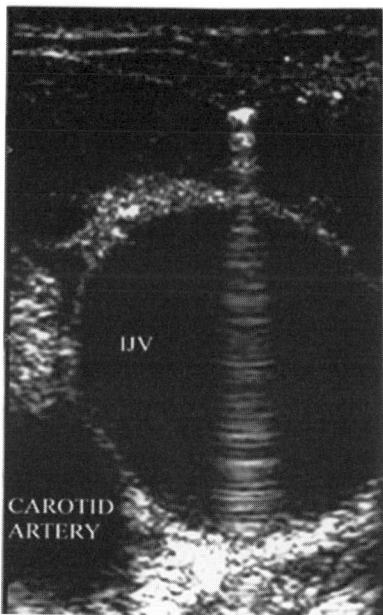
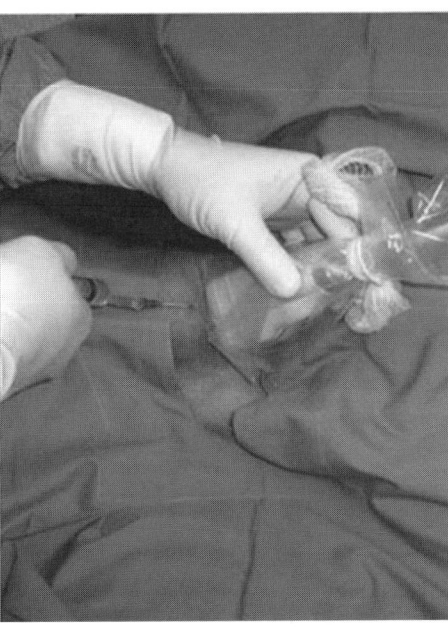

Figure 12.22 Technique for internal jugular vein (IJV) puncture and sonogram of needle near IJV. Note that the needle tip cannot be ascertained in this still picture.

optimized by Trendelenburg positioning, or by Valsalva maneuvering, or by pressing on the abdomen. The IJV is typically 1.5–2.5 cm under the skin surface and anterolateral to the carotid artery. The needle should be directed away from the carotid artery, and therefore the insertion point is usually anteromedial to the IJV (Fig. 12.22). The needle should be angled steeply into the neck in the direction of the IJV with the aim of contacting the vein in the plane of the ultrasound beam. The needle tip is seen initially displacing the anterior wall of the IJV. At this point, extravenous distension may be achieved by asking the patient to hold his or her breath in inspiration, or if the lungs are being ventilated by advancing during the inspiratory phase. A short, quick advancement or rotation of the needle may facilitate puncture of the anterior wall of the IJV, which may otherwise be pushed into contact with the posterior wall by pressure from the needle.

During the procedure the ultrasound probe should be manipulated by using small angulations to confirm that the needle tip is identified in the ultrasound beam. Movement of the anterior wall of the IJV alone is not sufficient to identify the tip, as some wall displacement occurs several centimeters from the puncture point. Once the needle tip is seen inside the vein and blood aspirated, a wire or cannula is inserted to complete the CVC by standard Seldinger techniques. Ultrasound scanning can reduce the risk of misplacement by imaging the wire or cannula within the vessel, using both short- and long-axis views.

Femoral venous puncture

The femoral vessels are identified below the inguinal ligament in short axis. The vein generally runs medial to the artery, although it is sometimes posterior. The femoral vein must be distinguished from the long saphenous vein, which is superficial, and the profunda femoral artery, which branches from the posterior aspect of the femoral artery. The femoral nerve may be seen lateral to the artery. The vein is targeted by a needle directed away from the femoral artery. As with the IJV, a short, quick advancement may facilitate puncture once the needle is positioned in contact with the vein.

Infraclavicular venous puncture

The subclavian vein is difficult to image in ultrasound in a probe position that guides needle puncture. The axillary vein, however, lies lateral to the first rib and may be imaged along its length in short or long axis. The axillary artery is relatively easy to mistake for the vein in long axis, as it runs immediately posterior, and the first rib and pleura are related deep to the medial end of the vein. By using the long-axis technique, the needle is introduced in plane from the lateral side under the length of the probe to the puncture site at the medial end of the vein (Fig. 12.23). The needle passes relatively perpendicular to the ultrasound beam, which facilitates tip visualization. Due to the width of the ultrasound beam, the needle may not be pointing as directly at the vein as may appear in the image, and it should be redirected if the superficial wall of the vein does not move in when needle appears to contact it. In the short-axis approach the artery and vein are easier to distinguish, and the needle can be directed confidently straight toward the vein. The needle tip, however, is harder to see and the angle of approach steeper, with the pleura in close proximity. Either technique requires caution and previous experience with other ultrasound-guided approaches.

Other vascular access

Large veins are usually identifiable in the cubital fossa and proximally in the arm. These may be identified in the short axis and cannulas placed under ultrasonic guidance using similar techniques as for larger veins. Similarly, arteries may be identified and cannulated. Short- and long-axis techniques may be used according to preference; it is often better to observe the needle for flashback rather than watching the ultrasound screen at the moment of vessel puncture.

Gastric volume assessment

Ultrasound may be used reliably to assess the gastric volume, which is particularly useful in patients with possible residual gastric contents, a common situation in trauma. A recent algorithm has been described using the measurement of the antral area with the patient in the right lateral position, where

it is located on ultrasound inferior and deep to the liver edge (Fig. 12.24).[23] Confidence should be gained using gastric ultrasound in routine practice before management decisions are made using the technique.

Summary

The past decade has seen an explosion in point-of-care ultrasound-based assistance in the management of trauma patients. The portability, availability, safety, and low cost of ultrasound imaging means that ultrasound examination can be used routinely to improve patient care. Simple procedures such as safer and faster vascular access; screening for pneumothorax, tamponade, and hemothorax; sophisticated pain management using neural blockade; and ultrasound-based injury assessment are techniques increasingly used in the emergency room, intensive care unit, and operating suite. Ultrasound skills are now an essential requirement for all practitioners in critical care specialties, to facilitate rapid and accurate trauma management.

Questions

(1) **Ultrasound of the brachial plexus identifies nerves as:**
   a. Anechoic nodules
   b. Hypodense granulated nodules
   c. Densely reflective
   d. Curved on longitudinal scan

(2) **Ultrasound of the radial nerve at the axilla shows it is related to the artery:**
   a. Posteriorly
   b. Superficially
   c. Anteriorly
   d. Within coracobrachialis

(3) **Surface ultrasound of the brachial plexus can identify all *except*:**
   a. Plexus sheath
   b. Nerve roots
   c. Injectate needle tip
   d. Lung

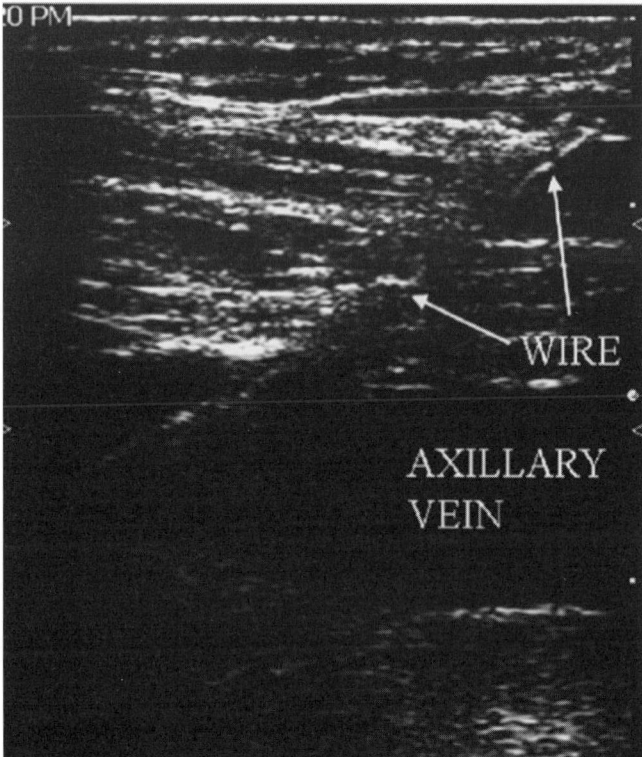

Figure 12.23 Seldinger wire placed in axillary vein in long-axis view (in-plane approach).

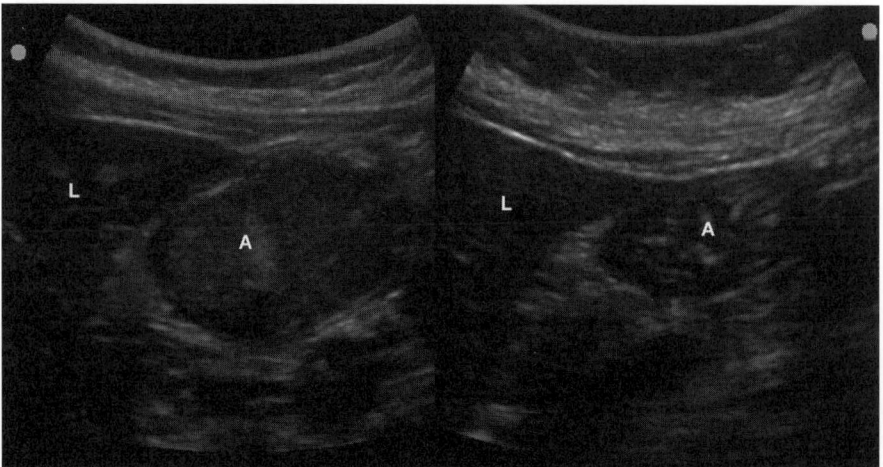

Figure 12.24 Comparison of empty antrum (∧, right) with antrum clearly containing gastric content (A, left). L, liver.

(4) Ulnar sparing during brachial plexus anesthesia is indicated by an ultrasound appearance of:
   a. Inferior trunk inferior to subclavian artery
   b. Inferior trunk superior to subclavian artery
   c. Superior trunk adjacent to subclavian artery
   d. Middle trunk lateral to anterior scalene

(5) The transverse process of C6:
   a. Lies lateral to the interscalene space
   b. Has the vertebral artery and vein posterior
   c. Has nerve roots lateral to it
   d. Is often used as a landmark for the supraclavicular approach

(6) In the axilla, on ultrasound:
   a. The axillary artery lies between coracobrachialis and biceps
   b. The axillary artery is surrounded by cords
   c. The median nerve lies anterior to the axillary artery
   d. The musculocutaneous nerve is located inferior to the axillary artery

(7) Light pressure can cause occlusion of:
   a. Veins
   b. Arteries
   c. Veins and arteries
   d. Neither veins nor arteries

(8) When cannulating the femoral artery, the order of structures on the patient's left side, from medial to lateral is:
   a. Nerve, vein, artery
   b. Nerve, artery, vein
   c. Vein, artery, nerve
   d. Vein, nerve, artery

(9) Which of the following transducers would be best to aid in the insertion of a PICC (peripherally inserted central catheter) line:
   a. 12 MHz phased-array transducer
   b. 15 MHz linear-array transducer
   c. 5 MHz phased-array transducer
   d. 4 MHz linear-array transducer

(10) Pneumothorax is suspected with:
   a. Presence of lung sliding
   b. Presence of A lines
   c. Absent lung sliding and B lines
   d. Absence of pleural line

Answers

(1) b
(2) a
(3) a
(4) a
(5) c
(6) c
(7) a
(8) c
(9) b
(10) c

References

1. Marhofer P, Harrop-Griffiths W, Kettner SC, Kirchmair L. Fifteen years of ultrasound guidance in regional anaesthesia: part 1. *Br J Anaesth* 2010; **104**: 538–46.

2. Plunkett AR, Brown DS, Rogers JM, *et al.* Supraclavicular continuous peripheral nerve block in a wounded soldier: when ultrasound is the only option. *Br J Anaesth* 2006; **97**: 715–17.

3. Barrington MJ, Watts SA, Gledhill SR, *et al.* Preliminary results of the Australasian Regional Anaesthesia Collaboration: a prospective audit of more than 7000 peripheral nerve and plexus blocks for neurologic and other complications. *Reg Anesth Pain Med* 2009; **34**: 534–41.

4. Orebaugh SL, Kentor ML, Williams BA. Adverse outcomes associated with nerve stimulator-guided and ultrasound-guided peripheral nerve blocks by supervised trainees: update of a single-site database. *Reg Anesth Pain Med* 2012; **37**: 577–82.

5. Peer S, Bodner G, Meirer R, Willeit J, Piza-Katzer H. Examination of postoperative peripheral nerve lesions with high-resolution sonography. *AJR Am J Roentgenol* 2001; **177**: 415–19.

6. Bodner G, Buchberger W, Schocke M, *et al.* Radial nerve palsy associated with humeral shaft fracture: evaluation with US – initial experience. *Radiology* 2001; **219**: 811–16.

7. Meissner M, Paun M, Johansen K. Duplex scanning for arterial trauma. *Am J Surg* 1991; **161**: 552–5.

8. Chapman GA, Johnson D, Bodenham AR. Visualisation of needle position using ultrasonography. *Anaesthesia* 2006; **61**: 148–58.

9. Franco CD. Connective tissues associated with peripheral nerves. *Reg Anesth Pain Med* 2012; **37**: 363–5.

10. Sandhu NS. Transpectoral ultrasound-guided catheterization of the axillary vein: an alternative to standard catheterization of the subclavian vein. *Anesth Analg* 2004; **99**: 183–7.

11. Royse CE, Sha S, Soeding PF, Royse AG. Anatomical study of the brachial plexus using surface ultrasound. *Anaesth Intensive Care* 2006; **34**: 203–10.

12. O'Donnell BD, Iohom G. An estimation of the minimum effective anesthetic volume of 2% lidocaine in ultrasound-guided axillary brachial plexus block. *Anesthesiology* 2009; **111**: 25–9.

13. Marhofer P, Schrogendorfer K, Koinig H, *et al.* Ultrasonographic guidance improves sensory block and onset time of three-in one blocks. *Anesth Analg* 1997; **85**: 854–7.

14. Chan VW, Nova H, Abbas S, *et al.* Ultrasound examination and localization of the sciatic nerve: A volunteer study. *Anesthesiology* 2006; **104**: 309–14.

15. Abdallah FW, Chan VW, Brull R. Transversus abdominis plane block: a systematic review. *Reg Anesth Pain Med* 2012; **37**: 193–209.

16. Hebbard PD, Barrington MJ, Vasey C. Ultrasound-guided continuous oblique

subcostal transversus abdominis plane blockade: description of anatomy and clinical technique. *Reg Anesth Pain Med* 2010; **35**: 436–41.

17. Børglum J, Jensen K, Christensen AF, *et al.* Distribution patterns, dermatomal anesthesia, and ropivacaine serum concentrations after bilateral dual transversus abdominis plane block. *Reg Anesth Pain Med* 2012; **37**: 294–301.

18. Allcock E, Spencer E, Frazer R, Applegate G, Buckenmaier C. Continuous transversus abdominis plane (TAP) block catheters in a combat surgical environment. *Pain Med* 2010; **11**: 1426–9.

19. Volpicelli G, Elbarbary M, Blaivas *et al*; International Liaison Committee on Lung Ultrasound (ILC-LUS) for International Consensus Conference on Lung Ultrasound (ICC-LUS). International evidence-based recommendations for point-of-care lung ultrasound. *Intensive Care Med* 2012; **38**: 577–91.

20. Tsang T, Enriquez-Sarano M, Freeman W, *et al.* Consecutive 1127 therapeutic echocardiographically guided pericardiocenteses: clinical profile, practice patterns, and outcomes spanning 21 years. *Mayo Clin Proc* 2002; **77**: 429–36.

21. National Institute for Clinical Excellence. *Guidance on the Use of Ultrasound Locating Devices for Placing Central Venous Catheters.* Technology Appraisal 49. London: NICE, 2002. http://guidance.nice.org.uk/TA49 (accessed July 2014).

22. Agency for Healthcare Research and Quality. *Evidence Report/Technology Assessment. No. 43. Making Health Care Safer: a Critical Analysis of Patient Safety Practices. Chapter 21. Ultrasound Guidance of Central Vein Catheterization.* http://archive.ahrq.gov/clinic/ptsafety/chap21.htm (accessed July 2014).

23. Perlas A, Mitsakakis N, Liu L, *et al.* Validation of a mathematical model for ultrasound assessment of gastric volume by gastroscopic examination. *Anesth Analg* 2013; **116**: 357–63.

Pharmacology of neuromuscular blocking agents and their reversal in trauma patients

François Donati

Objectives

(1) Describe the role of neuromuscular blocking agents for tracheal intubation and maintenance of relaxation in trauma patients.

(2) List key features of the pharmacology of depolarizing and nondepolarizing neuromuscular agents and their antagonists used in trauma patients.

(3) Formulate recommendations and define indications and contraindications for the use of neuromuscular blocking agents in different trauma settings.

Introduction

Neuromuscular blocking agents are given to trauma patients in two specific circumstances. First, they may be needed to facilitate tracheal intubation in the emergency department or prehospital environment to provide oxygenation and ventilation to the unstable patient (see Chapter 2). Second, neuromuscular blocking agents may be needed in an otherwise stable patient as an adjunct to other anesthetic drugs for emergency or elective surgery. In both cases, the major challenge is to choose the right drug for tracheal intubation. Neuromuscular blocking agents for maintenance of relaxation during surgery or mechanical ventilation are similar to those used in nontrauma cases, and the indications for reversal in trauma and nontrauma patients do not differ significantly.

Patients with recent trauma are likely to have hemodynamic instability. Thus, they may have an exaggerated response to sedative and hypnotic drugs. Ideally, these drugs should be titrated. However, trauma patients should be presumed to have a full stomach, and measures to prevent pulmonary aspiration of gastric contents should be applied. The management of tracheal intubation in the presence of a full stomach relies on the rapid sequence induction (RSI) technique, which involves the rapid administration of hypnotic drugs and a neuromuscular blocking agent. The technique may have to be modified in favor of titration of the hypnotic drug in hemodynamically unstable patients. The term *rapid sequence intubation* is commonly used when RSI is applied in the prehospital or emergency room setting.

Rapid sequence induction

Awake subjects have the protective reflexes to protect their tracheobronchial tree from foreign substances, notably from gastric contents that may find their way up through regurgitation or vomiting. In anesthetized, paralyzed, intubated patients, the trachea is isolated from the digestive system by a cuffed tracheal tube to prevent material in the oropharynx from gaining access to the lungs. The problem arises during the transition from the awake state to the anesthetized, paralyzed state, when protective reflexes may be blunted or abolished, while the airway is still not secured. The solution consists in minimizing the time between induction of anesthesia and insertion of a cuffed tracheal tube. The critical steps involved in RSI are summarized in Table 13.1 and explained below (see also Chapter 3).

Preoxygenation

If nitrogen is replaced by oxygen in the lungs, a normal adult without pulmonary disease can sustain 5–10 minutes of apnea if this is preceded by inhalation of 100% oxygen for 3–5 minutes.[1] Subjects with reduced functional residual capacity (FRC) or increased oxygen consumption (obesity, pregnancy, fever, hyperdynamic state) have a shorter period of apnea without desaturation. The purpose of preoxygenation is to provide adequate oxygenation during the interval between loss of consciousness and intubation. However, this time period is limited and RSI is not appropriate when a difficult airway is anticipated or if many attempts at intubation are made.

Rapid injection of drugs

Minimizing the time during which the airway is unprotected means that hypnotic drugs and neuromuscular blocking agents should be given rapidly. In addition, these drugs should be chosen so that their onset of action is as short as possible. This must be balanced against the risk of side effects such as hypotension.

Cricoid pressure

Unlike tracheal rings and the thyroid cartilage, which are not rigid posteriorly, the cricoid cartilage is rigid anteriorly and also posteriorly. The esophagus lies behind the cricoid

Trauma Anesthesia, 2nd Edition, ed. Charles E. Smith. Published by Cambridge University Press. © Charles E. Smith, 2015.

Table 13.1 Rapid sequence induction (RSI): critical steps

1. Preoxygenation with 100% O_2, ideally for 3–5 minutes
2. Rapid administration of a hypnotic drug and a neuromuscular blocking agent
3. Cricoid pressure and no manual ventilation (unless hypoxic or at risk for hypoxia)
4. When neuromuscular block is present, intubation of the trachea

cartilage, so that pressure applied anteriorly should normally compress the esophagus and prevent, to a certain extent, passage of gastric contents into the oropharynx. Application of cricoid pressure upon loss of consciousness, also called the Sellick maneuver, has had its detractors.[2] The right amount of pressure (20–30 N) should be applied by a well-trained assistant. Although the principle behind cricoid pressure appears logical, there is no compelling evidence that the risk of aspiration is reduced. Moreover, cricoid pressure may distort airway anatomy and impede the view of the glottis during intubation. Thus, cricoid pressure is not mandatory.

No manual ventilation

High inflation pressures generated by a bag and mask may allow gas into the stomach and increase the risk of regurgitation. Also, a distended stomach might press on the diaphragm and reduce lung volume. Therefore, bag-mask ventilation should be avoided during RSI. If, however, the patient is hypoxic or unable to be adequately preoxygenated, gentle manual bag-mask ventilation should be performed to prevent hypoxia. Properly applied cricoid pressure minimizes the risk of gastric distension during manual bag-mask ventilation when inflation pressures are less than 20 cmH_2O.

Intubation

The airway should be secured as soon as possible, but haste can be deleterious. Inadequate paralysis when laryngoscopy and intubation are performed might induce movement and coughing, with increased risk of aspiration. Warner *et al.* reported that inadequate paralysis at the time of intubation was present in as many as a third of the cases of aspiration that occurred at induction of anesthesia.[3] Thus, success of RSI depends on the administration of an adequate dose of neuromuscular blocking agent and on waiting long enough for complete paralysis to be manifest. To achieve this, neuromuscular monitoring is extremely useful.

Alternatives

There are few airway devices other than a cuffed tracheal tube that are indicated in trauma patients. Recent versions of supraglottic devices (laryngeal mask airways) have a relatively high sealing pressure and feature a drain tube to evacuate gastric fluid. However, these devices are not normally indicated in individuals with a full stomach, because they do not isolate the tracheobronchial tree as well as a tracheal tube. Awake tracheal

intubation may be the technique of choice, with or without the aid of a bronchoscope, especially in very unstable patients or in those with a difficult airway. However, a review of the literature suggests that, in most patients, the probability of intubation success is greater with RSI than with a technique involving only sedation. The failure rate may be as high as 15–20% when only light sedation is used, compared with 1–2% with RSI.[4]

Pharmacology with hypovolemia and depressed cardiac output

Drugs are usually thought of as being distributed in the body into one, two, or sometimes three compartments, from which they are excreted or metabolized. The effect of a drug is usually related to its concentration in the blood, or central compartment. This model fails to explain what happens in the seconds or minutes following intravenous injection of drugs and does not explain the behavior of drugs given for RSI, when an effect is expected within 1–2 minutes. Pharmacokinetics assumes instantaneous mixing of the drug in each compartment, starting right at the time of injection. In reality, a substance injected into a vein must reach the right side of the heart first, pass through the pulmonary circulation, get through the left side of the heart, and be distributed into the arteries before having access to the target organ. Thus, onset of action of drugs is associated with a certain time delay, which depends on how quickly the substance reaches the target organ. This is determined to a large extent by circulation time, which, in turn, depends on cardiac output. On the other hand, the drug concentration in the arterial blood will essentially depend on how much blood there is to dilute the drug.

If cardiac output is reduced, circulation time is increased. However, the drug will be diluted into a smaller volume of blood, because less blood goes through the heart as the drug is injected. This means that the concentration reaching the target organs will be greater if cardiac output is reduced than if it is normal. Similarly, initial concentrations will be greater if the patient is hypovolemic rather than normovolemic. A mathematical framework to describe what happens immediately after injection of a drug has been developed, and is now part of a special branch of pharmacokinetics, called front-end pharmacokinetics.[5] Studies have confirmed that hypovolemic subjects with reduced cardiac output are more sensitive to the effect of hypnotic drugs, but the effect takes longer to be manifest (see Chapter 7).[6]

For neuromuscular blocking agents, the same principles apply, but the net effect is different. Hypnotic drugs, such as propofol or thiopental, exert their action on the brain. When cardiac output decreases, blood flow to the vital organs, including the central nervous system, is relatively preserved, so that the brain receives a greater than normal proportion of cardiac output, and therefore a disproportionately large amount of drug. However, the site of action of neuromuscular blocking agents is at the neuromuscular junction in muscle tissue. Because the fraction of cardiac output irrigating muscle is reduced when cardiac output falls, in favor of vital organs, the amount of neuromuscular drug reaching its target might be less. However, the effect of reduced muscle blood flow is compensated for by the increased drug concentration in arterial blood, because of dilution of the drug into a small total blood volume. As a result, the required dose of neuromuscular blocking agent in hypovolemia and/or reduced cardiac output is not altered compared with normovolemia and normal cardiac output. However, the onset time, that is, the interval from injection until maximum neuromuscular blockade, is increased.[7]

Depolarizing agents
Mechanisms of action

Succinylcholine is the only depolarizing compound in clinical use. The mechanism of action of succinylcholine and other depolarizing agents is still poorly understood, but we know that, like acetylcholine, these drugs depolarize the muscle fiber at the endplate. However, contrary to acetylcholine, depolarizing drugs are not degraded by acetylcholinesterase. A persistent depolarization (longer than a few milliseconds) produces desensitization of acetylcholine receptors and/or inactivation of nearby sodium channels, the net effect of which is to prevent further acetylcholine activation and/or action potential generation in the muscle cell.

However, targets for succinylcholine action are not limited to the endplate, which contains a high density of receptors but occupies only a fraction of 1% of the area of the muscle cell membrane. Depolarizing agents also bind to extrajunctional receptors, which can be found at low density throughout the muscle membrane. In certain disease states, these receptors proliferate.[8] Because opening of any receptor, which the depolarizing agents produce at least once, causes potassium efflux from the cell, hyperkalemia is a feature of depolarizing blockade. In patients with a normal number of receptors, this increase in serum potassium is measurable (about 0.5 mEq/L), but insignificant clinically. In patients with an increased number of receptors, hyperkalemia may be catastrophic.[8,9]

Succinylcholine

Succinylcholine is used clinically not because of its depolarizing mechanism of action, but because it is the only neuromuscular blocking agent with rapid onset and rapid recovery. Its depolarizing nature carries many side effects, most of them minor, but some life-threatening. Succinylcholine also has many contraindications, most of them related to the depolarizing blockade it produces.

Plasma cholinesterase

The duration of succinylcholine blockade is only a few minutes thanks to metabolism by plasma cholinesterase, also called pseudocholinesterase or butyrylcholinesterase (Table 13.2). This enzyme is manufactured in the liver and released in plasma. Although similar to acetylcholinesterase, which hydrolyzes acetylcholine at the neuromuscular junction, the two enzymes are not strictly identical. Acetylcholinesterase does not hydrolyze succinylcholine. There are many genetic variants of plasma cholinesterase, and not all of them are associated with decreased activity of the enzyme.[10] Approximately 1 in 2000 individuals show a markedly decreased ability to metabolize succinylcholine, associated with neuromuscular blockade lasting 1–4 hours. The rest of the population shows a wide range of plasma cholinesterase activity, but enough to metabolize succinylcholine rapidly, so that the differences between individuals are not clinically apparent.

Table 13.2 Neuromuscular blocking agents: pharmacokinetics, metabolism, side effects

Agent	Elimination half-life	Excretion and metabolism	Major side effects
Succinylcholine	< 1 min with normal plasma cholinesterase	Plasma cholinesterase	See Table 13.4
Mivacurium	2 min (active isomers with normal plasma cholinesterase)	Plasma cholinesterase	Histamine release ($\geq$ 0.2 mg/kg)
Atracurium	20 min	Hofmann elimination Nonspecific esterase hydrolysis	Histamine release ($\geq$ 0.5 mg/kg)
Vecuronium	1–1.5 h	Liver uptake, metabolism, excretion Some renal elimination	None
Cisatracurium	25 min	Hofmann elimination Nonspecific esterase hydrolysis	None
Rocuronium	1–1.5 h	Liver uptake, metabolism, excretion Some renal elimination	None
Pancuronium	1–2 h	Liver metabolism, excretion Renal elimination	Tachycardia, hypertension
Doxacurium	1–2 h	Renal elimination	None

Pharmacology

After injection, succinylcholine first displays signs of its agonist properties at the neuromuscular junction. Disorganized muscle contractions can be observed, especially in young, muscular adults. These contractions, termed fasciculations, last for only a few seconds before flaccid paralysis is manifest. Dose–response relationships for succinylcholine can be obtained by plotting effect, defined as twitch depression at the thumb following ulnar nerve stimulation, versus dose given. For neuromuscular blocking agents, it is customary to determine the dose that corresponds, on average, to 95% twitch depression, or 95% block, and this dose is called the effective dose for 95% block, or ED_{95}.[11] The ED_{95} for succinylcholine is approximately 0.3 mg/kg (Table 13.3).[12] However, some patients need more to achieve the same degree of block. Also, the muscles of respiration, such as the diaphragm, are resistant to the effect of succinylcholine, that is, they require more than the muscles of the hand for an equal degree of paralysis.[13] As a result, the dose required to block all muscles in most, if not all, patients for tracheal intubation is greater than 0.3 mg/kg and is close to 1.0 mg/kg. Intubating conditions depend on dose. With 1.0 mg/kg, one can expect approximately 80% excellent conditions (no movement or cough). With 0.5 mg/kg, excellent conditions are found in only 50–60% of subjects.[14] The probability of

Table 13.3 Typical pharmacodynamic values for neuromuscular blocking agents

Agent	ED_{95} (mg/ kg)	Typical intubating doses (mg/ kg)	Onset (for 2 × ED_{95}) (min)	Duration (for 2 × ED_{95}) (min)
Ultra-short-duration agents				
Succinylcholine	0.3	1	1	8–10
Gantacurium*	0.19	0.6	1.5	8–10
Short-duration agents				
Mivacurium	0.1	0.2–0.25	3–5	15–25
Rapacuronium**	0.75	1.5–2.5	1–1.5	15–30
Intermediate-duration agents				
Atracurium	0.2	0.5	3–4	35–45
Vecuronium	0.05	0.1–0.15	3–4	35–45
Cisatracurium	0.05	0.15	5–7	40–45
Rocuronium	0.3	0.6–1.0	1.5–3	30–40
Long-acting agents				
Pancuronium	0.07	–	3–5	90–120
Doxacurium	0.025	–	7–10	90–120

ED_{95}, dose required to produce 95% twitch depression at the adductor pollicis. Derived from dose-response studies.
* Investigational drug.
** Withdrawn from market in 2001.

excellent conditions does not improve significantly if the dose is increased to 2 mg/kg.[15]

Onset and duration

In the vast majority of patients who metabolize succinylcholine normally, time to complete neuromuscular blockade as measured at the hand muscles after a 1 mg/kg dose is approximately 1 minute, and duration of action to return of normal twitch height is 10–12 minutes. Onset time is largely governed by circulatory factors. It is shorter in children and patients with a hyperdynamic circulation. It is prolonged in the elderly and low-output states, such as cardiac or hemorrhagic shock. Onset time is also shorter in central than in peripheral muscles. Thus, adequate conditions for tracheal intubation may be obtained before twitch response is abolished at the hand. The delay might be even greater if the response of foot muscles is monitored. Onset time is not markedly dose-dependent in the range of 0.5–2.0 mg/kg.[15] Duration shows marked interindividual variations for the same dose. Mean duration decreases or increases by only 2–3 minutes if the dose is halved or doubled, respectively.[14,15] Centrally located muscles, such as the diaphragm, recover faster than peripheral muscle. For example, the diaphragm starts to contract and breathing resumes 5 minutes, on average, after 1 mg/kg, 3–5 minutes before recovery is manifest at the hand.[16] However, variability of diaphragmatic recovery is wide.

Frequent side effects

Fasciculations are brief, disorganized contractions shortly after injection; they are the result of the brief agonist, acetylcholine-like action of succinylcholine. Mild (≤ 0.5 mEq/L) increase in potassium concentration occurs as a result of potassium efflux from the cells induced by activation of cholinergic receptors.[8] A contracture, or an increase in tension without nerve stimulation, may be seen in almost all muscles following succinylcholine, but the magnitude of this tension is usually too small to be seen. Myalgias are muscle pains occurring 24–48 hours after succinylcholine administration. Arrhythmias are common, and range from bradycardia due to vagal effect, to tachycardia, which is the result of catecholamine release. The side effects are listed in Table 13.4.

Uncommon side effects

In a small proportion of susceptible individuals, exaggerated contractures may be observed as masseter spasm, and may be of sufficient intensity to interfere with laryngoscopy and intubation. Succinylcholine may also precipitate malignant hyperthermia. Although masseter spasm may be an early manifestation of malignant hyperthermia, most cases of masseter spasm do not lead to malignant hyperthermia. Severe hyperkalemia, leading to cardiac arrhythmias and asystole, may be seen after succinylcholine in patients with extensive denervation and/or muscle injury.[9] This is observed after spinal cord injury, burns, extensive crush injuries, and muscle dystrophy. Milder versions of this phenomenon might occur in less extensive denervation, upper motor neuron lesions,

Table 13.4 Side effects of succinylcholine

Effect	Diminished by precurarization	Made worse by	Comments
Common side effects			
Fasciculations	Yes		Especially in muscular individuals
Myalgias	Yes		Especially in muscular and ambulatory individuals
Hyperkalemia	No	Burns, spinal cord trauma, crush injuries	Previously hyperkalemic patients might be at risk. Increased risk with acidosis
Bradycardia, asystole	No	More common in children or after second dose succinylcholine	Prevented by atropine
Catecholamine release	Yes		
Increased intraocular pressure	No	Light anesthesia, inadequate paralysis	
Increased intracranial pressure	Uncertain	Light anesthesia, inadequate paralysis	Magnitude of intracranial pressure increase is unlikely to be clinically significant. Secure airway, oxygenation, and ventilation of far greater importance after head injury
Rare side effects			
Malignant hyperthermia	No		
Masseter spasm	No		
Prolonged blockade	No		In patients with decreased plasma cholinesterase activity
Rhabdomyolysis	No	Muscle dystrophy, corticosteroid therapy	Risk of hyperkalemic cardiac arrest
Anaphylaxis	No		

other neurologic disease, immobility, steroid use, and preexisting hyperkalemia, as in renal failure. For most of these conditions, the common pathophysiologic mechanism is denervation-induced proliferation of extrajunctional receptors. In muscle disease, fragility of the muscle membrane is probably important. Considering the frequency of use, allergic or anaphylactic reactions have been reported for succinylcholine more than for any other drug used in anesthesia. Finally, patients with a genetic or acquired decrease in plasma cholinesterase activity have a prolonged response to the drug and may need to be ventilated for several hours after a usual dose of succinylcholine (Table 13.4).

Contraindications

Succinylcholine should not be given to patients with a documented history of malignant hyperthermia. Receptors in burns, spinal cord injury, and trauma with extensive muscle damage take a few days to proliferate, so succinylcholine should be avoided 24–48 hours after the injury.[8] The drug is probably safe again upon resolution of the initial injury. Succinylcholine should not be given in patients with muscle disease, especially muscle dystrophy, in subjects who have a history of an allergic reaction to the drug, or in those with a personal history of prolonged blockade after receiving either succinylcholine or mivacurium.

Special situations

In *pediatric* patients, the required mg/kg dose of succinylcholine increases with decreasing age. As much as 2 mg/kg is suitable in infants. Onset and duration are shorter in infants and children than in adults. Whereas adults often have tachycardia after succinylcholine, bradycardia, often leading to asystole, is frequent in infants and children. Pretreatment with atropine is effective (see Chapter 34).

In *obese* individuals, the same dose per kilogram actual body weight is recommended. Obese patients have a reduced volume of distribution per kilogram, because succinylcholine is water-soluble. However, plasma cholinesterase activity is increased in obese subjects. Both effects tend to cancel each other out.

Plasma cholinesterase activity is decreased in *liver disease*, *malnutrition*, and *pregnancy*. Patients with *myasthenia gravis* are resistant to the effects of succinylcholine and require more than the usual dose.

In children and adults, *repeat doses* of succinylcholine may cause bradycardia and asystole. Pretreatment with an anticholinergic, such as atropine 0.01 mg/kg, or glycopyrrolate 0.005 mg/kg, is indicated before administering a second dose of succinylcholine during RSI.

Controversies

There have been sporadic reports of intractable *cardiac arrests* associated with hyperkalemia in otherwise healthy children receiving succinylcholine. These events, which occurred chiefly in boys, have been attributed to undiagnosed muscle dystrophy.[9] These events have prompted some to recommend a ban of succinylcholine in the pediatric population, except in cases of emergency.

Succinylcholine has long been thought of as offering some kind of protection against *failed intubation*. Properly oxygenated lungs contain 1.5–2 L of oxygen, enough to sustain up to 8–10 minutes of apnea at a consumption rate of 200 mL/min. However, recent studies show that certain subjects (between 11% and 85%, depending on the study) given succinylcholine 1 mg/kg demonstrate a decrease in oxygen saturation before the diaphragm starts contracting again.[16–18] Clearly, oxygen desaturation can be seen in some patients, but the drug remains safer than other longer-acting agents in this regard.

Failure of the 1 mg/kg dose to protect against hypoxia has led some investigators to look for a better dose. With 0.56 mg/kg, acceptable intubating conditions were found in 95% of patients, which was considered acceptable, with shortening of the duration of neuromuscular blockade.[14] However, incidences of desaturation still occurred with 0.56 mg/kg.[16] Some patients were found to desaturate with just a fentanyl–propofol induction, without succinylcholine. Finding a perfect succinylcholine dose, which provides excellent intubating conditions and is associated with return of breathing before desaturation occurs, is an illusory goal. As failure at intubation occurs only in a small percentage of cases, priority should be given to adequate intubating conditions. The 1 mg/kg dose appears to be the best compromise.

A small dose of a nondepolarizing neuromuscular blocking agent given 2–4 minutes before succinylcholine is effective in the prevention of fasciculations and myalgia. This technique of *precurarization* has the potential to produce unpleasant symptoms in the awake patient. While diplopia and a general feeling of weakness are benign symptoms, difficulty swallowing or breathing are more serious, because they may indicate inability to protect one's airway against the possibility of pulmonary aspiration. A recent review of the literature shows that symptoms of muscle weakness are frequent in precurarization studies, but this may be all related to dose. Theoretical considerations and clinical studies suggest that the appropriate dose is one-tenth the ED_{95} of the precurarizing drug. Larger doses, amounting to 0.2–0.4 times the ED_{95}, should be avoided. With 0.1 times the ED_{95}, a larger dose of succinylcholine must be given (1.5–2 mg/kg) to

obtain the same onset and duration characteristics as with 1 mg/kg without precurarization.

Indications

Succinylcholine is used to obtain profound paralysis of short duration, and the need arises almost exclusively in the setting of securing the airway. In adults, the recommended dose for this indication is 1 mg/kg. Precurarization may be used to avoid fasciculations. A dose of no more than 0.03 mg/kg of rocuronium or equivalent should be given 2–3 minutes before succinylcholine. When precurarization is used, 1.5 or preferably 2 mg/kg of succinylcholine should be administered.

Nondepolarizing neuromuscular blocking agents

Mechanism of action

Nondepolarizing neuromuscular blocking agents bind to cholinergic receptors at the neuromuscular junction but do not produce activation. They compete with acetylcholine, which is released by the nerve terminal, for the same binding sites. In the absence of neuromuscular blocking agents, the amount of acetylcholine released with each nerve impulse is more than is needed to produce an endplate depolarization of sufficient magnitude to trigger a contraction. If impulses are generated by the nerve at a relatively high frequency (> 2 Hz), the amount of acetylcholine released with each impulse declines somewhat, but there is still enough release for the generation of a contraction. This "margin of safety" is essential for the production of sustained contractions.

With nondepolarizing neuromuscular blocking agents on board, many receptors are occupied, so the acetylcholine released might not be enough for a full contraction. If nerve impulses are generated at a high frequency, the amount of acetylcholine released decreases with each impulse. As a result, the contraction becomes weaker and weaker. This fade can be seen with a nerve stimulator when the train-of-four (2 Hz for 2 seconds) or tetanic (30–100 Hz for 5 seconds) are used. This is the basis of neuromuscular monitoring. The fade pattern observed with nondepolarizing blockade is analogous to that seen in myasthenia gravis. Train-of-four or tetanic fade is not seen with depolarizing agents (Fig. 13.1).

Characteristics of nondepolarizing neuromuscular blocking agents

Potency

Neuromuscular blocking agents are first characterized by their potency, which is determined by constructing dose–response curves. The force of contraction is measured at the adductor pollicis (thumb) in response to low-frequency stimulation (to avoid fade) of the ulnar nerve. The mean dose corresponding to 95% depression of twitch response (ED_{95}) can be obtained.[11] High-potency drugs have a low ED_{95}. Knowing the potency of drugs allows equipotent doses of different drugs to be compared.

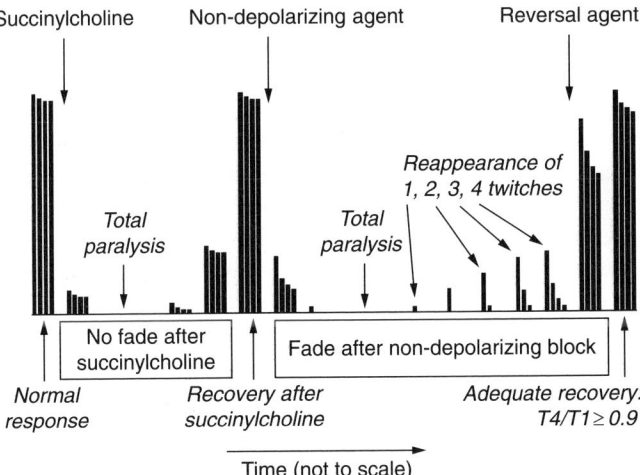

Figure 13.1 Neuromuscular monitoring during anesthesia for trauma. Succinylcholine is given for intubation. Upon recovery, a nondepolarizing agent is administered. An anticholinesterase drug is given to accelerate recovery. Train-of-four (stimulation at 2 Hz for 2 seconds) responses are represented against time. If succinylcholine is omitted in favor of a nondepolarizing agent, the sequence of events associated with succinylcholine does not occur.

Onset time

The time interval between injection of the drug and maximum blockade is called the *onset time*. In most circumstances, maximum blockade is 100%, as total paralysis is desired. Larger doses produce shorter onset times. When drugs are compared with one another, it is necessary to compare equipotent doses for meaningful comparisons. Usually, onset times are compared for doses equivalent to twice the ED_{95}.

Duration of action

Duration of neuromuscular blockade has to be measured until a key point in the recovery process. Investigators have agreed to define this key point as 25% first-twitch recovery, which happens to be approximately the time when four twitches start to be visible following train-of-four stimulation. In addition, reversal is more efficacious and reliable when given at 25% first-twitch recovery than when blockade is deeper. Larger doses produce longer-lasting paralysis.

Classification of nondepolarizing neuromuscular blocking agents

It is customary to classify neuromuscular blocking agents on the basis of their duration (Table 13.3). Again, it is necessary to make comparisons between equipotent doses of drugs, and the dose chosen for these comparisons is twice the ED_{95}. Although somewhat arbitrary, the following classification has proved useful.

Ultra-short-acting drugs

At present, there is no nondepolarizing neuromuscular blocking agent available for clinical use that is considered ultra-short-acting, with a duration of 8–12 minutes when a $2 \times ED_{95}$ dose is given. Succinylcholine is ultra-short-acting, but it is depolarizing.

Gantacurium is an investigational nondepolarizing compound that may fit the criteria for an ultra-short-acting agent. Its estimated ED_{95} is 0.12–0.19 mg/kg, and duration of action for twice the ED_{95} is less than 10 minutes in adults. It has some histamine-releasing properties. Gantacurium, if approved for clinical use, might become a succinylcholine replacement for tracheal intubation.

Short-acting drugs

Compounds with a duration of action in the 15- to 25-minute range belong to the short-acting category.

Mivacurium is a benzylisoquinolone derivative that is broken down by plasma cholinesterase, like succinylcholine, but unlike succinylcholine, it produces a nondepolarizing block. It is a mixture of three isomers (*trans–trans, cis–trans,* and *cis–cis*). Only the first two isomers are active at the neuromuscular junction, and these isomers have a plasma half-life of approximately 2 minutes.[19] The *cis–cis* isomer has a longer half-life (30 minutes), but it has virtually no neuromuscular blocking effect. The ED_{95} of mivacurium is approximately 0.1 mg/kg in patients with normal plasma cholinesterase. The duration of action for doses in the 0.15–0.25 mg/kg range is 15–25 minutes. As with succinylcholine, decreased plasma cholinesterase activity may be associated with a blockade lasting many hours, requiring mechanical ventilation of the lungs.

Mivacurium has a surprisingly long onset time, with complete blockade at the adductor pollicis taking 3–5 minutes after intubating doses (0.2–0.25 mg/kg). Thus, mivacurium is not recommended as a succinylcholine substitute for RSI. The other disadvantage of mivacurium is its propensity to release histamine in a dose-related fashion, at doses larger than or equal to 0.2 mg/kg. Mivacurium is indicated for short surgical procedures in patients who do not have a full stomach and in whom there is no anticipated difficulty with the airway. Mivacurium is no longer available in North America.

Rapacuronium is a nondepolarizing agent with a steroid nucleus. With 1.5–2.0 mg/kg, onset time approaches that of succinylcholine (1–1.5 minutes), and duration of action is in the 15- to 20-minute range. Rapacuronium enjoyed a brief period of popularity after it was released in the United States for clinical use. However, the drug was withdrawn in 2001, a year after its introduction, because of reports of severe bronchospasm in a small number of patients. The most likely mechanism for these reactions is preferential blockade of M_3 presynaptic muscarinic receptors in the lungs. These M_3 receptors normally put a brake on the activity of postsynaptic M_2 receptors, which produce bronchoconstriction.[20] Rapacuronium removes the brake in susceptible individuals, letting M_2 activity go unchecked.

Intermediate-acting drugs

Four nondepolarizing agents have a duration of action in the 30- to 45-minute range, when given in the $2 \times ED_{95}$ dose.

Atracurium is a benzylisoquinoline compound, like miva-curium. However, unlike mivacurium, it does not depend on plasma cholinesterase for its breakdown. Atracurium is degraded via two pathways, one of which is a nonenzymatic breakdown, called Hofmann elimination, a pH- and temperature-dependent process. Vials containing atracurium are acidified to prevent Hofmann elimination. The second pathway involves ester hydrolysis, via a group of enzymes called nonspecific esterases. These enzymes play a role in the breakdown of other drugs such as the β-blocker esmolol and the opioid remifentanil. Atracurium's unique mode of elimination provides a duration of action that is relatively independent of the function of traditional organs of elimination, such as the kidney and the liver. Elimination half-life of the drug is approximately 20 minutes, and is independent of age, end-organ function, and weight.

The ED_{95} of atracurium is 0.2–0.25 mg/kg, and recommended doses for intubation are 0.4–0.5 mg/kg. Duration of intubating doses is 35–45 minutes. Like mivacurium, atracurium releases histamine in a dose-related manner, with doses of 0.5 mg/kg and greater being associated with hypotension and tachycardia. Onset time is longer than for succinylcholine (3–4 minutes). Doses higher than 0.5 mg/kg are associated with an unacceptable incidence of histamine-related side effects. Thus, atracurium is not recommended for RSI. It may be used for maintenance of paralysis during anesthesia. The infusion rate is 3–7 μg/kg/min, or the equivalent in repeated bolus doses (0.1 mg/kg every 15–30 minutes).[21]

Hofmann elimination and ester hydrolysis both produce an end product called laudanosine, which is eliminated by the kidneys and has been found to produce seizures in high concentrations. Doses of atracurium normally required for anesthesia and surgery are not high enough to lead to laudanosine seizures. Theoretically, prolonged infusion of atracurium in the intensive care unit (ICU), especially in patients with altered renal function, might be associated with toxic laudanosine concentrations, but no case has been reported that linked atracurium with seizures in the ICU.[22]

Vecuronium is a compound with a steroid nucleus, like rapacuronium. After a bolus injection, the drug concentration in plasma falls rapidly due to redistribution, mainly to the liver. Vecuronium also undergoes some metabolism in the liver and is partially excreted unchanged by the kidney. Its elimination half-life is 1–2 hours. However, its duration of action is considerably less than the half-life would indicate, because vecuronium is extensively redistributed.[23]

The ED_{95} of vecuronium is 0.05 mg/kg, and doses of 0.1–0.15 mg/kg are recommended for intubation. Duration of action is heavily dose-dependent, ranging from 30–40 minutes after 0.1 mg/kg to 50–70 minutes after 0.15 mg/kg in young adults. Shorter durations are observed in children, and there is a longer duration of paralysis in the elderly. Hepatic failure and, to a lesser extent, renal failure are associated with a longer duration of action. Onset of action of vecuronium is 3–5 minutes for a 0.1 mg/kg dose. This interval can be shortened by increasing the dose, but at the expense of a prolonged duration of action. Fortunately, vecuronium is virtually devoid of cardiovascular side effects, even at doses as high as 0.4 mg/kg.

Vecuronium is not the drug of choice for RSI, at least in countries where the more rapidly acting rocuronium is available. Maintenance doses are typically 0.4–1 μg/kg/min when given by infusion,[21] or 0.02 mg/kg every 20–30 minutes.

Cisatracurium is one of the most potent isomers of atracurium, made up of approximately 10 isomers of different potencies. Hofmann elimination and ester hydrolysis, which both contribute to the degradation of atracurium, play the same role in the case of cisatracurium. The elimination half-life of cisatracurium is 20–25 minutes, and is independent of the patient's organs of elimination.[24]

The advantage of cisatracurium is its increased potency without an increase in the threshold for histamine side effects. The ED_{95} for neuromuscular block is 0.05 mg/kg, and histamine release does not occur unless the dose exceeds 0.4 mg/kg, which is rarely required clinically.[25] However, onset is long, 5–7 minutes for a $2 \times ED_{95}$ (0.1 mg/kg) dose, as is expected of potent drugs. Onset of action can be made shorter if the dose is increased to 0.15 or 0.2 mg/kg, at the expense of prolonged blockade. Duration of action increases from 40–45 minutes with 0.1 mg/kg to 60–75 minutes with 0.2 mg/kg.

Even high doses of cisatracurium do not provide a short enough onset time and adequate intubating conditions to recommend the drug for RSI. Cisatracurium may be used at induction of anesthesia if the patient does not have a full stomach, if there is no anticipated problem with management of the airway, and if the procedure is expected to last 1 hour or more, to match the expected duration of the recommended intubating dose (0.15 mg/kg). Lower doses are not recommended because of the long onset time. Infusion rates of 0.5–1.2 μg/kg/min,[26] or incremental doses of 0.02 mg/kg every 15–30 minutes, are recommended. Cisatracurium is also indicated when neuromuscular block is required in the ICU. Recovery is relatively rapid. Moreover, as the amount of drug administered is less than in the case of atracurium, the amount of laudanosine produced is less, and this virtually eliminates concerns with the seizure-producing effects of laudanosine.[22]

Rocuronium has a steroid nucleus, like vecuronium. Its pharmacokinetics are much like those of vecuronium, with an important redistribution phase after a bolus injection, followed by a slower elimination phase. Like vecuronium, distribution is mainly to the liver. Only part of the rocuronium dose is metabolized. The rest is excreted unchanged, chiefly in the bile and to a lesser extent by the kidney.[27] Elimination half-life is 1–2 hours, but duration of action of a $2 \times ED_{95}$ is much shorter (30–40 minutes).

The major pharmacologic difference between vecuronium and rocuronium is the ED_{95}. Rocuronium has one-sixth the potency of vecuronium, with an ED_{95} of 0.3 mg/kg. Because of its lack of potency, rocuronium has a faster onset of action than more potent drugs. At 0.6 mg/kg, complete neuromuscular block occurs in 1.5–2.5 minutes, about half the time required by an equipotent dose of vecuronium (0.1 mg/kg). Duration of action for that dose is 30–40 minutes. Thus, rocuronium is the nondepolarizing neuromuscular blocking agent of choice for tracheal intubation when succinylcholine is contraindicated or not desired.[28] However, rocuronium has a much longer duration of action than succinylcholine. If tracheal intubation is not successful after rocuronium administration, the selective binding agent sugammadex must be given to restore neurotransmission before onset of hypoxia. This option might not be possible if sugammadex is not immediately available.

Intubating conditions after rocuronium, 0.6 mg/kg, especially if laryngoscopy is started at 1 minute, are poorer than with succinylcholine, 1.0 mg/kg. For comparable intubating conditions, the rocuronium dose must be increased to 1.0 mg/kg, in which case onset becomes comparable to that of succinylcholine.[28] However, duration of action is increased to 60–75 minutes. Compared with young adults, onset time and duration of action are shorter in children and longer in the elderly. The duration of action of rocuronium may be prolonged in hepatic disease. Absence of renal function has only a modest effect on rocuronium duration of action. Rocuronium is virtually devoid of cardiovascular effects, up to a dose of 1.2 mg/kg.

Rocuronium is used to facilitate tracheal intubation, in doses varying between 0.6 and 1.2 mg/kg, depending on the quality of intubating conditions desired and the time one can afford to wait until laryngoscopy. In the presence of a full stomach, a high dose (> 0.9 mg/kg) is preferred because onset is rapid. Rocuronium is also used for maintenance of relaxation by infusion at a rate of 4–8 µg/kg/min,[26] or by bolus doses (0.1–0.2 mg/kg every 15–30 minutes).

Long-acting drugs

A disparate group of compounds is characterized by a long duration of action (> 60 minutes, usually 90–120 minutes). The older neuromuscular blocking agents, all of which have significant cardiovascular effects, fall into this category. In addition, some newer agents, which tend not to have cardiovascular side effects, also have a long duration of action. Representatives of the old group are *d*-tubocurarine, gallamine, pancuronium, alcuronium, and fazadinium. Doxacurium and pipecuronium are more recent. Long-acting drugs have fallen out of favor because they tend to be associated with a high incidence of residual paralysis.[29,30] Studies over the past 25 years or so have revealed a 50–75% incidence of residual paralysis in the recovery room, even with reversal agents, compared with 20–40% with intermediate blocking agents.[29,30] Thus, long-acting drugs should be given only to patients who are likely to have their lungs ventilated postoperatively, and even for this indication, their use might be associated with some drawbacks. For example, in cardiac surgery, it was found that extubation was delayed in patients who received pancuronium compared with rocuronium.[31] In the ICU, recovery may be very long after

stopping these agents. Only the most commonly used agents, pancuronium and doxacurium, are discussed here.

Pancuronium is a steroid-based molecule that does not exhibit the redistribution phase that vecuronium and rocuronium have. Elimination half-life and duration of action are thus similar (1–2 hours). Pancuronium is eliminated in the liver and the kidney. The ED_{95} is 0.07 mg/kg. Pancuronium is not recommended for tracheal intubation. Even modest doses produce hypertension and tachycardia. Maintenance doses are 0.01–0.02 mg/kg every 30–60 minutes.

Doxacurium is a potent benzylisoquinoline compound that depends chiefly on the kidney for its elimination. Terminal half-life and duration of action are similar to those of pancuronium. The ED_{95} is 0.025 mg/kg. Doxacurium is devoid of cardiovascular side effects. Because of its high potency, onset time is extremely slow (7–10 minutes), making doxacurium useless for tracheal intubation. Maintenance doses are 2–10 µg/kg per hour.

Reversal agents

Extubation criteria

After administration of neuromuscular blocking agents, recovery does not occur in all muscles simultaneously. The diaphragm is one of the first muscles to recover, and diaphragmatic movements can be detected relatively early. Abdominal muscles, which are essential for cough production, recover with a slight delay compared with the diaphragm.[32] Finally, muscles of the upper airway, which are needed to keep the airway patent, are last to recover.[33] This means that tidal volume breathing with a tracheal tube in place is not a sufficient criterion for readiness for extubation. Because the adequacy of upper airway muscles cannot be tested when the tracheal tube is in place, indirect measurements have to be made. It is generally agreed that a train-of-four ratio (height of fourth twitch divided by height of first twitch) greater than 0.9 at the adductor pollicis indicates recovery of respiratory function, including upper airway (Fig. 13.1).[29,30,33] To accelerate recovery, reversal agents are useful. These drugs are needed only when extubation is planned.

Anticholinesterase agents

The acetylcholinesterase inhibitors neostigmine, edrophonium, and pyridostigmine may be used for reversal of nondepolarizing neuromuscular blockade. Edrophonium is not available in many countries and pyridostigmine has a long onset of action. As a result, neostigmine is by far the most widely used acetylcholinesterase inhibitor. Neostigmine inhibits acetylcholinesterase, the enzyme that breaks down acetylcholine. Excess acetylcholine present at the neuromuscular junction competes with the neuromuscular agent present at the receptor, favoring transmission. Such a mechanism of action implies that there is a ceiling effect with these drugs: it is not possible to cause more than 100% inhibition of the enzyme.[34] This means that the degree of reversal produced by these drugs is limited, even at high doses. For this reason, reversal is usually ineffective when neuromuscular blockade is too deep. Rapid return of neuromuscular function only occurs when partial recovery is already apparent at the adductor pollicis muscle before injection of the anticholinesterase drug. The presence of at least two, and preferably four, responses to train-of-four stimulation is a prerequisite for adequate and effective reversal.[35]

Anticholinesterase agents have effects at all peripheral cholinergic synapses, so parasympathomimetic effects are expected. Severe bradycardia and asystole can be observed following injection of these drugs. To counteract these severe side effects, anticholinergic, antimuscarinic agents, such as atropine or glycopyrrolate, must be given. Neostigmine, edrophonium, and pyridostigmine penetrate the blood–brain barrier poorly, so they do not produce central cholinergic effects. Physostigmine, an anticholinergic drug that penetrates the blood–brain barrier, is not used as a reversal agent because of its central effects.

Neostigmine

The most commonly used reversal agent is neostigmine, in doses of 0.04–0.05 mg/kg. Doses of more than 0.07 mg/kg are not recommended. Peak effect is seen in 5–7 minutes.[34] Half-life is 1–2 hours, longer than the duration of action of intermediate-duration agents, and approximately the same as that of long-acting neuromuscular blocking drugs. Neostigmine should be used with the anticholinergic drugs atropine or glycopyrrolate, in doses amounting to one-half and one-quarter of the neostigmine dose, respectively.

Edrophonium

The recommended doses of edrophonium are 0.5–1 mg/kg. Peak effect occurs within 2 minutes. Half-life is like that of neostigmine.[34] Edrophonium is less effective than neostigmine for moderate blockade (less than four twitches visible or marked fade). The appropriate dose of atropine is 0.01 mg/kg, regardless of edrophonium dose.

Pyridostigmine

Peak effect of pyridostigmine is 10–15 minutes. Although the drug is as effective as neostigmine, its slow onset makes it less popular.

Selective binding agents

Another mechanism, selective binding of nondepolarizing agent molecules, has been proposed recently to accelerate recovery from neuromuscular blockade.

Sugammadex

Sugammadex is a relatively new compound that selectively binds rocuronium and, to a lesser extent, vecuronium and pancuronium. Chemically, it is a ring of eight sugars arranged in the form of a doughnut with a high affinity for rocuronium.

Sugammadex is excreted via the kidney either unbound or as a rocuronium–sugammadex complex. Sugammadex was released for clinical use in 2008 and has been approved in many countries, including Australia, Japan, and most of the European Union. At the time of writing, it was not available in the United States or Canada. Sugammadex provides rapid (2–3 minutes) and effective restoration of neuromuscular function, provided that the appropriate dose is given. Recovery is more rapid and more complete than with neostigmine.[36] Recommended doses are 2 mg/kg for "moderate" blockade, that is when two twitches have reappeared in the train-of-four, and 4 mg/kg for "deep" blockade, when no twitch response is seen and a response can be seen after a 50 Hz tetanus applied for 5 seconds (post-tetanic count or PTC of 1–2).[36] Unlike neostigmine, sugammadex is virtually free of cardiovascular effects, and it is effective even for profound blockade, provided that the appropriate dose is given. Sugammadex can be used as a rescue drug to reestablish neuromuscular function in case of a failed intubation. If used 3 minutes after high-dose rocuronium (1.2 mg/kg), sugammadex 16 mg/kg leads to full recovery of neuromuscular transmission in a mean of 3.2 minutes, for a total of 6.2 minutes from rocuronium administration. This is shorter than the mean 10.9-minute duration of succinylcholine block.[37]

Clinical use

The recommended sequence of events for a trauma patient suspected of having a full stomach is summarized in Table 13.5.

Intubation in the emergency setting

Neuromuscular blocking agents are used to facilitate tracheal intubation in unstable trauma patients who require airway management to improve oxygenation and ventilation. Large series demonstrate that success of tracheal intubation is greatly improved when neuromuscular blocking agents are given in this setting.[4] However, the potential for harm is greater when neuromuscular agents are given. If intubation and ventilation turn out to be impossible in an anesthetized, paralyzed patient, a fatal outcome is almost certain unless an alternative form of airway access can be obtained (e.g., laryngeal mask airway, transtracheal jet ventilation, cricothyroidotomy; see Chapter 3). If intubation is attempted in a mildly sedated, nonparalyzed patient, failure means no worsening of the patient's state. The decision to use neuromuscular blocking agents should be made by skilled personnel, after an adequate airway examination, and with due consideration to possible cervical spine injuries.

First-line drug

In the absence of any contraindication, the drug of choice is succinylcholine, because of its short onset and short duration of action. The drug should be given after proper preoxygenation and appropriate sedation. The usual dose is 1.0 mg/kg. Precurarization may be used, with special attention to the

Table 13.5 Suggested steps for rapid sequence induction (RSI)

Time (minutes)	Action
−3 to 0	Preoxygenation
−3 (optional)	Precurarization (0.03 mg/kg rocuronium or equivalent)
−1 (optional)	Small dose opioid
0	Induction agent
At loss of consciousness	Cricoid pressure*
	Neuromuscular blocking agent
	• succinylcholine 1 mg/kg if no precurarization, or
	• succinylcholine 2 mg/kg if precurarization, or
	• rocuronium 1 mg/kg
	No manual ventilation**
+1 to 1.5 (when blockade complete)	Laryngoscopy and intubation
After tracheal intubation	Release of cricoid pressure, confirm end-tidal CO_2

* Cricoid pressure may distort airway anatomy and impede the view of the glottis during intubation.
** Manual ventilation of the lungs using low inflation pressures (< 20 cmH$_2$O) is done if the patient is hypoxic or at risk for becoming hypoxic (modified RSI).

following: the precurarization dose should not cause any paralysis or discomfort of its own, and doses in excess of 10% of the ED$_{95}$ of the precurarizing agent should be avoided.[38] This corresponds to rocuronium 0.03 mg/kg or equivalent. When precurarization is used, the dose of succinylcholine should be increased by 50–100% to 1.5–2 mg/kg.

If sugammadex is readily available, rocuronium 1.0–1.2 mg/kg may be substituted for succinylcholine, even in patients with no contraindication for succinylcholine. However, an appropriate dose (16 mg/kg) of sugammadex should be stocked in a drawer next to the patient, not in a far-away emergency cart, and the dose should be calculated before rocuronium is given, so it is fresh in the minds of providers who manage the airway. Simulations have shown that if these conditions are not met, unacceptable delays may be introduced, putting the patient at risk of hypoxia.[39]

Raised intracranial pressure

The effects of succinylcholine on intracranial pressure (ICP) are uncertain. It appears that there is a modest increase in ICP with succinylcholine injected without precurarization, which has been attributed to the increase in the partial pressure of carbon dioxide (PaCO$_2$) following fasciculations. Precurarization seems to abolish this increase. However, it should be remembered that inadequate levels of anesthesia, inadequate paralysis, and multiple attempts at intubation are more likely to increase ICP than succinylcholine alone.

Open eye injury

Succinylcholine, but not nondepolarizing agents, raises intraocular pressure (IOP) by a few mmHg. This increase still persists after precurarization. As with ICP, inadequate anesthesia or paralysis is more likely to produce increased IOP than succinylcholine. The literature does not provide convincing evidence that succinylcholine has ever been associated with loss of an eye.[40] In open eye injuries, nondepolarizing agents are preferred, but inadequate anesthesia and struggling to secure the airway may be more detrimental to the patient than succinylcholine.

Full stomach

An RSI with cricoid pressure is recommended in patients with, or suspected of having, a full stomach. Such a technique is not 100% effective, however, and concerns have been raised about the ability of succinylcholine to raise intragastric pressure (IGP). This increase is related to fasciculations and is prevented by precurarization. However, succinylcholine raises gastric sphincter pressure, which cancels the IGP increase effect.

Burns

Receptor proliferation and succinylcholine-induced hyperkalemia occur 24–48 hours after injury. The extent of this phenomenon depends on the degree of injury and is not prevented by precurarization.[8] Succinylcholine is best avoided, unless the patient is seen within the first few hours after injury.

Spinal cord injury

The time course of receptor proliferation in cases of cord transection is much the same as in burns, so succinylcholine should be avoided unless the injury is recent. In the case of cervical injuries, fasciculations may, at least theoretically, move fractured vertebral fragments against each other, so precurarization is preferred if succinylcholine is used.

Extensive trauma

Hyperkalemia after extensive trauma has been reported after succinylcholine. This might be the direct consequence of extensive muscle damage, with associated leak of potassium out of the cells. Another mechanism for hyperkalemia is the acidosis commonly associated with hypovolemic shock. Both can be exacerbated by succinylcholine.

Alternatives to succinylcholine

If succinylcholine is contraindicated, rocuronium is the best alternative, because it has a faster onset of action than any other nondepolarizing agent.[28] A dose of 1 mg/kg is associated with better intubating conditions than 0.6 mg/kg, and this difference in dose might be important in cases of increased ICP or IOP. Duration of action of rocuronium (30–60 minutes) is much longer than that of succinylcholine (8–10 minutes). This is an important consideration when repeated neurologic examinations are planned on the patient, as such exams cannot be conducted in paralyzed individuals. In addition, sedation has to be provided for the duration of paralysis. It is possible that rocuronium will replace succinylcholine gradually as the first-line drug in trauma patients, as sugammadex use becomes more widespread. However, it must be emphasized that a large enough supply of sugammadex (16 mg/kg) must be within hand's reach, not stocked somewhere in the hospital. The high cost of sugammadex will probably prevent it from being available at all sites where intubations may be performed.

Tracheal intubation for anesthesia

In trauma patients who must undergo surgery, considerations for intubation are the same as in the emergency setting (see Intubation in the Emergency Setting, previously). The indications for a nondepolarizing neuromuscular blocking agent can be extended, however, because there is no possibility to assess the neurologic status and an anesthetic has to be given for the duration of surgery. Neuromuscular monitoring is extremely useful, and an example of its interpretation is depicted in Fig. 13.1. A thorough airway exam has to be performed to anticipate any difficulty with intubation (see Chapter 3). Of the nondepolarizing drugs, rocuronium has the fastest onset.

Maintenance of neuromuscular relaxation

During surgery, relaxation can be maintained with any intermediate-duration drug administered as intermittent boluses or by infusion (Fig. 13.1). The degree of relaxation required depends on the patient and the surgical procedure, but maintaining the train-of-four response at the adductor pollicis between zero and two visible twitches is usually adequate. Onset of action is not a concern for maintenance of relaxation, and the doses given are much lower than the threshold for cardiovascular effects. It is good practice to monitor signs of neuromuscular recovery after succinylcholine, if that drug was used for intubation, to rule out rare cases of prolonged paralysis due to plasma cholinesterase deficiency. The dose of nondepolarizing agent does not need to be as high as for intubation, because additional doses can be given if needed. A dose equivalent to the ED_{95} might be administered.

If extubation is planned immediately after surgery or shortly thereafter, intermediate-duration agents are preferred to long-acting agents because they provide flexibility of administration and a much reduced risk of postoperative paralysis.[29,31] If prolonged mechanical ventilation is planned after the surgical procedure, then long-acting drugs may be given. However, should relaxation be continued in the ICU with these drugs, recovery might be very long. For administration in the ICU, cisatracurium has the advantages of flexibility, titratability, and rapid recovery upon cessation of the infusion.

Recovery

Tracheal extubation should be performed only if the respiratory muscles, including those of the upper airway, have recovered. This occurs when the measured train-of-four ratio at the adductor pollicis is more than 0.9.[29,30] It should be remembered that visual or tactile evaluation of train-of-four responses fails to detect residual curarization for values of the train-of-four ratio as small as 0.3–0.4. Tetanic stimulation at 50 Hz is no better, so substantial paralysis may be present even if the tetanic response appears sustained.[41] Reversal with an anticholinesterase drug is therefore indicated unless a measurement device confirms that the train-of-four ratio is at least 0.9. Time alone is not a guarantee of recovery. Residual paralysis may be detected even 4 hours after $2 \times ED_{95}$ doses of rocuronium, atracurium, or vecuronium.[42]

Reversal with anticholinesterases should be attempted when sufficient spontaneous recovery is present, that is, when two, and preferably four, responses are observed after train-of-four stimulation.[35] If paralysis is too deep, early administration of reversal agents will not accelerate time to full recovery. In addition, recovery will be slow, so that the duration of "blind paralysis" will be increased. Blind paralysis occurs when visual or manual detection of paralysis is not possible (train-of-four ratio > 0.3–0.4) but when full recovery is not attained (train-of-four ratio ≤ 0.9).

Conclusions

Neuromuscular blocking agents are extremely useful in trauma patients who require an anesthetic. Succinylcholine is the drug of choice for tracheal intubation, because trauma patients usually have a full stomach and a rapid sequence induction is indicated. However, succinylcholine may be contraindicated as a result of the patient's condition or type of injury. Head, eye, spinal cord, burn, and crushing injuries require special attention. Rocuronium is the preferred nondepolarizing drug if succinylcholine is contraindicated. Availability of sugammadex may widen the indications for rocuronium. For maintenance of relaxation and recovery, the principles that are valid in elective patients usually apply in patients with traumatic injuries.

Questions

(1) A classic rapid sequence induction (RSI) typically involves all of the following, *except*:
   a. Preoxygenation
   b. Rapid injection of a hypnotic drug
   c. Bag-mask ventilation
   d. Injection of a neuromuscular blocking agent
   e. Cricoid pressure
(2) If a neuromuscular blocking agent is given to a patient with a decreased cardiac output:
   a. The dose should be reduced
   b. The dose should be increased

c. Time to maximum blockade is expected to be short

d. Time to maximum blockade is expected to be long

e. There is no marked change in dose or onset time

(3) Pharmacologic effects of succinylcholine include all of the following, *except*:

   a. Competitive antagonism at the postsynaptic receptor

   b. Depolarization of the endplate

   c. Inactivation of sodium channels

   d. Binding of extrajunctional receptors

   e. Potassium efflux from the muscle fiber

(4) Plasma cholinesterase activity is reduced in all of the following, *except*:

   a. In certain individuals who do not have the normal gene for plasma cholinesterase

   b. In obese individuals

   c. In patients with liver disease

   d. In malnourished subjects

   e. In pregnant women

(5) A small dose of a nondepolarizing neuromuscular blocking agent given before succinylcholine will likely:

   a. Increase the duration of succinylcholine blockade

   b. Abolish succinylcholine-induced hyperkalemia

   c. Prevent an increase in intraocular pressure

   d. Diminish the probability of fasciculations and postoperative myalgia

   e. Improve tracheal intubating conditions

(6) The nondepolarizing neuromuscular agent with the fastest onset time is:

   a. Mivacurium

   b. Atracurium

   c. Cisatracurium

   d. Vecuronium

   e. Rocuronium

(7) Termination of action of rocuronium depends mainly on:

   a. Plasma cholinesterase

   b. Nonspecific ester hydrolysis

   c. Redistribution

   d. Renal elimination

   e. Metabolism in liver

(8) A marked increase in sensitivity to nondepolarizing neuromuscular blocking agents is seen in:

   a. Burns

   b. Spinal cord injury

   c. Extensive trauma

   d. Myasthenia gravis

   e. Head injury

(9) If not contraindicated, succinylcholine is the drug of choice for tracheal intubation in trauma patients because:

   a. It has a fast onset and recovery

   b. It is a depolarizing drug

   c. It is metabolized by plasma cholinesterase

   d. It has few cardiovascular effects

   e. Its effect can be reversed by neostigmine

(10) Neostigmine:

   a. Penetrates the blood–brain barrier

   b. Has limited efficacy when blockade is deep

   c. Produces tachycardia

   d. Is more rapidly acting than edrophonium

   e. Binds irreversibly to nondepolarizing neuromuscular drugs

Answers

(1) c

(2) d

(3) a

(4) b

(5) d

(6) e

(7) c

(8) d

(9) a

(10) b

References

1. Edmark L, Kostova-Aherdan K, Enlund M, Hedenstierna G. Optimal oxygen concentration during induction of general anesthesia. *Anesthesiology* 2003; **98**: 28–33.

2. Brimacombe JR, Berry AM. Cricoid pressure. *Can J Anaesth* 1997; **44**: 414–25.

3. Warner MA, Warner ME, Weber JG. Clinical significance of pulmonary aspiration during the perioperative period. *Anesthesiology* 1993; **78**: 56–62.

4. Kovacs G, Law JA, Ross J, *et al.* Acute airway management in the emergency department by non-anesthesiologists. *Can J Anaesth* 2004; **51**: 174–80.

5. Krejcie TC, Avram MJ. What determines anesthetic induction dose? It's the front-end kinetics, doctor! *Anesth Analg* 1999; **89**: 541–4.

6. Shafer SL. Shock values. *Anesthesiology* 2004; **101**: 567–8.

7. Kuipers JA, Boer F, Olofsen E, Bovill JG, Burm AG. Recirculatory pharmacokinetics and pharmacodynamics of rocuronium in patients: The influence of cardiac output. *Anesthesiology* 2001; **94**: 47–55.

8. Martyn JA, Richtsfeld M. Succinylcholine-induced hyperkalemia in acquired pathologic states: Etiologic factors and molecular mechanisms. *Anesthesiology* 2006; **104**: 158–69.

9. Gronert GA. Cardiac arrest after succinylcholine: mortality greater with rhabdomyolysis than receptor upregulation. *Anesthesiology* 2001; **94**: 523–9.

10. Davis L, Britten JJ, Morgan M. Cholinesterase: its significance in anaesthetic practice. *Anaesthesia* 1997; **52**: 244–60.

11. Donati F. Neuromuscular blocking drugs for the new millennium: current practice, future trends–comparative pharmacology of neuromuscular

blocking drugs. *Anesth Analg* 2000; **90**: S2–6.

12. Smith CE, Donati F, Bevan DR. Dose–response curves for succinylcholine: Single versus cumulative techniques. *Anesthesiology* 1988; **69**: 338–42.

13. Smith CE, Donati F, Bevan DR. Potency of succinylcholine at the diaphragm and at the adductor pollicis muscle. *Anesth Analg* 1988; **67**: 625–30.

14. Naguib M, Samarkandi A, Riad W, Alharby SW. Optimal dose of succinylcholine revisited. *Anesthesiology* 2003; **99**: 1045–9.

15. Naguib M, Samarkandi AH, El Din ME, *et al.* The dose of succinylcholine required for excellent endotracheal intubating conditions. *Anesth Analg* 2006; **102**: 151–5.

16. Naguib M, Samarkandi AH, Abdullah K, Riad W, Alharby SW. Succinylcholine dosage and apnea-induced hemoglobin desaturation in patients. *Anesthesiology* 2005; **102**: 35–40.

17. Hayes AH, Breslin DS, Mirakhur RK, Reid JE, O'Hare RA. Frequency of haemoglobin desaturation with the use of succinylcholine during rapid sequence induction of anaesthesia. *Acta Anaesthesiol Scand* 2001; **45**: 746–9.

18. Heier T, Feiner JR, Lin J, Brown R, Caldwell JE. Hemoglobin desaturation after succinylcholine-induced apnea: a study of the recovery of spontaneous ventilation in healthy volunteers. *Anesthesiology* 2001; **94**: 754–9.

19. Lacroix M, Donati F, Varin F. Pharmacokinetics of mivacurium isomers and their metabolites in healthy volunteers after intravenous bolus administration. *Anesthesiology* 1997; **86**: 322–30.

20. Jooste EH, Sharma A, Zhang Y, Emala CW. Rapacuronium augments acetylcholine-induced bronchoconstriction via positive allosteric interactions at the M3 muscarinic receptor. *Anesthesiology* 2005; **103**: 1195–203.

21. Martineau RJ, St Jean B, Kitts JB, *et al.* Cumulation and reversal with prolonged infusions of atracurium and vecuronium. *Can J Anaesth* 1992; **39**: 670–6.

22. Fodale V, Santamaria LB. Laudanosine, an atracurium and cisatracurium metabolite. *Eur J Anaesthesiol* 2002; **19**: 466–73.

23. Miller RD, Rupp SM, Fisher DM, *et al.* Clinical pharmacology of vecuronium and atracurium. *Anesthesiology* 1984; **61**: 444–53.

24. Kisor DF, Schmith VD. Clinical pharmacokinetics of cisatracurium besilate. *Clin Pharmacokinet* 1999; **36**: 27–40.

25. Bryson HM, Faulds D. Cisatracurium besilate. A review of its pharmacology and clinical potential in anaesthetic practice. *Drugs* 1997; **53**: 848–66.

26. Miller DR, Wherrett C, Hull K, Watson J, Legault S. Cumulation characteristics of cisatracurium and rocuronium during continuous infusion. *Can J Anaesth* 2000; **47**: 943–9.

27. Khuenl-Brady KS, Sparr H. Clinical pharmacokinetics of rocuronium bromide. *Clin Pharmacokinet* 1996; **31**: 174–83.

28. Andrews JI, Kumar N, van den Brom RH, *et al.* A large simple randomized trial of rocuronium versus succinylcholine in rapid-sequence induction of anaesthesia along with propofol. *Acta Anaesthesiol Scand* 1999; **43**: 4–8.

29. Naguib M, Kopman AF, Ensor JE. Neuromuscular monitoring and postoperative residual curarisation: a meta-analysis. *Br J Anaesth* 2007; **98**: 302–16

30. Murphy GS, Brull SJ. Residual neuromuscular block: lessons unlearned. Part I: definitions, incidence, and adverse physiological effects of residual neuromuscular block. *Anesth Analg* 2010; **111**: 120–8.

31. Murphy GS, Szokol JW, Marymont JH, *et al.* Recovery of neuromuscular function after cardiac surgery: Pancuronium versus rocuronium. *Anesth Analg* 2003; **96**: 1301–7.

32. Kirov K, Motamed C, Dhonneur G. Differential sensitivity of abdominal muscles and the diaphragm to mivacurium: An electromyographic study. *Anesthesiology* 2001; **95**: 1323–8.

33. Herbstreit F, Peters J, Eikermann M. Increased upper airway collapsibility and blunted genioglossus muscle activity in response to negative pharyngeal pressure. *Anesthesiology* 2009; **110**: 1253–60.

34. Caldwell JE. Clinical limitations of acetylcholinesterase antagonists. *J Crit Care* 2009; **24**: 21–8.

35. Kirkegaard H, Heier T, Caldwell JE. Efficacy of tactile-guided reversal from cisatracurium-induced neuromuscular block. *Anesthesiology* 2002; **96**: 45–50.

36. Paton F, Paulden M, Chambers D, *et al.* Sugammadex compared with neostigmine/glycopyrrolate for routine reversal of neuromuscular block: a systematic review and economic evaluation. *Br J Anaesth* 2010; **105**: 558–67.

37. Lee C, Jahr JS, Candiotti KA, *et al.* reversal of profound neuromuscular block by sugammadex administered three minutes after rocuronium: a comparison with spontaneous recovery from succinylcholine. *Anesthesiology* 2009; **110**: 1020–5.

38. Schreiber JU, Lysakowski C, Fuchs-Buder T, Tramer MR. Prevention of succinylcholine-induced fasciculation and myalgia: A meta-analysis of randomized trials. *Anesthesiology* 2005; **103**: 877–84.

39. Bisschops MM, Holeman C, Huitink JM. Can sugammadex save a patient in a simulated 'cannot intubate, cannot ventilate' situation? *Anesthesia* 2010; **65**: 936–41.

40. Vachon CA, Warner DO, Bacon DR. Succinylcholine and the open globe: tracing the teaching. *Anesthesiology* 2003, **99**: 220–3.

41. Capron F, Fortier LP, Racine S, Donati F. Tactile fade detection with hand or wrist stimulation using train-of-four, double-burst stimulation, 50-hertz tetanus, 100-hertz tetanus, and acceleromyography. *Anesth Analg* 2006; **102**: 1578–84.

42. Debaene B, Plaud B, Dilly MP, Donati F. Residual paralysis in the PACU after a single intubating dose of nondepolarizing muscle relaxant with an intermediate duration of action. *Anesthesiology* 2003; **98**: 1042–8.

Chapter

14

Hypothermia in trauma

Eldar Søreide, Kristian Strand, and Charles E. Smith

Objectives

(1) Provide the reader with a thorough understanding of the clinical impact of hypothermia in trauma patients.

(2) Provide a clinically useful guide to the differentiation between mild, moderate, and severe trauma-associated hypothermia.

(3) Present the current knowledge on prevention and treatment of hypothermia in trauma victims, with a special focus on critical bleeding.

(4) Understand the mechanisms and the diagnosis and treatment of accidental hypothermia with and without asphyxia.

Introduction

The anesthesiologist can play many important roles in the trauma chain of survival (Fig. 14.1). In some systems, the contribution of the anesthesiologist is limited to perioperative care, while in other systems the anesthesiologist acts as a prehospital emergency physician, as a member of the hospital trauma team, and as a critical care physician. Independent of where and what role, hypothermia is a serious complication to trauma that deserves the anesthesiologist's full attention.[1–3] As hypothermia is generally considered detrimental for the patient, much focus has been on prevention. Despite this, hypothermia in trauma patients is still a common finding. There are many indications that hypothermia is still not managed in an optimal fashion.[3,4]

Based on promising animal results, some authors believe that rapidly induced extreme hypothermia ("hibernation") may play a future role in severe hemorrhagic shock during transport to definitive surgical care.[5,6] So far, this laboratory research has not changed clinical practice, and it probably will not do so in the near future. On the other hand, in patients with traumatic brain injury, induction of mild hypothermia (therapeutic hypothermia) has become a promising treatment modality.[7] Hypothermia may also develop without concurrent trauma (accidental hypothermia).[8,9] The aim of this chapter is to present an overview of our current understanding of hypothermia associated with trauma, with the main focus being on clinical management.

Thermoregulation and thermal management
Thermoregulation in humans

Thermoregulation allows core temperature to remain stable within a narrow temperature range despite large variations in environmental conditions.[10,11] In the thermoneutral zone (TNZ) the basal metabolic rate is producing enough heat to prevent a fall in core temperature, while not increasing it.[10,11] The insulation (clothing and other protective layers) is the most important factor defining the TNZ in humans (Figs. 14.2–14.4). Outside the TNZ, two main involuntary mechanisms will act to maintain a stable core temperature:

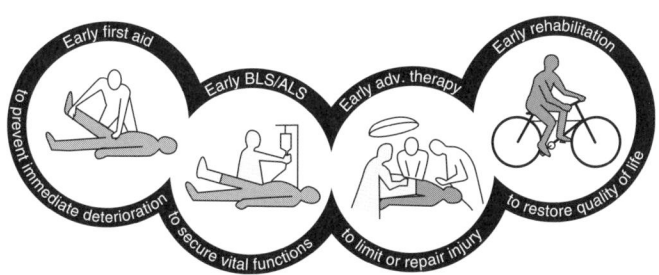

Figure 14.1 Trauma chain of survival. Reproduced with permission from Laerdal Medical Inc.

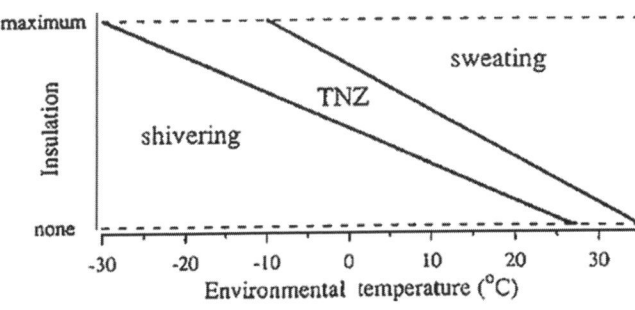

Figure 14.2 The insulation value of clothing determines the environmental range of the thermoneutral zone (TNZ). The greater the insulation, the lower the TNZ. Humans have the unique ability to alter their supracutanous insulation layer. (Reproduced with permission from Grahn 1997.[10])

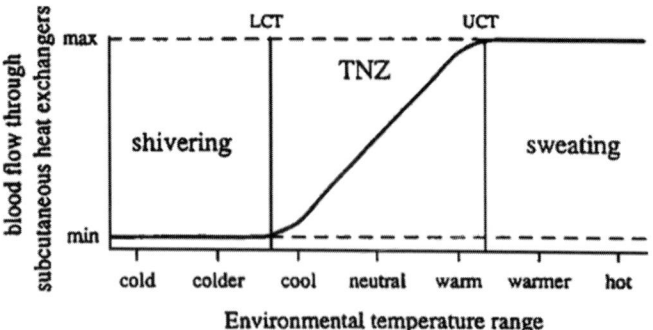

Figure 14.3 Environmental temperature and peripheral blood flow. Within the TNZ heat loss from the body is manipulated by adjusting vasomotor tone. Heat exchange between the body core and the environment is determined by the amount of blood flowing through the subcutaneous heat-exchange vascular structures located in the periphery. Arteriovenous anastomoses (AVAs) regulate blood flow through the subcutaneous layers. At the lower limit of the TNZ – the lower critical temperature (LCT) – all of the AVAs are closed and blood flow through the heat exchangers is minimal. At the upper limit of the TNZ – the upper critical temperature (UCT) – all of the AVAs are open and blood flow through the heat exchangers is maximal. (Reproduced with permission from Grahn 1997.[10])

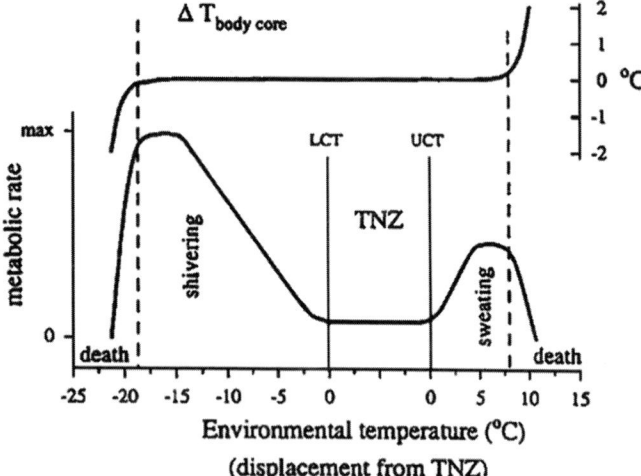

Figure 14.4 Environmental temperature and metabolic rate. Within the TNZ metabolic rate is low and constant; the individual thermoregulates by adjusting vasomotor tone to control heat loss from the thermal core. Above the UCT the individual must expend energy on heat loss (sweating) to maintain the desired temperature. Below the LCT the individual must increase the metabolic heat production (shivering) to compensate for the increased heat loss to the environment. If the capacity to compensate for the environment fails, body core temperature will fall (or increase) and eventually death will ensue. (Reproduced with permission from Grahn 1997.[10])

Table 14.1 Thermoregulation: behavioral and autonomic responses

System	Examples
Behavioral	1. Adjusting clothing 2. Modifying environmental temperature (heating, air conditioning) 3. Voluntary movements and timing of activities
Autonomic	1. Vasodilatation. Promotes either heat loss or heat gain depending on environmental conditions 2. Vasoconstriction. Cutaneous blood flow decreases to near zero in cold temperatures 3. Heart rate. Pulse is often higher for any given core temperature during heating than during cooling, thus increasing heat transfer via the blood 4. Piloerection. Increases insulation; slows heat exchange 5. Increased body fat. Fat conducts heat only one-third as fast as other tissues 6. Shivering. Increases heat production when the skin and/or body is cold 7. "Nonshivering" thermogenesis. Increases heat production without muscular activity. The principal heat producers are the liver, kidney, and brain via brown adipose tissue whose sole function is to produce heat in neonates 8. Evaporation. Increased amount of sweating

Modified from Kabbara A, Smith CE. Monitoring temperature. In Wilson WC, Grande CM, Hoyt DB, eds., *Trauma: Resuscitation, Anesthesia, and Critical Care*. New York, NY: Taylor & Francis, 2006.

The dominating afferent thermal signal to the brain comes from both nonthermospecific and thermospecific (cold or warm) receptors located in the skin and mucous membranes.[10] When the afferent thermal signals reach the hypothalamus (the control center), they are integrated with other information, which then result in an efferent response (cold or warm) (Figs. 14.2, 14.3). The exception is when the person is in the TNZ, also called the "set-point" temperature or the "interthreshold range."[10–12] This is the narrow range (0.4 °C) around the normal core temperature of 37.0 °C at which there is no efferent response. This set point may fluctuate with time of day, sex, and acclimation.

Both body morphology and age will influence the thermoregulatory response and capacity.[13–15] Infants and children cool much more quickly than adults because of their large surface area compared with their metabolic rate. On the other hand, external rewarming is much more effective in children. Chronic illness is one of the many factors predisposing individuals to the development of hypothermia (Table 14.2).

Effect of anesthesia and surgery (perioperative hypothermia)

Factors predisposing patients to perioperative hypothermia are the same as those predisposing conscious individuals to hypothermia (Table 14.2). However, induction of general anesthesia

shivering to produce heat, and sweating to eliminate heat (Figs. 14.2–14.4). From a metabolic point of view, both these autonomic mechanisms are costly to the body.

The most effective thermoregulatory response is behavioral (Table 14.1). For example, conscious humans respond to the surrounding conditions appropriately to avoid a decrease or increase in core temperature (e.g., clothing, seeking shelter). Another effective and metabolically inexpensive thermoregulatory response is the change in vasomotor tone in the arteriovenous shunt to either minimize heat loss through the skin or to increase it (Fig. 14.3).

Table 14.2 Predisposing factors for hypothermia

Mechanism	Examples
Impaired thermoregulation and decreased heat production	Drugs: alcohol, general and regional anesthesia, tricyclic antidepressants, phenothiazines, antipyretics Impaired neurologic state and mobility: e.g., brain injury, stroke, spinal cord injury, severe trauma, shock Extremes of age Autonomic nervous system dysfunction Chronic illness with hypometabolic features such as heart failure, hypothyroidism, adrenal disease, diabetes, malnutrition Severe sepsis (bacterial toxins)
Increased heat loss	Neonates and infants: increased body surface area to mass ratio Cold environmental temperature Exposure to windy and wet climate, submersion/immersion Poor socioeconomic status Burns Large blood loss Exposed abdominal and/or thoracic contents General and neuraxial anesthesia Geriatrics Thin body habitus Low skin-surface temperature prior to injury

Modified from Smith CE, Patel N. Hypothermia in adult trauma patients: anesthetic considerations. Part I. Etiology and pathophysiology. *Am J Anesthesiol* 1996; **23**: 283–90.

Thermoregulation, perioperative hypothermia

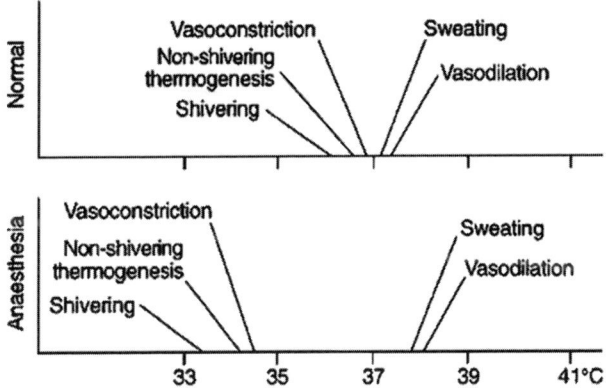

Figure 14.5 Activation of thermoregulatory effector responses is triggered at specific temperatures for a given individual ("threshold temperature"). Under general anesthesia, the thresholds for temperatures for activation of cold effector responses (including vasoconstriction and shivering) are lowered, whereas those for activation of warm responses (including sweating and vasodilatation) are increased. Thus, the interthreshold range is widened during general anesthesia to about 4 °C. (Reproduced with permission from Buggy & Crossley 2000.[12])

mean body temperature. As well, the greater the fluid requirement relative to body weight, the greater the potential drop in body temperature.

Epidural and spinal anesthesia also impair peripheral and central thermoregulation.[11,16] The initial vasodilatation in the conscious patient may cause the patient to feel warm, but a disturbing shivering may follow as the temperature falls. Although the mechanisms behind the disturbed thermoregulation are more complicated with regional than general anesthesia, the net effect is the same: a significant fall in core temperature.[11,16] Vasodilatation induced by regional anesthesia may, however, accelerate the temperature increase during rewarming.[11]

results in an immediate decrease in core temperature.[11,16] The first temperature fall (first phase of perioperative hypothermia) is due to anesthetic drug-induced vasodilatation causing heat distribution to the peripheral compartment.[17–20] All general anesthetics with the exception of ketamine affect the normal thermoregulatory responses in the same manner, but to different degrees.[11,14,16,21–26] This results in the "interthreshold range" expanding up to 4 °C (Fig. 14.5). The net effect is a rapid fall in core temperature (1–1.5 °C) during the first hour, followed by a slower decrease until the plateau phase when the thermoregulatory compensatory mechanisms kick in (primarily vasoconstriction). The surgical procedure further increases the risk for hypothermia if large body surface areas are exposed over a prolonged time. Moreover, replacement of shed blood with cold or inadequately warmed intravenous (IV) fluids and blood can significantly decrease body temperature.[11,14,16] The larger the gap between the temperature of the infused fluid and core temperature, the greater the drop in

Side effects of perioperative hypothermia in trauma

The general effect of cooling is that all body processes, including neuromuscular function,[1–3,27,28] slow down to the stage of depression and eventually death (Fig. 14.6). Even moderate degrees of hypothermia will produce clinically significant harmful effects in most organ systems, with worsened survival.[1–3,27,28] Both perioperative and trauma-associated hypothermia have a significant negative impact on outcome (Table 14.3).[1–3,11,29–32]

Although the general definition of hypothermia is a core temperature of less than 35 °C,[33] even milder deviations from the normal temperature may result in significant morbidity and mortality in surgical patients. For example, decreases in intraoperative temperatures to between 34 and 36 °C have been associated with complications such as shivering, postoperative wound infections, perioperative bleeding and transfusion requirements, cardiac events (myocardial ischemia,

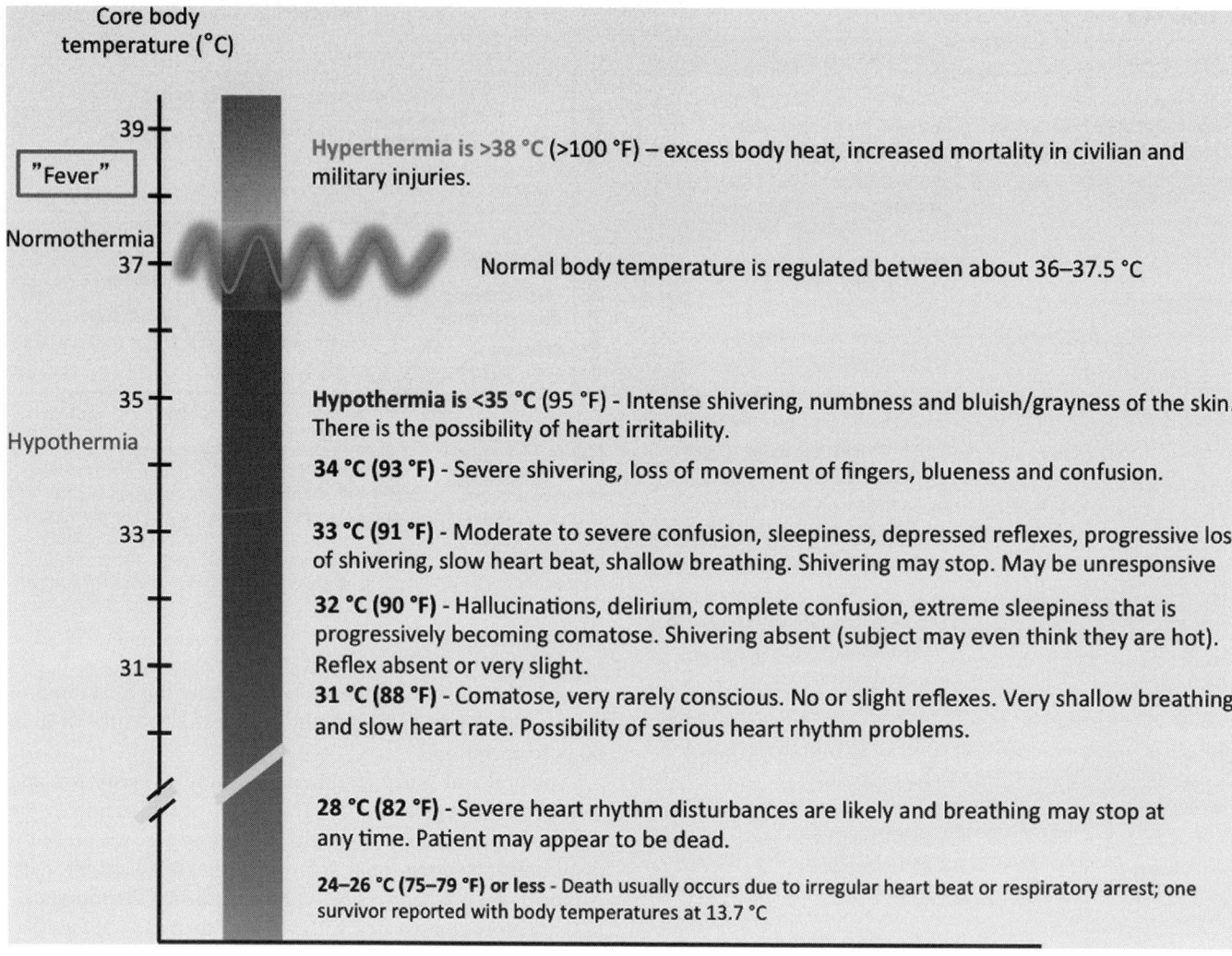

Figure 14.6 Pathophysiologic effects of alterations in core body temperature.

ventricular tachycardia), and prolonged hospital stay (Table 14.3).[11,29,32,34,35]

Importantly, the effects of all anesthetic drugs, including neuromuscular blocking drugs, are increased during hypothermia (Table 14.3).[11,32,36] There is a risk of prolonged neuromuscular blockade after standard doses of nondepolarizing relaxants. Neuromuscular function testing becomes increasingly difficult at low temperatures.[36]

Rewarming and maintaining normothermia: methods and equipment

Commercial rewarming equipment works by one of the following four mechanisms of heat transfer: convection, conduction, radiation, and evaporation (Table 14.4).[3,16] Convection represents heat transfer through air that is in contact with the body, and its efficiency is mostly determined by air velocity. Conductive heat transfer implies direct contact between two objects and depends on their characteristics. The rate of heat transfer from an object to fluid is 32 times

that of its transfer to air. Thus, cold and warm IV fluids are very effective in cooling and warming the patient, respectively. Radiation consists of heat transfer resulting from a temperature gradient, while evaporative heat transfer occurs with conversion of liquids (water, sweat) to the gaseous phase. The first three mechanisms are the most important in terms of heat loss, as well as for rewarming hypothermic patients.[1–3,11,16]

Various methods have been employed to rewarm patients and to prevent perioperative hypothermia. Active external warming, using both heating and reflective and convective air blankets, as well as radiant heat shields and fluid- and air-circulating warming blankets and mattresses, have been tested and employed in clinical practice.[12,14,16,37–43]

Forced-air warming (convective air blankets)

Considerable evidence exists demonstrating the safety and efficacy of forced-air warming devices, both in preventing and treating hypothermia and in preventing shivering during the perioperative period, as well as with accidental

Table 14.3 Pathophysiologic consequences and complications from perioperative and trauma-associated hypothermia

System affected	Examples
Impaired cardiorespiratory function	Cardiac depression Myocardial ischemia Arrhythmias Peripheral vasoconstriction Decreased tissue oxygen delivery Increased oxygen consumption during rewarming Blunted response to catecholamines Increased blood viscosity Acidosis Leftward shift of oxyhemoglobin dissociation curve
Impaired coagulation	Decreased function of coagulation factors Impaired platelet function
Impaired hepatorenal function and decreased drug clearance (anesthetics!)	Decreased hepatic blood flow Decreased clearance of lactic acid Decreased hepatic metabolism of drugs Decreased renal blood flow Cold-induced diuresis
Impaired resistance to infections (pneumonia, sepsis, wound infections) Impaired wound healing	Decreased subcutaneous tissue perfusion mediated by vasoconstriction (↑ s-norepinephrine) Anti-inflammatory effects and immunosuppression, including reduced T-cell-mediated antibody production and reduced nonspecific oxidative bacterial killing by neutrophils Decreased collagen deposition

Modified from Smith CE, Yamat RA. Avoiding hypothermia in the trauma patient. *Curr Opin Anaesthesiol* 2000; **13**: 167–74.

Table 14.4 Mechanisms of heat loss

Mechanism	Description
Radiation	The transfer of heat energy to or from a body by means of the emission or absorption of electromagnetic radiation.
Conduction	Transfer of heat energy between two solid objects in contact according to the thermal conductivity of the objects, area in contact, and thermal gradient • e.g., transfer of heat due to direct contact of skin and viscera with colder objects such as bed, spine backboard, and surrounding air • e.g., transfer of heat from patient's blood to unwarmed or inadequately warmed IV fluids.
Convection	Transfer of heat energy during the mass movement of gas or liquid.
Evaporation	Heat energy transferred during change of phase (water to gas): 58 kcal/g water evaporated from skin, respiratory tract, and viscera.
Redistribution	Redistribution of warmer core blood to the cooler periphery due to anesthetic agents (e.g., propofol, inhalational agents, alcohol intoxication). Subsequent heat loss by other mechanisms.

Modified from Smith CE, Patel N. Hypothermia in adult trauma patients: anesthetic considerations. Part I. Etiology and pathophysiology. *Am J Anesthesiol* 1996; **23**: 283–90; Wilson WC, Smith CE, Haan J, Elamin EM. Hypothermia and heat-related injuries. In Wilson WC, Grande CM, Hoyt DB, eds., *Trauma: Resuscitation, Anesthesia, and Critical Care*. New York, NY: Taylor & Francis, 2006.

hypothermia (Figs. 14.7, 14.8).[14,32,37,41,44,45] If a large enough surface area can be covered, these devices not only transfer heat across cutaneous surfaces, but also create a thermoneutral microenvironment so that all heat production goes to restoring body temperature. Thermoregulatory vasoconstriction, which separates and limits heat transfer between peripheral skin and central thermal compartments, limits the rate of rewarming using forced air.[46]

Other warming devices

Neither electric blankets using resistive heating nor radiant warmers using infrared radiation have become important methods for use during or after surgery.[32,41] Although both resistive heating and circulating water garments are effective in

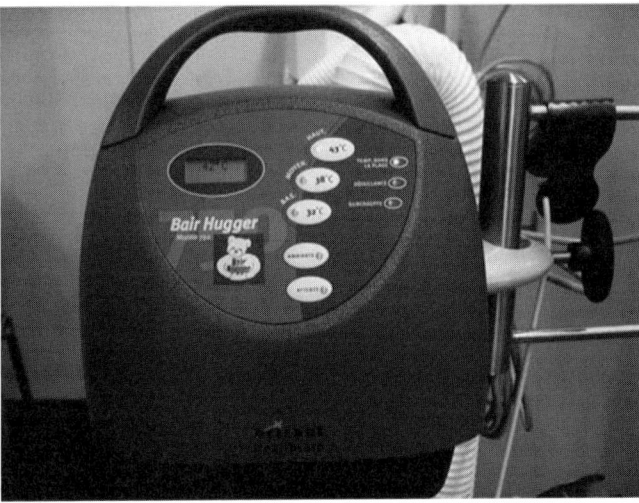

Figure 14.7 Convective warming device. Upper body convective (forced-air) warming device and hose. Heated air from the warming unit inflates a single-use blanket. The blanket design contains a series of hollow tubes with rounded upper surfaces and flattened lower surfaces joined in a parallel array. Once inflated, the blanket directs heated air onto the patient through exit ports in the blanket undersurface.

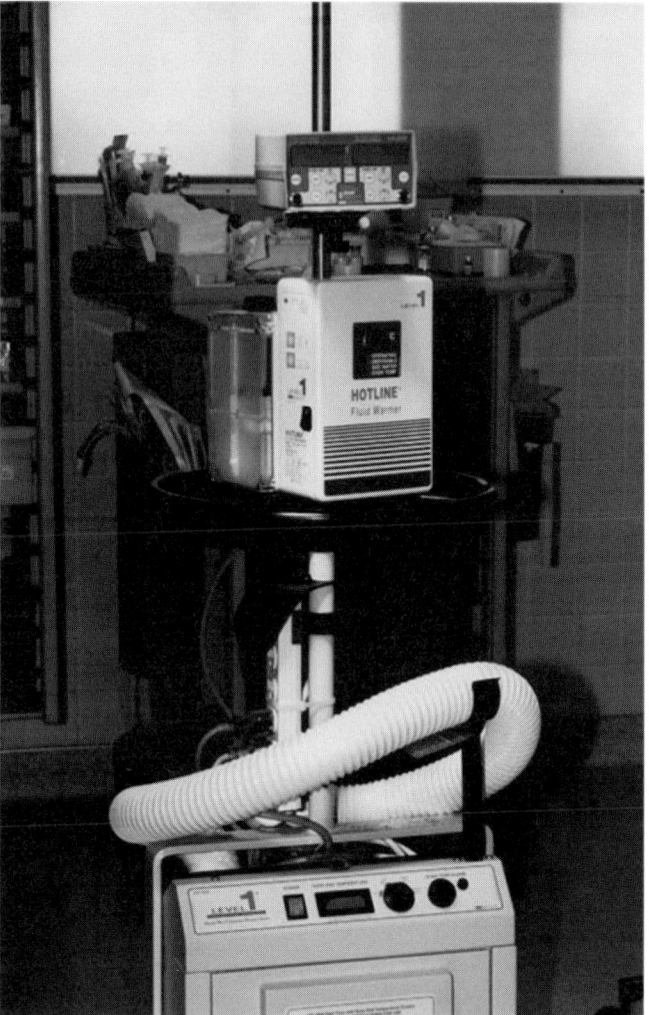

Figure 14.8 Convective warming device. The hypothermia station consists of a convective warming unit and a fluid warmer. The convective warming unit draws ambient room-temperature air through an ultrafine glass inlet filter. Filtered air is passed through a 0.2 μm outlet filter, heated, and delivered through a hose to the disposable blanket. The fluid warmer heats water to a 42 °C set point, and the warm water is then circulated through a disposable set that has a sterile central lumen for IV fluid administration surrounded by an outer layer through which the warm water circulates down one side and then back up to the heated reservoir, which prevents cool-down in the patient line. There is a four-outlet power strip and an adjustable hose-tree arm.

preventing intraoperative hypothermia, practical and economic issues have prevented their widespread use.[42,43] Alternatives to forced air may play a larger role in the field treatment of victims of accidental hypothermia and during trauma resuscitation of already cold and exposed patients.[3,47]

Fluid and blood warmers

Warm IV fluids minimize further heat loss while at the same time transferring significant amounts of heat to the core in patients requiring fluid and blood resuscitation. For example, 10 L of 40 °C fluid given to a 32 °C patient supplies 80 kcal, which is enough to increase core temperature in a 70 kg patient by 1.4 °C.[48] The thermal stress of infusing large volumes of room-temperature crystalloid and colloid or inadequately warmed blood and blood products can result in considerable decreases in mean body temperature.[3,16,32] The larger the difference between the temperature of the infused fluid and core temperature, the greater the decrease in body temperature. As well, the greater the fluid requirement relative to body weight, the greater the fall in body temperature.

The ability of fluid and blood warmers to safely deliver normothermic fluids over a wide range of flows is limited by several factors, including limited heat transfer capability of materials such as plastic, limited surface area of the heat exchange mechanism, inadequate heat transfer of the exchange mechanism at high flow rates, and heat loss after the IV tubing exits the warmer. Improvements in fluid warmer design, including higher set points, greater thermal capacity, air detection, and line pressure monitoring, allow the clinician to safely maintain thermal neutrality with respect to fluid management over a wide range of flows (Figs. 14.9–14.12).[49–54] Use of effective fluid-warming devices permits more efficient rewarming of hypothermic patients when combined with other methods such as forced air.[50]

Temperature monitoring

The most reliable temperature-monitoring sites are the distal esophagus, nasopharynx, tympanic membrane, and pulmonary artery (Table 14.5). These sites come closest to reflecting core temperature, which provides approximately 80% of thermal input to the hypothalamus. Core temperature can be estimated with reasonable accuracy by using intermediate sites such as sublingual (oral), rectal, and bladder temperatures, except during extreme thermal perturbations, when intermediate sites may lag behind core sites. Lag time is a function of both the magnitude of heat transferred and the time frame in which it is accomplished. Lag time reflects restricted perfusion to specific body temperature-monitoring sites and/or imperfect sensor placement.

Distal esophagus

Because of its proximity to the heart, distal esophageal thermometry is a highly accurate measure of core temperature. The thermistor is contained within an esophageal stethoscope, which is routinely used for monitoring heart and lung sounds during general anesthesia in tracheally intubated patients (Fig. 14.13). If the probe is not placed distally, temperature readings may be inaccurate. Distal placement is usually assured by listening for the loudest heart sounds. Continuous suction applied to a nasogastric tube will falsely lower esophageal temperature.

Nasopharynx

This site usually correlates well with other centrally measured temperatures. Nasopharyngeal temperature exceeded tympanic temperature during rewarming on cardiopulmonary bypass (CPB), which suggests that this site better reflects the

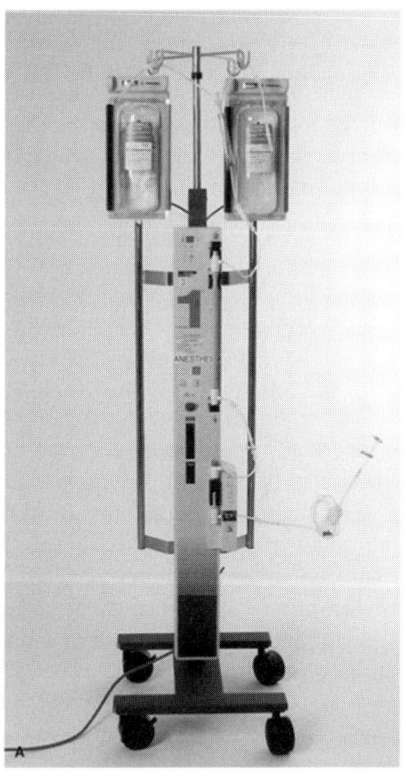
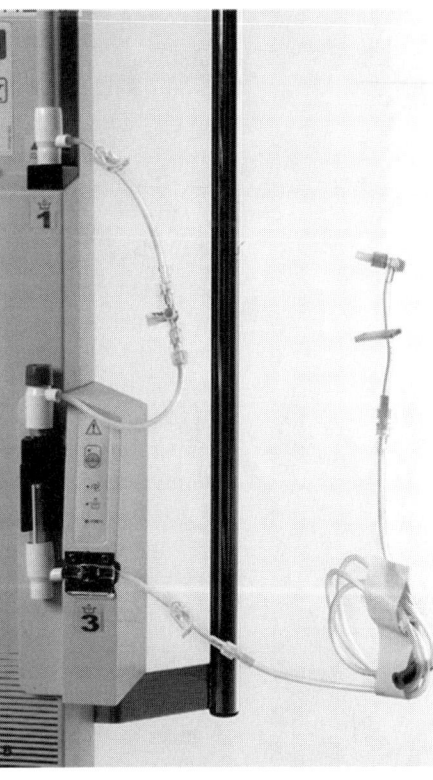

Figure 14.9 Rapid-infusion fluid-warming device. The device consists of a heater that warms water and circulates it through a pump and a heat-exchange segment with a central tube for water flow (countercurrent heat exchange technology). Fluid flows through the outer sheath, which surrounds the water core. (**A**) A pneumatic external compressor automatically squeezes the IV fluid or blood bag to increase flow. Normothermic fluid delivery is maintained at flows between 40 and 400 mL/min (20 °C input), and at flows between 40 and 300 mL/min (10 °C input). (**B**) The use of ultrasonic air detection coupled with automatic shutoff is a significant safety improvement. (Reproduced with permission from Avula et al. 2005.[53])

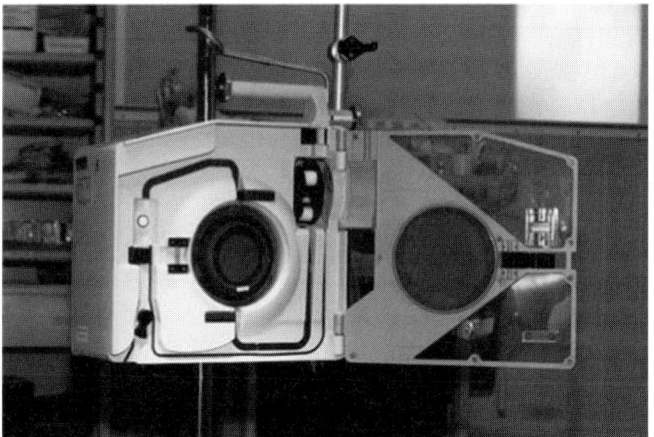

Figure 14.10 Rapid-infusion fluid warmer device. This device uses magnetic induction as a heat source. An integrated peristaltic pump eliminates the requirement for compression and pressurization of the fluid bag. The device contains two air detectors, an automatic air purge, and a line pressure sensor. There is redundant air detection, automatic air removal, and sensors to alert the operator when the system is out of fluid, or a line is obstructed. (Reproduced with permission from Smith CE, Kabbara A, Kramer RP, Gill I. A new IV fluid and blood warming system to prevent air embolism and compartment syndrome. *Trauma Care* 2001; **11**: 78–82.)

brain temperature.[55] Problems with this site include the risk of nasopharyngeal bleeding. Temperatures may vary between different probe positions. This site is relatively contraindicated in patients with severe midface or basilar skull fractures with cribriform plate disruption.

Tympanic membrane (ear)

The tympanic membrane is 3.5 cm from the hypothalamus, is perfused by the internal carotid artery, and can be readily monitored using a well-insulated thermocouple probe (thermistor) adjacent to the membrane itself. Cerumen or dried blood in the aural canal can result in a delayed response time. Tympanic membrane probes are contraindicated in patients with cerebrospinal fluid otorrhea and are easily dislodged during patient movement and transport. Measures may be inaccurate if the ears are cold or in the presence of otologic disease. It is important to distinguish the rather cumbersome but accurate method of applying a tympanic thermistor probe in the aural canal from the simpler to use, but less accurate, infrared aural canal thermometer.[56] Although very feasible for screening and prehospital use,[57,58] infrared aural canal thermometers are not considered appropriate for anesthesia and critical care use. Measurements from four products using this infrared technique were compared with tympanic thermistor measurements from the contralateral ear during CPB cooling.[56] None of the infrared thermometers was sufficiently precise for routine use. Indeed, the standard deviation of about 0.8 °C indicated that close to 70% of the measurements would span a range of 1.6 °C around the "true" thermistor value.

Pulmonary artery

The pulmonary artery (PA) catheter contains a distal thermistor used for cardiac output measurements (conservation of heat principle). Although the PA catheter provides a reliable

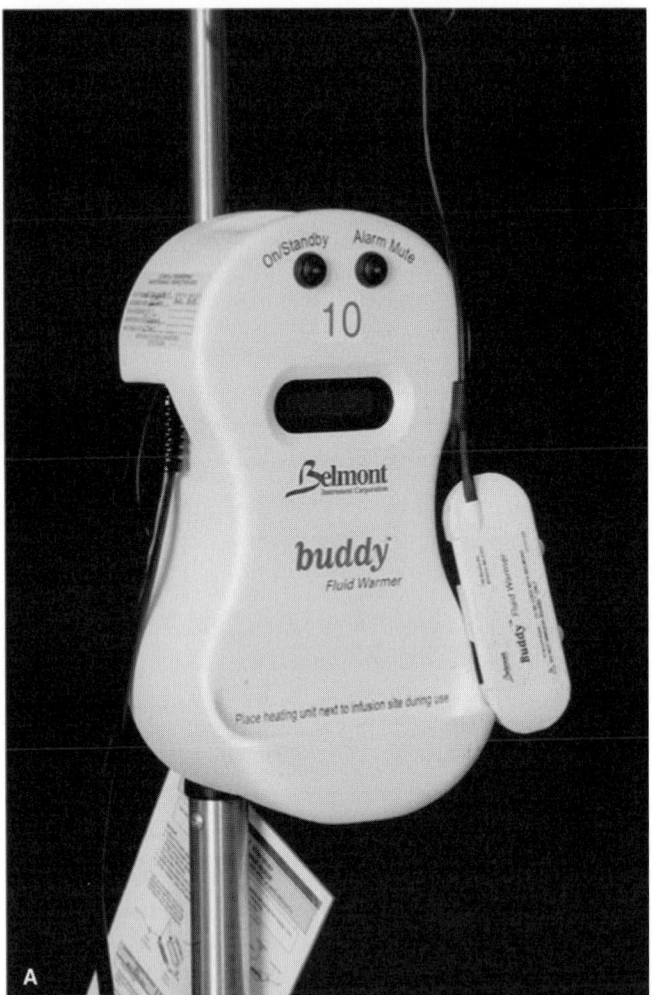

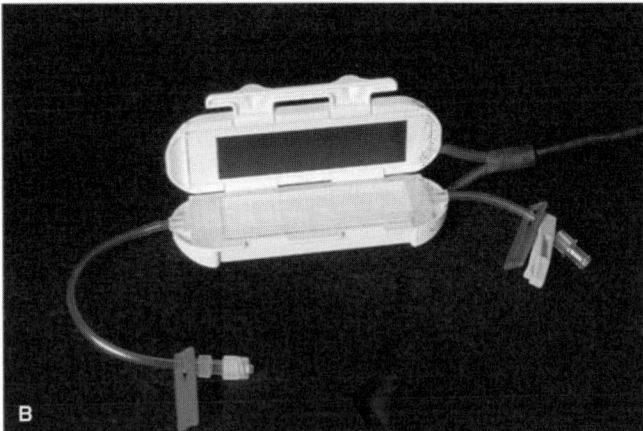

Figure 14.11 (**A**) Pediatric in-line fluid warmer disposable set and heating unit. The disposable set is attached close to the patient to minimize heat loss in the patient line. Priming volume is small (4 mL). (**B**) The disposable set has microporous membranes that vent air from crystalloid fluid. Air is released through the side vents of the set to minimize the risk of air embolism. (Reproduced with permission from Avula & Smith 2005.[54])

estimate of core temperature, it is too invasive to use this site for temperature measurement alone. In the absence of pulmonary blood flow during CPB, PA temperature is not accurate.

Sublingual

Sublingual temperature is lower than core temperature by about 0.5 °C. Correct placement of the thermometer is essential. Advantages are easy accessibility, familiarity, and noninvasiveness. Disadvantages are related to inaccurate readings due to noncompliance or rapid mouth breathing.

Rectum

Rectal temperature was long considered the "gold standard" for estimating core temperature (especially in children), and is about 0.1 °C higher than core temperature. Advantages are easy accessibility, low cost, and accurate readings. Because the rectum is a cavity, it can retain heat longer than other temperature sites. When a patient's temperature is rising or falling rapidly, the temperature in the rectum can lag behind by as much as an hour. This may be because the rectum contains no thermoreceptors and thus is heated or cooled as an effect of hypothalamic control, rather than in response to it. Other possible causes of inaccurate rectal readings are related to the insulating effect of fecal matter in the rectum and the heat produced by coliform bacteria.

Bladder

Bladder temperature can be measured by an indwelling urinary catheter containing a thermistor. If the patient's urinary catheter does not have a thermistor attached, it has to be changed to one that does. Low urinary flow may decrease the ability of this site to reliably estimate core temperature (e.g., shock, renal failure). Open pelvic and lower abdominal trauma may falsely lower temperature readings from this site.

Accidental hypothermia
Definitions and physiologic consequences

Accidental hypothermia has been defined as an unintentional decrease in core temperature below 35 °C. The thermoregulatory capacity for compensation will vary from person to person based on age, health status, and intake of drugs and alcohol (Tables 14.1, 14.2).[8,27,47] For the same cold exposure the thermoregulatory capacity of the person will determine when hypothermia sets in or the person merely remains "cold stressed" (feeling cold, shivering, vasoconstricted, with body temperature above 35.0 °C).[27,59]

The classic distinction between mild (35–32 °C), moderate (32–28 °C), and severe (< 28 °C) accidental hypothermia is still used.[60] When core temperature is not available, the Swiss system of grading can be used: Stage 1: conscious, shivering; stage 2: impaired consciousness, not shivering; stage 3: unconscious, not shivering, vital signs present; stage 4: no vital signs. This systems allows rescue workers to grade hypothermia based on clinical signs in the prehospital setting.[61]

Prolonged exposure to temperatures outside the TNZ causes hypothermia even in mild and hot climates. Hence, accidental hypothermia should not be considered an arctic or wilderness problem. Rather, it can occur in healthy persons

Table 14.5 Temperature monitoring sites in order of authors' preference

Core	Intermediate
Distal esophagus	Rectal
Nasopharynx	Bladder
Tympanic membrane (ear)	Sublingual (oral)
Pulmonary artery	Axilla

Modified from Kabbara A, Smith CE. Monitoring temperature. In Wilson WC, Grande CM, Hoyt DB, eds., *Trauma: Resuscitation, Anesthesia, and Critical Care.* New York, NY: Taylor & Francis, 2006.

exposed to ambient air temperatures, precipitation, and wind chill despite the initial protection by isolation and thermoregulatory compensation (increased heat production). Immersion or submersion in cold water accelerates the onset of hypothermia.[27,62,63] With intoxication and illness, hypothermia is well described in urban and warm surroundings. Hence, accidental hypothermia should always be part of the differential diagnosis in obtunded and collapsed patients. The diagnosis mandates only one single measure of decreased core temperature using a low-read thermometer.

Predisposing factors for involuntary cooling of the body and the thermoregulative countermeasures are shown in

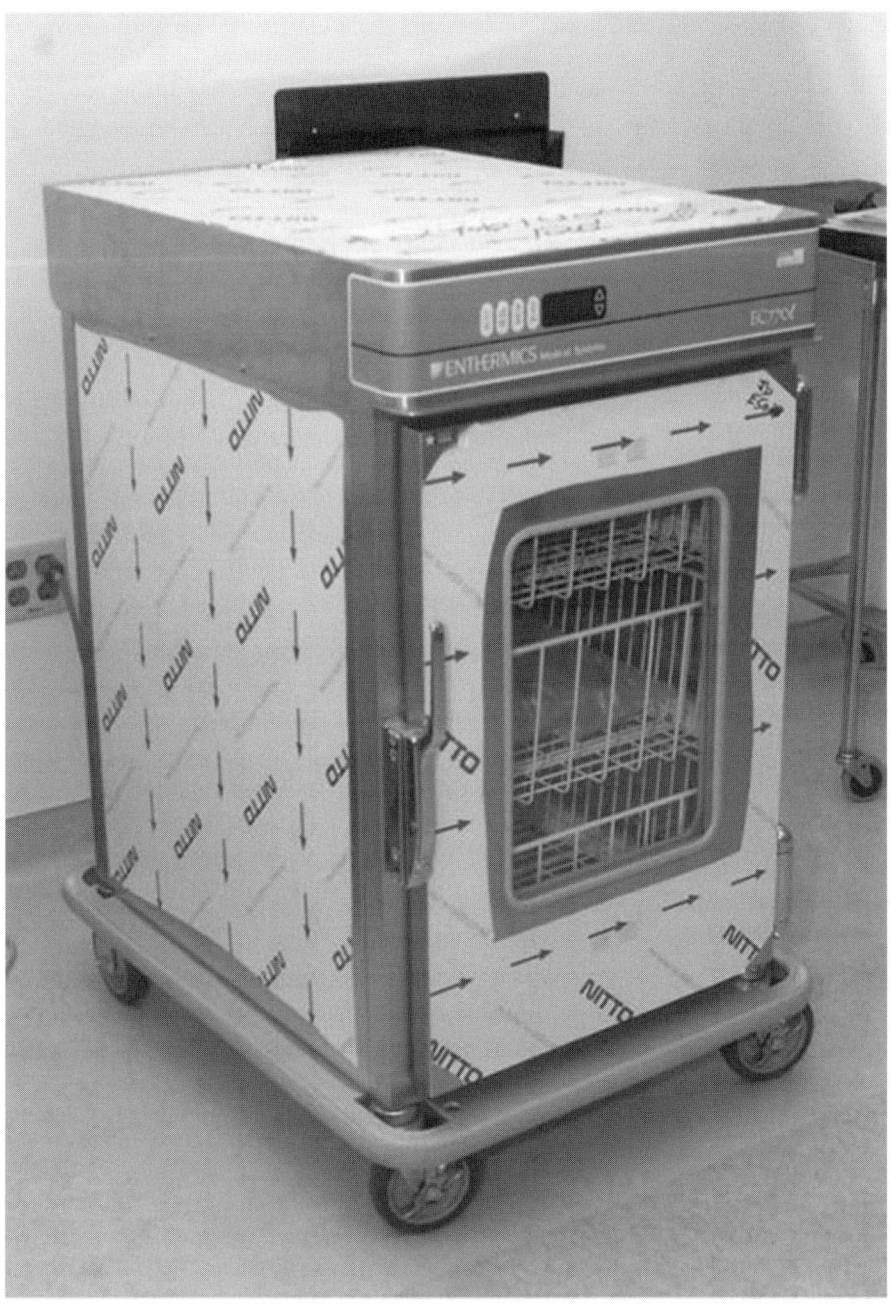

Figure 14.12 Fluid warming cabinet. The cabinet is warmed to 42 °C by using a low-heat-density electrothermal cable array to provide even heating of injection fluids. The stability of some solutions may vary according to temperature and duration of storage. Solution warm-up time varies depending on cabinet warmer load. The warming cabinet cannot be used for blood. (Reproduced with permission from Raymond CJ, Kroll A, Smith CE. Warming crystalloid fluid for intravenous infusion: how effective is a fluid warming cabinet? *Anesth Analg* 2006: **103**: 1605–6.)

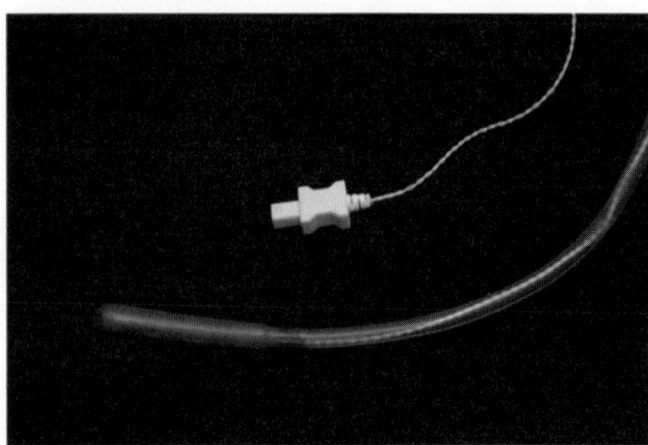

Figure 14.13 Distal esophageal thermometry. 18 Fr esophageal stethoscope with 400 series thermistor. The stethoscope is a latex-free single-use device that continuously measures core temperature in tracheally intubated patients. The esophageal stethoscope is positioned at the point of maximal heart sounds, and temperature is displayed on an electronic monitor. A 9 Fr size is available for pediatrics.

Tables 14.1 and 14.2 and Figures 14.2–14.4. From a therapeutic point of view, it is important to differentiate between mild/moderate and severe hypothermia,[27] between arrested and nonarrested hypothermic victims, and between asphyxiated and nonasphyxiated hypothermic arrest.[33,64]

In severe hypothermia, the initial slowing of the heart and supraventricular arrhythmias give way to ventricular fibrillation (VF) and finally asystole.[27,47] The respiratory rate slows dramatically, and the unconscious patient with dilated pupils may appear dead. The distinction between a dead person and a severely hypothermic patient becomes problematic. Therefore, the general consensus is that no hypothermic patient should be pronounced dead before "warm and dead."[2,27,33,64] An aggressive approach to rewarming is indicated. This approach, with prolonged cardiopulmonary resuscitation (CPR) and use of CPB, is resource-intensive and complicated, both from a logistical and from a therapeutic point of view.[33,65–67] Still, the merit is based on multiple successful cases of good neurologic outcome.

Treatment options in patients with mild, moderate, or severe accidental hypothermia with intact circulation

The degree of hypothermia will determine the most appropriate rewarming techniques. In mild hypothermia, transferring the patient from the cold environment to warm and protected surroundings, removing cold and wet clothes, drying the body surface, and blanket coverage is sufficient in most cases.[2,27] Under these circumstances, the body's own heat production will reverse the low temperature (passive external rewarming). If the patient is very uncomfortable or unable to spontaneously reverse the hypothermia, active external rewarming is indicated (Table 14.6).

In moderate hypothermia, active external rewarming is indicated. Forced-air warming is probably the most effective and practical method and can also be used in severe hypothermia, as long as there is an intact circulation (pulse present).[47,64,68] Other external rewarming methods include warm-water baths, heated blankets, heat lamps, heat packs, and reflective blankets. Infusion of warm IV fluids is important (Table 14.6).

In severe hypothermia, the pulse will become slow and irregular, and blood pressure may be unrecordable.[27,47] Since carotid pulses may be difficult to palpate, patients should be observed for spontaneous breathing or movements for at least 60 seconds. If signs of life are present (spontaneous movements or persistent breathing), the combination of rapid external/internal rewarming (Table 14.6), warm humidified oxygen by mask, and warm IV fluids to counteract the expansion of the vascular bed and to replace the fluids lost during cooling is sufficient.[27,33,69] Gentle handling is important in order to avoid rescue collapse. However, the small risk of inducing VF should not impede advanced airway management if indicated.[8,64] Depolarizing muscle relaxants should be withheld because of the risk of hyperkalemia.[70] Arrhythmias other than VF will revert spontaneously with normalization of temperature. In otherwise healthy patients, prognosis is excellent.[27,71] In moderate and severe hypothermia with an intact circulation, prognosis largely depends on the underlying diseases and causes of the hypothermia.[27,47,62] Reported in-hospital mortality varies from 10% to 40%, with numbers approximating 50% in those with severe underlying cardiopulmonary diseases.

At present, one rewarming method cannot be recommended over another in terms of outcome and efficacy. However, from a practical and safety point of view, we believe forced-air (convective) warming is a reasonable choice, even in the unconscious patient provided there is a perfusing rhythm, based on the following reports. In a randomized controlled trial of hypothermic patients with an average core temperature of 28.8 °C, forced-air warming increased core temperature by about 2.4 °C/hour versus 1.4 °C/hour in controls.[72] Both groups of patients received IV fluids warmed to 38 °C as well as warmed, humidified oxygen at 40 °C by inhalation. Koller *et al.* reported the use of forced-air warming in five patients with core temperature of less than 30 °C.[45] The outcome of all five patients was good without neurologic sequelae. Core temperature increased by approximately 1 °C/hour without any cardiac arrhythmias or core temperature afterdrop. Invasive methods should probably be reserved for the most severe cases or when there is cardiac instability refractory to medical management.[8] Such methods include intravascular rewarming with a balloon catheter, continuous arteriovenous rewarming (CAVR), and intracavital rewarming (thoracal or abdominal lavage).[73–75] It is important to continuously monitor core temperature to prevent an uncontrolled drop in temperature and to evaluate the efficacy of rewarming. Arrhythmias and hypotension may occur due to peripheral

Table 14.6 Rewarming methods and rates for injured patients

Category	Method	Comments	Rewarming rate (°C/h)
Passive external	Warmed blankets	Including head and neck, reduces evaporative heat loss, unsuccessful if there is loss of shivering	0.5–4
	Humidification of inspired air	Reduces evaporative heat loss, unsuccessful if there is loss of shivering	Variable
Active external	Convective (forced air)	Well studied and routinely used. Risk of temperature afterdrop and rewarming hypotension	1–2.5
	Warm blankets	Risks of burns, temperature afterdrop, and rewarming hypotension	Variable
	Warm-water immersion	Difficult to monitor patient, risk of temperature afterdrop and rewarming hypotension	2–4
Active internal	Warm (42 °C) humidified air	Low heat transport capacity	0.5–1.2
	Warm (42 °C) intravenous fluids	Especially useful in the resuscitation of hypothermic trauma victims, rapid infusion maximizes heat delivery	Variable
	Intravascular warming	Limited data in trauma, rapid initiation, automated temperature management.	1–4
	Body cavity lavage with warm fluid (gastric, bladder, colon, pleural, peritoneal)	Limited data, risk of mucosal injury, risk of aspiration with gastric lavage	Variable
Extracorporeal	Hemodialysis and hemofiltration	Widely available, rapid initiation, requires adequate blood pressure	2–3
	Continuous arteriovenous rewarming	Rapid initiation, trained perfusionist not required, less available, requires adequate blood pressure	3–4
	Cardiopulmonary bypass, extracorporeal membrane oxygenation	Provides full circulatory support, allows oxygenation, less available, requires trained perfusionist, delays in initiation	7–10

Modified from Aslam et al. 2006.[47]

vasodilatation, as well as from cool blood returning to the central circulation (afterdrop).[2,30,36] There is an increased need for IV fluids during the rewarming period. Normal saline may aggravate acidosis, and a more balanced crystalloid solution such as lactated Ringer's is indicated if large volumes are needed to achieve normovolemia.[76]

Accidental hypothermia may be associated with local cold-induced injuries.[27] These are most commonly seen in the extremities. They are classified as superficial (clear blisters) or deep (hemorrhagic blisters).[27] If refreezing is not a problem, local rewarming during transport should be started. Rubbing the frozen body part should not be done, as this may worsen the tissue damage. Further management beyond rapid rewarming in hot-water baths (40–42 °C) is still controversial.[27] Independent of the chosen approach, the need for prolonged hospital stay and repeated surgical procedures is frequent.

Treatment options in hypothermic cardiac arrest victims without a history of asphyxia

In hypothermic cardiac arrest victims, CPR should be commenced by using the same ventilation and compression ratios/rates as in normothermic patients (ratio 30:2; rate 100/min).[33] The general stiffness of the whole body will make CPR more complicated and a strange experience for the rescuer. There is a general consensus that vasoactive drugs and defibrillation are less effective if the core temperature is less than 30 °C, but existing European and American guidelines are not in agreement.[33,64] There is a lack of human evidence on the effect of vasopressors in severe hypothermia with cardiac arrest. Based on animal research, it seems reasonable to suggest up to three administrations of epinephrine and three defibrillation attempts even before reaching 30 °C.[64] Tracheal intubation is indicated in hypothermic cardiac arrest not only to secure an airway and to ventilate/oxygenate, but also to deliver warmed humidified oxygen/air (maximum, 42 °C).[64]

Survival after hours of resuscitation and weeks of intensive care has been reported even in patients with profound (< 20 °C) hypothermia.[66] Hence, in the absence of obvious lethal injuries or a completely frozen body making CPR impossible, patients with temperatures below 32 °C should be transported with ongoing CPR to a hospital capable of providing rapid invasive rewarming through the use of CPB or extracorporeal membrane oxygenation (ECMO) (Table 14.6).[8,33] There have been reports of improved outcomes by the use of venoarterial ECMO compared to traditional CPB.[77] This may be attributed to the ability of ECMO to provide life support for longer periods of time, since there may be persisting cardiopulmonary failure even after the restoration of spontaneous circulation. The management of such patients will require close cooperation between personnel specialized in cardiothoracic surgery, perfusion, cardiac anesthesia, and intensive care. Issues such as optimization of tissue perfusion, prevention of ischemia, and knowledge of the pathophysiology of reperfusion and microcirculation flow dysfunction need to be addressed (beyond the scope of this chapter). When transport to ECMO or CBP is not possible, thoracic lavage represents a reasonable alternative.[75]

Outcome depends on the temperature at the start of the resuscitation, the cause of the hypothermia, and underlying diseases. When analyzing the outcome of hypothermic cardiac arrest victims rewarmed with extracorporeal circulation, the critical factor was the presence or absence of asphyxia prior to the onset of hypothermia. For example, prognosis in victims rewarmed after immersion (as opposed to after drowning or avalanche) was good, with reported rates of intact survivors up to 60–70%.[9,33,65,67]

Treatment options in hypothermic cardiac arrest victims with a history of asphyxia

The association of hypothermia with asphyxia carries a poor prognosis. Because the prehospital clinical picture may be unclear, and prehospital signs such as dilated pupils and asystole have no prognostic value, every effort should be made to start immediate and adequate CPR.[33] In drowning cases, this is especially important. Even imperfect and simple bystander CPR may bring the patient back to life.

While submersion implies that the whole body has been under water, immersion only means being covered in water/fluid.[78] Hypothermia will develop with both immersion and submersion.[62] If the airway has been kept clear and over the water in immersed victims, hypothermia and subsequent cardiac arrest are not necessarily associated with asphyxia (primary hypothermia). In submersion, the situation is more complicated, as the general rule is that associated asphyxia and cardiac arrest carry a poor prognosis even if hypothermia develops. If submersion occurs in icy water, thereby inducing rapid cooling of the brain, the situation is quite different. Intact survivors have been described after up to 60-minute submersion periods, especially in children.[33]

CPR and advanced life support procedures in victims of drowning should follow the procedures presented for nonasphyxiated hypothermic cardiac arrest victims above. Post resuscitation, comatose survivors should probably be kept mildly hypothermic (32–34 °C) and mechanically ventilated for at least 24 hours.[79]

Avalanche victims constitute a special group.[33,65,68,70,77] Blunt trauma is the reason for death in up to one-third of avalanche victims, and early asphyxiation is also common.[70] Hypothermia is rarely the mechanism of death, but may become an important factor in those buried with an air pocket that allows respiration initially. Survival data from the European Alps have shown that the probability for survival in completely buried victims falls rapidly from 90% after 15 minutes burial time to 30% after 30 minutes.[80] Survival after 90 minutes is low. Canadian data show 77% survival at 10 minutes and 7% at 35 minutes. This is believed to be caused by higher incidences of trauma and denser snow in Canada. Local topographical factors (e.g., forest versus open terrain) will influence the likelihood of traumatic injuries. Triage and field management in avalanche accidents are notoriously difficult. The International Commission for Mountain Emergency Medicine published guidelines for the resuscitation of avalanche victims in 2001.[80] In the initial half hour, the focus should be on rapid extrication, immediate airway management, and CPR in lifeless victims to counteract asphyxia. When burial times exceed 35 minutes, treatment of hypothermia becomes more important. The maximum recorded cooling rate during burial is 9 °C/hour.[81] This means that a burial time of at least 35 minutes is needed to achieve a core temperature of 32 °C. Mechanical stimulation can provoke malignant arrhythmias (e.g., VF). Thus, gentle extrication with continuous ECG monitoring is warranted. The trachea of lifeless victims should be intubated, and if the core temperature is less than 32 °C, those found with an air pocket and clear airways should be transported with ongoing CPR to a hospital that is capable of providing extracorporeal rewarming with CPB or ECMO.[33,70] Serum potassium is regarded as the only valid prognostic marker. When serum potassium is more than 12 mmol/L, further CPR can be withheld.[8,70]

Trauma-associated hypothermia
Definitions, predisposing factors, and incidence

Despite decades of ongoing discussion and laboratory research on the possible protective effects of hypothermia in trauma patients,[2,5,6] the development of hypothermia is still considered detrimental.[1–3] Much discussion has centered on whether hypothermia is just a result of the shocked state itself, with low perfusion causing reduced metabolism and diminished heat production, or an imposed complication with an independent negative influence on prognosis. In their review of this topic, Hildebrand et al. concluded that accidental hypothermia in trauma victims is a very different situation from controlled, induced hypothermia (therapeutic) in trauma patients.[1] Laboratory research has shown beneficial effects of induced hypothermia during hemorrhagic shock despite the fact that hypothermia per se increases the bleeding tendency. Hypothermia has a definite anti-inflammatory effect, which can be used to ameliorate reperfusion injuries in various organs. While induced hypothermia with shivering prevention preserves body reserves of high-energy substrates, accidental hypothermia in trauma patients causes physiologic stress and

Table 14.7 An alternative proposal for classification of hypothermia in the trauma patient

General medical classification of hypothermia		Proposed trauma/ perioperative classification	
Category	°C	Class	°C
Mild	35–32	I	36–35
		II	34–32
Moderate	32–28	III	32–28
Severe	28	IV	28

Modified from Kirkpatrick et al. 1999.[2]

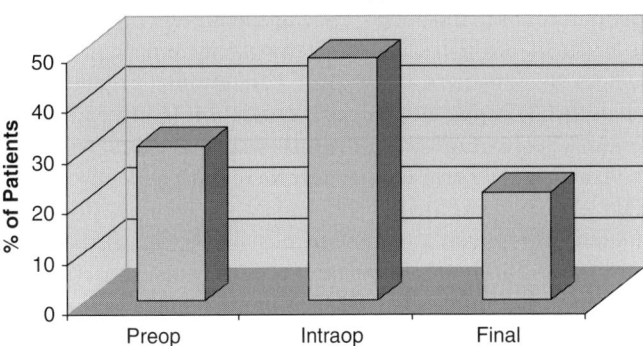

Figure 14.14 Incidence of hypothermia (< 36 °C) in 660 trauma patients requiring surgery within 24 hours of admission at MetroHealth Medical Center, Cleveland, Ohio. Preop, preoperative, intraop, intraoperative. (Presented at MetroHealth Research Exposition and Ohio Society of Anesthesiologists Annual Meeting, Sept, 2004.)

depletion of the same substrates, resulting in both increased morbidity and mortality.[1]

Nonintended hypothermia in trauma victims is still a common problem, occurring early during the resuscitative phase.[3] Due to the overall more negative effects of accidental hypothermia in trauma patients (increased bleeding and immunosuppression), the classic cutoff points have been redefined for the trauma population,[1–3] such that mild hypothermia corresponds to a core temperature between 34.0 and 35.9 °C; moderate hypothermia, 32 to 33.9 °C; and severe hypothermia, less than 32 °C. An alternative classification of hypothermia can be used with four classes (I–IV), as shown in Table 14.7.

In a prehospital study of trauma patients with accidental hypothermia, clinical symptoms pointing to hypothermia or other indicators (e.g., shivering) were noted in only 4.4% of hypothermic patients.[57] Little et al. also detected a lack of shivering response to hypothermia in traumatized patients immediately after injury.[82,83] The absence of shivering to compensate for the fall in core temperature is likely due to impaired thermoregulation after injury.[1,57,82] Shivering may also be abolished by general anesthesia.[84] Even without providing general anesthesia, the shivering threshold may be lowered by opioids and clonidine.[85] In animal research, the threshold hypothalamic temperature for onset of shivering was 34.8–36.4 °C in control animals, whereas after injury the threshold was lowered so that either no shivering occurred, or only slight shivering was observed at about 31 °C.[86] A similar impairment in the threshold for vasoconstriction may also occur after trauma. Possible mechanisms include reduced tissue oxygenation due to shock, central noradrenergic inhibition, central effects of hypotension and hypovolemia, and decrease in baroreceptor input to the brain.[82,83,86–88]

The incidences of hypothermia have been widely studied. The noted differences in incidences may be due to differences in (1) the trauma system and population itself (urban vs. rural, blunt injury vs. penetrating); (2) timing of temperature measurements (prehospital vs. emergency department vs. operating room [OR] vs. intensive care unit [ICU]); (3) technique of temperature measurement (core vs. intermediate site, thermocouple vs. infrared device); and (4) differences in trauma systems (thermal prevention methods vs. none, warmed IV fluids vs. unwarmed, immediate vs. delayed fluid resuscitation).

In one of the few prehospital studies, Helm et al. found that almost every second patient was hypothermic. Entrapped patients were at higher risk (98% vs. 35%; $p < 0.001$), as were patients older than 65 years ($p < 0.001$).[57] Using a tympanic infrared thermometer technique, Watts et al. showed that more than 60% of their trauma patients transported with air and ground ambulances had a subnormal temperature at initial assessment.[58] Fewer than 5%, however, had a temperature below 34 °C.

Studies from the emergency department (ED) also support the notion that hypothermia is prevalent. Luna et al. found that that about 66% of tracheally intubated trauma patients arrived in the ED hypothermic.[89] Hypothermia during the initial phase in the hospital was associated with severity of injury, number of transfusions needed, and time spent prehospital and in the ED. The overall incidence of admission hypothermia, defined as temperature ≤ 35 °C, was 5% in a study using data from a statewide trauma registry in Pennsylvania ($n = 38{,}520$ patients).[90] Even after adjustment for other factors, admission hypothermia was associated with a threefold increased odds ratio for fatal outcome. Perioperative hypothermia has been shown to occur in almost 50% of trauma patients requiring early surgery (Fig. 14.14). In a study of 2848 combat victims from Iraq, 18% of the victims were hypothermic (< 36 °C) at arrival in the Combat Support Hospital.[91] However, only 0.2% were severely hypothermic (< 32 °C) and 2% had a temperature between 32 and 34 °C (moderate hypothermia). Penetrating injury mechanism, a Glasgow Coma Scale (see Chapter 35, Table 35.1) less than 8, and shock (defined as systolic blood pressure < 90 mmHg) were independent predictors of hypothermia on arrival. Analyzing 38,550 trauma patients aged 18–55 years from the National Trauma Data Bank (American College of Surgeons), Shafi et al. found an 8.5% incidence of hypothermia at arrival in the ED.[92]

Hypothermic patients had the same age and sex distribution as the normothermic patients, but in general were more severely injured. In the French HypoTraum study independent risk factors of hypothermia (< 35 °C) in trauma patients were identified.[93] Intubation, reduced consciousness, higher Revised Trauma Scores, unclothing the patient, infusion fluid temperature, and mobile unit temperature were independently associated with hypothermia at ED arrival. In contrast to earlier studies, entrapment[57] or time of year did not reach statistical significance in the multivariate analysis. These disparities are probably due to a wide range of entrapment locations and absence of extreme temperatures in the HypoTraum study. While some risk factors seem quite universal, other factors may best be studied in the context of the location and organization of the prehospital trauma system at hand.

If not present at arrival, hypothermia may develop and worsen during the stay in the ED and OR (Fig. 14.14). The etiology, predisposing factors, and pathophysiology are the same as for other major surgery patients (Tables 14.1–14.3). During initial resuscitation and surgical procedures, exposure of the patient, immobilization, and use of anesthesia, combined with suboptimal thermal protection, will soon render the trauma patient hypothermic. Unfortunately, despite everything that has been written on the subject, there is still a distinct impression that thermal management of trauma patients is suboptimal.[3,4]

Clinical implications, prevention, and rewarming options

The negative clinical consequences of hypothermia in trauma victims are well defined[1–3] and are particularly linked to coagulopathy and immunosuppression (Table 14.3). Although a link between hypothermia and reduced survival seems to have been established, the effect of isolated, mild hypothermia (33–36 °C) on coagulation is controversial.[94,95] Even though such a direct effect on coagulation may be negligible, there is an acceptance of the additive negative effects of acidosis and other trauma-related coagulopathic disturbances leading to clinical bleeding in patients presenting with temperatures below 34 °C. As core temperature falls below 32 °C, mortality from traumatic hemorrhage is markedly increased, but treatment should by no means be seen as futile. In contrast to earlier studies, analysis of the 2004 National Trauma Data Bank showed a survival of almost 60% in patients with temperature below 32 °C.[96] There is, however, a need for more data on the subgroup of trauma survivors with very low temperatures.

Separating the effects of hypothermia on outcome from other markers of severity has proved difficult. Studies of large cohorts of trauma patients have shown hypothermia (< 35 °C) to be an independent predictor of morbidity and mortality. Incidences of infections overall, pneumonia, renal failure, and acute respiratory distress syndrome (ARDS) have all been shown to increase with hypothermia.[96] In studies using multivariate analysis on retrospective data, there will always be a question whether the statistical association found also implies a causal link. An alternative view is that hypothermia merely reflects the magnitude of injury, shock, and bleeding.[97] In a study of 5197 patients from the German Trauma Registry (DGU), the authors found that temperature was not an independent predictor of mortality when hemorrhage/coagulopathy was included in their model.[98] However, such efforts to separate the impact of hypothermia from other closely linked manifestations of trauma may prove less than useful in clinical practice. Perioperative hypothermia and hypothermia on arrival to the ICU or during the first ICU hour should always be considered a danger sign, and every measure should be taken to counteract a fall in body temperature in trauma patients, both prior to and after arrival at the hospital.

Prevention is always better than treatment, including during intrahospital transport.[99] Reducing the incidence of hypothermia in the prehospital setting is possible by implementing guidelines focusing on basic measures of heat-loss prevention. By limiting external hemorrhage, removing wet clothing, providing wrapping and warm blankets, and active warming of resuscitation fluids, the American military reduced the proportion of hypothermic admissions from 7% to 1%.[100] Heat conservation during transport is possible through minimizing exposure and covering or wrapping the body by a number of methods, but data on specific measures of temperature management during transport are limited. In one of the very few studies of prehospital intervention to maintain normothermia in trauma victims, Watts et al. found that the use of chemical hot packs increased body temperature during transport.[58] Neither passive rewarming and reflective blankets nor warmed IV fluids alone caused the same increase in temperature. Thomassen et al. found initial wrapping with a vapor-tight layer and an additional dry insulating layer (Hibler's method) to be superior to bubble wrap or woolen blankets alone in healthy volunteers.[101] Hibler's method provided increased skin temperatures, lower metabolic rates, and better thermal comfort. An anterior heat pad was clinically tested in a small randomized trial on awake trauma patients by Lundgren et al.[102] Although a small increase in temperature was achieved, the difference was not significant. Even though the effect on temperature may be modest, the application of active surface warming during transport still has a potential clinical relevance since it may reduce shivering strain on the metabolism. Prehospital anesthesia may abolish shivering, leading to an accentuation of hypothermia.[84] In anesthetized, unconscious, or severely injured patients with long transport times, active warming may prove valuable. Scheck et al. have demonstrated that the application of a resistive heating blanket preserves temperature compared to woolen blankets in the intrahospital transport of critically ill trauma patients.[99]

Limiting heat loss through prompt, external bleeding control will reduce the need for fluids later on. Even beyond the principle of permissive hypotension, judicious use of IV fluids is important, because cold fluids may have a profound effect on body temperature. In general, active modes of temperature

Table 14.8 Suggested management of different levels of hypothermia in trauma victims

Phase of care	Hypothermia type/class			
	Mild		Moderate	Severe
	Class I	Class II	Class III	Class IV
Prehospital/ emergency department/ICU	Standard measures ± active external warming	Active external warming	Extracorporeal measures	Extracorporeal measures
Intraoperative	Standard measures ± active external warming	Active internal warming (intracavitary irrigation)	Extracorporeal measures ± intracavitary methods	Extracorporeal measures ± intracavitary mettiods
Permissibility of further surgery?	Definitive surgery allowed	Damage control	Damage control	Damage control

Modified from Kirkpatrick *et al.* 1999.[2]

Standard measures to be instituted in all serious trauma patients encompass but are not limited to measures recognized as passive external methods (warm environment, blankets, covers), warmed intravenous fluids, warmed inspired gases if intubated, convective warming blankets.

Extracarporeal methods to be utilized with appropriate personnel and institutional support: continuous arteriovenous rewarming, venovenous rewarming with centrifugal vortex pump, arteriovenous rewarming with centrifugal vortex pump, standard cardiopulmonary bypass, hemodialysis circuits with heated dialysate. DHCA, deep hypothermic circulatory arrest (only with severe injuries and appropriate support).

management such as warm fluids, fluid warmers, and body heating are warranted, but their availability in the prehospital setting is hampered by many practical, logistical, and financial barriers.

In-hospital, convective forced-air warming devices are very useful in a wide variety of locations (ED, OR, ICU, post-anesthesia care unit), and if a large enough surface area can be covered, these devices create a thermoneutral microenvironment such that all heat production goes to restoring core temperature.[4,32,49,51,52,103] It is recognized that it may be somewhat difficult to apply these devices to the trauma patient in the ED because of the requirement for patient exposure. This fact underlines the need to keep the stay in the ED as short as possible.

Other warming methods are also available in trauma patients (Tables 14.6, 14.8). Heated humidification of the breathing circuit will prevent respiratory-gas-related heat loss and can add heat to the patient. Delivery of warm, humidified gas has been shown to increase core temperature by 0.5–0.65 °C per hour in injured, hypothermic patients,[104,105] and should be used as an integrated part of a combined approach to treat or prevent hypothermia.[32] Although mostly used for accidental hypothermia patients, active, internal rewarming (Tables 14.6, 14.8) restores normothermia at a faster rate than surface methods and has been associated with more rapid normalization of cardiac output and ECG, and a decreased risk of rewarming shock in trauma-associated severe hypothermia.[48,106,107] These methods of core rewarming are generally appropriate for severely hypothermic patients, but may also be useful for moderately hypothermic patients (32–34 °C) with cardiovascular instability.

CPB (Tables 14.6, 14.8) is the most effective means of rewarming severely hypothermic patients, but requires systemic heparinization.[2,3,27,47,74] Relative contraindications to CPB include asphyxia, severe traumatic injury (risk of bleeding), and greatly elevated potassium levels (> 12 mmol/ L). The development of smaller, portable, percutaneous ECMO systems with heparinized circuits has the potential to reduce practical and logistical barriers in providing effective rewarming in selected trauma patients.[108] Peritoneal or pleural lavage with heated crystalloid at an exchange rate of 6 L/min may increase core temperature at a rate of 2–3 °C per hour, and has been shown to be beneficial in patients sustaining environmental or exposure hypothermia.[2,3,27,47,75,109]

Another technique involves the connection of a percutaneously placed femoral arterial line to a countercurrent fluid warmer (Tables 14.6, 14.8).[48,106] The patient's blood volume flows through the warmer and returns to the patient by large-bore venous tubing so a fistula is created through the heating warmer (Fig. 14.15). This technique, known as continuous arteriovenous rewarming (CAVR), has been shown to rapidly rewarm mildly hypothermic patients. In the initial experience of 16 patients treated with CAVR, core rewarming to 35 °C was accomplished in 39 minutes, and to 36 °C in 66 minutes.[106] Advantages of CAVR include no requirement for heparinization, rapid reversal of hypothermia, decreased total fluid requirements, decreased organ failure, and decreased length of ICU stay. The CAVR technique provided a continuous transfusion of heat to the patient as long as systolic blood pressure was more than 80 mmHg. The risks of CAVR consist mainly of those related to percutaneous cannulation of the femoral vessels.[106]

There are very few randomized controlled studies of rewarming trauma patients. Gentillelo *et al.* compared CAVR with standard rewarming in a randomized prospective trial of 57 trauma patients arriving in the ICU hypothermic (core temperature ≤ 34.5 °C).[107] There was a marked decrease in fluid requirement, a significantly faster rewarming rate, and lower early mortality in patients receiving CAVR (7% with CAVR vs. 43% with standard rewarming), but survival to

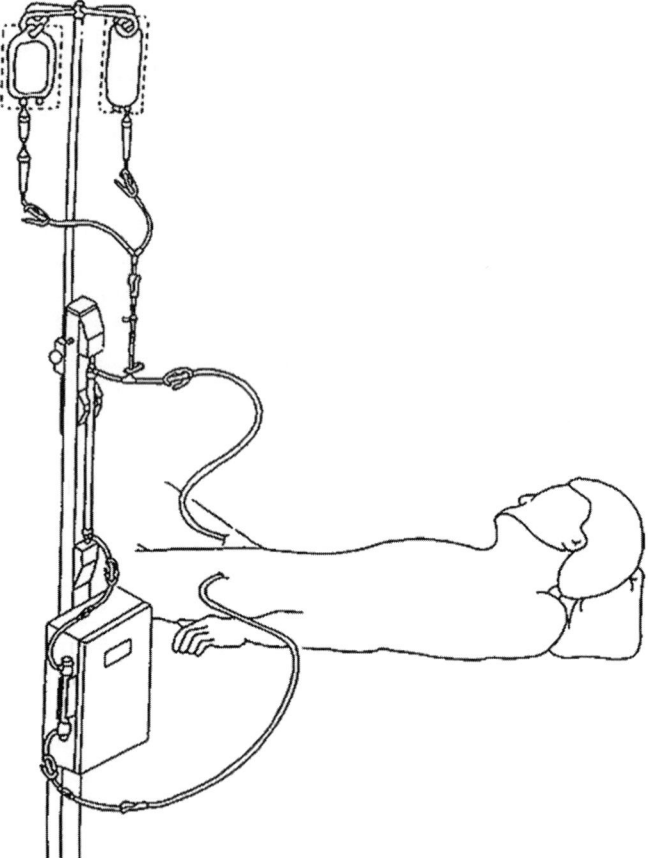

Figure 14.15 Schematic depiction of the continuous arteriovenous rewarming (CAVR) device that uses percutaneously placed femoral arterial and venous catheters and the patient's own blood pressure to create an arteriovenous fistula that diverts a portion of the cardiac output through a compact, heparin-bonded heat exchanger. (Reproduced with permission from Gentilello et al. 1992.[106])

discharge was not significantly different between groups (66% survival with CAVR vs. 50% with standard rewarming). This study illustrates the problems with such studies, and how short-term effects may be deleted by later problems in the ICU. Still, the study supports the notion that hypothermia should be treated aggressively in trauma patients. The methods used (Tables 14.6, 14.8) will vary with the circumstances, and with the experience and available resources of the local trauma team.

Surgery and anesthesia are two major risk factors for causing or exacerbating hypothermia in trauma. Forced-air warming and warm fluids are considered to be standard measures of heat-loss prevention, but the efficacy of forced air may be reduced by the area available for application. If forced-air warming is not feasible because of the size and location of the surgical procedure, underbody resistive heating with pressure relief, gel-pad warming, and underbody convective forced-air warming may provide alternatives.[42] Increasing OR temperature to > 24 °C is a simple and often overlooked method of heat conservation, and higher ambient temperatures (e.g., ≥ 27 °C) have been suggested. In an observational study,

Inaba and coworkers did not find ambient OR temperatures to reduce the incidence of perioperative hypothermia in trauma patients when other aggressive measures of temperature management were employed.[110] Radiant lamps may prove useful, especially in burn surgery, but their effectiveness will depend on their proximity to the patient and the tolerance of the OR staff. Irrigating fluids should be warmed to 36 °C. Most importantly, in damage control surgery operating time should be kept as short as possible in order to avoid the deadly triad of hypothermia, acidosis and coagulopathy.[95,98,111]

Summary and conclusions

Hypothermia as a complication of major surgery and anesthesia is well known to the anesthesiologist. Life-threatening hypothermia without trauma may also develop (accidental hypothermia). Hypothermia often complicates the management of patients with blunt or penetrating trauma and is associated with increased morbidity and mortality. Early control of bleeding and prevention of further heat loss are key factors to avoid the lethal triad of hypothermia, acidosis, and coagulopathy. Standard measures to prevent and/or treat hypothermia include warmed IV fluids and blood products, increased ambient temperatures, and convective forced-air warming systems. Other measures may be used depending on the severity of hypothermia, the clinical situation, and available resources and equipment. During all trauma resuscitation situations, it is important for the anesthesiologist to use his or her experience from major surgical patients, and to pay close attention to temperature management in trauma patients.

Questions

(1) True or false? Reliable temperature-monitoring sites are the distal esophagus, nasopharynx, and pulmonary artery.

(2) True or false? In healthy humans, the core temperature remains stable within a narrow temperature range despite large variations in environmental conditions.

(3) Regarding methods and equipment for rewarming and maintaining normothermia:
   a. Conduction represents heat transfer through air that is in contact with the body, and its efficiency is mostly determined by air velocity
   b. Convective heat transfer implies direct contact between two objects and their characteristics
   c. Commercial rewarming equipment (e.g., convective forced-air, fluid warmer) is generally not effective in preventing perioperative hypothermia
   d. Evaporative heat transfer occurs with conversion of liquids (water, sweat) to the gaseous phase

(4) Identify the correct statement regarding side effects of perioperative hypothermia:
   a. Decreases in core temperatures to between 34 and 36 °C have not been associated with increased

complications such as cardiac events (myocardial ischemia, ventricular tachycardia)

b. Decreases in core temperatures to between 34 and 36 °C have not been associated with increased complications such as perioperative bleeding and transfusion requirements

c. Decreases in core temperatures to between 34 and 36 °C have not been associated with a significant increase in postoperative complications such as wound infections

d. The general effect of cooling is that all body processes, including neuromuscular function, slow down to the stage of depression and eventually death

e. Moderate degrees of hypothermia are generally indicated for trauma patients

(5) Regarding the effects of anesthesia and surgery on perioperative hypothermia, identify the correct statement:

a. Induction of general anesthesia results in a gradual decrease in core temperature

b. All general anesthetics with the exception of ketamine affect the normal thermoregulatory responses in the same manner

c. Replacement of shed blood with cold or inadequately warmed IV fluids and blood can rarely decrease body temperature

d. Epidural and spinal anesthesia have negligible effects on peripheral and central thermoregulation

(6) A 64-year-old woman with stable angina is undergoing urgent exploratory laparotomy with general anesthesia following blunt trauma. Blood loss is 2 L and a fluid warmer was not available. At the end of the 3.5-hour surgery you note that her core temperature is 34.8 °C. Which of these statements is true?

a. She is not at increased risk of postoperative wound infection

b. She is not at increased risk of postoperative ventricular tachycardia and unstable angina

c. She is at increased risk of postoperative shivering and prolonged peripheral vasoconstriction

d. The most likely cause of her low temperature is monitoring error

(7) Intraoperative hypothermia can be safely minimized by:

a. Maintaining OR temperature at 19 °C

b. Warming crystalloid solutions to 36 °C prior to IV administration and using convective forced-air warming

c. Warming refrigerated blood products to 36 °C in a microwave oven prior to IV administration

d. Warming crystalloid solutions to 55 °C prior to IV administration

(8) Regarding avalanche victims, identify the correct statement:

a. Early asphyxiation is uncommon

b. The probability of survival is unrelated to burial time

c. In lifeless victims, the focus should be on rapid extrication and immediate airway management and CPR rather than rewarming

d. Serum potassium is not a prognostic marker

Questions 9 and 10 refer to the following case: A 70-year-old female is brought to your emergency department after a motor vehicle crash with prolonged extrication. She has an obvious deformity of her left proximal femur and multiple abrasions over her left chest. BP is 150/60 mmHg; pulse 92 bpm; respirations 8; oxygen saturation 98% on nonrebreather; rectal temperature 33 °C.

(9) Concerning hypothermia in this patient:

a. Rewarming methods should be instituted during the secondary survey and IV fluids should be warmed

b. Hypothermia is likely to be beneficial, due to cerebral and myocardial protection

c. Thermoregulation is usually normal after injury

d. Severity of hypothermia is not associated with severity of injury

(10) Concerning thermal management in this patient:

a. Coagulopathy and immunosuppression are unlikely with this degree of hypothermia

b. Exposure of the patient may further aggravate hypothermia

c. Treatment of this degree of hypothermia is futile, since mortality is markedly increased

d. Infusion of unwarmed crystalloid fluids is unlikely to aggravate hypothermia

Answers

(1) True
(2) True
(3) d
(4) d
(5) b
(6) c
(7) b
(8) c
(9) a
(10) b

References

1. Hildebrand F, Giannoudis PV, van Griensven M, Chawda M, Pape HC. Pathophysiologic changes and effects of hypothermia on outcome in elective surgery and trauma patients. *Am J Surg* 2004; **187**: 363–71.

2. Kirkpatrick AW, Chun R, Brown R, Simons RK. Hypothermia and the trauma patient. *Can J Surg* 1999; **42**: 333–43.

3. Tsuei BJ, Kearney PA. Hypothermia in the trauma patient. *Injury* 2004; **35**: 7–15.

4. Wooten C, Schultz P, Sapida J, Laflamme C. Warming and treatment of mild hypothermia in the trauma resuscitation room: an intervention algorithm. *J Trauma Nurs* 2004; **11**: 64–6.

5. Alam HB, Pusateri AE, Kindzelski A, *et al.* Hypothermia and hemostasis in severe trauma: a new crossroads workshop report. *J Trauma Acute Care Surg* 2012; **73**: 809–17.

6. Tisherman SA. Hypothermia and injury. *Curr Opin Crit Care* 2004; **10**: 512–19.

7. Sadaka F, Veremakis C. Therapeutic hypothermia for the management of intracranial hypertension in severe traumatic brain injury: a systematic review. *Brain injury* 2012; **26**: 899–908.

8. Brown DJ, Brugger H, Boyd J, Paal P. Accidental hypothermia. *N Engl J Med* 2012; **367**: 1930–8.

9. Silfvast T, Pettila V. Outcome from severe accidental hypothermia in Southern Finland: a 10-year review. *Resuscitation* 2003; **59**: 285–90.

10. Grahn D. The physiology of mammalian temperature homeostasis. In Smith C, Grande C, eds., *Hypothermia in Trauma: Deliberate or Accidental*. Baltimore, MD: International Trauma Anesthesia Critical Care Society (ITACCS), 1997, pp. 1–6.

11. Szmuk P, Ezri T, Sessler DI, Stein A, Geva D. Spinal anesthesia speeds active postoperative rewarming. *Anesthesiology* 1997; **87**: 1050–4.

12. Buggy DJ, Crossley AW. Thermoregulation, mild perioperative hypothermia and postanaesthetic shivering. *Br J Anaesth* 2000; **84**: 615–28.

13. Szmuk P, Rabb MF, Baumgartner JE, *et al.* Body morphology and the speed of cutaneous rewarming. *Anesthesiology* 2001; **95**: 18–21.

14. Taguchi A, Kurz A. Thermal management of the patient: where does the patient lose and/or gain temperature? *Curr Opin Anaesthesiol* 2005; **18**: 632–9.

15. Kurz A, Sessler DI, Narzt E, Lenhardt R, Lackner F. Morphometric influences on intraoperative core temperature changes. *Anesth Analg* 1995; **80**: 562–7.

16. Sessler DI. Perioperative heat balance. *Anesthesiology* 2000; **92**: 578–96.

17. Belani K, Sessler DI, Sessler AM, *et al.* Leg heat content continues to decrease during the core temperature plateau in humans anesthetized with isoflurane. *Anesthesiology* 1993; **78**: 856–63.

18. Frank SM, Beattie C, Christopherson R, *et al.* Epidural versus general anesthesia, ambient operating room temperature, and patient age as predictors of inadvertent hypothermia. *Anesthesiology* 1992; **77**: 252–7.

19. Glosten B, Hynson J, Sessler DI, McGuire J. Preanesthetic skin-surface warming reduces redistribution hypothermia caused by epidural block. *Anesth Analg* 1993; **77**: 488–93.

20. Sessler DI, Moayeri A. Skin-surface warming: heat flux and central temperature. *Anesthesiology* 1990; **73**: 218–24.

21. Kurz A, Go JC, Sessler DI, *et al.* Alfentanil slightly increases the sweating threshold and markedly reduces the vasoconstriction and shivering thresholds. *Anesthesiology* 1995; **83**: 293–9.

22. Kurz A, Sessler DI, Annadata R, *et al.* Midazolam minimally impairs thermoregulatory control. *Anesth Analg* 1995; **81**: 393–8.

23. Ozaki M, Sessler DI, Matsukawa T, *et al.* The threshold for thermoregulatory vasoconstriction during nitrous oxide/sevoflurane anesthesia is reduced in the elderly. *Anesth Analg* 1997; **84**: 1029–33.

24. Ikeda T, Kazama T, Sessler DI, *et al.* Induction of anesthesia with ketamine reduces the magnitude of redistribution hypothermia. *Anesth Analg* 2001; **93**: 934–8.

25. Ikeda T, Kim JS, Sessler DI, *et al.* Isoflurane alters shivering patterns and reduces maximum shivering intensity. *Anesthesiology* 1998; **88**: 866–73.

26. Ikeda T, Sessler DI, Kikura M, *et al.* Less core hypothermia when anesthesia is induced with inhaled sevoflurane than with intravenous propofol. *Anesth Analg* 1999; **88**: 921–4.

27. Biem J, Koehncke N, Classen D, Dosman J. Out of the cold: management of hypothermia and frostbite. *CMAJ* 2003; **168**: 305–11.

28. Heier T, Caldwell JE. Impact of hypothermia on the response to neuromuscular blocking drugs. *Anesthesiology* 2006; **104**: 1070–80.

29. Frank SM, Beattie C, Christopherson R, *et al.* Unintentional hypothermia is associated with postoperative myocardial ischemia. The Perioperative Ischemia Randomized Anesthesia Trial Study Group. *Anesthesiology* 1993; **78**: 468–76.

30. Frank SM, Fleisher LA, Breslow MJ, *et al.* Perioperative maintenance of normothermia reduces the incidence of morbid cardiac events: a randomized clinical trial. *JAMA* 1997; **277**: 1127–34.

31. Frank SM, Higgins MS, Breslow MJ, *et al.* The catecholamine, cortisol, and hemodynamic responses to mild perioperative hypothermia: a randomized clinical trial. *Anesthesiology* 1995; **82**: 83–93.

32. Sessler DI. Complications and treatment of mild hypothermia. *Anesthesiology* 2001; **95**: 531–43.

33. Soar J, Perkins GD, Abbas G, *et al.* European Resuscitation Council Guidelines for Resuscitation 2010 Section 8. Cardiac arrest in special circumstances: Electrolyte abnormalities, poisoning, drowning, accidental hypothermia, hyperthermia, asthma, anaphylaxis, cardiac surgery, trauma, pregnancy, electrocution. *Resuscitation* 2010; **81**: 1400–33.

34. Frank SM, Fleisher LA, Olson KF, *et al.* Multivariate determinants of early postoperative oxygen consumption in elderly patients. Effects of shivering, body temperature, and gender. *Anesthesiology* 1995; **83**: 241–9.

35. Schmied H, Kurz A, Sessler DI, Kozek S, Reiter A. Mild hypothermia increases blood loss and transfusion requirements during total hip arthroplasty. *Lancet* 1996; **347**: 289–92.

36. Heier T, Clough D, Wright PM, *et al.* The influence of mild hypothermia on the pharmacokinetics and time course of action of neostigmine in anesthetized volunteers. *Anesthesiology* 2002; **97**: 90–5.

37. Brauer A, English MJ, Steinmetz N, *et al.* Comparison of forced-air warming systems with upper body blankets using a copper manikin of the human body. *Acta Anaesthesiol Scand* 2002; **46**: 965–72.

38. Camus Y, Delva E, Bossard AE, Chandon M, Lienhart A. Prevention of hypothermia by cutaneous warming with new electric blankets during

abdominal surgery. *Br J Anaesth* 1997; **79**: 796–7.

39. Camus Y, Delva E, Just B, Lienhart A. Leg warming minimizes core hypothermia during abdominal surgery. *Anesth Analg* 1993; **77**: 995–9.

40. Camus Y, Delva E, Sessler DI, Lienhart A. Pre-induction skin-surface warming minimizes intraoperative core hypothermia. *Journal of clinical anesthesia* 1995; **7**: 384–8.

41. Torossian A. Thermal management during anaesthesia and thermoregulation standards for the prevention of inadvertent perioperative hypothermia. *Best Pract Res Clin Anaesthesiol* 2008; **22**: 659–68.

42. Egan C, Bernstein E, Reddy D, *et al.* A randomized comparison of intraoperative PerfecTemp and forced-air warming during open abdominal surgery. *Anesth Analg* 2011; **113**: 1076–81.

43. Taguchi A, Ratnaraj J, Kabon B, *et al.* Effects of a circulating-water garment and forced-air warming on body heat content and core temperature. *Anesthiology* 2004; **100**: 1058–64.

44. Goheen MS, Ducharme MB, Kenny GP, *et al.* Efficacy of forced-air and inhalation rewarming by using a human model for severe hypothermia. *J Appl Physiol* 1997; **83**: 1635–40.

45. Koller R, Schnider TW, Neidhart P. Deep accidental hypothermia and cardiac arrest–rewarming with forced air. *Acta Anaesthesiol Scand* 1997; **41**: 1359–64.

46. Ereth MH, Lennon RL, Sessler DI. Limited heat transfer between thermal compartments during rewarming in vasoconstricted patients. *Aviat Space Environ Med* 1992; **63**: 1065–9.

47. Aslam AF, Aslam AK, Vasavada BC, Khan IA. Hypothermia: evaluation, electrocardiographic manifestations, and management. *Am J Med* 2006; **119**: 297–301.

48. Gentilello LM, Cortes V, Moujaes S, *et al.* Continuous arteriovenous rewarming: experimental results and thermodynamic model simulation of treatment for hypothermia. *J Trauma* 1990; **30**: 1436–49.

49. Smith C. Trauma and hypothermia. *Curr Anaesth Crit Care* 2001; **12**: 87–9.

50. Smith CE, Desai R, Glorioso V, *et al.* Preventing hypothermia: convective and intravenous fluid warming versus convective warming alone. *J Clin Anes* 1998; **10**: 380–5.

51. Smith CE, Patel N. Hypothermia in adult trauma patients: anesthetic considerations. Part II. Prevention and treatment. *Am J Anesthesiol* 1997; **24**: 29–36.

52. Smith CE, Yamat RA. Avoiding hypothermia in the trauma patient. *Curr Opin Anaesthesiol* 2000; **13**: 167–74.

53. Avula RR, Kramer R, Smith CE. Air detection performance of the level 1 H-1200 fluid and blood warmer. *Anesth Analg* 2005; **101**: 1413–16.

54. Avula RR, Smith CE. Air venting and in-line intravenous fluid warming for pediatrics. *Anesthesiology* 2005; **102**: 1290.

55. Stone JG, Young WL, Smith CR, *et al.* Do standard monitoring sites reflect true brain temperature when profound hypothermia is rapidly induced and reversed? *Anesthesiology* 1995; **82**: 344–51.

56. Imamura M, Matsukawa T, Ozaki M, *et al.* The accuracy and precision of four infrared aural canal thermometers during cardiac surgery. *Acta Anaesthesiol Scand* 1998; **42**: 1222–6.

57. Helm M, Lampl L, Hauke J, Bock KH. [Accidental hypothermia in trauma patients. Is it relevant to preclinical emergency treatment?] *Anaesthesist* 1995; **44**: 101–7.

58. Watts DD, Roche M, Tricarico R, *et al.* The utility of traditional prehospital interventions in maintaining thermostasis. *Prehosp Emerg Care* 1999; **3**: 115–22.

59. Søreide E, Grahn DA, Brock-Utne JG, Rosen L. A non-invasive means to effectively restore normothermia in cold stressed individuals: a preliminary report. *J Emerg Med* 1999; **17**: 725–30.

60. Danzl DF, Pozos RS. Accidental hypothermia. *N Engl J Med* 1994; **331**: 1756–60.

61. Durrer B, Brugger H, Syme D; International Commission for Mountain Emergency Medicine. The medical on-site treatment of hypothermia: ICAR-MEDCOM recommendation. *High Alt Med Biol* 2003; **4**: 99–103.

62. Bierens JJ, Uitslager R, Swenne-van Ingen MM, van Stiphout WA, Knape JT. Accidental hypothermia: incidence, risk factors and clinical course of patients admitted to hospital. *Eur J Emerg Med* 1995; **2**: 38–46.

63. Lonning PE, Skulberg A, Abyholm F. Accidental hypothermia: review of the literature. *Acta Anaesthesiol Scand* 1986; **30**: 601–13.

64. Vanden Hoek TL, Morrison LJ, Shuster M, *et al.* Part 12: cardiac arrest in special situations: 2010 American Heart Association Guidelines for Cardiopulmonary Resuscitation and Emergency Cardiovascular Care. *Circulation* 2010; **122**: S829–61.

65. Farstad M, Andersen KS, Koller ME, *et al.* Rewarming from accidental hypothermia by extracorporeal circulation: a retrospective study. *Eur J Cardiothorac Surg* 2001; **20**: 58–64.

66. Gilbert M, Busund R, Skagseth A, Nilsen PA, Solbo JP. Resuscitation from accidental hypothermia of 13.7 degrees C with circulatory arrest. *Lancet* 2000; **355**: 375–6.

67. Walpoth BH, Walpoth-Aslan BN, Mattle HP, *et al.* Outcome of survivors of accidental deep hypothermia and circulatory arrest treated with extracorporeal blood warming. *N Engl J Med* 1997; **337**: 1500–5.

68. Kornberger E, Schwarz B, Lindner KH, Mair P. Forced air surface rewarming in patients with severe accidental hypothermia. *Resuscitation* 1999; **41**: 105–11.

69. Giesbrecht GG, Hayward JS. Problems and complications with cold-water rescue. *Wilderness Environ Med* 2006; **17**: 26–30.

70. Brugger H, Durrer B, Elsensohn F, *et al.* Resuscitation of avalanche victims. Evidence-based guidelines of the international commission for mountain emergency medicine (ICAR MEDCOM): intended for physicians and other advanced life support personnel. *Resuscitation* 2013; **84**: 539–46.

71. Silfvast T, Tiainen M, Poutiainen E, Roine RO. Therapeutic hypothermia after prolonged cardiac arrest due to non-coronary causes. *Resuscitation* 2003; **57**: 109–12.

72. Steele MT, Nelson MJ, Sessler DI, *et al.* Forced air speeds rewarming in accidental hypothermia. *Ann Emerg Med* 1996; **27**: 479–84.

73. Taylor EE, Carroll JP, Lovitt MA, *et al.* Active intravascular rewarming for hypothermia associated with traumatic injury: early experience with a new technique. *Proc (Bayl Univ Med Cent)* 2008; **21**: 120–6.

74. Kirkpatrick AW, Garraway N, Brown DR, *et al.* Use of a centrifugal vortex blood pump and heparin-bonded circuit for extracorporeal rewarming of severe hypothermia in acutely injured and coagulopathic patients. *J Trauma* 2003; **55**: 407–12.

75. Plaisier BR. Thoracic lavage in accidental hypothermia with cardiac arrest–report of a case and review of the literature. *Resuscitation* 2005; **66**: 99–104.

76. Todd SR, Malinoski D, Muller PJ, Schreiber MA. Lactated Ringer's is superior to normal saline in the resuscitation of uncontrolled hemorrhagic shock. *J Trauma* 2007; **62**: 636–9.

77. Ruttmann E, Weissenbacher A, Ulmer H, *et al.* Prolonged extracorporeal membrane oxygenation-assisted support provides improved survival in hypothermic patients with cardiocirculatory arrest. *J Thoracic Cardiovasc Surg* 2007; **134**: 594–600.

78. Szpilman D, Bierens JJ, Handley AJ, Orlowski JP. Drowning. *N Engl J Med* 2012; **366**: 2102–10.

79. Polderman KH, Rijnsburger ER, Peerdeman SM, Girbes AR. Induction of hypothermia in patients with various types of neurologic injury with use of large volumes of ice-cold intravenous fluid. *Crit Care Med* 2005; **33**: 2744–51.

80. Brugger H, Durrer B, Adler-Kastner L, Falk M, Tschirky F. Field management of avalanche victims. *Resuscitation* 2001; **51**: 7–15.

81. Oberhammer R, Beikircher W, Hormann C, *et al.* Full recovery of an avalanche victim with profound hypothermia and prolonged cardiac arrest treated by extracorporeal re-warming. *Resuscitation* 2008; **76**: 474–80.

82. Little RA, Stoner HB. Body temperature after accidental injury. *Br J Surg* 1981; **68**: 221–4.

83. Little RA, Stoner HB, Randall P, Carlson G. An effect of injury on thermoregulation in man. *Q J Exp Physiol* 1986; **71**: 295–306.

84. Langhelle A, Lockey D, Harris T, Davies G. Body temperature of trauma patients on admission to hospital: a comparison of anaesthetised and non-anaesthetised patients. *Emerg Med J* 2012; **29**: 239–42.

85. Weant KA, Martin JE, Humphries RL, Cook AM. Pharmacologic options for reducing the shivering response to therapeutic hypothermia. *Pharmacotherapy* 2010; **30**: 830–41.

86. Stoner HB. Effect of injury on the responses to thermal stimulation of the hypothalamus. *J Appl Physiol* 1972; **33**: 665–71.

87. Stoner HB. The role of catecholamine in the effects of trauma on thermoregulation, studied in rats treated with 6-hydroxydopamine. *Br J Exp Pathol* 1977; **58**: 42–9.

88. Stoner HB, Marshall HW. Localization of the brain regions concerned in the inhibition of shivering by trauma. *Br J Exp Pathol* 1977; **58**: 50–6.

89. Luna GK, Maier RV, Pavlin EG, *et al.* Incidence and effect of hypothermia in seriously injured patients. *J Ttrauma* 1987; **27**: 1014–18.

90. Wang HE, Callaway CW, Peitzman AB, Tisherman SA. Admission hypothermia and outcome after major trauma. *Crit Care Med* 2005; **33**: 1296–301.

91. Arthurs Z, Cuadrado D, Beekley A, *et al.* The impact of hypothermia on trauma care at the 31st combat support hospital. *Am J Surg* 2006; **191**: 610–14.

92. Shafi S, Elliott AC, Gentilello L. Is hypothermia simply a marker of shock and injury severity or an independent risk factor for mortality in trauma patients? Analysis of a large national trauma registry. *J Trauma* 2005; **59**: 1081–5.

93. Lapostolle F, Sebbah JL, Couvreur J, *et al.* Risk factors for onset of hypothermia in trauma victims: The HypoTraum study. *Crit Care* 2012; **16**: R142.

94. Thorsen K, Ringdal KG, Strand K, *et al.* Clinical and cellular effects of hypothermia, acidosis and coagulopathy in major injury. *Br J Surg* 2011; **98**: 894–907.

95. Hess JR, Brohi K, Dutton RP, *et al.* The coagulopathy of trauma: a review of mechanisms. *J Trauma* 2008; **65**: 748–54.

96. Martin RS, Kilgo PD, Miller PR, *et al.* Injury-associated hypothermia: an analysis of the 2004 National Trauma Data Bank. *Shock* 2005; **24**: 114–18.

97. Shapiro MB, Jenkins DH, Schwab CW, Rotondo MF. Damage control: collective review. *J Trauma* 2000; **49**: 969–78.

98. Trentzsch H, Huber-Wagner S, Hildebrand F, *et al.* Hypothermia for prediction of death in severely injured blunt trauma patients. *Shock* 2012; **37**: 131–9.

99. Scheck T, Kober A, Bertalanffy P, *et al.* Active warming of critically ill trauma patients during intrahospital transfer: a prospective, randomized trial. *Wien Klin Wochenschr* 2004; **116**: 94–7.

100. Eastridge BJ, Jenkins D, Flaherty S, Schiller H, Holcomb JB. Trauma system development in a theater of war: experiences from Operation Iraqi Freedom and Operation Enduring Freedom. *J Trauma* 2006; **61**: 1366–72.

101. Thomassen O, Faerevik H, Osteras O, *et al.* Comparison of three different prehospital wrapping methods for preventing hypothermia–a crossover study in humans. *Scand J Trauma Resus Emerg Med* 2011; **19**: 41.

102. Lundgren P, Henriksson O, Naredi P, Bjornstig U. The effect of active warming in prehospital trauma care during road and air ambulance transportation – a clinical randomized trial. *Scand J Trauma Resus Emerg Med* 2011; **19**: 59.

103. Smith C, Grande CM, eds. Hypothermia in trauma: deliberate or accidental. *Trauma Care* 2004; **14** (2): 45–91.

104. Guild WJ. Rewarming via the airway (CBRW) for hypothermia in the field? *J R Nav Med Serv* 1978; **64**: 186–93.

105. Lloyd EL. Accidental hypothermia treated by central rewarming through the airway. *Br J Anaesth* 1973; **45**: 41–8.

106. Gentilello LM, Cobean RA, Offner PJ, Soderberg RW, Jurkovich GJ. Continuous arteriovenous rewarming: rapid reversal of hypothermia in critically ill patients. *J Trauma* 1992; **32**: 316–25.

107. Gentilello LM, Jurkovich GJ, Stark MS, Hassantash SA, O'Keefe GE. Is hypothermia in the victim of major trauma protective or harmful? A randomized, prospective study. *Ann Surg* 1997; **226**: 439–47.

108. Morita S, Inokuchi S, Yamagiwa T, *et al.* Efficacy of portable and percutaneous cardiopulmonary bypass rewarming versus that of conventional internal rewarming for patients with accidental deep hypothermia. *Crit Care Med* 2011; **39**: 1064–8.

109. Kjaergaard B, Bach P. Warming of patients with accidental hypothermia using warm water pleural lavage. *Resuscitation* 2006; **68**: 203–7.

110. Inaba K, Berg R, Barmparas G, *et al.* Prospective evaluation of ambient operating room temperature on the core temperature of injured patients undergoing emergent surgery. *J Trauma Acute Care Surg* 2012; **73**: 1478–83.

111. Blackbourne LH. Combat damage control surgery. *Crit Care Med* 2008; **36**: S304–10.

Chapter

15

Pharmacologic management of acute pain in trauma

Shalini Dhir, Rakesh V. Sondekoppam, and Sugantha Ganapathy

Objectives

(1) Evaluate pain management modalities in the acutely injured patient.

(2) Review the pharmacology of acetaminophen (paracetamol), nonsteroidal anti-inflammatory drugs (NSAIDs), opioids, tramadol, local anesthetics, and ketamine in trauma patients.

(3) Discuss the role of antidepressants, anticonvulsants, benzodiazepines, α_2 agonists, N-methyl-D-aspartate (NMDA) receptor antagonists, and entonox for acute pain in trauma.

(4) Discuss the role of multimodal analgesia for trauma patients.

Introduction

The widely accepted definition of pain was developed by a taxonomy task force of the International Association for the Study of Pain: "Pain is an unpleasant sensory and emotional experience that is associated with actual or potential tissue damage or described in such terms."[1] Managing pain can be challenging in most scenarios, and providing adequate pain relief forms a vital part in the initial management of trauma. Inadequate analgesia in acute situations can have deleterious effects on the immune system, healing process, and autonomic activity and can lead to the development of a chronic pain state (see Chapter 17). Although the majority of the medications used have been evaluated mainly for acute postoperative pain, with lesser evidence specifically for posttraumatic pain, they are effective when used for the latter purpose. A concern is that the contribution of analgesic agents to preemptive analgesia may not be applicable in posttraumatic situations, since the insult has already occurred.

Physiology of pain transmission relevant to pain pharmacology

In simple terms, the pain pathway consists of the peripheral nociception, the spinal transmission (dorsal horn), and the supraspinal sensory region (brain). The whole pathway is not only adaptable but also dynamic. The fast pain, also known as nociceptive pain since it exists as long as the nociceptive stimulus is present, is carried by Aδ fibers, whereas the slow pain, also known as pathophysiological pain, is transmitted by the C fibers.

The fast pain fibers (5–30 m/s) carrying pain sensation from the periphery synapse at laminae I, V, and X of the dorsal horn, and the secondary neurons relay it to the posterior thalamic nuclei via the neospinothalamic tract, and from there to the sensory cortex. The slow pain component should protect the injured area, but this response is thought to flare up pathologically, resulting in chronic pain. The free endings sense the nociceptive stimuli carried by the C fibers (< 1 m/s) to laminae II and III (substantia gelatinosa) of the dorsal horn, from where they relay at the medial thalamic nuclei via the paleospinothalamic tract and further into the sensory cortex. Local anesthetics act on the dorsal horn sensory neurons of the spinal cord to produce analgesia.

The integration of excitatory and inhibitory influences on the pain pathway occurs at the dorsal horn, which can be seen as the first processing center and is a target for pain pharmacology. While opioids potentiate the influence of descending endogenous opioid pathways, $\alpha 2$ agonists and neostigmine act by increasing the noradrenergic influence on the pain pathway. Midazolam is thought to act by increasing the GABAergic tone on the dorsal horn neuron at the specific spinal level.

The pain pathway has projections to the limbic system through connections to the reticular formation, the periaqueductal gray matter, and the hypothalamus, and may lead to behavioral and endocrine responses following pain. Pain sensation and subsequent responses have memory, and the response to a given input changes based on previous experience. In short, the plasticity of the pain pathway can be explained based on both central and peripheral sensitization. While peripheral sensitization can be simply explained in terms of increased neurotransmitter release and posttranslational modulation (at the level of receptor and secondary messenger response) in peripheral neurons, usually following a sustained stimulus, the central sensitization is a little more complex, with the involvement of spinal and supraspinal structures. In the supraspinal mechanisms, rostroventral medulla, anterior cingulate gyrus, and amygdala are important, having both excitatory and inhibitory influence on the dorsal root ganglion, and the balance between excitatory and inhibitory influences is managed by local circuitry. At the level of the spinal cord dorsal horn, the three mechanisms that result in sensitization include the wind-up phenomenon, spinal long-term potentiation (LTP), and classic central sensitization.

The first mechanism involves the stimulation of AMPA (2-amino-3-(3-hydroxy-5-methyl-isoxazol-4-yl)propanoic acid) receptors following repeated stimulation, which removes voltage-dependent Mg^{2+} block of NMDA (N-methyl-D-aspartate) receptors and also activates voltage-gated Ca^{2+} channels, thereby generating plateau potentials. With sustained stimulus, the Aβ fibers are also able to mount the wind-up phenomenon.

In the gate theory proposed by Melzac and Wall, the sensory inputs from pain fibers (nociceptive sensation) and Aβ fibers (fine touch and pressure) coalesce on the wide dynamic rage (WDR) neurons in the dorsal horn, where both of them stimulate the pain pathway.[2] Inhibitory interneurons from the substantia gelatinosa rolandi (SGR) inhibit the firing of WDR neurons. These inhibitory interneurons are stimulated by Aβ neurons and are inhibited by Aδ and C fibers. Normally, stimulation of Aβ fibers of the given dermatome gates the pain signals at SGR. But in chronic pain there is a phenotypic switch in Aβ fibers terminating on the WDR, which not only increase the neurotransmitter release to the WDR neurons, but also start de novo synthesis of substance P (normally produced by primary afferents) and thus increase the impulse intensity on the WDR neurons. In the wind-up phenomenon, repeated stimulation of nociceptive afferents leads to a progressive and frequency-dependent increase in the excitability of dorsal horn neurons.

The other two mechanisms of long-term potentiation and central sensitization are similar in that they define the membrane potential of the second-order neurons following sustained stimulus. They can be excitatory, wherein the resting membrane potential is more depolarized than normal (–70 mV), or depressive, wherein it is slightly hyperpolarized (–85 mV). The second similarity is that LTP and central sensitization are both preferentially induced in dorsal horn projection neurons that express the NK_1 receptor. The difference between LTP and central sensitization lies in the fact that LTP is homosynaptic while central sensitization is heterosynaptic. Thus central sensitization contributes to receptive field enlargement (thought to be the basis of secondary allodynia) by involvement of adjacent neurons while LTP does not. In addition to these mechanisms, a decrease in γ-aminobutyric acid (GABA) inhibitory tone also contributes to the development and maintenance of central sensitization. Thus, AMPA, NK_1, NMDA, and GABA are all potential targets for prevention and treatment of pain.

Epidemiology of traumatic pain

According to World Health Organization (WHO) statistics, injuries are the number one cause of the global burden of death and disability in age groups below 60 years.[3] The economic impact in terms of lifetime costs and lost productivity is staggering. In the United States, as of 2000, the incidence of medically treated injuries was as high as 50 million per year, with an estimated lifetime cost of $406 billion. This incidence, although decreasing over the years, is still a significant burden.[4] Acute and chronic pain following injury is also a significant component of this burden. Although the exact incidence of severe traumatic injury is not known, CDC (Centers for Disease Control and Prevention) estimates in 2010 showed more than 17 million hospitalizations and over 37 million medically consulted injury episodes (www.cdc.gov/nchs/fastats/injury.htm).

Traumatic injury occurs most often in young adults (in the third or fourth decade), with a higher incidence in males than in females. The type of injury depends on the geographical location studied, and there is further regional variation. In a recent study by the Resuscitation Outcome Consortium (ROC) investigators covering nine North American cities, blunt trauma was more common than penetrating trauma, and the variety differed between the centers.[5] It is worthwhile to know the type of trauma and preexisting sensitization of pain pathways in order to prioritize the pain management, since patients having burns or thoracic, musculoskeletal, or abdominal trauma, and those with preexisting chronic pain or opioid dependence, need more support tthan those with head or spine injury. The incidence of pain following trauma is in the range of 35–70%,[6] but unfortunately evidence suggests that a surprisingly high number of patients receive inadequate pain relief following trauma, both in hospital (49%)[7,8] and in the prehospital setting (43%).[9]

There are also sex differences in pain reporting, especially in acute pain conditions, with women being more sensitive to pain than men.[10] This may be due to hormonal, psychosocial, and associated factors influencing pain pathways and the descending modulation systems. Estrogen influences the central and peripheral nervous system pain pathways and also affects endogenous opioid systems,[11] and dopaminergic[12] and serotonergic components[13] of the nociceptive processing. The evidence in this regard is not straightforward. In experimental models, systemically administered estradiol has been shown to decrease pain sensitivity, whereas centrally administered estradiol has been found to increase pain sensitivity. The situation is more complex in traumatic pain, since estradiol has varying influences on the inflammatory response, which itself contributes to nociception. Very high estrogen levels are known to decrease inflammation, but on the other hand very low levels may be proinflammatory.[14] The estrogen also has a similar variable influence on peripheral pain receptors (C fibers and $TRPV_1$ receptors).[15] There can be sex differences in the 5-HT_3 and NMDA systems also, which may further contribute to these differences in pain. Hence, at present, it can be concluded that although the exact direction is variable, the hormonal influences are thought to be contributory to the sex differences in pain sensitivity.

Pathophysiology of stress response to injury and pain

Pain is a protective response. This reflex response has an effect on multiple systems in the body. These include an exaggerated stress response, sleep deprivation, altered glucose homeostasis, increased sympathetic nervous system activation, and altered gastrointestinal, renal, and endocrine function. The stress response produced has effects on various organ systems additionally, such as cardiovascular, immune, endocrine, and respiratory systems. Thus, the stress response to injury is a complex hormonal and neurologic phenomenon. In a trauma patient, the consequences of this response are multifactorial. There is usually a rise in catecholamines, growth hormone, cortisol, renin, antidiuretic hormone (vasopressin), enkephalins, and endorphins, resulting in tachycardia, hypertension, decreased renal and splanchnic blood flow, and decreased glomerular filtration rate, among others. A predominant catabolic response results in alteration in glucose homeostasis, leading to hyperglycemia and decreased glucose turnover (insulin resistance). There is also increased endogenous glucose production (gluconeogenesis and glycogenolysis). It is difficult to separate the role of trauma in the stress response from that of pain, but providing analgesia has been documented to blunt the endocrine response to pain, that is, adrenocorticotrophic hormone, antidiuretic hormone, and enkephalins. The aim of pain management in trauma is to reduce the stress response as much as possible and to provide the patient with pain relief while maintaining cardiovascular stability and tissue homeostasis.

Pain management in trauma

Safe and balanced analgesia is one of the cornerstones of trauma management. Pain management in trauma can be complex and has to be tackled by using a multimodal approach.

Pain scoring is very important in the trauma setting. The key to effective pain management is thorough and appropriate assessment. Caregivers often underestimate the pain level experienced by patients, resulting in undertreatment of pain. Assessment of pain using the visual analog scale (VAS) or verbal reporting score can be very unreliable because it requires patient cooperation. Further, ratings are known to be different between patients, nurses, and doctors, and they are also found to be different in the same patient when recorded at admission and its subsequent recall. Although assessment of pain scores has been inadequate in many circumstances, a 2004 study showed that proper assessment of pain scores improves analgesia administration in acute trauma.[16] Though these assessment tools are routinely used, they may often be ineffective for caregivers to recognize discomfort and pain. Patients might be intubated, paralyzed, and/or unable to communicate, adding a level of complexity to pain management.

Kelly has shown that a nurse-managed intravenous (IV) narcotic policy induces a remarkable improvement in pain management in the emergency department.[17] Usage of pharmacologic and nonpharmacologic interventions has proven to be effective in various stages of pain management in trauma. The key is to treat the pain as early and as adequately as possible to avoid the formation of a chronic pain state and development of posttraumatic stress disorder.

The American Geriatric Society has published guidelines for the management of pain in older persons. They reiterate the importance of subjective reports: "The most accurate and reliable evidence of the existence of pain and its intensity is the patient's report."[18] Elderly patients, like other adults, require aggressive pain assessment and management (see Chapter 36).

In children, additional factors may modify assessment of pain, a major factor being psychologic response to acute trauma and repeated interventions (see Chapter 34). Trauma often results in separation of children from parents, accentuating the difficulty in evaluating and treating pain.

Many trauma victims will be precluded from any oral intake in anticipation of potential surgery, thus ruling out any oral medications. Parenteral access may be difficult in a vasoconstricted patient. By far the most common reason for inadequate management of pain is the fear of masking signs and symptoms of organ injury and altering circulatory stability.

Pharmacologic measures: analgesic drugs

Table 15.1 summarizes the characteristics of a range of analgesic drugs used for the management of acute pain in trauma.

Acetaminophen (paracetamol)

Acetaminophen (also known as paracetamol) was first synthesized by Morse in 1878 and first used clinically by von Mering in 1887. Acetaminophen became popular following the concerns of nephrotoxicity of phenacetin, its metabolic predecessor. Acetaminophen is the most commonly prescribed drug for acute pain.[19] Despite its long use and popularity, acetaminophen lacks a clear mechanism of action. From the animal models, the site of action of acetaminophen seems to be the central nervous system (CNS), and hence it is devoid of any anti-inflammatory action.

Flower and Vane showed that acetaminophen inhibited cyclooxygenase (COX) activity in dog brain.[20] Though two isoenzymes of COX are known, neither isoenzyme is sensitive to acetaminophen at therapeutic concentrations. Based on canine studies, a COX-3 inhibition was proposed,[21] but this has been disproved in humans.[22] The most likely mechanism suggested is that acetaminophen may block activity of COX-2 by reducing the active oxidized form of enzyme to an inactive form.[23] A third mechanism has also been proposed. Experimental data suggest that acetaminophen antinociception involves CNS opioid networks.[24] This is associated with a decrease of dynorphin levels in the frontal cortex that is

Table 15.1 Pharmacologic modalities for acute pain management in trauma

Type of drug	Mechanism of action	Routes	Drugs	Specific advantages	Disadvantages
Opioids	Action on opioid receptors (μ, κ, δ) Agonist Antagonist Partial agonist Mixed agonist/antagonist	PO, SC, IV, IM, IT, IA, buccal, inhaled, nasal, rectal, transmucosal, transdermal, locally into wound	Morphine Meperidine Codeine Fentanyl Hydromorphone Oxycodone Methadone Pentazocine Buprenorphine	Multiple routes Ease of administration Profound analgesia	Depends on route Respiratory depression Ileus Itching Hypotension Dependence/withdrawal
Acetaminophen (paracetamol)	Lacks clear mechanism COX inhibition in CNS+ endothelial cells COX-3 inhibition activates CB_1 cannabinoid receptor	PO, rectal, suppository, liquid suspension, IV*, IM	Marketed as generic or as Panadol, Tylenol, Anacin-3, Tempra, Datril, and others	Multiple routes Relatively safe profile Ease of administration May be formulated with opioids (oxycodone, hydrocodone) or propoxyphene (Darvocet) Antipyretic	Ceiling effect Hepatotoxicity at high doses
Nonsteroidal anti-inflammatory drugs (NSAIDs)	COX inhibition LOX/COX inhibition	PO, IA, IV, IM, IA, transdermal, intranasal, rectal	Ketorolac Diclofenac Ibuprofen Acetaminophen Coxibs	Powerful first-line analgesics Prevent central sensitization Preemptive analgesia Opioid-sparing	↓ Bone fusion, healing Gastric ulceration Renal, platelet dysfunction
Phencyclidine derivatives	NMDA receptor inhibition	IV, IT, IM, rectal	Ketamine	Amnesia Intense analgesia Hemodynamic stability	Secretions PONV Agitation ↑ ICP/IOP Hallucinations
Mixed	Weak μ agonist Inhibition of 5-HT and norepinephrine reuptake 5-HT release	PO, IV*, IA*, epidural*	Tramadol	Low abuse potential	Interaction with anticoagulants/antiepileptics
Local anesthetics	Block of neuronal sodium channel	IT, epidural, PNB, IV, S/C, IA, topical	Lidocaine Bupivacaine Ropivacaine Prilocaine	Short/long acting	Systemic toxicity Methemoglobinemia
Tricyclic antidepressants	Inhibition of neuronal reuptake of serotonin, norepinephrine, histamine, NMDA, and cholinergic receptors,	PO	Imiprimine Doxepin Desipramine Amitriptyline Nortriptyline	Neuropathic pain Opioid-sparing Control of anxiety/stress Antidepressant	Delayed onset of action Ileus Agitation Hypertension Arrhythmia
Anticonvulsants	Hyperpolarization ↓ Neuronal firing Release of substance P, norepinephrine, glutamate	PO	Gabapentin Pregabalin	Neuropathic pain Opioid-sparing Preemptive analgesia Synergy with COX-2	Sedation Dizziness Confusion Ataxia

Table 15.1 (cont.)

Type of drug	Mechanism of action	Routes	Drugs	Specific advantages	Disadvantages
a_2 Agonists	↑ Aactivation of inhibitory pathways ↓ Release of substance P	PO, IV*, IT*, IM*, transdermal	Clonidine Dexmedetomidine	Synergy with opioids Sedation	Hypotension Bradycardia Hyperglycemia
Benzodiazepines	↑ GABA receptor activity ↑ Chloride ion conduction Inhibition of action potential	PO, IV, IM, IT, rectal, buccal, nasal, inhaled	Diazepam Midazolam Lorezepam	Opioid-sparing Sedation Anxiolysis Multiple routes	Respiratory depression
Entonox	Unclear	Inhaled	50:50 mixture of N_2O and O_2	Conscious sedation Anxiolysis Quick-acting	Regurgitation Nausea Excitability Special equipment Closed head injury Pneumothorax

COX, cyclooxygenase; GABA, γ-aminobutyric acid; 5-HT, 5-hydroxytryptamine; IA, intraarticular; ICP, intracranial pressure; IM, intramuscular; IOP, intraocular pressure; IT, intrathecal; IV, intravenous; LOX, lipooxygenase; N_2O, nitrous oxide; NMDA, N-methyl-D-aspartate; NSAIDs, nonsteroidal anti-inflammatory drugs; O_2, oxygen; PNB, peripheral nerve block; PO, oral; PONV, postoperative nausea and vomiting; SC, subcutaneous.
* Not available in all countries.

prevented by κ-receptor antagonists,[25] and that the analgesic activity of acetaminophen may partially depend on dynorphin release.[26] More recently it has been discovered that acetaminophen undergoes a two-step transformation in the CNS to produce a compound known as AM404 (N-arachidonoylaminophenol), which inhibits the reuptake of anandamide[27] with subsequent stimulation of cannabinoid 1 (CB_1) receptors.[28] Although acetaminophen is thought to improve cannabinoid/vanilloid tone in the brain and in dorsal root ganglia, animal models suggest that AM404 may be important for the prevention of chronic pain[29] and less effective for acute visceral pain.[30] The endocannabinoids are metabolized to arachidonic acid mainly by the enzyme fatty acid amide hydrolase and monoacylglycerol lipase and secondarily by COX-2, lipooxygenase, and CYP isoforms. Acetaminophen and NSAIDs are thought to act by decreasing endocannabinoid metabolism through COX inhibition. Recent evidence points to the interaction of acetaminophen (or its active metabolite in the CNS, AM404) with multiple neurotransmitter systems including the serotonergic system, opioidergic (μ and κ receptors), noradrenergic, cholinergic, and nitric acid (NO)-synthase systems, and suggests that the final common pathway is the modulation of pain at the spinal and supraspinal levels.[31] Advantages of acetaminophen include the antipyretic action seen with NSAIDs without their gastrointestinal, renal, or antiplatelet side effects.

The main advantage of acetaminophen is its relatively safe profile compared with the anti-inflammatory drugs. Because of its nonacidic chemistry and lower affinity with plasma proteins, it has minimal unwanted effects and does not accumulate in the gastrointestinal, renal, and hematopoietic systems in therapeutic doses. It can be administered in enteral and, recently, in parenteral forms. The parenteral form is a prodrug of acetaminophen. Because of its profile, it can be used in pediatric and adult populations without much concern, although dosing needs to be adjusted according to weight to have reliable efficacy. In all, it is a very useful adjuvant in acute pain management.

Acetaminophen has been shown to be effective in the treatment of moderate pain associated with minor surgical procedures. A meta-analysis of single-dose oral acetaminophen showed effectiveness for moderate to severe acute postoperative pain,[32] but in another meta-analysis of single intravenous dose, effective analgesia was seen for around 4 hours in only 37%.[33] Acetaminophen must be considered as a safe alternative to NSAIDs for the relief of mild to moderate pain in elderly patients, and in patients with kidney disease, hypertension, or congestive heart failure.

Intravenous administration is the route of choice when oral administration is not possible or when rapid analgesia is required after surgery. IV preparations (propacetamol and acetaminophen) are available in many countries now. Both acetaminophen and propacetamol, when given in a 15-minute infusion, are fast-acting analgesic agents (faster median time to reach T_{max} and C_{max}) and are more effective in terms of onset of analgesia than oral preparations.[34] The C_{max} threshold for potential hepatotoxicity is above 150 mg/L, which is not seen with IV infusion of 15 minutes' duration. 2 g of IV propacetamol is hydrolyzed by plasma esterases within 7 minutes of administration to 1 g of acetaminophen.[35] The recommended dose of IV acetaminophen injection in adults is 1 g (7.5 mg/kg q 4–6 h for weight < 10 kg, and 15 mg/kg for weight < 10 kg q 4–6 h), though pharmacokinetic and pharmacodynamic findings suggest that better analgesia could be obtained with a 2 g starting dose.[36] The IV formulations (1 g/100 mL) are not recommended for children age < 2 years, and a weight-based strategy should be employed for age 2–12 years.[37] Patients who weigh < 50 kg should not receive the entire 100 mL vial of IV acetaminophen, and the contents of this single-use vial should be administered within 6 hours of opening it.[38]

Acetaminophen is important as an adjuvant to opioid analgesia, as it decreases total opioid consumption in surgical and trauma intensive care. In a meta-analysis of acetaminophen and propacetamol for postoperative analgesia, their overall opioid-sparing property was around 30% at 4 hours and 16% over 6 hours, compared with placebo. [39] The meta-analysis also noted that acetaminophen did not decrease opioid related adverse effects. It is worth remembering that acetaminophen has a ceiling effect at the oral dose of 1 g/dose[40] and possibly at an IV dose of 15 mg/kg,[41] as further dose increases do not produce increases in analgesic activity but may only risk hepatotoxicity.[42] Patients should avoid taking more than the recommended dose (4 g/day in adults or 90 mg/kg/day for infants and older children).

Acetaminophen has the disadvantage of requiring four doses per day to maintain therapeutic serum levels. The recent introduction of sustained-release (SR) acetaminophen has reduced this requirement to three doses per day.[43] The other disadvantages of IV acetaminophen, apart from the need for frequent dosing, include the requirement of a 100 mL infusion for each dose, which may be difficult in the volume-restricted, the need for a 15-minute infusion, the need to reconstitute propacetamol from the powdered form, and pain on injection, which is seen in up to 23% of patients.[37]

Rectal suppositories of acetaminophen are available. However, there is wide variation in bioavailability following rectal administration. Studies have demonstrated the need for higher loading doses (40 mg/kg) to achieve target plasma concentrations of 10 mg/L after rectal administration. Rectal administration of drugs is contraindicated in neutropenic patients (risk of sepsis) and in those with ulcerative or acute inflammatory conditions of the rectum or anus. Despite erratic bioavailability, the rectal route is particularly attractive for use in children, who may be uncooperative, have poor venous access, have delayed/erratic gastric emptying, or can take nothing by mouth (NPO) following trauma.

Cormack et al. have shown that a single rectal dose of acetaminophen (40 mg/kg) in children with liver disease is probably a safe and satisfactory analgesic alternative.[44] Despite a low incidence of adverse effects, acetaminophen has potential for hepatotoxicity and is thought to be responsible for at least 42% of acute liver failure cases at tertiary care centers and one-third of the deaths in the United States.[45] Under normal circumstances, approximately 90% of the drug is metabolized in the liver through a conjugation with glucuronides and sulfates and about 5% is metabolized by cytochrome P450 2E1 (CYP2E1) isozymes to N-acetyl-p-benzo-quinone imine (NAPQI), which is the hepatotoxic metabolite and requires glutathione for detoxification. If an excessive dose of acetaminophen is administered, the primary metabolic pathway is saturated, resulting in increased production of the toxic metabolite and further hepatotoxicity. Acute liver failure can develop within 24–36 hours after ingestion of excessive amounts of the drug (in excess of 5 g/24 h),[46] but this can be prevented if the glutathione stores are replenished by the administration of the antidote N-acetylcysteine (NAC) within the same period. With an increase in the prescription and over-the-counter (OTC) medication sales of acetaminophen, alone and in combination with various other drugs, there has been an increase in the incidence of liver damage. Hence, in June 2009, the US Food and Drug Administration (FDA) public advisory committee focused to address these problems by limiting the OTC content of acetaminophen, to standardize the range of OTC liquid concentrations, and to eliminate prescription combinations or enforce a boxed warning on the labels of these products.[47] We not only should use acetaminophen cautiously in patients with altered liver function, but also need to reduce the dose in high-risk populations such as those fasting or malnourished; concurrently abusing alcohol; having a genetic predisposition; being older than 40 years; and concomitantly using CYP inducers such as phenytoin, isoniazid, and some antiretrovirals including ritonavir and zidovudine.[48,49]

Nitroparacetamol (nitroacetaminophen) is a new nitric oxide-releasing version of acetaminophen with analgesic and anti-inflammatory properties, though the exact molecular mechanism of these actions is not clear.[50] Animal models suggest reduced liver damage in overdose situations, and nitroparacetamol may be a safer alternative to acetaminophen. It is also known to suppress synthesis of several proinflammatory cytokines, and it may in fact be a useful therapy in acetaminophen-induced liver damage.[51]

A summary of the current role of acetaminophen when given alone is that it is a drug efficacious for mild pain, but that it may provide inadequate analgesia in moderate to severe pain. Hence the FDA approval of its use for the management of mild to moderate pain, management of moderate to severe pain with adjunctive opioid analgesics, as a part of multimodal pain management, and for the reduction of fever. When combined with opioids it reduces opioid requirement, but this reduction does not appear sufficient to reduce opioid-induced adverse effects. Further, based on the clinical and economic evidence currently available, intravenous acetaminophen is best considered in the limited number of patients who cannot receive drugs orally or rectally and who cannot tolerate other parenteral nonopioid analgesic or antipyretic agents, rather than as a substitute for oral or rectal preparations.[52]

Nonsteroidal anti-inflammatory drugs (NSAIDs)

The history of NSAIDs dates back to the times of Hippocrates (400 BC), when the use of willow bark extract for treating fever and inflammation was documented. The active ingredient of

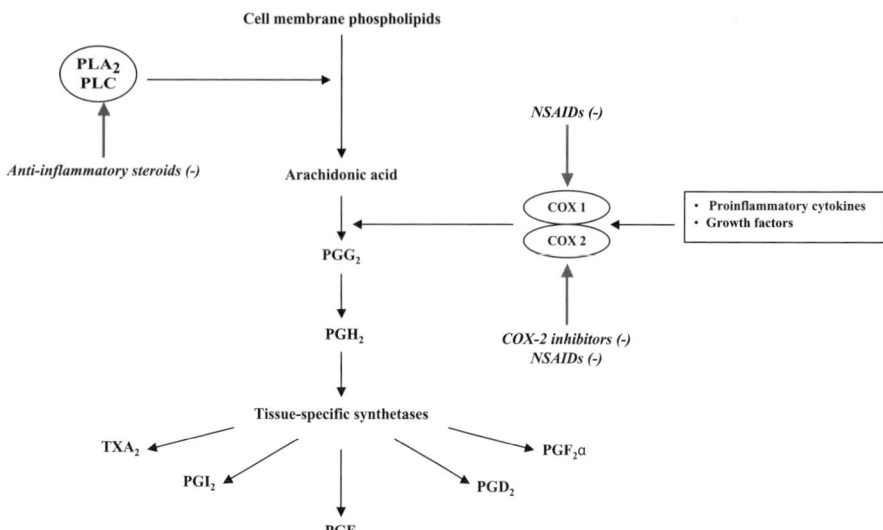

Figure 15.1 The action of nonsteroidal anti-inflammatory drugs (NSAIDs). COX, cyclooxygenase; PLA$_2$, phospholipase A$_2$; PG, prostaglandin; TXA$_2$, thromboxane A$_2$.

the willow bark (salicin) was identified in the seventeenth century, and the mass production of salicylic acid began in 1860 by the Kolbe Company in Germany. This was followed by the introduction of a more palatable form of salicylic acid, acetylsalicyclic acid (aspirin) by Bayer in 1899, which was followed in turn by the discovery of other compounds.[53] Today an estimated 70 million prescriptions for NSAIDs are written annually, accounting for an annual turnover of $6.8 billion worldwide.

John Vane discovered the mechanism of action of aspirin and other NSAIDs.[54] Nonselective NSAIDs are powerful inhibitors of COX and a first-line treatment for many painful conditions. They act by inhibiting prostaglandin synthesis, predominantly at peripheral sites but also in the CNS (Fig. 15.1). There are several categories of COX enzymes. Some are involved in physiologic functions of the body while others are expressed on initiation of injury. Drugs that inhibit this class of enzymes play an important role in pain management. They are effective in moderate to severe pain. The main disadvantage of COX inhibitors is the effect they have on gastrointestinal (GI), renal, and platelet function due to their acidic nature and their high binding to plasma proteins. They also inhibit wound healing and bone fusion, thereby limiting their use. NSAIDs are relatively contraindicated in pregnant women, because of concerns about fetal effects (such as premature closure of the ductus arteriosus).

COX-2-selective inhibitors (coxibs) offer the peripheral pain-relieving benefits of nonselective NSAIDs but with fewer adverse GI effects.[55] It has been suggested that they may ameliorate postoperative pain by preventing the development of central sensitization. In addition to their selectivity for the COX-2 isoenzyme overall, unique differences among the coxibs, such as plasma half-life, may impart certain clinical advantages.[56]

Samad and colleagues have demonstrated significant upregulation of COX-2 in CNS parenchyma in response to acute peripheral inflammatory pain.[57] Increased synthesis of prostaglandins is known to increase neuronal excitability and may play a role in CNS remodeling.

Rofecoxib, lumiracoxib, and celecoxib are all COX-2 selective inhibitors that have been investigated. In humans, plasma rofecoxib enters the cerebrospinal fluid (CSF) with a CSF/plasma concentration ratio of approximately 15%.[58] This finding suggests that rofecoxib is able to penetrate and possibly reduce CNS responses to locally synthesized prostaglandin E$_2$ (PGE$_2$). Unfortunately, this drug was withdrawn from the market because of concerns of increased cardiovascular risk due to selective COX-2 inhibition that altered the balance between thromboxane A$_2$ (TxA$_2$) and prostacyclin (PGI$_2$) thereby increasing the possibility of a thrombotic event.[59,60] The previously available drug lumiracoxib (Prexige, Novartis Pharmaceuticals) has also been withdrawn from the market because of concerns over liver toxicity. Currently, only celecoxib (Celebrex) is available in North America, with a black box warning indicating a risk of adverse cardiovascular events. Although the COX-2 inhibitors decrease GI-related adverse events, with the recent reduced costs of proton-pump inhibitors, nonspecific COX inhibitors can be used comparably.[61] The use of selective COX-2 inhibitors does not reduce the renal adverse effects seen with long-term use, since both COX-1 and COX-2 are constitutively expressed in various parts of the nephrons that are crucial to the vascular distribution and functioning of the nephron.[62]

Coxibs may be synergistic with acetaminophen in providing pain relief. The effects of rofecoxib and celecoxib alone and in combination with acetaminophen were compared, and it was found that rofecoxib and celecoxib in combination with acetaminophen produced a significant reduction in fentanyl use and a significant improvement in patient satisfaction.[55]

Reduction of algesic flare

Partly because of the specific action of COX-2 on PGE_2, COX-2-selective inhibitors can be used immediately prior to surgery, as well as postoperatively, thereby preventing algesic flare and resulting peripheral and central sensitization.[63] Ideally, these drugs have been documented to provide better analgesia when given preemptively. Unfortunately, in the trauma situation one may not be able to derive benefit from their preemptive effects.

Although they provide excellent adjuvant analgesia with multimodal technique, in the trauma situation, with its associated stress, one has to keep in mind the combined effect of stress and NSAIDs on gastric mucosa. Trauma is often associated with hemodynamic disturbances and/or sepsis, which may play a causal role in acute kidney injury as well as stress ulcers. NSAIDs have to be administered taking these factors into consideration. Higher rates of myocardial infarction with prolonged NSAID or COX-2 use have been suggested in some studies, although data are presently conflicting.[64]

In their analysis of 114 randomized trials, Zhang et al. showed that rofecoxib increased the risk of renal events and arrhythmia, though the exact mechanisms remain uncertain.[65]

Because prostaglandins and leukotrienes are critical in inflammation, pharmaceutical companies are developing dual cyclooxygenase and 5-lipoxygenase (LOX) enzyme inhibitors. Experimental data with licofelone (a dual LOX/COX inhibitor) indicate that it shares the antipyretic, analgesic, anti-inflammatory, and antiplatelet activities of conventional NSAIDs and also exhibits antiallergic properties. In animal studies, it appears to induce less gastrointestinal damage. The safety of this drug remains to be proved in humans.[66] It has been shown to provide analgesic efficacy similar to celecoxib but with fewer GI side effects.[55]

Protective strategies include the co-prescription of gastroprotective drugs such as misoprostol or a proton-pump inhibitor with NSAIDs. Addition of a proton-pump inhibitor to celecoxib confers extra protection for patients aged 75 years or older.[67] Prophylaxis with proton-pump inhibitors has been recommended in patients receiving long-term treatment with COX-2 inhibitors and who are at high ulcer-bleeding risk.[68] Normal doses of H_2 antagonists do not effectively prevent NSAID-induced gastric ulceration, and in fact may mask warning symptoms.[69]

Ketorolac is available for parenteral use and provides opioid-sparing effects.[70] It has an advantage in patients for whom the oral route is not available/feasible. Use of parenteral ketorolac should be restricted to no more than 5 days in adults with severe postsurgical pain.[71] A variety of delivery systems have been tried in experimental set-ups for the delivery of NSAIDs apart from the oral, intramuscular, and intravenous formulations. These were developed due to the shorter therapeutic half-life of the drugs given by the traditional routes (ranging from 5.5 hours to 8 hours) necessitating repeated doses and also increasing the chances of adverse events such as gastrointestinal upset and bleeding. Although a variety of sustained drug delivery systems, including transoral, nasal, transdermal, and parenteral depot formulations, have been in development over the past three decades for NSAIDs, most of them have never been evaluated in the clinical setting and have been confined to either in-vivo or in-vitro lab settings. The expert opinion on ketorolac summarises the attempts at the development of these drug formulations.[72] In one study, a diclofenac patch was found to be effective and safe for the treatment of blunt impact injuries.[73]

There have been extensive efforts to improve the safety of NSAIDs while maintaining or improving their efficacy, but this has met with limited clinical success, and no newer NSAIDs have been introduced to the market in almost a decade. The novel molecules evaluated can be summarized as those intended to make the NSAIDs safer or to make them more efficacious. The former group include LOX/COX inhibitors, nitric oxide donors, and H_2S donors, all of which were designed to decrease gastrointestinal adverse events. The latter group include the nanoformulated NSAIDs, which are designed to increase the potency and efficacy of NSAIDs. Many of the attempts to make NSAIDS safer have resulted in a drug with lesser clinical efficacy without any additional safety benefit over conventional NSAIDs – best exemplified by the NO-NSAID (nitric oxide donor NSAID) naproxcinod, which resulted in more orthostatic hypotension and inferior analgesia without reducing NSAID-related adverse events compared to naproxen.[74] Thus, a rational drug design does not always translate to the necessary clinical benefit, and this may be the reason for the failure of many of the tested novel NSAIDs such as flavocoxid (LOX/COX inhibitor), naproxcinod (NO/COX inhibitor), cimicoxib (NO/COX-2 inhibitor), and prostaglandin synthase inhibitors (mPGES-1 inhibitors) to make it to clinical practice. Nanoformulated NSAIDs with greater potency and faster peak plasma concentration are currently in preclinical development, and their final place in the NSAID armamentarium will be determined in the coming years.

Role of coxibs in bone and wound healing

Concerns about the use of coxibs and their effects on bone and wound healing have been raised. Most of these concerns were based on studies on nonselective NSAIDs in animal models.[75] A variety of experimental models of bone, ligament, and tendon repair have assessed the effects for selective and nonselective COX inhibitors in animals with variable intra- and interspecies outcomes, which limits extrapolation of animal data to humans.[76] It has been demonstrated in rat models that NSAIDs (both traditional and COX-2-specific) following rotator cuff repair significantly inhibit bone-to-tendon healing.[77] However, these results need to be verified in larger animal as well as human models before drawing firm conclusions. In humans, two large-scale trials have shown that continuous use of acetaminophen and NSAIDs but not aspirin or opioids leads to increased fracture rates.[78,79] The exact mechanism is not known and none of the above drugs affected bone mineral density in any trials. The probable mechanism is thought to involve the endocannabinoid stimulation by NSAIDs and acet-aminophen, which indirectly controls the sympathetic nervous system and hence the bone metabolism, but definitive evidence for causation is lacking.[80–82]

Opioids

Opioids have been the cornerstone of acute pain management for centuries. They are the first line of drugs used for analgesia in a trauma situation.

Their potent analgesic effects are due to action on the opioid receptors. Opioid receptors are ubiquitous. There is increased expression at the peripheral site after injury.[83] They are present in different locations in the CNS, vas deferens, spinal cord, gastrointestinal tract, lungs, and synovium. There are central and peripheral opioid receptors, although the effects of peripheral receptors are still not entirely clear. The opioids are thought to act in a variety of ways ranging from membrane hyperpolarization to voltage-gated ion channels to G-protein-mediated suppression of adenylyl cyclase. These receptors are classfied as mu (μ), kappa (κ), delta (δ), and epsilon (ϵ) depending on the agonists associated with the receptors. The most common receptors are μ and κ. These receptors are also associated with some of the undesirable side effects such as nausea, vomiting, sedation, and respiratory depression. Opioids have also been classified as pure, partial agonists, and partial antagonists, depending on the affinity to these receptors, resulting in differing side-effect profiles.

In general, opioids are thought to reduce the affective response to nociception. They also alter the psychical response to pain. Patients may still feel some pain, but they report being comfortable.

Opioids significantly decrease pain scores, especially in thoracic injuries, though at the expense of a few significant side effects.[84] Carefully titrated systemic opioids continue to be the most commonly applied pain management treatment, either by fixed dosing or by patient-controlled analgesia (PCA) techniques.[85] Alternately, intravenous opioids can be titrated to the degree of pain by using a sliding scale of physiological parameters and a pain scale to prevent under-dosing or overdosing of medications, but this can be labor-intensive. Neuraxial opioids, especially epidural opioids, offer a relatively safe method of providing good analgesia, as shown in studies of postoperative pain management of thoracic injuries.[86] Neuraxial opioids provide superb analgesia at a much smaller dose. Thus, opioids remain the mainstay of analgesia in trauma. However, there have been changes in how they are currently utilized, prescribed, and administered.

Opioids can be administered via several routes, making them versatile in clinical application. The traditional well-known routes of administration include oral, subcutaneous, intramuscular, intravenous, intrathecal, and epidural, while nasal,[87] transmucosal,[88] buccal,[89] transdermal,[90] inhaled,[91] intraarticular,[92] and local injection into the wound[93] are alternative routes that have been mostly investigated and tested in animal models, with only transdermal preparations being commercially available currently. The transmucosal route has the advantage of avoiding first-pass metabolism, thus resulting in a quicker onset. Slow-release preparations are particularly useful in managing pain for an extended period following trauma.

Fulda *et al.* studied nebulized morphine and found that it could be used safely and effectively to control posttraumatic thoracic pain, and that it provided equivalent pain relief with less sedative effect when compared with intravenous morphine.[94] The inhalational route for opioids, which offers the attraction of first-pass metabolism of the drug and a large lung surface area for rapid absorption, has been in investigation for some time now.[91] Subsequent clinical evaluation of the products showed unreliable or low bio-availability compared to the intravenous route.[95,96] However, a recent study showed similar pharmacokinetics of inhaled fentanyl (Staccato fentanyl) to that of the intravenous formulation.[97]

A patient-controlled transdermal system (IONSYS, Ortho-McNeil Pharmaceutical, Inc., Raritan, NJ) with fentanyl uses an imperceptible low-intensity direct current to transfer fenta-nyl on demand across the skin into the systemic circulation (Fig. 15.2). It can be applied to the patient's upper arm/chest and is designed to manage moderate to severe pain requiring opioid analgesia.[98] While fentanyl patches are effective for long-term pain relief, their role in acute management is limited because it takes 24 hours to achieve the full effect. Controlled transdermal delivery patches of fentanyl[99] and buprenorphine have been associated with a lower incidence of constipation and, in the case of transdermal buprenorphine, CNS side effects as compared with systemic opioids.[100]

Wound infiltration with morphine can reduce the inci-dence of both immediate and chronic pain following surgery. Peripheral morphine administration can inhibit the release of proinflammatory neuropeptides in peripheral tissues. Three opioid receptors (μ, δ, κ) have been demonstrated in peripheral nerve endings and have been shown to be responsible for mediating peripheral antinociception.[101,102] Periarticular opioid infiltration alone[103] or as part of a multimodal drug injection regime[104] has been shown to provide significant analgesia, reduce the requirements for PCA, and improve patient satifaction.

As PCA requires dedicated IV access, some of the nontra-ditional routes may be particularly useful, especially in the pediatric population.

Undesirable side effects of opioids include sedation, altered sensorium, and cognitive dysfunction, which may make moni-toring of the CNS difficult. Respiratory depression and result-ant hypoxia may accentuate the hypoxia associated with diffuse lung injury. Nausea and vomiting are side effects that most patients dislike. The GI side effects can be decreased with the use of newer peripheral opioid antagonists such as alvimo-pan or methylnaltrexone without decreasing the central anal-gesic efficacy of the opioids.[105]

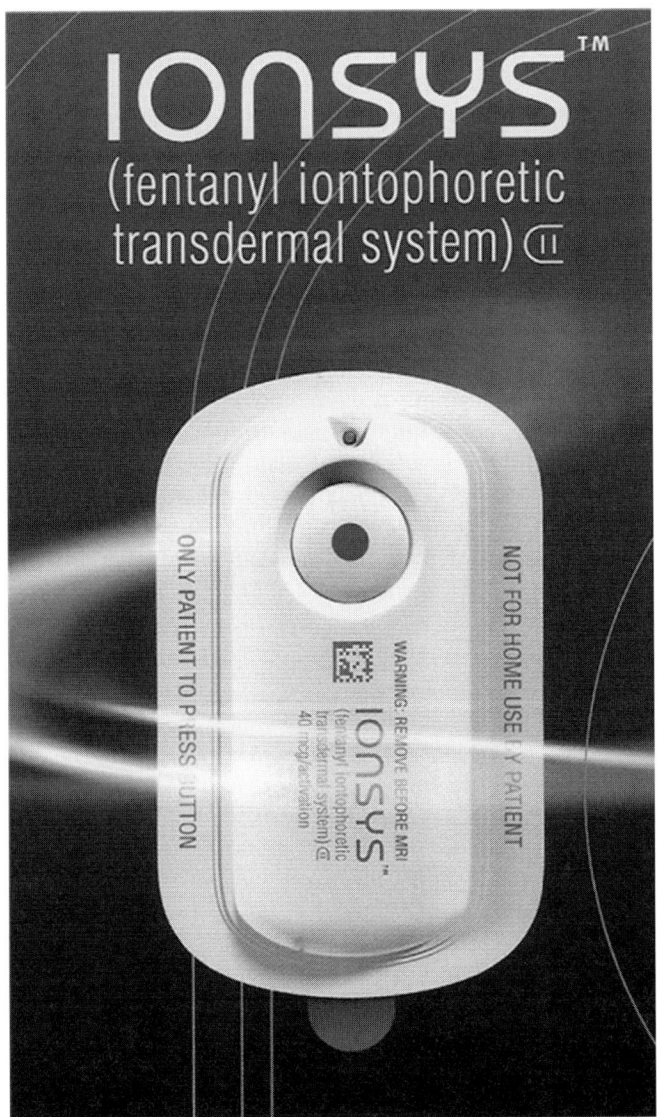

Figure 15.2 Patient-controlled transdermal system: IONSYS (Ortho-McNeil Pharmaceutical, Inc., Raritan, NJ). The system transfers fentanyl on demand across the skin into the systemic circulation. With permission from Ortho-McNeil.

Opioids have been implicated in acute colonic pseudo-obstruction or Ogilivie's syndrome,[106] which is a potentially fatal condition characterized by clinical and radiographic appearance of colonic obstruction in the absence of an anatomically obstructing lesion. Opioid drugs can cause increased frequency of nonpropulsive phasic contractions, ablate propulsive migration contractions, and promote water reabsorption, thus increasing the duration of postoperative ileus.[107] This, combined with prior vascular insufficiency, may contribute to ischemia and colonic distension, precipitating Ogilivie's syndrome. Reduction of predisposing factors, good bowel care, early oral diet, early mobilization, good hydration, and opioid rotation are very important in preventing acute colonic pseudo-obstruction.[108] Early detection and aggressive treatment are essential.

Available evidence suggests that there is a significant and underappreciated risk of serious injury from PCA and neuraxial opioids in the postoperative period. While the risk is notably higher in the patient population at risk, there is still a low but unpredictable incidence of life-threatening opioid-induced respiratory depression in young and healthy patients. Despite concerns about costs, the Anesthesia Patient Safely Foundation advocates the routine use of continuous postoperative respiratory monitoring (pulse oximetry and continuous measurement of respiratory rate) in at-risk patients receiving PCA or neuraxial opioids.[109]

The effects of opioids on the immune system are complex. In brief, both acute and chronic opioid treatment affects innate and adaptive immunity[110] These effects will have immense therapeutic consequences. Morphine has been shown to mediate these effects by acting directly both on receptors present on the immune cells and on centrally mediated pathways. There seems to be general agreement that opioid treatment compromises host defense.

The disease of addiction affects approximately 10% of the general population, though its prevalence may be higher in certain subpopulations.[111] Both active and recovering addiction may complicate the use of medications, such as opioids, which are important in the management of pain. There is a persistent misunderstanding among healthcare providers, regulators, and the general population regarding the nature and manifestations of addiction, which may result in undertreatment of pain. This is further complicated by a true addiction potential with extended use.

Traditionally, oral long-acting opioids have been used for chronic pain. In a prospective analysis, Illgen *et al.* showed that oral administration of long-acting opioids may provide an opioid-sparing effect.[112] It has been postulated that oral long-acting opioids provide a better route to control moderate to severe acute pain by providing steady levels of medication and convenience, avoiding peaks and troughs and gaps in pain control during sleep.

Off-label nebulization of opioids has been used as an alternative method of treatment for minor procedures in patients who would be at risk of systemic adverse effects.[113] However, more research is needed in evaluating this route of administration.

The future of opioid pharmacology will target decreasing opioid-related side effects and opioid tolerance or opioid-induced hyperalgesia. Opioid-induced glial cell activation via nonstereoselective binding to toll-like receptor 4 (TLR4) in the brain is thought to result in undesired effects such as tolerance, withdrawal, respiratory depression, and hyperalgesia, and hence agents such as ibudilast (AV-411), which has TLR4-like activity and suppresses glial cell activity, are in development.[114]

Tramadol

Tramadol is an unusual agent whose analgesic activity is mediated through two different mechanisms. When first used clinically, it was thought to be a centrally acting opioid of the aminocyclohexanol group.[115] While the side-effect profile of tramadol resembled that of a μ-receptor agonist, the binding affinity for the receptor was weak and the analgesic effect was only partially reversed by naloxone. Later on, the multimodal nature of the drug was revealed, and this was attributed to the inhibition of serotonin (5-hydroxytryptamine) and norepinephrine uptake, coupled with presynaptic stimulation of serotonin release.

Tramadol apparently lacks abuse potential, although the possibility of dependence with long-term use cannot be entirely excluded. It has only one pharmacologically active metabolite (of 11 identified). Patients with genetic cytochrome P450 3A4 (CYP3A4) enzyme deficiency may show a reduced response to the drug. Though the data available are conflicting, it may have interaction with oral anticoagulants and antiepileptics and should be avoided in epileptic patients.[116]

Tramadol exerts anti-inflammatory action without directly affecting the enzymes in the generation of arachidonic acid metabolites. The pharmacodynamic profile of tramadol is therefore completely different from that of NSAIDs, including COX-2 inhibitors.

Intraarticular tramadol has been used to provide effective and reliable pain control following arthroscopic knee surgery.[117]

As an additive for intravenous regional anesthesia, tramadol has a limited role. Though its addition may decrease the time to onset of sensory block, it does not decrease tourniquet pain or prolong postoperative analgesia.[118]

Tramadol appears to have local anesthetic properties similar to prilocaine[119] and lidocaine,[120] though the incidence of local adverse effects may preclude its use as a local anesthetic.

Intravenous tramadol 50–150 mg is equivalent in analgesic efficacy to morphine 5–15 mg. However, parenteral preparations of tramadol are not available in North America.

Epidural tramadol appears to be a comparable and safe alternative to epidural morphine in thoracic surgery patients,[121] though the duration of pain relief is shorter.

Tapentadol

Tapentadol, a centrally acting drug with dual mode of action, has been approved in the United States as an immediate-release formulation for the relief of moderate to severe acute pain in patients 18 years or older. It has μ-opioid receptor agonist and norepinephrine reuptake inhibitor activity and is supposed to have a lesser GI side-effect profile as compared to conventional opioids. The immediate-release formulation (50, 75, and 100 mg) is approved for use in acute pain, but data regarding its use in post-trauma patients is lacking. Its oral absorption is rapid, it has a $t_{1/2}$ of ~4 hours, and it is primarily excreted renally. Since the metabolism of tapentadol does not produce active metabolites, no dosing adjustment is necessary for patients with mild to moderate renal impairment or mild hepatic impairment. Its use in severe hepatic or renal impairment is not recommended presently because of lack of data in these patients, whereas in patients with moderate hepatic

impairment it can be instituted in 50 mg every 8 hours with an increase in the intervals between dosing.

In clinical trials, tapentadol IR (50–100 mg every 4–6 hours) provided an analgesic effect that was comparable to that of oxycodone IR (10 or 15 mg every 4–6 hours) in moderate to severe acute (post-orthopedic surgical or musculoskeletal) pain. It was also associated with significant reductions in the incidences of nausea, vomiting, and constipation compared with oxycodone IR therapy. The side-effect profile includes concerns of respiratory depression, especially in elderly or debilitated patients, and in those with known severe respiratory illness. Tapentadol should not be used concurrently with monoamine oxidase inhibitors or serotonin reuptake inhibitors because of the risk of hemodynamic lability and a risk of serotonin syndrome.[122] Nausea and gastrointestinal side effects (18–35%), although less than noted with oxycodone (35–63%), are the most common adverse effects associated with immediate-release tapentadol.[123] At higher doses of tapentadol (75–100 mg), rates of nausea are similar to those of oxycodone.[124] Tapentadol is an expensive medication in comparison to the currently prescribed opioids like oxycodone and hydromorphone.

Ketamine

Ketamine is a phencyclidine derivative. It is a noncompetitive inhibitor at *the* N-methyl-D-aspartate (NMDA) receptor. It is thought to have an agonistic action at opioid receptors and an antagonistic action at muscarinic receptors. Its uniqueness comes from producing a dissociative state causing amnesia and intense analgesia with preservation of vital brainstem functions and hemodynamic stability. Ketamine produces a clinical state of lack of response to pain or other noxious stimuli while maintaining stability of respiratory and cardiovascular functions. It provides profound amnesia and analgesia. It has been shown to reduce hyperalgesia caused by opioids when used perioperatively and also to decrease opioid requirements.[125] A 50:50 mixture of propofol and ketamine (ketofol) has been used to provide analgosedation for minor procedures in the emergency department following trauma.[126]

The drawbacks with ketamine are excessive secretions, agitation on recovery, its ability to raise intracranial and intraocular pressures, and hallucinations (thought to be lessened by concomitant administration of benzodiazepines). For these reasons, ketamine has to be used with caution in an acute trauma patient who may have a head injury. Despite this, it is a very useful drug for treating burn pain, for dressing changes, and for minor procedures such as wound debridement. This is particularly useful in the triage area in the field to extricate patients from a trauma site where securing an airway may be difficult or equipment is lacking. Ketamine has been shown to be an effective analgesic for trauma and burn patients, including in the prehospital setting.[127]

Low-dose ketamine infusions have been used as an opioid adjuvant with a loading dose of 0.25–0.5 mg/kg followed by a continuous infusion in the range of 50–500 μg/kg/h for post-operative analgesia and for the reduction of exogenous opioid-induced hyperalgesia,[128] and this can also be utilized for trauma patients. The use of ketamine has also been shown to decrease secondary hyperalgesia, and combining it with morphine has been found to prevent the wind-up phenomenon,[129] since NMDA pathways are primarily involved in opioid-induced hyperalgesia and opioid tolerance. It is imperative to rule out head injury, raised ICP or IOP, recent myocardial infarction, poorly controlled hypertension, or congestive cardiac failure prior to administering ketamine.

Local anesthetics

Local anesthetics act by producing a reversible blockade of the sodium channel in the nerve cell. This hyperpolarizes the nerve cell and prevents impulse transmission. There is a variety of short-acting, long-acting, and rapid-onset/offset local anesthetics available. The common routes of administration are peripheral and neuraxial (see Chapter 16).

Intravenous lidocaine has been found to have preventive effects on postoperative pain,[130] to reduce post-amputation pain[131] and visceral pain,[132] as well as to control complicated unrelieved acute post-surgical pain. Systemic administration of lidocaine has been used to relieve neuropathic pain[133] at and below the level of injury (centrally acting effect of sodium channel blockade).[134] The safety of intravenous lidocaine for analgesia is far from assured by small studies such as those currently available, and there is a possibility of accumulation of lidocaine in the blood during the period of infusion, even at low doses.[135] Intravenous lidocaine is appealing as a simple and inexpensive method to gain the same benefits as more invasive and costly techniques, but we currently lack large studies to define its safety and efficacy in trauma situation.

Local anesthetics are very useful in burn treatment, where topical application has proved effective for superficial burns.[136] Commonly used topical anesthetics require 30–60 minutes to provide effective anesthesia. In order to improve the permeation of local anesthetics across the skin, a variety of technologies have been evaluated in the experimental set-up in the past, including passing a small ionic current (direct current) across the skin to facilitate the passage of ionic local anesthetic through the skin (iontophoresis), magnetic current (magnetophoresis), ultrasound (sonophoresis), short high-voltage pulses to create aqueous pores in the skin (electroporation). Iontophoresis is probably the only one that made a brief appearance in clinical practice, in the form of the Needle Buster, Numby Stuff, and LidoSite devices, which are no longer available commercially. Clinical studies show better permeation of LA and good clinical effect within 2 minutes when a combination of technologies like sonophoresis and iontophoresis are used, compared to 10 minutes for iontophoresis alone.[137]

There are reports of local anesthetic toxicity, mainly in children, observed following topical application to mucous membranes.[138] Recently, liposomal bupivacaine, a novel multivesicular formulation, has been finding increasing application for managing postoperative pain, and it may soon find its utility in field trauma and in the hospital. It is designed for rapid absorption with peak plasma concentrations at 1 hour of administration followed by a prolonged release of around 96 hours. Hence it is designed for providing long-lasting analgesia following a single intraoperative administration into the surgical wound. The evidence so far in nonpregnant adult patients is that it provides analgesia of about 72 hours' duration after administration of ≤ 266 mg, with a reduction in opioid consumption.[139] The incidence of adverse events may increase if ≥ 266 mg has been used.[140]

Antidepressants

Tricyclic antidepressants (TCAs) have a long history of use in neuropathic pain conditions. They can reduce pain, alleviate depression, and facilitate sleep in patients with trauma injuries (see Chapter 17). Tricyclic antidepressants act by preventing the neuronal reuptake of serotonin and norepinephrine. They are thought to modulate the descending nociceptive pathways and thus alleviate the pain resulting from injury. The antidepressants have quite a different clinical pharmacologic profile when used in pain management, as opposed to endogenous depression. Randomized controlled trials provide strong evidence that TCAs can treat neuropathic pain, with their analgesic effect being independent of their antidepressant action.[141] They may provide an opioid-sparing effect and reduce opioid requirement. This could be very beneficial in the narcotic-dependent patient who has sustained trauma. Many patients with trauma go through tremendous psychologic stress and anxiety, which may accentuate pain perception. Preoperative anxiety has been documented to be a single factor associated with repeated bolus requests with PCA; thus it is imperative to control anxiety in trauma patients.

Amitriptyline can be used in low doses (10–25 mg initially). However, the onset of action takes a few days. Side effects like anticholinergic effects and sedation are mostly dose-dependent and can limit antidepressant use.

Antidepressants exhibit a number of pharmacologic mechanisms, including norepinephrine and serotonin modulation, direct and indirect effects on opioid receptors, inhibition of histamine, cholinergic, and NMDA receptors, and inhibition of ion-channel activity.[142] Although it is not entirely clear which mechanisms produce analgesia and to what extent, the available animal and clinical trials data indicate that antidepressants are effective in treating many types of pain. These drugs can be administered only orally and have limited application in acute trauma situations, while being very useful as an adjuvant in the management of post-trauma pain.

Some TCAs can result in prolonged QT interval,[143] arrhythmia,[144] paralytic ileus,[145] and Ogilvie's syndrome.[146] The serotonin–norepinephrine reuptake inhibitors are safer to use than TCAs and are a better option in patients with cardiac disease.[147] They are considered moderately effective for pain of neuropathic origin. However, their side effects (agitation, gastrointestinal disturbances, and hypertension) have to be kept in mind.

Anticonvulsants

Various anticonvulsants have been tried in treating pain, especially neuropathic pain. Anticonvulsants act by causing hyperpolarization and decreasing spontaneous neuronal firing in the CNS. Until recently, anticonvulsants were not thought to be useful in acute conditions. However, similar to nerve injury, tissue injury is known to produce neuroplastic changes, leading to spinal sensitization and the expression of stimulus-evoked hyperalgesia and allodynia. Pharmacologic effects of anticonvulsant drugs that may be important in the modulation of these neural changes include suppression of sodium-channel, calcium-channel, and glutamate receptor activity at peripheral, spinal, and supraspinal sites. Although several anticonvulsant drugs potentiate the inhibitory neurotransmitter GABA, which plays a role in pain modulation,[148] analgesic effects of GABAergic anticonvulsants such as benzodiazepines and barbiturates are not reliably observed. The anticonvulsant gabapentin is a structural analog of GABA and binds to the $\alpha2\delta$ subunit of voltage-dependent calcium channels, thus preventing the release of nociceptive neurotransmitters including glutamate, substance P, and norepinephrine. It has been shown to reduce hyperalgesia following intradermal capsaicin injection.[149]

Many reports are available on the efficacy of gabapentin and its prodrug, pregabalin. Gabapentin has been found to be very successful in treating neuropathic pain and postsurgical, posttraumatic pain.[150,151] In trauma, it could be useful in treating/preventing neuropathic pain. It has a favorable side-effect profile but may be associated with sedation, dizziness, headache, abnormal thinking or confusion, and ataxia, which may be dose-related. Hepatic enzyme induction is low, thus minimizing significant drug interactions. Preemptive analgesia with gabapentin has been found to reduce VAS scores and opioid requirements.[152] While it is unlikely that the analgesic efficacy of any currently available anticonvulsant is sufficient to eliminate the need for opioids, anticonvulsants may, like NSAIDs, exert an opioid-sparing effect. Available evidence suggests that anticonvulsants might decrease opioid consumption either by enhancing opioid analgesia[153] or by suppressing mechanisms of opioid tolerance or withdrawal.[154]

Pregabalin is an $\alpha2\delta$ ligand that is structurally related to gabapentin without known activity at the GABA or benzodiazepine receptors. It prevents calcium flux by presynaptically inhibiting excitatory neurotransmitters, including glutamate, substance P, and calcium gene-related peptide. It has analgesic, anticonvulsant, and anxiolytic activity.

At present, only oral forms of these drugs are available. Bioavailability of gabapentin is dose-dependent, being higher at lower doses. As more drug is administered, less is available.

Pregabalin has a more linear pharmacokinetic effect and has been documented to be a superb anxiolytic,[155,156] a feature that can play a pivotal role in pain management.

The most common side effects with long-term use of $\alpha2\delta$ ligands are dizziness, somnolence, and peripheral edema.[157] These drugs are eliminated via the renal route, so one has to be careful about renal function/creatinine clearance to determine the dosing.

α_2 Agonists

α_2 Receptors play an important role in pain modulation. The modes of action proposed are increased activation of descending inhibitory pathways via the locus ceruleus, direct inhibitory effect on neuronal firing at receptor sites in the substatia gelatinosa, and a reduction in release of substance P.[158] Clonidine is the most important α_2-receptor agonist with analgesic and sedative properties currently available for clinical use, and it may be useful in trauma pain. Interestingly, it was originally investigated as a nasal decongestant, but associated hypotension and sedation made it unsuitable. Since then, it has been used as a centrally acting antihypertensive agent, as treatment for acute drug withdrawal, for prevention of shivering after general anesthesia, as well as for reducing anesthetic requirements. Studies have shown clonidine to reduce perioperative analgesic requirements, prolong the duration of local anesthetics, and enhance opioid analgesia. Clonidine can be administered by oral, intravenous, transdermal, intramuscular, and neuraxial routes.

Mechanisms of action of α_2-adrenergic receptor agonists include synergy with opioids, since both receptors have a similar distribution throughout the brain,[159] and are coupled with the cyclic GMP effector system.[160] Nitric oxide synthetase is also found in similar locations on the spinal cord, and antinociception from α_2-adrenergic receptor agonists may be partially dependent on nitric oxide synthesis.[161] The sedative effects of α_2 agonists may also decrease pain perception.[162] Despite a large body of evidence from both in-vivo and in-vitro studies, the exact neuroprotecitve mechanisms of α_2-adrenergic receptor agonists have been confined to laboratory experiments.[163] As the α_{2a}-adrenergic receptor is more important in pain modulation, attention has been focused on dexmedetomidine (D-enantiomer of medetomidine), which has $\alpha_2:\alpha_1$ selectivity ratio of 1620:1 (compared with 220:1 for clonidine).[164] Dexmedetomidine has shown promising activity in human trials,[165] but not without side effects. It may have an important role to play in trauma patients whose critical condition may preclude the use of other analgesics. Nasal dexmedetomidine has been evaluated for sedation in children, and it has been found to be comparable to midazolam.[166]

Some trauma patients may not tolerate the hypotension and bradycardia associated with these drugs.[167] α_2-Adrenergic receptor agonists can cause hyperglycemia in humans.[168] The mechanism is thought to involve postsynaptic α_2-adrenergic receptor stimulation of pancreatic β-cells, which inhibit insulin release. However, attenuation of sympathoadrenal response to trauma and stress can inhibit this hyperglycemic response.[169] Dexmedetomidine when used for analog-sedation in patients with traumatic brain injury may have the benefit of neuroprotection, but the evidence for this is sparse at present.

Benzodiazepines

Benzodiazepines have effects on sedation, anxiolysis, and muscle relaxation but do not have any analgesic properties. Although many researchers have shown that anxiety exacerbates pain, the data for this are not confirmative. When a benzodiazepine is used in conjunction with opioids, the opioid dose required to produce analgesia is reduced. In a study on burn patients, the dose of opioid required was significantly reduced by concomitant administration of lorazepam.[170] It has an important role in treating highly strung, anxious patients. Reducing their anxiety level may help in altering their perception of pain. Caution must be exercised when using benzodiazepines with opioids, as their effects are synergistic. Common drugs used in emergency departments are midazolam and diazepam. Midazolam is usually preferred because of its shorter duration of action (60–90 minutes), to avoid any untoward side effects. The most effective route of administration is intravenous. In children with poor or no IV access, oral, rectal, inhaled,[171] buccal,[172] and nasal[173] midazolam have proved effective.

Intrathecal midazolam has been used clinically. The rationale for the use of intrathecal midazolam focuses on the awareness that it is an agonist at the benzodiazepine binding site on a subunit of the pentameric $GABA_A$ receptor,[174] causing spinally mediated analgesia. Current reports suggest that the use of midazolam in a dose not exceeding 1–2 mg at concentrations not exceeding 1 mg/mL, delivered either alone or as an intrathecal adjuvant, has positive effects on perioperative and chronic pain therapy and is not accompanied by an increase in the incidence of adverse events.[175]

Entonox

Entonox is a 50:50 mixture of oxygen and nitrous oxide. It provides safe and effective analgesia without loss of consciousness for moderately painful trauma-related procedures. Its use is usually in an awake, cooperative patient. It is practically PCA with a mask or mouthpiece through an on-demand valve. Entonox produces analgesia and anxiolysis about 20 seconds after inhalation, with peak effects occurring within 2 minutes. It is pleasant to inhale but may cause drowsiness, excitability, or paresthesia. The main disadvantage is nausea, and there is a risk of regurgitation in a trauma patient with a potential full stomach. Cardiovascular side effects are minimal. Entonox should be avoided in patients with altered sensorium, bowel obstruction, pneumothorax, head injury, chronic obstructive pulmonary disease, decompression sickness, or air embolism. Nevertheless, it is a good first aid method of pain relief for mild to moderate pain and minor procedures such as

manipulations and fracture reductions, in both adults[176] and children.[177]

Exposure of staff in and outside operating room areas could be high, as environmental control measures are difficult to apply. Chronic exposure to nitrous oxide may be associated with high homocysteine plasma levels and decreased DNA synthesis, thereby increasing the risk of clinical depression, reduced fertility, and increased pregnancy loss, though some of these concerns were dispelled in a large study.[178]

Special equipment, with mask or mouthpiece and demand valve, is needed. As patient cooperation is required for effective administration, critically ill and/or uncooperative patients are not good candidates for the use of Entonox.

Methoxyflurane

The anesthetic agent popular in the 1960s and 1970s (until its dose-dependent nephrotoxicity made it unpopular) is seeing a newer utility in providing pain relief to trauma victims when used in subanesthetic concentrations. Methoxyflurane is approved for field trauma in a self-administered pen like inhalation device (Penthrox Inhaler) in Australia and New Zealand. It delivers a concentration of 0.2–0.4%, and this concentration has shown good pain relief and patient satisfaction at 5 and 10 minutes in both adult[179] and pediatric populations.[180] It is indicated for self-administration to conscious hemodynamically stable patients with trauma and associated pain, and it has also been tried for procedural pain as seen in burn patients.[181] The current inhalers consist of a plastic tube with a unidirectional valve. A 3 mL solution of methoxflurane saturates the polypropylene wick contained within the device. Due to the concerns of nephrotoxicity, the recommended daily dose is 6.0 mL, with a maximum of 15 mL per week. Minor side effects include sedation, hallucinations, vomiting, confusion, dizziness, cough, and rarely headache. The quality of analgesia is inferior to that of intravenous opioids but comparable to that of nitrous oxide.[182]

Specific types of trauma
Thoracic injuries

Thoracic trauma, especially blunt chest wall trauma, is a leading cause of mortality and morbidity.[183] Pain management in thoracic trauma is often inadequate, because ventilatory compromise worries most treating healthcare professionals. The elderly population has the highest morbidity from thoracic trauma.[184] Adequate analgesia is one of the most important determinants of morbidity in elderly patients. Opioids, neuraxial more than systemic, have been found to be very effective with fewer side effects. Local anesthetics through neuraxial, paravertebral, or intercostal nerve blocks have been shown to be useful (see Chapter 30).

Many chest injuries may be associated with lung and cardiac injuries, making the patient vulnerable to major hemodynamic changes. Thus, opioid administration has to be titrated in a deliberate fashion. Often, patients with thoracic injuries may be on ventilatory support, making administration of opioids less risky.

Burn injuries

A sizeable proportion of burn patients end up having chronic pain. This is as a result of wind-up and secondary hyperalgesia caused by sensitized nerve endings exposed by the burn. A process of central sensitization occurs, and eventually a neuropathic pain state develops.[185] A multimodal approach is therefore required to manage the various stages of burn pain. In the acute phase, the patient has intravascular blood volume depletion, exaggerating the hemodynamic responses to IV opioid medications (see Chapters 39 and 40). Eventually, repeated visits to the operating room and lack of venous access may pose additional problems with pain management. Invariably, these patients end up receiving chronic opioid therapy, which can also result in dependence and opioid-induced hyperalgesia.

Topical anesthetics

Traditional burn care consists of topical antimicrobial agents applied to a burn that has been debrided of devitalized skin. Although very effective in protecting against surface infections, antimicrobial agents are usually applied frequently to maintain their effectiveness. For children, these dressing changes can be associated with significant anxiety. While some agents (silver sulfadiazine) are less irritating, most applications are quite painful. Usage of topical local anesthetics to reduce this discomfort is a known technique. Topical lidocaine applied to skin harvest sites produces analgesic effects and reduces narcotic requirements in burn patients undergoing repeated graft procedures.[186] Systemic toxicity from topical application of local anesthetics has been reported, especially seizures in children.[187] Intravenous lidocaine has been reported to provide some benefit in burns. Topical application of EMLA cream (eutectic mixture of 2.5% lidocaine and 2.5% prilocaine) is useful, but there have been reports of CNS toxicity[188] and methemoglobinemia[189] on excessive application.

During the healing phase of burns, local anesthetics in combination with antihistamines have been used successfully to treat the intense itching that can be present.

Opioids

Opioids still are the mainstay for the treatment of burns worldwide. Their potency and analgesic efficacy make them the first-choice drugs. The intravenous route of administration by PCA has been found to be most effective in providing adequate pain relief. The flexibility, ease of use, less dependency on medical personnel, and reduction in resource utilization make it a more effective system. The worries about altered pharmacokinetics and plasma drug level because of a catabolic state and altered plasma protein levels have not panned out. The commonly used technique involves a constant background

opioid infusion along with an on-demand bolus. Burn patients have higher opioid requirements and may be tolerant to opioids. When switching over to oral medications, equianalgesic doses of long-acting opioids need to be added along with nonopioid adjuvants. The opioid methadone has antagonistic effects on NMDA and serotonin reuptake and thus provides an ideal enteral formulation.

Nonopioid adjuvants

NSAIDs can be used to treat burn pain, but the main worry is their effect on renal function and GI mucosa. Acetaminophen might be a preferred drug in such a situation because of its favorable side-effect profile. Regular administration, rather than as-needed (PRN), is preferred. Acetaminophen alone can provide good control of baseline pain.

Ketamine, as described earlier, is a potent analgesic and amnesic. Its CNS effects could limit its use but it has been found to be very useful in opioid-resistant patients. Conscious sedation with rectally applied ketamine and midazolam allows safe and painless dressing changes after burn injuries in children.[190]

Benzodiazepine or other major tranquilizers can be useful for anxiolysis. The emotional aspect and psychologic issues surrounding pain treatment enhance the perception of pain. These drugs have been effective in such cases. Lorezepam is a preferred agent because of its relatively clean metabolic pathway (glucuronidation).

Antihistamines are standard treatment in burn centers.[191] The reason is intense pruritus during the healing phase. The C fibers, which are polymodal, transmit the itching sensation that is often more irritating than pain. The sedative effect of the antihistamines can be useful in augmenting sleep and relieving anxiety, and possibly result in some decrease in narcotic requirement.[192] Gabapentin has been shown to be effective in relieving itching in burn patients.[193]

Regional anesthesia with nerve blocks for isolated burn injuries can be helpful but is limited to few instances. Epidurals and intrathecal analgesia appear attractive, but the increased incidence of catheter colonization and risk of infection is a real possibility.

Pediatric trauma

The major challenges of pediatric trauma are the psychological component, lack of IV access, and difficulty in assessing pain (see Chapter 34). Studies have shown that more than one-third of pediatric trauma victims have intense to severe pain in the prehospital setting,[194] and these children tend to be undermedicated after trauma because of a global fear of overdose.[195] There is mounting evidence that adequately treating pain in children is not only safe but can also improve outcomes.[196] Although various subjective and objective pain scales have been designed to assess pain in various age groups (Wong-Baker FACES scale: quantifies pain by series of faces ranging from a happy face at 0, "no hurt," to a crying face at 10, "hurts worst"; Poker Chips scale: quantifies pain in "pieces of hurt" with more poker chips representing more pain; FLACC scale: Face, Legs, Activity, Cry, Consolability scale; VAS: visual analog scale; NRS: numerical rating scale), a combination of physiological parameters like heart rate, respiration, and blood pressure along with pain scales is helpful in assessing pain and differentiating it from anxiety.

During transport from the scene of accident, parenteral analgesics should be used in severely injured children. Intramuscular and/or low-dose opioid infusions provide reasonable pain relief during undressing, mobilization, and fracture reduction. NSAIDs are known to provide good-quality analgesia in the emergency department with pain from acute musculoskeletal injuries.[197] Falanga et al. have shown that in children, the use of a nurse-controlled algorithm for pain relief is safe and effective, as it focuses on regular combined analgesia, frequent pain assessment, and a standardized therapeutic decision.[198] Ketamine, usually with a benzodiazepine, can also be used for procedural pain relief. It is crucial to give traumatized children support and reassurance, to minimize fear. Objective pain scales or physiologic and behavior scales can be used in children for pain assessment.

Nerve blocks may be appropriate for children both in the acute care setting and before painful procedures (see Chapter 34).

Multimodal analgesia

Multimodal analgesia is a concept that uses two or more agents throughout the pain cycle. High enough doses of individual agents will achieve good results, but the multimodal approach maximizes the benefits while minimizing the adverse effects using synergistic agents.

As pain varies in intensity and duration according to degree of bony/soft tissue damage, need for physiotherapy, need for ambulation, preexisting condition, and individual pain threshold, there can be no single recipe for pain control. The guiding principle is that a balance of agents will provide optimal pain control. The goals are to maximize the positive aspects of treatment and limit the side effects. In this strategy, coxibs can be used to reduce peripheral and central sensitization, local anesthetics and opioids can be used during and immediately after surgical procedures, and an agent such as ketamine can be introduced as an NMDA-receptor antagonist to minimize central sensitization. This results in additive or synergistic analgesia with superior pain control, lower total doses, fewer side effects, and attenuated stress response.

A stepwise multimodal pain therapy similar to the WHO ladder can be followed wherein NSAIDs and acetaminophen, along with local wound infiltration, are commonly used for mild pain, with the addition of intermittent opioids for moderate pain and the further inclusion of peripheral nerve blocks and modified-release opioids for severe pain.

Nonpharmacologic approaches

Psychologic support is a major part of initial acute trauma/burn treatment, and also of the rehabilitation phase. Alleviating anxiety, decreasing fear, and ensuring a reasonable sleep pattern play a crucial role. In the long term, nightmares and posttraumatic stress disorder are quite common following trauma. Counseling plays an indispensable part in minimizing the sequelae from this. Hypnosis, relaxation techniques, biofeedback, and acupuncture have all been reported to decrease the intensity of burn pain.[199]

TENS (transcutaneous electrical nerve stimulation) is a valuable and fast-acting pain treatment under difficult circumstances, including out-of-hospital rescue, and it lacks side effects. It has been shown to reduce pain scores, anxiety, heart rate, and blood pressure related to transport after traumatic hip fractures.[200] The only limiting factors are the need for proper application of the device and patients having implanted electronic devices such as pacemakers, defibrillators, or spinal cord or deep brain stimulators.

Microamperage current treatment has shown significant reduction in pain scores and biologic markers for pain and proinflammatory cytokines, as well as an increase in serum cortisol and β-endorphin release in fibromyalgia associated with cervical spine trauma.[201] This may hold promise.

Conclusions

The management of pain plays a pivotal role in the treatment of trauma patients. The ideal goal for most patients appears to be minimizing pain, achieving an arousable state by avoiding excessive sedation, and allowing evaluation of pain and neurologic function. It has become increasingly clear that prompt and proper pain control can have a positive impact on outcomes. Early mechanical measures such as fixation of fractures and repositions of dislocations are important in pain management. While drugs are important in acute pain management, reassurance, empathy, and explanations about the condition and its likely course have an equally vital role to play.[202]

Questions

(1) Concerning pain and the stress response after trauma, which of the following is correct?
   a. A predominant anabolic response occurs
   b. There is usually a rise in catecholamines and cortisol
   c. Hypoglycemia is common due to increased levels of insulin
   d. Splanchnic blood flow is increased

(2) With regard to pain management, which of the following is correct?
   a. Caregivers frequently overestimate the pain level experienced by patients
   b. A tracheally intubated patient cannot report pain
   c. Pain scores such as the visual analog scale are inaccurate and therefore should not be used

d. The most accurate and reliable evidence of pain is from the patient

(3) **Considering the use of acetaminophen in trauma, which of the following is correct?**
   a. It is effective for moderate pain after minor surgery
   b. It is contraindicated in elderly patients because of gastrointestinal side effects
   c. It impairs wound healing
   d. It reduces bone fusion

(4) **Concerning the use of nonsteroidal anti-inflammatory drugs (NSAIDs) in trauma, which of the following is correct?**
   a. Nonselective NSAIDs act predominantly at COX-3 receptors
   b. They are not effective for treating moderate pain after surgery
   c. There are fewer gastrointestinal and antiplatelet side effects with selective COX-2 inhibitors (e.g., coxibs)
   d. In adults with moderate to severe postsurgical pain, there is no opioid-sparing effect with ketorolac

(5) **Regarding the use of opioids and other drugs in trauma patients, which of the following is correct?**
   a. Neuraxial opioids are generally avoided after thoracic surgery because of the risk of epidural hematoma
   b. Transmucosal opioids cannot be used because the increased first-pass metabolism in trauma patients decreases their efficacy
   c. Multimodal analgesia using local anesthetics, ketamine, NSAIDs, and opioids results in inferior pain control and more side effects than single-modal therapy (one agent only)
   d. Clonidine reduces analgesic requirements and can prolong the effect of local anesthetics

(6) **Which of the following statements regarding chronic pain is true?**
   a. The fast pain pathway is involved in flare-up and chronic pain
   b. Pain fibers traveling through the paleospinothalamic tract are involved in slow pain
   c. The integration of pain signals first occurs at the posterior or medial thalamic nuclei
   d. The pain pathway has connections to the limbic system, which is responsible for the neuroendocrine response
   e. Pain sensation does not have memory

(7) **Which of the following statements is false concerning pain perception following trauma?**
   a. Hormonal differences partly explain sexual differences in pain perception
   b. Estradiol has different pain modulation properties depending on whether it is acting centrally or peripherally

c. NMDA (*N*-methyl-D-aspartate) and 5-HT$_3$ pathways are not responsible in differences in pain perceptions
   d. The incidence of pain following trauma varies widely between 35% and 70%
   e. A high percentage of patients receive inadequate pain relief following trauma

(8) **All of the following are components of the stress response following traumatic pain, *except*:**
   a. Rise in catecholamines, growth hormone, cortisol, renin, antidiuretic hormone
   b. Increased secretion of enkephalins and endorphins
   c. Tachycardia, hypertension, and decreased splanchnic blood flow
   d. Increased glomerular filtration rate
   e. Predominant catabolic response

(9) **Which of the following statements regarding tapentadol is *false*?**
   a. It is a μ-opioid receptor agonist and norepinephrine reuptake inhibitor
   b. Tapentadol should not be used concurrently with monoamine oxidase inhibitors
   c. At higher doses of tapentadol, rates of nausea are similar to those of oxycodone
   d. Tapentadol is more economical than currently prescribed oral opioids
   e. Nausea and gastrointestinal side effects are the most common adverse effects

(10) **Which statement regarding ketamine is true?**
   a. Ketamine is a competitive inhibitor at the N-methyl-D-aspartate (NMDA) receptor
   b. Ketamine may decrease secondary hyperalgesia, and when combined with morphine has been shown to prevent the wind-up phenomenon
   c. Ketamine does not cause excessive secretions and agitation on recovery
   d. Ketamine is thought to have an antagonistic action at opioid receptors and an agonist action at muscarinic receptors

Answers

(1) b
(2) d
(3) a
(4) c
(5) d
(6) d
(7) c
(8) d
(9) d
(10) b

References

1. Taxonomy of pain syndromes. In Charlton JE, ed. *Core Curriculum for Professional Education in Pain*. Seattle, WA: IASP Press, 2005.

2. Melzack R, Wall PD. Pain mechanisms: a new theory. *Science* 1965; **150**: 971–9.

3. Peden M, McGee K, Krug E, eds. *Injury: a Leading Cause of the Burden of Disease, 2000*. Geneva: World Health Organization, 2002.

4. Corso P, Finkelstein E, Miller T, Fiebelkorn I, Zaloshnja E. Incidence and lifetime costs of injuries in the United States. *Inj Prev* 2006; **12**: 212–18.

5. Minei JP, Schmicker RH, Kerby JD, *et al.* Severe traumatic injury: regional variation in incidence and outcome. *Ann Surg* 2010; **252**: 149–57.

6. Jennings PA, Cameron P, Bernard S. Epidemiology of prehospital pain: an opportunity for improvement. *Emerg Med J* 2010; **28**: 530–1.

7. Guru V, Dubinsky I. The patient vs. caregiver perception of acute pain in the emergency department. *J Emerg Med* 2000; **18**: 7–12.

8. Heins JK, Heins A, Grammas M, *et al.* Disparities in analgesia and opioid prescribing practices for patients with musculoskeletal pain in the emergency department. *J Emerg Nurs* 2006; **32**: 219–24.

9. Albrecht E, Taffe P, Yersin B, *et al.* Undertreatment of acute pain (oligoanalgesia) and medical practice variation in prehospital analgesia of adult trauma patients: a 10 yr retrospective study. *Br J Anaesth* 2013; **110**: 96–106.

10. Fillingim RB, King CD, Ribeiro-Dasilva MC, Rahim-Williams B, Riley JL 3rd. Sex, gender, and pain: a review of recent clinical and experimental findings. *J Pain* 2009; **10**: 447–85.

11. Ji Y, Murphy AZ, Traub RJ. Estrogen modulation of morphine analgesia of visceral pain in female rats is supraspinally and peripherally mediated. *J Pain* 2007; **8**: 494–502.

12. Herrero JF, Laird JM, Lopez-Garcia JA. Wind-up of spinal cord neurones and pain sensation: much ado about something? *Prog Neurobiol* 2000; **61**: 169–203.

13. Nakai A, Kumakura Y, Boivin M, *et al.* Sex differences of brain serotonin synthesis in patients with irritable bowel syndrome using alpha-[11C] methyl-L-tryptophan, positron emission tomography and statistical parametric mapping. *Can J Gastroenterol* 2003; **17**: 191–6.

14. Straub RH. The complex role of estrogens in inflammation. *Endocr Rev* 2007; **28**: 521–74.

15. Bereiter DA, Cioffi JL, Bereiter DF. Oestrogen receptor-immunoreactive neurons in the trigeminal sensory system of male and cycling female rats. *Arch Oral Biol* 2005; **50**: 971–9.

16. Silka PA, Roth MM, Moreno G, Merrill L, Geiderman JM. Pain scores improve analgesic administration patterns for trauma patients in the emergency department. *Acad Emerg Med* 2004; **11**: 264–70.

17. Kelly AM. A process approach to improving pain management in the emergency department: development and evaluation. *J Accid Emerg Med* 2000; **17**: 185–7.

18. AGS Panel on Persistent Pain in Older Persons. The management of persistent pain in older persons. *J Am Geriatr Soc* 2002; **50** (6 Suppl): S205–24.

19. Sachs CJ. Oral analgesics for acute nonspecific pain. *Am Fam Phys* 2005; **71**: 913–18.

20. Flower RJ, Vane JR. Inhibition of prostaglandin synthetase in brain explains the antipyretic activity of paracetamol (4-acetamidophenol). *Nature* 1972; **240**: 410–11.

21. Chandrasekharan NV, Dai H, Roos KLT, *et al.* COX-3, a cyclooxygenase-1 variant inhibited by acetaminophen and other analgesic/antipyretic drugs: cloning, structure and expression. *Proc Natl Acad Sci USA* 2002; **99**: 13926–31.

22. Kis B, Snipes JA, Busija DW. Acetaminophen and the cyclooxygenase-3 puzzle: sorting out facts, fictions, and uncertainties. *J Pharmacol Exp Ther* 2005; **315**: 1–7.

23. Lucas R, Warner TD, Vojnovic I, Mitchell JA. Cellular mechanisms of acetaminophen: role of cyclo-oxygenase. *FASEB J* 2005; **19**: 635–7.

24. Herrero JF, Headly PM. Reversal by naloxone of the spinal antinociceptive actions of a systemically administered NSAIDs. *Br J Pharmacol* 1996; **118**: 968–72.

25. Sandrini M, Romualdi P, Vitale G *et al.* The effect of a paracetamol and morphine combination on dynorphin A levels in the rat brain. *Biochem Pharmacol* 2001; **61**: 1409–16.

26. Bujalska M. Effect of non-selective and selective opioid receptor antagonists on antinociception action of acetaminophen. *Pol J Pharma* 2004; **56**: 539–45.

27. Di Marzo V, Deutsch DG. Biochemistry of the endogenous ligands of cannabinoid receptors. *Neurobiol Dis* 1998; **5**: 386–404.

28. Bertollini A, Ferrari A, Ottani A, *et al.* Paracetamol: new vistas of an old drug. *CNS Drug Rev* 2006; **12**: 250–75.

29. Mallet C. Endocannabinoid and serotonergic systems are needed for acetaminophen-induced analgesia. *Pain* 2008; **139**: 190–200.

30. Mallet C. TRPV1 in brain is involved in acetaminophen-induced antinociception. *PLoS ONE* 2010; **5**: 127–48.

31. Smith HS. Potential analgesic mechanisms of acetaminophen. *Pain Physician* 2009; **12**: 269–80.

32. Barden J, Edwards J, Moore A, *et al.* Single dose oral paracetamol (acetaminophen) for postoperative pain (Cochrane review). *Cochrane Database Syst Rev* 2004; (1): CD004602.

33. McNicol ED, Tzortzopoulou A, Cepeda MS, *et al.* Single-dose intravenous paracetamol or propacetamol for prevention or treatment of postoperative pain: a systematic review and meta-analysis. *Br J Anaesth* 2011; **106**: 764–75.

34. Moller PL, Sindet-Pedersen S, Petersen CT, *et al.* Onset of acetaminophen analgesia: comparison of oral and intravenous routes after third molar surgery. *Br J Anaesth* 2005; **94**: 642–8.

35. Anderson BJ, Pons G, Autret-Leca E, Allegaert K, Boccard E. Pediatric intravenous paracetamol (propacetamol) pharmacokinetics: a population analysis. *Paediatr Anaesth* 2005; **15**: 282–92.

36. Juhl GI, Norholt SE, Tonnesen E, *et al.* Analgesic efficacy and safety of intravenous paracetamol (acetaminophen) administered as a 2 g starting dose following third moral surgery. *Eur J Pain* 2006; **10**: 371–7.

37. Ofirmev [package insert]. San Diego, CA: Cadence Pharmaceuticals, 2010.

38. Pasero C, Stannard D. The role of intravenous acetaminophen in acute pain management: a case-illustrated review. *Pain Manag Nurs* 2012; **13**: 107–24.

39. Shaikh N, Kettern MA, Ali Ahmed AH, Louon A. Morphine sparing effect of proparacetamol in surgical and trauma intensive care. *Middle East J Emerg Med* 2006; **6** (2): 28–30.

40. Skoglund LA, Skjelbred P, Fyllingen G. Analgesic efficacy of acetaminophen 1000 mg, acetaminophen 2000 mg, and the combination of acetaminophen 1000 mg and codeine phosphate 60 mg versus placebo in acute postoperative pain. *Pharmacotherapy* 1991; **11**: 364–9.

41. Hahn TW, Mogensen T, Lund C, *et al.* Analgesic effect of IV paracetamol; possible ceiling effect of paracetamol in postoperative pain. *Acta Anaesthesiol Scand* 2003; **47**: 138–45.

42. Vitols S. Paracetamol hepatotoxicity at therapeutic doses. *J Intern Med* 2003; **253**: 95–8.

43. Bacon TH, Hole JG, North M, Burnett I. Analgesic efficacy of sustained release paracetamol in patients with osteoarthritis of the knee. *Br J Clin Pharmacol* 2002; **53**: 629–36.

44. Cormack CRH, Sudan S, Anderson R, *et al.* The pharmacokinetics of a single rectal dose of paracetamol (40 mg/kg) in children with liver disease. *Paediatr Anaesth* 2006; **16**: 417–23.

45. Larson AM, Polson J, Fontana RJ, *et al.* Acetaminophen-induced acute liver failure: results of a United States multicenter, prospective study. *Hepatology* 2005; **102**: 822–31.

46. Dal Pan GJ. *Acetaminophen: Background and Overview.* Silver Spring, MD: US Food and Drug Administration, Office of Surveillance and Epidemiology, Center for Drug Evaluation and Research; 2009. www.fda.gov/downloads/AdvisoryCommittees/Committees%20MeetingMaterials/Drugs/DrugSafetyandRiskManagementAdvisoryCommittee/UCM175767 (accessed July 2014).

47. Woodcock J. A difficult balance: pain management, drug safety, and the FDA. *N Engl J Med* 2009; **361**: 2105–7.

48. Larrey D. Epidemiology and individual susceptibility to adverse drug reactions affecting the liver. *Semin Liver Dis* 2002; **22**: 145–55.

49. Schilling A, Corey R, Leonard M, Eghtesad B. Acetaminophen: old drug, new warnings. *Cleve Clin J Med* 2010; **77**: 19–27.

50. Moore PK, Marshall M. Nitric oxide releasing acetaminophen (nitroactaminophen). *Dig Liver Dis* 2003; **35** (Suppl 2): S49–60.

51. Anderson BJ, Palmer GM. Recent developments in the pharmacological management of pain in children. *Curr Opin Anaesthesiol* 2006; **19**: 285–92.

52. Yeh YC, Reddy P. Clinical and economic evidence for intravenous acetaminophen. *Pharmacotherapy* 2012; **32**: 559–79.

53. Vane JR. The fight against rheumatism: from willow bark to COX-1 sparing drugs. *J Physiol Pharmacol* 2000; **51**: 573–86.

54. Vane JR. Inhibition of prostaglandin synthesis as a mechanism of action for aspirin-like drugs. *Nat New Biol* 1971; **43**: 232–5.

55. Watson DJ, Harper SE, Zhao PL, *et al.* Gastrointestinal tolerability of the selective cyclooxygenase-2 (COX-2) inhibitor rofexoxib compared with nonselective COX-1 and COX-2 inhibitors in osteoarthritis. *Arch Intern Med* 2000; **160**: 2998–3003.

56. Sinatra R. Role of COX-2 inhibitors in the evolution of acute pain management. *J Pain Symptom Manage* 2002; **24**: S18–27.

57. Samad TA, Moore KA, Sapirstein A, *et al.* Interleukin-1 beta-mediated induction of COX-2 in the CNS contributes to inflammatory pain hypersensitivity. *Nature* 2001; **410**: 471–5.

58. Buvanendran A, Kroin JS, Tuman KJ, *et al.* Cerebrospinal fluid and plasma pharmacokintetics of the cycloxygenase 2 inhibitor rofexoxib in humans: single and multiple oral drug administration. *Anesth Analg* 2005; **100**: 1320–4.

59. Mukherjee D, Nissen SE, Topol EJ. Risk of cardiovascular events associated with selective COX-2 inhibitors. *JAMA* 2001; **286**: 954–9.

60. Solomon DH, Schneeweiss S, Glynn RJ, *et al.* Relationship between selective cyclooxygenase-2 inhibitors and acute myocardial infarction in older adults. *Circulation* 2004; **109**: 2068–73.

61. Chen YF, Jobanputra P, Barton P, *et al.* Cyclooxygenase-2 selective non-steroidal anti-inflammatory drugs (etodolac, meloxicam, celecoxib, rofecoxib, etoricoxib, valdecoxib and lumiracoxib) for osteoarthritis and rheumatoid arthritis: a systematic review and economic evaluation. *Health Technol Assess* 2008; **12**: 1–278.

62. W Ye, H Zhang, E Hillas, *et al.* Expression and function of COX isoforms in renal medulla: evidence for regulation of salt sensitivity and blood pressure. *Am J Renal Physiol* 2006; **290**: F542–9.

63. Hawkey CJ, Glitton X, Hoexter G, Richard D, Weinstein WM. Gastrointestinal tolerability of lumiracoxib in patients with osteoarthritis and rheumatoid arthritis. *Clin Gastroenterol Hepatol* 2006; **4**: 57–66.

64. Mehallo CJ, Drezner JA, Bytomski JR. Practical management: nonsteroidal antiinflammatory drug (NSAID) use in athletic injuries. *Clin J Sport Med* 2006; **16**: 170–4.

65. Zhang J, Diang EL, Song Y. Adverse effects of cyclooxygenase 2 inhibitors on renal and arrhythmia events. *JAMA* 2006; **296**: 1619–32.

66. Bannwarth B. Is licofelone, a dual inhibitor of cyclooxygenase and 5-lipoxygenase, a promising alternative in anti-inflammatory therapy? *Fundam Clin Pharmacol* 2004; **18**: 125–30.

67. Rahme E, Barkun AN, Toubouti Y, *et al.* Do proton-pump inhibitors confer additional gastrointestinal protection in patients given celecoxib? *Arthritis Rheum* 2007; **57**: 748–55.

68. Chan F, Wong V, Suen B, *et al.* Combination of a cyclooxygensase-2 inhibitor and a proton-pump inhibitor for prevention of recurrent ulcer bleeding in patients at very high risk: a double-blind, randomized trial. *Lancet* 2007; **369**: 1621–6.

69. Singh G, Rosen Ramey D. NSAID induced gastrointestinal complications: the ARAMIS perspective-1997, Arthritis, Rheumatism and Aging Medical Information System. *J Rheumatol Suppl* 1998; **51**: 8–16.

70. Chen JY, Wu GJ, Mok MS, *et al.* Effect of adding ketorolac to intravenous morphine patient-controlled analgesia

on bowel function in colorectal surgery patients: a prospective, randomized, double-blind study. *Acta Anaesthesiol Scand* 2005; **49**: 546–51.

71. Stephens JM, Pashos CL, Haider S, Wong JM. Making progress in the management of postoperative pain: a review of the cyclooxygenase-2 specific inhibitors. *Pharmacotherapy* 2004; **24**: 1714–31.

72. Sinha VR, Kumar RV, Singh G. Ketorolac tromethamine formulations: an overview. *Expert Opin Drug Deliv* 2009; **6**: 961–75.

73. Predel HG, Koll R, Pabst H, *et al.* Diclofenac patch for topical treatment of acute impact injuries: a randomized, double blind, placebo controlled, multicentre study. *Br J Sports Med* 2004; **38**: 318–23.

74. Spaulding J, Li F. Naproxcinod: FDA efficacy and safety review. May 12, 2010. http://www.fda.gov/downloads/ AdvisoryCommittees/ CommitteesMeetingMaterials/Drugs/ ArthritisAdvisoryCommittee/ UCM212679.pdf (accessed September 2014).

75. Dimar JR, Ante WA, Zhang YP, Glassman SD. The effects of nonsteroidal anti-inflammatory drugs on posterior spinal fusion in rat. *Spine* 1996; **21**: 1870–6.

76. Radi ZA, Khan NK. Effect of cyclooxygenase inhibition on bone, tendon and ligament healing. *Inflamm Res* 2005; **54**: 358–66.

77. Cohen DB, Kawarmura S, Ehteshami JR, Rodeo SA. Indo-methacin and celecoxib impair rotator cuff tendon-to-bone healing. *Am J Sports Med* 2006; **34**: 362–9.

78. Williams LJ, Pasco JA, Henry MJ, *et al.* Paracetamol (acetaminophen) use, fracture and bone mineral density. *Bone* 2011; **48**: 1277–81.

79. Vestergaard P, Hermann P, Jensen JE, Eiken P, Mosekilde L. Effects of paracetamol, non-steroidal anti-inflammatory drugs, acetylsalicylic acid, and opioids on bone mineral density and risk of fracture: results of the Danish Osteoporosis Prevention Study (DOPS). *Osteoporos Int* 2012; **23**: 1255–65.

80. Tam J, Trembovler V, Di Marzo V, *et al.* The cannabinoid CB1 receptor regulates bone formation by modulating adrenergic signaling. *FASEB J* 2008; **22**: 285–94.

81. Ofek O, Karsak M, Leclerc N, *et al.* Peripheral cannabinoid receptor, CB2, regulates bone mass. *Proc Natl Acad Sci USA* 2006; **103**: 696–701.

82. Tam J, Ofek O, Fride E, *et al.* Involvement of neuronal cannabinoid receptor CB1 in regulation of bone mass and bone remodeling. *Mol Pharmacol* 2006; **70**: 786–92.

83. Yaksh TL. Pharmacology and mechanisms of opioid analgesic activity. *Acta Anaesthesiol Scand* 1997; **41** (1pt 2): 94–111.

84. Mackersie RC, Karagianes TG, Hoyt DB, Davis JW. Prospective evaluation of epidural and intravenous administration of fentanyl for pain control and restoration of ventilatory function following multiple rib fractures. *J Trauma* 1991; **31**: 443–9.

85. Evans E, Turley N, Robinson N, Clancy M. Randomized controlled trial of patient controlled analgesia compared with nurse delivered analgesia in an emergency department. *Emerg Med J* 2005; **22**: 25–9.

86. George MJ. The site of action of epidurally administered opioids and its relevance to postoperative pain management. *Anaesthesia* 2006; **61** (7): 659–64.

87. Dale O, Hjortkjaer R, Kharasch ED. Nasal administration of opioids for pain management in adults. *Acta Anaesthesiol Scand* 2002; **46**: 759–70.

88. Mercadante S, Villari P, Ferrera P, *et al.* Transmucosal fentanyl vs. intravenous morphine in doses proportional to basal opioid regimen for episodic breakthrough pain. *Br J Cancer* 2007; **96**: 1828–33.

89. Simpson DM, Xie F, Messina J. Fentanyl buccal tablet (FBT) in the treatment of breakthrough pain in opioid tolerant patients with chronic neuropathic pain: randomized, placebo controlled study. *Eur J Pain* 2007; **11**: 84.

90. Viscusi ER, Reynolds L, Chung F, Atkinson LE, Khanna S. Patient-controlled transdermal fentanyl hydrochloride vs. intravenous morphine pump for postoperative pain. *JAMA* 2004; **291**: 1333–41.

91. Farr SJ, Otulana BA. Pulmonary delivery of opioids as pain therapeutics. *Adv Drug Deliv Rev* 2006; **58**: 1076–88.

92. Rosseland L, Solheim N, Stubhaug A. Intra-articular morphine in acute pain

trials. *Reg Anesth Pain Med* 2007; **32**: 176–7.

93. Kotwal RS, O'Connor KC, Johnson TR, *et al.* A novel pain management strategy for combat casualty care *Ann Emerg Med* 2004; **44**: 121–7.

94. Fulda GJ, Giberson F, Fagraeus L, Angood PB, Gentilello LM. A prospective randomized trial of nebulized morphine compared with patient-controlled analgesia morphine in the management of acute thoracic pain. *J Trauma* 2005; **59**: 383–90.

95. Higgins MJ, Asbury AJ, Brodie MJ. Inhaled nebulised fentanyl for postoperative analgesia. *Anaesthesia* 1991; **46**: 973–6.

96. Worsley MH, MacLeod AD, Brodie MJ, Asbury AJ, Clark C. Inhaled fentanyl as a method of analgesia. *Anaesthesia* 1990; **45**: 449–51.

97. Macleod DB, Habib AS, Ikeda K, *et al.* Inhaled fentanyl aerosol in healthy volunteers: pharmacokinetics and pharmacodynamics. *Anesth Analg* 2012; **115**: 1071–7.

98. Sinatra R. The fentanyl HCl patient-controlled transdermal system (PCTS): an alternative to intravenous patient-controlled analgesia in the postoperative setting. *Clin Pharmacokinet* 2005; **44** (Suppl 1): 1–6.

99. Allan L, Richarz U, Simpson K, *et al.* Transdermal fentanyl versus sustained release oral morphine in strong-opioid naive patients with chronic low back pain. *Spine (Phila Pa 1976)* 2005; **30**: 2484–90.

100. Kress HG. Clinical update on the pharmacology, efficacy and safety of transdermal buprenorphine. *Eur J Pain* 2009; **13**: 219–30.

101. Stein C. Peripheral mechanisms of opioid analgesia. *Anesth Analg* 1993; **339**: 182–9.

102. Stein C, Millan MJ, Shippenberg TS, Peter K, Hertz A. Peripheral opioid receptors mediating antinociception in inflammation. Evidence for involvement of mu, delta and kappa receptors. *J Pharmacol Exp Ther* 1989; **248**: 1269–75.

103. Stein C, Comisel K, Haimeri E, *et al.* Analgesic effects of intraarticular morphine after arthroscopic knee surgery. *N Engl J Med* 1991; **325**: 1123–6.

104. Busch CA, Shore BJ, Bhandari R, *et al.* Efficacy of periarticular multimodal

drug injection in total knee arthroplasty. *J Bone Joint Surg* 2006; **88:** 959–63.

105. Ahlbeck K. Opioids: a two-faced Janus. *Curr Med Res Opin* 2011; **27:** 439–48.

106. Ogilvie H. Large-intestine colic due to sympathetic deprivation: a new clinical syndrome. *Br Med J* 1948; **2:** 671–3.

107. Rogers M, Cerda JJ. The narcotic bowel syndrome. *J Clin Gastroenterol* 1989; **11:** 132–5.

108. Brill S, McCartney CJL, Weksler N, Chan VWS. Acute colonic pseudo-obstruction (Ogilvie's syndrome), lower limb arthroplasty and opioids. *Acute Pain* 2003; **5:** 45–50.

109. Weinger MB. Dangers of postoperative opioids. *APSF Newslett* 2006–2007; **21** (4): 61–8.

110. Roy S, Want J, Kelschenbach, Koodie L, Martin J. Modulation of immune function by morphine: implications for susceptibility to infection. *J Neuroimmune Pharmacol* 2006; **1:** 77–89.

111. Savage S. Assessment for addiction in pain-treatment settings. *Clin J Pain.* 2002; **18:** S28–38.

112. Illgen RL, Pellino TA, Gordon DB, Butts S, Heiner JP. Prospective analysis of a novel long-acting oral opioid analgesic regimen for pain control after total hip and knee arthroplasty. *J Arthroplasty* 2006; **21:** 814–20.

113. Shirk MB, Donahue KR, Shirvani J. Unlabeled uses of nebulized medications. *Am J Health Syst Pharm* 2006; **63:** 1704–16.

114. Hutchinson MR, Zhang Y, Shridhar M, *et al.* Evidence that opioids may have toll-like receptor 4 and MD-2 effects. *Brain Behav Immun* 2010; **24:** 83–95.

115. Bamigbade TA, Langford RM. The clinical use of tramadol hydrochloride. *Pain Rev* 1998; **5:** 155–82.

116. Gardner JS, Blough D, Drinkard CR, *et al.* Tramadol and seizures: a surveillance study in a managed car population. *Pharmacotherapy* 2000; **20:** 1423–31.

117. Akinci S, Saricaoglu F, Atay O, Doral M, Kanbak M. Analgesic effect of intra-articular tramadol compared with morphine after arthroscopic knee surgery. *Arthroscopy* 2005; **21:** 1060–5.

118. Langlois G, Estebe JP, Gentili ME, *et al.* The addition of tramadol to lidocaine does not reduce tourniquet and postoperative pain during IV regional anesthesia. *Can J Anaesth* 2002; **49:** 165–8.

119. Altunkaya H, Ozer Y, Kargi E, Babuccu O. Comparison of local anaesthetic effects of tramadol with prilocaine for minor surgical procedures. *Br J Anaesth* 2003; **90:** 320–2.

120. Pang WW, Mok MS, Chang DP, *et al.* Local anesthetic effects of tramadol, metaclopromide and lidocaine following intradermal injection. *Reg Anesth Pain Med* 1998; **23:** 580–3.

121. Turker G, Goren S, Bayram S, Sahin S, Korfali G. Comparison of lumbar epidural tramadol and lumbar epidural morphine for pain relief after throracotomy: a repeated dose study. *J Cardiothorac Vasc Anesth* 2005; **19:** 468–74.

122. Erlich DR, Bodine W. Tapentadol (nucynta) for treatment of pain. *Am Fam Physician* 2012; **85:** 910–11.

123. Daniels S, Casson E, Stegmann JU, *et al.* A randomized, double-blind, placebo-controlled phase 3 study of the relative efficacy and tolerability of tapentadol IR and oxycodone IR for acute pain. *Curr Med Res Opin* 2009; **25:** 1551–61.

124. Etropolski M, Kelly K, Okamoto A, Rauschkolb C. Comparable efficacy and superior gastrointestinal tolerability (nausea, vomiting, constipation) of tapentadol compared with oxycodone hydrochloride. *Adv Ther* 2011; **28:** 401–17.

125. Kissin I, Bright CA, Bradley EL. The effect of ketamine on opioid-induced acute tolerance: can it explain reduction of opioid consumption with ketamine–opioid analgesic combinations? *Anesth Analg* 2000; **91:** 1483–8.

126. Willman EV. Andolfatto G. A prospective evaluation of "ketofol" (ketamine/propofol combination) for procedural sedation and analgesia in the emergency department. *Ann Emerg Med* 2007; **49:** 23–30.

127. Jennings PA, Cameron P, Bernard S. Ketamine as an analgesic in the pre-hospital setting: a systematic review. *Acta Anaesthesiol Scand* 2011; **55:** 638–43.

128. Berti M, Baciarello M, Troglio R, Fanelli G. Clinical uses of low-dose ketamine in patients undergoing surgery. *Curr Drug Targets* 2009; **10:** 707–15.

129. McGuinness SK, Wasiak J, Cleland H, *et al.* A systematic review of ketamine as an analgesic agent in adult burn injuries. *Pain Med* 2011; **12:** 1551–8.

130. Koppert W, Weigand M, Neumann F, *et al.* Perioperative intravenous lidocaine has preventive effects on postoperative pain and morphine consumption after major abdominal surgery. *Anesth Analg* 2004; **98:** 1050–5.

131. Conlay L. Analgesic effects of intravenous lidocaine and morphine on post amputation pain: a randomized double blind, active placebo controlled, crossover trial. *Surv Anesthesiol* 2004; **48** (1): 43.

132. Tanaka T, Okano S, Tsukui R, *et al.* Continuous low dose intravenous lidocaine is effective for visceral pain secondary to peritoneal carcinomatosis in terminally cancer patients. ASCO Annual Meeting Proceedings Part 1. *J Clin Oncol* 2006; **24:** 8533.

133. Tremont-Lukats IW, Challapalli V, McNicol ED, Lau J, Carr DB. Systemic administration of local anesthetics to relieve neuropathic pain: a systemic review and metanalysis. *Anesth Analg* 2005; **101:** 1738–49.

134. Finnerup N, Biering-Sorensen F, Johannesen I, *et al.* Intravenous lidocaine relieves spinal cord injury pain: a randomized controlled trial. *Anesthesiology* 2005; **102:** 1023–30.

135. Kaba A, Laurent SR, Detroz BJ, *et al.* Intravenous lidocaine infusion facilitates acute rehabilitation after laparoscopic colectomy. *Anesthesiology* 2007; **106:** 11–18.

136. Palmeri TL, Greenhalgh DG. Topical treatment of pediatric patients with burns: a practical guide. *Am J Clin Derm* 2002; **3:** 529–34.

137. Spierings ELH, Brevard JA, Katz NP. Two-minute skin anesthesia through ultrasound pretreatment and iontophoretic delivery of a topical anesthetic: a feasibility study. *Pain Med* 2008; **9:** 55–9.

138. Mofenson HC, Caraccio TR, Miller H, Greensher J. Lidocaine toxicity from topical mucosal application. *Clin Pediatr* 1983; **22:** 190–2.

139. Dasta J, Ramamoorthy S, Patou G, Sinatra R Bupivacaine liposome injectable suspension compared with bupivacaine HCl for the reduction of opioid burden in the postsurgical

setting. *Curr Med Res Opin* 2012; **28**: 1609–15.

140. Hu D, Onel E, Singla N, Kramer WG, Hadzic A. Pharmacokinetic profile of liposome bupivacaine injection following a single administration at the surgical site. *Clin Drug Investig* 2013; **33**: 109–15.

141. Paneral AE, Monza G, Movilia P, Francucci BM, Tiengo M. A randomized within-patient crossover placebo-controlled trial on the efficacy and tolerability of the tricyclic antidepressants chlorimipramine and nortryptyline in central pain. *Acta Neurol Scand* 1990; **82**: 34–8.

142. Carter GT, Sullivan MD. Antidepressants in pain management. *Curr Opin Investig Drugs* 2002; **3**: 454–8.

143. Vieweg WVR, Weed MA. Tricyclic antidepressants, QT interval prolongation and torsade de pointes. *Psychosomatics* 2004; **45**: 371–7.

144. Ray W, Meredith S, Thapa PB, Hall K, Murray KT. Cyclic antidepressants and the risk of sudden cardiac death. *Clin Pharm Ther* 2004; **75**: 234–41.

145. Cappell MS. Colonic toxicity of administered drugs and chemicals. *Am J Gastroenterol* 2004; **99**: 1175–90.

146. Hayes JR, Bojral S, McCarthy MC. Gastrointestinal effects of tricyclic antidepressants: Ogilvie's syndrome. *Psychosomatics* 1987; **28**: 442–3.

147. Attal N, Cruccu G, Haanpaa M et al. EFNS guidelines in pharmacological treatment of neuropathic pain. *Eur J Neurol* 2006; **13**: 1153–69.

148. Orii R, Obashi Y, Haldar S, et al. GABAergic interneurons at supraspinal and spinal levels differentially modulate the antinociceptive effects of nitrous oxide in Fischer rats. *Anesthesiology* 2003; **98**: 1223–30.

149. Gottrup H, Juhl G, Kristensen AD, et al. Chronic oral gabapentin reduces elements of central sensitization in human experimental hyperalgesia. *Anesthesiology* 2004; **101**: 1400–8.

150. Sihoe AD, Lee TW, Wan IY, Thung KH, Yim AP. The use of gabapentin for post-operative and post-traumatic pain in thoracic surgery patients. *Eur J Cardiothorac Surg* 2006; **29**: 795–9.

151. Coderre TJ, Kumar N, Lefebvre CD, Yu JS. Evidence that gabapentin reduces neuropathic pain by inhibiting the spinal release of glutamate. *J Neurochem* 2005; **94**: 1131–9.

152. Seib RK, Paul JE. Preoperative gabapentin for postoperative analgesia: Meta-analysis. *Can J Anaesth* 2006; **53**: 461–9.

153. Gilron I, Bailey JM, Tu D, et al. Morphine, gabapentin or their combination for neuropathic pain. *N Engl J Med* 2005; **352**: 1324–34.

154. Gilron I. The role of anticonvulsant drugs in postoperative pain management: A bench to bedside perspective. *Can J Anaesth* 2006; **53**: 562–71.

155. Dahl JB, Mathiesen O, Moiniche S. "Protective premedication": an option with gabapentin and related drugs? A review of gabapentin and pregabalin in the treatment of post-operative pain. *Acta Anaesthesiol Scand* 2004; **48**: 1130–6.

156. Pandey A, Feltner D, Jefferson J, et al. Efficacy of the novel anxiolytic pregabalin in social anxiety disorders: a placebo-controlled, multicenter study. *J Clin Psychopharmacol* 2004; **24**: 141–9.

157. Beghi E. Efficacy and tolerability of the new antiepileptic drugs: comparison of two recent guidelines. *Lancet Neurol* 2004; **3**: 618–21.

158. MacPherson RD. The pharmacological basis of contemporary pain management. *Pharmcol Therapeut* 2000; **88**: 163–85.

159. Khan ZP, Ferguson CN, Jones RM. Alpha-2 and imidazoline receptor agonists. *Anaesthesia* 1999; **54**: 146–65.

160. Vulliemoz Y, Virag L, Whittington RA. Interaction of alpha-2-adrenergic and opioid receptor with the cGMP system in the mouse cerebellum. *Brain Res* 1998; **813**: 26–31.

161. Xu Z, Li P, Tong C, et al. Location and characteristics of nitric oxide synthetase in sheep spinal cord and its interaction with alpha(2)-adrenergic and cholinergic anti-nociception. *Anesthesiology* 1996; **84**: 890–9.

162. Bernard JM, Hommeril JL, Passuti N, Pinaud M. Postoperative analgesia by intravenous clonidine. *Anesthesiology* 1991; **75**: 577–82.

163. Daqing M, Rajakumaraswamy N, Maze M. α$_2$-Adrenoceptor agonists: shedding light on neuroprotection? *Br Med Bull* 2005; **71**: 77–92.

164. Virtanen R, Savola JM, Sano V, Nyman L. Characterization of selectivity, specificity and potency of medetomidine as alpha-2 adrenoreceptor agonist. *Eur J Pharmacol* 1988; **150**: 9–14.

165. Arain SR, Ruehlow RM, Uhrich TD, Ebert TJ. The efficacy of dexmedetomidine versus morphine for postoperative analgesia after major inpatient surgery. *Anesth Analg* 2004; **98**: 153–8.

166. Talon MD, Woodson LC, Sherwood E, Aarsland A, McRae L. Nasal dexmedetomdine is comparable to midazolam as preoperative sedative in children. *Anesthesiology* 2007; **107**: A1398.

167. Devabhakthuni S, Pajoumand M, Williams C, et al. Evaluation of dexmedetomidine: safety and clinical outcomes in critically ill trauma patients. *J Trauma* 2011; **71**: 1164–71.

168. Lyons FM, Bew S, Sheeran P, Hall GM. Effects of clonidine on pituitary hormonal response to pelvic surgery. *Br J Anaesth* 1997; **78**: 134–7.

169. Mukhtar AM, Obayah EM, Hassona AM. The use of dexmedetomidine in pediatric cardiac surgery. *Anesth Analg* 2006; **103**: 52–6.

170. Patterson DR, Ptacek JT, Carrougher GJ, Sharar SR. Lorezepam as an adjunct to opioid analgesics in the treatment of burn pain. *Pain* 1997; **72**: 367–74.

171. Kaabachi O, Ouezini R, Koubaa W, Ghrab B. Comparative study between mask nebulization and oral administration of midazolam in children. *Anesthesiology* 2007; **107**: A1095.

172. Scott R. Buccal midazolam as rescue therapy for acute seizures. *Lancet Neurol* 2005; **4**: 592–3.

173. Harbord MG, Kyrkou NE, Kay D, Coulthard KP. Use of intranasal midazolam to treat acute seizures in paediatric community settings. *J Paediatr Child Health* 2004; **40**: 556–8.

174. Whiting PJ. GABA-A receptor subtype in the brain: a paradigm for CNS drug delivery. *Drug Discov Today* 2003; **8**: 445–50.

175. Yaksh TL, Allen JW. The use of intrathecal midazolam in humans: a case study process. *Anesth Analg* 2004; **98**: 1536–45.

176. Goh PL, Lee SW, Goh SH. Analgesia for adult distal radius fracture manipulation in the emergency department: demand valve nitrous oxide compared with intravenous regional anaesthesia. *Hong Kong J Emerg Med* 2002; **9**: 181–7.

177. Wilson MJ, Hunter JB. Supracondylar fractures of the humerus in children-wire removal in the outpatient setting. *Injury Extra* 2006; **37**: 313–15.

178. Burm AGL. Occupational hazards of inhalational anaesthetics. *Best Pract Res Clin Anaesthesiol* 2003; **17**: 147–61.

179. Buntine P, Thom O, Babl F, Bailey M, Bernard S. Prehospital analgesia in adults using inhaled methoxyflurane. *Emerg Med Australas* 2007; **19**: 509–14.

180. Babl FE, Jamison SR, Spicer M, Bernard S. Inhaled methoxyflurane as a prehospital analgesic in children. *Emerg Med Australas* 2006; **18**: 404–10.

181. Wasiak J, Mahar PD, Paul E, *et al.* Inhaled methoxyflurane for pain and anxiety relief during burn wound care procedures: an Australian case series. *Int Wound J* 2014; **11**: 74–8.

182. Grindlay J, Babl FE. Review article: Efficacy and safety of methoxyflurane analgesia in the emergency department and prehospital setting. *Emerg Med Australas* 2009; **21**: 4–11.

183. Ziegler AW, Agarwal NN. Morbidity and mortality of rib fractures. *J Trauma* 1994; **37**: 975–9.

184. Bergeron E, Lavoie A, Clas D, *et al.* Elderly trauma patients with rib fractures are at a greater risk of death and pneumonia. *J Trauma* 2002; **54**: 478–85.

185. Schneider JC, Harris NL, El Shami A, *et al.* A descriptive review of neuropathic-like pain after burn injury. *J Burn Care Res* 2006; **27**: 524–8.

186. Jellish WS, Gamelli RL, Furry PA, McGill VL, Fluder EM. Effect of topical local anesthetic application to skin harvest sites for pain management in burn patients undergoing skin-grafting procedures. *Ann Surg* 1999; **229**: 115–20.

187. Wehner D, Hamilton GC. Seizures following application of local anesthetics to burn patients. *Ann Emerg Med* 1984; **13**: 456–8.

188. Rincon E, Bakern RL, Iglesias AJ, Duarte AM. CNS toxicity after topical application of EMLA cream with molluscum contagiosum. *Pediatr Emerg* 2000; **16**: 252–4.

189. Hahn IH, Hoffman RS, Nelson LS. EMLA induced methemogobinemia and systemic topical anesthetic toxicity. *J Emerg Med* 2004; **26**: 85–8.

190. Heinrich M, Wetzstein V, Muensterer OJ, Till H. Conscious sedation: Off label use of rectal S(+) ketamine and midazolam for wound dressing changes in paediatric heat injuries. *Eur J Pediatr Surg* 2004; **14**: 235–9.

191. Summer G, Puntillo K, Miaskowski C, Green P, Levine J. Burn injury pain: the continuing challenge. *J Pain* 2007; **8**: 533–48.

192. Baker RA, Zeller RA, Klein RL, *et al.* Burn wound itch control using H1 and H2 antagonists. *J Burn Care Rehabil* 2001; **22**: 263–8.

193. Mendham JE. Gabapentin for the treatment of itching produced by burns and wound healing in children: a pilot study. *Burns* 2004; **30**: 851–3.

194. Galinski M, Picco N, Hennequin B, *et al.* Out-of-hospital emergency medicine in pediatric patients: prevalence and management of pain. *Am J Emerg Med* 2011; **29**: 1062–6.

195. Jacob E, Puntillo KA. Variabiltiy of analgesic practices for hospitalized children on different pediatric speciality units. *J Pain Symptom Manage* 2000; **20**: 59–67.

196. Cohen SP, Christo PJ, Moroz L. Pain management in trauma patients. *Am J Phys Med Rehabil* 2004; **83**: 142–61.

197. Clark E, Plint AC, Correll R, Gaboury I, Passi B. A randomized controlled trial of acetaminophen, ibuprofen and codeine for acute pain relief in children with musculoskeletal trauma. *Pediatrics* 2007; **119**: 460–7.

198. Falanga IJ, Lafrenaye S, Mayer SK, Tetrault JP. Management of acute pain in children: safety and efficacy of a nurse-controlled algorithm for pain relief. *Acute Pain* 2006; **8**: 45–54.

199. Patterson DR, Hoffman HG, Weichman SA, Jensen MP, Sharar SR. Optimizing control of pain from severe burns: a literature review. *Am J Clin Hypn* 2004; **47**: 43–54.

200. Lang T, Barker R, Steinlechner B, *et al.* TENS relieves acute posttraumatic hip pain during emergency transport. *J Trauma* 2007; **62**: 184–8.

201. McMakin CR, Gregory WM, Phillips TM. Cytokine changes with microcurrent treatment of fibromyalgias associated with cervical spine trauma. *J Bodywork Move Ther* 2005; **9**: 169–76.

202. Ducharme J. Emergency pain management: a Canadian Association of Emergency Physicians (CAEP) consensus document. *J Emerg Med* 1994; **12**: 855–66.

Chapter

16

Regional anesthesia

Shalini Dhir, Ranjita Sharma, and Sugantha Ganapathy

Objectives

(1) Discuss the mechanisms of acute pain after trauma.

(2) Evaluate posttraumatic pain modalities.

(3) Describe the use of regional anesthesia for trauma patients, including brachial plexus blocks, epidurals, and lower limb blocks.

Introduction

Trauma is a major cause of mortality throughout the world, and pain is the most common symptom reported by patients admitted to the emergency room.[1] Specific protocols have been developed to treat all pain-related complications, such as chronic pain and posttraumatic stress disorder,[2] making anesthesiologists more involved in the management of trauma patients.[3] Improved pain management in the trauma patient not only increases comfort and reduces patient suffering but has also been demonstrated to reduce the rate of tracheal intubation and morbidity and to improve short- and long-term outcomes.[4–7]

The Joint Commission on Accreditation of Healthcare Organizations in 2001 stated that "unrelieved pain has physical and psychological effects," that the patient's right to pain management should be respected and supported, and that pain must be assessed in all patients.[8]

Effective and early pain management following trauma is important to decrease the stress response and the resulting inflammatory response, hypercoagulopathy, multiorgan dysfunction, catabolism, and posttraumatic stress syndrome.

Polytrauma involves injuries to multiple organs, often requiring emergent or urgent surgeries. The involvement of the central nervous system (CNS) and the cardiorespiratory system, as well as peripheral limbs, results in significant pain for the patient. There is inadequate time to deal with such severe pain, because of the need for life-saving surgical procedures. Caregivers are often worried about masking clinical signs of major organ injury involving the CNS, abdomen, and chest viscera. Caregivers at the emergency site or in emergency rooms may be inadequately trained on the pain management modalities that are currently available. For a long time, regional blocks were not adequately exploited in the emergency room for pain management, but the trend is currently changing.

Pain mechanisms

The stress response following multiple trauma is far greater than that after elective surgery.[9] Activation of the hypothalamic–pituitary–adrenal (HPA) axis and the sympathoadrenal system (SAS), with the release of cortisol and catecholamines, activation of the renin–angiotensin system, impaired coagulation, and altered immune response, accounts for major portions of mortality, morbidity, and cost in trauma patients.[10] Untreated pain may additionally contribute to an undesirable neuroendocrine response. Peripheral inflammation causes induction of cyclooxygenase-2 (COX-2),[11] leading to release of prostanoids that sensitize peripheral nociceptive terminals and produce localized pain hypersensitivity.[12] In the acute phase, this includes release of substances such as serotonin, bradykinin, hydrogen ions, potassium, and acute-phase reactants, causing excitation of afferent fibers. These fibers converge on the substantia gelatinosa, where spinal antinociceptive modulation is expected to occur. Increased pain impulses arriving at the substantia gelatinosa, as well as expanded expression of nociceptive input from Aβ fibers, result in spinal cord wind-up. Wind-up refers to an increase in pain sensitivity and intensity over time. This is a frequency-dependent increase in the excitability of spinal cord neurons, evoked by repeated stimulation of afferent C fibers. Peripheral inflammation also generates pain hypersensitivity in neighboring uninjured tissue (secondary hyperalgesia). There is substantial evidence that rostral ventromedial medulla (RVM) on cells may be responsible for contributing to the descending facilitatory influences that result in secondary hyperalgesia in persistent pain states[13] and increased neuronal excitability in the spinal cord (central sensitization) (Fig. 16.1).[14,15]

Apart from this route of spinal excitation, release of cytokines such as interleukin 1β (IL-1β) results in increased expression of COX-2 receptors and messenger RNA in the spinal cord. Release of mediators such as cytokines, purines, leukotrienes, neuropeptides, nitric oxide, and nerve growth factors may contribute to the chronic pain state by forcing the spinal cord into a state of hyperexcitability sustained by intrinsic mechanisms.[16]

Untreated pain can increase the adverse effects that trauma has on normal physiologic functions such as ventilation, hemodynamics, and gastrointestinal and renal function. Further compromise of these already impaired functions can result in increased mortality and morbidity.[17]

Whipple *et al.* assessed pain treatment in patients with multiple trauma wounds, and found that although 81% of nurses and 95% of house staff considered pain to be adequately managed, 74% of patients rated their pain as moderate or severe.[18] Adequate treatment of pain in trauma patients has been shown to reduce morbidity and improve short- and long-term outcomes.[19–21] Thus, it is important to manage pain after trauma adequately. Most studies involving trauma patients are based on surgical trauma, and care must be taken in extrapolating these findings to patients involved in accidental trauma. Nevertheless, it is becoming increasingly apparent that the proper treatment of pain is essential to optimize outcomes in trauma victims.[22]

Posttraumatic pain therapies

An ideal method of pain management is one that is safe and simple, provides predicable analgesia, and does not interfere with respiration or hemodynamics (Table 16.1). While many patients with multiple injuries, especially those with severe head or thoracic injuries, require endotracheal intubation and deep sedation, patients with isolated extremity injuries are often stable, awake, and sufficiently ventilating. Patients with traumatic injuries often require multiple physical examinations, diagnostic imaging studies, and treatment procedures

Table 16.1 Desired characteristics of an ideal analgesic technique in trauma

Safe
Simple
Predictable
Extended analgesia
Minimal hemodynamic disturbance
Minimal respiratory disturbance
No interference with neurological monitoring
High degree of patient acceptance
Minimal complications
Reduces chronic pain
Economical
Minimal effect on immunity

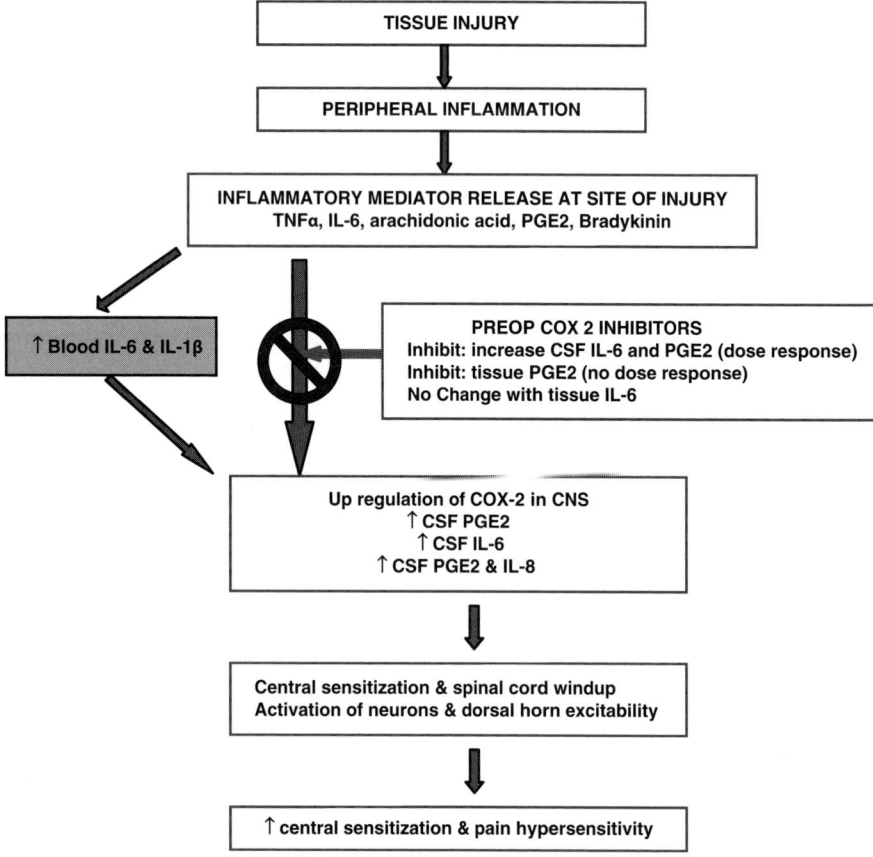

Figure 16.1 Diagrammatic representation of pain modulation with injury. (Modified from: Samad TA, Moore KA, Sapirstein A, *et al.* Interleukin-1 beta-mediated induction of COX-2 in the CNS contributes to inflammatory pain hypersensitivity. *Nature* 2001; 410: 471–5; Buvanendran A, Kroin JS, Berger RA, *et al.* Upregulation of prostaglandin E2 and interleukins in the central nervous system and peripheral tissue during and after surgery in humans. *Anesthesiology* 2006; **104**: 403–10.)

during their stay in the emergency room. Such care requires multiple transports from one location to another, as well as multiple patient transfers from the stretcher to the x-ray table to the examination table, all of which can cause severe discomfort and necessitate pain relief.

The most common approach to pain management in trauma patients in the civilian emergency room is the use of intravenous (IV) opioids. This approach has advantages and disadvantages and is primarily based on the perception of quick and easy application compared with performing regional anesthesia. Trauma patients typically have IV access placed early on in the course of their emergency care, thereby facilitating this primary route of pain treatment.

In addition, many trauma patients have multiple injuries, making such systemic pain relief more applicable than regional anesthesia. Another barrier to regional anesthesia as the primary pain control method in the emergency department is the required training and expertise of the physician who is performing the procedure, including the availability of equipment and experienced providers such as anesthesiologists.

Many trauma patients in the emergency room often require not only background analgesia, but also additional sedation/analgesia to facilitate therapeutic procedures such as wound suturing, foreign body removal, fracture or joint reduction, cast application, or specialized examinations. While it is common practice to use local anesthetic infiltration or field blocks for closing small wounds, patients with more complicated injuries or who require more complex interventions often receive a combination of IV opioids and benzodiazepines.

If such brief sedation is neither feasible nor sufficient to facilitate the procedure, patients may require treatment in the operating room, where they may receive general anesthesia or regional anesthesia by an anesthesiologist. Since the patient must ideally be NPO for several hours prior to general anesthesia or deep sedation, in an effort to reduce aspiration risk, significant delays can result, prolonging the time the patient must stay in the emergency room while consuming precious space and staff resources.

Titration of IV opioids and sedatives can be challenging in trauma patients. Common side effects include hypotension, respiratory depression, nausea, and vomiting. Moderate sedation, deep sedation, and general anesthesia all require more intense cardiorespiratory and neurologic monitoring, both during the procedure and in the postprocedure recovery period, compared with patients undergoing regional anesthesia.

While patients undergoing regional anesthesia still require monitoring, the need for more intense monitoring for potentially fatal opioid-induced respiratory depression is lessened. In the emergency room, where nursing staff may sometimes care for several patients simultaneously, it is often not possible to closely monitor patients to the same intensity as they are monitored in a post-anesthesia care unit. Further complicating hemodynamic assessments in this setting, patients with multiple trauma, including long-bone fractures, can have significant occult blood loss.

Many trauma patients, especially young patients, are able to compensate for blood loss through vasoconstriction, a subtle decrease in blood pressure, and an increase in heart rate. However, administration of sedatives or opioids in such patients can cause profound vasodilatation and diminish the body's compensatory mechanisms for blood loss, resulting in severe and unexpected hypotension. As an alternative to IV analgesia and sedation, regional anesthesia offers potential advantages in this setting (Table 16.2).

While not all trauma patients are candidates for regional anesthesia, selected patients may benefit from regional anesthesia as either the primary or the adjunctive secondary mode of background pain treatment, or for procedural pain relief.

Table 16.2 Advantages and limitations of regional anesthesia

Advantages	Limitations/disadvantages
Opioid-sparing/eliminating	Need for trained personnel
↓ Nausea	Need for special equipment
↓ Paralytic ileus	Time required to initiate
↓ Immunosuppression	Possible difficulty in positioning
Improved dynamic pain relief	Neurostimulation pain
↓ Blood loss	Local anesthetic toxicity
↓ Incidence of thromboembolism	Possible failure
↓ Monitoring intensity	Nerve injuries
↓ Sedation	Diaphragm weakness
↓ Resources	Pneumothorax
↓ Phantom limb pain	Motor weakness
↓ Recrudescence of CRPS	Catheter malfunction
↓ Chronic pain syndromes	? Masking compartment syndrome
↓ Vasospasm	↓ Mobility with lower limb block
↓ Pulmonary morbidity	
↓ Cognitive dysfunction	
↓ Infective complications	
Fetomaternal safety	
Economical	
Extendable	
Smooth transitional analgesia	
Improved patient satisfaction	
Early discharge/bypass PACU	
Home regional possible	

CRPS, complex regional pain syndrome; PACU, post-anesthesia care unit.

While various regional techniques have been practiced for decades in the perioperative surgical setting, they are often underutilized in many anesthesia departments, and even more so in emergency departments. This may be due to the shortage of trained providers capable of performing regional anesthesia techniques, or to a lack of knowledge regarding the usage of these techniques and/or equipment.

Regional anesthesia offers some flexibility with respect to the duration of pain relief that can be obtained. Depending on the specific local anesthetic chosen, a single-shot peripheral nerve block or even infiltration anesthesia (i.e., field block) can provide analgesia both during and after a procedure for periods ranging from approximately 2 to 12 hours. In addition, a correctly placed nerve block catheter and the use of continuous infusion of local anesthetics can provide analgesia for several days, facilitating multiple examinations, transport, and physical rehabilitation by keeping the patient pain-free.

Peripheral nerve block catheters have been shown to be especially useful for repeated surgical procedures, as they can be dosed repeatedly, avoiding the need for the patient to undergo multiple general anesthetics or repeated needle sticks for serial nerve block procedures. While many techniques for regional anesthesia can be performed after brief training and practice (e.g., field block), other techniques such as nerve plexus blocks require specialized training and considerable experience, and should preferably be performed by anesthesiologists trained in regional anesthesia.

Furthermore, some regional techniques carry particular safety risks and require a back-up plan and equipment to induce general anesthesia and secure the airway in case of an emergency. The American Society of Anesthesiologists (ASA) has developed guidelines for providing such care in non-operating-room anesthetizing locations, including when nerve block procedures are being performed in the emergency room.[23]

Compared to deep sedation by IV sedatives and opioids, regional anesthesia has a superior safety profile and a more predictable effect, especially in hypovolemic patients or in patients with a history of drug or alcohol abuse. In patients abusing illicit drugs or prescription opioids, the amount of opioid analgesia required to treat these patients is unpredictable, resulting in either undertreated patients or patients who receive far more opioids than they actually require.

The latter group is particularly at risk for respiratory compromise due to airway obstruction and/or depression of respiratory drive. A successful regional nerve block procedure in these patients achieves decreased motor and sensory function that is not affected by previous substance abuse, will generally not affect respiratory drive, and will give excellent pain relief even in patients tolerant to high doses of opioids.

A peripheral nerve block also offers advantages in extremity-injured patients who require frequent neurological evaluation, such as patients with concomitant head or spinal cord trauma. In contrast to systemic sedatives, which can complicate the evaluation of neurological function, a peripheral nerve block can be applied to a single limb or body region to facilitate such evaluations.

In a German study of 100 patients with acute femoral fractures receiving either a femoral nerve block or IV analgesia, significant pain relief was achieved in both groups; however, the global pain scores in the regional anesthesia group were significantly lower than in the IV analgesia group.[24]

Prehospital and emergency room management in adult trauma

The primary aim during the acute treatment of patients with traumatic injuries is to stabilize vital functions, diagnose life-threatening conditions, avoid worsening of injuries, and facilitate transport to Level I trauma centers (see Chapter 2). Most often, pain management takes a low priority in such a scenario. Ideally, after resuscitation, airway control, cervical spine immobilization (if indicated), and vascular access, pain management should begin.

Pain control procedures may include simple measures such as rewarming, communication, fracture splinting, and oxygenation, as well as pharmacologic agents given systemically.

Prehospital pain management

Regional analgesia can benefit a patient in the prehospital setting if patients are selected appropriately and a correct technique is chosen. In a trauma patient with crush injuries, fractures, and burns limited to a limb, nerve blocks can provide an attractive pain management alternative to systemic opioids without hemodynamic instability. A baseline neurologic examination is mandatory to rule out any neurologic contraindications to regional anesthesia.

For upper limb injuries, the brachial plexus can be blocked at various locations depending on the site of injury. A portable nerve stimulator or ultrasound is needed for a high degree of success. The axillary approach is easy and free from hazardous side effects such as pneumothorax, and has been used to provide effective analgesia such as when the arm is trapped in machinery.

In France, the femoral nerve block is extremely popular in the prehospital setting because it is simple, quick, and safe.[25] It has become routine for transport of adult and pediatric patients with fractured femoral shafts and is being taught to the majority of physicians involved in prehospital care.

Other distal nerve blocks such as ankle, digital, or wrist are possible but not usually put into practice. Intercostal nerve blocks are helpful in the prehospital setting to relieve pain in thoracic trauma and reduce opioid requirements. There is a potential risk of pneumothorax as well as local anesthetic toxicity due to rapid absorption.

Interpleural analgesia is also useful, especially when a chest tube is already in situ. Because of the need for spinal column protection, neuraxial blocks are not an option at the triage site, although they may be considered once the patient is in the hospital.

Personnel performing these blocks must be appropriately trained and have adequate experience in a hospital setting before attempting blocks in a field setting. After the block, the limb needs to be immobilized and padded to avoid fracture displacement and further trauma during transport.

Regional anesthesia: concerns in trauma patients

Informed consent

Obtaining informed consent may be challenging due to various factors such as distressed patient and altered sensorium. Since peripheral nerve blocks offer substantial benefits, alternative paths to obtaining consent may be indicated.

If patients are not able to provide consent, one of the following options may prove feasible:

- Obtain consent from a proxy or family member.
- Consider a two-physician consent in emergency cases, should benefits of regional blockade be expected to be substantial.
- Postpone peripheral nerve block procedure until consent can be obtained.

Hemodynamic instability

Depending upon the type and site of injury, there can be substantial hemodynamic instability in trauma patients. In such scenarios, the addition of a regional anesthetic can further contribute to hypotension, especially if the technique is associated with extensive sympathectomy.

Regional blockade can also unmask relative hypovolemia by blunting the patient's normal sympathomimetic stress response.

The following strategy appears appropriate in cases of existing hemodynamic instability or suspected hypovolemia:

- Avoid neuraxial blockade.
- Select a peripheral nerve block technique with no or low risk of significant sympathectomy.
- If circumstances allow, normalize the patient's volume status.

Coagulation status

There are well-recognized guidelines from the American Society of Regional Anesthesia and Pain Medicine (ASRA) regarding the performance of neuraxial regional anesthetic techniques in patients receiving prophylactic or therapeutic anticoagulation.[26] However, relatively little is known regarding the use of regional anesthetic techniques in patients in whom the coagulation status has been altered by trauma and significant blood loss requiring aggressive fluid replacement.

In such scenarios the following precautions should be considered:

- Carefully weigh benefits of regional anesthesia versus risks of hematoma formation.
- Consider using ultrasound to decrease the risk of accidental puncture of blood vessels adjacent to nerve structures.
- Consider choosing "shallow" nerve block approaches over "deeper" techniques to allow for the ability to compress the site in case of accidental puncture of blood vessels.
- Consider application of ASRA guidelines for any nerve block catheter in close proximity to the spine (e.g., lumbar plexus or paravertebral nerve block) in order to avoid untoward outcomes, such as epidural hematoma formation.

Traumatic nerve injury

Occasionally, a trauma patient will present with traumatic nerve injuries. This may complicate the decision to perform a regional anesthetic technique, since the question may later arise whether nerve damage preexisted or was caused or exacerbated by the regional anesthetic.

A strategic approach to balance these concerns includes the following:

- Examine patient for preexisting nerve damage prior to performing a regional anesthesia technique.
- Review surgical notes for evidence of nerve injury.
- Document discussion with person providing consent, any abnormal findings and discussion with surgical colleagues (in case of discrepancy between your assessment and their findings).
- Do not perform regional technique if patient has signs of neuraxial or complex plexus injury.

Risk of infection

Infection and sepsis are feared complications in any severely injured patient. The anesthesiologist should take careful precautions in order to minimize the risk of infection, as follows:

- Use aseptic technique for any single-shot technique, and full barrier precautions for any continuous catheter placement.
- Do not introduce nerve block needles or place continuous catheters in areas where the skin is not intact.

Compartment syndrome

Of great concern to orthopedic surgeons is the development of a compartment syndrome. For early detection and timely intervention, surgeons rely on the patient as a monitor to alert healthcare personnel by reporting significant ischemic pain in the involved extremity.

Consequently, surgeons have expressed significant concerns over whether peripheral nerve blocks, especially nerve block catheters, may mask a compartment syndrome. Similar concerns were raised when other advances in perioperative pain management, such as patient-controlled analgesia (PCA), were introduced into clinical practice.

However, ischemic pain is usually not well controlled by peripheral nerve blockade. Indeed, discrepancies between an apparently functioning nerve block and new-onset patient complaints of pain have frequently alerted the medical staff to a developing underlying problem.

There is no convincing evidence that PCA opioids or regional analgesia delay the diagnosis of compartment syndrome, provided patients are adequately monitored. Regardless of the type of analgesia used, a high index of clinical suspicion, ongoing assessment of patients, and compartment pressure measurement are essential for early diagnosis.[27]

Suggestions to address the concerns of performing peripheral nerve blocks in patients at risk for compartment syndrome are as follows:

- Identify patients at risk together with the surgical colleagues.
- Educate colleagues regarding ischemic pain.
- Consider additional methods of monitoring such as measurement of compartment pressures.
- Consider short-acting local anesthetics for the initial block, place a nerve block catheter, and infuse with normal saline (this will create a "free interval" to allow for assessment). After surgical clearance (e.g., 24 hours postoperative), bolus catheter with local anesthetic and start local anesthetic infusion.
- If the peripheral nerve is blocked with long-acting local anesthetic or a nerve block catheter is placed in patients at risk, notify the surgeon immediately if there is new onset of pain or apparent discrepancy between expected and achieved levels of pain control.

Regional techniques in trauma (see also Chapter 12)

Upper limb nerve blocks

Nerve plexus blocks take advantage of anatomic locations where peripheral nerves are grouped closely together before they divide into smaller branches innervating the extremities. Thus, a plexus block enables the physician to completely anesthetize a selected extremity with a smaller and safer amount of local anesthetic. Depending on the choice of local anesthetic, the pain relief from a single-shot procedure can last up to 12 hours. Since the plexus block anesthetizes all innervating nerves into an extremity, this technique can provide excellent pain relief for even the most severe extremity injuries (e.g., amputation). The plexus block can also be augmented by placement of a catheter to provide long-term analgesia by a continuous infusion of local anesthetic.

A variety of brachial plexus blocks can be used to anesthetize the upper extremity. The brachial plexus is formed by the ventral rami of the spinal nerves arising from C5 to T1, with minor contribution from C4 and T2. Moving in a distal fashion, the spinal nerves first coalesce into trunks, then separate into divisions, and subsequently reorganize as cords high in the axilla. The cords then form the named terminal nerves lower in the axilla (radial, median, ulnar, axillary and musculocutaneous nerves). In relation to the brachial artery at this level, the radial nerve lies posterior, the median nerve lies lateral, and the ulnar nerve lies medial. These relationships to the artery may, however, change with arm position. The brachial plexus is typically blocked at one of four anatomic locations: interscalene, supraclavicular, infraclavicular, or axillary regions.

Interscalene brachial plexus block

The interscalene approach to the brachial plexus can anesthetize the entire upper extremity, but is most suitable for procedures above the elbow since the lower cervical nerves can easily be missed, resulting in a failed ulnar nerve block.

Indications

- soft tissue injuries of the upper arm or shoulder
- reduction of humerus fractures
- shoulder dislocations
- acromioclavicular joint repair
- clavicle fractures

Anatomy

The nerves are quite superficial (only 1–2 cm deep) between the anterior and middle scalene muscles, just behind the posterior border of the sternocleidomastoid muscle. The nerves at this location may have a dural sheath that can lead to epidural extension of the drug. They have scanty connective tissue, and therefore the incidence of nerve damage is high in this location. The phrenic nerve and the cervical sympathetic chain both are close by, and it is possible to block these with large volumes of local anesthetics.

Technique

With the patient in a supine position and the head slightly turned towards the contralateral side, the brachial plexus is identified with the ultrasound probe in the following fashion. A transverse (short-axis) view can be obtained with a depth of 3 cm and frequency of 12–15 MHz. The probe is placed parallel to the clavicle at the level of the cricoid cartilage. Scanning from medial to lateral will identify the carotid artery, the internal jugular vein, the sternocleidomastoid muscle, the anterior scalene muscle, the nerve roots (hypoechoic), and the middle scalene muscle (Fig. 16.2).

The vertebral artery, which is normally visualized below C6, also appears hypoechoic. Color flow may be used to distinguish the artery from the nerve roots. If the nerve root visualization appears difficult, a scan of the supraclavicular region can be utilized to identify the divisions of the brachial plexus lateral to the subclavian artery (grouping of small hyperechoic circles with hypoechoic centers, often described as a bunch of grapes). The divisions of the brachial plexus can be followed in a cephalad direction until the nerve roots are

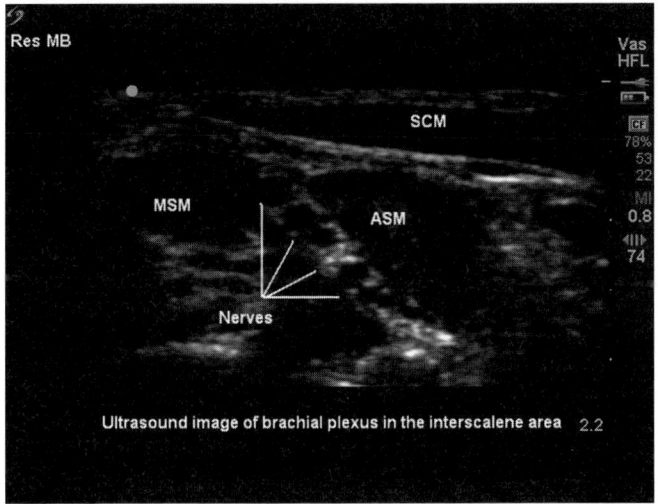

Ultrasound image of brachial plexus in the interscalene area 2.2

Figure 16.2 Interscalene block for shoulder surgery. ASM, anterior scalene muscle; MSM, middle scalene muscle; SCM, sternocleidomastoid muscle.

identified. Individual nerve roots can be confirmed with nerve stimulation. The usual volume of local anesthetic is between 10 and 25 mL.

Special considerations in trauma

- The interscalene approach commonly results in paresis of the ipsilateral phrenic nerve, and it may be contraindicated in patients with respiratory problems from other injuries.
- Possible paresis of the recurrent laryngeal nerve will result in hoarseness, and an ipsilateral sympathetic block can produce Horner's syndrome (ptosis, miosis, anhydrosis, and unilateral conjunctival engorgement of the face on the same side). The resulting anisocoria can raise diagnostic confusion in the emergency room, particularly in patients with traumatic brain injury.
- For optimal block performance, one needs to rotate the neck to the contralateral side, which may not be possible in patients with neck trauma or cervical spine injury necessitating an off-plane approach when using ultrasound.
- A fractured clavicle may also distort the anatomy in this area, making traditional techniques more difficult to use. The fracture or its surgical management may also be associated with arterial injury[28] or neurological injury,[29] as well as with air embolism.[30]
- Accidental intravascular injection or epidural/intrathecal spread may be particularly undesirable in a hemodynamically unstable patient.
- Swelling at the site of the block as well as skin lacerations may make fixation of the catheter more difficult and increase the potential for catheter infection.
- A previously placed central venous catheter (e.g., internal jugular vein) on the side to be blocked may impede the interscalene block insertion.

Supraclavicular block

With the advent of ultrasound, this block has regained popularity because of the proximity of the plexus to the skin and the relatively small volumes of local anesthetic required to block the entire arm. All divisions of the brachial plexus are in close proximity, resulting in a fast-onset dense arm block.

Indications

Surgical procedures of the upper arm, elbow, forearm, and hand.

Anatomy

The divisions of the brachial plexus and the subclavian artery lie superior to the first rib and are located posterior and lateral to the artery. The subclavian vein lies medial to the artery and is separated by the anterior scalene muscle. The pleura is located inferior and posterior to the plexus and can be as close as 1–2 cm.

Technique

A transverse (short-axis) view can be obtained with a depth setting of 4 cm and a frequency of 12–15 MHz with the patient supine and the head turned to the contralateral side (Fig. 16.3). The probe is placed in the supraclavicular fossa. After identifying the subclavian artery, the divisions of the brachial plexus can be seen just lateral to the artery. The approach is in a lateral-to-medial direction with an in-plane technique as it is critical to have real-time visualization of the needle tip to avoid accidental pleural puncture. The usual volume of local anesthetic is 20–30 mL. It is important to do a pre-procedure scan and use color Doppler to identify vessels.

Special considerations in trauma

- If the patient already has a drained pneumothorax on the ipsilateral side, the risk with this block is not exaggerated.
- If the patient has a contralateral chest injury, there is increased risk of pneumothorax in the uninjured lung.
- Ultrasound visualization can become difficult and painful in the presence of a clavicle or rib fracture.
- Stone et al. described a series of supraclavicular brachial plexus blocks performed under ultrasound guidance by emergency medicine physicians for procedures where procedural sedation would usually have been performed, but either could not be safely performed or would have delayed care. The authors reported excellent pain control and procedural ease without associated complications, and concluded that an ultrasound-guided supraclavicular brachial plexus block is a useful alternative to procedural sedation.[31]

Infraclavicular block

Indications

Surgical procedures of the upper arm, elbow, forearm and hand.

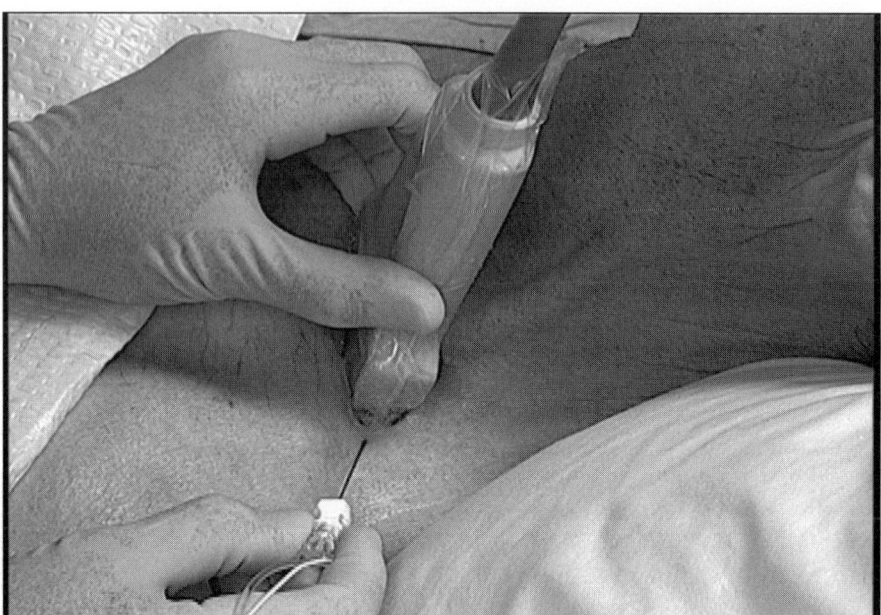

Figure 16.3 Ultrasound-guided supraclavicular block. *A black and white version of this figure will appear in some formats. For the color version, please refer to the plate section.*

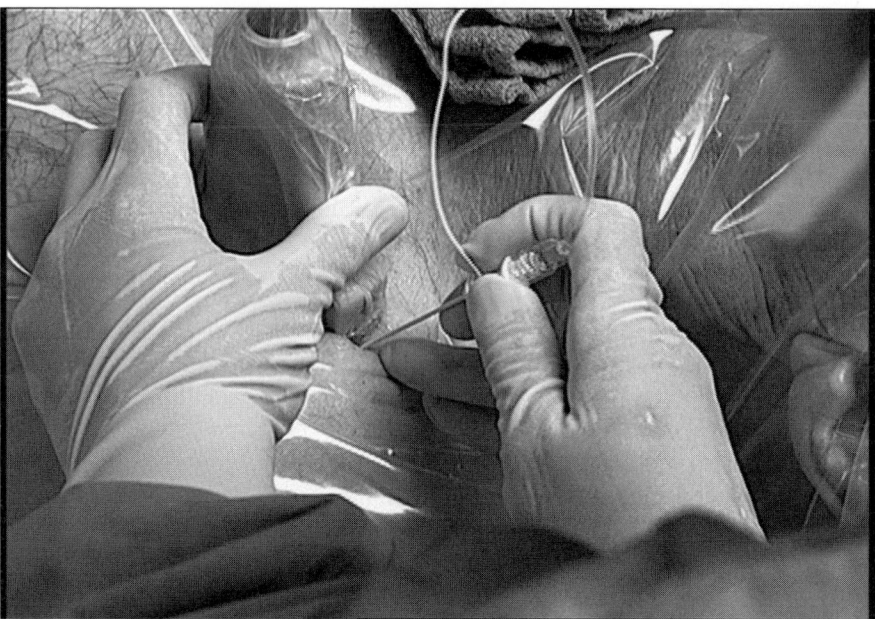

Figure 16.4 Ultrasound-guided infraclavicular block. *A black and white version of this figure will appear in some formats. For the color version, please refer to the plate section.*

Anatomy

The infraclavicular block is performed below the clavicle, where the axillary vessels and the cords of the brachial plexus lie deep to the pectoralis muscles, just inferior and slightly medial to the coracoid process. The three cords – lateral, medial, and posterior – surround the axillary artery and are named for their usual position relative to the axillary artery.

Technique

The block is performed with the patient in a supine position. The head is turned away from the side to be blocked. This block is particularly advantageous if arm abduction is not possible. Scanning usually begins just medial to the coracoid process and inferior to the clavicle (Fig. 16.4). The probe transducer is positioned in the parasagittal plane to identify the axillary artery. The axillary artery is typically seen at between 3 and 5 cm depth. The needle is inserted in plane from the cephalad aspect, with the insertion point just inferior to the clavicle. The needle is aimed towards the posterior aspect of the artery and passes through the pectoralis major and minor muscles. The injectate should spread cephalad and caudad to cover the lateral and medial cords in a "U" shape around the artery.

Special considerations in trauma

- The infraclavicular area is particularly convenient to initiate a continuous catheter block, requiring minimal or no movement of the injured arm.
- The risk of pneumothorax is significantly less with this approach (compared to the supraclavicular approach).
- This block also lends itself to more secure catheter fixation as well as the use of ultrasound for initiation of the block.
- This block can also be used for managing the complex regional pain syndrome of the upper limb following trauma.
- The infraclavicular approach is quite useful in the trauma patient, especially with cervical spine injury, as it can be performed with the head and neck in the neutral position.
- There is no impairment of respiratory function, as there is reduced incidence of phrenic nerve involvement.

Axillary block

Although axillary block was once considered the least successful approach to the brachial plexus, ultrasound and multi-stimulation techniques have made this an attractive option for hand and forearm trauma.

Indications

Procedures on the forearm and hand.

Anatomy

The terminal branches of the brachial plexus are blocked at this level. The median, ulnar, and radial nerves surround the axillary artery. The musculocutaneous nerve is visualized in the belly of the coracobrachialis muscle. Multiple anatomical variations in terms of nerve location in relation to the axillary artery have been described. Use of a peripheral nerve stimulator (PNS) may help confirm the identity of the nerve.

Technique

With the patient in a supine position and the arm abducted to 90 degrees, the probe is placed perpendicular to the arm as high as possible in the axilla. A short-axis view can be obtained with a frequency of 12–15 MHz at a depth of 3 cm. Nerves may have a round or oval shape and may have a honeycomb appearance (Fig. 16.5). Identification of the axillary vein by relieving pressure on the probe is important to prevent accidental intravascular injection. Nerve identity can be confirmed by electrical stimulation. A total of 5–10 mL of local anesthetic around each nerve should provide adequate surgical anesthesia.

Special considerations in trauma

- Because the artery is in a compressible location, use of this block is particularly attractive in a patient with coagulopathy.
- This block may be difficult in the presence of vascular injury or graft in the axillary area.

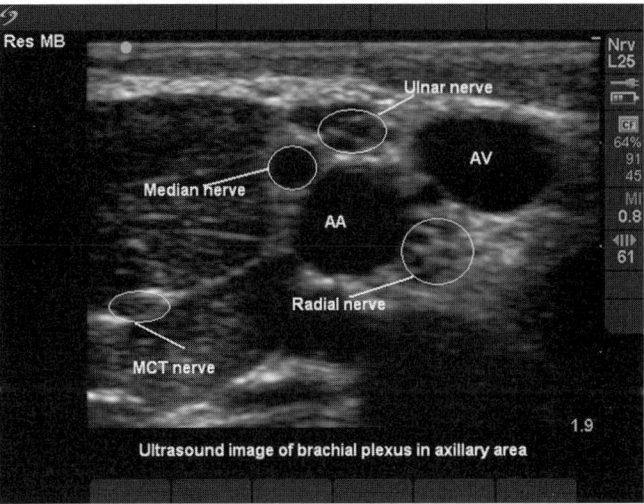

Figure 16.5 Ultrasound image of axillary area. AA, axillary artery; AV, axillary vein; MCT, musculocutaneous.

- There is a need to abduct the arm and manipulate its position, which may not be possible in certain cases.
- Compared with other brachial plexus techniques, the axillary approach does not carry the risk of pneumothorax or Horner's syndrome. However, it does require higher volumes of local anesthetics.

Blocks at the elbow

Indications

Hand procedures. May be used to supplement incomplete brachial plexus blocks.

Anatomy and technique

The three nerves that supply the hand and the cutaneous nerves that supply the forearm can be blocked at the elbow using a high-frequency ultrasound probe and a depth of 2–3 cm to obtain a short-axis view of the nerves. 5–10 mL of local anesthetic around each nerve is sufficient for a successful block.

The median nerve lies medial to the brachial artery at the elbow. The artery can be identified easily with ultrasound, and the median nerve is seen very close to it (Figs. 16.6, 16.7).

The radial nerve lies between the brachioradialis and brachialis muscles and superficial to the radial head. With the arm in flexed position at the elbow, the nerve is identified superficial to the humerus and can be blocked (Fig. 16.8).

The ulnar nerve lies within the olecranon groove. It should be blocked either proximal to the olecranon groove or over the volar aspect of the forearm, but never in the groove itself. Injection in the tight ulnar sulcus can cause pressure-induced neurapraxia and/or needle-induced nerve injury.[32] If the arm is abducted and externally rotated with the hand held in supination, key anatomical landmarks are identified easily (Fig. 16.9).

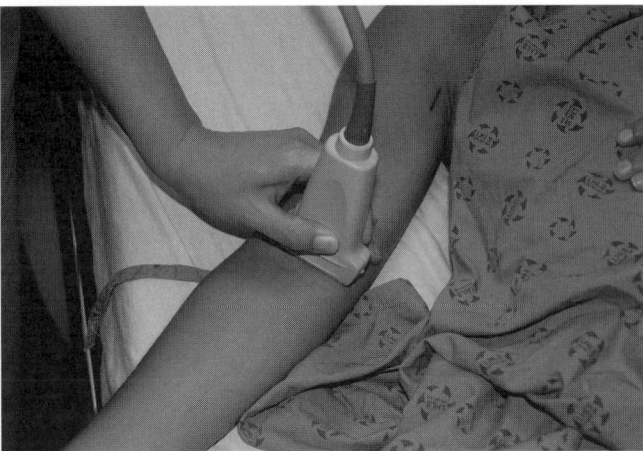

Figure 16.6 Scanning of median nerve at the elbow. *A black and white version of this figure will appear in some formats. For the color version, please refer to the plate section.*

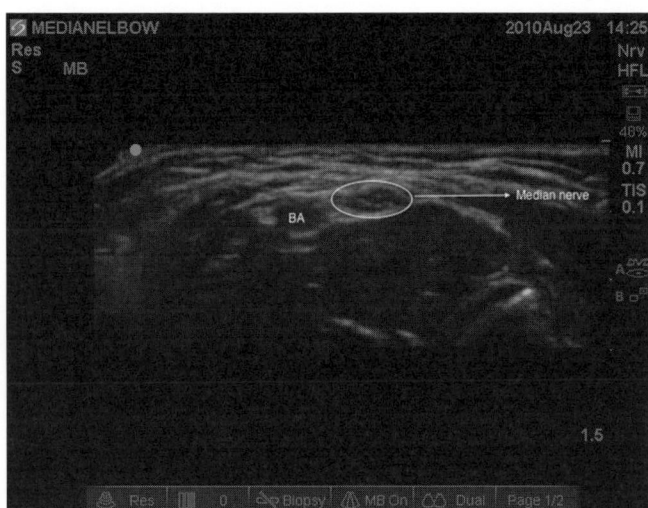

Figure 16.7 Ultrasound image of median nerve at the elbow. BA, brachial artery.

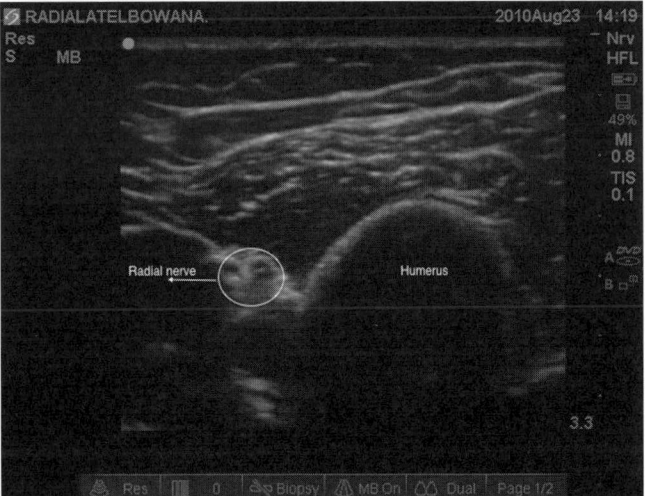

Figure 16.8 Ultrasound image of radial nerve at the elbow.

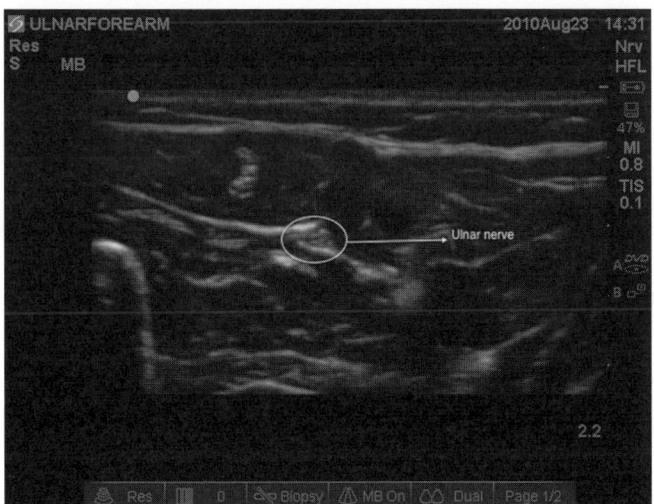

Figure 16.9 Ultrasound image of ulnar nerve in the forearm.

Special considerations in trauma

- These blocks are quite safe and easy under an ultrasound for hand injuries involving the digits.

Wrist blocks

The radial, median, and ulnar nerves can be blocked at the wrist either to supplement an incomplete block or for distal hand surgeries requiring individual nerve blocks only. Often, these techniques can be used to provide analgesia following internal fixation of digits and soft tissue injuries. Again, these blocks can be done elegantly using ultrasonography with minimal local anesthetic.

Lower limb nerve blocks

Nerve blocks of the lumbar plexus

In patients with unilateral lower limb trauma who are not candidates for epidural blockade, nerve blocks of the lumbar plexus can provide excellent pain relief for surgery of femur

fractures,[33] hip fractures,[34] tibial plateau fractures,[35] and ankle fractures.[36]

The major peripheral nerves in the lower extremity include the sciatic and femoral nerves. The sciatic nerve originates from the lumbosacral plexus and terminates in the tibial and common peroneal nerves. The sciatic nerve provides sensory innervation to the femur, posterior thigh, lateral aspect of the lower leg, ankle, and foot. It also provides articular branches to the hip, knee, and ankle. The femoral nerve originates from the lumbar plexus and terminates in the saphenous nerve. It innervates most of the femur and proximal medial tibia, all the flexors of the hip, the extensors of the knee, the muscles of the anterior compartment of the thigh, and the skin of the anterior thigh and anteromedial aspect of the lower leg. It also gives articular branches to the hip and knee joints.

Positioning may be a challenge in trauma patients when planning a posterior approach to either of these nerves. Judicious use of IV analgesics may be beneficial when positioning the patient.

Psoas compartment block

The lumbar plexus can be blocked from a posterior approach. It is also called the psoas compartment block, because the final positioning of the needle is within the body of the psoas muscle through which the lumbar plexus traverses. The most consistent approach is thought to be a block of the entire lumbar plexus with a single injection. It is useful for providing consistent anesthesia in the distributions of the femoral, lateral femoral cutaneous, and obturator nerves. The psoas compartment block reduces intraoperative blood loss, provides quality analgesia, and improves functional outcome. The block of the sacral plexus is inconsistent,[37] but allows less motor block and early ambulation.[38]

Special considerations in trauma

- Complications of this deep block include epidural spread, spinal anesthesia,[39] peritoneal injection, IV injection,[40] renal injury,[41] urinary retention, flank bleeding, and infection.
- The psoas compartment is a deep block. It can be technically challenging to perform.
- In contrast to all other peripheral blocks, this block should be treated similarly to neuraxial block with regard to coagulopathy.[26]
- Positioning for this block in a traumatized patient may be difficult.
- A peripheral nerve stimulator is required, which is uncomfortable in patients with trauma.

Continuous lumbar plexus blocks provide analgesia after a variety of operations including hip and knee arthroplasty, open reduction and internal fixation of acetabular fractures, open reduction and internal fixation of femur fractures, and anterior cruciate ligament (ACL) reconstruction.[42]

Femoral nerve block

Indications for a femoral block include analgesia for femoral shaft fractures, ACL repairs, and tibia plateau fractures. It is known to reduce pain scores.[43] It is an easy block to teach and learn, and it provides good analgesia for patients with femoral fractures.[44]

The continuous femoral nerve block provides improved analgesia after major ligament reconstructions following trauma.[45] The use of stimulating catheters has been documented to improve the accuracy of catheter placement as well as success with this block.[46] However, insertion of stimulating catheters may be painful in a traumatized patient. We use a combination of ultrasound and PNS to reduce local anesthetic requirements and improve success with this block. Motor blockade of the quadriceps may pose problems with ambulation and may predispose to falls.

Special considerations in trauma

- It is a superficial block that can be done with caution even in patients with coagulopathy.

- The patient remains supine, so the block can easily be done in suspected spine injury patients.
- It is an easy block to teach and learn.
- It provides good analgesia for patients with femoral fractures.

Fascia iliaca block

The indications for this block are the same as for the femoral nerve block, and continuous blocks have been described for analgesia after femur fracture repair, skin graft harvesting, and ACL repair. The catheter location may be unpredictable.[47] In 1989, Dalens and colleagues described this technique initially without the use of a nerve stimulator with a high success rate in anesthetized children.[48] Contrary to common belief, neither femoral nor fascia iliaca blocks anesthetize other nerves in this area predictably. Thus, a trauma patient may still perceive some pain in the areas supplied by the obturator, sciatic, and lateral femoral cutaneous nerves, and one should be prepared to provide rescue analgesia or block these nerves separately.

Saphenous nerve block

This block is often combined with a sciatic block to provide analgesia for the medial aspect of the foot in patients with ankle or forefoot fractures, and to prevent tourniquet pain. The saphenous nerve is a purely sensory nerve and does not contribute to the bony innervation of the foot. It may be blocked in the subsartorial canal, where a catheter may be inserted to provide continuous analgesia.

Sciatic nerve block

This block can be done at various levels of the sciatic nerve either anteriorly or posteriorly. Analgesia to the posterior thigh and most of the lower leg can be provided by sciatic nerve block. The posterior approach as described by Labat remains one of the most popular and reliable. The patient has to be positioned in the Sims position for initiating this block. If patient positioning is difficult because of trauma, an alternative anterior approach may be selected or the leg may be splinted. Clinical, cadaveric, and magnetic resonance imaging (MRI) studies have shown that internal rotation of the limb increases chances of success of the anterior approach by rotating the lesser femoral trochanter out of the way, allowing for accurate needle advancement.[49] The anterior approach allows one to perform a sciatic nerve block in the supine position in patients who cannot be positioned on the side with flexion of hip and knee. The inaccessibility of the sciatic nerve from the anterior approach may cause block failures in a high percentage of patients.[50] In this approach, the landmarks may be painful to palpate, and there is potential for injuring the femoral nerve as the needle is advanced toward the sciatic nerve (Fig. 16.10).

A block of the sciatic nerve before it divides in the popliteal fossa is called a popliteal sciatic block, and it is excellent for operations on the lower leg, ankle, and foot. This block allows

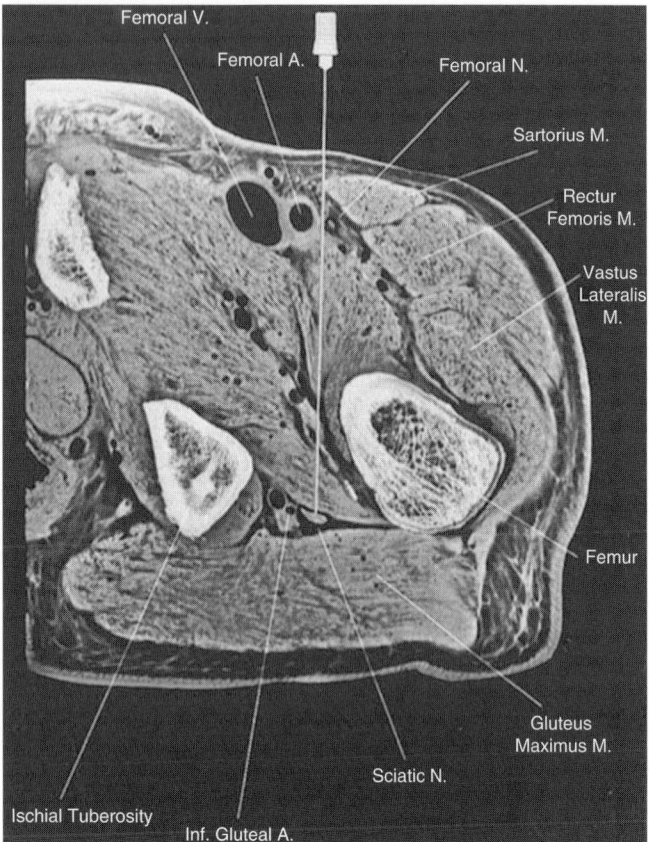

Figure 16.10 Anterior approach to sciatic nerve.

patients to ambulate using crutches as it avoids proximal hamstring motor weakness. The block has been performed bilaterally without problems.[51] Blockade of the femoral nerve or its components such as the saphenous nerve is required for analgesia of the tourniquet area and medial ankle. Continuous infusion of local anesthetic via a popliteal sciatic nerve block in an ambulatory setting for planned surgery has been shown to reduce pain scores, opioid consumption, and sleep disturbances.[52]

Ankle block

The ankle block is a combination of individual nerve blocks around the ankle and can be done easily with a low rate of complications and a high rate of success. The ultrasound-guided ankle block is a reliable and accurate anesthetic technique for forefoot surgery.[53,54] This block can be used for operations on the foot such as fracture of toes, soft tissue injuries, removal of foreign body, amputations, and debridement. It is a relatively easy and safe block to perform, but multiple punctures are involved. A single case of compartment syndrome after revision of forefoot arthroplasty under ankle block has been reported.[55] However, prompt surgical intervention prevented long-term sequelae in this case. This complication reinforces the fact that careful postoperative observation is mandatory when regional blocks are used for trauma patients.

Intravenous regional anesthesia

Intravenous regional anesthesia (IVRA) is also called Bier's block. It is simple to administer, reliable, cost-effective, and ideal for short operative procedures on extremities. Although all local anesthetic drugs have been used with good success, cardiotoxic drugs such as bupivacaine can lead to cardiovascular collapse in the emergency room when used for fracture reductions.[56] It is prudent to use drugs such as lidocaine and prilocaine for this block. Various authors have advocated addition of adjuvants such as opioids, nonsteroidal anti-inflammatory drugs (NSAIDs), tramadol, clonidine, and muscle relaxants to the local anesthetic for IVRA to improve block efficacy, decrease tourniquet pain, and prolong duration of post-deflation analgesia.[57] The use of ropivacaine 0.375% in forearm IVRA provides an effective method of anesthesia for outpatient hand surgery with superior postoperative analgesic effect compared with the use of lidocaine 0.5%, as shown in a randomized controlled trial,[58] though ropivacaine is known to have some cardiodepressant effects as well.

IVRA does require exsanguination of the limb with a tight Esmarch bandage, which may be very uncomfortable in an injured limb. It is commonly used in emergency rooms, with a high degree of success and safety. However, unplanned deflation of the tourniquet can result in local anesthetic toxicity. It is not a suitable technique for prolonged or repeated procedures. Lower limb IVRA is not commonly used, possibly because of lack of clinical experience, difficulty in locating veins in the foot/ankle, thigh tourniquet pain, and the requirement for large volumes of local anesthetic.

Fracture infiltrations

The principle of this technique is to desensitize the periosteum in the region of fracture by injection of local anesthetic into the fracture hematoma. It is a simple technique to perform. Risks include infection, rapid absorption of local anesthetic, significant increase in pressure in the carpal tunnel,[59] and neurologic complications resulting from scarring and fibrosis secondary to this increase in pressure.[60]

Head and neck nerve blocks

Various nerves can be blocked in the head and neck region for trauma-associated pain. More than 80% of patients reported good pain relief following occipital nerve blocks for post-concussion headaches.[61] Bilateral infraorbital nerve blocks have been shown to provide excellent analgesia in lip and sinus surgery,[62] and the technique can be applied to facial laceration repairs.[63] Direct infiltration of local anesthetic into the face is very painful and requires multiple injections. The entire sensory apparatus of the face is supplied by the trigeminal nerve and several cervical branches. There exist many patterns of nerve distribution anomaly, cross-innervation, and individual patient variation. However, by following basic techniques, it is possible to achieve pain control of the major dermatomes of the head and neck.[64]

The stellate ganglion block is a selective block of the cervical sympathetic chain that affects the ipsilateral head, neck, upper extremity, and upper part of thorax. Blockade of the stellate ganglion is an established and highly effective diagnostic and therapeutic procedure for management of certain acute and chronic pain syndromes of the upper limb and thorax, and for vascular insufficiency,[65] but the inability to assess the pupillary changes can confound neurologic monitoring in head-injured patients. Convulsions are a recognized complication arising from inadvertent intraarterial injection during stellate ganglion block.[66] The stellate ganglion block decreases cerebral vascular tone without affecting the capacity of cerebral blood vessels to react to the changes in carbon dioxide or to autoregulate. This may have a therapeutic role in patients where cerebral insufficiency can be attributed to cerebral vasospasm.[67] This block may be used to provide sympathetic block of the upper limb following vascular injury repairs and complex regional pain syndrome.[68]

Epidural opioids

Although it is recognized that epidural opioids are not "magic bullets," they are a significant component of contemporary prevention and treatment of postoperative pain in patients who have undergone upper abdominal or thoracic surgery and selected orthopedic procedures.[69] Typically, combinations of very low concentrations of long-acting local anesthetics with a lipid-soluble opioid provide near-ideal clinical conditions such as low pain scores, stable hemodynamics, and minimum motor block. Motor block, however little, can affect neurologic monitoring in a trauma patient. Motor function can be preserved by omitting local anesthetics from the epidural regime entirely. Local anesthetic-free, opioid-based epidural analgesia may hold this promise. However, delayed respiratory depression, pruritus, incomplete analgesia, and urinary retention must be kept in mind. Aggravation of preexisting or subclinical neurologic deficit is also possible with neuraxial intervention.[70]

Documentation of block procedure and orders

It is important to document the block procedure in a standardized format. Documentation is an excellent communication tool between caregivers. Meticulous documentation is also necessary because some trauma patients may be involved in litigation pertaining to their injury. Attorneys may critically look upon any additional injury resulting from the regional blocks. In our hospital, we use a standard form (Fig. 16.11), though electronic charting is gaining popularity worldwide. This form incorporates the risks explained, the sedation administered, the details of the procedure, and the common adverse events (such as paresthesia, pleural puncture, intravascular injection, and pain on injection). A standardized form is also used for orders (Fig. 16.12).

Specific patient considerations
Pediatric patients

Nerve blocks may be appropriate for children in an acute setting, including intercostal and interpleural blocks for chest trauma and peripheral nerve blocks for limb fractures. As patient cooperation is necessary for nerve blocks, heavy sedation and/or general anesthesia may be necessary to initiate some of the blocks (see Chapter 34).

Upper limb blocks in children can be used for laceration repairs, closed reduction, or open surgical repair. Caudal and epidural blocks are not recommended in trauma patients with lumbar spine injuries or severe dehydration. Femoral–sciatic nerve blocks have been shown to provide superior-quality analgesia and reduced opioid requirements for knee surgery in children.[71] Foot and ankle surgery in children is very painful postoperatively. Continuous popliteal nerve blocks provide excellent postoperative analgesia and are associated with less urinary retention, nausea, and vomiting compared with epidural blocks for foot and ankle surgery.[72] Continuous peripheral nerve blocks with the help of elastomeric pumps in children have been shown to provide excellent analgesia with no adverse events.[73] Greater auricular nerve blocks for ear surgery in children have been shown to provide better or equivalent parent/child satisfaction than morphine.[74] With the increasing utility of ultrasound, the placement of paravertebral blocks has increased for both intraoperative and postoperative pain relief in the pediatric population. There has been a shift from a paradigm of block placement as an alternative to neuraxial anesthesia in patients with comorbid conditions to a primary form of analgesia, with increasing success.[75,76] Despite all of these findings, application of these techniques in injured pediatric patients, unfortunately, is lacking.

The diagnosis of acute compartment syndrome in children can be challenging because of the difficulty with cooperation. The classic symptoms of compartment syndrome (five P's: pain, pressure, paresthesia, paralysis, pulselessness) may be unobtainable. Adjunctive diagnostic tests such as invasive intracranial pressure (ICP) measurement may help guide treatment. However, the entire clinical picture must be considered, especially in infants. Early fasciotomy is pivotal.[77]

Pregnant patients

In the pregnant patient with trauma, regional blocks can play an important role, as they do not jeopardize maternal hemodynamic stability and fetal well-being. Many peripheral injuries can be managed entirely with regional anesthesia and analgesia, with minimal effects on the mother or the fetus.

Geriatric patients

In patients with isolated orthopedic injuries, regional anesthesia becomes a viable consideration. There is insufficient evidence to conclude whether anesthetic technique influences mortality, cardiovascular morbidity, duration of surgery, or

St JOSEPH's HEALTH CARE LONDON

REGIONAL BLOCK PROCEDURE RECORD

DRAFT

DATE: _____ UNIT: _____
(YYYY/MM/DD)

PROCEDURE: _____

KEY: NKA = No Known Allergies   N/A = Not Applicable

PRE-PROCEDURE

ALLERGIES: ☐ NKA   ☐ Yes Specify (drug, food, tape, dyes, latex, other) and reactions: _____

HISTORY: _____

RISKS OF BLOCK EXPLAINED: ☐ Bruising and Infection   ☐ Nerve Damage (temporary/permanent)   ☐ Failure
☐ Dural Puncture   ☐ Pleural Puncture   ☐ PDPH   ☐ IV Injection and Seizure   ☐ Total Spinal   ☐ LA Toxicity

PRE-OPERATIVE MULTIMODAL ANALGESIA: ☐ Acetaminophen (_____ mg)   ☐ Celecoxib/Indocid (_____ mg)
☐ Gabapentin/pregabalin (_____ mg)   ☐ OxyContin ® (_____ mg)   ☐ Other: _____ (_____ mg)

EQUIPMENT PRESENT : AIRWAY: ☐ Airway Adjuncts   ☐ Bag-Valve-Mask   ☐ Suction
BREATHING: ☐ Oxygen   ☐ Pulse Oximeter   ☐ Naloxone (CO_2 monitor optional)   ☐ Flumazenil
CIRCULATION: ☐ Cardiac Monitor   ☐ BP Monitor   ☐ Patent I.V.   ☐ Crash Cart available

MEDICATION RECORD

TIME	MEDICATION	DOSE

EPIDURAL / PERIPHERAL NERVE BLOCK PROCEDURE

APPROACH: _____   ☐ Left ☐ Right

PREPARATION: ☐ Povidine-Iodine   ☐ Chlorhexidine   ☐ Other: _____

POSITION: ☐ Supine ☐ Prone ☐ LLD ☐ RLD ☐ Sitting

EPIDURAL LEVEL: _____   **EPIDURAL DEPTH:** _____   **LORA / LORS**

NEEDLE: ☐ Pajunk ☐ Arrow   ☐ Other: _____

Size: ☐ 22 G ☐ 18/17 G Tuohy   ☐ Other: _____

Length: ☐ 40 mm ☐ 50 mm ☐ 80 mm ☐ 90 mm ☐ 100 mm ☐ 110 mm   ☐ Other: _____

SPINAL LEVEL: _____   **Needle:** ☐ Whitacre 25 G / 22 G   ☐ 22 G Quincke   ☐ Other: _____

PVB: ☐ Left ☐ Segments _____   ☐ Right ☐ Segments _____

Catheter: ☐ Left ☐ Right   Length at skin: _____ cm

BLOCK KIT:
☐ Arrow Stimucath 4 cm   ☐ Arrow Stimucath 8 cm   ☐ Other: _____
☐ Pajunk Stimucath 50 mm   ☐ Pajunk Stimucath 100 mm   ☐ Pajunk Stimucath 110 mm   ☐ Other: _____

TECHNIQUE: ☐ PNS: _____   ☐ Ultrasound

Motor Response(s): _____   Current (mA): _____

CATHETER: ☐ Stimulating ☐ Non-stimulating ☐ Flextip   Depth at skin: _____ cm   Tunnelled: ☐ Yes ☐ No

DRUG(S)	CONCENTRATION	VOLUME	EPINEPHRINE	INJECTION	THROUGH
			1/ 00,000	☐ Needle	☐ Catheter
			1/ 00,000	☐ Needle	☐ Catheter
			1/ 00,000	☐ Needle	☐ Catheter
			1/ 00,000	☐ Needle	☐ Catheter
			1/ 00,000	☐ Needle	☐ Catheter
			1/ 00,000	☐ Needle	☐ Catheter
			1/ 00,000	☐ Needle	☐ Catheter

FORM NUMBER (2007/01/26)

Figure 16.11 Form used for block procedure.

incidence of deep venous thrombosis (DVT) and pulmonary embolus (PE) in the setting of routine thromboprophylaxis (see Chapter 36). Blood loss may be reduced in patients receiving regional rather than general anesthesia for hip procedures.[78] If minimal sedation is given, mental status and respiratory function can be well preserved. Elderly patients with isolated upper extremity fractures are often good candidates for regional anesthesia. However, careful evaluation and documentation of the preoperative neurologic status of the affected limb is critical.[79]

EPIDURAL/ PERIPHERAL NERVE BLOCK PROCEDURE (continued)

IV Injection: ☐ Yes ☐ No   Pleural Puncture: ☐ Yes ☐ No

Pain on Injection: ☐ Yes ☐ No   Dural Puncture: ☐ Yes ☐ No

Resistance on Injection: ☐ Yes ☐ No   Ultrasound Spread: ☐ Adequate ☐ Not visualised

Paresthesia: ☐ Yes ☐ No

BLOCK: ☐ Adequate ☐ Inadequate ☐ Failed ☐ Not assessed

SUPPLEMENTAL BLOCK(s): _____

_____

_____

_____

POST PROCEDURE STATUS

Airway patent and stable: ☐ Yes ☐ No _____

Respirations at rest are quiet and regular or similar to pre-procedure: ☐ Yes ☐ No _____

Blood pressure and pulse +/-20% of pre-procedure level: ☐ Yes ☐ No _____

Return to pre-procedure level of consciousness: ☐ Yes ☐ No _____

Motor activity as pre-procedure: ☐ Yes ☐ No _____

Pain: - none or minimal ☐ Yes ☐ No _____

    - controlled with analgesic ☐ Yes ☐ No _____

Inpatient discharged/transferred to: _____ at _____ h.

Outpatient discharged/transferred to: _____ at _____ h.

Accompanied by (name(s) and status): _____

COMMENTS: _____

_____

_____

_____

_____

_____

_____

_____

_____

_____

_____

_____

_____

_____

_____

_____

_____

_____

_____

_____

_____

_____

_____

EPIDURAL/PERIPHERALNERVE BLOCK PROCEDURE DONE BY: PRINTED NAME/ SIGNATURE OF ANESTHETIST:	**DATE** (YYYY/MM/DD):	**TIME:**
PROCEDURE ASSISTED BY: PRINTED NAME/ SIGNATURE OF ANESTHETIST:	**DATE** (YYYY/MM/DD):	**TIME:**

FORM NUMBER (2007/01/26)

Figure 16.11 *(cont.)*

Occurrence of postoperative delirium is associated with increased perioperative morbidity and mortality.[80] A systematic review and meta-analysis advocates the use of regional anesthesia wherever possible, especially in people otherwise vulnerable to developing cognitive dysfunction.[81]

Special trauma types
Blunt chest trauma

Chest wall trauma is a strong indicator of severe internal injury, especially with rib fractures. Severe thoracic injuries compromise respiratory mechanics, increase the incidence of

London Health Sciences Centre

DEPARTMENT OF ANESTHESIA & PERIOPERATIVE MEDICINE

REGIONAL PAIN MANAGEMENT
PREPRINTED ORDER

APPROVED

☐ SSH   ☐ UH   ☐ VH   ☐ SJHC

KEY: R - REQUISITIONED   P-PROCESSED (KARDEX)   P&T 2002/11/26

NON-MEDICATION ORDERS	R	P	MEDICATION ORDERS	P

Venous access required.
Refer to Protocol for Regional Anesthesia/Analgesia for monitoring/assessment guidelines
Report:
  - progressive change in neurologic status (motor/sensory)
  - inadequate analgesia
Inform anesthesiologist prior to initiation of anticoagulant therapy
			MEDICATION ALLERGIES AND REACTIONS:
			_____
			_____
			_____
			_____
			_____	

ADULT:
Administer O2: ☐ mask   ☐ nasal prongs
☐ @ ___ litres/min ☐ ___ % ☐ other _____
If SaO2 <92% report to the Department of Anesthesiology & Perioperative Medicine Acute Pain Service:
  - respiratory rate of 8/minute or below
  - sedation score of 3 or 4 (according to protocol)
  - systolic blood pressure <80 mmHg
			☐ **REGIONAL**
			☐ **PATIENT CONTROLLED REGIONAL ANALGESIA**
			OPIOIDS/SEDATIVES ARE NOT HELD
			TYPE OF BLOCK
			☐ Axillary ☐ Lumbar Plexus
			☐ Femoral ☐ Popliteal
			☐ Interscalene ☐ Paravertebral
			☐ Infraclavicular ☐ Sciatic
			☐ Inter-Pleural ☐ Supracalvicular
			☐ Intercostal ☐ Other
			☐ bupivacaine ___ % ☐ ropivacaine ___ %
			☐ Other: _____
			to infuse @ ___ mL/hr
			PCRA Dose ___ ☐ mg ☐ mcg ☐ mL
			☐ Delay ___ minutes
			Patient activated timed infusion ___ hrs
			Maximum hourly dose ___ ☐ mg ☐ mcg ☐ mL	

PAEDIATRIC: Weight: ___ kg
Administer O2: ☐ mask   ☐ nasal prongs
☐ @ ___ litres/min ☐ ___ % ☐ other _____
If SaO2 <92% report to the Department of Anesthesiology & Perioperative Medicine Acute Pain Service:
  - respiratory rate: 5 - 13years - 14/minute or below
  - respiratory rate: 14 - 18years - 10/minute or below
  - sedation score of 3 or 4 (according to protocol)
  - systolic blood pressure <70 mmHg unless otherwise stated: ___ mmHg
			ANTIEMETICS:
			☐ ondansetron ___ mg I.V. q ___ hr p.r.n.
			☐ metoclopramide ___ mg I.V. q ___ hr p.r.n.
			☐ dimenhydrinate ___ mg I.V. q ___ hr p.r.n.
			☐ prochlorperazine ___ mg I.V. q ___ hr p.r.n.
			
			FOR PRURITUS:
			☐ diphenhydramine ___ mg I.V./p.o. q ___ hr p.r.n.
			☐ Other: _____
			
			OTHER MEDICATIONS:
			_____
			_____
			_____
			_____
			_____
			_____	

PRESCRIBER'S PRINTED NAME / SIGNATURE / CONTACT#:		DATE (YYYY/MM/DD):	TIME:
PROCESSOR'S INITIALS:	DATE (YYYY/MM/DD): TIME:	RN INITIALS: DATE (YYYY/MM/DD):	TIME:

NS5008 (Rev. 2002/12/19)

Distribution: WHITE - Chart   CANARY - Pharmacist   PINK - Nurse

Figure 16.12 Form used for block orders.

pulmonary infections, exacerbate underlying lung injury and preexisting lung disease, and predispose to respiratory failure. The cornerstone of management is early institution of effective pain relief.[82]

Kerr-Valentic *et al.* showed that despite intensive pain therapy, patients with rib fractures are still in pain 30 days after injury.[83] To reduce mortality and morbidity, aggressive pain management is mandatory in chest trauma patients.[84]

Karmakar *et al.*, in a prospective, nonrandomized case series, described how continuous thoracic paravertebral block not only provided pain relief but also improved respiratory parameters and oxygenation.[85] Moon *et al.* showed that epidural analgesia significantly reduced pain with chest wall excursion compared with PCA.[86] The route of analgesia did not affect the catecholamine response. However, serum levels of IL-8 (the proinflammatory chemoattractant implicated in acute lung injury) were significantly reduced in patients receiving epidural analgesia on days 2 and 3. This may have important clinical implications, because lower levels of IL-8 may reduce infectious or inflammatory complications in the trauma patient. Tidal volume and maximal inspiratory force also improved with epidural analgesia by day 3. These results demonstrate that epidural analgesia is superior to PCA in providing analgesia, improving pulmonary function, and modifying the immune response in patients with severe chest injury. A recent meta-analysis suggested that thoracic epidural analgesia (TEA) decreased postoperative cardiac morbidity and mortality. TEA appears to ameliorate gut injury in major surgery as long as the systemic hemodynamic effects of TEA are adequately controlled.[87]

In patients where an epidural is not considered a good choice, interpleural analgesia may be an alternative technique. The interpleural block is easy to perform when clear landmarks are present, and usually involves the placement of a continuous catheter for infusion.[88] The main complication of interpleural analgesia is pneumothorax, the incidence of which is less than 5%. Local anesthetic toxicity can occur after repeated boluses. The chest tube should be clamped after a bolus for the block to be effective, which might not be practical in a patient with thoracic trauma.[89]

Intercostal nerve blocks are relatively simple to perform and are effective in managing rib fracture pain.[90] However, problems with such blocks are inconsistent analgesia due to the single-shot technique and the requirement for multiple punctures at various levels with the risk of pneumothorax, high blood levels of local anesthesia, and lack of effect on visceral pain. Respiratory function improves after intercostal nerve blocks. Paravertebral blockade is a versatile regional technique that can be done by an ultrasound-guided approach.[91] Continuous thoracic paravertebral infusion of local anesthesia has been shown to provide pain relief, as well as a sustained improvement in respiratory parameters and oxygenation in patients with multiple rib fractures.[92]

Hip and femoral fractures

In a randomized controlled trial, Fletcher *et al.* demonstrated that the femoral block provided analgesia more quickly than IV morphine in patients with femoral neck fractures.[93] They also demonstrated that it was possible to teach district hospital emergency medical staff to perform femoral blocks successfully and safely in a short period of time despite minimal experience in regional anesthesia. These blocks also reduce

perioperative blood loss during orthopedic surgery.[94] They can also be used to position the patient for spinal anesthesia for femoral neck fractures.[95]

Burn injuries

Major burn injuries are devastating, and often require prolonged hospital stay and major psychological and physical rehabilitation (see Chapters 39 and 40). These patients need frequent dressing changes and wound debridement, and it is well known that the patient's assessment of pain is different from the healthcare provider's assessment. For example, half of all burn patients reported inadequate analgesia for dressing changes.[96] A large number of burn patients will go on to develop chronic pain. Aggressive pain management is therefore of the utmost importance in such patients, to improve outcomes and reduce the risk of developing chronic neuropathic pain.

Regional techniques are limited in patients with a large percentage of burn area. The burn and donor sites may extend beyond the area that can be covered by a single block. However, the use of continuous epidural, continuous nerve blocks, and subcutaneous infiltration has been described.[97,98] Thoracic and lumbar epidural anesthesia techniques may be used for dressing changes involving the chest and abdomen. Brachial plexus blockade may be used for the upper extremity.

The potential for catheter-related infections may be high in this subpopulation. Fixation of the catheter may pose a major problem. For burns limited to a limb, continuous nerve blocks with the insertion of a catheter are an attractive option for pain control as well as for dressing changes and frequent wound debridement. Though the use of dilute solutions (0.125% bupivacaine) can provide excellent analgesia, higher concentrations (0.5% bupivacaine) may be required for the analgesic needs of dressing change.[99]

Phantom limb and stump pain

Management of amputation-related pain is extremely important. Almost all amputees experience stump pain immediately after surgery.[100] This is expected after major surgery, and if no contraindication exists it is best managed by continuous epidural or continuous nerve block catheters. The pain that persists beyond the expected healing time after amputation is defined as persistent stump pain, and the prevalence varies between studies.[101,102] Causes of stump pain are multifactorial and include ischemia, surgical trauma, inflammation, skin infection, osteomyelitis, bone spurs, scar tissue, referred pain, neuromata, and ill-fitting prostheses leading to skin ulcers and infection. Deafferentation, CNS neuroplasticity, and unknown peripheral mechanisms are among the etiologies. Treatment of stump pain is the treatment of its causes. Phantom limb pain is, however, a different entity, with a prevalence varying from 2% to almost 98%.[103] Some studies have shown a beneficial preemptive effect of epidural analgesia for preventing phantom limb pain.[104] Perineural catheters for amputation surgery provide good analgesia.

In a study by Flor et al., amputation stump anesthesia produced by brachial plexus blockade abolished all aspects of cortical reorganization that could be identified by neuroelectric source imaging, while at the same time it virtually eliminated the current experience of phantom limb pain.[105] The combination of long-term regional analgesia with prolonged block of N-methyl-D-aspartate receptors appears to be a promising preventive strategy for phantom limb pain following traumatic amputations.[106] Because of the well-documented benefits of surgical and postoperative analgesia in preventing phantom pain, epidural for lower limb and regional nerve blocks for upper limb should be strongly considered for all planned amputations.

Traumatic brain injury

Traumatic brain injury (TBI) is a common cause of pain and disability. The prevalence of pain (acute and chronic) largely depends on the severity of TBI. In patients with mild TBI (e.g., head injuries without loss of consciousness), persistent neck pain and occipital headaches can be a major source of disability.[107] For patients with posttraumatic cervicogenic headaches, radiofrequency denervation of medial branches innervating the cervical facet joints may provide long-term relief.[108] Moderate to severe TBI can result in extensor hypertonic spasticity of lower limbs, which can contribute to chronic pain. Intrathecal baclofen infusions in this setting may provide good results in adults[109] as well as in children.[110] A disadvantage of these techniques is the repeated requirement for refills.

Nerve-agent intoxication

The use of regional anesthesia for conventional injuries and nerve-agent intoxication needs some consideration. Peripheral nerve blocks do not aggravate hemodynamic instability secondary to an already unstable and dysfunctional autonomic system induced by nerve agents. Care must be taken to avoid sympatholytic activity with the blocks in the presence of the parasympathetic overactivity that comes with nerve agents. Amide local anesthetics such as bupivacaine, ropivacaine, and lidocaine are preferred, as esters are degraded by plasma cholinesterase, which is inhibited by the nerve agent.[111] Neuraxial blockade should be used cautiously in view of the anticipated coagulopathy that can accompany nerve-agent intoxication[112] and the poorly defined extent of sympathetic blockade with such blocks.

Complex regional pain syndrome

Complex regional pain syndrome (CRPS) is an uncommon consequence of trauma or illness affecting a limb with nerve injury (CRPS I) or without nerve injury (CRPS II). Prevention of CRPS is based on the importance of efficient preoperative, intraoperative, and postoperative analgesia and anesthesia (see also Chapter 17).[113] Continuous brachial plexus blocks may be feasible and effective interventional techniques for the management of CRPS type I of upper extremities.[114] The majority of CRPS occurs after trauma or orthopedic procedures or both. It has been recommended that CRPS patients undergoing surgery should avoid general anesthesia, because the disease process might be "rekindled by surgery under general anesthesia."[115] Two types of regional anesthetic techniques are available, namely a sympathetic nerve block and a combined somatic and sympathetic nerve block. Sympathetic nerve blocks are chosen when the patient has marked improvement after a diagnostic sympathetic block. A somatic plus sympathetic block is used in patients who do not respond to the diagnostic sympathetic block. Physical therapy should be initiated immediately after the block. A series of daily or every-alternate-day blocks using local anesthetic agents is usually required for 1–3 weeks.[116] It has been postulated that if CRPS is mediated in part by an increase in the density of voltage-sensitive sodium channels in an injured axon, then desensitization via regional blockade is essential.[117]

Adequate perioperative analgesia, limitation of operative time, limitation of tourniquet time, and use of regional anesthetic technique are recommended for secondary prevention of CRPS I.[118] In one review article, after a search of 41 randomized controlled trials, only bisphosphonates appeared to offer clear benefits for patients with CRPS. Improvement has been reported with dimethyl sulfoxides, steroids, epidural clonidine, intrathecal baclofen, and spinal cord stimulation.[119]

Digit reimplantation

Vasospasm may be devastating, causing irreversible damage to the replanted limb. Blocking the stellate ganglion decreases the sensitivity of the sympathetic system to developing vasospasm due to intrinsic or extrinsic causes. It provides baseline security for avoiding and reversing ongoing vasospasm.[120] Continuous brachial plexus blockade is effective in improving vascular flow and perfusion, reducing vasospasm, and providing sympathetic blockade, as well as in managing postoperative pain. This block should be considered whenever an anastomosis is performed in the upper extremity.[121,122] There is a single report of "steal phenomenon" occurring after axillary block in a toe-to-finger transfer in which the blood flow was markedly reduced in the implanted digit[123] due to sympathetic blockade denervation, but this has been not been subsequently proven.[124]

Nerve localization techniques
Nerve stimulators

Use of peripheral nerve stimulators to initiate continuous regional blocks can be painful, and thus alternative methods of initiating these blocks may have to be used.

Table 16.3 Pharmacological adjuvants to local anesthetics: advantages and disadvantages

Drug	Advantages	Disadvantages
Epinephrine	Exposes neural tissue to LA for longer period ↓ Peak plasma level of LA ↑ Duration/quality of blocks Helps in detection of IV injection	Neural/spinal ischemia Fatal arrhythmia on IV injection
Clonidine	↑ Duration of LA action Prolongs postop analgesia ↓ Plasma LA level at higher doses	Sedation Bradycardia Hypotension Not useful in CPNB
Ketamine	Prolongs analgesia Manage opioid induced hyperalgesia Prehospital analgesia Hemodynamic stability Multiple routes of application	Psychomimetic action Nausea Salivation No protection from aspiration No LA effect in PNB
Opioids	Easy to administer Multiple routes of administration Prolongs analgesia with neuraxial application	Lack efficacy in PNB Nausea and vomiting Sedation Immunosuppression Gut effects Interfere with monitoring
Sodium bicarbonate	↑ pH of LA faster onset (5 min)	Precipitation ↓ PNB intensity ↓ Duration of block
Tramadol	↓ Immunosuppression Anti-inflammatory effect	Nausea Weak analgesic
Verapamil	Potentiates neuraxial block ↓ Need of supplemental analgesics	No prolongation of block
Hyaluronidase	Better spread of LA ↑ Onset of block	↓ Duration of block
Neostigmine	Prolongs analgesia with IVRA	Nausea and vomiting
NSAIDs	Prolongs analgesia with IVRA Multimodal analgesic advantage	GI side effects Renal dysfunction Bronchoconstriction Platelet dysfunction
COX-2 inhibitors	Central and peripheral analgesia Multimodal analgesic advantage Synergy with other analgesics	Cardiac and renal dysfunction
Muscle relaxants	Muscle relaxation in IVRA	Paresis on tourniquet release

COX, cyclooxygenase; CPNB, continuous peripheral nerve block; IV, intravenous; IVRA, intravenous regional anesthesia; LA, local anesthetic agent; NSAIDs, nonsteroidal anti-inflammatory drugs; PNB, peripheral nerve block; Postop, postoperative; PVB, paravertebral block.

Ultrasound guidance

The usefulness of ultrasound in localizing nerves and plexus cannot be overemphasized (see Chapter 12). Studies have found that ultrasound guidance is superior to nerve stimulation, and this was attributed to the ability to visualize the nerves, needle path, and local anesthetic spread in real time.[125] Marhofer *et al.* compared the use of ultrasound guidance with nerve stimulation during femoral nerve block, and found that ultrasound was superior to nerve stimulation as they were able to visualize local anesthetic administration during the injection.[126] They also found that they could use smaller volumes, and that the latency period was shorter.[127] Most clinicians will report an almost 50% reduction in the amount of local anesthetic for all blocks when using ultrasound.[128]

Pharmacologic adjuvants in regional anesthesia

In traumatized patients with unstable hemodynamics, one should carefully consider the risk–benefit ratio of adding drugs to regional blocks, since many adjuvants are of questionable efficacy and have side effects that may confound patient safety (Table 16.3)

Vasoconstrictors

Epinephrine is often added to facilitate detection of intravascular injection. The addition of epinephrine is known to prolong the duration and quality of most blocks. It causes vasoconstriction of the perineural vessels, thereby resulting in decreased uptake, which in turn exposes the neural tissue to the local anesthetic for a longer period. Additionally, plasma levels rise less steeply, which reduces the risks of systemic toxicity. Various concentrations have been used (2.5–5 μg/mL). Although 2.5 μg/mL epinephrine prolongs the block to the same extent as 5 μg/mL concentration, it has minimal effect on nerve blood flow[129] and is therefore recommended. The addition of epinephrine to long-acting local anesthetics with vasoconstrictive properties such as ropivacaine may not increase the block duration but it may still help in the detection of intravascular injection.[130] Epinephrine may also produce analgesia through α₂-adrenergic mechanism.[131] Epinephrine is likely safe when applied to nerve bundles with intact barrier mechanisms, but it may accentuate injury in the event of barrier disruption or decreased neural blood flow.

Clonidine

Clonidine has been investigated as an adjuvant in peripheral nerve blocks. Although it has been shown to increase the duration of local anesthetic action and prolong postoperative analgesia when included in single-injection nerve blocks,[132] it has not shown any clinical benefit in continuous perineural infusions.[133] Side effects such as hypotension, decreased heart rate, and sedation may occur. The side-effect profile of clonidine is dose-dependent and usually does not occur at doses ≤ 1.5 μg/kg.

The addition of clonidine to mepivacaine 1% and to bupivacaine 0.5% resulted in a very impressive block prolongation but did not lead to an additional block-prolonging effect when used with ropivacaine. Both bupivacaine and lidocaine produced vasodilatation in human skin, but ropivacaine decreased skin blood flow. As ropivacaine had intrinsic vasoconstricting properties not mediated by an activation of α_2-adrenergic receptors, this could have explained why the addition of clonidine did not result in any benefit.[134]

A systematic review of the intrathecal use of clonidine as an adjunct to local anesthetic found that it prolonged the duration of the sensory blockade by approximately 1 hour and the time to first analgesic request by around 100 minutes. The time to establish the block was unchanged, but the duration of motor blockade was prolonged. The addition of clonidine resulted in a greater incidence of hypotension. The optimal dose for intrathecal use could not be established, but there was a linear relationship between clonidine doses of between 15 and 150 μg and the time to regression of the sensory block. The clinical significance of these changes is open to question, and further work is needed to establish whether intrathecal clonidine offers an advantage over an increased dose of local anesthetic alone.[135]

Dexmedetomidine

Dexmedetomidine is a highly selective α_2-adrenergic receptor agonist that has an α_2:α_1 selectivity ratio seven times greater than that of clonidine.[136] It is a unique drug with sedative, anxiolytic, and analgesic properties. A study comparing intrathecal dexmedetomidine with intrathecal clonidine in patients undergoing transurethral urological surgery found that dexmedetomidine offered no additional benefit in terms of duration of sensory blockade or postoperative analgesia requirements.[137] Dexmedetomidine does not seem to provide prolonged postoperative analgesia when used as an additive to a local anesthetic in total IV anesthesia.[138,139] However, its neuroprotective properties (seen in experimental models and clinical setting) have been reported. Dexmedetomidine may also be a valuable adjuvant when regional anesthesia is used.[140]

Ketamine

The peripheral analgesic effect of ketamine may be explained by blocking of sodium and potassium currents in peripheral nerves[141] as well as central antinociception through a noncompetitive antagonism at the N-methyl-D-aspartate receptor.[142] However, it may also enhance analgesia through interaction with spinal opioid receptors and α_2-adrenergic receptors.[143] Local anesthetic properties of ketamine have also been reported,[144] but it does not seem to enhance sensory or motor blockade in peripheral nerve blocks.[145] Doses of 2–3 mg/mL have been used.

Ketamine has a special role in patients with debilitating heat allodynia and positive cognitive symptoms via its action on the central pain pathway. As an adjuvant in sympatholytic blocks it has a targeted action without significant neuropsychiatric side effects. There is a report of three patients with CRPS type II following gunshot wounds experienced debilitating central sensitization, heat/mechano-allodynia, and cognitive symptoms ("vicarious pain"). Each of these three patients experienced dramatic relief with the addition of ketamine as an adjuvant to the sympathetic blocks after conventional therapy failed.[146]

Opioids

Intrathecal[147] and epidural[148] opioids were first administered to human subjects in 1979, and since that time they have been proven to provide effective and prolonged analgesia.

This improvement in analgesia has to be balanced against the high incidence of undesirable side effects including respiratory depression (which may occur several hours after initial administration), nausea, vomiting, pruritus, and urinary retention.[149] Liposomally encapsulated preparations of morphine are now available that can provide analgesia for up to 48 hours after administration.[150] Because of the gradual-release mechanism, this technology can allow larger epidural doses to be given, providing analgesia for a greater period of time. Improved pain scores and decreased opioid consumption have been demonstrated for up to 48 hours after lower abdominal surgery.[151]

A review article examining the efficacy of adding opioids to local anesthetics for brachial plexus blocks considered 10 trials involving 413 patients. The opioids included morphine, fentanyl, sufentanil, alfentanil, butorphanol, and buprenorphine. Overall, six were supportive and four negative. The authors concluded that there was little evidence for any analgesic benefit of using opioid analgesics in brachial plexus block over systemic administration.[152] Epineural buprenorphine has been shown to prolong postoperative analgesia from an interscalene block more effectively than intramuscular buprenorphine, which suggests that buprenorphine acts at a peripheral nervous system site of action.[153]

Peripheral opioid effects have been shown with intraarticular injection and with wound infiltration, but the clinical relevance of peripheral opioid receptors is uncertain. Various reviews of the role of opioids in peripheral nerve block have concluded that their analgesic effects are not clinically significant.[154]

Sodium bicarbonate

Local anesthetics cross the cell membrane as uncharged molecules. Increasing the pH of a local anesthetic solution closer to the pKa increases the number of uncharged molecules in the solution. This may facilitate the movement of local anesthetic agent across the nerve sheath and membrane, resulting in a faster onset of anesthesia.[155] Studies that do show a benefit at most show a decreased latency of less than 5 minutes. However, there is evidence that adding sodium bicarbonate to local anesthetic solution may decrease the block intensity and duration of plexus anesthesia.[156] One must therefore decide whether a few minutes of onset time is significant enough to warrant its use.

Other adjuvants

Tramadol, a centrally acting analgesic with peripheral local anesthetic effects,[157] has been shown to moderately increase block duration.[158,159]

Neostigmine has been used successfully in labor analgesia.[160,161] In peripheral nerve blocks, it does not seem to improve sensory or motor block qualities, though there are conflicting reports on its efficacy.[162,163] It is associated with a 30% incidence of gastrointestinal side effects.[164] Neostigmine (60–500 µg) has been used as an adjunct for epidural use and has produced improved postoperative analgesia with a low incidence of nausea and vomiting, but with an increase in sedation.[165]

Though ophthalmic surgeons use hyaluronidase commonly, it has been shown not to hasten block onset, reduce the incidence of failed block, or affect local anesthetic blood concentration, but it does shorten block duration.[166]

To date, there have been no double-blind studies evaluating NSAIDs as adjuvants for nerve blocks, although intraarticular ketorolac[167] and tenoxicam[168] have been shown to provide some postoperative analgesia. The usefulness of NSAIDs as adjuvants to local anesthesia may depend on the presence of inflammation at the site, and this may explain the controversial issue of usefulness of NSAIDs in IVRA. When used as an adjunct to brachial plexus blockade, the addition of adenosine 10 mg to a prilocaine and lidocaine mixture made no difference to the onset or offset of sensory blockade, and did not extend the duration of analgesia.[169]

Prostaglandins are produced from virtually all tissues in response to trauma. NSAIDs may produce analgesia indirectly by attenuation of the hyperalgesic state caused by sensitization of afferent nerve fibers by prostaglandins.[170]

Nondepolarizing muscle relaxants have been added to local anesthesia in IVRA to improve operative conditions and provide postoperative analgesia, but this has not shown much promise.[171]

For IVRA, there is good evidence to recommend adding ketorolac to improve postoperative analgesia, and clonidine to improve postoperative analgesia and prolong tourniquet tolerance.[172]

Complications of regional techniques

As with any procedure, regional blocks are associated with side effects and complications (Table 16.4). These range from less serious and common to extremely rare and life-threatening. Many patients report at least one side effect after axillary block, such as soreness, transient numbness, or bruising.

Auroy and colleagues prospectively evaluated serious complications after more than 21,000 peripheral nerve blocks in a 5-month period in France.[173] The estimated number of serious complications per 10,000 nerve blocks was as follows: death, 0–2.6; cardiac arrest, 0.3–4.1; nerve injury, 0.5–4.8; seizures, 3.9–11.2.

Peripheral nerve injury is a potential complication of regional anesthesia. It may present as residual weakness, hypoesthesia, or permanent paresis. Data from a recent review of published studies suggest that the incidence of neurologic symptoms following peripheral nerve block varies depending on the anatomic location, ranging from 0.03% for supraclavicular block to 0.3% for femoral blocks to 3% for interscalene blocks.[174] Causes of peripheral nerve injury include needle/catheter-induced mechanical trauma, perineural edema, and local anesthetic neurotoxicity. There are no randomized trials to support the ability of various needles and bevel types to prevent nerve injury. Contrary to common belief, Steinfeldt *et al.* concluded in their study that neither the pencil point nor the short beveled needle can be designated a less traumatic device.[175]

Role of paresthesia

Elicitation of paresthesia during the nerve block has been implicated in nerve injury, although this finding has not been confirmed in prospective studies.[176]

Role of epinephrine

Epinephrine is considered safe when it is applied to nerves with intact blood flow. However, if the neural blood flow is disrupted (intraneuronal injection, chemotherapy-exposed nerves, atherosclerosis, or diabetic neuropathy), injury can be accentuated.[177] In conditions of trauma, disruption or reduction of neural blood flow can occur, especially in the presence of severe hypotension and use of vasopressors and inotropes. Use of epinephrine together with local anesthetic solutions in such circumstances may possibly be detrimental.

Role of local anesthetic neurotoxicity

Even though local anesthetics have been widely used with great safety, they can be neurotoxic under certain circumstances, such as with high concentrations, prolonged exposure, use of

Table 16.4 Complications associated with regional anesthesia

Complication	Incidence	Steps to reduce incidence	Early detection
Infection Colonization	1–1.9% 28–57%	Aseptic precautions Antibiotics Bacterial filters for extended blocks Prevent hub disconnection (Fig. 16.11)	Daily inspection Early removal Culture on suspicion
Bruising	6.7–19.1%	Gentle technique	
Nerve injury	0.02–8%	Ultrasound-guided blocks Pressure relief valve with injection Modified techniques Inject via catheter ↓ Epinephrine	Resistance on injection Pain on injection Ultrasound examination
Accidental IV injection		Ultrasound guidance Add epinephrine to LA Cardiac monitoring Fractionate dosing Aspirate frequently	Ultrasonography ↑ HR with 3–5 mL injection Neurological symptoms
Failure	2–20%	Ultrasound guidance Inject via catheter Stimulating catheter	Establish block via catheter
Local anesthetic toxicity	0.01–0.2%	Use minimum effective dose Beware of total dose Add epinephrine to LA Special medical problems: renal and hepatic	Tremulousness, twitching and slurred speech
Pneumothorax	0.04–0.15%	Ultrasound guidance Closed system of injection	Vigilance Aspiration prior to injection
Diaphragm paresis	100% with ISB	↓ Dose and concentration of LA Posterior approach	Hypoxia Shortness of Breath
Motor weakness	variable	Lower concentration of local anesthetic ↓ Basal rate Patient controlled analgesia	Monitor/adjust rate and concentration
Hematoma	variable	Ultrasound guidance Use of alternate blocks e.g: axillary	Aspiration of needle/catheter Application of pressure
Horner's syndrome	10–15%	↓ Volume of LA	
Compartment syndrome	rare	Lowest effective anesthetic concentration Prophylactic fasciotomy Delayed closure	Vigilance Compartment pressure measurement
Epidural spread	1–5% with PVB	Slow injection Fractionate dosing	↑ Resistance to injection
Catheter malfunction	20–25%	Tunneling (Fig. 16.8) Catheter and hub fixation (Fig. 16.9) Liquid adhesive to entry site (Fig. 16.10)	Warn patient to report pain and leak Daily inspection

HR, heart rate; IV, intravenous; LA, local anesthetic.

epinephrine, or intraneuronal injection. It has been suggested that high intraneuronal pressures may be involved in the injury mechanisms.[178] This might have implications in an injured patient who is hypovolemic and hypotensive and is receiving vasopressors and inotropic drugs to support blood pressure.

Role of peripheral nerve stimulators

Nerve stimulators have been in use for more than 45 years to improve block success rate. However, there are no randomized controlled studies in humans to show that they improve patient safety. It has been shown that motor response is inconsistent despite the needle being in close proximity to the nerve[179] or indeed in the nerve.[180] Such concerns are further validated by reports of nerve injury after low-current ($< 0.5\,mA$) electrical stimulation.[181] Thus, peripheral nerve stimulators may contribute to some neurotrauma.

Vascular injury

Deep plexus blocks in coagulopathic patients should be based on careful risk–benefit analysis and performed cautiously, especially if an expanding hematoma cannot be accessed. Transient vascular insufficiency is a known complication of peripheral nerve blocks, as vasospasm may occur after vascular puncture or as a result of local anesthetic. Medial brachial fascial compartment syndrome is a definite entity after brachial plexus blocks.[182] Evolution of neurologic deficit takes some time to develop (4 hours to 3 days). Without intervention, it can lead to axon loss and sensory and motor deficit. A preexisting traumatic or vascular injury must be considered when planning peripheral nerve blockade in trauma patients.

Diaphragm weakness

The phrenic nerve lies very close to the interscalene groove and is easily blocked during the interscalene approach to the brachial plexus. In one study, the incidence of hemidiaphragmatic paresis was 100% after interscalene block.[183] The supraclavicular approach to the brachial plexus has a lower but unpredictable incidence of hemidiaphragmatic weakness. Although unilateral diaphragmatic weakness does not cause significant effects in healthy subjects, it may be deleterious in patients with chest trauma or contralateral pneumothorax, or in patients who would not be able to tolerate reduction in pulmonary function.

Pneumothorax

Pneumothorax is a serious complication of the supraclavicular brachial plexus block. It can also occur after interscalene, and rarely after infraclavicular, approaches. The incidence also depends on the experience of the person doing the block. Symptoms can be delayed in presentation and must be kept in mind whenever there is chest discomfort 6–12 hours after the block. The use of ultrasound may help decrease the risk of pneumothorax from brachial plexus blockade. Pneumothorax can also occur after intercostal nerve block and paravertebral block.

Intravascular injection

Most plexuses are in the vicinity of vascular structures, and intravascular injection can occur even with careful technique. Signs and symptoms of local anesthetic toxicity may include circumoral numbness, ringing in the ears, metallic taste in mouth, hypotension and/or changes in heart rhythm. Intraarterial injection can cause sudden convulsions, arrhythmias, and cardiac arrest. Careful multiple aspirations, slow fractionated injections, and constant vigilance are of the utmost importance. Addition of epinephrine helps to detect accidental intravascular injection. The total dose of local anesthesia should be reduced in patients with a compromised metabolism, to minimize the risk of systemic toxicity. Availability of intralipid emulsion for treatment of local anesthetic cardiac toxicity cannot be overemphasized. The American Society of Regional Anesthesia (ASRA) has developed a series of recommendations addressing the management of local anesthetic toxicity. The ASRA practice advisory on local anesthetic toxicity is published in the society's official publication *Regional Anesthesia and Pain Medicine*, and can be downloaded from the journal website.[184]

Horner's syndrome

Proximity of the cervical sympathetic chain to the brachial plexus can lead to Horner's syndrome (ptosis, miosis, anhydrosis, and unilateral conjunctival engorgement) with interscalene as well as supraclavicular approaches in up to 90% of patients.[185] Due to ipsilateral pupillary changes, neurologic monitoring in head-injured patients can be confusing. Hoarseness can occur after interscalene block due to ipsilateral paresis of recurrent laryngeal nerve and can delay detection of impending airway edema following trauma.

Compartment syndrome

Compartment syndrome may occur anywhere that the muscles are enclosed by fascia. Common sites after trauma are the lower leg and forearm. Increased pressure within the compartment compromises the circulation and function of tissues (see Chapters 27 and 28). Since one of the primary presenting symptoms of compartment syndrome is pain, many trauma surgeons and anesthesiologists worry that regional anesthesia may mask the symptoms of early compartment syndrome after trauma and after major extremity surgery. Indeed, there are plenty of anecdotes about regional anesthesia and analgesia masking compartment syndrome. Others believe that the ischemic pain of compartment syndrome breaks through an analgesic peripheral nerve block. Nonetheless, the potential for losing a limb in a patient because of delayed intervention deters many anesthesiologists from doing these blocks in the traumatized patient. Samet and Dutton reviewed the implications of regional anesthesia and compartment syndrome.[186] They noted that the majority of patients had fasciotomy during their initial surgery, and a significant number had fasciotomy within 24 hours of injury. None of the fasciotomies were performed for symptoms of pain. This makes one wonder if we should deny the trauma patient this modality of analgesia. Diagnosing compartment syndrome requires a high index of suspicion, performance of serial examinations, and careful documentation of changes over time.[187] Prophylactic fasciotomies, delayed closure, and measurement of compartment pressure should hopefully allow this excellent modality of analgesic intervention to be made more available to trauma patients.

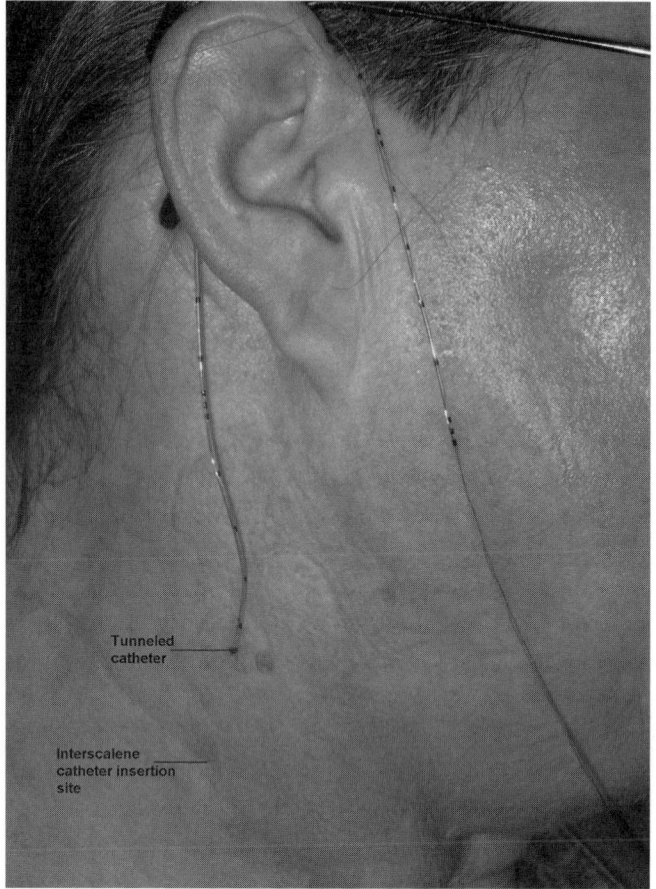

Figure 16.13 Tunneling of catheter. *A black and white version of this figure will appear in some formats. For the color version, please refer to the plate section.*

Labels in figure: Tunneled catheter; Interscalene catheter insertion site

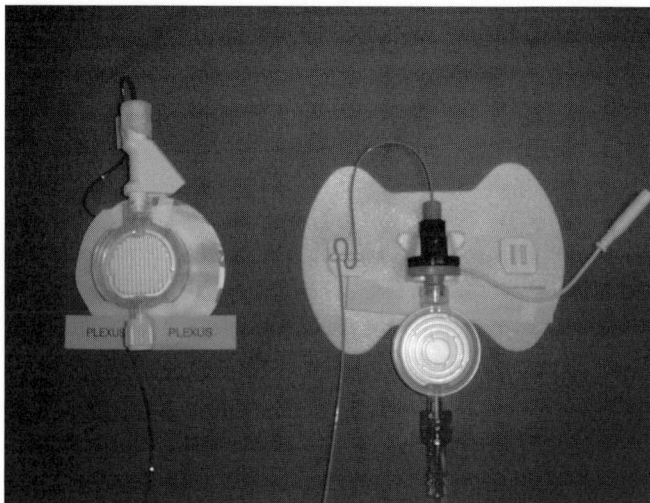

Figure 16.14 Catheter fixation devices.

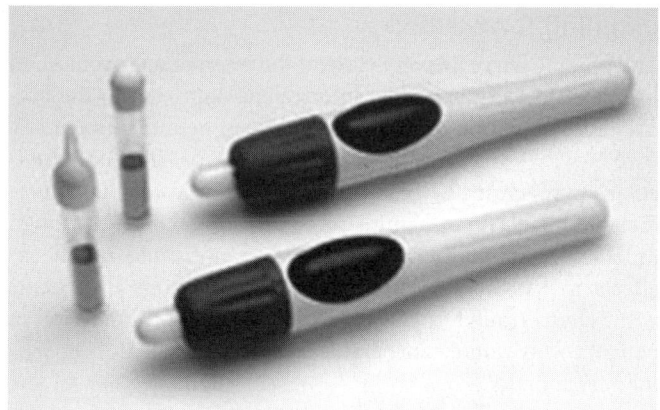

Figure 16.15 Liquid skin adhesives.

Infections

There are no reports of infections after single-injection blocks. However, bacterial colonization of indwelling femoral catheters is known to occur as early as 48 hours postoperatively.[188] Though the rate of colonization was frequent in this study, the risk of bacterial infections was found to be small. Immediate catheter removal, catheter culture, and psoas muscle imaging were recommended in case of suspected infection. There have been case reports of psoas muscle abscess complicating femoral nerve block catheters and requiring antibiotic therapy and drainage.[189] Adherence to strict aseptic guidelines as published by the American Society of Regional Anesthesia and Pain Medicine, the American Society of Anesthesiologists, and the Royal College of Anaesthetists may reduce the risk of infectious complications.[190]

Technical issues

Continuous peripheral nerve block is commonly used for surgical anesthesia and postoperative analgesia. It is an evolving and exciting area of clinical research and technologic advancement. It has been used effectively in combat casualties to extend the duration of analgesia during evacuation and convalescence (see Chapter 38).[191] Technical problems with catheters and devices are of importance when considering continuous peripheral nerve blocks. For example, a catheter tip design that increases adhesion to surrounding tissue in an intensely inflammatory environment could increase the potential for injury with removal, particularly in long-term catheters. Capdevila *et al.* carried out a prospective analysis of 1416 patients and found that nearly 18% had technical problems with catheters and devices.[192] Problems consisted of kinked, blocked, displaced, and leaking catheters as well as malfunctioning pumps. In the authors' experience, accidental withdrawal or pulling out at the end of surgery with the drapes is a frequent cause of unwanted termination of therapy. Tunneling of the catheter (Fig. 16.13), adequate catheter fixation devices (Fig. 16.14), application of liquid skin adhesives (Fig. 16.15), prevention of hub disconnection (Fig. 16.16), and use of "surgeon-proof" dressing have proved very successful in our center (Fig. 16.17).

Limitations of regional analgesia in trauma

Personnel and training

The most significant factor that is likely to deter the use of regional techniques in trauma in the early phase is lack of trained individuals in the acute trauma area. Many emergency medicine physicians lack adequate training in regional anesthesia.

Patient condition

Apart from lack of available trained personnel, patients may be hypovolemic in the acute trauma phase, precluding the use of neuraxial techniques. Patients may develop coagulopathy due to massive transfusion and/or multisystem organ failure, making neuraxial blocks unsafe. Multiorgan trauma may also be associated with cervical, thoracic, and/or lumbar spine injury, making positioning of the patient for the block difficult or impossible. Neuraxial local anesthetics should be used with caution in trauma patients with cardiac arrhythmias.

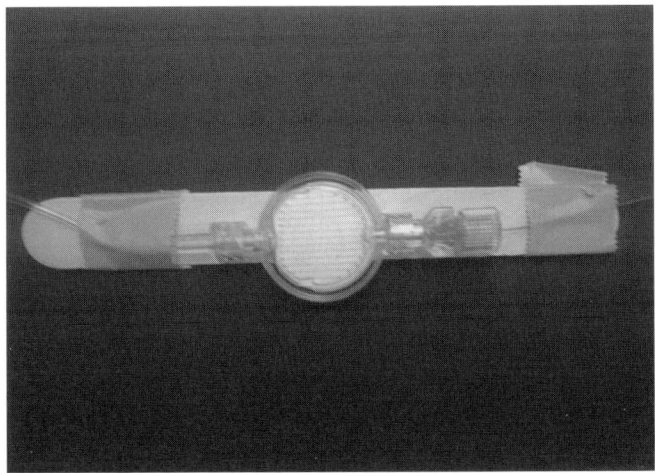

Figure 16.16 Fixation to prevent hub disconnection.

Accidental intravascular injections are poorly tolerated in the setting of coexisting cardiac disease, such as blunt cardiac injury and myocardial contusion. Intoxicated patients, and those with altered sensorium from other causes, will not be able to consent to or cooperate with the initiation of various regional blocks. Alteration in hepatic blood flow, preexisting hepatic insufficiency, or liver injury may alter local anesthetic pharmacokinetics and pharmacodynamics.

Informed consent

In many institutions, separate regional anesthesia consent is not obtained, as it is implied when the patient agrees to the surgical procedure. This is currently a topic for discussion in many countries. Addition of regional blocks may be perceived as interventions beyond what is required for the surgical procedure. In the acute trauma scenario, many patients with multiple injuries may not be in a condition to give informed consent, and therefore it may have to be obtained from the legal guardian. Further, consents obtained when the patient is in severe pain and/or under the effect of sedatives may not be considered valid.

Patients who undergo planned procedures following trauma, such as for a fractured humerus or ankle, may not have consent issues. Patients should be provided with enough information about the blocks and the potential risks of regional anesthesia and the alternative therapies that are available to manage their pain. A sample of the form that we use in our institution is shown in Figure 16.18. The patient's signature is not required on this form. Often, audiovisual aids can be used to inform patients about the details of regional blocks and their risks.

Patient follow-up

Patients receiving continuous regional analgesia either at the hospital or at home require proper follow-up to ensure safety and efficacy of the intervention. The acute pain team most often provides follow-up of inpatients. It is important to

(A)

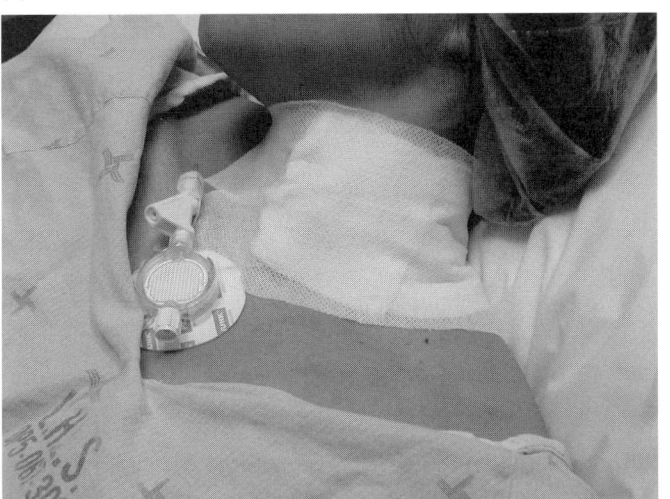

(B)

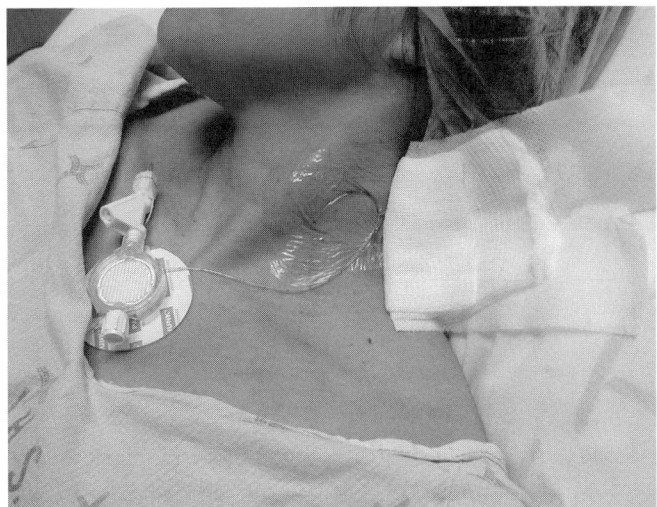

Figure 16.17 Surgeon-proof dressing. *A black and white version of this figure will appear in some formats. For the color version, please refer to the plate section.*

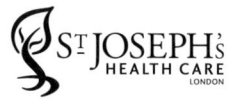

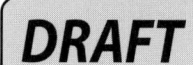

Department of Anesthesia

**PRE-OPERATIVE CONSULTATION
FOR REGIONAL ANESTHESIA &
PAIN MANAGEMENT**

Scheduled Surgery: _____ Date of Surgery: _____
                                                                                                    (YYYY/MM/DD)

Date of Consultation: _____ Time: _____
                                        (YYYY/MM/DD)

Name of Anesthesiologist: _____

Did the patient have blocks for previous surgeries: ☐ Yes   ☐ No

Pre-operative (previous and current) medical problems: _____
_____
_____
_____

Contraindications to regional block: ☐ Yes   ☐ No

If yes, specify: _____
_____
_____

Type of block discussed:

☐ Axillary
☐ Continuous catheter
☐ Epidural
☐ Infraclavicular
☐ ISB
☐ Lumbar plexus
☐ Paravertebral
☐ PCA
☐ Popliteal
☐ Sciatic
☐ Spinal
☐ Supraclavicular
☐ Ultrasound guided block

Risks explained:

☐ Bruising
☐ Diaphragm weakness
☐ Epidural spread
☐ Failure
☐ Horner's
☐ Infection
☐ LA toxicity
☐ Nerve damage permanent
☐ Nerve damage temporary
☐ Pneumothorax
☐ Seizure and CV collapse
☐ Vascular injection
☐ Other: _____

Suitable for home regional discharge?   ☐ Yes   ☐ No
_____

Patient has seen the educational video?   ☐ Yes   ☐ No   _____

I have given explanation about the regional block procedure and the potential risks. Alternative therapy has
been explained to the patient. All questions have been answered. Patient agrees to have the block procedure.

Printed Name/Signature of Anesthetist: _____

Has O.R. Bookings been informed to add anesthesia information on the O.R. list?   ☐ Yes   ☐ No

FORM NUMBER (2006/12/06)   **COPY DISTRIBUTION:**   WHITE - Patient's Chart;   CANARY - O.R. Block Room

Figure 16.18 Block consent form.

have personnel trained in regional anesthesia on the team to provide the best continuity of care. Postoperative block orders have to be clear and precise, with instructions regarding patient-administered and nurse-administered boluses. When multiple catheters are used, it is mandatory to be specific about each block infusion order. One has to be cognizant of the total local anesthetic administered to reduce the chances of local anesthetic toxicity. When using multiple catheters, we allow only one block to have the patient-controlled modality. No patient should be given more than one hand-held button to self-administer pain therapy.

Recommended monitoring during continuous regional analgesia includes pain scores during rest and activity, extent of motor and sensory blockade, pulse oximetry saturations, clinical evidence of local anesthetic toxicity, and inspection of the catheter site for infection. A sample of the monitoring sheet used at our institution is shown in Fig. 16.19. If the catheter site looks inflamed or infected, the catheter should be removed and the tip sent for culture and sensitivity. Consideration should be given to continuing the perioperative antibiotic for longer periods if the block is continued for more than 48 hours.

It is important to educate nurses and physiotherapists involved in the care of the patients prior to running a regional-block-based pain management program. This is often provided with the help of periodic in-service training to the team as well as the use of self-learning packages. Physiotherapists will have to take into consideration the weakness in certain groups of muscles, such as the quadriceps with femoral nerve block, to provide safe physiotherapy to patients without the risk of accidental falls or dislocations.

Home regional analgesia

Patients who are discharged home with a regional block should be given written and verbal instructions prior to discharge.

These instructions should contain details of contact personnel in case of problems, as well as a description of what to anticipate from the therapy (Fig. 16.20). These instructions could include details on how to remove the block catheter if the patient or the caregiver is given responsibility for the process. If neither is comfortable removing the block catheter, arrangements should be made with home-care nurses to provide this service, or instructions regarding a return visit to the hospital for removal of the catheter should be given. The instructions should also include care of the limb that will be numb and weak. Patients should be advised to contact the hospital in case they perceive an increase in pain despite the block. This may be an early sign of compartment syndrome or displaced catheter. One must ensure that patients who are discharged home with regional blocks have a capable chaperone to troubleshoot in case of emergency. The patients should be advised to return to the hospital emergency room if they are unable to contact the regional/acute pain team. Thus, it is very important to have a team of anesthesiologists and nurses available 24 hours a day, 7 days a week.

All patients who have received a regional block should be contacted by the team on postoperative days 1, 7, and 30 to gather information on the adequacy of pain control, transitional pain with oral analgesics, and early as well as delayed complications. Patients who report persistent paresthesia or ongoing neurologic deficits should be brought back to the hospital for detailed evaluation, documentation, and follow-up.

Patients who develop neurologic deficits should have early electromyography and nerve conduction studies on both the operated and the nonoperated limb to document baseline deficits that may impact etiology, therapy, and follow-up.[193] Studies of the nonoperated limb may sometimes reveal preexisting neurologic deficits of unrelated etiology (e.g., diabetic neuropathy). This is particularly important, as many diabetic patients with subtle evidence of neuropathy often require much higher currents with PNS or fail to develop a motor response during the initiation of the block.[194]

Many institutions have a database to effect evidence-based changes to the program. One has to factor in the need for nursing and database personnel in the business plan for such a service. If such personnel make telephone contacts, there should be a mechanism set to refer the patients with ongoing problems to the anesthesiologists involved in the regional block care of the patient, thus closing the loop of care. Pending establishment of the database, one can have a ledger where all blocks performed are entered, with the follow-up data, to ensure continuity of care.

Recent advances

Efforts have been made to prolong the duration of action of a single dose of local anesthetic block by using slow-release local anesthetics, such as liposomal preparations entrapped in multilamellar devices.[195] Biodegradable bupivacaine-containing polymer microcapsules have produced local anesthetic with a duration of up to 7 days in animals,[196] and addition of dexamethasone within these capsules further extended the duration.[197] Kopacz et al. performed intercostal nerve blocks with bupivacaine microcapsules in healthy volunteers and demonstrated a block that lasted for 96 hours.[198] These formulations are still experimental and are not yet practical or safe for routine human use.[199]

Ultrasound for peripheral nerve block has gained popularity worldwide. It has the potential to become standard care in the near future (see Chapter 12).

Opioids in trauma and food for thought

There have been reports about the deleterious effects of opioid analgesics in unstable trauma patients. The exacerbation of hemodynamic instability has been raised as a potential reason to avoid or limit opioid use in such patients.[200] Molina et al. questioned the use of opioids in trauma using an animal model because of possible harmful effects.[201] The authors reported that hemorrhaged animals treated with morphine had a blunted pressor response, aggravated hemodynamic instability, and increased 48-hour mortality rates. They also reported that morphine compromised the immune defense mechanisms that may increase the risk of infection.

Further developments are needed to provide safer medications and techniques for trauma patients. Long-acting local anesthetics and the introduction of ultrasound to aid in the performance of peripheral nerve blocks are promising examples.

LONDON Health Sciences Centre

St JOSEPH's HEALTH CARE LONDON

DRAFT

ACUTE PAIN MANAGEMENT BEDSIDE MONITORING RECORD

☐ SSS ☐ UC ☐ WC ☐ SJHC

_____
Approval Signature / Date

CURRENT DATE:			DATE STARTED:		
YYYY	MM	DD	YYYY	MM	DD

☐ **PCA** ☐ **EPIDURAL** ☐ **Continuous Infusion** Drug/s _____

Dose _____ Delay _____ Basal (Continuous) _____ Max. Hourly Dose _____

☐ **OTHER:** _____ Drug _____ Rate _____

SEDATION SCALE:
0 Alert
1 Occasionally drowsy
2 Frequently drowsy, easy to arouse
3 Somnolent, difficult to arouse
4 Unarousable
"S" Sleeping

PAIN SCALE:
0 - No Pain   10 - Worst Pain
FLACC
Refer to guidelines on back of record.
Sensory blockade guidelines on back of record

MOTOR BLOCKADE (Right/Left)

Lower
0 - Able to Raise Extended Leg off Bed
1 - Able to Flex Knee and Ankle
2 - Able to Flex Ankle Only
3 - Unable to Flex Hip, Knee or Ankle

Upper
0 - Able to approximate thumb & 5th finger
1 - Unable to approximate thumb & index finger
2 - Unable to flex biceps
3 - Unable to extend triceps

SIDE EFFECTS:
N - Nausea   P - Pruritus
0 None
1 Mild, No Rx Needed
2 Moderate, Rx Effective
3 Severe, Rx Not Effective

TIME	RESPIRATORY RATE	SEDATION SCALE	PAIN SCORE REST	PAIN SCORE ACTIVITY	MOTOR BLOCK ☐ UPPER ☐ LOWER R	L	SENSORY BLOCKADE	SIDE EFFECTS	BALANCE IN SYRINGE	TOTAL HOURLY	INJECTIONS ATTEMPTS	BOLUS OR CHANGES	INITIALS
0700-0800													
0800-0900													
0900-1000													
1000-1100													
1100-1200													
1200-1300													
1300-1400													
1400-1500													
1500-1600													
1600-1700													
1700-1800													
1800-1900													
1900-2000													
2000-2100													
2100-2200													
2200-2300													
2300-2400													
2400-0100													
0100-0200													
0200-0300													
0300-0400													
0400-0500													
0500-0600													
0600-0700													

8460-5608 (Rev. 2004/03/22)

PLEASE TURN OVER →

Figure 16.19 Block monitoring form.

GUIDELINES FOR ASSESSMENT

GUIDELINES FOR TESTING SENSORY BLOCKADE / DERMATOME CHART:

Check cold sensation using an alcohol/ chlorhexidine swab or an ice cube q4h x 24 hours of epidural therapy, then q12h at the beginning of each shift (and as required, while on epidural infusion). Document the level that the patient can no longer feel cold, as well as areas that have reduced sensation. (Refer to self-directed learning package for additional information).

Pain Scale: > 7 years of age

In addition to the 0 - 10 pain scale, ask the patient:
1) Are you comfortable at rest?   Yes or No
2) Are you comfortable with activity?   Yes or No

The patient's responses are to be documented in the "Comments" section below.

FLACC Scale: Non verbal & < 7 years of age

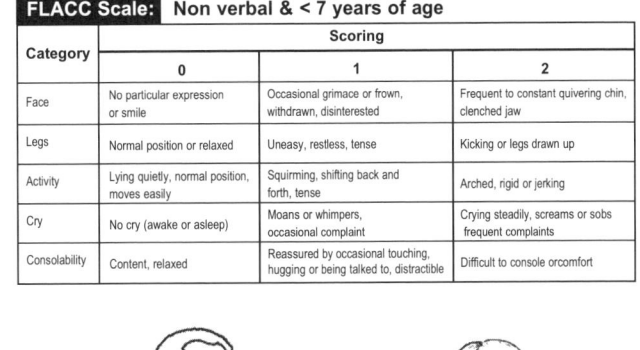

Category	Scoring		
	0	1	2
Face	No particular expression or smile	Occasional grimace or frown, withdrawn, disinterested	Frequent to constant quivering chin, clenched jaw
Legs	Normal position or relaxed	Uneasy, restless, tense	Kicking or legs drawn up
Activity	Lying quietly, normal position, moves easily	Squirming, shifting back and forth, tense	Arched, rigid or jerking
Cry	No cry (awake or asleep)	Moans or whimpers, occasional complaint	Crying steadily, screams or sobs frequent complaints
Consolability	Content, relaxed	Reassured by occasional touching, hugging or being talked to, distractible	Difficult to console or comfort

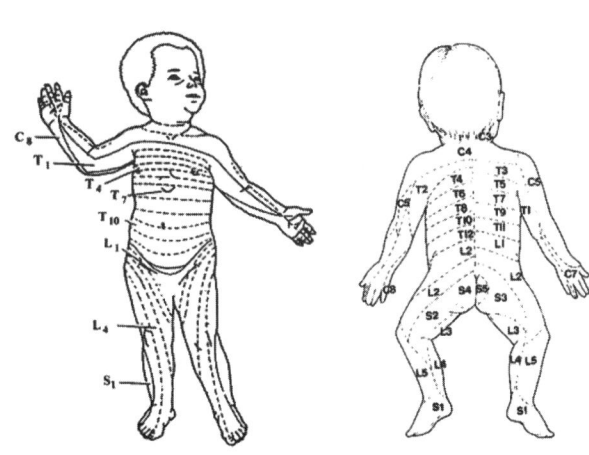

Document epidural site checks and removal in the **COMMENTS** section below.

TIME	COMMENTS	INITIALS

Figure 16.19 *(cont.)*

Instructions for Patient Controlled Regional Analgesia (Infraclavicular Block)   **Figure 16.20** Block instructions.

The infusion pump connected to your block tube contains local anesthetic freezing called Ropivacaine. The pump is set to continuously deliver _____mls of local anesthetic near the nerves. If you start to feel mild discomfort in your hand, you can give an additional 4 mls of the local anesthetic by pressing the hand held button. You may press this button as often as every 1 hour. Please give yourself the boluses while you are in bed. The 300 mL of freezing given to you will last approximately 40 hours.

A small amount of seepage around the catheter insertion site is normal.

If you have moderate to severe pain in the operated hand in spite of the boluses, please call Dr. _____ immediately.

Please take the following precautions:

Make sure you have a responsible adult in the room when you give your bolus.

Stop the pump if you get a metallic taste in your mouth or you feel funny in your head when the bolus is running. Call Dr._____(519) XXXXXXX pager XXXXX immediately.

Your blocked arm will be numb and weak. Have as ling to hold your arm up as long as the block is continued.

Please keep the elbow of the blocked arm on a pillow while in bed to avoid pressure damaging the nerve behind your "funny bone" in the elbow.

Alcohol, driving, handling of fire and machinery are prohibited while you receive the block.

As your operated arm will be numb, you can accidentally hurty our self if you spill hot liquids such as coffee or tea on the blocked area. Take extreme care to look after the numb weak arm.

If you notice any pain on injection during the bolus or redness in the blocked area, kindly call Dr. _____

Please take the pain pills prescribed for you if as needed. The block is used in addition to the oral pain killers that you are prescribed. Severe pain while the block is effective is not normal. Report to Dr. _____ if this happens.

Please come to St Joseph's Health Care on _____ at _____ hours to the PACU on the first floor. Dr._____will meet you there to remove the catheter and take back the pump.

Your caregiver at home may remove the catheter once the pump is empty. This should be done while you are comfortably lying in bed. The caregiver should wash the hands with soap and water. Remove the sticky drape covering the block site. Hold the catheter where it enters the skin between the thumb and index finger and gently pull the catheter out. This should not hurt. Once the catheter is out make sure the blue or black tip is seen. Cover the area with a band aid.

If you perceive any pain during the removal, do not remove the catheter and call Dr_____at_____

Questions

(1) **Pain has:**
   a. No effects on the patient
   b. Physical effects on the patient
   c. Psychological effects on the patient
   d. Both physical and psychological effects on the patient

(2) **Pain leads to:**
   a. Release of prostanoids and cytokines
   b. Localized hypersensitivity
   c. Spinal cord wind-up
   d. Neuronal excitability
   e. All of the above

(3) **When assessing pain:**
   a. Nurses and physicians assess patients' pain adequately
   b. Only nurses assess patients' pain accurately
   c. Only physicians assess patients' pain accurately
   d. Neither nurses nor physicians assess patients' pain adequately

(4) **Regional blocks can help in:**
   a. Airway protection during transfer of patients from a triage area
   b. Preventing posttraumatic neuropathic pain states
   c. Providing surgical anesthesia as well as postoperative analgesia
   d. Repeated dressing changes and debridements
   e. All of the above

(5) **Femoral blocks:**
   a. Are safe, simple, and quick
   b. Are easy to teach and learn
   c. Can provide pain control for prehospital patient transfer
   d. Can be used in children as well as adults
   e. All of the above

(6) **Continuous regional techniques should be done:**
   a. In the field situation
   b. In the ambulance
   c. In the emergency room
   d. In the operating room
   e. In the emergency and operating rooms

(7) **For shoulder and upper arm analgesia, the best block is:**
   a. Axillary block
   b. Interscalene block
   c. Infraclavicular block
   d. Lumbar plexus block

(8) **Problems with supraclavicular block include:**
   a. Pneumothorax
   b. Diaphragmatic weakness
   c. Horner's syndrome
   d. All of the above
   e. None of the above

(9) **Regarding the use of adjuvants with local anesthetics:**
   a. Adjuvants should be used in all trauma patients
   b. Adjuvants should be used in no trauma patients
   c. Careful selection of patients is needed
   d. Only opioids can be used
   e. Only epinephrine can be used

(10) **For nerve localization techniques in trauma:**
   a. Ultrasound is a not a good option, as it requires equipment and training

b. Use of a peripheral nerve stimulator is mandatory
c. Ultrasound guidance is a relatively new technique which is superior to other available nerve-seeking techniques
d. Nerve localization techniques are rarely required when doing regional blocks in trauma patients

Answers

(1) d
(2) e
(3) d
(4) e
(5) e
(6) e
(7) b
(8) d
(9) c
(10) c

References

1. Cordell WH, Keene KK, Giles BK, *et al.* The high prevalence of pain in emergency medical care. *Am J Emerg Med* 2002; **20**: 165–9.

2. Cuthbertson BH, Hull A, Strachan M, *et al.* Post-traumatic stress disorder after critical illness requiring general intensive care. *Intensive Care Med* 2004; **30**: 450–5.

3. Gregoretti C, Decaroli D, Miletto A, *et al.* Regional anesthesia in trauma patients. *Anesthesiology Clin* 2007; **25**: 99–116.

4. Bulger EM, Edwards Thomas, Klotz PRN, *et al.* Epidural analgesia improves outcome after multiple rib fractures. *Surgery* 2004; **2**: 426–30.

5. Osinowo OA, Zahrani M, Softah A. Effect of intercostal nerve block with 0.5% bupivacaine on peak expiratory flow rate and arterial oxygen saturation in rib fractures. *J Trauma* 2004; **56**: 345–7.

6. Davidson EM, Ginosar Y, Avidan A. Pain management and regional anaesthesia in the trauma patient. *Curr Opin Anaesthesiol* 2005; **18**: 169–74.

7. Cohen SP, Christo PJ, Moroz L. Pain management in trauma patients. *Am J Phys Med Rehabil* 2004; **83**: 142–61.

8. Joint Commission on Accreditation of Healthcare Organizations. *Comprehensive Accreditation Manual for Hospitals.* Chicago, IL: JCAHO, 2001.

9. Cohen SP, Christo PJ, Moroz L. Pain management in trauma patients. *Am J Phys Med Rehabil* 2004; **83**: 142–61.

10. Marik PE, Flemmer M. The immune response to surgery and trauma: implications for treatment. *J Trauma Acute Care Surg* 2012; **73** (4): 801–8.

11. Vane JR, Bakhle YS, Botting RM. Cyclooxygenases 1 and 2. *Annu Rev Pharmacol Toxicol* 1998; **38**: 97–120.

12. McCleskey EW, Gold MS. Ion channels of nociception. *Annu Rev Physiol* 1999; **61**: 835–56.

13. Fishman SM, Ballantyne JC, Rathmell JP. *Bonica's Management of Pain*, 4th edition. Philadelphia, PA: Lippincott, Williams & Wilkins, 2010, Chapter 5, pp. 56–7.

14. Woolf CJ, Salter MW. Neuronal plasticity: increasing the gain in pain. *Science* 2000; **288**: 1765–8.

15. Yaksh TL, Hua XY, Kalcheva I, *et al.* The spinal biology in humans and animals of pain states generated by persistent small afferent input. *Proc Natl Acad Sci USA* 1999; **96**: 7680–6.

16. Omergovic M, Duric A, Muratovic N, *et al.* Metabolic response to trauma and stress. *Medicinski Arhiv* 2003; **57**: 57–60.

17. Cohen SP, Christo PJ, Moroz L. Pain management in trauma patients. *Am J Phys Med Rehabil* 2004; **83**: 142–61.

18. Whipple JK, Lewis KS, Quebbeman EJ, *et al.* Analysis of pain management in critically ill patients. *Pharmacotherapy* 1995; **15**: 592–9.

19. Bulger EM, Edward T, Klotz P, Jurkovich V. Epidural analgesia improves outcome after multiple rib fractures. *Surgery* 2004; **136**: 426–30.

20. Matot I, Oppenheim-Eden A, Ratrot R, *et al.* Preoperative cardiac events in elderly patients with hip fracture randomized to epidural or conventional analgesia. *Anesthesiology* 2003; **98**: 156–63.

21. Cohen SP, Christo PJ, Moroz L. Pain management in trauma patients. *Am J Phys Med Rehabil* 2004; **83**: 142–61.

22. Malchow RJ, Black IH. The evolution of pain management in the critically ill trauma patient: Emerging concepts from the global war on terrorism. *Crit Care Med* 2008; **36**: S346–57.

23. Statement on nonoperating room anesthetizing locations. *Standard and Practice Parameters.* ASA House of Delegates, 15 October (2003), amended 22 October (2008).

24. Gille J, Gille M, Gahr R, Wiedemann B. Acute pain management in proximal femoral fractures: femoral nerve block (catheter technique) vs systemic pain therapy using a clinic internal

organization model. *Anaesthesist* 2006; **55**: 414–22.

25. Telion C, Carli P. Prehospital and emergency room pain management for the adult trauma patient. *Tech Regional Anesth Pain Manag* 2002; **6** (1): 10–18.

26. Horlocker TT, Wedel DJ, Rowlingson JC, *et al*. Regional anesthesia in the patient receiving antithrombotic or thrombolytic therapy: American Society of Regional Anesthesia and Pain Medicine evidence-based guidelines (third edition). *Reg Anesth Pain Med* 2010; **35**: 64–101.

27. Rao S, Gatlin M, Gebhard RE. Regional anesthesia for trauma. In Varon AJ, Smith C, eds., *Essentials of Trauma Anesthesia*. Cambridge: Cambridge University Press, 2012, pp. 95–115.

28. Shackford SR, Connolly JF. Taming of the screw: a case report and literature review of limb-threatening complications after plate osteosynthesis of a clavicularnonunion. *J Trauma* 2003; **55**: 840–3.

29. Ring D, Holovacs T. Brachial plexus palsy after intramedullary fixation of a clavicle fracture: a report of three cases. *J Bone Joint Surg Am* 2005; **87**: 1834–7.

30. Bain GI, Eng K, Zumstein MA. Fatal air embolus during internal fixation of the clavicle: a case report. *JBJS Case Connect* 2013; **3** (24): 1–4.

31. Stone MB, Wang R, Price DD. Ultrasound-guided supraclavicular brachial plexus nerve block vs procedural sedation for the treatment of upper extremity emergencies. *Am J Emerg Med* 2008; **26** (6): 706–10.

32. McCahon RA, Bedforth NM. Peripheral nerve block at the elbow and wrist. *Contin Educ Anaesth Crit Care Pain* 2007; **7**: 42–4.

33. Enneking FK, Chan V, Greger J, *et al*. Lower extremity peripheral nerve blockade: essentials of our current understanding. *Reg Anesth Pain Med* 2005; **30**: 4–35.

34. Capdevilla X, Macaire P, Dadure C, *et al*. Continuous psoas compartment block for postoperative analgesia after total hip arthroplasty: New Landmarks, technical guidelines and clinical evaluation. *Anesth Analg* 2002; **94**: 1606–13.

35. Chelly JE, Delaunay L. A new anterior approach to the sciatic nerve block. *Anesthesiology* 1999; **91**: 1655–60.

36. Meier G, Buettner J. Blocks at the knee. In *Peripheral Regional Anesthesia: an Atlas of Anatomy and Techniques*, 2nd edition. Stuttgart: Georg Thieme, 2007, Chapter 11.

37. Mannion S. Psoas compartment block. *Contin Educ Anaesth Crit Care Pain* 2007; **7**: 162–6.

38. Ilfeld BM, Ball ST. Gearen PF, *et al*. Ambulatory continuous posterior lumbar plexus block after hip arthroplasty. *Anesthesiology* 2008; **109**: 491–501.

39. Auroy Y, Benhanou D, Bargues L. Major complications of regional anesthesia in France. *Anesthesiology* 2002; **97**: 1274–80.

40. Huet O, Eyrolle LJ, Mazoit JX, Ozier YM. Cardiac arrest after injection of ropivacaine for posterior lumbar plexus blockade. *Anesthesiology* 2003; **99**: 1451–3.

41. Aida S, Takahashi H, Shimoji K. Renal subcapsular hematoma after lumbar plexus block. *Anesthesiology* 1996; **84**: 452–5.

42. Grant SA, Nielsen KC, Greengrass RA, Steele SM, Klein SM. Continuous peripheral nerve block for ambulatory surgery. *Reg Anesth Pain Med* 2001; **26**: 209–14.

43. William BA, Kentor ML, Vogt M, *et al*. Femoral sciatic nerve blocks for complex outpatient knee surgery are associated with less postoperative pain before same day discharge. *Anesthesiology* 2003; **98**: 1206–13.

44. Triner W, Levine J, Lai S-Y, McErlean M. Femoral nerve block for femoral fractures. *Ann Emerg Med* 2005; **45**: 679.

45. Dauri M, Polzoni M, Fabbi E, *et al*. Comparison of epidural, continuous femoral block and intraarticular analgesia after anterior cruciate ligament reconstruction. *Acta Anaesthesiol Scand* 2003; **47**: 20–5.

46. Enneking FK, Chan V, Greger J, Hadzic A, *et al*. Lower extremity peripheral nerve blockade: essentials of our current understanding. *Reg Anesth Pain Med* 2005; **30**: 4–35.

47. Ganapathy S, Wasserman RA, Watson JT, *et al*. Modified continuous femoral three-in-one block for postoperative pain after total knee arthroplasty. *Anesth Analg* 1999; **89**: 1197–202.

48. Dalens B, Vanneuville G, Tanguy A. Comparison of fascia iliaca compartment block with the 3-in-1 block in children. *Anesth Analg* 1989; **69**: 705–13.

49. Al-Haddad MF, Coventry DM. Major nerve blocks of the lower limb. *BJA CEPD Rev* 2003; **3**: 102–5.

50. Ericksen ML, Swenson JD, Pace NL. The anatomic relationship of the sciatic nerve to the lesser trochanter: Implications for anterior sciatic nerve block. *Anesth Analg* 2002; **95**: 1071–4.

51. Geffen GJV, Scheuer M, Muller A, Garderniers J, Gielen M. Ultrasound guided bilateral continuous sciatic nerve blocks with stimulating catheters for postoperative pain relief after bilateral lower limb amputations. *Anaesthesia* 2006; **61**: 1204–7.

52. Ilfeld BM, Morey TE, Wang RD, Enneking FK. Continuous popliteal sciatic nerve block for postoperative pain control at home: A randomized, doubleblinded, placebo-controlled study. *Anesthesiology* 2002; **97**: 959–65.

53. Lopez AM, Sala-Blanch X, Magaldi M, *et al*. Ultrasound-guided ankle block for forefoot surgery-the contribution of the saphenous nerve. *Reg Anaesth Pain Med* 2012; **37** (5): 544–57.

54. Chelley JE. *Peripheral Nerve Blocks: a Color Atlas*, 3rd edition. Philadelphia, PA: Lippincott, Williams & Wilkins, 2008. Chapter 15.

55. Middleton RW, Varian JP. Tourniquet paralysis. *Aust N Z J Surg* 1974; **44**: 124–7.

56. Heath ML. Deaths after intravenous regional anaesthesia. *Br Med J* 1982; **285**: 913–14.

57. Choyce A, Peng P. A systemic review of adjuncts for intravenous regional anesthesia for surgical procedures. *Can J Anaesth* 2002; **49**: 32–45.

58. Peng PWH, Coleman MM, Macartney CJL, *et al*. Comparison of anesthetic effect between 0.375% Ropivacaine versus 0.5% lidocaine in forearm intravenous regional anesthesia. *Reg Anesth Pain Med* 2002; **27**: 595–9.

59. Kongsholm J, Olerud C. Carpal tunnel pressure in the acute phase after Colles' fracture. *Arch Orthop Trauma Surg* 1986; **105**: 183–6.

60. Kongsholm J, Olerud C. Neurological complications of dynamic reduction of

Colles' fractures without anesthesia compared with traditional manipulation after local infiltration anesthesia. *J Orthop Trauma* 1987; **1**: 43–7.

61. Hecht JS. Occipital nerve blocks in postconcussive headaches: a retrospective review and report of ten patients. *J Head Trauma Rehab* 2004; **19**: 1.

62. Bernard JM, Pereon Y. Nerve stimulation for regional anesthesia of the face. *Anesth Analg* 2005; **101**: 589–91.

63. Budac S, Suresh S. Emergent facial lacerations repair in children: nerve blocks to the rescue. *Anesth Analg* 2006; **102**: 1901–2.

64. Shiffman MA, Mirrafati SJ, Lam SM, Cueteaux CG. *Simplified Facial Rejuvenation*. Berlin: Springer, 2008. Chapter 2, pp. 27–8.

65. Menon R, Swanepoel A. Sympathetic blocks. *Contin Educ Anaesth Crit Care Pain* 2010; **10**: 88–92.

66. Mahli A, Coskun D, Akcali DT. Aetiology of convulsions due to stellate ganglion block: a review and report of two cases. *Eur J Anaesth* 2002; **19**: 376–80.

67. Gupta MM, Bithal PK, Dash HH, Chaturvedi A, Mahajan RP. Effects of stellate ganglion block on cerebral haemodynamics as assessed by transcranial Doppler ultrasonography. *Br J Anaesth* 2005; **95**: 669–73.

68. van Eijs F, Stanton-Hicks M, Van Zundert J, *et al.* Complex Regional Pain Syndrome. *Pain Practice* 2011; **11**: 70–87.

69. Chestnut DH. Efficacy and safety of epidural opioids for post-operative analgesia. *Anesthesiology* 2005; **102**: 221–3.

70. Aldrete JA, Reza-Medina M, Daud O, *et al.* Exacerbation of preexisting neurological deficit by neuraxial anesthesia: a report of 7 cases. *J Clin Anesth* 2005; **17**: 304–13.

71. Tran KM, Ganley TJ, Wells L, *et al.* Intraarticular bupivacaine–clonidine–morphine vs femoral–sciatic nerve block on pediatric patients undergoing anterior cruciate ligament reconstruction. *Anesth Analg* 2005; **101**: 1304–10.

72. Dadure C, Bringuier S, Nicolas F, *et al.* Continuous epidural block vs. continuous popliteal nerve block for postoperative pain relief after major pediatric surgery in children: a prospective comparative randomized study. *Anesth Analg* 2006; **102**: 744–9.

73. Dadure C, Pirat P, Raux O *et al.* Perioperative continuous peripheral nerve blocks with disposable infusion pumps in children: a prospective descriptive study. *Anesth Analg* 2003; **97**: 687–90.

74. Santhanam S, Barcelona SL, Young NM, *et al.* Postoperative pain in children undergoing tympanomastoid surgery: Is regional block better than opioids? *Anesth Analg* 2002; **94**: 859–62.

75. Bhalla T, Sawardekar A, Dewhirst E, Jagannathan N, Tobias JD. Ultrasound-guided trunk and core blocks in infants and children. *J Anesth* 2013; **27**: 109–23.

76. Karmakar MK, Booker PD, Franks R, Pozzi M. Continuous extrapleural paravertebral infusion of bupivacaine for post thoracotomy analgesia in young infants. *Br J Anaesth* 1996; **76**: 811–15.

77. Erdös J, Dlaska C, Szatmary P, *et al.* Acute compartment syndrome in children: a case series in 24 patients and review of the literature. *International Orthopaedics (SICOT)* 2011; **35**: 569–75.

78. Macfarlane AJR, Prasad GA, Chan VWS, Brull R. Does regional anesthesia improve outcome after total hip arthroplasty? A systemic review. *Br J Anaesth* 2009; **103** (3): 335–45.

79. Deiner S, Silverstein JH, Abrams KJ. Management of trauma in the geriatric patient. *Curr Opin Anaesthesiol* 2004; **17**: 165–70.

80. Bilotta F, Doronzio A, Stazi E, *et al.* Early postoperative cognitive dysfunction and postoperative delirium after anaesthesia with various hypnotics: study protocol for a randomised controlled trial – The PINOCCHIO trial. *Trials* 2011; **12**: 170.

81. Mason SE, Noel-Storr A, Ritchie CW. The impact of general and regional anesthesia on the incidence of post-operative cognitive dysfunction and post-operative delirium: a systematic review with metaanalysis. *J Alzheimers Dis* 2010; **22** (Suppl 3): 67–79.

82. Karmakar M, Ho AMH. Acute pain management of patients with multiple fractured ribs. *J Trauma Injury Infect Crit Care* 2003; **54**: 615–25.

83. Kerr-Valentic MA, Arthur MM, Mullins RJ, *et al.* Rib fracture pain and disability: can we do better? *J Trauma* 2003; **54**: 1058–63.

84. Gratch DM, McMurtrie. Pain management in chest trauma. *Semin Cardiothorac Vasc Anesth* 2002; **6**: 113–25.

85. Karmakar MK, Critchley LA, Ho AM, *et al.* Continuous thoracic paravertebral infusion of bupivacaine for pain management in patients with multiple fractured ribs. *Chest* 2003; **123**: 424–31.

86. Moon MR, Luchette FA, Gibson SW, *et al.* Prospective, randomized comparison of epidural versus parenteral opioid analgesia in thoracic trauma. *Ann Surg* 1999; **229**: 684–91.

87. Freise H, Van Aken HK. Risks and benefits of thoracic epidural anaesthesia. *Br J Anaes* 2011; **107**: 859–68.

88. Finucane BT. *Complications of Regional Anesthesia*, 2nd edition. New York, NY: Springer, 2007. Chapter 7, p. 14.

89. Karmakar MK, Ho AMH. Acute pain management of patients with multiple fractured ribs. *J Trauma* 2003; **54**: 615–25.

90. Osinowo OA, Zahrani M, Softah A. Effect of intercostal nerve block with 0.5% bupivacaine on peak expiratory flow rate and arterial oxygen saturation in rib fractures. *J Trauma* 2004; **56**: 345–7.

91. Marhofer P, Kettner SC, Hajbok L, Dubsky P, Fleischmann E. Lateral ultrasound-guided paravertebral blockade: an anatomical-based description of a new technique. *Br J Anaes* 2010; **105**: 526–32.

92. Karmakar MK, Chui PT, Joynt GM *et al.* Thoracic paravertebral blocks for management of pain associated with multiple fractured ribs in patients with concomitant lumbar spine trauma. *Reg Anesth Pain Med* 2001; **26**: 169–73.

93. Fletcher AK, Rigby AS, Heyes FL. Three in one femoral block as analgesia for fractured neck of femur in the emergency department: a randomized controlled trial. *Ann Emerg Med* 2003; **41**: 227–33.

94. Guay J. Postoperative pain significantly influences postoperative blood loss in patients undergoing total knee replacement. *Pain Med* 2006; **7**: 476.

95. Sia S, Pelusio F, Barbagli R, Rivituso C. Analgesia before performing a spinal block in the sitting position in patients with femoral shaft fracture: a comparison between femoral nerve block and intravenous fentanyl. *Anesth Analg* 2004; **99**: 1221–4.

96. Choiniere M, Melzack R, Girard N, *et al.* Comparison between patients' and nurses' assessment of pain and medication efficacy in severe burn injuries. *Pain* 1990; **40**: 143–52.

97. Tobias JD. Indications and application of epidural anesthesia in a pediatric population outside perioperative period. *Clin Pediatr (Phila)* 1993; **32**: 81–5.

98. Gallagher G, Rae CP, Kinsella J. Treatment of pain in severe burns. *Am J Clin Dermatol* 2000; **1**: 329–35.

99. Tarantino D. Burn pain and dressing changes. *Tech Reg Anesth Pain Manag* 2002; **6** (1): 33–8.

100. Nikolajsen LJ, Jensen TS. A comprehensive overview of factors that contribute to phantom limbs, and treatment options. In Koltzenburg M, McMahon SB, eds., *Wall and Melzack's Textbook of Pain*. Amsterdam: Elsevier, 2005, pp. 961–71.

101. Nikolajsen L. Phantom limb pain. In Stannard CF, Kalso E, Ballantyne J, eds., *Evidence Based Chronic Pain Management*. Chichester: Wiley Blackwell 2010, 237–47.

102. Woodhouse A. Phantom limb sensation. *Clin Exp Pharmacol Physiol* 2005; **32**: 132–4.

103. Flor H, Nikolajsen L, Jensen TS. Phantom limb pain: A case of maladaptive CNS plasticity? *Nat Rev Neurosci* 2006; **7**: 873–81.

104. Rathmell JP, Kehlet H. Do we have the tools to prevent phantom limb pain? *Anesthesiology* 2011; **114**: 1021–4.

105. Flor H, Elbert T, Knecht S, *et al.* Phantom-limb pain as a perceptual correlate of cortical reorganization following arm amputation. *Nature* 1995; **357**: 482–4.

106. Kiefer RT, Wiech K, Topfner S, *et al.* Continuous brachial plexus analgesia and NMDA-receptor blockade in early phantom limb pain: a report of two cases. *Pain Med* 2002; **3**: 156–60.

107. Beeter JT, Guilmette T, Sparadeo F. Sleep and pain complaints on symptomatic traumatic brain injury and neurologic populations. *Arch Phys Med Rehabil* 1996; **77**: 1298–301.

108. Sapir DA, Gorup JM. Radiofrequency medial branch neurotomy in litigant and non litigant patients with cervical whiplash. *Spine* 2001; **26**: E268–73.

109. Phillips K, Pitt V, O'Connor D, Gruen RL. Interventions for managing skeletal muscle spasticity following traumatic brain injury (Protocol). *Cochrane Database Syst Rev* 2011; (1): CD008929.

110. Galland B.C, Elder D.E, Taylor B.J. Interventions with sleep outcome for children with cerebral palsy or a post traumatic brain injury: a systematic review. *Sleep Med Rev* 2012; **16**: 561–73.

111. Warltier DC. Practical guidelines for acute care of victims of bioterrorism. *Anesthesiology* 2002; **97**: 989–1004.

112. Anderson P.D. Bioterrorism: toxins as weapons. *J Pharm Pract.* 2012; **25**: 521–9.

113. Perez R.S, Zollinger P.E, Dijkstra. Evidence based guidelines for complex regional pain syndrome type 1. *BMC Neurol* 2010; **10**: 20.

114. Toshniwal G, Sunder R, Thomas R, Dureja GP. Management of complex regional pain syndrome type I in upper extremity-evaluation of continuous stellate ganglion block and continuous infraclavicular brachial plexus block: a pilot study. *Pain Med* 2012; **13**: 96–106.

115. Rocco AG. Sympathetically maintained pain may be rekindled by surgery under general anesthesia. *Anesthesiology* 1993; **79**: 865.

116. Sebastin SJ. Complex regional pain syndrome. *Indian J Plast Surg* 2011; **44**: 298–307.

117. Jenson MG, Sorensen RF. Early use of regional and local anesthesia in a combat environment may prevent the development of complex regional pain syndrome in wounded combatants. *Mil Med* 2006; **171**: 396–8.

118. Perez R, Zollinger P, Dijkstra P, *et al.* Evidence based guidelines for complex regional pain syndrome-1. *BMC Neurol* 2010; **10**: 20.

119. Tran D, Duong S, Bertini P, Finlayson R. Treatment of CRPS: a review of evidence. *Can J Anaesth* 2010; **57**: 149–66.

120. Zor F, Ozturk S, Usyilmaz S, Sengezer M. Is stellate ganglion blockade an option to prevent early arterial vasospasm after digital microvascular procedures? *Plast Reconstr Surg* 2006; **117**: 1059–60.

121. Kurt E, Ozturk S, Isik S, Zor F. Continuous brachial plexus blockade for digital replantation and toe to hand transfers. *Am Plast Surg* 2005; **54**: 24–7.

122. Assmann N, McCartney CJ, Tumber PS, Chan VW. Ultrasound guidance for brachial plexus localization and catheter insertion after complete forearm amputation. *Reg Anesth Pain Med* 2007; **32** (1): 93.

123. Van der Werff JF, Medici G, Hovius SE, Kusuma A. Axillary plexus blockade in microvascular surgery, a steal phenomenon? *Microsurgery* 1995; **16** (3): 141–3.

124. Lumenta DB, Haslik W, Beck H, *et al.* Influence of brachial plexus blockade on oxygen balance during surgery. *Anesth Analg* 2011; **113**: 199–201.

125. Sites BD, Brull R. Ultrasound guidance in peripheral regional anesthesia: philosophy, evidence based medicine and techniques. *Curr Opin Anaesth* 2006; **19**: 630–9.

126. Marhofer P, Schrogendorfer K, Koinig H, *et al.* Ultrasonographic guidance improves sensory block and onset times of three-in-one blocks. *Anesth Analg* 1997; **85**: 854–7.

127. Marhofer P, Schrogendorfer K, Wallner T, *et al.* Ultrasonography guidance reduces the amount of local anesthetic for 3-in-1 blocks. *Reg Anesth Pain Med* 1998; **23**: 584–8.

128. Warman P, Nicholls B. Ultrasound-guided nerve blocks: efficacy and safety. *Best Pract Res Clin Anaesthesiol* 2009; **23**: 313–26.

129. Neal JM. Effects of epinephrine in local anesthetics on the central and peripheral nervous systems: Neurotoxicity and neural blood flow. *Reg Anesth Pain Med* 2003; **28**: 124–34.

130. Weber A, Fournier R, Van Gessel E, Riand N, Gamulin Z. Epinephrine does not prolong the analgesia of 20 mL ropivacaine 0.5% or 0.2% in a femoral

three-in-one block. *Anesth Analg* 2001; **93**: 1327–31.

131. Forster JG, Rosenberg PH. Clinically useful adjuvants in regional anaesthesia. *Curr Opin Anaesthesiol* 2003; **16**: 477–86.

132. Iskandar H, Guillaume E, Dixmerias F, *et al.* The enhancement of sensory blockade by clonidine selectively added to mepivacaine after midhumeral block. *Anesth Analg* 2001; **93**: 771–5.

133. Ilfeld BM, Morey TE, Thannikary LJ *et al.* Clonidine added to a continuous interscalene ropivacaine perineural infusion to improve postoperative analgesia: A randomized, double blind controlled study. *Anesth Analg* 2005; **100**: 1172–8.

134. Erlacher W, Schuschnig C, Koinig H, *et al.* Clonidine as adjuvant for mepivacaine, ropivacaine and bupivacaine in axillary, perivascular brachial plexus block. *Can J Anaesth* 2001; **48** (6): 522–5.

135. Wiles M, Nathanson M. Local anaesthetics and adjuvants: future developments. *Anaesthesia* 2010; **65** (Suppl. 1): 22–37.

136. Virtanen R, Savola JM, Saano V, Nyman I. Characterization of the selectivity, specificity and potency of medetomidine as an α_2-adrenoceptor agonist. *Eur J Pharmacol* 1988; **150**: 9–14.

137. Kanazi GE, Aouad M.T, Jabbour-Kloury SI, *et al.* Effect of low-dose dexmedetomidine or clonidine on the characteristics of bupivacaine spinal block. *Acta Anaesthesiol Scand* 2006; **50**: 222–7.

138. Esmaoglu A, Mizrak A, Akin A, Turk Y, Boyaci A. Addition of dexmedetomidine to lidocaine for intravenous regional anaesthesia. *Eur J Anaesth* 2005; **22**: 447–51.

139. Arslan G, Yeter H, Suslu H, *et al.* Addition of dexmedetomidine to prilocaine for intravenous regional anesthesia. *Reg Anesth Pain Med* 2006; **31**: 67

140. Mantz J, Josserand J, Hamada S. Dexmedetomidine: new insights. *Eur J Anaesth* 2011; **28**: 3–6.

141. Brau ME, Sander F, Vogel W, *et al.* Blocking mechanisms of ketamine and its enantiomers in enzymatically demyelinated peripheral nerve as revealed by single-channel experiments. *Anesthesiology* 1997; **86**: 394–404.

142. Carlton SM, Hargett GL, Coggeshall RE. Localization and activation of glutamate receptors in unmyelinated axons of rat glabrous skin. *Neurosci Lett* 1995; **197**: 25–8.

143. Pekoe GM, Smith DJ. The involvement of opiate and mono-aminergic neuronal systems in the analgesic effects of ketamine. *Pain* 1982; **12**: 57–73.

144. Weber WV, Jawalekar KS, Jawalekar SR. The effect of ketamine on the nerve conduction in isolated sciatic nerves of the toad. *Neurosci Lett* 1975; **1**: 115–20.

145. Lee IO, Kim WK, Kong MH, *et al.* No enhancement of sensory and motor blockade by ketamine added to ropivacaine interscalene brachial plexus blockade. *Acta Anaesthesiol Scand* 2002; **46**: 821–6.

146. Sunder RA, Toshniwal G, Dureja GP. Ketamine as an adjuvant in sympathetic blocks for management of central sensitization following peripheral nerve injury. *J Brachial Plexus Peripheral Nerve Injury* 2008; **3**: 22.

147. Wang JK, Nauss LA, Thomas JE. Pain relief by intrathecally applied morphine in man. *Anesthesiology* 1979; **50**: 149–51.

148. Morgan M. The rational use of intrathecal and extradural opioids. *Br J Anaesth* 1989; **63**: 165–88.

149. Chaney MA. Side effects of intrathecal and epidural opioids. *Can J Anaes* 1995; **42**: 891–903.

150. Wiles MD, Nathanson MH. Local anaesthetics and adjuvants: future developments. *Anaesthesia* 2010; **65** (Suppl. 1): 22–37.

151. Gambling D, Hughes T, Martin G, Horton W, Manvelian G. A comparison of Depodur, a novel, single-dose extended-release epidural morphine, with standard epidural morphine for pain relief after lower abdominal surgery. *Anesth Analg* 2005; **100**: 1065–74.

152. Murphy DB, McCartney CJL, Chan VWS. Novel analgesic adjuncts for brachial plexus block: A systematic review. *Anesth Analg* 2000; 1122–8.

153. Behr A, Freo U, Ori C, Westermann B, Alemanno F. Buprenorphine added to levobupivacaine enhances postoperative analgesia of middle interscalene brachial plexus block. *J Anesth* 2012: **26**: 746–51.

154. Neal JM, Hebl JR, Gerancher JC, Hogan QH. Brachial plexus anesthesia: essentials of our current understanding. *Reg Anesth Pain Med* 2002; **27**: 402–28.

155. Joseph RS, McDonald SB. Facilitating the onset of regional anesthetic blocks. *Tech Reg Anesth Pain Manag* 2004; **8**: 110–13.

156. Murphy DB, McCartney CJL, Chan VWS. Novel analgesic adjuncts for brachial plexus block: a systematic review. *Anesth Analg* 2000; **90**: 1122–8.

157. Tsai YC, Chang PJ, Jou IM. Direct tramadol application on sciatic nerve inhibits spinal somatosensory evoked potentials in rats. *Anesth Analg* 2001; **92**: 1547–51.

158. Kapral S, Gollmann G, Waltl B, *et al.* Tramadol added to mepivacaine prolongs the duration of an axillary brachial plexus blockade. *Anesth Analg* 1999; **88**: 853–6.

159. Robaux S, Blunt C, Viel E, *et al.* Tramadol added to 1.5% mepivacaine for axillary brachial plexus block improves postoperative analgesia dose-dependently. *Anesth Analg* 2004; **98**: 1172–7.

160. Benhamou D. Are local anesthetics needed for local anesthesia? *Anesthesiology* 2004; **101**: 271–2.

161. Roelants F, Lavand'homme PM: Epidural neostigmine combined with sufentanil provides balanced and selective analgesia in early labor. *Anesthesiology* 2004; **101**: 439–44.

162. Van Elstraete AC, Pastureau F, Lebrun T, Mehdaoui H. Neostigmine added to lidocaine axillary plexus block for postoperative analgesia. *Eur J Anaesth* 2001; **18**: 257–60.

163. Bouderka MA, Al-Harrar R, Bouggad A, Harti A. Neostigmine added to bupivacaine in axillary plexus block: which benefit? *Ann Franc Anesth Reanim* 2003; **22**: 510–13.

164. Bouaziz H, Paqueron X, Bur ML, *et al.* No enhancement of sensory and motor blockade by neostigmine added to mepivacaine axillary plexus block. *Anesthesiology* 1999; **91**: 79–83.

165. Kaya FN, Sahin S, Owen MD, Eisenach JC. Epidural neostigmine produces analgesia but also sedation in women after cesarean delivery. *Anesthesiology* 2004; **100**: 381–5.

166. Keeler JF, Simpson KH, Ellis FR, Kay SP. Effect of addition of hyaluronidase to bupivacaine during axillary brachial plexus block. *Br J Anaesth* 1992; **68**: 68–71.

167. Gupta A, Axelsson K, Allvin R, *et al.* Postoperative pain following knee arthroscopy: the effects of intra-articular ketorolac and/or morphine. *Reg Anesth Pain Med* 1999; **24**: 225–30.

168. Talu GK, Ozyalcin S, Koltka K, *et al.* Comparison of efficacy of intraarticular application of tenoxicam, bupivacaine and tenoxicam: bupivacaine combination in arthroscopic knee surgery. *Knee Surg Sports Traumatol Arthrosc* 2002; **10**: 355–60.

169. Apan A, Basar H, Ozcan S, Buyukkocak U. Combination of adenosine with prilocaine and lignocaine for brachial plexus block does not prolong postoperative analgesia. *Anaesth Intensive Care* 2003; **31**: 648–52.

170. Clerc S, Vuilleumier H, Frascarolo P, Spahn DR, Gardaz JP. Is the effect of inguinal field block with 0.5% Bupivacaine on postoperative pain after hernia repair enhanced by addition of ketorolac or S(+) ketamine? *Clin J Pain* 2005; **21**: 101–5.

171. Kurt N, Kurt I, Aygunes B, *et al.* Effects of adding alfentanil or atracurium to lidocaine solution for intravenous regional anaesthesia. *Eur J Anaesthesiol* 2002; **19**: 522–5.

172. Choyce A, Peng P. A systemic review of adjuncts for intravenous regional anesthesia for surgical procedures. *Can J Anaesth* 2002; **49**: 32–45.

173. Auroy Y, Narchi P, Messiah A, *et al.* Serious complications related to regional anesthesia. Results of a prospective survey in France. *Anesthesiology* 1997; **87**: 479–86.

174. Hadzic A. *Hadzic's Peripheral Nerve Blocks and Anatomy for Ultrasound-Guided Regional Anaesthesia*, 2nd edition. New York, NY: McGraw-Hill, 2010. Chapter 10 pg 127–138.

175. Steinfeldt T, Nimphius W, Wurps M, *et al.* Nerve perforation with pencil point or short bevelled needles: histological outcome. *Acta Anaesthesiol Scand* 2010; **54**: 993–9.

176. Neal JM, Hebl JR, Gerancher JC, Hogan QH. Brachial plexus anesthesia: essentials of our current understanding. *Reg Anesth Pain Med* 2002; **27**: 402–28.

177. Neal JM. Effects of epinephrine in local anesthetics on the central and peripheral nervous systems: Neurotoxicity and neural blood flow. *Reg Anesth Pain Med* 2003; **28**: 124–34.

178. Hadzic A, Dilberovic F, Shah S *et al.* Combination of intraneural injection and high injection pressure leads to fascicular injury and neurologic deficits in dogs. *Reg Anesth Pain Med* 2004; **29**: 417–23.

179. Urmey WF, Stanton J. Inability to consistently elicit a motor response following sensory paresthesia during interscalene block administration. *Anesthesiology* 2002; **96**: 552–4.

180. Tsai T, Vuckovic I, Eldan K, Kucuk-Alija D. Intensity of the stimulating current is not a reliable indicator of intraneural needle placement. *Reg Anesth Pain Med* 2008; **33**: 207–10.

181. Benumof JL. Permanent loss of cervical spinal cord function associated with interscalene block performed under general anesthesia. *Anesthesiology* 2000; **93**: 1541–4.

182. Tsao BE, Wilbourn AJ. Infraclavicular brachial plexus injury following axillary regional block. *Muscle Nerve* 2004; **30**: 44–8.

183. Urmey WF, Talts KH, Sharrock NE. One hundred percent incidence of hemidiaphragmatic paresis associated with interscalene brachial plexus anesthesia as diagnosed by ultrasonography. *Anesth Analg* 1991; **72**: 498–503.

184. Neal JM, Bernards CM, Butterworth JF, *et al.* ASRA practice advisory on local anesthetic systemic toxicity. *Reg Anesth Pain Med* 2010; **35**: 152–61. http://journals.lww.com/rapm/Fulltext/2010/03000/ASRA_Practice_Advisory_on_Local_Anesthetic.7.aspx (accessed September 2014).

185. Cousins MJ, Carr DB, Horlocker TT, Bridenbaugh PO. *Cousin's and Bridenbaugh's Neural Blockade in Clinical Anesthesia and Pain Medicine*, 4th edition. Philadelphia, PA: Lippincott, Williams & Wilkins, 2009. Chapter 13, pp. 316–42.

186. Samet RE, Dutton RP. Diagnosing compartment syndrome: implications of regional anesthesia. *Anesthesiology* 2006; **105**: A885.

187. Olson SA, Glasgow RR. Acute compartment syndrome in lower extremity musculoskeletal trauma. *J Am Acad Orthop Surg* 2005; **13**: 436–44.

188. Cuvillon P, Ripart J, Lalourcey L, *et al.* The continuous femoral nerve block catheter for postoperative analgesia: Bacteria colonization, infectious rate and adverse effects. *Anesth Analg* 2001; **93**: 1045–9.

189. Adam F, Jaziri S, Chauvin M. Psoas abscess complicating femoral nerve block catheter. *Anesthesiology* 2003; **99**: 230–1.

190. Hebl JR, Niessen AD. Infectious complications of regional anesthesia. *Curr Opin Anaesthesiol* 2011; **24**: 573–80.

191. Buckenmaier CC III, Auton AA, Flournoy WS. Continuous peripheral nerve block catheter tip adhesion in a rat model. *Acta Anaesthesiol Scand* 2006; **50**: 694–8.

192. Capdevila X, Pirat P, Bringuier S *et al.* Continuous peripheral nerve blocks in hospital wards after orthopedic surgery. *Anesthesiology* 2005; **103**: 1035–45.

193. Horlocker TT. Neurological complications of neuraxial and peripheral blockade. *Can J Anaesth* 2001; **48** (6): R1–8.

194. Sites BD, Gallagher J, Sparks M. Ultrasound-guided popliteal block demonstrates an atypical motor response to nerve stimulation in 2 patients with diabetes mellitus. *Reg Anesth Pain Med* 2003; **28**: 479–82.

195. Grant GJ, Barenholz Y, Bolotin EM, *et al.* A novel liposomal bupivacaine formulation to produce ultralong acting analgesia. *Anesthesiology* 2004; **101**: 133–7.

196. Curley J, Castillo J, Hotz J, *et al.* Prolonged regional nerve blockade: injectable biodegradable bupivacaine/polyester microspheres. *Anesthesiology* 1996; **84**: 1401–10.

197. Castillo J, Curley J, Hotz J, *et al.* Glucocorticoids prolong rat sciatic nerve blockade in vivo from

bupivacaine microspheres. *Anesthesiology* 1996; **85**: 1157–66.

198. Kopacz DJ, Lacouture PG, We D, *et al.* The dose response and effects of dexamethasone on bupivacaine microcapsules for intercostals

blockade (T9 to T11) in healthy volunteers. *Anesth Analg* 2003; **96**: 576–82.

199. Grant SA. The Holy Grail: long-acting local anaesthetics and liposomes. *Best Pract Res Clin Anaesthesiol* 2002; **16**: 345–52.

200. Holaday JW. Opiate antagonists in shock and trauma. *Am J Emerg Med* 1984; **2** (1): 8–12.

201. Molina PE, Zambell KL, Zhang P, *et al.* Hemodynamic and immune consequences of opiate analgesia after trauma/haemorrhage. *Shock* 2004; **21**: 526–34.

Chapter

17

Posttrauma chronic pain

David Ryan, Yashar Eshraghi, and Kutaiba Tabbaa

We must all die. But that I can save him from days of torture, that is what I feel as my great and ever new privilege. Pain is a more terrible lord of mankind than even death himself.
Albert Schweitzer

Objectives

(1) Discuss the pathophysiology and treatment of complex regional pain syndrome (CRPS).
(2) Evaluate and manage a range of other posttraumatic pain conditions, including posttraumatic headache, whiplash, and phantom limb pain.
(3) Review the incidence, classification, and management of pain after spinal cord injury.

Introduction

Although advances in trauma care have led to improved survival for victims of major trauma, these patients frequently survive with chronic disability and pain. A prospective cohort study of 201 trauma surgical patients found that only one-third did not develop chronic pain at 7 months, while one-third had developed significantly debilitating chronic pain at the same interval.[1] Likewise, studies of chronic pain populations have shown that a significant percentage of these patients have a history of trauma or surgery. Clearly, chronic pain is a common and potentially devastating consequence of trauma. In this chapter we will review chronic pain syndromes in the trauma patient, after considering the historical and current clinical approach to the chronic pain patient.

A brief history of pain

Pain has been viewed throughout history as a punishment for sins, and it has been associated with mystical beliefs for thousands of years. The Mediterranean region appears to have given birth to some of the first civilizations that relied on a mixture of religious ritual, potion, and therapeutic procedures to treat illness and pain. Our earliest evidence of a priest–physician is the *asu* from Mesopotamia (3000 BC). These original inhabitants of the Mediterranean not only sought relief through divine intervention, but developed elixirs from opium poppy, one of the earliest and most enduring of all medicines in recorded history.[2]

Although Asian civilizations originated independently, these societies also developed a similar spiritual, medicinal, and procedural approach to pain. Writings from Indian physicians (1000 BC) classify medicines into three categories: magical and spiritual acts, those ingested, and those resulting from mental discipline. Chinese acupuncture dates back to 2600 BC and is based on the concept of correcting spirit meridian imbalance. In addition, a wide range of Chinese herbal remedies was also employed. Although opium came late to China, acupuncture has been continually practiced for millennia and is playing an ever greater role in the modern treatment of chronic pain.[2]

Early Western civilization developed a more practical scientific approach to illness and pain that was codified in the writings of the Greek physician Galen in about AD 200. He organized the teachings of Hippocrates, promoted the study of anatomy, and expanded the use of medication.[2] This methodology stagnated during the Middle Ages as faith replaced reason in face of the devastating wars and plagues that marked this era.[3] By the Renaissance, scientific inquiry was embraced once more, opening the door for the development of modern pain theory and practice.

The modern era of chronic pain management has not simply been an evolution and refinement of scientific techniques. As was true in the early civilizations of both the West and the East, the complexity of chronic pain requires a multidisciplinary approach including an understanding of the cultural, psychological, and even religious context in which it is experienced. Although the ancients addressed these issues mostly through mystical practices, modern practice employs

---

Trauma Anesthesia, 2nd Edition, ed. Charles E. Smith. Published by Cambridge University Press. © Charles E. Smith, 2015.

what has been termed the comprehensive pain management approach. The remainder of this chapter will be dedicated to a discussion of the modern understanding and treatment of chronic pain resulting from trauma. However, many aspects of modern treatment have been employed since the beginning of civilization.

The role of pain in protecting the individual

Although pain has been largely thought of as a punishment from God, throughout much of history, modern medicine has proved a far more utilitarian role for pain. The value of pain becomes evident when we consider congenital pain insensitivity syndrome (Fig. 17.1). Individuals born without the ability to perceive pain do not benefit from the warning that pain provides. They suffer trauma without concern and infection goes unnoticed. Children born with this disease have reduced life expectancy and experience significant morbidity, including loss of limb and vision as well as early death. Pain conditions us not only to avoid trauma but also to react to situations that are harmful to our being. Ultimately, acute pain is protective and purposeful.

Defining chronic pain

The terminology used in the field of pain not only provides a vocabulary to describe painful phenomena but also reflects a framework from which to understand pain (Table 17.1). The International Association for the Study of Pain (IASP) defines pain as "an unpleasant sensory and emotional experience associated with actual or potential tissue damage, or described in terms of such damage."[4] Chronic pain can then be viewed as pain that has outlived its usefulness. This is in contrast to the traditional temporal definition of chronic pain as pain that lasts for more than 3–6 months. Most pain management practitioners prefer to define chronic pain from the functional point of view, given that it is less arbitrary and relates more to the physiology of pain.

Pain sensation is classified by pathophysiologic mechanisms. *Somatic pain* is pain that arises from damage or trauma to tispsue (e.g., bone, tendons). *Neuropathic pain* is defined by the IASP as "Pain initiated or caused by a primary dysfunction in the nervous system."[4] Most common pain syndromes are a mixture of somatic and neuropathic pain components.

Either perspective must look beyond the functional role of pain and allow for the fact that pain is actually an experience that may or may not result from direct or ongoing tissue damage. Such a viewpoint is essential to understanding, diagnosing, and treating chronic pain. Though acute painful trauma is a common initiating event that leads to chronic pain, many neuroscientists believe chronic pain to be a neurogenic disease with a significant genetic predisposition that presents after an acute trauma. Others believe that undertreated acute pain results in chronic pain conditions. Further research is needed to clarify the components of chronic pain that may be amenable to genetic treatment.

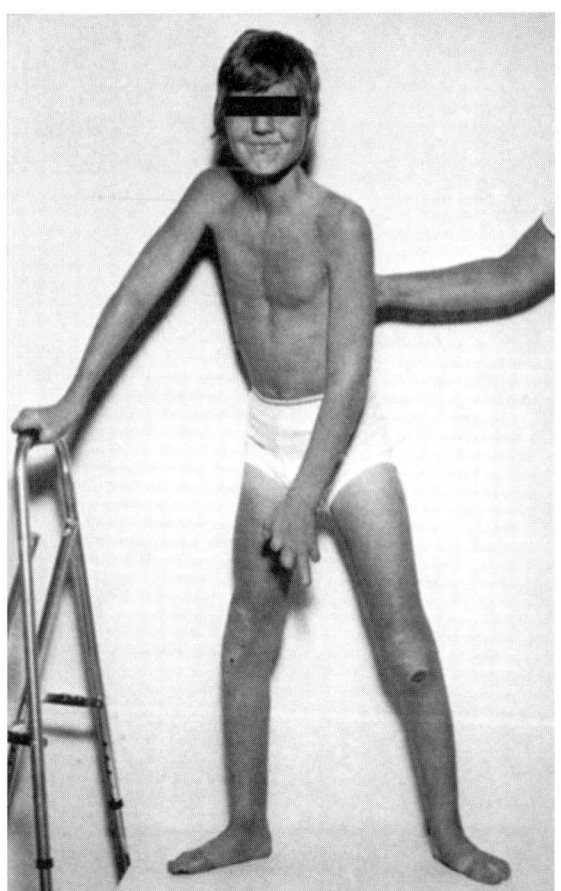

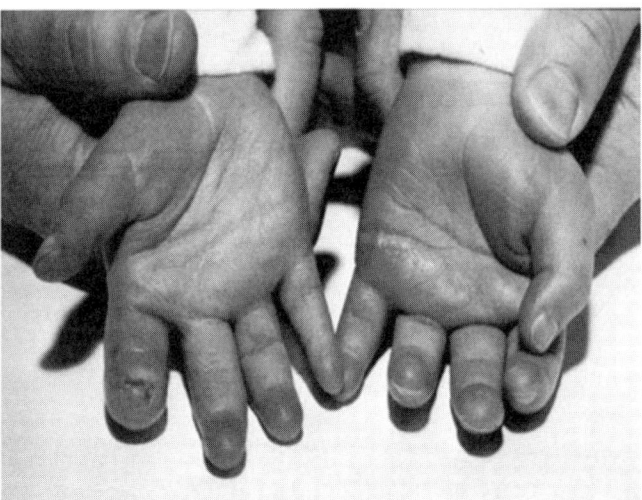

Figure 17.1 Children born with congenital insensitivity to pain often suffer severe trauma and deformity at an early age due to lack of nociceptive perception of tissue injury. (Courtesy of Michael H. Ossipov, PhD, University of Arizona.)

Evaluation of the chronic pain patient

Any patient presenting with chronic pain after trauma requires a complete evaluation without prejudice based on the history of trauma. The purpose of this evaluation is to obtain clues to the possible etiology, which may be related to the trauma, and

Table 17.1 Pain terms and definitions

Pain	An unpleasant sensory and emotional experience associated with actual or potential tissue damage, or described in terms of such
Neuropathic pain	Pain initiated or caused by a primary lesion or dysfunction in the nervous system
Central pain	Pain initiated or caused by a primary lesion or dysfunction in the central nervous system
Allodynia	Pain due to a stimulus that normally does not provoke pain
Causalgia	A syndrome of sustained burning pain, allodynia, and hyperpathia after a traumatic nerve lesion, often combined with vasomotor and sudomotor dysfunction and later trophic changes
Dysesthesia	An unpleasant, abnormal sensation, whether spontaneous or evoked
Hyperalgesia	An increased response to a stimulus that normally is painful
Hyperpathia	A painful syndrome that is characterized by an abnormally painful reaction to a stimulus, especially a repetitive stimulus, as well as an increased threshold
Hypoesthesia	Diminished sensation or numbness
Neuralgia	Pain in the distribution of a nerve or nerves
Neuropathy	A disturbance or pathologic change in a nerve; in one nerve, mononeuropathy; in several nerves, mononeuropathy multiplex; if diffuse and bilateral, polyneuropathy
Nociceptor	A receptor preferentially sensitive to a noxious stimulus
Noxious stimulus	One that is damaging to normal tissues
Paresthesia	An abnormal sensation, whether spontaneous or evoked

Adapted from (a) Milch R. Neuropathic pain: implications for the surgeon. *Surg Clin N Am* 2005; **85**: 225–36; (b) Merskey H, Bogduk N. *Classification of Chronic Pain*, 2nd edition. Seattle, WA: IASP Press, 1994.

	None	Mild	Moderate	Severe
Throbbing	0)_____	1)_____	2)_____	3)_____
Shooting	0)_____	1)_____	2)_____	3)_____
Stabbing	0)_____	1)_____	2)_____	3)_____
Sharp	0)_____	1)_____	2)_____	3)_____
Cramping	0)_____	1)_____	2)_____	3)_____
Gnawing	0)_____	1)_____	2)_____	3)_____
Hot-burning	0)_____	1)_____	2)_____	3)_____
Aching	0)_____	1)_____	2)_____	3)_____
Heavy	0)_____	1)_____	2)_____	3)_____
Tender	0)_____	1)_____	2)_____	3)_____
Splitting	0)_____	1)_____	2)_____	3)_____
Tiring-exhausting	0)_____	1)_____	2)_____	3)_____
Sickening	0)_____	1)_____	2)_____	3)_____
Fearful	0)_____	1)_____	2)_____	3)_____
Punishing-cruel	0)_____	1)_____	2)_____	3)_____

Rate the intensity of your pain on the two scales below. Make a mark on the line to indicate where your pain falls between *No pain* and *Worst possible pain* and then circle the appropriate number on the second scale.

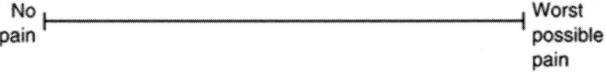

No pain |——————————————————————————————| Worst possible pain

Circle the one of the following words that best describes your current pain:

    0 No pain
    1 Mild
    2 Discomforting
    3 Distressing
    4 Excruciating

Figure 17.2 Short-form McGill Pain Questionnaire. This form includes 15 descriptors from the original McGill Pain Questionnaire; 11 are sensory, 4 are affective, and all are rated on a scale from none to complete. A present pain intensity and visual analog scale are also included. This short form correlates well with the original McGill questionnaire. (From Edwards RR. Pain assessment. In Benzon HT, Raja SN, Molloy RE, Liu SS, Fishman SM, eds., *Essentials of Pain Medicine and Anesthesia*, 2nd edition. London: Elsevier Churchill Livingstone, 2005, pp. 29–34, with permission.)

to develop an appropriate treatment plan based on the diagnosis. The history and physical exam are the beginning of this process.

The history should focus on a description of the pain as well as the past medical and surgical history. The short-form McGill Pain Questionnaire can be used as a quantitative assessment tool to help differentiate somatic from neuropathic as well as affective components of a patient's pain (Fig. 17.2). Pain physicians gain a multidimensional perspective on the patient's pain experience by using questionnaires such as this as well as assessments of functionality. The McGill Pain Questionnaire has been validated and shown to be reliable across cultures, age groups, and patient populations. In addition, duration, location, distribution, and referral patterns, relieving and exacerbating conditions, as well as associated symptoms, give clues to the origin of pain.

Although details will be discussed in the later sections on pain syndromes, the description of pain can help identify the possible causes. For example, chronic pain in the cranium of a trauma patient needs to be evaluated for headache, including, but not limited to, etiologies related to head injury. Headache could originate from the occipital nerve, migraine, or traumatic brain injury, all of which will have various presentations. Radicular neuropathic pain may radiate in a pattern consistent with a particular nerve or nerve root. Such pain commonly presents as numbness with qualities of tingling or burning.[5] Axial pain that does not radiate suggests pain related to the vertebral structures. A patient who describes skin color changes related to his or her pain may be describing vasomotor abnormalities related to autonomic involvement. A thorough description of the patient's pain is an invaluable part of the overall evaluation.

The patient's medical and surgical histories are critical as well. The diabetic patient may have suffered trauma but has continued pain as a result of poor wound healing, occult osteomyelitis, or diabetic neuropathy, all of which will have associated history and findings. Surgical history is equally informative. Poorly controlled postoperative pain has been shown to lead to increased incidence of some chronic pain syndromes and may be a contributing factor. Trauma patients often have had orthopedic and spinal surgeries. Postlaminectomy syndrome is a common cause of chronic pain independent of the trauma history. Patients with a short gut syndrome secondary to resection following trauma or otherwise will not properly benefit from time-released oral narcotics. Medical history may also affect treatment modality. The anticoagulated patient with atrial fibrillation should not undergo any procedure involving placement of needles near the spine until coagulation is normalized and a plan for re-anticoagulation is in place. As is true in any specialty, the patient's history is critical to the overall management of the chronic pain patient.

The physical exam further narrows the differential diagnosis. Emphasis will be on the neurologic musculoskeletal exam, especially the motor and sensory findings of the area involved. Temperature differences and muscular atrophy in addition to sudomotor (sweat) changes may give clues to precipitation of complex regional pain syndrome (CRPS). Extremity weakness is of particular concern in that this suggests potential nerve compression at the root or level of the cord. Magnetic resonance imaging (MRI) and nerve conduction studies may be warranted to rule out the need for surgical intervention.

Posttraumatic chronic pain patients can present with a wide variety of complaints. In any case, the initial evaluation should focus not only on trying to identify the pathology, but also on ruling out unlikely, yet devastating, causes of pain. For example, in the patient with lower back pain, it is necessary to consider cauda equina syndrome, osteomyelitis, and vertebral compression fractures. Review of systems should include questioning about bowel and bladder problems in order to rule out cauda equina syndrome. A history of fever, prior infection, or immune suppression may warrant a workup for osteomyelitis. A history of fall or osteoporosis suggests that a plain film would be appropriate to evaluate possible compression fracture. When ordering diagnostic tests, it is especially important to clarify to the patient the reasons for such tests. Often imaging will show degenerative findings and changes that

may not explain the patient's pain. Further interventional tests such as discography or facet joint injections may be necessary.

Psychosocial variables are important factors that contribute to a patient's pain. Not only can emotional factors such as anxiety and depression have a negative impact on treatment and response, but a history of physical, sexual, or substance abuse, work history, and status of any pending lawsuits or workman's compensation claims can play a major role in developing the patient's treatment plan. These components of the patient's history will help guide a comprehensive pain management program.

Initial evaluation of the posttrauma patient may suggest a variety of chronic pain syndromes. Subsequent sections will discuss a variety of the chronic pain syndromes that occur in this patient population.

Complex regional pain syndrome (CRPS)

Causalgia, the most terrible of all tortures which a nerve wound may inflict ... Its favorite site is the foot or hand ... Its intensity varies from the most trivial burning to a state of torture, which can hardly be credited, but reacts on the whole economy, until the general health is seriously affected.

(S. W. Mitchell, 1872[6])

Definition

Trauma can result in a variety of pain disorders. One of the most perplexing is CRPS, which describes a constellation of symptoms most often seen in patients following injury or surgery. The prevalence of CRPS following fractures has been reported to be between 0.03% and 37%, with no distinct correlation between the severity of trauma and the degree of CRPS symptoms (Fig. 17.3).[7–14] These symptoms include pain (often out of proportion to that expected from the initial trauma), sensory abnormalities (allodynia, hypoalgesia,

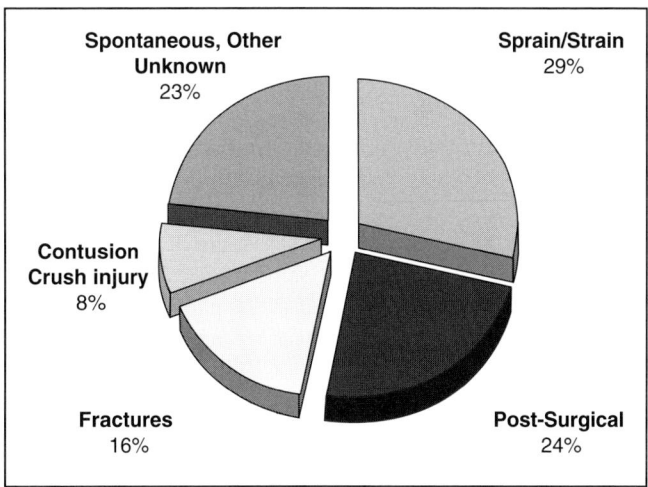

Figure 17.3 Epidemiology of complex regional pain syndrome (CRPS). A majority of patients develop CRPS after injury or surgery. (From Allen G. Epidemiology of complex regional pain syndrome: a retrospective chart review of 134 patients. *Pain* 1999; **80**: 539–44, with permission.)

Table 17.2 Examples of terms now incorporated into complex regional pain syndrome (CRPS)

Causalgia
Reflex sympathetic dystrophy
Sudeck's atrophy
Shoulder–hand syndrome
Sympathetically maintained pain
Sympathalgia

Adapted from: (a) Hartick C. Pain due to trauma including sports injuries. In Gay SM, ed., *Practical Management of Pain*, 2nd edition. St Louis, MO: Mosby-Year Book, 1992, pp. 409–33; (b) Binder A, Schattschneider J, Baron R. Complex regional pain syndrome type I (reflex sympathetic dystrophy). In Waldman SD, ed., *Pain Management*, Philadelphia, PA: Saunders Elsevier, 2007, pp. 283–301.

hyperalgesia), edema, dysregulation of temperature, blood flow, and sweating, as well as trophic changes to skin and subcutaneous tissues. Active and passive movement limitations (including tremor) are often present as well.[15]

The first report of symptoms similar to CRPS perhaps dates back to 1864, when Silas Weir Mitchell described his observation of peripheral nerve injuries in soldiers during the American Civil War.[16] Historically, many terms that reference these symptoms have been used to depict this condition (Table 17.2).[17,18] Previously, the two subtypes of CRPS have been referred to as reflex sympathetic dystrophy and causalgia. Because these terms have lost their clinical utility, in 1994 the IASP developed the term CRPS to emphasize the following clinical characteristics:

- *complex*: multiple and varied clinical features, as noted above
- *regional*: majority of cases involve a region of the body, usually an extremity
- *pain*: cardinal feature, often out of proportion to original insult, and essential to the diagnosis

Patient evaluation

The current taxonomy maintains the two subtypes: CRPS I (previously reflex sympathetic dystrophy) is the more common and is distinguished on the basis that the pattern of pain does not follow a particular nerve distribution. CRPS II (previously causalgia) has all the same features as CRPS I with the exception that the distribution of pain is related to a particular nerve lesion. These nerves are generally large nerves of the extremities. The diagnosis of CRPS is essentially clinical and is achieved by thorough physical examination and medical history. The latest available diagnostic criteria have been published by the IASP in 2007 (the "Budapest criteria": Table 17.3). Application of these criteria may provide the diagnosis with sensitivity (0.85) and specificity (0.69). In addition, the Veldman criteria, the IASP criteria, and the Bruehl criteria can be

Table 17.3 Proposed clinical diagnostic criteria for CRPS (the Budapest criteria)

General definition of the syndrome

CRPS describes an array of painful conditions that are characterized by a continuing (spontaneous and/or evoked) regional pain that is seemingly disproportionate in time or degree to the usual course of any known trauma or other lesion. The pain is regional (not in a specific nerve territory or dermatome) and usually has a distal predominance of abnormal sensory, motor, sudomotor, vasomotor, and/or trophic findings. The syndrome shows variable progression over time.

To make the clinical diagnosis, the following criteria must be met

1. Continuing pain, which is disproportionate to any inciting event
2. Must report at least one symptom in three of the following four categories
   Sensory: reports of hypoesthesia and/or allodynia
   Vasomotor: reports of temperature asymmetry and/or skin color changes and/or skin color asymmetry
   Sudomotor/edema: reports of edema and/or sweating changes and/or sweating asymmetry
   Motor/trophic: reports of decreased range of motion and/or motor dysfunction (weakness, tremor, dystonia) and/or trophic changes (hair, nail, skin)
3. Must display at least one sign at time of evaluation in two or more of the following categories:
   Sensory: evidence of hyperalgesia (to pinprick) and/or allodynia (to light touch and/or temperature sensation and/or deep somatic pressure and/or joint movement)
   Vasomotor: evidence of temperature asymmetry (> 1 °C) and/or skin color changes and/or asymmetry
   Sudomotor/edema: evidence of edema and/or sweating changes and/or sweating asymmetry
   Motor/trophic: evidence of decreased range of motion and/or motor dysfunction (weakness, tremor, dystonia) and/or trophic changes (hair, nail, skin)
4. There is no other diagnosis that better explains the signs and symptoms

For research purposes, diagnostic decision rule should be at least one symptom in all four categories and at least one sign (observed at evaluation) in two or more sign categories.
Reproduced from Harden RN, *et al.* Validation of proposed diagnostic criteria (the "Budapest Criteria") for complex regional pain syndrome. *Pain* 2010; **150**: 268–74.

utilized. The IASP diagnostic criteria for each subtype are listed in Table 17.4.[4,19,20]

CRPS is considered a subset of neuropathic pain.[21] In evaluating patients with this condition, other neuropathic pain syndromes and causes of pain must be ruled out, including peripheral neuropathies, infection, inflammation, and vasospasm. Although CRPS II is distinguished by a definable nerve injury, as the diagnostic criteria suggest, CRPS is distinct from most neuropathic pain in that features of autonomic dysregulation are present. The most notable of these findings are edema, temperature discrepancy between affected and unaffected limbs (> 1 °C), and sudomotor (sweating)

Table 17.4 International Association for the Study of Pain (IASP) diagnostic criteria for complex regional pain syndrome – CRPS I and CRPS II

CRPS I (reflex sympathetic dystrophy)	CRPS II (causalgia)
1. The presence of an initiating noxious event, or a cause of immobilization 2. Continuing pain, allodynia, or hyperalgesia with which the pain is disproportionate to any inciting event 3. Evidence at some time of edema, changes in skin blood flow, or abnormal sudomotor activity in the region of the pain 4. This diagnosis is excluded by the existence of conditions that would otherwise account for the degree of pain and dysfunction	1. The presence of continuing pain, allodynia, or hyperalgesia after a nerve injury, not necessarily limited to the distribution of the injured nerve 2. Evidence at some time of edema, changes in skin blood flow, or abnormal sudomotor activity in the region of the pain 3. This diagnosis is excluded by the existence of conditions that would otherwise account for the degree of pain and dysfunction

Reproduced from: (a) Stanton-Hicks M. Complex regional pain syndrome. *Anesthesiol Clin N Am* 2003; **21**: 733–44; (b) Janig W, Stanton-Hicks M. Reflex sympathetic dystrophy: a reappraisal. *Progress in Pain Research and Management*. Seattle: IASP Press, 1996, vol. 6.

abnormalities.[22] Although diagnosis is clinical, assessments directed at autonomic aspects of CRPS include thermography, quantitative sudomotor axon reflex test, and sympathetic nerve blocks. Other studies targeted at narrowing the differential diagnosis or identifying tissue, motor, and sensory changes include radiographs, bone scintigraphy, electromyography, nerve conduction testing, and quantitative sensory testing. Objective and timely means of accurately diagnosing CRPS are critical, because treatment outcomes are more favorable in the early stages. Keeping in mind that these studies cannot rule out CRPS, the use of indirect measures of autonomic function such as thermography, which correlates with microvascular blood flow, not only provides a means of physiologically staging the disease, but also enables the clinician to monitor its response to treatment. Staging can be difficult, given that the rate of disease progression is variable. However, quantifiable testing helps overcome these challenges.[23]

The role of the autonomic nervous system in CRPS is variable. Sympathetically maintained pain is relieved by either systemic adrenergic antagonist medication (e.g., phentolamine) or neurolysis of the sympathetic ganglion (stellate ganglion and lumbar plexus blocks, Fig. 17.4). Although sympathetic blocks are used to aid in the diagnosis and treatment of CRPS, not all patients meeting the criteria for the syndrome respond to sympathectomy. This has led to further subclassification of pain in CRPS as either sympathetically maintained pain or sympathetically independent pain.

Sympathetically maintained pain can be present in any neuropathic pain syndrome. Patients with sympathetically maintained pain respond favorably to treatment with sympathetic blocks. Pain that does not respond favorably to treatment with a sympathetic block is termed *sympathetically independent pain*. Sympathetically independent pain is much more refractory to treatment, and prognosis is poor.[23]

Sympathetically maintained pain does not respond uniformly to varying sympatholytic interventions. For example, patients who respond classically to a regional or peripheral nerve block may experience no relief from phentolamine. Although these clinical phenomena need to be discussed when considering the pathophysiology and mechanisms of pain in CRPS, one must keep in mind that there is no pathognomonic test for diagnosing sympathetically maintained pain. The significance in determining the presence of sympathetically maintained pain is not for diagnosis of CRPS, but rather to establish the viability of sympatholysis as a treatment option. Given the importance of initiating treatment early, identifying CRPS pain that is responsive to sympatholytic treatment by any means needs to be a priority in the initial workup in these patients.[23]

Pathophysiology

The pathophysiology of this disease is still unclear. Most pain researchers believe CRPS is developed and maintained by abnormalities in the central and peripheral nervous systems. The peripheral component is evidenced by peripheral sensitization of primary nociceptive afferent neurons associated with sympathetic efferent coupling, upregulation of ion channels and adrenergic receptors, and increased concentrations of neuropeptides. Inflammatory cells such as macrophages and mast cells are implicated by inflammatory changes associated with CRPS, but whether their role is primary or secondary remains controversial.[15,23]

The central component is explained by changes in the region of the dorsal horn containing wide-dynamic-range neurons. Mechanisms of central sensitization resulting in increased perception of pain could include spontaneous firing of the wide-dynamic-range neuron as well as amplification of ascending signals or insufficient descending inhibitory signals. Multiple neurotransmitters, receptors, and cytokines have been implicated, including glutamate, magnesium, glycine, substance P, γ-aminobutyric acid (GABA), neurokinin, serotonin, α_2 receptors, μ receptors, and prostaglandin.[24]

Additional central mechanisms implicated in CRPS involve the sympathetic nervous systems and cortical processing. Loss of thermoregulatory reflexes and increased sudomotor activity are reversed by sympathetic block. These phenomena suggest that the central sympathetic nervous system is responsible. Functional MRI and positron emission tomography (PET) scan studies suggest that the cortical processing of pain sensation is altered in CRPS. Acerra and Moseley propose that allodynia and paresthesia may be mediated by the brain in experiments demonstrating dysynchiria, the phenomenon of eliciting pain or parasthesia in an affected limb while watching a mirror image of the healthy limb being touched.[25] Future therapies directed at spinal as well as cortical targets of the central nervous system may prove valuable.

Treatment

The primary goal in treating patients with CRPS is to preserve the function of the affected region of the body. Early diagnosis and initiation of medical therapy combined with directed physiotherapy and psychologic therapy is the mainstay of conservative treatment. A successful outcome depends largely on aggressive pain control and physical therapy focused on desensitization and maximizing functionality. Although rehabilitation is critical to the treatment of CRPS, flexibility in employing the most appropriate therapeutic modality that supports further improvement at any given time is recommended by published expert guidelines.[22] Nonpharmacological treatment modalities require active involvement of the patient within the treatment concept. Early physiotherapy is crucial to prevent complications such as atrophy and contractures. The beneficial effects of mirror therapy and transcutaneous electric nerve stimulation (TENS) have been reported in some studies.[26–29]

Multiple medications have been postulated for the treatment of CRPS. A large dose of oral steroids in the early stages is advocated by some specialists, while the traditional approach to CRPS treatment includes tricyclic antidepressants, antiepileptic medications, and calcium-channel or β-blockers. α₂ Agonists (e.g., clonidine) as well as N-methyl-D-aspartate (NMDA) receptor antagonists (e.g., ketamine and dextromethorphan) have been shown to be effective in the treatment of central sensitization (Table 17.5).[23]

New pharmacological agents such as tumor necrosis factor alpha (TNF-α) antibodies, free radical scavengers, GABA agonists (baclofen), calcitonin, bisphosphonates, mannitol, and vasodilating drugs (e.g., verapamil, ketanserin) have been introduced recently in the treatment of CRPS. There is great need for further randomized controlled studies to understand the role of these medications in the management of CRPS.[30–43]

(A)

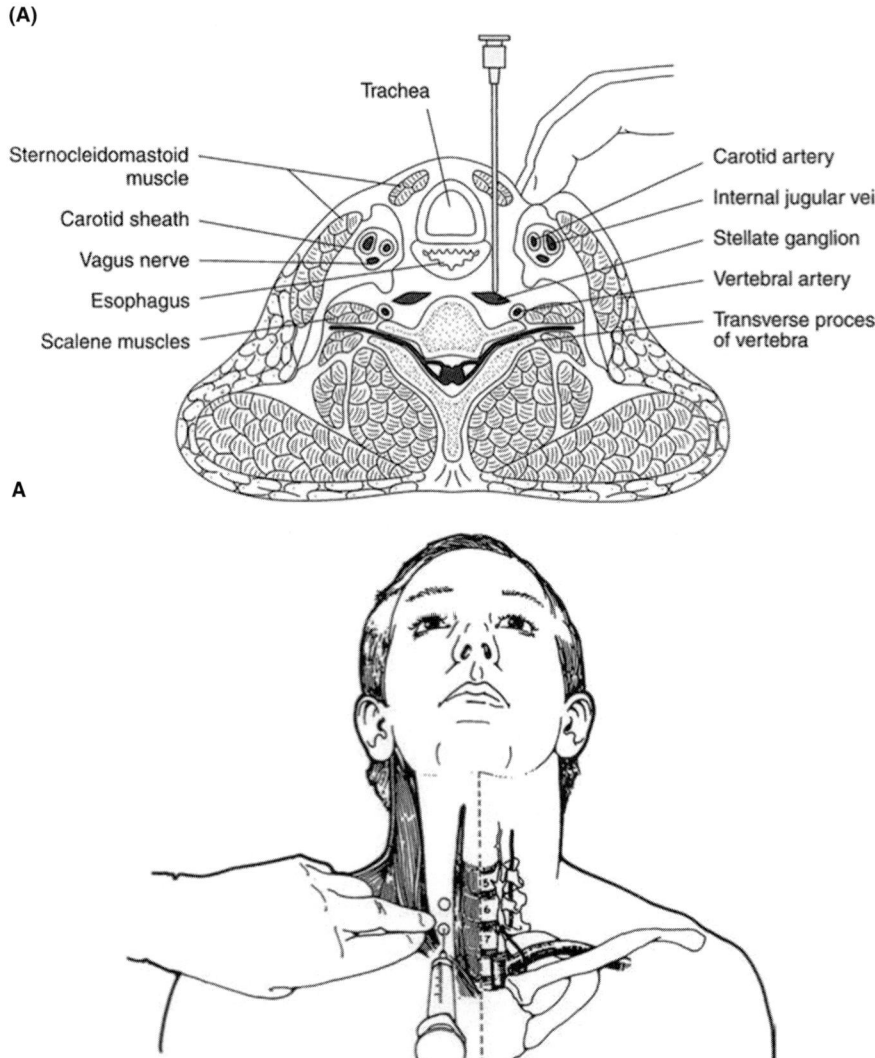

Figure 17.4 Examples of stellate ganglion and lumbar plexus blocks. (**A**) An axial view of the clinically relevant anatomy in placing the stellate ganglion block. (**B**) Demonstration of the technique that involves retracting the carotid sheath and advancing toward the transverse process of C6 or C7 then withdrawing 2–3 mm prior to aspiration. Aspiration is done in two planes prior to a 1 mL test dose in order to avoid intravascular injection of the vertebral and subclavian artery. (**C**) Representation of the innervation of the lumbar plexus, which originates between L1/L2 and L5/S1 and ultimately forms the major branches of the plexus, which include the genitofemoral nerve through the obturator nerve. (**D**) Demonstration of the lumbar plexus block technique that involves advancing the needle 4 cm lateral to the spine at the level of the iliac crest. (From: (A) Morgan GE, Mikhail MS, Murray MJ. Clinical Anesthesiology, 4th edition. New York: McGraw–Hill, 2006, p 385, figure 18.16. (B) Barash PG, Cullen BF, Stoelting RK. Clinical Anesthesia, 5th edition. Philadelphia: Lippincott, Williams & Wilkins, 2006, p 736, figure 26.22. (C and D) Hadzic AJ, Vloka ID. Peripheral Nerve Blocks. New York: McGraw–Hill, 2004, pp. 219–23, figures 18.2 and 18.7, with permission.)

Interventional management

Regional anesthetic techniques, including sympathetic blocks, have been successfully utilized in the treatment of CRPS. Sympathetic blocks are very effective in the subset of patients with sympathetically maintained pain. By definition, these blocks are completely ineffective in the subset of patients with sympathetically independent pain. Single-shot and continuous regional blocks are effective modalities of treatment in appropriate cases. Epidural and intrathecal infusions have been successfully utilized in the management of pain in resistant cases. Combinations of opioid, local anesthetic, clonidine, and baclofen have been used as well. Implantable therapies such as spinal cord stimulators and intrathecal delivery devices are very successful in treating highly resistant and selective groups of patients (Fig. 17.5). These implantable devices have proven to be of long-term benefit. It is important to realize that all these modalities require effective psychologic and physical rehabilitation in order to be successful.

Table 17.5 Oral and parenteral drugs used in the treatment of complex regional pain syndrome (CRPS)

Oral
Nonsteroidal anti-inflammatory drugs
Steroids
Antidepressants
Tricyclic antidepressants
Serotonin reuptake inhibitors
Anticonvulsants
Calcium-channel blockers
α_2 Agonists
Parenteral
Bretylium
Steroids
α_2 Agonists

Reproduced from Teasdall RD. Complex regional pain syndrome (reflex sympathetic dystrophy). *Clin Sports Med* 2004; **23**: 145–55, with permission from Elsevier.

Posttraumatic abdominal pain

Trauma patients often suffer abdominal injury and require surgery that can result in chronic abdominal pain. This pain can manifest as a neuropathic entrapment syndrome or a more generalized abdominal pain. The patient with a neuropathic entrapment syndrome will experience pain in the distribution of the involved nerve such as the ilioinguinal or intercostal nerves. Conservative medical treatment involves neuropathic membrane stabilizers such as gabapentin, antidepressants, opioids, and TENS. Abdominal pressure message can serve to desensitize the entrapped nerves of the abdominal wall and release adhesions. Injection with local anesthetic and steroid may also release adhesions around the nerve while providing relief. Interventional treatment may begin with radiofrequency ablation or cryotherapy. As a last resort,

(B)

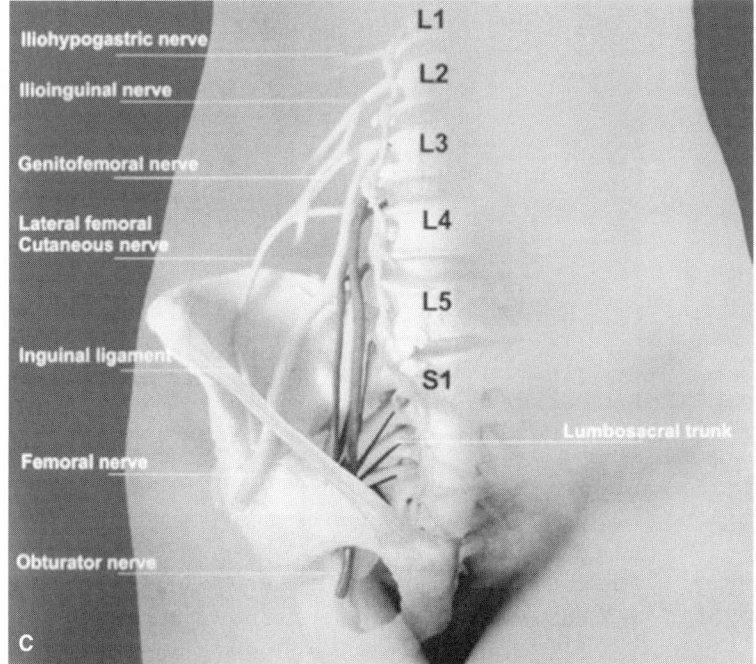

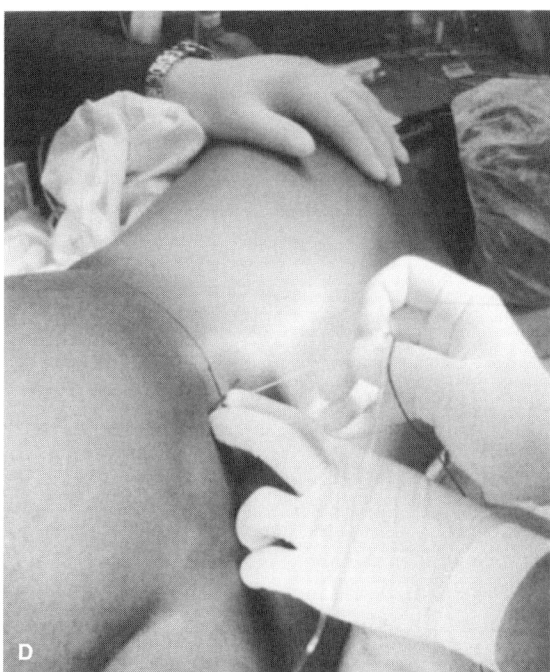

Figure 17.4 (cont.)

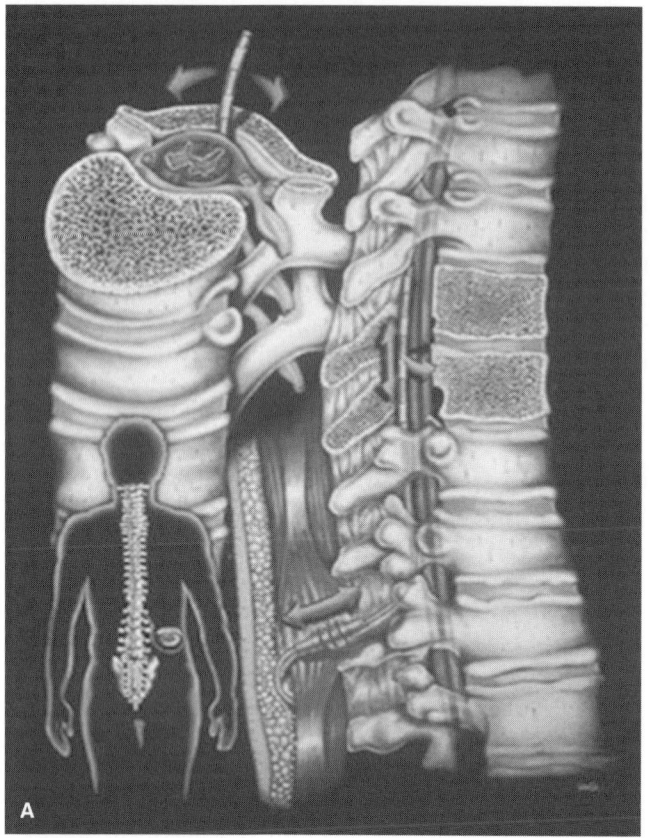

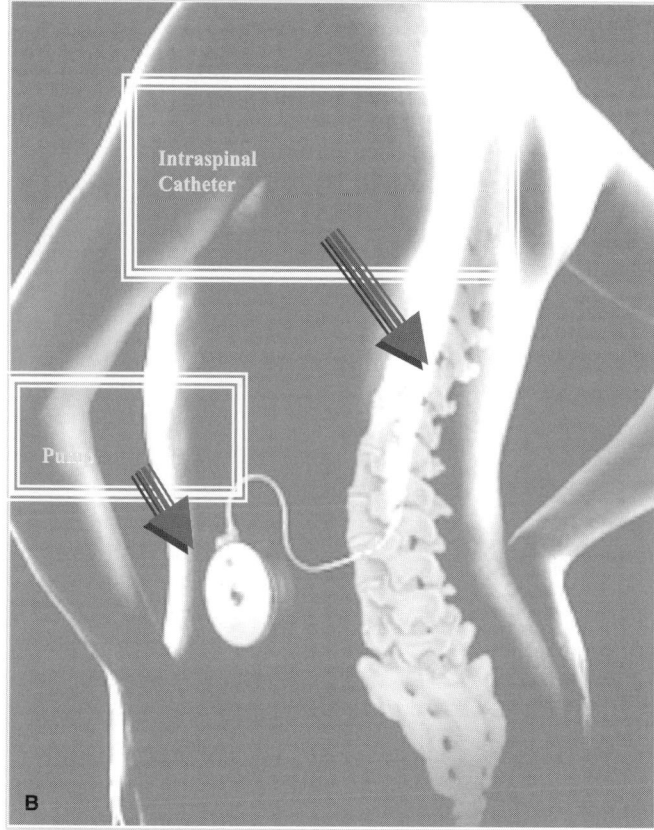

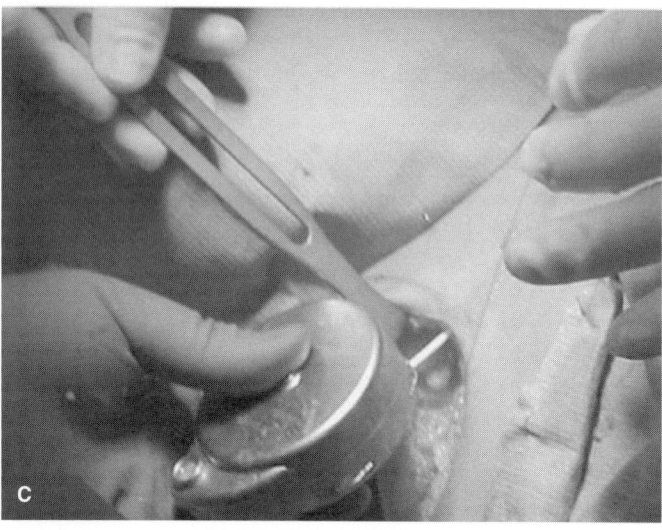

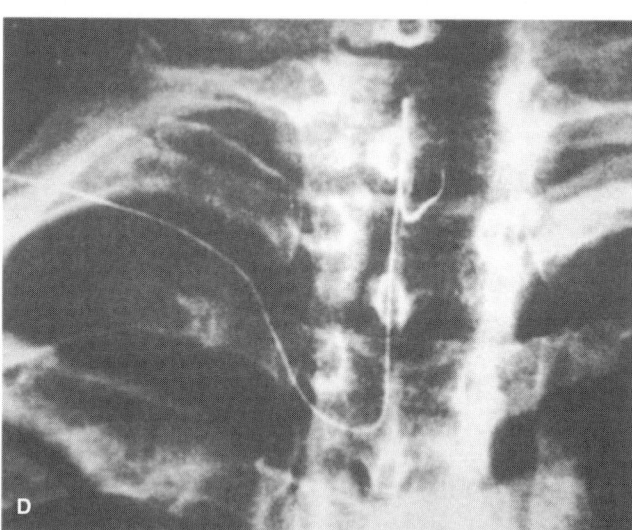

Figure 17.5 Implantable devices are often effective in treating severe and refractory pain conditions, including CRPS and other neuropathic pain syndromes. Due to their invasive nature, associated complications, and expense, these devices are typically third-line treatments. (**A**) Implanted spinal cord stimulator and the course of the lead in the epidural space. (**B**) The course of an implanted intrathecal pump. (**C**) The implantation of an intrathecal pump. (**D**) Radiograph of a patient with an implanted intrathecal pump. (A and B from Medtronic, with permission.)

placement of a peripheral nerve stimulator over the affected area, with an implanted generator, may be attempted and has yielded excellent results (Fig. 17.5).

Posttraumatic abdominal pain can manifest as regional pain confined to one quadrant or as generalized pain throughout the entire abdomen. This is an idiopathic chronic abdominal pain that is diagnosed by exclusion of identifiable sources

such as obstruction, pseudocyst, abscess, or chronic adhesions. These patients can suffer for an extended period of time while undergoing multiple diagnostic tests and failed treatments. Such pain is considered a visceral neuropathic disease, involves autonomic pathways, and is only diagnosed by exclusion.

In general, visceral pain is described by patients in vague terms such as a dull cramping pain without a precise point of origin that is not relieved by bowel movement or affected by eating habits. Initially, the source of abdominal pain is visceral, peritoneal, or referred.[44] However, visceral nociceptors differ from somatic in that they are sparsely distributed with a larger receptive field. Representation of these nociceptors is poor in the primary somatosensory cortex relative to representation in the secondary somatosensory cortex, cingulate, and insular cortex. This distribution of cerebral representation possibly explains the association of visceral pain with an intense emotional quality but imprecise localization.[45]

The neuroanatomy of visceral pain at the level of the spinal cord needs to be understood when considering treatment options. Afferent nociceptors are slow C fibers that follow sympathetics to the dorsal horn in a pattern generally corresponding to embryonic gut formation. As a result the region of pain correlates with the sympathetic preaortic ganglia as follows: celiac with epigastrium (foregut), superior mesenteric with the periumbilical region (midgut), and the inferior mesenteric with the lower abdominal quadrants (hindgut).[46] Pelvic visceral afferents project to S2 through S4.[45] Similar to CRPS, posttraumatic chronic visceral pain can respond to sympathetic blockade, because visceral afferents pass through these ganglia. However, visceral pain is not necessarily a symphathetically maintained pain.

Treatment of this pain includes conservative medical management along with psychologic therapy and interventional techniques applied as indicated. Medical treatment is the same as for neuropathic pain (Table 17.5), including membrane stabilizers, antidepressants, and opioids supported with behavioral modification techniques. Interventional treatment includes regional anesthesia, diagnostic sympathetic blocks, followed by neurolytic blocks utilizing radiofrequency techniques or chemicals such as dehydrated alcohol or phenol, in addition to implantable devices such as spinal cord stimulators or intrathecal delivery systems.

Diagnostic regional blocks of visceral afferents at identifiable nerve roots that relieve pain give information as to the neuroanatomy involved. This information can be used to determine the value of interventions, such as neurolytic bilateral splenic nerve blocks, celiac plexus blocks, or superior hypogastric plexus blocks.[45] Spinal cord stimulators may have difficulty capturing abdominal pain; however, if successful, they are very effective in providing relief. Intrathecal pump administration of a cocktail including an opioid, an α_2 agonist, baclofen, and local anesthetic has demonstrated efficacy.

It is important to realize that trauma patients with abdominal pain require special consideration. Patients who have experienced bowel resection (short gut syndrome) will not adequately absorb medications properly, especially the extended-release formulations. It should be additionally emphasized that careful follow-up of these patients and repeated evaluation are essential in order to detect any complications of the original illness during early rather than late stages.

Traumatic brain injury

Approximately 30% of trauma patients experience traumatic brain injury (TBI: see Chapters 20 and 21)). Even trivial trauma can result in long-term sequelae. Headache and cognitive and psychologic impairment are some of the major symptoms. More than half of TBI patients report chronic pain, with headache being the most common. Although trauma that causes damage to the central nervous system can lead to pain in limbs or other parts of the body, this discussion will focus on pain associated with the head and neck. Reviews of TBI describe a spectrum of insults ranging from mild head injury, whiplash, and concussion to moderate or severe TBI. Mild head injury is often referred to as mild TBI. Mild TBI has varying definitions but is defined by one source as "a traumatically induced physiological disruption of brain function" with any period of loss of consciousness, memory loss around the time of trauma, any change in mental state, and focal neurologic deficits of any duration. The American Academy of Neurology defines concussion as a "trauma-induced alteration in mental status that may or may not involve loss of consciousness." It also grades concussion from 1, which is confusion without loss of consciousness, to 3, which is head trauma with loss of consciousness. These injuries are most commonly caused by motor vehicle collisions (MVCs: 42%) followed by falls, assault, and sports injuries.[47]

The sources of pain following TBI can be divided into intracranial and extracranial categories. Any tissue containing nociceptors is a potential source of such pain. The nociceptive intracranial structures include the cerebral arteries, the fifth, ninth, and tenth cranial nerves, the dural arteries, and the dura mater at the base of the brain. Extracranial sources of pain include skeletal muscle, tendons, joints, cancellous bone, skin, mucous membranes, fascia, periosteum, and peripheral nerves.[48] Therefore, head injury can also result in trauma to extracranial structures such as cervical ligaments, the temporomandibular joint (TMJ), and peripheral nerves without causing brain injury. Whether pain arises from intracranial or extracranial structures, all are included in most discussions of posttraumatic headache. Of note, the incidence of posttraumatic headache is inversely proportional to the severity of head injury. Between 30% and 90% of patients with mild head injury are reported to develop posttraumatic headache.[49] The most recent criteria established by the International Headache Society for posttraumatic headache is onset within 7 days of the incident (which is an arbitrary designation).[49] There is a clinical concept that patients with mild TBI have a higher prevalence of chronic pain syndrome than patients with moderate to severe TBI. The etiology of this difference is not well understood. However, patients with more severe TBI might have more difficulty presenting or describing their symptoms, which could lead to underestimation of the occurrence of chronic pain following TBI.[50]

Mechanisms of posttraumatic headache may involve injury to tissue or may result from physiologic changes secondary to

TBI. Cerebral blood flow is noted to be decreased and asymmetric in posttraumatic headache patients when compared with migraineurs and normal controls. Migraine headache and TBI share many common biochemical alterations in neuropeptides such as substance P, glutamate, excitatory neurotransmitters, serotonin, as well as loss of calcium homeostasis and development of magnesium deficiency. The trigeminovascular system is thought to be involved in the development of migraine and is possibly triggered by mild TBI. Most posttraumatic headaches are of a mixed variety involving pain likely due to direct or indirect tissue damage along with a component of vasoactive or migraine-type headache.[47]

The primary posttraumatic headache types are similar to tension headache, migraine, and cluster headache. Tension headache is involved in 85% of posttraumatic headaches and is similar to the nontraumatic type with band-like or cap-like tightening, with variable duration and maybe a dull aching component. These headaches are most responsive to nonsteroidal anti-inflammatory drugs (NSAIDs). Many patients with migraine-like headache respond to migraine therapeutics. Researchers have proposed that TBI may trigger migraine in genetically susceptible individuals who previously may not have experienced migraines. Cluster headaches that are rapid in onset and of short duration are rare in posttraumatic headache.[15,32]

Posttraumatic headache may include pain resulting from injury to structures of the head. One example is whiplash, which involves hyperextension followed by flexion of the neck and can result in cervical muscle injury, occipital neuralgia, and TMJ pain.[32] TMJ pain results from hyperextension of the mandibular joint with mastoid muscle tenderness, limited jaw opening, and popping or clicking at the joint. True articular pathology must be ruled out but is rare. This is often a myofascial pain responsive to trigger point injections in the muscles of mastication.[51] Occipital neuralgia is pain in the distribution of either the greater or lesser occipital nerves, which may be from entrapment of these nerves or a referred myofascial pain. Palpation of the occipital nerves may reproduce this pain. If Tinel's sign is present, occipital nerve block may be effective.[52] Cervicogenic headaches refer to any headache originating from cervical soft tissue or bony structures. Within the trigeminocervical nucleus C2, C3, and C4 and trigeminal terminal afferents are in close proximity. Noxious stimuli of cervical structures can activate the trigeminal nucleus, as well as the trigeminovascular system, generating referred pain to frontal and anterior portions of the head.[47] C2–C3 joint pain refers to the upper neck and occipital region. Neurolysis of the median branch from the dorsal rami with local anesthetic is one treatment option. Radiofrequency ablation is also employed but is more controversial.[51] Head trauma can also cause myofascial pain responsive to trigger-point injections.

Medical therapy in posttraumatic headache depends somewhat on whether the headache is constant or intermittent. Rebound headache can result from the continued use or excessive use of prophylactic analgesics, caffeine, and abortive medications. Generally if the headache is constant and/or of a musculoskeletal nature, NSAIDs and acetaminophen are very effective, with opioids and migraine-specific agents used as abortive therapy as necessary. Migraine medications include serotonin receptor agonists and ergot derivatives. Midrin (combination of acetaminophen, dichloralphenazone, and isometheptene) is also a unique formulation effective in migraine-type headache. β-Blockers and calcium-channel blockers have been used for migraine prophylaxis. Muscle relaxants have little role in chronic posttraumatic headache. Posttraumatic headaches of a chronic nature are difficult to treat and require a therapeutic plan tailored to the specific symptoms and comorbidities of each patient.[51]

Phantom limb pain

Phantom limb sensation is a common sensory phenomenon in amputees. Phantom limb sensation may last weeks to a month without contributing to a pain syndrome. On the other hand, phantom limb pain is a condition associated with excruciating pain felt by the patient in the amputated extremity. The prevalence of phantom pain varies between 50% and 80%, with severe pain being reported in approximately 5% of patients.[53,54]

Most researchers believe that phantom limb pain is a form of neuropathic pain that develops in the first week of injury. The mechanisms of this pain are believed to be central, with multiple neurotransmitters involved. It is essential to differentiate between phantom limb pain and stump pain, which is localized to a neuroma formation around severed nerves.

Although neuropathic pain has generally been considered to be nonresponsive to opioid treatment, recent studies demonstrate that higher-than-standard doses can be effective.

Interventional management including regional and sympathetic blocks has been effective in a subset of this population. Spinal cord stimulators have shown some promise in modifying pain signaling and decreasing pain sensation. All treatment modalities, whether medical or interventional, should be accompanied by aggressive psychotherapy, biofeedback, and imagery.[55]

Vertebral fracture

Life expectancy in developed countries has increased dramatically. As the number of individuals leading active lives into their ninth decade has grown, so has the incidence of trauma-related injury among the elderly (see Chapter 36). The incidence of vertebral fracture is around 750,000 in the United States each year. Those older than 50 years of age have up to a 25% lifetime risk of suffering at least one vertebral fracture.[56,57]

Vertebral fracture in the elderly results not only from effects of aging on bone that render it susceptible to fracture at lower levels of mechanical force than younger bone, but also from the increased prevalence of osteoporosis as a coexisting disease. Falls from standing are by far the most common cause of trauma-related injury in the elderly. Evidence suggests that for patients older than 70 years, MVCs are second to falls as a cause of traumatic injury. In the elderly, injuries from car crashes are more severe, though the pattern of injury is similar to that of their younger counterparts. Given that vertebral fractures are a common cause of chronic back pain in the elderly and are generally related to mild or unnoticed trauma, this subset of the trauma population is at an even greater risk for vertebral fractures. Trauma patients presenting with back pain, especially elderly trauma patients, should be thoroughly evaluated for vertebral fracture and triaged accordingly.[58,59]

Acute vertebral fracture is treated aggressively in the trauma bay. Of note, elderly trauma patients are twice as likely to have cervical spine injury on radiographic imaging. High cervical injury is more common in patients who have fallen from a low height, while low cervical injury predominates in MVC patients.[58] Any associated neurologic deficit is treated with an appropriate surgical modality. However, isolated vertebral compression fracture without neurologic deficit is a source of intractable back pain. Early evaluation with the appropriate radiographic studies is essential in evaluating the stability of the fracture. Bed rest and spinal bracing, in addition to proper pain control, are the main treatment options. The majority of these patients recover uneventfully without any sequelae. Those who do not recover continue to experience intractable axial pain with or without radiation. Several interventional techniques have been described for treatment of vertebral fracture, including intercostal block, percutaneous radiofrequency treatment, pulsed radiofrequency treatment of the dorsal root ganglion or intercostal nerves, and spinal cord stimulation (SCS).

Postprocedural pain is the most frequent adverse effect of interventional treatment. Surgical interventions have not proven to offer adequate treatment. In response to this therapeutic void, vertebroplasty and kyphoplasty have been developed as minimally invasive techniques that increase fracture stability and strengthen structure, and they have also been shown to provide more effective pain relief than conservative management.[60–62]

Chronic pain from vertebral fractures in patients with osteoporosis is thought to be due to vertebral deformity, paraspinal muscle spasm, alteration in spinal alignment, or arthritic changes in the area of the fracture.[63] Interventional treatments such as vertebroplasty or kyphoplasty are targeted at stabilizing or restoring spinal architecture, and they have been shown to be most effective in patients with severe focal pain and confirmation of recent fracture on imaging. One review of case reports in patients with osteoporosis found relief in 67–100% of patients undergoing these procedures.[64] Vertebroplasty is the older technique, developed in the 1980s, and involves fluoroscopically guided percutaneous injection of a low-viscosity, slow-curing cement under pressure into the collapsed vertebral body, providing stability and pain relief but without restoring body height. Kyphoplasty, on the other hand, involves placement of a cannula into the vertebral body under fluoroscopy to facilitate insertion of an inflatable bone tamp that creates a cavity to be filled with a viscous bone cement, reducing the vertebral fracture and restoring some of the vertebral body height in the process (Fig. 17.6). The creation of a cavity has advantages beyond restoring vertebral body height and reducing some of the morbidity associated with that loss of height. The most significant benefit is that extravasation of a monomer is less likely with kyphoplasty because more viscous, partially polymerized cement is able to be injected under lower pressure into the cavity, which has also reduced the fractures, further decreasing the possibility of leakage and systemic absorption.[65] Complications from leakage can include nerve root compression, pulmonary emboli, and, rarely, cauda equina syndrome.[66]

The mechanism of action of pain relief with vertebroplasty and kyphoplasty is not entirely clear. The most intuitive explanation is that mechanical fixation and stabilization of the fracture leads to pain relief. However, in one review, pain relief is not correlated with quantity of cement injected. These authors suggest evidence that neurotoxic effects of polymethyl methacrylate may cause nociceptive denervation within the bone matrix of the vertebral body.[67] Another proposed mechanism is redistribution of the axial load away from the cortices of the vertebral body back to the center, allowing forces to be transmitted in a more physiologically normal pattern.[65] Some authors reported improved functional recovery in a multicenter randomized controlled trial following kyphoplasty, with a lower complication rate compared with nonsurgical management.[68–70] On the other hand, other studies demonstrated no advantage in patients who underwent vertebroplasty in comparison with a sham procedure. Controversy persists over the efficacy of vertebroplasty. Some experts have abandoned the use of vertebroplasty for the treatment of vertebral fracture, while others question the quality of the results of trials that showed no superior benefit for vertebroplasty.[71–74]

Contraindications to vertebroplasty and kyphoplasty in the trauma patient with an acute vertebral compression fracture include an asymptomatic stable fracture, complete vertebral body collapse, local osteomyelitis or diskitis, systemic bacterial infection, coagulopathy, and cardiopulmonary pathology. Relative contraindications include burst fractures, severe but not complete vertebral compression, radicular signs, or spinal canal narrowing greater than 20%. As mentioned above, in patients who suffer from chronic back pain from vertebral fracture and do not obtain relief from conservative management nor are able to benefit from these percutaneous techniques, placement of an intrathecal pump is the treatment of last resort.[65,66]

Spinal cord injury

Among the most challenging chronic pain conditions encountered in the trauma patient population are those that occur in individuals who have suffered spinal cord injury. Trauma is

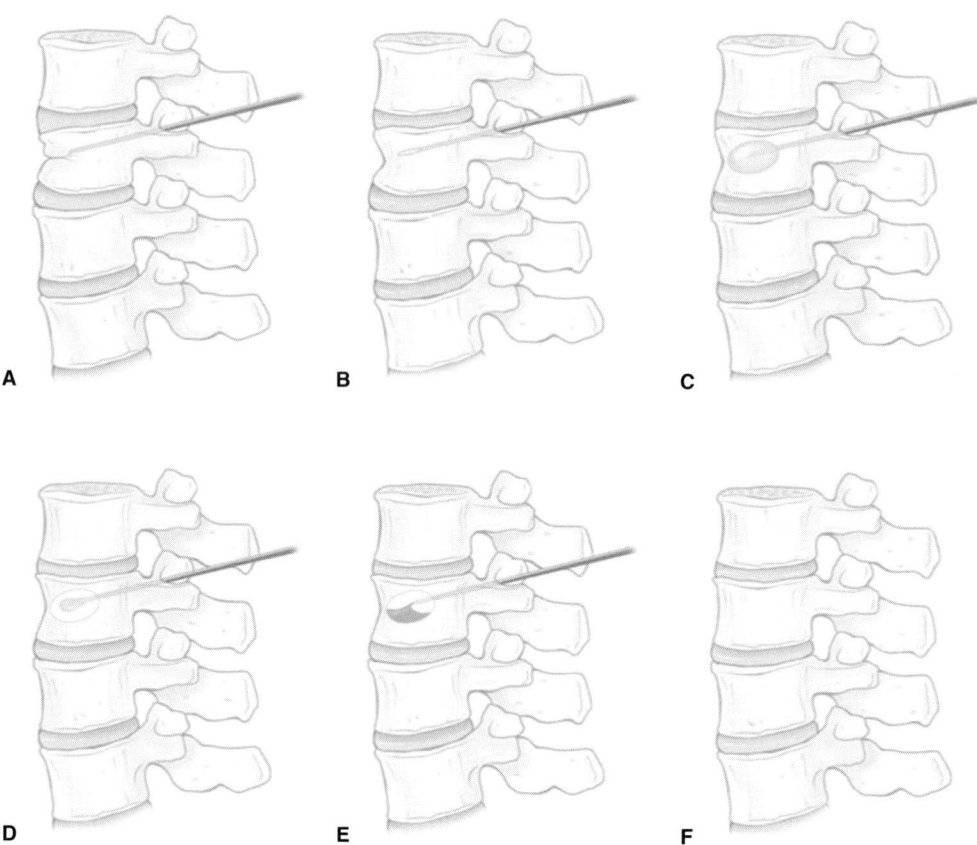

Figure 17.6 Kyphoplasty. (**A**) The blunt dissector and the working cannula are introduced using a pedicular approach. (**B**) The deflated balloon tamp is passed down the working cannula under fluoroscopic control. (**C**) Inflation of the balloon tamp and reduction of the fracture. (**D**) Deflation of the balloon tamp. (**E**) Application of the cement. (**F**) Removal of the working cannula. (From Daniel S, Daisuke T, Isador HL. Kyphoplasty: vertebral augmentation for compression fractures. *Clin Geriatr Med* 2006; **22**: 535–44, with permission.)

the leading cause of spinal cord pain, with MVCs responsible for more than 60–70% of spinal cord injury-related chronic pain.[75] The reported incidence of chronic pain following spinal cord injury varies greatly, with most surveys suggesting that 65–80% of patients experience chronic pain.[76] There is a strong relationship between pain and functional disability of the patients who suffer from spinal cord injury.[77,78] Treatment is frustrated by a lack of quality data on mechanism-specific outcomes for treatment modalities. Efforts to improve treatment outcomes have focused on adopting a useful classification system of spinal cord injury pain types. The IASP Spinal Cord Injury Task Force has proposed a three-tiered classification system that initially divides spinal cord injury pain into nociceptive and neuropathic types (Table 17.6). In tier 2, nociceptive pain is subdivided into musculoskeletal or visceral pain, while neuropathic pain is categorized by pain above, at, or below lesion level. In tier 3, specific structures or pathology are identified. Such taxonomy helps organize the approach to the patient with spinal cord injury-related chronic pain, and an algorithm for the treatment of spinal cord injury has been proposed by Siddall and others based on this classification system.[79]

Tier 1 focuses on basic mechanisms of pain. Nociceptive pain originates from damaged tissues that trigger peripheral myelinated Aδ and unmyelinated C nociceptor fibers. These high-threshold fibers are activated in response to high-intensity thermal, mechanical, or chemical stimulation. Such pain is likely to be in a region of normal sensation, to be identifiable, and to have a dull, aching quality. Musculoskeletal pain, including damage to ligaments, inflammation, as well as overuse and muscle spasm, all can be sources of nociceptive pain. Examples of visceral causes include etiologies such as renal calculi, sphincter dysfunction, and dysreflexic headache. It should be noted that the quality of visceral pain may be affected by the level of spinal cord lesion. For example, patients with tetraplegia may experience even more vague symptoms than those reviewed in the earlier section on abdominal pain. If the workup is negative or therapies directed at visceral etiology fail, then classifying the patient's pain as neuropathic is appropriate.[80,81]

Neuropathic pain is the other major category in the tier 1 classification. Sensory loss and abnormal pain perception are characteristic in spinal cord injury. In terms of the proposed treatment algorithm, neuropathic pain is discriminated from nociceptive pain in that it occurs in an area of abnormal sensation. Descriptors are not diagnostic but often include terms such as burning, electric shock, or shooting pain.

Table 17.6 Spinal cord injury pain typing and classification as proposed by the International Association for the Study of Pain (IASP)

Broad type (tier 1)	Broad system (tier 2)	Specific structures/ pathology (tier 3)
Nociceptive	Musculoskeletal	Bone, joint, muscle trauma or inflammation; mechanical instability; muscle spasm; secondary overuse syndromes
	Visceral	Renal calculus; bowel, sphincter dysfunction; dysreflexic headache
Neuropathic	Above level	Compressive mononeuropathies; complex regional pain syndromes
	At level	Nerve root compression (including cauda equina); syringomyelia; spinal cord trauma/ischemia (transitional zone, etc.); dual level cord and root trauma (double-lesion syndrome)
	Below level	Spinal cord trauma/ischemia

From Siddall PJ, Yezierski RP, Loeser JD. Pain following spinal cord injury: clinical features, prevalence, and taxonomy. *IASP Newslett* 2000; **3**: 3–7. http//www.iasp-pain.org/TC00–3.html.

Authors on the subject have noted that, while reviews of spinal cord injury mechanisms of neuropathic pain focus on central sensitization/plasticity, similar mechanisms of central plasticity are involved in both nociceptive and central neuropathic pain.[80–82] Animal and human experimental models provide evidence that structural and neurochemical changes interact to produce an array of dysesthesias including painful sensations. In response to injury or transection, trophic substances induce neuronal remodeling at the spinal and thalamic level resulting in plastic changes. Factors contributing to central pain may include neuronal destruction from excitatory amino acids as well as hypofunction of inhibitory monoaminergic, GABAergic, and opioid systems. Proposed mechanisms for spontaneous and evoked pain include upregulation of neuronal activity. The central neuropathic changes are discussed in a review by Eide.[80,81]

Tier 2 evaluation of neuropathic pain is based on the level of pain relative to the spinal cord injury. Pain *above the level of injury* suggests a condition not specific to spinal cord injury such as CRPS or peripheral nerve compression. Spinal cord injury patients, however, are at greater risk for developing CRPS. Evaluation includes physical exam and electrophysiologic studies, as well as MRI.[81] Based on this evaluation, appropriate treatments may include nerve decompression or sympathetic block.

At-level neuropathic pain is defined as pain occurring within two segments above or below the level of injury. This pain is associated with allodynia and hyperesthesia, and may be due to injury to the nerve root or the spinal cord. Distinguishing radicular symptoms due to nerve root injury, spinal instability, and facet joint or disk compression may be assisted by imaging and electrophysiologic studies. However, treatment options are different for nerve root pain compared with pain from spinal cord injury. Therefore, the clinician needs to keep this differential in mind when evaluating and treating the patient.

Syringomyelia is also a possibility in cases of delayed onset of pain. This is associated with a constant burning pain, allodynia, hyperalgesia, and progressive sensory loss in a limb. Muscle wasting is common. Motor loss is possible. The syndrome of syrongomyelia is caused by tubular cavitation developing in the spinal cord. MRI is diagnostic, and treatment is decompression. Syrinx can also be involved in above-level pain.[81]

Below-level neuropathic pain is true central pain and is characterized by diffuse spontaneous and/or evoked pain below the level of the lesion. Other terms for this condition include central dysesthesia syndrome, phantom pain, and deafferentation pain. The only evaluation of benefit is MRI to rule out syrinx or to investigate changing symptoms. To date, treatment options of at-level and below-level neuropathic pain targeted at the mechanisms outlined above are limited. First-line treatment in the chronic neuropathic pain patient is gabapentin, based on positive results in randomized controlled trials.[83–85] On the other hand, another randomized controlled trial was not able to show any significant advantage from treatment with gabapentin.[86] Some trials reported results supporting the effectiveness of pregabalin in the management of neuropathic pain in patients with spinal cord injury.[87,88] Evidence is mixed for use of tricyclic antidepressants or weak opioids such as tramadol as a second line of treatment.[81] Table 17.7 outlines third-line treatment options along with type of evidence, drawbacks, and indications.

Evidence for invasive treatments such as spinal cord stimulators is limited to case reports, but these do offer relief for some patients with incomplete lesions and at-level neuropathic pain.[89] Intrathecal administration of morphine and clonidine has been shown to be efficacious in patients with spasticity as well as at-level and below-level pain.[90–93] Both of these treatments are initiated in selected patients with a trial. If the trial is effective, then a permanent device is implanted. Experimental invasive treatments with limited evidence of efficacy include deep brain stimulation, motor cortex stimulation, dorsal root entry zone lesions, and cordotomy.[81,94–99] Surgical options may provide only temporary relief and result in additional deficits.

Conclusions

Treatment of the trauma patient with chronic pain involves many conditions including CRPS, posttraumatic headache, phantom limb pain, and pain from spinal cord injury. After evaluation and appropriate diagnostic studies, treatment is

Table 17.7 Third-line therapies in the treatment of spinal cord injury, with level of evidence, limitations, and specific indications

Treatment	Level of evidence	Disadvantages and side effects	Specific indications
Pregabalin	Unpublished RCT	Somnolence, dizziness, asthenia, dry mouth, edema, constipation	
Opioids	+ve cases	Constipation, drowsiness, tolerance, dependence	
Mixed serotonin–norepinephrine reuptake inhibitors	+ve cases	Hypertensive effects, gastrointestinal disturbance, dry mouth, reduced appetite, sweating	
Mexiletine	–ve RCT	Gastrointestinal upset, cardiovascular, hematologic disturbance, skin reactions	
Topiramate	+ve RCT	Drowsiness, dizziness, ataxia, anorexia, fatigue, gastrointestinal upset	
Lamotrigine	–ve RCT	Potentially life-threatening skin rash, hepatic effects, diplopia, blurred vision, dizziness	
Dronabinol	+ve cases	Dizziness, drowsiness, irritability	
Older anticonvulsants	–ve RCT	(valproate) Drowsiness, dizziness, liver dysfunction, hematologic effects	
Acupuncture	+ve cases	Invasive, Effectiveness for below-level neuropathic pain in SCI uncertain	
Intravenous ketamine	+ve RCT	Short-term relief, invasive, dysphoria	
Intravenous propofol	+ve RCT	Short-term relief, invasive, hypotension, arrhythmias, bradycardia	
Intravenous alfentanil	+ve RCT	Short-term relief, invasive, respiratory depression, bradycardia, sedation, hypotension, nausea, vomiting	
Intravenous morphine	+ve RCT	Short-term relief, invasive, respiratory depression, sedation, hypotension, nausea, vomiting	Effectiveness demonstrated for mechanical allodynia in SCI
Intrathecal baclofen	+ve RCT	Invasive, reports of increased or "unmasked" neuropathic pain in SCI	Stronger evidence for spasm-related pain
Intrathecal morphine and Clonidine	+ve RCT	Invasive tolerance, hypotension, respiratory depression, drowsiness	
Subarachnoid lignocaine	+ve RCT	Invasive, central nervous system disturbance	
Spinal cord stimulation	+ve cases	Invasive	At-level neuropathic pain, incomplete SCI
Deep brain stimulation	+ve cases	Invasive, intracranial hemorrhage	
Motor cortex stimulation (transcranial)	+ve cases	Short-term effect	
Motor cortex stimulation (epidural)	+ve cases	Invasive	
DREZ	+ve cases	Invasive, risk of further deficits	At-level neuropathic pain
Cordotomy	+ve cases	Invasive, risk of further deficits	

Note that these include most of the treatment options mentioned for many of the other neuropathic pain conditions such as CRPS and phantom limb pain. While the level of evidence and specific indications do not apply, the disadvantages and side effects do.

DREZ, dorsal root entry zone; RTC, randomized controlled trial; –ve or +ve, evidence indicates drug superior (+ve) or no more effective (–ve) when compared with placebo (RCT) or reported as beneficial (+ve cases); SCI, spinal cord injury.

Modified from Siddall PJ, Middleton JW. A proposed algorithm for the management of pain following spinal cord injury. *Spinal Cord* 2006; **44**: 67–77.

initiated to preserve function and relieve pain. Physical therapy and rehabilitation are important factors in overcoming pain in many of these conditions. Pain often interferes with accomplishing the goal of rehabilitation. A comprehensive pain management approach focuses not only on the rehabilitation effort, but also on the psychological conditions faced by chronic pain patients, such as depression. Thus, treatment should be directed at quality-of-life issues in order to obtain the best possible outcomes for chronic pain patients.[81]

Questions

(1) Concerning pain in medicine, identify the correct statement:
   a. Acute pain is protective and purposeful
   b. Congenital pain insensitivity is associated with normal life expectancy
   c. Most common pain syndromes do not involve neuropathic pain
   d. Somatic pain is defined as pain initiated or caused by a primary dysfunction in the nervous system

(2) True or false? The patient's medical and surgical histories are critical in evaluating the chronic pain patient.

(3) Concerning complex regional pain syndrome (CRPS), identify the correct statement:
   a. Pain is in proportion to that expected from the injury
   b. Causalgia is a better term to describe the pain findings
   c. The distribution of pain does not necessarily follow a particular nerve distribution in CRPS I
   d. There is no relation between CRPS and neuropathic pain

(4) Treatment of complex regional pain syndrome consists of:
   a. large doses of intravenous opioids and avoidance of nonsteroidal anti-inflammatory agents (NSAIDs)
   b. pain control, physical therapy to improve function, and psychological therapy
   c. sympathetic blocks and avoidance of physical therapy
   d. implantable devices and motor cortex stimulation, and avoidance of psychological therapy

(5) Identify the correct statement concerning posttraumatic abdominal pain:

   a. Chronic abdominal pain may develop after surgery
   b. Identifiable sources such as obstruction, pseudocyst, abscess, and adhesions need to be excluded
   c. Diagnostic regional blocks are useful in determining neuroanatomy
   d. All of the above are correct statements

(6) True or false? Phantom limb pain is somatic in origin and often involves neuroma formation around severed nerves.

(7) True or false? High cervical injury is more common in patients who have fallen from a low height, while low cervical injury predominates in motor vehicle accident patients.

(8) What is the first-line treatment for the chronic neuropathic pain patient following spinal cord injury?
   a. Gabapentin
   b. Opiods
   c. Baclofen
   d. Ketamine

(9) What is the most common complication of interventional treatment for chronic pain following vertebral fracture?
   a. Pneumothorax
   b. Infection
   c. Hematoma
   d. Postprocedural pain

(10) True or false? Intrathecal administration of morphine and clonidine is not efficacious in spinal cord injury patients with spasticity.

Answers

(1) a
(2) True
(3) c
(4) b
(5) d
(6) False
(7) True
(8) a
(9) d
(10) False

References

1. Gehling M. Persistent pain after elective trauma surgery. *Acute Pain*, 1999; **2** (3): 110–14.

2. Madigan SR. History and current status of pain management. In Raj PP, ed., *Practical Management of Pain*, 2nd edition. St. Louis, MO: Mosby Year Book, 2000, pp. 3–15.

3. Meldrum M. A capsule history of pain management. *JAMA* 2003; **290**: 2470–5.

4. Merskey H, Bogduk N. *Classification of Chronic Pain*, 2nd edition. Seattle, WA: IASP Press, 1994, pp. 209–14.

5. Irving, G.A., Contemporary assessment and management of neuropathic pain. *Neurology* 2005; **64** (12 Suppl 3): S21–7.

6. Mitchell SW. *Injuries of the Nerves and Their Consequences.* Philadelphia, PA: JB Lippincott, 1872.

7. Stanton-Hicks M, Jänig W, Hassenbusch S, *et al.* Reflex sympathetic dystrophy: changing concepts and taxonomy. *Pain* 1995; **63**: 127–33.

8. Atkins RM, Duckworth T, Kanis JA. Features of algodystrophy after Colles' fracture. *J Bone Joint Surg Br* 1990; **72**: 105–10.

9. Atkins RM, Duckworth T, Kanis JA. Algodystrophy following Colles' fracture. *J Hand Surg Br* 1989; **14**: 161–4.

10. Bickerstaff DR, Kanis JA. Algodystrophy: an under-recognized complication of minor trauma. *Br J Rheumatol* 1994; **33**: 240–8.

11. Dijkstra PU, Groothoff JW, ten Duis HJ, Geertzen JH. Incidence of complex regional pain syndrome type I after fractures of the distal radius. *Eur J Pain* 2003; **7**: 457–62.

12. Field J, Atkins RM. Algodystrophy is an early complication of Colles' fracture. What are the implications? *J Hand Surg Br* 1997; **22**: 178–82.

13. Raja SN, Grabow TS. Complex regional pain syndrome I (reflex sympathetic dystrophy). *Anesthesiology* 2002; **96**: 1254–60.

14. Sarangi PP, Ward AJ, Smith EJ, Staddon GE, Atkins RM. Algodystrophy and osteoporosis after tibial fractures. *J Bone Joint Surg Br* 1993; **75**: 450–2.

15. Jänig W, Baron R. Complex regional pain syndrome: mystery explained? *Lancet Neurol* 2003; **2**: 687–97.

16. Mitchell SW, Morehouse GR, Keen WW. *Gunshot Wounds and Other Injuries of Nerves.* New York, NY: Lippincott, 1864.

17. Hartick C. Pain due to trauma including sports injuries. In Gay SM, ed., *Practical Management of Pain*, 2nd edition. St Louis, MO: Mosby-Year Book, 1992, pp. 409–33.

18. Binder A, Schattschneider J, Baron R. Complex regional pain syndrome type I: reflex sympathetic dystrophy. In Waldman SD, ed., *Pain Management.* Philadelphia, PA: Saunders Elsevier, 2007, pp. 283–301.

19. Veldman PH, Reynen HM, Arntz IE, Goris RJ. Signs and symptoms of reflex sympathetic dystrophy: prospective study of 829 patients. *Lancet* 1993; **342**: 1012–16.

20. Bruehl S, Harden RN, Galer BS, *et al.* External validation of IASP diagnostic criteria for complex regional pain syndrome and proposed research diagnostic criteria. International Association for the Study of Pain. *Pain* 1999; **81**: 147–54.

21. Milch RA. Neuropathic pain: implications for the surgeon. *Surg Clin North Am* 2005; **85**: 225–36.

22. Stanton-Hicks M. Complex regional pain syndrome. *Anesthesiol Clin North America* 2003; **21**: 733–44.

23. Teasdall RD, Smith BP, Koman LA. Complex regional pain syndrome (reflex sympathetic dystrophy). *Clin Sports Med* 2004; **23**: 145–55.

24. Woolf CJ, Mannion RJ. Neuropathic pain: aetiology, symptoms, mechanisms, and management. *Lancet* 1999; **353**: 1959–64.

25. Acerra NE, Moseley GL. Dysynchiria: watching the mirror image of the unaffected limb elicits pain on the affected side. *Neurology* 2005; **65**: 751–3.

26. McCabe CS, Haigh RC, Ring EF, *et al.* A controlled pilot study of the utility of mirror visual feedback in the treatment of complex regional pain syndrome (type 1). *Rheumatology (Oxford)* 2003; **42**: 97–101.

27. Moseley GL. Graded motor imagery is effective for long-standing complex regional pain syndrome: a randomised controlled trial. *Pain* 2004; **108**: 192–8.

28. Moseley GL. Graded motor imagery for pathologic pain: a randomized controlled trial. *Neurology* 2006; **67**: 2129–34.

29. Robaina FJ, Rodriguez JL, de Vera JA, Martin MA. Transcutaneous electrical nerve stimulation and spinal cord stimulation for pain relief in reflex sympathetic dystrophy. *Stereotact Funct Neurosurg* 1989; **52**: 53–62.

30. Maihöfner C, Seifert F, Markovic K. Complex regional pain syndromes: new pathophysiological concepts and therapies. *Eur J Neurol* 2010; **17**: 649–60.

31. van Hilten B, van de Beek WJ, Hoff JI, Voormolen JH, Delhaas EM. Intrathecal baclofen for the treatment of dystonia in patients with reflex sympathetic dystrophy. *N Engl J Med* 2000; **343**: 625–30.

32. Huygen FJ, Niehof S, Zijlstra FJ, van Hagen PM, van Daele PL. Successful treatment of CRPS 1 with anti-TNF. *J Pain Symptom Manage* 2004; **27**: 101–3.

33. Bernateck M, Rolke R, Birklein F, *et al.* Successful intravenous regional block with low-dose tumor necrosis factor-alpha antibody infliximab for treatment of complex regional pain syndrome 1. *Anesth Analg* 2007; **105**: 1148–51.

34. Zuurmond WW, Langendijk PN, Bezemer PD, *et al.* Treatment of acute reflex sympathetic dystrophy with DMSO 50% in a fatty cream. *Acta Anaesthesiol Scand* 1996; **40**: 364–7.

35. Zollinger PE, Tuinebreijer WE, Breederveld RS, Kreis RW. Can vitamin C prevent complex regional pain syndrome in patients with wrist fractures? A randomized, controlled, multicenter dose-response study. *J Bone Joint Surg Am* 2007; **89**: 1424–31.

36. Zollinger PE, Tuinebreijer WE, Kreis RW, Breederveld RS. Effect of vitamin C on frequency of reflex sympathetic dystrophy in wrist fractures: a randomised trial. *Lancet* 1999; **354**: 2025–8.

37. Perez RS, Zuurmond WW, Bezemer PD, *et al.* The treatment of complex regional pain syndrome type I with free radical scavengers: a randomized controlled study. *Pain* 2003; **102**: 297–307.

38. Perez RS, Kwakkel G, Zuurmond WW, de Lange JJ. Treatment of reflex sympathetic dystrophy (CRPS type 1): a research synthesis of 21 randomized clinical trials. *J Pain Symptom Manage* 2001; **21**: 511–26.

39. Gobelet C, Waldburger M, Meier JL. The effect of adding calcitonin to physical treatment on reflex sympathetic dystrophy. *Pain* 1992; **48**: 171–5.

40. Bickerstaff DR, Kanis JA. The use of nasal calcitonin in the treatment of post-traumatic algodystrophy. *Br J Rheumatol* 1991; **30**: 291–4.

41. Adami S, Fossaluzza V, Gatti D, Fracassi E, Braga V. Bisphosphonate therapy of reflex sympathetic dystrophy syndrome. *Ann Rheum Dis* 1997; **56**: 201–4.

42. Varenna M, Zucchi F, Binelli L, *et al.* Intravenous pamidronate in the treatment of transient osteoporosis of the hip. *Bone* 2002; **31**: 96–101.

43. Perez RS, Pragt E, Geurts J, *et al.* Treatment of patients with complex regional pain syndrome type I with mannitol: a prospective, randomized, placebo-controlled, double-blinded study. *J Pain* 2008; **9**: 678–86.

44. Flasar MH, Goldberg E. Acute abdominal pain. *Med Clin North Am* 2006; **90**: 481–503.

45. Bicanovsky LK, Lagman RL, Davis MP, Walsh D. Managing nonmalignant chronic abdominal pain and malignant bowel obstruction. *Gastroenterol Clin North Am* 2006; **35**: 131–42.

46. Adolph MD, Benedetti C. Percutaneous-guided pain control: exploiting the neural basis of pain sensation. *Gastroenterol Clin North Am* 2006; **35**: 167–88.

47. Packard RC. Epidemiology and pathogenesis of posttraumatic headache. *J Head Trauma Rehabil* 1999; **14**: 9–21.

48. Walker WC. Pain pathoetiology after TBI: neural and nonneural mechanisms. *J Head Trauma Rehabil* 2004; **19**: 72–81.

49. Evans RW. Post-traumatic headaches. *Neurol Clin* 2004; **22**: 237–49, viii.

50. Nampiaparampil DE. Prevalence of chronic pain after traumatic brain injury: a systematic review. *JAMA* 2008; **300**: 711–19.

51. Bell KR, Kraus EE, Zasler ND. Medical management of posttraumatic headaches: pharmacological and physical treatment. *J Head Trauma Rehabil* 1999; **14**: 34–48.

52. Krusz JC. Aggressive interventional treatment of intractable headaches in the clinic setting. *Clin Fam Pract* 2005; **7**: 545–65.

53. Nikolajsen L. Phantom limb. In McMahon S, Koltzenburg M, eds., *Wall & Melzack's Textbook of Pain*, 5th edition. London: Churchill-Livingstone. 2006, pp. 961–71.

54. Jensen TS, Krebs B, Nielsen J, Rasmussen P. Phantom limb, phantom pain and stump pain in amputees during the first 6 months following limb amputation. *Pain* 1983; **17**: 243–56.

55. Wilder-Smith CH, Hill LT, Laurent S. Postamputation pain and sensory changes in treatment-naive patients: characteristics and responses to treatment with tramadol, amitriptyline, and placebo. *Anesthesiology* 2005; **103**: 619–28.

56. Melton LJ, Thamer M, Ray NF, *et al.* Fractures attributable to osteoporosis: report from the National Osteoporosis Foundation. *J Bone Miner Res* 1997; **12**: 16–23.

57. Jones G, White C, Nguyen T, *et al.* Prevalent vertebral deformities: relationship to bone mineral density and spinal osteophytosis in elderly men and women. *Osteoporos Int* 1996; **6**: 233–9.

58. Aschkenasy MT, Rothenhaus TC. Trauma and falls in the elderly. *Emerg Med Clin North Am* 2006; **24**: 413–32, vii.

59. Winters ME, Kluetz P, Zilberstein J. Back pain emergencies. *Med Clin North Am* 2006; **90**: 505–23.

60. Stolker RJ, Vervest AC, Groen GJ. The treatment of chronic thoracic segmental pain by radiofrequency percutaneous partial rhizotomy. *J Neurosurg* 1994; **80**: 986–92.

61. Fuchs S, Erbe T, Fischer HL, Tibesku CO. Intraarticular hyaluronic acid versus glucocorticoid injections for nonradicular pain in the lumbar spine. *J Vasc Interv Radiol* 2005; **16**: 1493–8.

62. Burchiel KJ, Anderson VC, Brown FD, *et al.* Prospective, multicenter study of spinal cord stimulation for relief of chronic back and extremity pain. *Spine (Phila Pa 1976)* 1996; **21**: 2786–94.

63. Tamayo-Orozco J, Arzac-Palumbo P, Peón-Vidales H, Mota-Bolfeta R, Fuentes F. Vertebral fractures associated with osteoporosis: patient management. *Am J Med* 1997; **103**: 44S–48S.

64. Watts NB, Harris ST, Genant HK. Treatment of painful osteoporotic vertebral fractures with percutaneous vertebroplasty or kyphoplasty. *Osteoporos Int* 2001; **12**: 429–37.

65. Shedid D, Togawa D, Lieberman IH. Kyphoplasty: vertebral augmentation for compression fractures. *Clin Geriatr Med* 2006; **22**: 535–44.

66. Heran MK, Legiehn GM, Munk PL. Current concepts and techniques in percutaneous vertebroplasty. *Orthop Clin N Am* 2006; **37**: 409–34.

67. Niv D, Gofeld M, Devor M. Causes of pain in degenerative bone and joint disease: a lesson from vertebroplasty. *Pain* 2003; **105**: 387–92.

68. Rohlmann A, Klockner C, Bergmann G. [The biomechanics of kyphosis]. *Orthopade* 2001; **30**: 915–18.

69. Lee JS, Kim KW, Ha KY. The effect of vertebroplasty on pulmonary function in patients with osteoporotic compression fractures of the thoracic spine. *J Spinal Disord Tech* 2011; **24**: E11–15.

70. Wardlaw D, Cummings SR, Van Meirhaeghe J, *et al.* Efficacy and safety of balloon kyphoplasty compared with non-surgical care for vertebral compression fracture (FREE): a randomised controlled trial. *Lancet* 2009; **373**: 1016–24.

71. Buchbinder R, Osborne RH, Ebeling PR, *et al.* A randomized trial of vertebroplasty for painful osteoporotic vertebral fractures. *N Engl J Med* 2009; **361**: 557–68.

72. Kallmes DF, Comstock BA, Heagerty PJ, *et al.* A randomized trial of vertebroplasty for osteoporotic spinal fractures. *N Engl J Med* 2009; **361**: 569–79.

73. Rousing R, Andersen MO, Jespersen SM, Thomsen K, Lauritsen J. Percutaneous vertebroplasty compared to conservative treatment in patients with painful acute or subacute osteoporotic vertebral fractures: three-months follow-up in a clinical randomized study. *Spine (Phila Pa 1976)* 2009; **34**: 1349–54.

74. Miller FG, Kallmes DF. The case of vertebroplasty trials: promoting a culture of evidence-based procedural medicine. *Spine (Phila Pa 1976)* 2010; **35**: 2023–6.

75. Nicholson BD. Evaluation and treatment of central pain syndromes. *Neurology* 2004; **62** (5 Suppl 2): S30–6.

76. Siddall PJ, McClelland JM, Rutkowski SB, Cousins MJ. A longitudinal study of the prevalence and characteristics of pain in the first 5 years following spinal cord injury. *Pain* 2003; **103**: 249–57.

77. Jensen MP, Kuehn CM, Amtmann D, Cardenas DD. Symptom burden in persons with spinal cord injury. *Arch Phys Med Rehabil* 2007; **88**: 638–45.

78. Siddall PJ. Management of neuropathic pain following spinal cord injury: now and in the future. *Spinal Cord* 2009; **47**: 352–9.

79. Vierck CJ, Siddall P, Yezierski RP. Pain following spinal cord injury: animal models and mechanistic studies. *Pain* 2000; **89**: 1–5.

80. Eide PK. Pathophysiological mechanisms of central neuropathic pain after spinal cord injury. *Spinal Cord* 1998; **36**: 601–12.

81. Siddall PJ, Middleton JW. A proposed algorithm for the management of pain following spinal cord injury. *Spinal Cord* 2006; **44**: 67–77.

82. Dubner R, Basbaum AI. Spinal dorsal horn plasticity following tissue or nerve injury. In Wall PD, Melzack R, eds., *Textbook of Pain*. Edinburgh: Churchill Liningstone, 1994, pp. 225–42.

83. Levendoglu F, Ogün CO, Ozerbil O, Ogün TC, Ugurlu H. Gabapentin is a first line drug for the treatment of neuropathic pain in spinal cord injury. *Spine (Phila Pa 1976)* 2004; **29**: 743–51.

84. Tai Q, Kirshblum S, Chen B, *et al.* Gabapentin in the treatment of neuropathic pain after spinal cord injury: a prospective, randomized, double-blind, crossover trial. *J Spinal Cord Med* 2002; **25**: 100–5.

85. Putzke JD, Richards JS, Kezar L, Hicken BL, Ness TJ. Long-term use of gabapentin for treatment of pain after traumatic spinal cord injury. *Clin J Pain* 2002; **18**: 116–21.

86. Rintala DH, Holmes SA, Courtade D, *et al.* Comparison of the effectiveness of amitriptyline and gabapentin on chronic neuropathic pain in persons with spinal cord injury. *Arch Phys Med Rehabil* 2007; **88**: 1547–60.

87. Siddall PJ, Cousins MJ, Otte A, *et al.* Pregabalin in central neuropathic pain associated with spinal cord injury: a placebo-controlled trial. *Neurology* 2006; **67**: 1792–800.

88. Vranken JH, Dijkgraaf MG, Kruis MR, *et al.* Pregabalin in patients with central neuropathic pain: a randomized, double-blind, placebo-controlled trial of a flexible-dose regimen. *Pain* 2008; **136**: 150–7.

89. Cioni B, Meglio M, Pentimalli L, Visocchi M. Spinal cord stimulation in the treatment of paraplegic pain. *J Neurosurg* 1995; **82**: 35–9.

90. Middleton JW, Siddall PJ, Walker S, Molloy AR, Rutkowski SB. Intrathecal clonidine and baclofen in the management of spasticity and neuropathic pain following spinal cord injury: a case study. *Arch Phys Med Rehabil* 1996; **77**: 824–6.

91. Gatscher S, Becker R, Uhle E, Bertalanffy H. Combined intrathecal baclofen and morphine infusion for the treatment of spasticity related pain and central deafferentiation pain. *Acta Neurochir Suppl* 2002; **79**: 75–6.

92. Siddall PJ, Gray M, Rutkowski S, Cousins MJ. Intrathecal morphine and clonidine in the management of spinal cord injury pain: a case report. *Pain* 1994; **59**: 147–8.

93. Siddall PJ, Molloy AR, Walker S, *et al.* The efficacy of intrathecal morphine and clonidine in the treatment of pain after spinal cord injury. *Anesth Analg* 2000; **91**: 1493–8.

94. Hosobuchi Y. Subcortical electrical stimulation for control of intractable pain in humans. Report of 122 cases (1970–1984). *J Neurosurg* 1986; **64**: 543–53.

95. Kumar K, Toth C, Nath RK. Deep brain stimulation for intractable pain: a 15-year experience. *Neurosurgery* 1997; **40**: 736–46.

96. Nguyen JP, Lefaucheur JP, Decq P, *et al.* Chronic motor cortex stimulation in the treatment of central and neuropathic pain. Correlations between clinical, electrophysiological and anatomical data. *Pain* 1999; **82**: 245–51.

97. Edgar RE, Best LG, Quail PA, Obert AD. Computer-assisted DREZ microcoagulation: posttraumatic spinal deafferentation pain. *J Spinal Disord* 1993; **6**: 48–56.

98. Nashold BS, Bullitt E. Dorsal root entry zone lesions to control central pain in paraplegics. *J Neurosurg* 1981; **55**: 414–19.

99. Sindou M, Mertens P, Wael M. Microsurgical DREZotomy for pain due to spinal cord and/or cauda equina injuries: long-term results in a series of 44 patients. *Pain* 2001; **92**: 159–71.

Chapter

18

Damage control in severe trauma

Michael J. A. Parr and Ulrike Buehner

Objectives

(1) Understand the concept of damage control surgery (DCS).

(2) Understand that reversal of the lethal triad (trauma triad of death) requires aggressive intervention for improved outcome.

(3) Understand staged physiological restoration (the four phases of the damage control process).

Introduction

The management of the multiply injured patient has been revolutionized during the past century. Advances in prehospital care, resuscitation, interventional radiology, and intensive care medicine have all contributed to better trauma outcomes. The damage control process of abbreviated laparotomy with rapid control of hemorrhage and contamination has proved to be effective to combat the physiologic failure associated with severe blunt and penetrating injury.

This chapter reviews some of the key issues of damage control surgery, highlighting the importance of a multidisciplinary team approach to optimize trauma patient management.

Damage control surgery (DCS) is abbreviated surgery performed on selected critically injured patients. Definitive operative management is accomplished in a stepwise fashion based on the patient's physiologic tolerance; the objective is to gain time to stabilize the severely traumatized patient and to optimize his or her physiologic state before definitive repair. Rather than restoring anatomic integrity, the rationale for DCS is to minimize the metabolic insults of coagulopathy, hypothermia, and acidosis. Each of these three factors tends to exacerbate the others and interact to produce a downward metabolic spiral: the "bloody vicious cycle."[1] The concept of DCS originally emerged from collective experience with major abdominal injuries. Over the past decade, other surgical subspecialties have adopted the DCS concept successfully, and it has also served to define damage control resuscitation shock management (see Chapter 4).

Historical background

The fundamentals of damage control laparotomy were first described by Pringle in 1908 and modified by Halsted in 1913, who described packing liver injuries with a planned return to theater following stabilization of the patient.[2,3] In 1983, Stone et al. popularized the technique of abdominal packing and rapid temporary closure for patients with major intraoperative coagulopathy.[4] This proved to be life-saving in previously nonsalvageable situations. Rotondo et al. refined the technique and demonstrated a survival advantage in selected patients.[5] Recently, the three-stage approach described by Rotondo et al. has been amended to a four-stage process:

(1) early recognition of patients requiring damage control

(2) salvage operation for hemorrhage and contamination control

(3) intensive care management

(4) operation for definitive repair and reconstruction

Damage control surgery

The overriding principles of DCS are:

(1) control hemorrhage

(2) prevent contamination

(3) limit sepsis

(4) protect from further injury

Limited or staged procedures are aimed at prevention of metabolic failure. In the severely traumatized patient prehospital and emergency department (ED) times should be minimized. Unnecessary investigations that will not immediately affect patient management should be deferred. These patients should be transferred rapidly to an operative/interventional suite without repeated attempts to restore circulating volume. They require emergent control of hemorrhage and simultaneous vigorous resuscitation with blood and clotting factors (Fig. 18.1). The ability to co-locate operative, imaging, and interventional capabilities in the one location has led to the introduction of the RAPTOR suite (resuscitation with angiography, percutaneous techniques, and operative repair) capable of advancing the damage control approach to trauma.[6]

Table 18.1 Room and equipment preparation

Increase ambient room temperature
Monitoring equipment on standby
Intravenous lines/transducers primed
Warmed intravenous fluids
Level 1 or similar rapid infusion device
Blood warmers
Forced-air warming device
Humidified and warmed gas delivery
Documentation

Table 18.2 Patient scenarios for damage control consideration

Penetrating abdominal injury with systolic blood pressure < 90 mmHg
High-velocity gunshot or blast injury
Polytrauma with major abdominal injury
Compound pelvic fracture with associated abdominal injury
Multiple casualties and limited resources
Military situations

Table 18.3 Predictive indicators for damage control surgery

Major hemorrhage: > 10 units of packed red blood cells
Severe wound contamination
High injury severity score and prolonged shock
An evolving lethal triad of: • Hypothermia: core temperature < 34 °C • Acidosis: pH < 7.2 or base deficit ≥ 8 • Coagulopathy: aPTT > 60 seconds

aPTT, activated partial thromboplastin time.

Table 18.4 Indications for damage control surgery

Inability to achieve hemostasis
Inaccessible major venous injury
Time-consuming procedure in the presence of suboptimal resuscitation
Management of extraabdominal life-threatening injury
Reassessment of intraabdominal contents
Inability to close abdomen due to visceral edema/risk of intraabdominal hypertension (IAH)

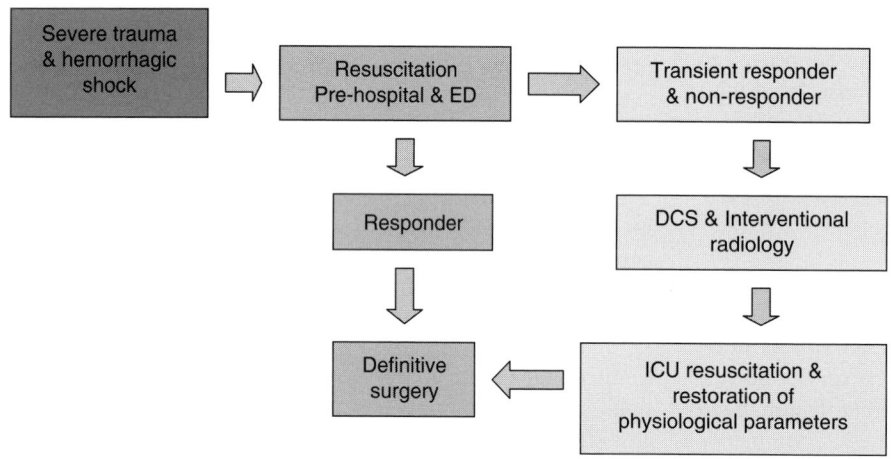

Figure 18.1 Resuscitation and damage control surgery.

Prior preparation prevents poor performance and outcome. To ensure this, early communication between trauma team members, surgical subspecialties, and operating room staff, intensive care unit (ICU), blood bank, and the radiology department are vitally important for effective and timely resuscitation and damage control. In response, the resuscitation room in the emergency department, the operating/interventional room, and ICU bed space should be prepared for receiving the patient (Table 18.1). Key factors for patient selection are listed in Tables 18.2 and 18.3. Emphasis should be on the early implementation of damage control principles guided by the patient's injuries and physiology (Table 18.4), as some of the indicators will predict the need for DCS too late in the resuscitation process.

The trauma triad of death

Hypovolemia as a result of exsanguinating hemorrhage leads to hypothermia, coagulopathy, and metabolic acidosis, known as the triad of death. It has also been described as "the bloody vicious cycle" (Fig. 18.2). Each factor exacerbates the others, leading to a downward spiral and death. Once metabolic

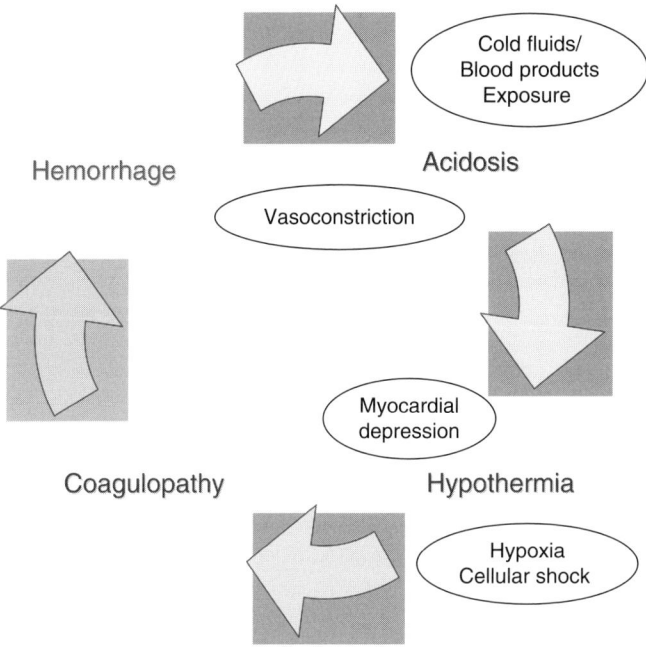

Figure 18.2 The bloody vicious cycle.

failure has become established, it is extremely difficult to control hemorrhage and correct the physiologic derangement.

Hypothermia

Hypothermia is a marker of profound injury and is also deleterious. It is often the inevitable result of severe exsanguinating injury and subsequent massive resuscitative effort.[7] Severe hemorrhage causing hypovolemia leads to tissue hypoperfusion in the body. This means diminished oxygen delivery at the cellular level and reduced heat generation. Clinically, hypothermia is important if the body temperature drops below 36 °C for more than 4 hours.[8] It can lead to cardiac arrhythmias, decreased cardiac output, increased systemic vascular resistance, and left shift of the oxyhemoglobin dissociation curve, and can induce coagulopathy by inhibition of the clotting cascade.[9] The immune system is also impaired at low temperature. Temperatures of less than 34.5 °C are associated with an increased prevalence of multiorgan dysfunction and increased need for vasopressor and inotropic support. At temperatures below 32 °C mortality approaches 100%.[10] The trauma team should take every measure to prevent worsening of hypothermia, which is aggravated by heat loss either by conduction or convection due to environmental factors, impaired thermogenesis, exposure, and transfusion of cold fluids in the emergency room or operating room.

Passive external rewarming techniques include removal of wet clothing and simple covering of the patient to minimize convective heat loss.[11] Active external rewarming techniques include fluid-circulating heating blankets, convective warm air blankets, and radiant warmers. Active core-rewarming techniques include warmed airway gases, heated peritoneal or

pleural lavage, warmed intravenous fluid infusion, and extracorporeal rewarming.

Coagulopathy

Coagulopathy has been shown to be present in approximately 25–35% of major trauma patients on admission to the emergency room. If present on admission, there is an associated doubling of mortality. This represents a serious problem for major trauma patients, and hemorrhage accounts for 40% of all trauma-related deaths. Coagulopathy forces a strategy of early and rapid hemostatic treatment to prevent exsanguination.[12-15] The pathogenesis of acute traumatic coagulopathy is complex and multifactorial,[16] but this initial clotting derangement is particularly associated with major injury and shock and precedes fluid resuscitation. Every aspect of the normal clotting mechanism is affected in a cold acidotic exsanguinating patient. Coagulopathy associated with major injury and shock is then compounded by hemodilution from blood losses replaced with colloid or crystalloid, massive blood transfusion, progressive hypothermia and acidosis; consumption of coagulation factors and platelets in clot formation; primary or secondary fibrinolysis related to endothelial damage and/or clot formation.

Prioritizing reversal of the coagulopathy has led to the development of massive transfusion protocols with proactive strategies of replacement of red blood cells (RBCs), plasma, and platelets in near-physiological ratios (see Chapter 6). There is increasing evidence that the new recommendation of a higher plasma/platelets to RBC ratio can significantly reduce hospital mortality in a dose–response relationship.[17-19] Thrombocytopenia is particularly common in patients who receive transfusion volumes in excess of 1.5 times their blood volume. After replacement of one blood volume, only about 35–40% of platelets remain in circulation. In addition, the release of mediators after tissue trauma activates multiple humoral systems, including the coagulation, fibrinolysis, complement, and kallikrein cascades. These in turn have wide-ranging effects on neutrophils, macrophages, platelets, and other cellular elements, which provoke a multitude of changes in the body's hemostatic mechanisms. These same mechanisms are implicated in the development of the systemic inflammatory response syndrome (SIRS) and multiple organ failure.[20]

Certain injuries, in particular, are known to interfere with the coagulation system. Brain injuries have been shown to lead to coagulopathy, caused in part by release of brain tissue thromboplastins after neuronal injury.[21,22] Similarly, long-bone fractures may be associated with hemostatic disorders.[23]

In acidosis, endothelial sloughing and subsequent activation of factor XII results in activation of procoagulant substances that may trigger disseminated intravascular coagulation (DIC). This process leads to an imbalance of procoagulant and anticoagulant activity, resulting in overstimulation of coagulation. The initial response to trauma also includes release of both platelet-activating factor and arachidonic acid from cell membrane triglycerides. Both are inflammatory mediators and cause a wide spectrum of inflammatory responses. The balance between thromboxane and prostacyclin is affected in the hypothermic state, resulting in platelet dysfunction. Recently, it has become clear that one of the key factors in SIRS is endothelial injury precipitating aberrant coagulation. The endothelial impairment secondary to trauma and the interaction with the coagulation cascade and platelet activation leads to reduction in antithrombin III and fibrinogen levels, thus enhancing fibrinolysis. This is rapidly followed by a hyperactive and dysfunctional fibrinolytic system. In the multiple-trauma setting, bleeding from puncture wounds and multiple injuries further aggravates the coagulopathic status, contributing to hypothermia.[24]

Tranexamic acid (TXA) has recently been evaluated in the CRASH-2 study, a large randomized placebo-controlled trial of the effects of antifibrinolytic treatment on death, vascular occlusive events, and transfusion requirement among trauma patients. Patients were randomly allocated to receive a loading dose of 1 g of TXA over 10 minutes, followed by an intravenous infusion of 1 g over 8 hours, or matching placebo. The results show that the early administration of TXA to trauma patients with, or at risk of, significant bleeding reduces the risk of death from hemorrhage with no apparent increase in fatal or nonfatal vascular occlusive events. All-cause mortality was significantly reduced with TXA when given within 3 hours of injury.[25,26]

Clinical evidence suggests that prevention of coagulopathy is superior to its treatment. Early and intensive therapy with plasma or clotting factors and platelets appears to be associated with better outcomes when accompanied by hemorrhage control.[18] Therefore therapy for patients with coagulopathy after major trauma should be rapidly initiated (Table 18.5). Medical management begins with ensuring that adequate help and equipment (e.g., fluid warmers, pressure bags, and rapid infusors) are available for the rapid administration of warmed fluid, blood, and blood products. The blood bank should be informed as early as possible of large transfusion requirements and activation of the massive transfusion protocol (MTP). The benefits of an MTP are multifold: ease of use, rapid blood product availability during DCS and intensive care, and the higher plasma and platelet doses appear to be associated with reduced blood use and improved outcomes (see Chapter 7). The fixed volume ratios will also allow the number of administered units of RBCs to be used as surrogates for blood loss and primary treatment effect.[18] A single phone call for activation should result in the expedited delivery of blood products to the patient. The ongoing availability of blood products needs to be confirmed, particularly for hospitals at a distance from the central blood transfusion service.

The rheologic effect of anemia (bleeding time is inversely related to hematocrit) is compounded by thrombocytopenia less than 100,000/μL, resulting in a prolonged bleeding time.[27] During continued hemorrhage, and especially if head injury is

Table 18.5 Strategies to correct coagulopathy

Consider tranexamic acid
Reverse hypothermia
Maintain effective circulating blood volume and oxygenation
Reverse anticoagulants (prothrombin concentrate, FFP, vitamin K)
Replace coagulation factors with FFP (approximately 1:1:1 RBC: FFP:platelet ratio)
Keep platelets > 100,000/μL
Replace fibrinogen if < 1.5 g/L with cryoprecipitate or fibrinogen concentrate
Reverse hypocalcemia with calcium (10 mmol)
Consider use of rFVIIa
Consider hemostatic adjuncts to promote coagulation/reduce fibrinolysis (e.g., aminocaproic acid, tranexamic acid, and desmopressin)
Repeat coagulation tests and blood count to guide therapy

FFP, fresh frozen plasma; RBC, red blood cells; rFVIIa, recombinant factor VIIa.

present, the hematocrit should be maintained at more than 30% and the platelet count at more than 100,000/μL. Platelet counts of less than 100,000/μL can be anticipated when between 1 and 1.5 blood volumes have been replaced. Initially, platelets will be given empirically and repeated according to ongoing blood loss, transfusion requirement, and platelet counts. When faced with massive transfusion and DCS, aiming for an early platelet count greater than 100,000/μL will provide a margin of safety. With resolution of the acidosis, coagulopathy, and hypothermia, lower platelet counts (50,000–75,000/μL) may be a more suitable level to aim for. The requirement for fresh frozen plasma (FFP) is less predictable, because the labile factors V and VIII have wide normal ranges, and levels down to 20% of normal may not result in coagulopathy if the hematocrit and platelet count are maintained.[27] However, in massive transfusion (defined as the replacement of one blood volume in 24 hours) FFP should be given early and empirically, because any delay in blood component therapy for confirmation of coagulopathy by laboratory tests would be detrimental to the outcome (see Chapter 7). The transfusion of clotting factors and platelets is essential until the consumptive process resolves. The time-consuming nature of current coagulation tests (40 minutes) compromises the optimal treatment of bleeding. For clotting factors an additional 30 minutes is added for thawing and transport. During this time the entire blood volume of the bleeding trauma patient may have been exchanged, making the laboratory results obsolete. Furthermore, coagulopathy in the hypothermic patient is often underestimated by standard coagulation tests performed at 37 °C, and hence an abnormal coagulation profile may not be revealed.[28–31]

In recent years, viscoelastic point-of-care (POC) methods that assess the speed of clotting and quality of the clot, such as thromboelastometry (e.g., TEG, ROTEM) are being used successfully to guide hemostatic therapy. Increasing evidence is emerging that goal-directed coagulation management using real-time assessment of coagulation function via POC rapid thromboelastography can improve outcome. In addition, fibrinogen is increasingly viewed as the coagulation factor that is the first to become critically low in cases of major hemorrhage. Therefore aiming at functional fibrinogen levels as assessed by elastometry appears reasonable.[1,32–34] If POC coagulation monitoring is not available, 10 units of cryoprecipitate (or equivalent fibrinogen concentrate) should be given as fibrinogen replacement early in the resuscitation process. Clinicians should be aware that in the presence of artificial colloids such as hydroxyethyl starch (HES) or gelatin, the most often used fibrinogen measurement method, the Clauss method, significantly overestimates fibrinogen concentration.[35]

As a general rule, blood components are administered until the prothrombin time (PT) and activated partial thromboplastin time (aPTT) reach less than 1.25 times control levels, the platelet count is more than a 100,000/μL, and the fibrinogen level is greater than 1.5–2.0 g/L, and/or bleeding is controlled. Some abnormalities may be acceptable, however, provided bleeding is controlled and the risks of rebleeding are small. After meticulous surgical control of hemorrhage has been attempted, in selected patients residual diffuse bleeding may respond to antifibrinolytics (TXA, and aminocaproic acid) and the vasopressin analog (desmopressin). Another recent study on Military Application of Tranexamic acid in Trauma Emergency Resuscitation (MATTERs) assessed the effect of its administration on total blood-product use, thromboembolic complications, and mortality. The use of TXA with blood-component-based resuscitation resulted in improved coagulopathy and survival, a benefit that was most prominent in patients requiring massive blood transfusions.[36] Aprotinin, a serum protease inhibitor, has been effective in reducing blood loss in major cardiothoracic surgery, major orthopedic surgery, and orthotopic liver transplantation but currently has therapeutic license issues in many countries.[37] Desmopressin can be used to treat bleeding in patients with congenital or acquired defects of platelet function. The true roles of these two agents in the major trauma setting have not been evaluated in suitable trials; therefore, there is little information available on their safety and efficacy.

Recombinant factor VIIa (rFVIIa) is currently licensed for use in hemophiliacs with antibodies to factor VII. At present, its use in trauma and hemorrhage is on a "compassionate" basis. The first published account of the use of rFVIIa in trauma was published by Kenet in 1999.[38] She describes the successful use of rFVIIa in a soldier with traumatic coagulopathy following a high-velocity gunshot. The safety and efficacy of rFVIIa as potential adjunct to treatment of coagulapathy in severely injured trauma patients with life-threatening bleeding has been evaluated in the CONTROL trial.[39,40] This phase 3 trial was the largest prospective trauma trial to date. It was terminated early due to the unexpectedly low mortality rate (less than half that predicted), which meant that the study was underpowered for its primary endpoints. Consequently, the trial did not demonstrate a mortality benefit, only a trend towards less frequent multiorgan failure and acute respiratory distress syndrome (ARDS). The use of rFVIIa was associated with a significant reduction in blood-product requirements (median of 2.6 units) in bleeding trauma patients. The evidence-based protocolized approach of the trial is likely to have had a major beneficial effect on the survival of all bleeding patients in the study. With regard to patient safety, two large randomized controlled trauma trials have demonstrated no increase in thrombotic effects where patients received rFVIIa rather than placebo.[40,41] Recombinant FVIIa was originally developed as a prohemostatic agent for the treatment of bleeding episodes in hemophiliac patients. It is almost identical in structure and activity to human factor VII and its mode of action.[42] rFVII becomes active after forming a complex with tissue factor, located in the subendothelium and hence only exposed to circulating blood after vessel injury. Formation of the tissue factor–rFVIIa complex initiates activation of factor IX and X, inducing thrombin activation and faster formation of the fibrin clots at the site of vascular injury. Recombinant FVIIa has been used as rescue therapy in moribund trauma patients in whom standard procedures had failed to correct bleeding.[38,43,44]

Acidosis

Metabolic acidosis describes any decrease in body pH not caused by excess carbon dioxide but attributed to increased hydrogen ion concentration. It is a reliable indicator of tissue hypoxia and primarily the end result of reduced oxygen-carrying capacity and/or decreased effective cardiac output (Fig. 18.2). The acidosis may be due to ischemia or necrosis from direct tissue injury or hemorrhage. Profound hypoperfusion causes decreased cellular substrate delivery and necessitates conversion to anaerobic metabolism. This in turn leads to lactic acid synthesis, which is potentiated by trauma-induced catabolism. Lactic acidosis may be aggravated by impaired lactate clearance due to a secondary hepatic ischemic injury post trauma.

Lactic acidosis that is not cleared after 48 hours is associated with a mortality rate of greater than 85%.[45] Ongoing acidosis after volume resuscitation and blood pressure restoration is a grave prognostic sign. Metabolic acidosis impairs hepatic blood flow and alters the normal coagulation process, contributing to hemostatic and coagulation system disorders. The associated base deficit is a valuable indicator of shock and fluid requirements as well as a predictor of mortality after trauma.[46] Base deficit is defined as the amount of base required by a liter of whole arterial blood to normalize the pH to 7.4 at PCO_2 of 5.3 kPA (40 mmHg), thereby reflecting the severity of acidosis. The correction of this acidosis requires control of hemorrhage and optimization of oxygen delivery, initially by blood and fluid administration. Inotropic or vasopressor support should only be considered if the patient does not respond adequately to volume and RBC replacement because of myocardial depression at a pH less than 7.2.[27] The need for inotropes and vasopressors correlates with poor outcomes for these patients.

There is little evidence-based research documenting the benefits of bicarbonate administration for the correction of a metabolic acidosis. Conversely, deleterious effects have been widely described in the literature.[47] Bicarbonate therapy is inappropriate when tissue hypoperfusion or necrosis is present. Bicarbonate cannot cross the cell membrane without dissociation; consequently the increase in $PaCO_2$ may result in intracellular acidosis and depression of myocardial cell function. The associated decrease in plasma ionized calcium may also cause a decrease in myocardial contractility. Convincing evidence in humans that bicarbonate improves myocardial contractility or increases responsiveness to circulating catecholamines is lacking. Two studies comparing saline and bicarbonate in patients with pH $\geq$ 7.13–7.15 failed to reveal any difference in hemodynamics and vasopressor requirements between equimolar concentrations of bicarbonate in normal saline with either therapy.[48,49] The respiratory compensation of the acidosis puts a large burden on the respiratory system, and continued ventilatory support is required. Some patients will have established acute kidney injury, and the early commencement of renal replacement therapy may benefit

these patients to achieve a faster correction of their acidosis and to restore an optimal metabolic environment. Persistent acidosis may represent reduced cardiac output, reduced oxygen delivery, or abnormal oxygen utilization. It emphasizes the need for continuous monitoring, repeated objective assessment, and setting appropriate resuscitation endpoints.[27]

Interventional radiology (see also Chapter 11)

Modern trauma care involves a multidisciplinary approach to patients with complex injuries. The traditional role of radiology has been primarily diagnostic and noninvasive. The past decade has seen major advances in interventional radiology, such that therapeutic angiographic techniques now form an essential part of trauma care.[50–52] The goal of angiography in severely injured patients is to identify and treat arterial hemorrhage in a minimally invasive fashion, with preservation of organ function and tissue. Transcatheter arterial embolization (TAE) has been reported to be rapid and effective for the control of arterial pelvic bleeding (Figs. 18.3–18.6) and hepatic injury.[53] Hemodynamic instability has now become only a relative contraindication. Balloon occlusion of the distal aorta for bleeding pelvic fractures and the proximal aorta for cross-clamping is well established. An evolving new treatment concept in severe trauma is RAPTOR (resuscitation with angiography, percutaneous techniques, and operative repair), which combines emergent percutaneous therapies, open interventions, resuscitation, and critical care in one physical location, the RAPTOR suite, merging trauma bay, angiography suite, operating room, and intensive care unit.[6] This novel concept achieves successful treatment of hemorrhagic shock

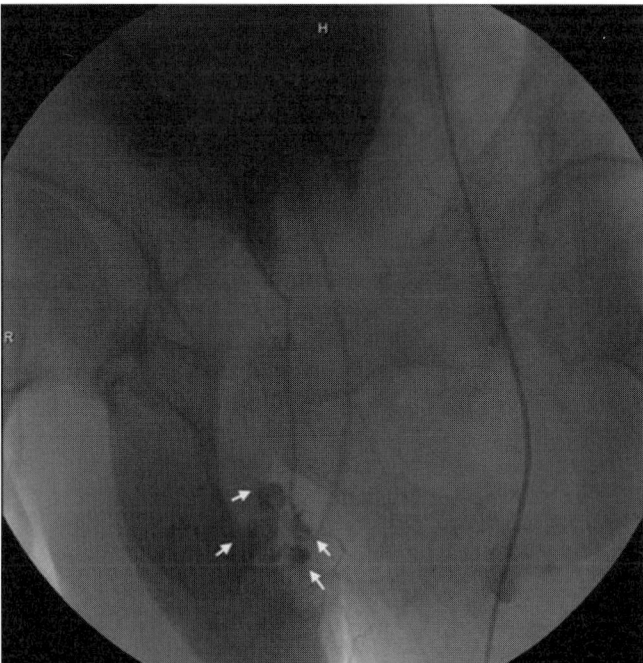

Figure 18.3 Native preembolization image of right internal iliac artery demonstrating an area of active bleeding (white arrows) at the external pudendal runoff.

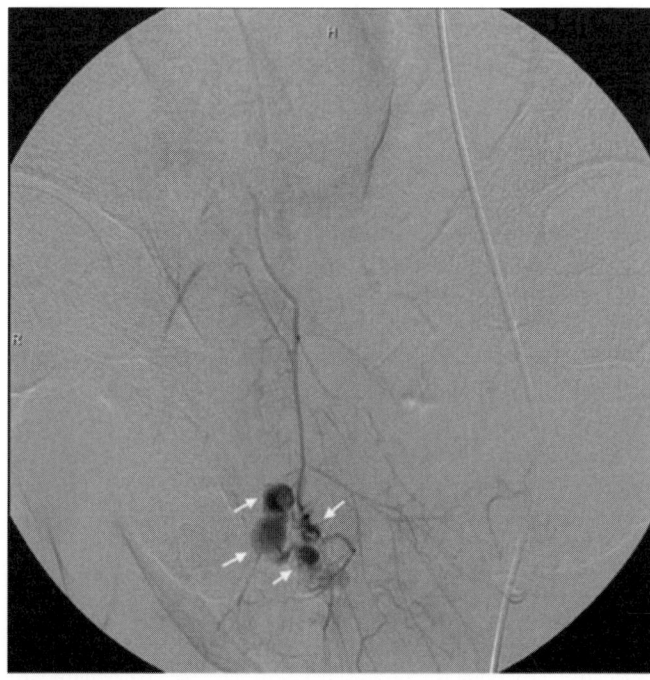

Figure 18.4 Same image as Figure 18.3, but subtracted view.

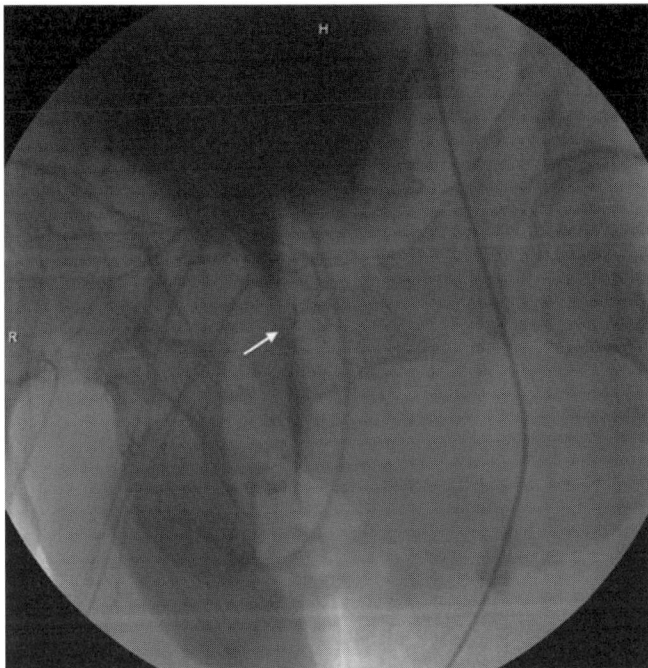

Figure 18.5 Native postembolization image of right internal iliac artery with two steel coils in situ (white arrow).

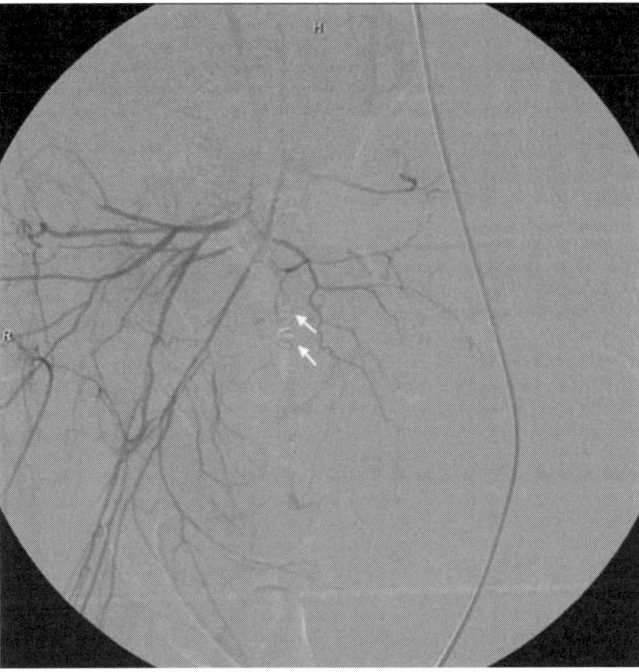

Figure 18.6 Same image as Figure 18.5, but subtracted view.

by expedient localization and arrest of bleeding by the on-site team without the inherently risky transfer of patients from one area to another, while still providing ongoing quality resuscitation.[54,55]

The percutaneous trauma interventions fall into two groups:

(1) emergent procedures aimed at arresting hemorrhage (e.g., intravascular balloon occlusion with or without embolization), performed by the trauma surgeon

(2) urgent interventions used to repair damaged vessels (i.e., stent grafting), performed by clinicians with experience in angiographic techniques

TAE is the intentional occlusion of an artery by deposition of thrombogenic materials directly into the vessel via an angiographic catheter under remote control. A contrast blush at CT and angiography indicates active arterial bleeding and the need for embolization. Angiography before damage control laparotomy may be indicated to control retroperitoneal pelvic hemorrhage in hemodynamically unstable patients who have insufficient intraperitoneal blood loss to account for the hemodynamic instability. Angiography after damage control laparotomy should be considered when a nonexpanding, inaccessible hematoma is found at operation in a patient with a coagulopathy. Extensive surgical exploration of the retroperitoneum may exacerbate blood loss, especially when a coagulopathy coexists. Hence interventional radiology can be part of both the initial phase of damage control (abbreviated resuscitative surgery for control of hemorrhage and contamination) and in the later phase (reexploration of definitive management of injuries).

For these reasons, the interventional radiology suite needs to change from a routine diagnostic area to an acute resuscitation area. This move involves a combination of infrastructure and protocol changes, such as installing multipurpose hemodynamic monitors, obtaining a dedicated ventilator, stocking the room with resuscitation equipment, and purchasing fluid warmers. Safe patient transfer to the angiography suite requires a coordinated approach between intensive care, surgical, and radiology staff.

Hemorrhage associated with pelvic trauma, with or without pelvic fracture, is common. Early transcatheter embolization, within 3 hours of presentation, has been shown to lower the mortality rate. Overall, angiography is required in fewer than 10% of patients with pelvic trauma. When angiography is performed, extravasation (blush) is seen in approximately 50% of these patients, warranting transcatheter embolization.

The traditional treatment of blunt splenic trauma has consisted of surgical splenectomy. The trend to splenic salvage through nonoperative management recognizes the important role of the spleen in preventing overwhelming sepsis by the encapsulated organisms such as pneumococcus. Helical CT can predict which hemodynamically stable patients may fail nonoperative management if extravasation or posttraumatic splenic vascular injury is demonstrated. These patients should be referred for transcatheter embolization of the spleen.[56,57]

Analogous to splenic injury, the trend in blunt hepatic trauma is nonoperative management of the hemodynamically stable patient. Overall, the nonoperative success rate has been reported to be as high as 89–98%. Patients who are hemodynamically stable but show ongoing signs of hemorrhage (which occurs in 3% of patients) or have documented extravasation on CT of the liver should undergo conventional angiography of the liver. If these patients have angiographic extravasation, pseudoaneurysm, arteriovenous fistula, or arteriobiliary fistula, transcatheter embolization of the abnormal site should be performed.[58,59] In trauma, the two embolic agents of choice are metallic coils and gelatin sponges. Detachable coils include mechanical and electrolytic mechanisms of detachment. These are ideal for occluding an aneurysm sac and can be retrieved if placement is suboptimal. Gelatin sponges are temporary occluding agents. The artery often recanalizes within weeks to months. Gelatin sponges are useful when a more distal occlusion is necessary or when multiple collateral channels are present.

The four phases of DCS

Figure 18.7 shows the four phases of the damage control process.

Phase 1. Emergency department
Initial assessment and primary resuscitation

The primary goal of this phase is the rapid assessment of the multiply injured patient by the emergency medical services at the scene and expedient transfer to the nearest trauma center. Time is imperative once the team assesses a patient's injury pattern and physiology as critical (Table 18.6), to then initiate damage control principles.[60] As soon as exsanguinating hemorrhage is identified in the primary survey, a speedy transition from the emergency room to the operating room for hemorrhage control is essential. Important steps in this phase include obtaining large-bore intravenous access, rapid sequence intubation for airway control, naso- or orogastric tube placement, urinary catheter and chest tube placement, early rewarming maneuvers, and early controlled blood product resuscitation within the context of damage control resuscitation through activation of the massive transfusion protocol (Table 18.7).

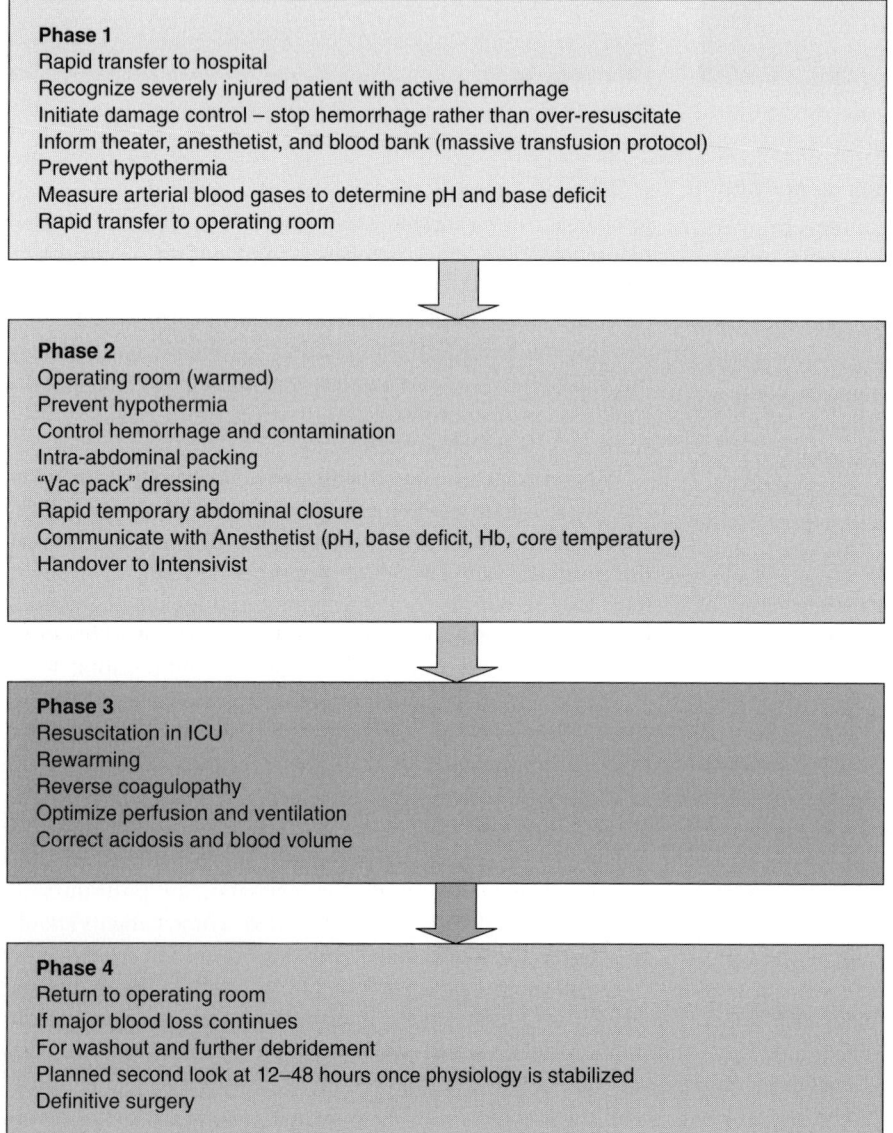

Figure 18.7 The four phases of the damage control process.

Phase 1
Rapid transfer to hospital
Recognize severely injured patient with active hemorrhage
Initiate damage control – stop hemorrhage rather than over-resuscitate
Inform theater, anesthetist, and blood bank (massive transfusion protocol)
Prevent hypothermia
Measure arterial blood gases to determine pH and base deficit
Rapid transfer to operating room

Phase 2
Operating room (warmed)
Prevent hypothermia
Control hemorrhage and contamination
Intra-abdominal packing
"Vac pack" dressing
Rapid temporary abdominal closure
Communicate with Anesthetist (pH, base deficit, Hb, core temperature)
Handover to Intensivist

Phase 3
Resuscitation in ICU
Rewarming
Reverse coagulopathy
Optimize perfusion and ventilation
Correct acidosis and blood volume

Phase 4
Return to operating room
If major blood loss continues
For washout and further debridement
Planned second look at 12–48 hours once physiology is stabilized
Definitive surgery

Table 18.6 Rapid identification of exsanguinating hemorrhage

Monitoring/observations
Clinical examination/primary survey ABCDE
Essential investigations • X-ray: chest, pelvis, C-spine (or CT C-spine) • FAST • Bloods: crossmatch, coagulation, FBC, U&E, glucose, ABG

ABG, arterial blood gas; FAST, focused assessment with sonography for trauma; FBC, full blood count; U&E, urea and electrolytes.

Table 18.7 Initial treatment in the emergency department

Airway/RSI/intubation/oxygenation
Intravenous access/arterial line
Intravenous fluid resuscitation – according to hemodynamics
Blood products – pRBCs, FFP, platelets, cryoprecipitate
Inotropes/vasopressors
Warming/maintaining body temperature
Communicate with OR and ICU teams, blood bank
Rapid transfer to RAPTOR suite or operating room

FFP, fresh frozen plasma; ICU, intensive care unit; OR, operating room; pRBCs, packed red blood cells; RAPTOR, resuscitation with angiography, percutaneous techniques, and operative repair[6]; RSI, rapid sequence induction/intubation.

Table 18.8 Essential equipment for damage control surgery (DCS)

Abdominal tray (self-contained abdominal wall retractors, laparotomy packs)
Vascular tray (aortic crossclamp, Spencer Wells forceps)
Thoracic tray (sternal saw, thoracostomy tubes)
Balloon catheters of various sizes
Operating room towels
Topical hemostatic agents
Adhesive plastic
Suction drains

Table 18.9 Aims of damage control surgery (DCS)

Control of hemorrhage
Control of contamination
Thorough exploration of abdomen
Intraabdominal packing
Temporary closure

Phase 2. Operating room: DCS

The goal of phase 2 of damage control is to stop hemorrhage, limit contamination and subsequent inflammatory response, and achieve temporary abdominal wall closure to protect viscera and reduce heat loss. The operating room must have essential equipment ready (Table 18.8). The patient should be positioned supine on the operating table with the upper extremities at right angles. The anterior chest wall should be kept free of leads and tubing if a median sternotomy or resuscitative left thoracotomy is needed.

The optimal method of vascular control and resuscitation in patients with life-threatening, extrathoracic torso hemorrhage remains debated. Guidelines recommend emergency department thoracotomy (EDT) with aortic clamping, although transabdominal clamping followed by vascular control and direct vascular control (DVC) without aortic clamping are alternatives. Although aortic clamping increases central and cerebral perfusion, DVC results in less physiologic derangement.[61] The surgical incision should not be delayed for insertion of monitoring devices (arterial and central venous catheters). In view of the large body surface exposure, a heating mattress may be more practical for heat conservation than a forced-air warming device. In cases of abdominal hemorrhage, the abdomen should be quickly explored. If the patient has had a previous midline laparotomy, a bilateral

subcostal incision can give rapid access to the peritoneal cavity away from the anticipated midline adhesions, which can then be separated quickly under direct vision. Once in the abdomen, a large handheld abdominal wall retractor (or a self-retaining retractor such as a Bookwalter or Balfour) can create space for extensive packing of all four quadrants. Removal of packs should occur sequentially, beginning in the areas least likely to harbor the source of major hemorrhage. This provides space to pack the bowels away from the areas of bleeding and maximizes exposure. Exposure is the key step in the abbreviated repair of abdominal vascular injuries.[62] Packing alone is adequate for some vascular, specifically venous, injuries. If the injury is amenable, rapid arterial or venous ligation is the treatment of choice. Almost every abdominal vessel can be ligated with limited morbidity.[63] However, ligation of the main aorta, external iliac arteries, and proximal superior mesenteric artery are associated with life-threatening tissue and/or bowel ischemia. Intraaortic balloon occlusion of the thoracic aorta has been successfully attempted in hemodynamically unstable patients with missile injuries of the abdomen, facilitating operative control of hemorrhage and patient discharge in a functional status.[65]

After controlling the hemorrhage, the next priority is to limit contamination (Table 18.9). Controlling spillage of intestinal contents and urine from hollow viscus injuries is crucial prior to repacking of the abdomen, with focus on raw surface areas that can become the source of massive blood loss in the coagulopathic patient. In the damage control situation, no intestinal anastomoses are performed. Packing should provide adequate tamponade without compromising venous return to the heart or distal arterial supply.[3]

Abdominal closure is the final step in the initial laparotomy. Temporary closure aims to contain abdominal viscera, prevent hypothermia, control abdominal secretions, and prevent intraabdominal hypertension (IAH) and abdominal compartment syndrome (ACS). The formal closure of the abdominal fascia after damage control laparotomy has been associated with an increased risk of ACS, acute respiratory distress syndrome (ARDS), and multiple organ failure (MOF). All result from postoperative reperfusion injury and ongoing capillary leakage, causing intestinal and abdominal wall edema. Several techniques have been suggested for abdominal closure. The simplest option is a rapid whipstitch to the abdominal wall using a large nylon suture. This, however, is not the preferred technique because it results in tissue tension and IAH.[65] Often, the increased capillary permeability of traumatic shock and concurrent fluid resuscitation produce significant visceral edema. If extensive edema is present, a modified VAC (vacuum pack) or commercial VAC can be applied.

Complex hepatic, retroperitoneal, pelvic, or deep muscle injuries may not be amenable to operative control, or may require lengthy exploration in a coagulopathic patient. Interventional radiology (IR) may be needed to achieve hemodynamic stability.[66] Early communication with the IR team is important to maintain damage control strategies. Pelvic fractures are characterized by a high mortality rate due to frequently associated critically uncontrollable hemorrhagic shock. Often patients are too unstable to undergo a hemostatic procedure, such as angioembolization, and only damage control maneuvers such as pelvic packing can be attempted. Intraaortic balloon occlusion (IABO) may help to stabilize the patient, allowing subsequent hemostatic procedures.[67] A decision for IABO should be made as soon as possible when the patient becomes critically unstable. Physicians must be aware of the risk of shock at the time of balloon deflation and the possibility to perform embolization with the balloon still inflated. IABO can be life-saving by controlling temporarily critical bleeding to "buy time" for angioembolisation in severely injured patients. Endovascular treatment of blunt aortic injuries using thoracic aortic endografts has led to decreased blood loss and resuscitation requirements compared to open repairs, and has translated into improved outcomes.[68,69] Operative control of the pelvic space can be achieved through either a transperitoneal approach at the time of laparotomy, using a midline or Pfannenstiel incision, or an extraperitoneal approach. The former is the quicker approach, enabling access to the aorta and distal vasculature along with the hollow viscera within that region. The extraperitoneal approach allows access to the external iliac vasculature for suprainguinal arterial control and for packing the preperitoneal space. The latter is a useful adjunct to managing venous bleeding in complex fractures once bony stabilization had been achieved.

Adherence to clinical damage control principles can be associated with improved survival, as demonstrated by the systematic analysis of global differences in causes, management, and survival after severe trauma, based on data collected in the CONTROL trial (clinicaltrials.gov NCT00184548).[39] This was a prospective, randomized, double-blinded, multicenter (100 hospitals in 20 countries) comparison of rFVIIa with placebo in severe trauma with refractory bleeding. In keeping with findings of other studies, predictors of 90-day mortality were age $\geq$ 60 years, male sex, admission lactate $\geq$ 5 mmol/L, hemoglobin < 10 g/dL or RBC $\geq$ 10 units from admission to 24 hours. Patients with this level of transfusion requirement had an almost sevenfold odds of death compared with lower transfusion levels.

Complications of DCS: abdominal compartment syndrome

With the widespread success of damage control laparotomy, ACS has emerged as a significant problem. Recent studies have identified ACS as an independent predictor of MOF, and demonstrate that the prevention of ACS decreases the incidence of MOF.[70–72] Recently the second World Congress on Abdominal Compartment Syndrome (WCACS, www.wsacs. org) agreed on the following consensus ACS definition: the presence of both

(1) sustained increase in intraabdominal pressure (IAP) greater than 20 mmHg with or without an abdominal perfusion pressure (APP) less than 60 mmHg; and

(2) single or multiple organ system failure, which was not previously present.

Primary ACS (formerly termed surgical, postoperative, or abdominal) is defined as a condition associated with injury or disease in the abdominopelvic region that frequently requires surgical or angioradiologic intervention, or a condition that develops following abdominal surgery. Examples are the following: abdominal organ injuries that require surgical repair or damage control surgery secondary to peritonitis, bleeding pelvic fractures, or other causes of massive retroperitoneal hematomas and liver transplantation.

Secondary ACS (formerly termed medical or extraabdominal) refers to conditions that do not originate from the abdominopelvic region, such as sepsis and capillary leak, major burns, and other conditions requiring massive fluid resuscitation.[73–77] Shock and ischemia will result in globally increased capillary permeability because of activation of inflammatory cells and release of mediators, especially in the setting of reperfusion injury.[76,78,79] There are no abdominal injuries to draw the clinician's attention to the abdomen. Recognition is often delayed. Here, abdominal content is increased by bowel edema and ascites.[78] Pertinent factors affecting fluid volume of the abdomen after goal-directed shock resuscitation[80,81] have been identified as the rate of infusion, type of fluid infused, magnitude of capillary leak, and the colloid oncotic pressure. The importance of prompt hemorrhage control for blood loss can therefore never be emphasized enough.

Recurrent ACS (formerly termed tertiary) refers solely to the condition where ACS develops following prophylactic or therapeutic surgical or medical treatment of primary or secondary ACS.

The pathophysiology of ACS

Intraabdominal pressure is primarily determined by the volume of the viscera and the intracompartmental fluid. The abdominal cavity has a great tolerance to fluctuating volumes with little rise in IAP. Adaptation can occur over time, as seen in patients with ascites, large ovarian tumors, and pregnancy. The causes of acutely increased IAP are usually multifactorial. Common causes are:

- trauma and intraabdominal hemorrhage
- abdominal surgery
- retroperitoneal hemorrhage
- peritonitis (pancreatitis, recurrent abscess)
- massive fluid resuscitation (5 L of fluid in a 24-hour period)
- ileus

Independent risk factors

Both primary and secondary ACS are early events and herald impending MOF. Organ dysfunction that typifies ACS can occur at urinary bladder pressures (UBP) < 25 mmHg, whereas some patients with UBP ≥ 25 mmHg do not develop any symptoms. Hence, the decision for decompression is not only based on UBP measurements, but also takes into account potential risk factors for ACS, such as severe hemorrhagic shock, damage control laparotomy, fascial closure after damage control laparotomy, and decreased (gastric mucosal) interstitial pH. Balogh *et al.* found that primary and secondary ACS patients developed the same symptoms and predecompression physiology, but their injury pattern, resuscitation, and hospital times were different.[72] Primary ACS predictors upon ICU admission appeared to be hypothermia, low hemoglobin concentration, and a high base deficit, whereas secondary ACS predictors included a large crystalloid fluid infusion volume and impaired renal function.

Prevention

Prevention starts early in the resuscitation process with identification of the patient at risk of ACS. Continuing crystalloid loading in the face of ongoing hemorrhage sets the stage for the bloody vicious cycle. Therefore, the first step is to extend standardized shock resuscitation to the ED, OR, and IR suites.

This should prevent indiscriminate crystalloid loading. Blood transfusions should be used preferentially, and, in exsanguinating hemorrhage, early FFP administration is recommended to minimize dilutional coagulopathy.[82,83] Hemorrhage control is paramount. With damage control laparotomy, novel hemorrhage control techniques such as the application of topical fibrin sealant materials can be important adjuncts to reduce the need for bulky packing. Hypothermia, an independent predictor of primary ACS, should be prevented by infusion of warm fluids/blood, use of forced-air warming devices, and

heated, humidified air in ventilated patients. The timely minimally invasive stabilization of long-bone and pelvic fractures reduces blood loss and prevents further amplification of the inflammatory response. The concept of damage control orthopedics focuses primarily on hemorrhage control and other life-saving measures. Complex reconstructive work is delayed until the patient is better able to withstand the additional trauma.[35,84–87]

Treatment

The primary treatment is decompressive laparotomy to increase the volume of the abdominal cavity and decrease abdominal contents by evacuating retained blood and removal of unnecessary packs. In selected patients, an alternative is to decrease abdominal volume by peritoneal drainage: for example, drainage of ascites in burn patients and nonoperative management of liver injuries (biliary drainage). In case of a decompressive laparotomy, the next treatment challenge will be the "open abdomen." Recent experience with vacuum-assisted wound closure indicated early fascial closure to be achieved in more than 85% of these patients with minimal complications.[88]

Phase 3. Intensive care unit: secondary resuscitation

Secondary resuscitation takes place in the intensive care unit (Table 18.10). Early communication with the ICU team regarding details of the trauma, current resuscitation, and surgical intervention is important in order to prepare for optimal care of the patient. The primary goal of this phase is the prevention of the trauma triad of death: hypothermia, coagulopathy, and acidosis. This may include preparing an isolation room to high ambient temperature, preparing warming devices, obtaining warm fluids, and setting up special equipment (e.g., ventilator and/or dialysis machine). The major immediate concern after initial laparotomy is the correction of hypothermia by extensive rewarming techniques. Heat loss during major trauma laparotomy may be as high as 4.6 °C per hour despite aggressive attempts to limit heat loss.[89] Hypothermia, or core temperatures less than 35 °C, can affect all systems of the body. Of primary concern in the trauma patient are platelet dysfunction and disruption of the

Table 18.10 Key goals of intensive care

Rewarming
Correct coagulopathy
Optimize hemodynamics (fluid/blood product transfusion)
Ventilatory support
Nutritional support
Abdominal compartment syndrome (ACS) monitoring
Injury identification (secondary/tertiary survey)
Safe transfer to radiology for diagnostic or therapeutic purposes

Table 18.11 Monitoring endpoints of resuscitation

Core temperature (core–peripheral gradient)
Coagulation
Arterial base deficit
Lactate concentration
Mixed venous hemoglobin O_2 saturation
Oxygen delivery index
Gastric mucosal pH

Table 18.12 Secondary complications

Systemic inflammatory response syndrome (SIRS)
Disseminated intravascular coagulopathy (DIC)
Secondary abdominal compartment syndrome (ACS)
Multiorgan dysfunction syndrome/multiple organ failure (MODS/MOF)
Acute lung injury/acute respiratory distress syndrome (ALI/ARDS)
Ventilator-associated pneumonia (VAP)/nosocomial infection
Wound infection
Deep venous thrombosis/pulmonary embolus (DVT/PE)

Table 18.13 Surviving trauma guidelines

Damage control	
F	Feeding
A	Analgesia
S	Sedation break for more rapid ventilation weaning
T	Thromboprophylaxis
H	Head up 30–45°
U	Ulcer prophylaxis
G	Glucose control
+	
	Intraabdominal pressure (IAP) measurement
	Protective ventilatory strategies
	Restrictive transfusion after resuscitation
	Tertiary survey
Antibiotic guidelines	
M	Microbiology guides therapy wherever possible
I	Indications should be evidence-based
N	Narrowest spectrum required
D	Dosage appropriate to the site and type of infection
M	Minimize duration of therapy
E	Ensure monotherapy in most situations

coagulation cascade. Despite aggressive replacement of clotting factors and platelets, normal coagulation may not occur until the core temperature exceeds 34 °C.[30]

Monitoring resuscitation endpoints

The response to therapy is monitored initially by observing vital signs and urine output. However, even in young trauma patients, these signs may be unreliable and fail to demonstrate significant cardiac depression.[90] These patients may therefore benefit from more invasive monitoring (e.g., SvO_2 and PA catheter) or other noninvasive (e.g., echocardiography) repeated assessments of cardiac filling and cardiac contractility. Other resuscitative endpoints include serum lactate and base deficit, mixed oxygen saturation, and gastric mucosal pH (Table 18.11).[91]

Communication

Critically important for the management of DCS and an optimal outcome for the severely injured patient is early and effective communication between the treating teams. The comprehensive assessment of all injuries, the timely availability of blood products, the coordinated return to the operating room for definitive care or urgent interventions to save life depends on clear communication between the emergency physicians, surgeons, anesthetists, intensivists, radiologists, hematologists, nurses, and laboratory staff. This is often overlooked, and it is an area of trauma care that can be improved.

ICU strategies to reduce complications

Given the critical condition of DCS patients, it is not surprising that the overall mortality rate is high (12–67%) and complications are frequent (Table 18.12).[11] However, many complications are predictable and can be reduced by the implementation of strategies during the intensive care phase that are analogous to the Surviving Sepsis Campaign guidelines but applied to severe trauma ("surviving trauma guidelines") (Table 18.13).

All patients should have IAP measured to recognize early the development of IAH and ACS. Stress ulcer prophylaxis with an H_2-blocker or proton-pump inhibitor should be commenced on admission to ICU.

Enteral nutrition is also protective but may be better delayed until the acidosis is corrected and the splanchnic perfusion is considered adequate. Compression stockings and calf compressors alone will provide deep venous thrombosis (DVT) prophylaxis until the coagulopathy is corrected and low-dose subcutaneous heparin therapy is safely added.

These patients are at high risk of ARDS, because of chest trauma, aspiration, large intravenous fluid administration, or transfusion-related acute lung injury (TRALI), in which case a lung-protective ventilatory strategy will be appropriate.[92] Positioning the patient head-up will reduce the incidence of nosocomial pneumonia. Antimicrobial prophylaxis should be kept to a minimum.[93–95] The rational, targeted use of antibiotics for proven infections in conjunction with infection control measures is important to prevent bacterial resistance.

General nursing and pressure-area care must be meticulous, and neuromuscular blocking agents should, in general, be avoided because of the risk of prolonged neuromuscular blockade and critical illness neuromyopathy following discontinuation. Any longer-term neuromuscular blockade should be regularly assessed with train-of-four monitoring.

Injuries can be missed in the secondary survey because the signs and symptoms were masked by other injuries, drugs, alcohol, or an altered level of consciousness. Therefore, a tertiary survey should be performed within 24 hours to ensure that all injuries have been identified, and the priorities of interventions and ongoing management are agreed on.[96,97]

Phase 4. Operating room: definitive surgery

The primary objectives of phase 4 are definitive organ repair and fascial closure if possible (Table 18.14). Physiologic homeostasis is usually only achieved after 24–36 hours, even with aggressive ICU management. Generous irrigation of the abdominal cavity is important prior to careful removal of the packs, taking special care of raw surfaces so that clotting is not disrupted. The reexploration of the abdomen allows a reassessment of the repairs made during damage control phase 2 and helps to identify missed injuries. Formal vascular repairs are now performed and intestinal continuity restored. Once all repairs are completed, formal abdominal closure without tension is the final step in the planned reoperation sequence.[60] However, persistent edema within the retroperitoneum, bowel wall, and abdominal wall can make primary closure impossible at this stage.

If the bowels are above the level of the skin when viewed from across the operating table a low-tension primary closure is unlikely. In this case, the fascia should be left open and the vacuum-pack dressing applied. The patient returns to ICU. Aggressive diuresis for the next few days should help to decrease bowel and body wall edema. Most open abdomens

Table 18.14 Aims of definitive surgery

Timing critical (window period 36–48 hours post trauma)
Abdominal packs are removed
Thorough exploration for hidden injuries
Restoration of gastrointestinal continuity
Formal vascular repair
Provision for enteral feeding (jejunostomy or gastrostomy)
Washout with warmed isotonic fluid
Attempt at primary definitive closure
Abdominal wall reconstruction
Plastic surgery (skin grafts, free flap)

can be primarily closed in 7–10 days, especially if intraabdominal infection is absent.

Conclusions

Damage control surgery is a significant advance in trauma patient management. It involves a move from attempting definitive repair of all injuries to focused hemorrhage and contamination control and delayed definitive repair. This principle is based on the recognition that more patients die of the triad of hypothermia, coagulopathy, and acidosis than of a failure to complete operative repairs.[27] If the patient is to survive, definitive surgery has to wait until physiologic homeostasis has been achieved. The correction of the physiologic parameters should occur over a period of hours in the ICU and result in reversal of metabolic failure. A multidisciplinary approach with excellent communication is needed to optimize outcome.

Questions

(1) Damage control surgery is:
   a. Definitive surgery performed on the severely traumatized patient
   b. Abbreviated surgery performed on every severely traumatized patient
   c. A way of gaining time to optimize the physiologic state of the severely traumatized patient before definitive surgical repair
   d. Minor surgery performed on selected critically injured patients
   e. A concept that emerged from the collective experience with major thoracic injuries

(2) The "lethal triad" is a term used to describe the metabolic insults of:
   a. Hypoxia, hypovolemia, hypothermia
   b. Hypothermia, hypercoagulopathy, acidosis
   c. Coagulopathy, hypoglycemia, hypovolemia
   d. Coagulopathy, acidosis, hypothermia
   e. Hemorrhage, hypothermia, hypoxia

(3) Regarding the abdominal compartment syndrome (ACS):
   a. Decompressive laparotomy is the last resort
   b. Secondary ACS is usually recognized early
   c. Primary and secondary ACS lead to the same symptoms because of their similar mechanism
   d. Normothermia, low hemoglobin concentration, and high base deficit are predictors of secondary ACS
   e. Recurrent ACS develops following surgical or medical treatment of primary or secondary ACS

(4) Hypothermia in multitrauma patients can result in:
   a. Cardiac arrhythmias and delta waves on the ECG
   b. Reduced systemic vascular resistance
   c. Right shift of the oxyhemoglobin dissociation curve
   d. Hypercoagulopathy
   e. Greater than 95% mortality at temperatures less than 32 °C

(5) Coagulopathy:
  a. After trauma is occasionally attributed to dilution with intravenous fluid therapy, massive blood transfusion, hypothermia, and acidosis
  b. Is frequently caused by brain injuries
  c. Results after replacement of one adult blood volume because only 20% of platelets remain in the circulation
  d. Results from the release of mediators after tissue trauma which also lead to the development of SIRS and multiple organ failure
  e. Should routinely be managed with antifibrinolytic agents

(6) With regard to acidosis in trauma:
  a. Metabolic acidosis is an unreliable indicator of tissue hypoxia
  b. Lactic acidosis not cleared after 48 hours is associated with a mortality rate of about 50%
  c. Ongoing acidosis after restoration of volume and blood pressure has a poor prognosis
  d. Trauma-induced catabolism prevents lactic acid synthesis
  e. Tissue hypoxia leads to aerobic metabolism resulting in lactic acid synthesis

(7) Concerning the damage control process:
  a. It has five distinct phases
  b. Phase 2 is resuscitation in ICU
  c. Phase 3 is definitive surgery
  d. Patients for DCS should be rapidly transferred to the OR without repeated attempts to restore circulating volume
  e. Principles include sepsis limitation and immediate restoration of all anatomical integrity

(8) With regard to interventional radiology:
  a. It is contraindicated in the initial phase of damage control, especially in the coagulopathic patient
  b. Transcatheter arterial embolization (TAE) can provide rapid effective control of arterial pelvic bleeding and hepatic injury
  c. A contrast blush at angiography indicates a venous bleed and need for embolization
  d. Splenectomy is the preferred method of hemorrhage control in blunt splenic injuries

  e. Two embolic agents of choice are plastic coils and gelatin sponges

(9) Which of the following statements about DCS complications is correct?
  a. At the initial laparotomy complications are reduced when the abdomen is formally closed regardless of intraabdominal pressure
  b. Intraabdominal pressure is primarily determined by the volume of the viscera and intracompartmental fluid
  c. ACS can be defined as a urinary bladder pressure greater than 25 mmHg
  d. In recent studies ACS has been refuted as an independent predictor of multiorgan failure
  e. Primary ACS predictors include massive blood transfusion and impaired renal function

(10) Regarding resuscitation on ICU:
  a. All severely injured patients should have intraabdominal pressure measured in order to recognize the development of ACS early
  b. The first priority is correction of acidosis with bicarbonate administration
  c. Early administration of parenteral nutrition improves outcome
  d. Normalization of coagulation may not occur until core temperature reaches 36 °C despite administration of clotting factors and platelets
  e. The gastric mucosal pH should be monitored in all patients

Answers

(1) c
(2) d
(3) e
(4) e
(5) d
(6) c
(7) d
(8) b
(9) b
(10) a

References

1. Kashuk JL, Moore EE, Sawyer M, et al. Postinjury coagulopathy management: goal-directed resuscitation via POC thromboelastography. Ann Surg 2010; 251: 604–14.

2. Pringle J. Notes on the arrest of hepatic haemorrhage due to trauma. Ann Surg 1908; 48: 541–9.

3. Halsted W. Ligature and suture material: the employment of fine silk in preference to catgut and the advantages of transfixing tissues and vessels in controlling hemorrhage – also an account of the introduction of gloves, gutta-percha tissue and silver foil. JAMA 1913; 60: 1119–26.

4. Stone HH, Strom PR, Mullins RJ. Management of the major coagulopathy with onset during laparotomy. Ann Surg 1983; 197: 532–5.

5. Rotondo MF, Schwab CW, McGonigal MD et al. Damage control: an approach for improved survival in exsanguinating penetrating abdominal injury. J Trauma 1993; 35: 375–83.

6. Ball CG, Kirkpatrick AW. The RAPTOR: resuscitation with angiography, percutaneous techniques and operative repair. Can J Surg 2011; 54: E3–4.

7. Rotondo MF, Zonies DH. Damage control sequence and underlying logic. Surg Clin N Am 1979; 77: 761–77.

8. Slotman G, Jed F, Burchard K. Adverse effects of hypothermia in post-operative patients. *Am J Surg* 1985; **149**: 495.

9. Frank SM, Beattie C, Christopherson R, *et al.* Unintentional hypothermia is associated with postoperative myocardial ischaemia. *Anaesthesiology* 1992; **78**: 468–76.

10. Patt A, McCroskey BL, Moore EE. Hypothermia-induced coagulopathies in trauma. *Surg Clin N Am* 1988; **68**: 775–85.

11. Shapiro MB, Jenkins DH, Schwab CW, Rotondo MF. Damage control: a collective review. *J Trauma* 2000; **49**: 969–78.

12. Brohi K, Singh J, Heron M, *et al.* Acute traumatic coagulopathy. *J Trauma* 2003; **54**: 1127–30.

13. Maegele M, Lefering R, Yucel N, *et al.* Early coagulopathy in multiple injury: an analysis from the German Trauma Registry on 8724 patients. *Injury* 2007; **38**: 298–304.

14. Schoechl H, Nienaber U, Hofer G, *et al.* Goal-directed coagulation management of major trauma patients using thromboelastometry (ROTEM®)-guided administration of fibrinogen concentrate and prothrombin complex concentrate. *Crit Care* 2010; **14**: R55.

15. Spahn DR, Cerry V, Coats TJ, *et al.* Management of bleeding following major trauma: a European guideline. *Crit Care* 2007; **11**: R17.

16. Hess JR, Brohi K, Dutton RP, *et al.* The coagulopathy of trauma: a review of mechanisms. *J Trauma* 2008; **65**: 748–54.

17. Dente CJ, Shaz BH, Nicholas JM, *et al.* Improvements in early mortality and coagulopathy are sustained better in patients with blunt trauma after institution of a massive transfusion protocol in a civilian level 1 trauma center. *J Trauma* 2009; **66**: 1616–24.

18. Malone DL, Hess JR, Fingerhut A. Massive transfuion practices around the globe and a suggestion for a common massive transfusion protocol. *J Trauma* 2006; **60**: S91–6.

19. Mohan D, Milbrandt EB, Alarcon LH. Black Hawk Down: the evolution of resuscitation strategies in massive traumatic hemorrhage. *Crit Care* 2008; **12**: 305.

20. Schlag G, Redl H. Mediators in trauma. *Acta Anaesthesiol Belg* 1987; **38**: 281–91.

21. Hulka F, Mullins RJ, Frank EH. Blunt brain injury activates the coagulation process. *Arch Surg* 1996; **131**: 923–7.

22. Olsen JD, Kaufmann HH, Moake J, *et al.* The incidence and significance of haemostatic abnormalities in patients with head injuries. *Neurosurgery* 1989; **24**: 825–32.

23. Hofmann S, Huemer G, Kratochwill C. Pathophysiologie der Fettembolie in der Orthopaedie und Traumatologie. *Orthopaede* 1995; **24**: 84–93.

24. Wetzel RC, Burns RC. Multiple trauma in children: critical care overview. *Crit Care Med* 2002; **30**: 468–77.

25. CRASH-2 collaborators. Effects of tranexamic acid on death, vascular occlusive events, and blood transfusion in trauma patients with significant hemorrhage (CRASH-2): a randomized placebo-controlled trial. *Lancet* 2010; **376**: 23–32.

26. CRASH-2 collaborators. The importance of early treatment with tranexamic acid in bleeding trauma patients: an exploratory analysis of the CRASH-2 ranomized controlled trial. *Lancet* 2011; **377**: 1096–101,1101.e1–2.

27. Parr MJA, Alabdi T. Damage control surgery and intensive care. *Injury* 2004; **35**: 713–22.

28. Gubler KD, Gentilello LM, Hassantash SA, *et al.* The impact of hypothermia on dilutional coagulopathy. *J Trauma* 1994; **36**: 847–51.

29. Lynn M, Jeroukhimov I, Klein Y, *et al.* Updates in the management of severe coagulopathy in trauma patients. *Intensive Care Med* 2002; **28**: 241–7.

30. Reed RL, Bracey AW, Hudson JD, *et al.* Hypothermia and blood coagulation: dissociation between enzyme activity and clotting factor levels. *Circ Shock* 1990; **32**: 141–52.

31. Rohrer MJ, Natale AM. Effect of hypothermia on the coagulation cascade. *Crit Care Med* 1992; **20**: 1402–5.

32. Enriquez LJ, Shore-Lesseron L. Point-of-care coagulation testing and transfusion algorithms. *Br J Anaesth* 2009; **103**: 14–22.

33. Spahn DR, Ganter MT. Towards early individual goal-directed coagulation management in trauma patients. *Br J Anaesth* 2010; **105**: 103–5.

34. Stinger HK, Spinella PC, Perkins JG, *et al.* The ratio of fibrinogen to red cells transfused affects survival in casualties receiving massive transfusions at an army combat support hospital. *J Trauma* 2008; **64** (2 Suppl): S79–85.

35. Pape A, Weber CF, Stein P, *et al.* ROTEM and multiplate = a suitable tool for POC? *ISBT Science Series* 2010; **5**: 161–8.

36. Morrison JJ, Dubose JJ, Rasmussen TE, *et al.* Military Application of Tranexamic acid in Trauma Emergency Resuscitation (MATTERs) study. *Arch Surg* 2012; **147**: 113–19.

37. Bedirhan MA, Turna A, Yagan N, *et al.* Aprotinin reduces postoperative bleeding and the need for blood products in thoracic surgery: results of a randomised double-blind study. *Eur J Cardiothoracic Surg* 2001; **20**: 1122–7.

38. Kenet G, Walden R, Eldad A, *et al.* Treatment of traumatic bleeding with recombinant factor VIIa. *Lancet* 1999; **354**: 1879.

39. Christensen MC, Parr M, Tortella BJ, *et al.* Global differences in causes, management, and survival after severe trauma: the recombinant activated Factor VII Phase 3 trauma trial. *J Trauma* 2010; **69**: 344–52.

40. Hauser CJ, Boffard K, Dutton R, *et al.* Results of the CONTROL trial: efficacy and safety of recombinant activated factor VII in the management of refractory traumatic hemorrhage. *J Trauma* 2010; **69**: 489–500.

41. Boffard KD, Riou B, Warren B, *et al.* NovoSeven Trauma Study Group. Recombinant factor VIIa as adjunctive therapy for bleeding control in severely injured trauma patients: two parallel randomized placebo-controlled double-blind clinical trials. *J Trauma* 2005; **59**: 8–15.

42. Bernstein DE, Jeffers L, Erhardtsen E, *et al.* Recombinant factor VIIa corrects prothrombin time in cirrhotic patients: a preliminary study. *Gastroenterology* 1997; **113**: 1930–7.

43. Lynn M, Jeroukhimov I, Jewelewicz D, *et al.* Early use of recombinant factor VIIa improves mean arterial pressure and may potentially decrease mortality in experimental haemorrhagic shock: a pilot study. *J Trauma* 2002; **52**: 703–7.

44. Martinowitz U, Kenet G, Segal E, *et al.* Recombinant activated factor VII for adjunctive haemorrhage control in trauma. *J Trauma* 2001; **51**: 431–9.

45. Abramson D, Scalea TM, Hitchcock R, *et al.* Lactate clearance and survival following injury. *J Trauma* 1993; **35**: 584–9.

46. Davis JW, Parks SN, Kaups KL, *et al.* Admission base deficit predicts transfusion requirements and risk of complications. *J Trauma* 1996; 4: 764–74.

47. Mixock BA, Falk JL. Lactic acidosis in critical illness. *Crit Care Med* 1992; **20**: 80–92.

48. Cooper DJ, Walley KR, Wiggs BR, *et al.* Bicarbonate does not improve hemodynamics in critically ill patients who have lactic acidosis: a prospective, controlled clinical study. *Ann Intern Med* 1990; **112**: 492–8.

49. Mathieu D, Neviere R, Billiard V, *et al.* Effects of bicarbonate therapy on hemodynamics and tissue oxygenation in patients with lactic acidosis: a prospective, controlled clinical study. *Crit Care Med* 1991; **19**: 1352–6.

50. Britt LD, Weireter LJ, Cole FJ. Newer diagnostic modalities for vascular injuries: The way we were, the way we are. *Surg Clin N Am* 2001; **81**: 1263–97.

51. Kushimoto S, Arai M, Aiboshi J, *et al.* The role of interventional radiology in patients requiring damage control laparotomy. *J Trauma* 2003; **54**: 171–6.

52. Prior JP, Braslow B, Reilly PM *et al.* The evolving role of interventional radiology in trauma care. *J Trauma* 2005; **59**: 102–4.

53. Carrillo EH, Spain DA, Wohltmann CD, *et al.* Interventional techniques are useful adjuncts in non operative management of hepatic injuries. *J Trauma* 2000; **46**: 619–24.

54. Morozumi J, Homma H, Ohta S, *et al.* Impact of mobile angiography in the emergency department for controlling pelvic fracture hemorrhage with hemodynamic instability. *J Trauma* 2010; **68**: 90–5.

55. Zealley IA, Chakraverty S. The role of interventional radiology in trauma. *BMJ* 2010; **340**: c497.

56. Sclafani SJ, Shaftan GW, Scalea TM, *et al.* Non-operative salvage of computed tomography-diagnosed splenic injuries: utilisation of angiography for triage and embolisation for haemostasis. *J Trauma* 1995; **39** (5): 818–25.

57. Shanmuganathan K, Mirvis SE, Boyd-Kranis R. Nonsurgical management of blunt splenic injury: use of CT criteria to select patients for splenic arteriography and potential endovascular therapy. *Radiology* 2000; **217**: 75–82.

58. Ciraulo DL, Luk S, Palter M, *et al.* Selective hepatic arterial embolization of grade IV and V blunt hepatic injuries: an extension of resuscitation in the non operative management of traumatic hepatic injuries. *J Trauma* 1998; **45**: 353–8.

59. Hagiwara A, Yukioka T, Ohta S, *et al.* Nonsurgical management of patients with blunt hepatic injury: Efficacy of transcatheter arterial embolization. *Am J Roentgenol* 1997; **169** (4): 1151–6.

60. Braslow B. Damage control in abdominal trauma: how a progressive-step approach and delayed repairs can actually improve outcomes. *Contemp Surg* 2006; **62** (2): 65–74.

61. White JM, Cannon JW, Stannard A, *et al.* Direct vascular control results in less physiologic derangement than proximal aortic clamping in a porcine model of non-compressible extrathoracic torso hemorrhage. *J Trauma* 2011; **71**: 1278–86.

62. Kashuk KL, Moore EE, Millikan JS, Moore JB. Major abdominal vascular trauma: a unified approach. *J Trauma* 1982; **22**: 672–9.

63. Feliciano DV. Abdominal vascular injury. In Mattox KL, Feliciano DV, Moore EE, eds., *Trauma*, 5th edition. New York, NY: McGraw-Hill, 2004, pp. 755–77.

64. Gupta BK, Khaneja SC, Flores L, *et al.* The role of intra-aortic balloon occlusion in penetrating abdominal trauma. *J Trauma* 1989; **29**: 861–5.

65. Sugrue M, D'Amours SK, Joshipura M. Damage control surgery and the abdomen. *Injury Int J Care Injured* 2004; **35**: 642–8.

66. Feliciano DV, Mattox KL, Burch JM, *et al.* Packing for control of hepatic hemorrhage. *J Trauma* 1986; **26**: 738–43.

67. Martinelli T, Thony F, Declety P. Intra-aortic balloon occlusion to salvage patients with life-threatening hemorrhagic shocks from pelvic fractures. *J Trauma* 2010; **68**: 942–8.

68. Kauvar DS, White JM, Johnson CA, *et al.* Endovascular versus open management of blunt traumatic aortic disruption at two military centers: comparison of in-hospital variables. *Military Medicine* 2009; **174**: 869–73.

69. Propper BW, Alley JB, Gifford SM, *et al.* Endovascular treatment of blunt aortic injury in Iraq: extension of innovative endovascular capabilities to the modern battlefield. *Ann Vasc Surg* 2009; **23**: 687.e19–22.

70. Balogh Z, McKinley BA, Cocanour CS, *et al.* Supra-normal trauma resuscitation causes more cases of abdominal compartment syndrome. *Arch Surg* 2003; **138**: 637–43.

71. Balogh Z, McKinley BA, Cox CS, *et al.* Abdominal compartment syndrome: the cause or effect of post injury organ failure. *Shock* 2003; **20** (6): 483–92.

72. Balogh Z, McKinley BA, Holcomb JB, *et al.* Both primary and secondary abdominal compartment syndrome (ACS) can be predicted early and are harbingers of multiple organ failure. *J Trauma* 2003; **54**: 848–61.

73. Balogh Z, McKinlay BA, Cocanour CS, *et al.* Secondary abdominal compartment syndrome: an elusive complication of traumatic shock resuscitation. *Am J Surg* 2002; **184**: 538–43.

74. Biffl WL, Moore EE, Burch JM, *et al.* Secondary abdominal compartment syndrome is a highly lethal event. *Am J Surg* 2001; **182**: 645–8.

75. Ivy ME, Atweh NA, Palmer J, *et al.* Intraabdominal hypertension and abdominal compartment syndrome in burn patients. *J Trauma* 2000; **49**: 387–91.

76. Kopelman T, Harris C, Miller R, *et al.* Abdominal compartment syndrome inpatients with isolated extraperitoneal injuries. *J Trauma* 2000; **49**: 744–9.

77. Maxwell RA, Fabian TC, Croce MA, *et al.* Secondary abdominal compartment syndrome: an underappreciated manifestation of severe hemorrhagic shock. *J Trauma* 1999; **47**: 995–9.

78. Kirkpatrick AW, Balogh Z, Ball CG, *et al.* The secondary abdominal compartment syndrome: Iatrogenic or unavoidable? *J Am Coll Surg* 2006; **202**: 668–79.

79. Malbrain MLNG, Chiumello D, Pelosi P, *et al.* Incidence and prognosis of intraabdominal hypertension in a mixed population of critically ill

patients: a multiple center epidemiological study. *Crit Care Med* 2005; **33**: 315–22.

80. McKinley BA, Valdivia A, Moore FA. Goal orientated-shock resuscitation for major torso trauma: what are we learning? *Curr Opin Crit Care* 2003; **9**: 292–9.

81. Moore FA, McKinley BA, Moore EE. The next generation in shock resuscitation. *Lancet* 2004; **363**: 1988–96.

82. Biffl WL, Smith WR, Moore EE, *et al.* Evolution of a multidisciplinary clinical pathway for the management of unstable patients with pelvic fractures. *Ann Surg* 2001; **233**: 843–50.

83. Hirshberg A, Dugas M, Banez EI, *et al.* Minimizing dilutional coagulopathy in exsanguinating hemorrhage: a computerized simulation. *J Trauma* 2003; **54**: 454–63.

84. Harwood PJ, Giannoudis PV, van Griensven M, *et al.* Alterations in the systemic inflammatory response after early total care and damage control procedures for femoral shaft fracture in severely injured patients. *J Trauma* 2005; **58**: 446–54.

85. Heetveld MJ, Harris I, Schlaphoff G, *et al.* Guidelines for the management of hemodynamically unstable pelvic fracture patients. *ANZ J Surg* 2004; **74**: 520–9.

86. Hildebrand F, Giannoudis P, Krettek C, *et al.* Damage control: extremities. *Injury Int J Care Injured* 2004; **35**: 678–89.

87. Taeger G, Ruchholtz S, Waydhas C, *et al.* Damage control orthopedics in patients with multiple injuries is effective, time saving and safe. *J Trauma* 2005; **59**: 408–15.

88. Suliburk JW, Ware DN, Cocanour CS, *et al.* Vacuum assisted wound closure provides early fascial closure of open abdomens after severe trauma. *J Trauma* 2003; **55** (6): 1155–60.

89. Burch JM, Denton JR, Noble RD. Physiologic rationale for damage control surgery. *Surg Clin N Am* 1997; **77**: 779–82.

90. Sauaia A, Moore FA, Moore EE, *et al.* Epidemiology of trauma deaths: a reassessment. *J Trauma* 1995; **38**: 185–93.

91. Tisherman SA, Barie P, Bokhari F, *et al. Clinical Practice Guideline: Endpoints of Resuscitation.* Eastern Association for the Surgery of Trauma, 2003 (www.east.org, Oct 2006).

92. Acute Respiratory Distress Syndrome Network. Ventilation with lower tidal volumes as compared with traditional tidal volumes for acute lung injury and the acute respiratory distress syndrome. *N Engl J Med* 2000; **342**: 1301–8.

93. Dellinger EP. Antibiotic prophylaxis in trauma: penetrating abdominal injuries and open fractures. *Rev Infect Dis* 1991; **13** (Suppl): 847.

94. Dellinger EP, Wertz MJ, Lennard ES, *et al.* Efficacy of short course antibiotic prophylaxis after penetrating intestinal injury: a prospective randomized trial. *Arch Surg* 1986; **121**: 23–30.

95. Nichols RL, Smith JW, Robertson JD, *et al.* Prospective alterations in therapy for penetrating abdominal trauma. *Arch Surg* 1993; **128**: 55.

96. Grossman MD, Born C. Tertiary survey of the trauma patient in the intensive care unit. *Surg Clin N Am* 2000; **80**: 805–24.

97. Janjua KJ, Sugrue M, Deane SA. Prospective evaluation of early missed injuries and the role of tertiary trauma survey. *J Trauma* 1998; **44** (6): 1000–6.

Mechanical ventilation of the patient following traumatic injury

Roman Dudaryk, Earl Willis Weyers, and Maureen McCunn

Objectives

(1) Describe the impact of trauma on the respiratory system.

(2) Explain the rationale for using lung-protective strategies in the injured patient.

(3) Evaluate the role of less conventional modes of mechanical ventilation in trauma.

(4) Discuss the influence of common trauma-related conditions on the approach to mechanical ventilation.

Physiologic effects of trauma on respiratory system

Pulmonary trauma and aggressive resuscitation can lead to edema, bleeding, and resultant inflammation within the alveolar spaces. The response to injury represents a continuum from subclinical elevation in inflammatory markers to acute lung injury (ALI) to acute respiratory distress syndrome (ARDS).

The physiological effects of trauma on the respiratory system can be looked at in the context of the lung's ability to repair and regenerate. The lung is an intricate organ and requires interactions between over 40 different cell lines to affect development or repair.[1] The intricacy of these structural and repair mechanisms can impact how well the pulmonary system can restore itself. It is important to understand the difference between regeneration and lung repair. Normally, the lung tissue only performs low levels of cell regeneration and has the innate ability to activate a rapid cycle of regeneration in response to acute injury. Repair can lead to scar formation, fibrosis, and repopulation of pulmonary segments with epithelium that does not function well.

Dysregulated repair of injured alveolar epithelial cells results in a process of proliferation, matrix production, and fibrosis leading to changes in the mechanical environment of the individual alveoli.[2] This dysregulated repair process becomes a vicious cycle promoting yet more maladaptation as the lung attempts to repair itself.[1]

At the microscopic level, alveolar function can be thought of in terms of tissue deformation. Tissue deformation, in turn, can be expressed in terms of mechanical strain. Methods using real-time fluorescence microscopy and tomography are being utilized to examine volume changes with differential pressures at the level of the alveolus. These studies have indicated that the redistribution of volume in the context of the liquid-filled versus air-filled alveolar interface is heterogeneous, and this may be behind overdistension injury associated with lung edema in the acute and chronic phases of pulmonary trauma. Researchers are close to being able to link mechanical strain or stress in cell cultures and genetic alterations that promote regeneration versus repair. These gene expressions within the alveolar epithelium are ultimately what guide the preferred adaptive response to injury.

- A key question to be asked is, can physicians intervene to promote this process over a potentially dysfunctional repair process using lung-protective ventilation strategies?
- Additionally, can interventions be performed in the setting of acute lung trauma, in the operating room, in the intensive care unit (ICU), and throughout the perioperative period?

Current evidence from cardiac and noncardiac surgical patients with ALI and ARDS demonstrates that lung-protective ventilation strategies create a favorable microenvironment for the pulmonary tissue. This favorable microenvironment could, in turn, promote *regeneration* over the *repair* processes during and after periods of tissue trauma.

ARDS nomenclature and definitions have been recently revised, and the term ALI has been replaced by mild ARDS (Table 19.1).[3] In clinical practice, and in the scientific literature, however, the older nomenclature still prevails. For the purpose of this review we will therefore continue to refer to ALI rather than mild ARDS.

Lung-protective ventilation strategies: intraoperative implications in the trauma patient, and practical approach

A basic understanding of ventilator modes and phase variables is required to assist the practitioner in deciding between different ventilator modes and lung-protective ventilation strategies. For proprietary reasons, manufacturers' nomenclatures

Table 19.1 Berlin definition and classification of ARDS[3]

Timing	Within 1 week of a known clinical insult or new or worsening respiratory symptoms
Chest imaging	Bilateral opacities – not fully explained by effusions, lobar/lung collapse
Origin of edema	Respiratory failure not fully explained by cardiac failure or fluid overload. Need objective assessment (e.g., echocardiography) to exclude hydrostatic edema if no risk factors are present
Oxygenation (severity of ARDS) by PaO$_2$/FiO$_2$ ratio with PEEP $\geq$ 5 cmH$_2$O	
Mild	200–300
Moderate	100–200
Severe	< 100

Table 19.2 Comparison of "TLC" phase variables of mechanical ventilation in common ventilatory modes

Ventilatory mode	Trigger (patient or time)	Limit (flow or pressure)	Cycle (volume, pressure, or time)
Assist control/ volume control	Patient	Flow	Volume
Assist control/ pressure control	Patient	Pressure	Time
Pressure support	Patient	Pressure	Flow
Airway pressure release ventilation	Time	Pressure	Time

Table 19.3 Preferred combinations of FiO$_2$ and PEEP[6]

FiO$_2$	PEEP (cmH$_2$O)
30%	5
40%	5,8
50%	8,10
60%	10
70%	10,12,14
80%	14
90%	14,16,18
100%	18,20,22,24

for similar modes of ventilation are not the same between ventilators.

The elements that can be manipulated in different ventilator modes are the phase variables. Phase variables are divided into the "TLCs" – trigger, limit, and cycle. An understanding of what the ventilator is doing to (or for) the patient in terms of these phase variables or "TLCs" is fundamental to making better decisions for treatment (Table 19.2).

The overall goal of trauma patient management is aimed at avoiding hypoxia and secondary tissue injury leading to lactic acidosis, free radical formation, and inflammatory mediator release with resultant local or distant tissue damage. In the setting of trauma, mechanical ventilation is frequently initiated for reasons other than respiratory system compromise, such as traumatic brain injury (TBI), severe hypovolemic shock, intoxication, agitation, or combativeness.

The prevailing cause of death after traumatic injury continues to be injury involving the central nervous system, with rates that range from 21.6% to 71.5%. Mortality associated with isolated respiratory failure in traumatic injury is far less common (1.9–8%). Although the overall causes of mortality have changed very little since the 1980s, there have been significant improvements in terms of decreased mortality due to hemorrhage and exsanguination.[4,5] Lung-protective ventilation strategies are aimed at reducing volume and pressures that are delivered to the lungs. Ventilation protocols typically include tidal volumes (Vt) of 6–8 mL/kg of predicted body weight (PBW) regardless of the mode chosen for operation. PBW is calculated in men and women as follows:

Male : PBW $= 50 + 0.91$(height in centimeters $- 152.4$)
Female : PBW $= 45.5 + 0.91$(height in centimeters $- 152.4$)

Tidal volumes on the lower end of the scale, closer to 4–6 mL/ kg PBW, may be more beneficial at achieving adequate Vt and lowering distending pressures.

- KEY POINT: Lung-protective ventilation strategies consist of using a lower Vt of 4–6 mL/kg PBW, liberal application

of positive end-expiratory pressure (PEEP) (Table 19.3) and limiting plateau pressures (Pplat) to less than 30 cmH$_2$O.[6,]

Relative hypoxemia – that is, lower than expected arterial oxygen tension (PaO$_2$) levels for a given inspired percentage of oxygen delivered (FiO$_2$) – declining PaO$_2$/FiO$_2$ ratios, and atelectasis are common events under general anesthesia and in the operative management of trauma. However, subsequent studies have looked at intraoperative ventilation strategies applied in patients with or without ALI, and have discovered that anesthesiologists avoid applying protective ventilation strategy as advocated (tidal volumes were too high, peak and plateau pressures were not being routinely monitored).[7]

The true incidence of ALI or subclinical ALI is likely to be underreported in the general surgical patient population. Therefore, it is safe to assume that occurrences in the trauma patient population are indeed very high, and patients should be treated as such. Numerous studies have evaluated and validated the development of ALI in settings where traditional patterns of intraoperative ventilation strategies have favored treatment of atelectasis with larger Vt and lower PEEP.[8] Furthermore, examination of ARDS development in patients more than 48 hours after the onset of mechanical ventilation has revealed strong associations between high Vt, high peak airway pressure, and high PEEP.[9] This management has been found to be counterproductive and places unnecessary shear stresses on alveolar units.

Prevention of perioperative lung injury becomes especially important in patients who may have subclinical or frank lung injury due to trauma, transfusion-related acute lung injury (TRALI), or massive resuscitation. Studies focused on markers of lung injury have demonstrated increases in ALI related to duration of nonprotective mechanical ventilation.[8]

A recently published prospective randomized trial of low-tidal-volume mechanical ventilation in patients undergoing moderate and high-risk abdominal surgery demonstrated significantly decreased incidence of respiratory events and decreased hospital stay in the low-volume (6–8 mL/kg) group. This level 1 evidence further consolidates the importance of lung-protective ventilation strategies for intraoperative management of high-risk surgical patients.[10]

Based on the prevailing body of evidence, anesthesiologists have a clear role to play both in treating pulmonary trauma/injury effectively and in avoiding further pulmonary damage. Key application of lung-protective ventilation strategies will favor pulmonary processes that lead to adaptive repair and regeneration, avoiding maladaptive remodeling.

Clinical pearls that can be generally applied to protect the lungs include:

- Vt should be based on PBW (patient height is an important parameter) from the onset of mechanical ventilation.
- Vt and plateau pressures should be carefully monitored.

- Liberal PEEP should be used to improve oxygenation.
- Moderate hypercapnia is usually well tolerated in the trauma setting (with the exception of patients with elevated intracranial pressure, ICP).
- Volutrauma should not be induced with the ventilator or the bag-mask. The bag-mask should be compressed with one hand, at a frequency of 10–14 breaths per minute. This approach will deliver adequate Vt and minute ventilation, allowing sufficient time for exhalation, and will help to avoid auto-PEEP.

Monitoring of mechanical ventilation in the setting of trauma

In order to deliver adequate ventilation assistance to a patient, the ventilator has to establish a pressure gradient to produce gas flow. When considering the distending pressure of the complete respiratory system, the plateau pressure should be measured at end inspiration. This equates to the inspiratory alveolar pressure or plateau pressure at end inspiration during an inspiratory hold maneuver (Pplat) (Fig. 19.1).[11] An inspiratory hold maneuver of this type is obtained most accurately in an anesthetized, paralyzed patient. Hence, intraoperative assessments of pulmonary mechanics can prove invaluable prior to the transition to intensive care. The safe upper limit of this Pplat has not been defined in patients with ARDS/ALI. Based on available data, it can be concluded that the lower the Pplat, the lower the mortality. Evidence-based practice suggests that Pplat should be < 30 cmH$_2$O.[12]

Mortality reductions are tightly correlated with maintenance of a lower Pplat from the onset of mechanical ventilator therapy. Yet Pplat and the change in Pplat responsible for gas flow fulfills the relationship of two separate though linked elements. Plateau pressure changes (ΔPplat) represent the pressure required to insufflate the lung (ΔP_L) and the chest

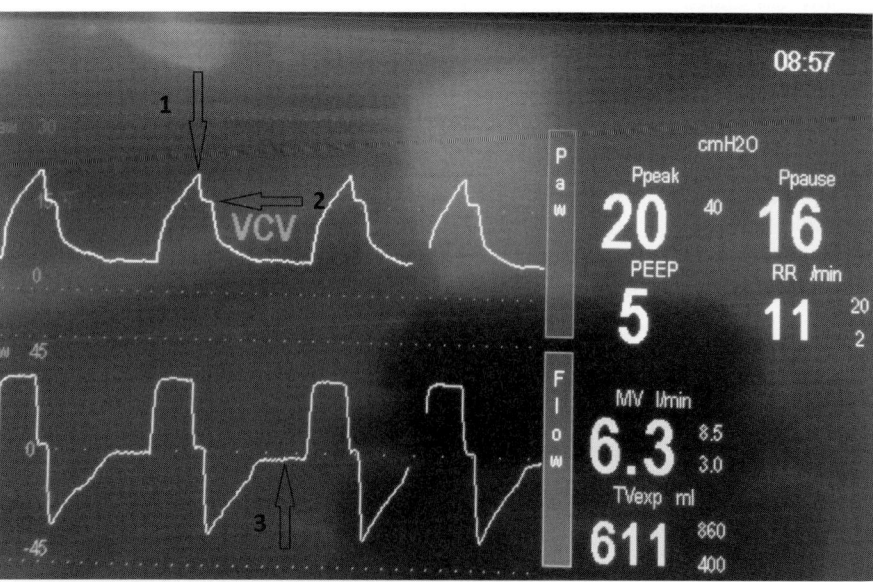

Figure 19.1 Volume-controlled ventilation. (1) Peak inspiratory pressure, PIP. (2) End-inspiratory pressure (plateau pressure, Pplat). Lung-protective strategy should target Pplat < 30 cmH$_2$O. Significant difference between PIP and Pplat may indicate airway resistance problems such as mucous plugs, clots, obstructed ETT, bronchospasm. (3) Flow curve returns back to baseline before next breath is delivered, suggesting no dynamic hyperinflation (auto-PEEP) present.

wall (ΔP_{CW}).[11] In other words, $\Delta Pplat = \Delta P_L + \Delta P_{CW}$, and therefore the Pplat that is usually monitored depends on both lung and chest wall characteristics. The mechanics of these separate elements can be profoundly deranged when afflicted with thoracic trauma. Transpulmonary pressure telemetry can be obtained by the use of an esophageal balloon catheter, with esophageal pressure used as a surrogate for pleural pressure, but this is not widely available.[13]

Measuring Pplat enables monitoring and estimation of the static respiratory system compliance ($C_{rs} = C_{lung} + C_{chestwall}$). C_{rs} is clearly associated with determinations of the volume of aerated tissue in ALI/ARDS.[11]

In terms of assessing the adequacy of mechanical ventilation, the gold standard is the arterial blood gas and the arterial carbon dioxide tension, $PaCO_2$ (see Chapter 9). Noninvasive end-tidal CO_2 ($P_{ET}CO_2$) can be used in almost all trauma and perioperative environments as a surrogate or estimate of true $PaCO_2$ via its approximation of alveolar CO_2 tension (P_ACO_2).[14] Physiological dead space is the sum of all of the components of tidal volume not participating in gas exchange, and it equals anatomical dead space plus alveolar dead space – this limits our estimation of the true $PaCO_2$. A larger $PaCO_2$ to $P_{ET}CO_2$ gradient means increasing alveolar dead space – this may indicate hypovolemia and regional ventilation/perfusion mismatching in a trauma patient. $P_{ET}CO_2$ is a misleading guide for the adequacy of ventilation in the trauma setting[15] and is only useful if examined in the context of a known $PaCO_2$. The true value of $P_{ET}CO_2$ is used for confirmation of endotracheal intubation and also as a later marker of cardiac output status.

Hyperventilation and hypocapnia are also prevalent in the prehospital setting of traumatic injury and can be particularly detrimental in terms of TBI (see Chapter 21). Considering the above limitations of $P_{ET}CO_2$, ventilation requirements should be addressed as part of a goal-directed therapeutic approach to balance an optimum ventilation strategy for the injuries of the patient.[16]

Conventional modes of mechanical ventilation in the trauma operating room

Volume-controlled ventilation (VCV) is the most widely used mode in the operating room. Tidal volume (Vt), respiratory rate, PEEP, and FiO_2 are the known variables set by the operator. This mode of ventilation guarantees delivery of a set Vt and minute ventilation, with one important caveat to keep in mind: the mechanical breath will be terminated if the peak inspiratory pressure (PIP) set on the ventilator's alarm is reached. In trauma settings, patients may have drastically reduced compliance due to pulmonary edema, ARDS, abdominal compartment syndrome, or surgical retractor placement. In the majority of anesthesia machines, the PIP alarm is set at 40 cmH_2O. If this threshold is reached during the inspiratory phase before delivering an adequate Vt, the mechanical breath will be terminated and hypoventilation and hypoxemia may

occur. At the same time, the activation of the PIP alarm must be investigated for causes of increased PIPs: obstruction, bronchospasm, and pneumothorax need to be ruled out. After initial stabilization, ventilator settings have to be optimized and the primary reason for PIP increase has to be sought and addressed.

Pressure-controlled ventilation (PCV) may be used less often in the setting of trauma operating rooms at some centers. Vt delivered during PCV is variable and depends on lung and chest wall compliance, in addition to airway resistance. As pulmonary compliance may change through the case, a patient may be either hypoventilated (abdominal compartment syndrome, pulmonary edema, and blood in the airway), or the lung hyperinflated (release of surgical retractors, decompression laparotomy). More importantly, the ventilator should not be switched from VCV into PCV mode solely because of PIP elevation without a search for the underlying cause of elevated PIP. PCV can be used in the operating room in the case of severe ARDS, as it may provide better gas exchange due to improved gas flow distribution and higher mean alveolar pressure, although these benefits are largely theoretical.[16] This has to be done with an understanding of the above-mentioned caveats.

The inspiratory/expiratory (I/E) ratio is a useful parameter that is frequently overlooked. I/E ratio will affect the inspiratory flow rate, which in turn will affect the peak airway pressure. The time of the respiratory cycle spent in "inspiration" will directly affect the mean airway pressure and oxygenation. This can be practically used for the trauma patient with severe ARDS and poor lung compliance. That is, a longer inspiratory time will increase mean airway pressure and improve PaO_2. Caution should be used if attempting the maneuver in volume-depleted patients, since the increase in mean airway pressure may result in decreased preload followed by hypotension. It has not been shown to have an outcome advantage as compared to increasing the PEEP, but it is a useful tool in a patient with refractory hypoxemia.

Weaning from mechanical ventilation

The plan for discontinuation of mechanical ventilation should be addressed at the same time as a decision for postoperative ventilator support has been made. Initiation of pressure-support ventilation should be done as soon as possible in the postoperative period. Pressure support should be titrated to ensure appropriate tidal volumes (6 mL/kg) and acceptable minute ventilation. Transition to pressure-support ventilation has numerous benefits. There is hemodynamic profile improvement due to decrease in intrathoracic pressure. Gas exchange improves due to a decrease in ventilation/perfusion (V/Q) mismatch. There is better patient/ventilator synchrony and a decreased need for sedation.[17] Even short periods of controlled mechanical ventilation (24–48 hours) may lead to diaphragmatic dysfunction and prolonged respiratory failure. However, there are trauma patients who will require controlled mechanical ventilation and cannot be switched to spontaneous modes immediately: TBI, hemodynamic instability with shock and ongoing resuscitation, and severe ARDS are a few examples.

The duration of the weaning process is determined by the degree of lung pathology affecting gas exchange as well as resolution of other, nonrespiratory causes that may require mechanical ventilation. Many trauma patients necessitate so-called "discretionary" intubation on arrival. They are combative and dangerous to themselves and medical staff due to intoxication or antisocial behavior. These patients can be extubated as soon as the diagnostic workup is completed, if they are cooperative during a spontaneous breathing trial (SBT).[18]

The SBT is the most widely accepted approach to liberation from mechanical ventilation. It should be attempted on a daily basis on all mechanically ventilated patients, unless contraindicated (hemodynamic instability, acute phase of TBI). The SBT is a part of the "ABCDE" bundle that emerged recently as the most comprehensive and evidence-based tool of weaning. ABCDE stands for Awakening and Breathing Coordination, Delirium monitoring and management, and Early mobility. This multidisciplinary approach involving SBT, delirium screening and treatment, early mobilization, and physical therapy has been shown to significantly shorten duration of mechanical ventilation, decrease mortality, and improve long-term functional outcomes.[3]

SBTs can be done with low levels of pressure support (5–7 cmH$_2$O) or unassisted breathing via T-piece. Each approach has its advantages and disadvantages. Pressure-support trials allow monitoring of tidal volumes and minute ventilation during SBT, which can help to diagnose early respiratory decompensation. Occasionally, even the low levels of pressure support used during SBT can be significant for debilitated patients. After complete discontinuation of pressure support on extubation, this subgroup may deteriorate, necessitating reestablishment of mechanical ventilation. T-piece trials do test the ability to maintain adequate ventilation without *any* support, but the patient has to be closely monitored for clinical signs of respiratory failure (tachypnea, tachycardia, diaphoresis, etc.), as tidal volumes and minute ventilation cannot be assessed. Numerous indices have been used to predict successful liberation from mechanical ventilation. The rapid shallow breathing index or f/TV ratio is the most frequent index employed, with 105 being a cutoff for termination of SBT. However, a multicenter prospective double-blinded study invalidated the use of this parameter. In fact, incorporation of the f/TV ratio in the decision-making algorithm was associated with prolonged mechanical ventilation without concurrent decrease in extubation failure or incidence of tracheostomy.[19] There are various institution-dependent algorithms for liberation from mechanical ventilation. Implementation of an algorithm-driven approach executed by respiratory therapists and ICU nurses has been shown to decrease the duration of mechanical ventilation.[20]

Less conventional methods of mechanical ventilation

APRV (airway pressure release ventilation)

APRV might be the ideal modality in patients who have suffered blunt thoracic trauma with pulmonary contusions and significant atelectasis. It is a time-triggered, pressure-limited, and time-cycled mode of ventilation that allows the patient to breathe spontaneously throughout the ventilator cycle.[21] The bulk of the ventilatory cycle is spent in high pressure (P$_{high}$), with a release period at the low pressure (P$_{low}$). The time in each phase is controlled with the T$_{high}$ and T$_{low}$ duration setting. Spontaneous breathing can occur throughout this entire ventilatory cycle; if the patient does not breathe spontaneously, APRV functions like a pressure-limited and time-cycled mode.

This mode can provide optimal recruitment of collapsed, atelectatic lung in hypoxemic patients who require careful control of peak airway pressures. Indications for APRV in trauma can be morbid obesity, pregnancy, segmental/lobar atelectasis, and ALI/ARDS patients with requirements for high FiO$_2$ or PEEP. The amount of ventilator support is determined by controlling the duration of CPAP (continuous positive airway pressure) and the tidal volume (Vt) desired. Breathing spontaneously may be more comfortable for the patient and may result in lower requirements for deep sedation. Negative hemodynamic disruptions are also likely to improve, along with better mean airway pressures and recruitment of alveoli. Reductions in peak airway pressure, improved PaO$_2$/FiO$_2$ ratios, and improved release tidal volumes may be noted in these patients on APRV ventilation.[21]

HFOV (high-frequency oscillation ventilation)

HFOV is a subtype of high-frequency ventilation (HFV) and functions by using a piston pump to oscillate at a very high frequency (180–600 breaths per minute or 3–10 Hz) with fresh gas flow delivered at 30–60 L/min. This functionally results in the rapid delivery of very small tidal volumes with application of high mean airway pressures (Fig. 19.2). The higher mean airway pressures are thought to prevent cyclical de-recruitment of alveoli, and the small tidal volumes delivered prevent alveolar overdistension.[22] Unlike other methods of HFV, the HFOV piston return stroke leads to active exhalation or expiration of gases. Active expiration potentially reduces air trapping.

HFOV has been utilized in patients with severe pulmonary contusions, ALI/ARDS, and smoke inhalation injury. HFOV is considered to be a rescue mode when more conventional modalities have failed. In particular, HFOV should be considered early for patients with both severe pulmonary contusions and ARDS. Significant improvements in PaO$_2$/FiO$_2$ ratio, pulmonary compliance and oxygenation index have been noted in these patients.[23]

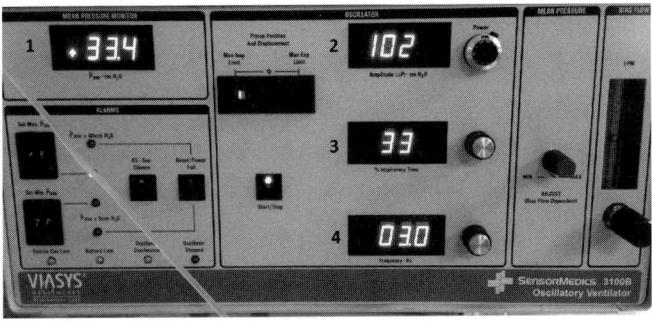

Figure 19.2 HFOV ventilator with common settings displayed. (1) Mean airway pressure, which is set by operator and determines oxygenation. (2) Airway pressure amplitude, delta P (power): adjusted by respiratory therapist to get visible chest "wiggle." May increase spontaneously if ETT obstruction is present. (3) Percentage of inspiratory time: usually left at 33% in adults. (4) Frequency, an often misunderstood parameter. Frequency has to be decreased if there is CO_2 retention – opposite to conventional ventilator.

Table 19.4 Etiology of ARDS. Note: most of the common causes are very frequent in trauma settings.

Direct insult	Indirect insult
Common	**Common**
Aspiration pneumonia	Sepsis
Pneumonia	Severe trauma
	Shock
Less common	**Less common**
Inhalational injury	Acute pancreatitis
Pulmonary contusions	Cardiopulmonary bypass
Fat emboli	Transfusion-related acute lung injury (TRALI)
Near drowning	Disseminated intravascular coagulation (DIC)
Reperfusion injury	Burns
	Head injury

Two recent randomized prospective clinical trials comparing HFOV to conventional lung-protective strategy ventilation failed to show any clinical improvement. One trial showed no improvement in morbidity and 28-day mortality in the HFOV group, and the other had to be terminated prematurely due to higher mortality in the HFOV group. These recent data raise significant concerns regarding the use of HFOV in the adult population.[24,25]

Role of noninvasive positive-pressure ventilation (NIPPV) in trauma patients

Noninvasive CPAP or bilevel airway pressure (BiPAP) has been widely adopted in emergency departments and intensive care units across the globe for the treatment of acute respiratory failure resulting from chronic obstructive pulmonary disease (COPD) exacerbation or pulmonary edema due to congestive heart failure.[26,27]

There are circumstances when CPAP or BiPAP would be a preferred method of ventilatory support for trauma patients as well. Appropriate patent selection is crucial for the success of an NIPPV trial, and for patient safety. Patients who have traumatic brain injury, facial trauma, intoxication, or obtundation, or who are at risk of aspiration, should have their airway secured with an endotracheal tube. In general, a patient who is not conscious enough to understand instructions should not be started on NIPPV.

Hypoxic respiratory failure due to pulmonary contusion is a well-established indication for CPAP therapy in trauma patients. CPAP therapy – in combination with thoracic epidural analgesia – has also been shown to improve outcomes in flail chest trauma victims. It helps by improving ventilation/perfusion ratio and preventing atelectasis, thus leading to improvement in oxygenation. It also enhances pain relief by creating stenting of the rib fracture segments and minimizing their movements. It significantly reduces the incidence of hospital-acquired pneumonia.[28,29]

Close observation, monitoring, and noted improvement in oxygenation are needed to justify continuation of an NIPPV trial. If there is no improvement in oxygenation within 2 hours of NIPPV initiation, endotracheal intubation should be strongly considered.

Special considerations in trauma patients that may influence choice of the mode of mechanical ventilation

Acute respiratory distress syndrome (ARDS)

Trauma is one of the most common etiologies of ARDS (Table 19.4). It may develop due to direct pulmonary insult – aspiration, pneumonia, severe lung contusion (pulmonary ARDS) – or due to indirect damage to the alveolar membranes by inflammatory mediators via the systemic circulation (extrapulmonary ARDS). Severe injury triggers a complex inflammatory response involving all the components of the immune system. This systemic inflammatory response syndrome, SIRS, with continued uncontrolled release of inflammatory mediators and neutrophil infiltration in the lung, clinically manifests as acute lung injury (ALI) or ARDS.

A lung-protective ventilation strategy has been a cornerstone of the management of ALI/ARDS. The overall goal of this strategy is to prevent or to minimize ventilator-induced lung injury (VILI), which is caused by excessive pressure (barotrauma), excessive volume (volutrauma), and repetitive opening and closing of the alveoli (atelectrauma) (Fig. 19.3). It has been shown that this approach is frequently underutilized in the perioperative period. All trauma patients on mechanical ventilation in the ICU or the operating room should be strongly considered as candidates for lung-protective ventilation strategy.

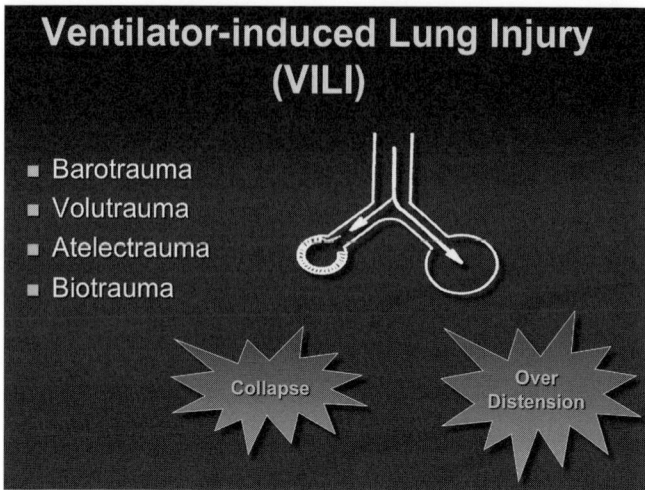

Figure 19.3 The concept of ventilator-induced lung injury.

A lung-protective ventilation strategy is based on two main principles:

- *Lung protection* – refers to ventilation with tidal volume of 4–6 mL/kg of *ideal body weight,* targeting plateau airway pressure, Pplat of less than 30 cmH$_2$O. Pplat serves as a surrogate estimate of intraalveolar pressure. It is important to remember that trauma patients with decreased chest wall or abdominal compliance, such as that seen with abdominal compartment syndrome, obesity, or circumferential burns, may need higher Pplat targets. In those patients, Pplat elevation above 30 cmH$_2$O will be due to contributions from chest wall compliance and increased intraabdominal pressure – and thus the transpulmonary pressure gradient would be unchanged. At the present time there is no reliable and widely accepted technique to measure transpulmonary gradient and to isolate the pulmonary tissue compliance from the total static compliance represented by Pplat. It largely remains a bedside clinical estimate at best.

- *Lung recruitment* – refers to prevention of atelectasis using an "open lung" concept. Unlike tidal volume, the initial level of PEEP remains the subject of debate. In the majority of studies initial levels in the range of 8–15 cmH$_2$O have been used, and adjusted according to arterial blood gas and oxygen saturation (Table 19.2).

Fat embolism syndrome (FES)

FES has an incidence varying from 3% to 29% in trauma patients with long-bone fractures.[30] This syndrome is frequently underdiagnosed and may also be seen in patients with soft tissue disruption/avulsion. Subclinical manifestations most likely are more frequent, especially in patients undergoing intramedullary nailing. The classic clinical triad of respiratory distress with hypoxia, petechial rash of upper torso and conjunctivae, and encephalopathy is noted in 20–50% of the patients.[31] However, the absence of these findings does not rule out FES. The temporary relationship of a decrease in

oxygen saturation during manipulation at the fracture site remains the most likely clue to this syndrome.

FES should be high on the differential list if intraoperative hypoxemia and decreased oxygen saturation develop during an orthopedic procedure. Treatment is supportive and mandates application of lung-protective ventilation with limited Pplat and increased levels of PEEP to prevent secondary lung injury intraoperatively as well as in the postoperative period.[32]

Pneumothorax

Pneumothorax is one of the most common entities found in trauma, and it can have significant implications for mechanical ventilation. If unnoticed it may expand during positive-pressure ventilation, leading to tension pneumothorax and cardiopulmonary collapse. Therefore, clinicians should maintain a high level of suspicion of this pathology regardless of previous imaging studies. Portable chest radiography has been shown to have poor sensitivity for the detection of occult pneumothorax by trauma teams in up to 76% of the cases, compared with computed tomography (see Chapter 11).[33] However, rapid diagnosis of pneumothorax can be obtained with ultrasound examination (see Chapter 11).

A small pneumothorax, even on positive-pressure ventilation, does not always warrant chest tube placement. There are numerous retrospective studies looking at occult pneumothoraces during positive-pressure ventilation that have been successfully managed without chest tube placement.[34] The anesthesiologist must always be vigilant to the early signs of tension pneumothorax. Simultaneous elevation of PIP and Pplat should prompt an immediate investigation of expanding pneumothorax. If there is simultaneous new-onset hypotension, tracheal deviation (may need to remove anterior of C collar to observe this), or an absence of contralateral breath sounds, immediate tube thoracostomy should be considered, even prior to imaging studies.

If a thoracostomy tube is already present, it should be connected to low continuous suction and examined for air leaks when the patient arrives in the operating room. Patency of the drainage system should be maintained throughout the procedure to avoid expansion of the pneumothorax. A chest tube in situ does not guarantee that a residual pneumothorax may not be present, or that a tension pneumothorax may not develop secondarily.

Bedside thoracic ultrasonography is emerging as a highly efficient method of diagnosis of pneumothorax in the operating room, compared with portable chest x-ray or clinical exam.[35]

Chest wall injury: fractures

Fractures of the ribs, scapula, and sternum can lead to significant limitations of respiration. These injuries can also be indicators of underlying thoracic, abdominal, or cranial injuries. Rib fractures are the most frequently encountered traumatic chest injury (see Chapter 30). Additionally, patients with rib fractures are likely to experience significant pulmonary dysfunction and posttraumatic pneumonia.[36] Single rib fractures require less specific management of ventilation strategies.

Aggressive multimodal pain management should be initiated in these patients (see Chapters 15 and 16) with the goal of avoiding endotracheal intubation and mechanical ventilation. Avoidance of endotracheal intubation after isolated chest trauma and rib fractures has been associated with better outcomes in comparison with pain control in combination with NIPPV.

Adequate pain relief is essential in patients with rib fractures to improve functional residual capacity, enable adequate clearing of secretions, and prevent atelectasis. By doing so, respiratory failure and mechanical ventilation can be prevented. Posttraumatic pneumonia in these patients is common and is associated with a 4% mortality. Patient-controlled analgesia with morphine via intravenous pump delivery has been compared to nebulized morphine. The investigators discovered equivalent analgesia with less sedation experienced with intravenous delivery.[36] Isolated rib fractures and analgesia may be managed with a continuous epidural catheter. Unfortunately, polytrauma seldom lends itself to such an ideal circumstance, in which just a single injury needs to be treated. Flail chest presents as a compromised thoracic cage with rib fractures in multiple locations. Mortality rates can be particularly high in these cases, and even higher in elderly patients with a flail chest. Development of a subsequent pneumothorax related to displaced rib fractures must always be suspected in a patient without chest tubes in place whenever positive-pressure ventilation is considered.

Pulmonary contusion

Pulmonary contusion occurs frequently in the setting of blunt thoracic trauma where enough kinetic energy is transmitted through the thorax into the lung tissue (see Chapter 30). A review of data from a trauma registry in Texas estimated that up to 27% of patients with polytrauma were found to have pulmonary contusions.[28] Thoracic injuries among pediatric patients are less frequent, because children have more compliant ribs and a lower incidence of rib fractures; however, the incidence of pulmonary contusion in this group is as high as 50% (see Chapter 34). The physical exam signs of tachypnea, rhonchi, wheezes, or hemoptysis may be preliminary findings in a patient afflicted with severe pulmonary contusion.

Physiological derangements related to ventilation/perfusion mismatch, increasing intrapulmonary shunt, lung edema, and lost compliance are seen in segmental lung contusion. These entities can manifest as hypoxemia and hypercarbia (usually peaks at 72 hours) followed by an increased work of breathing.[28] Visible changes may not be apparent on chest x-ray for at least 4–6 hours, and they usually resolve within 7 days. Management of pulmonary contusion is mostly supportive with the routine use of recruitment maneuvers, permissive hypercapnia, conservative fluid management, appropriate PEEP, and lung-protective ventilation strategy. Rarely, cases of unilateral lung contusion, intratracheal bleeding, and air leaks will require bronchial blockers or double-lumen tubes (see Chapter 33). These cases may require one-lung ventilation or a tailored dual-lung ventilation strategy.[21]

Hemothorax

Rupture of intercostal vessels and subsequent bleeding are responsible for the majority of hemothoraces. Chest tube placement and the rate of blood loss will determine the most likely immediate steps in management. Massive hemothorax is regarded to be the rapid accumulation of over 1500 mL of blood in the thorax, or one-third or more of a patient's blood volume. Blood loss at or above these volumes may indicate that emergent surgical thoracotomy is required.[37] Chest tube drainage and patency should be closely monitored intraoperatively by the anesthesia team in a polytrauma patient undergoing surgery for other injuries. If an increase in thoracostomy tube output or a significant decrease in static compliance is noted, the surgical team should be notified regarding the possibility of intrathoracic bleeding. If the chest tube output is smaller, the decision for surgery is based on the clinical status of the patient rather than the rate of continued blood loss from the thorax. Although less common with hemothorax than with tension pneumothorax, tracheal deviation may still be seen.

Diaphragmatic rupture

Violated diaphragmatic domes (more likely significant with blunt trauma) lead to abdominal contents passing into the thoracic cavity with subsequent compression of the pulmonary (and cardiovascular) structures, leading to problems with gas exchange. The diagnosis of diaphragmatic rupture should be kept in mind as a possible explanation for hypoxia developing while on mechanical ventilation after blunt trauma with an absence of significant thoracic injuries. The liver may be protective with right-sided diaphragmatic injury, but injury on the left almost always necessitates surgical repair. Defects greater than 6 cm in size are considered to be significant and are more likely to occur on the left side.[38]

Implications of massive transfusion for mechanical ventilation

Massive transfusion may lead to the acute onset of pulmonary edema intraoperatively, manifesting itself with progressive hypoxemia, decreased lung compliance, and/or frothy sputum coming from the endotracheal tube. This can be due to either acute manifestation of transfusion-related acute lung injury (TRALI) or transfusion-associated circulatory overload (TACO). TACO has clinical manifestations similar to TRALI but a different mechanism: it develops secondary to circulatory overload. An elevated left atrial pressure distinguishes TACO from TRALI. A rapid infuser should be used judiciously during the massive transfusion protocol to minimize the risk of TACO. Treatment is supportive, with frequent suctioning and an intraoperative lung-protective ventilation strategy. High levels of PEEP, in excess of 20 cmH$_2$O, may be required to ensure adequate oxygen saturation. An oxygen saturation (SpO$_2$) level of greater than 88% may be adequate in these circumstances, unless the patient has a known traumatic brain injury.[39]

Mechanical ventilation in trauma patients with bronchopleural fistulas

Bronchopleural fistula (BPF) is an infrequent complication of thoracic trauma but is challenging in terms of the management of mechanical ventilation. BPF implies presence of communication between proximal or distal airways and the pleural space via a defect in visceral pleura. It may initially present as pneumothorax and should be treated with tube thoracostomy.

The clinical diagnosis is frequently made in the operating room when a patient with a tube thoracostomy is placed on positive-pressure ventilation and develops a persistent air leak (usually > 100 mL per breath), with frequent cycling of the ventilator and inability to fill up the bellows despite an increase in gas flow. A significant air leak leads to a decrease in minute alveolar ventilation, the loss of PEEP, and the resultant development of hypoxemia and respiratory acidosis.

There is no universally accepted ventilation strategy for patients with BPF. In general, mean airway pressure should be kept at minimum, creating the lowest possible pressure gradient and minimizing air leak across the fistula. Some experts favor pressure-controlled ventilation, as it gives the ability to control the pressure gradient more precisely compared to volume-control modes. CO$_2$ retention may occur but is usually not a problem, as CO$_2$ clearance often parallels the degree of leak.[40]

If the size of the leak makes positive-pressure ventilation technically not feasible, lung isolation should be performed. If BPF is present on the left side, a right main stem bronchus intubation with a single-lumen endotracheal tube may be an alternative, or may serve as a temporizing measure while getting ready for placement of a double-lumen tube or bronchial blocker.

In some cases, HFOV targeting the lowest mean airway pressure that provides acceptable oxygenation has been used with success. One lung ventilation and ECMO (extracorporeal membrane oxygenation) are last-resort modalities that have been utilized on a case-by-case basis.[41]

Abdominal compartment syndrome and ventilation of the trauma patient

Abdominal compartment syndrome (ACS) has a profound impact on pulmonary mechanics and gas exchange. A decrease in static lung compliance is noted by the simultaneous increase in Pplat and PIP. The anesthesiologist should promptly communicate this finding to the surgical team.

Decompressive laparotomy remains a mainstay of the definitive therapy. Patients frequently develop significant atelectasis due to compression of dependent areas of the lung by the intraabdominal contents. A high level of clinical suspicion and monitoring of bladder pressure is the key to timely diagnosis and intervention.[42]

When the patient returns to the operating room for abdominal closure, the baseline peak airway pressure should be noted and the ventilator should be switched to volume-control mode. Peak and plateau pressures should be monitored closely as closure progresses, and the surgical team should be notified of significant elevation of those pressures.[43]

Traumatic brain injury

Maintenance of adequate oxygenation and ventilation – seemingly trivial recommendations – are extremely important measures in improving the outcome after TBI (see Chapters 20 and 21). Hyperventilation to induce hypocarbia is no longer recommended for routine use in the setting of TBI because it leads to vasospasm and may increase the size of ischemic penumbra (and exacerbate secondary injury).[44] Low normal PaCO$_2$ is the goal of mechanical ventilation. Hyperventilation should be only used as a temporizing measure when there is a deterioration of neurological status (see Chapter 21).

Although patients with TBI were excluded from major ARDS network trials, newer data suggest that lung-protective ventilation strategies can be safely used in these patients. An increased level of PEEP in the range of 10–15 cmH$_2$O (below ICP levels) has not been shown to impair venous return from the brain and reduce cerebral perfusion pressure. In fact, PEEP may lead to resolution or prevention of atelectasis, which would decrease pulmonary artery pressure because of reversal of hypoxic pulmonary vasoconstriction, leading to a decrease in the right atrial pressure and improvement of venous drainage from the cranium. Therefore, titration of PEEP in a polytrauma patient should be individualized, ideally with the aid of continuous ICP monitoring if severe TBI and ARDS are present at the same time.

Considerations for transport of the trauma patient on mechanical ventilation

Intrahospital transport of the mechanically ventilated trauma patient is almost a universal event. The majority of adverse events during transport are related to mechanical ventilation and airway problems.

Bag-mask ventilation is the most frequent modality chosen in a majority of the centers, because of ease and portability. It has several caveats. There is a possibility of auto-PEEP or dynamic hyperinflation with aggressive bag ventilation when the bag is squeezed with both hands at a high rate. Dynamic hyperinflation resulting in decreased venous return has been demonstrated to be an underrecognized preventable cause of severe hypotension and sometimes cardiac arrest.[45] This may be more critical in trauma patients, who frequently are hypovolemic and therefore may be more prone to the development of hemodynamic compromise from dynamic hyperinflation.

A PEEP valve should always be used and set at levels similar to the mechanical ventilator setting used prior to transport; this will prevent the derecruitment of alveoli and the development of atelectasis.

Portable mechanical ventilators are gaining popularity. They have the ability to deliver a preset tidal volume and minute ventilation similar to ventilators used in the operating room. The use of portable transport ventilators is particularly beneficial in the settings of ARDS and TBI, when it is imperative to maintain oxygenation and CO_2 clearance. Capnography should be used if available for transport. It confirms correct placement of the endotracheal tube and provides an indirect estimate of cardiac output.

Patients with severe ARDS receiving newer modes of ventilation such as APRV or HFOV require special attention. If a patient on APRV has to be transported to the OR, it may be prudent to try either volume- or pressure-control modes of ventilation – prior to transport – in combination with high PEEP (targeting the same mean airway pressure as in APRV mode). Alternatively, the patient can be transported to the OR on the ICU ventilator, maintaining APRV settings. Patients on HFOV can also safely be transported to the OR with appropriate monitoring. Total intravenous anesthesia should then be used for these patients, because the delivery of volatile agents is not technically feasible.[46]

Summary

Lung injury following trauma is common, and can be exacerbated by shock, massive resuscitation, aspiration, fracture mobilization, and inappropriate mechanical ventilation settings. Anesthesiologists can minimize lung injury by being vigilant to low tidal volume ventilation, appropriate PEEP, and alternative modes of mechanical ventilation. Attention to ventilator indices of worsening lung compliance will allow the practitioner to institute "lung protection."

Questions

(1) Dysregulated repair of pulmonary tissue leads to:
   a. Low levels of cell regeneration
   b. No change to the mechanical environment of the alveoli
   c. The process of proliferation, matrix production, and fibrosis
   d. No change in pulmonary compliance and elastic recoil

(2) All of the following concerning pulmonary contusions are true, *except*:
   a. They are more common in blunt trauma setting
   b. They need supportive treatment with recruitment maneuvers, permissive hypercapnia, conservative

fluid management, appropriate PEEP, and lung-protective ventilation strategy
   c. Chest x-ray changes are not visible for 4–6 hours post injury
   d. They are more common in adults than in pediatric thoracic injuries

(3) When considering the distending pressure of the complete respiratory system we should analyze the inspiratory alveolar pressure or plateau pressure. At what point in the ventilation cycle should this measurement be taken?
   a. At end inspiration during the regular ventilation cycle
   b. At the beginning of inspiration during the regular ventilation cycle
   c. At end inspiration during an inspiratory hold maneuver
   d. At the beginning of inspiration during an inspiratory hold maneuver

(4) An increasing $PaCO_2$ to $P_{ET}CO_2$ gradient can be indicative of the following in the trauma patient:
   a. Regional ventilation/perfusion mismatching and hypovolemia
   b. Increasing anatomical dead space
   c. Increasing alveolar dead space
   d. Both a and c
   e. None of the above

(5) Which of the following trauma patients is an appropriate candidate for noninvasive positive-pressure ventilation (NIPPV)?
   a. A patient with traumatic brain injury (TBI)
   b. An awake, alert patient with blunt chest trauma, pulmonary contusions, and hypoxemia
   c. A patient with facial trauma and pulmonary contusions
   d. An obtunded trauma patient with suspected alcohol intoxication with a respiratory rate of 18 breaths per minute

(6) Fat embolism syndrome (FES) is associated with all of the following *except*:
   a. Petechial rash on upper torso
   b. Encephalopathy
   c. Multiple rib fractures
   d. Respiratory distress and hypoxemia

(7) Which of the following elements should be considered when preparing to transport a trauma patient?
   a. Careful avoidance of aggressive "bagging" and dynamic hyperinflation
   b. Use of a PEEP valve with bag ventilation set at similar levels to mechanical ventilator
   c. End-tidal capnography
   d. Status of any thoracostomy tubes and drainage systems requirements
   e. All of the above

(8) What is the upper limit for plateau pressure in a lung-protective ventilation strategy?
   a. 26 cmH$_2$O
   b. 28 cmH$_2$O
   c. 30 cmH$_2$O
   d. 32 cmH$_2$O
   e. 40 cmH$_2$O

(9) What changes in peak inspiratory pressure (PIP) and plateau airway pressure (Pplat) would be expected in tension pneumothorax?
   a. Pplat increased, PIP unchanged
   b. Pplat unchanged, PIP increased
   c. PIP increased, Pplat increased
   d. PIP increased, Pplat decreased
   e. PIP decreased, Pplat decreased

(10) A patient with chest tube thoracostomy is taken to the OR for exploratory laparotomy. The ventilator is set in a volume-control mode. During the case there is a progressive decrease in oxygen saturation and an increase in ETCO$_2$ and respiratory acidosis, as well as frequent cycling of the ventilator. Which intervention should be done next?
   a. Increase PEEP
   b. Increase fresh gas flow
   c. Increase tidal volume and respiratory rate
   d. Change to pressure-control mode with lowest possible delta P that will provide adequate ventilation

Answers

(1) c
(2) d
(3) c
(4) d
(5) b
(6) c
(7) e
(8) c
(9) c
(10) d

References

1. Beers MF, Morrisey EE. The three R's of lung health and disease: repair, remodeling, and regeneration. *J Clin Invest* 2011; **121**: 2065–73.

2. Roan E, Waters CM. What do we know about mechanical strain in lung alveoli? *Am J Physiol Lung Cell Mol Physiol* 2011; **301**: L625–35.

3. ARDS Definition Task Force. Acute respiratory distress syndrome: the Berlin definition. *JAMA* 2012; **307**: 2526–33.

4. Pfeifer R, Tarkin IS, Rocos B, Pape HC. Patterns of mortality and causes of death in polytrauma patients: has anything changed? *Injury* 2009; **40**: 907–11.

5. Shackford SR, Mackersie RC, Davis JW, Wolf PL, Hoyt DB. Epidemiology and pathology of traumatic deaths occurring at a level I trauma center in a regionalized system: the importance of secondary brain injury. *J Trauma* 1989; **29**: 1392–7.

6. Acute Respiratory Distress Syndrome Network. Ventilation with lower tidal volumes as compared with traditional tidal volumes for acute lung injury and the acute respiratory distress syndrome. *N Engl J Med* 2000; **342**: 1301–8.

7. Blum JM, Maile M, Park PK, et al. A description of intraoperative ventilator management in patients with acute lung injury and the use of lung protective ventilation strategies. *Anesthesiology* 2011; **115**: 75–82.

8. Slinger P. Perioperative lung injury. *Best Pract Res Clin Anaesthesiol* 2008; **22**: 177–91.

9. Gajic O, Frutos-Vivar F, Esteban A, Hubmayr RD, Anzueto A. Ventilator settings as a risk factor for acute respiratory distress syndrome in mechanically ventilated patients. *Intensive Care Med* 2005; **31**: 922–6.

10. Futier E, Constantin JM, Paugam-Burtz C. A trial of intraoperative low-tidal-volume ventilation in abdominal surgery. *N Engl J Med* 2013 **369**: 428–37.

11. Zanella A, Bellani G, Pesenti A. Airway pressure and flow monitoring. *Curr Opin Crit Care* 2010; **16**: 255–60.

12. Hager DN, Brower RG. Customizing lung-protective mechanical ventilation strategies. *Crit Care Med* 2006; **34**: 1554–5.

13. Talmor D, Sarge T, Malhotra A, et al. Mechanical ventilation guided by esophageal pressure in acute lung injury. *N Engl J Med* 2008; **359**: 2095–104.

14. Hiller J, Silvers A, McIlroy DR, Niggemeyer L, White S. A retrospective observational study examining the admission arterial to end-tidal carbon dioxide gradient in intubated major trauma patients. *Anaesth Intensive Care* 2010; **38**: 302–6.

15. Bulger EM, Maier RV. Prehospital care of the injured: what's new. *Surg Clin North Am* 2007; **87**: 37–53, vi.

16. Lessard MR, Guerot E, Lorino H, Lemaire F, Brochard L. Effects of pressure-controlled with different I: E ratios versus volume-controlled ventilation on respiratory mechanics, gas exchange, and hemodynamics in patients with adult respiratory distress syndrome. *Anesthesiology* 1994; **80**: 983–91.

17. Thille AW, Cabello B, Galia F, Lyazidi A, Brochard L. Reduction of patient–ventilator asynchrony by reducing tidal volume during pressure-support ventilation. *Intensive Care Med* 2008; **34**: 1477–86.

18. Barr J, Fraser GL, Puntillo K, et al. Clinical practice guidelines for the management of pain, agitation, and delirium in adult patients in the intensive care unit. *Crit Care Med* 2013; **41**: 263–306.

19. Tanios MN, Nevins ML, Hendra KP, et al. A randomized, controlled trial of the role of weaning predictors in clinical decision making. *Crit Care Med* 2006; **34**: 2530–5.

20. Kollef MH, Shapiro SD, Silver P, et al. A randomized, controlled trial of protocol-directed versus physician-directed weaning from mechanical ventilation. *Crit Care Med* 1997; **25**: 567–74.

21. Myers TR, MacIntyre NR. Respiratory controversies in the critical care setting. Does airway pressure release ventilation offer important new advantages in mechanical ventilator support? *Respir Care* 2007; **52**: 452–8.

22. Chan KP, Stewart TE, Mehta S. High-frequency oscillatory ventilation for adult patients with ARDS. *Chest* 2007; **131**: 1907–16.

23. Funk DJ, Lujan E, Moretti EW, et al. A brief report: the use of high-frequency oscillatory ventilation for severe pulmonary contusion. *J Trauma* 2008; **65**: 390–5.

24. Ferguson ND, Cook DJ, Guyatt GH, et al. High-frequency oscillation in early acute respiratory distress syndrome. *N Engl J Med* 2013; **368**: 795–805.

25. Young D, Lamb SE, Shah S, et al. High-frequency oscillation for acute respiratory distress syndrome. *N Engl J Med* 2013; **368**: 806–13.

26. Scala R, Bartolucci S, Naldi M, Rossi M, Elliott MW. Co-morbidity and acute decompensations of COPD requiring non-invasive positive-pressure ventilation. *Intensive Care Med* 2004; **30**: 1747–54.

27. Mariani J, Macchia A, Belziti C, et al. Noninvasive ventilation in acute cardiogenic pulmonary edema: a meta-analysis of randomized controlled trials. *J Card Fail* 2011; **17**: 850–9.

28. Cohn SM, Dubose JJ. Pulmonary contusion: an update on recent advances in clinical management. *World J Surg* 2010; **34**: 1959–70.

29. Magret M, Amaya-Villar R, Garnacho J, et al. Ventilator-associated pneumonia in trauma patients is associated with lower mortality: results from EU-VAP study. *J Trauma* 2010; **69**: 849–54.

30. Shaikh N. Emergency management of fat embolism syndrome. *J Emerg Trauma Shock* 2009; **2**: 29–33.

31. Fabian TC, Hoots AV, Stanford DS, Patterson CR, Mangiante EC. Fat embolism syndrome: prospective evaluation in 92 fracture patients. *Crit Care Med* 1990; **18**: 42–6.

32. Habashi N, Andrews P. Ventilator strategies for posttraumatic acute respiratory distress syndrome: airway pressure release ventilation and the role of spontaneous breathing in critically ill patients. *Curr Opin Crit Care* 2004; **10**: 549–57.

33. Akoglu H, Akoglu EU, Evman S, et al. Utility of cervical spinal and abdominal computed tomography in diagnosing occult pneumothorax in patients with blunt trauma: Computed tomographic imaging protocol matters. *J Trauma Acute Care Surg* 2012; **73**: 874–9.

34. Moore FO, Goslar PW, Coimbra R, et al. Blunt traumatic occult pneumothorax: is observation safe? Results of a prospective, AAST multicenter study. *J Trauma* 2011; **70**: 1019–23.

35. Husain LF, Hagopian L, Wayman D, Baker WE, Carmody KA. Sonographic diagnosis of pneumothorax. *J Emerg Trauma Shock* 2012; **5**: 76–81.

36. Keel M, Meier C. Chest injuries: what is new? *Curr Opin Crit Care* 2007; **13**: 674–9.

37. Kortbeek JB, Al Turki SA, Ali J, et al. Advanced trauma life support, 8th edition, the evidence for change. *J Trauma* 2008; **64**: 1638–50.

38. Adegboye VO, Ladipo JK, Adebo OA, Brimmo AI. Diaphragmatic injuries. *Afr J Med Med Sci* 2002; **31**: 149–53.

39. Renaudier P, Rebibo D, Waller C, et al. Pulmonary complications of transfusion (TACO-TRALI). *Transfus Clin Biol* 2009; **16**: 218–32.

40. Litmanovitch M, Joynt GM, Cooper PJ, Kraus P. Persistent bronchopleural fistula in a patient with adult respiratory distress syndrome. Treatment with pressure-controlled ventilation. *Chest* 1993; **104**: 1901–2.

41. Ha DV, Johnson D. High frequency oscillatory ventilation in the management of a high output bronchopleural fistula: a case report. *Can J Anaesth* 2004; **51**: 78–83.

42. Carr JA. Abdominal compartment syndrome: a decade of progress. *J Am Coll Surg* 2013; **216**: 135–46.

43. Young AJ, Weber W, Wolfe L, Ivatury RR, Duane TM. One elevated bladder pressure measurement may not be enough to diagnose abdominal compartment syndrome. *Am Surg* 2013; **79**: 135–9.

44. Gianino JW, Afuwape LO. Evidence-based guidelines for the management of traumatic brain injury. *Mo Med* 2012; **109**: 384–7.

45. Myles P. Dynamic hyperinflation and cardiac arrest. *Anaesth Intensive Care* 1994; **22**: 316–17.

46. Walia G, Jada G, Cartotto R. Anesthesia and intraoperative high-frequency oscillatory ventilation during burn surgery. *J Burn Care Res* 2011; **32**: 118–23.

Figure 18. Mechanical ventilation following traumatic injury.

Chapter

20

Head trauma: surgical issues

Shoji Yokobori, Khadil Hosein, and M. Ross Bullock

Objectives

(1) Review the pathophysiology of primary and secondary brain injuries.

(2) Discuss the indications for surgical and intensive care treatment for intracranial hypertension, and mass lesion management in traumatic brain injury (TBI) patients.

Introduction

A wealth of basic and clinical research exists regarding the treatment of severe traumatic brain injury (TBI). However, despite much research effort, the prognosis for severe TBI patients remains poor. In the United States, an estimated 1.4 million people still suffer a TBI each year.[1] Worldwide, TBI is recognized as the leading cause of mortality and morbidity in young adults.[2] Globally, TBI stands out as a major worldwide health and socioeconomic problem.

The most important factor which determines the prognosis of TBI patients is the severity of the "primary" brain injury. Additional delayed "secondary" brain damage is set in progress, and continues from the time of traumatic impact in TBI patients, and the two combine to determine outcome.

Primary brain injury itself is mostly not amenable to treatment. Consequently, the strategy of primary TBI treatment should be prevention, such as use of helmets and vehicle modification (see Chapter 41). Treatment strategy for TBI should be the surgical management of TBI together with intensive care to prevent additional secondary brain injury. An adequate understanding of the pathophysiology, mechanisms, and operative indications is needed for neurointensivists and anesthesiologists to optimally manage these patients. The definition and classification of TBI is also important for targeted TBI treatments. For optimal and "seamless" TBI care, all neuroclinicians have to share a common language for a universal concept of TBI treatment strategies.

In this chapter, we first focus on the pathophysiology of primary and secondary brain injuries. We then discuss the indications for surgical and intensive care treatment for intracranial hypertension, and mass lesion management in TBI patients. Whenever possible, we have placed the management

discussion in the context of current guidelines on the management of severe TBI,[3] and the surgical management of TBI.[4–8]

Pathophysiology of TBI
Classification of TBI: primary and secondary, focal and diffuse

As mentioned above, primary injury is due to the unavoidable direct mechanical forces occurring at the time of traumatic insult. Secondary injury is derived from complications initiated by the primary injury and includes potentially avoidable entities such as hypoxic/ischemic injury, cerebral edema, alterations of vascular permeability, metabolic dysfunction, diminished cerebral circulation, and inflammation. Almost all clinical TBI treatments have been aimed at modulating these secondary injury mechanisms.

Both primary and secondary brain injury can be further classified according to whether the mechanism is focal or diffuse (Table 20.1). The distinction between focal and diffuse injuries is historically derived from the absence or presence of radiographic mass lesions on computed tomography (CT).

Table 20.1 A neuropathological classification of traumatic brain injury (TBI)

	Diffuse injury	Focal injury
Primary brain injury	Diffuse axonal injury	Focal cortical contusion
	Petechial white matter hemorrhage with diffuse vascular injury	Intracerebral hemorrhage Extracerebral hemorrhage
Secondary brain injury	Delayed neuronal injury	Delayed neuronal injury
	Diffuse brain swelling	Focal brain swelling
	Diffuse ischemic injury	Focal ischemic injury
	Diffuse hypoxic injury	Focal hypoxic injury
	Diffuse metabolic dysfunction	Regional metabolic dysfunction

In TBI cases, several types of injury coexist at the same time (e.g., nerve and vessel injury, diffuse and focal injury).

Trauma Anesthesia, 2nd Edition, ed. Charles E. Smith. Published by Cambridge University Press. © Charles E. Smith, 2015.

This distinction has now evolved to consider the pathological mechanisms imparted by the trauma in regions local to and remote from the point of impact. Although these classifications are widely accepted, most TBIs consist of a heterogeneous mixture of focal and diffuse damage, with intermingling of pathological processes (Table 20.1).

Diffuse brain injury

Diffuse axonal injury: representative of diffuse brain injury

The best example of primary diffuse injury is diffuse axonal injury (DAI). DAI was first defined as a clinical, pathological syndrome in patients who were unconscious from the time of trauma, with histopathological evidence of axonal damage in many white matter areas of the brain, and without major intraparenchymal lesions – the "retraction balls" scar on silver stain.

DAI is now recognized to typically involve a more progressive response involving a transient, traumatically induced, neurochemical disruption of the axonal membrane over 24 hours in humans allowing for uncontrollable calcium influx.[9] These mechanisms induce a subsequent failure of axoplasmic transportation, pooling of intraaxonal contents ("retraction balls"), and separation of the axon from its distal part. This disconnection occurs over 24–72 hours from the traumatic impact and is termed delayed or secondary axotomy.

At the molecular level, calcium influx initiates calpain activation and mitochondrial injury/swelling with cytochrome *c* release and caspase activation,[10] which continues to further exacerbate axonal injury and apoptosis.[11] These ion-channel-mediated changes directly influence the neural function. Arrest of axonal flow leads to proximal Wallerian degeneration over weeks to months after the event. Distally, the axon degenerates, fragments, and disappears, thereby resulting in deafferentation of the affected neuronal fields. The functional influences of this mechanism may include seizures, with excitatory electric potentials because of lack of inhibitory effects, spasticity, intellectual decline, and unmodulated behavior patterns. When this process is widespread and Wallerian degeneration destroys a great number of neurons, the whole brain becomes atrophic, with ventriculomegaly and, in the worst case, a persistent vegetative state.

Brain swelling

Brain swelling occurs in almost all patients with severe TBI, and to a lesser extent in 5–10% of those with moderate injuries.[12] This high incidence is a major reason for neurointensive care management for these patients. Brain swelling may cause delayed intracranial hypertension and death, and this is a major reason why aggressive management improves outcome. The delayed morbidity and death associated with severe TBI was once thought to be largely correlated with the extent of posttraumatic edema. The causes of brain swelling after severe head injury are multifactorial. There is now clear evidence that the majority of early brain edema, both global and focal, is cytotoxic rather than vasogenic. In humans studied with both gadolinium-enhanced magnetic resonance imaging (MRI) and pertechnetate-enhanced single-photon emission CT (SPECT) scans, vasogenic edema with opening of the blood–brain barrier is only seen at later time points around contusions, and not at all in patients with diffuse nonfocal injuries.[13–15] Vasogenic edema probably becomes important around focal contusions on the second through the 10th–15th post-TBI day.

Focal brain injuries

Focal brain injuries may be associated with a breach of the cranial coverings, such as a compound fracture. Usually they are the result of the stationary cranium being struck by moving objects with relatively small mass such as sticks, baseball bats, or golf clubs. Impacts of focal injury themselves do not usually cause prolonged unconsciousness, but they may cause permanent focal neurological deficits due to the immediate focal injury, or death due to delayed consequences of cerebral contusion or intracranial hematoma. Much more commonly, however, contusions occur with diffuse brain injury when the rapidly decelerating cranium strikes a surface within a crashing motor vehicle.

Cortical contusion and traumatic intracerebral hemorrhage

Focal cortical contusion is usually caused by mechanical forces which damage the blood vessels (veins, arteries, or larger capillaries) and other neural structures of the parenchyma (neural and glial cells). Contusions typically develop on the inferior surface of the brain, but some may be due to hemorrhagic lesions in the deeper structures of the brain – so-called "gliding contusions" associated with DAI.[16] Contusions often increase in size over hours to days owing to the evolving events related to the interplay of hemorrhage, vasogenic edema, and ischemic necrosis.

Traumatic intracerebral hemorrhages (ICH) are defined as hematomas 2 cm or larger not in contact with the surface of the brain, and they are present in 15% of autopsy cases of severe head injury. The pathology of ICH is due to rupture of the intrinsic blood vessels, typically in deep white matter tracts or basal ganglia (single or multiple), at the time of impact. Damage to multiple small blood vessels may result in the coalescence of many smaller hemorrhages. Hemorrhage sometimes will expand with time, and the rate and extent of increase in volume are related to factors such as the type and size of injured vessel, blood pressure, and the underlying bleeding tendency. Delayed traumatic ICH is one of the causes of neurological deterioration after TBI, and increased intracranial hemorrhage has been reported in up 51% of patients on repeated CT scan in the first 24 hours.[17] Delayed ICH can occur in severe TBI patients as well as patients who have sustained even relatively mild injuries. Hematomas may be discovered within hours or days to weeks after the injury. Several biomarkers have been proposed to better understand enlargement of delayed ICH (e.g., thrombomodulin, which is also located in the surface of the endothelium in the arteries[17]).

Epidural hematoma

Epidural hematoma, occurring between the dura and skull, occurs in about 2% of all types of head injury and in up to 15% of fatal head injuries. Increased use of CT after TBI reveals small asymptomatic epidural hematoma in an increasing number of cases. The clots are most frequently found in the temporoparietal regions, where the middle meningeal arteries have been damaged by fracture (Fig. 20.1).[18]

The ultimate size of the hematoma depends on the diameter of the vessels injured and how tightly the dura is adherent to the skull. The dura mater of infants is firmly adherent to the developing skull, and the meningeal vessels are not embedded in the skull, as is often the case in later life. Because of this, epidural hematomas are not common in children under the age of 2 years. Deformation of the more elastic skulls of adolescents or young adults may strip the dura mater from the bone, and thus produce an epidural hematoma more easily than in younger adults. With increasing age, the meningeal vessels become embedded in bone, and are at a greater risk of being damaged with skull fractures.

The clinical hallmark of epidural hematoma patients is the experience of a "lucid interval." This occurs typically after trivial or mild injury, but results in delayed coma, due to brain compression. On the other hand, one-third of patients have other significant brain injuries such as cerebral contusions, subdural hematomas, and lacerations. Such patients may experience no lucid interval and be unconscious from the time of impact.

Subdural hematoma

Subdural hematomas (SDH) are usually caused by rupture of the veins that bridge the subdural space, where they connect the superior surface of the cerebral hemispheres to the sagittal sinus. Thin bilateral films of blood in the subdural space are common in acute fatal head injury, and in about 13% of cases the hematoma is "pure" with very little evidence of other brain damage. Because blood can spread freely throughout the subdural space, SDHs tend to cover the entire hemisphere and are more extensive than epidural hematomas, usually 200–300 mL, versus 60–100 mL for epidural hematoma (Fig. 20.2). Some SDHs are arterial in origin, with the hemorrhage stemming from a cortical artery, and they typically occur with contusions.

The reported mortality rate of traumatic SDH varies from 30% to 90%, with the lower mortality rates occurring in patients who are operated on within 4 hours of injury.[19]

The severity of the underlying brain injury determines the outcome even when surgery has been done promptly. Outcome has been correlated with neuropathologic studies, showing ischemic brain damage in the hemisphere underlying the hematoma. An important factor leading to this ischemic damage is raised intracranial pressure (ICP) producing impaired cerebral perfusion. Increasing ICP reduces the volume of cerebral blood circulation. Removal of the SDH

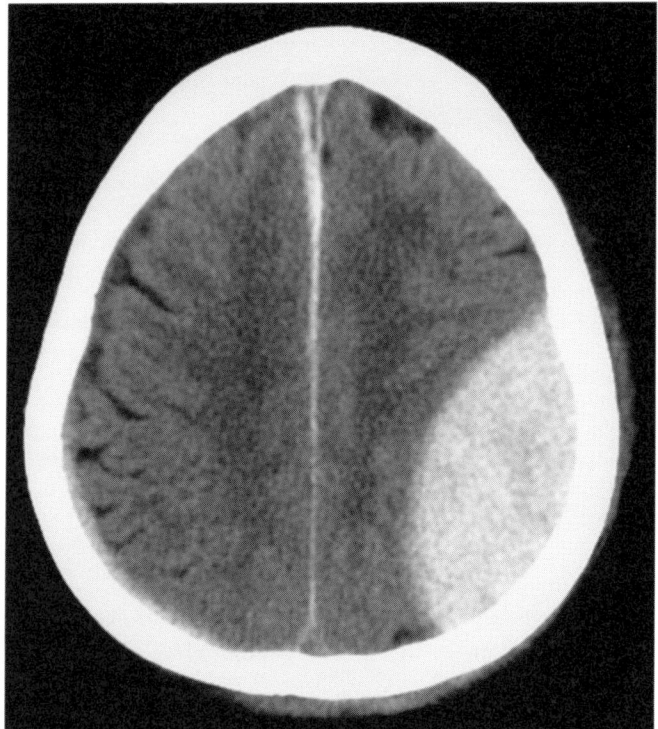

Figure 20.1 CT of epidural hematoma. Epidural hematomas usually present a convex shape because their expansion stops at skull sutures, where the dura is attached to the skull more tightly. This shape is sometimes called a "lentiform hemorrhage."

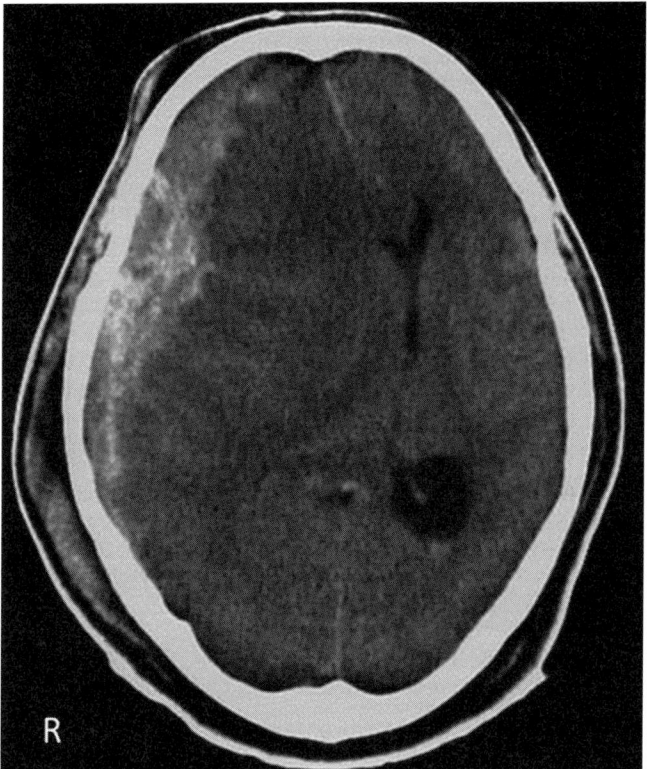

Figure 20.2 CT of acute subdural hematoma (SDH). In acute SDH, the hemorrhage spreads below the inner layer of the dura, and is thus not constrained, and can spread over the entire hemisphere (subdural space). This crescent-shaped clot is the most likely pattern in CT scan.

may result in the immediate reversal of global ischemia. This abrupt reduction of a mass lesion sometimes induces a reperfusion injury.[20–22] Previous experimental and clinical studies have shown that SDH and its removal may be considered as an ischemia/reperfusion injury.[23,24]

Indications for surgical management in TBI

In 2006, *Guidelines for the Surgical Management of Traumatic Brain Injury* was published by the Joint of Congress of Neurological Surgeons and the Brain Trauma Foundation.[4–8] The publication was the product of an extensive review of the literature. Five primary complications of TBI warranting

surgical consideration were identified: (1) traumatic parenchymal lesions, (2) epidural hematomas, (3) SDHs, (4) posterior fossa mass lesions, and (5) depressed cranial fractures (Table 20.2).

Intraparenchymal hemorrhage and contusions[4]
Indications for surgery

- Patients with parenchymal mass lesions and signs of progressive neurological deterioration referable to the lesion, medically refractory intracranial hypertension, or signs of mass effect on CT scan should be treated operatively.

Table 20.2 Indications for surgical management and intracranial pressure (ICP) monitoring for traumatic brain injury (TBI) patients

Type of injury	Indications	Procedures/methods
Intraparenchymal hemorrhage and contusions	Parenchymal mass lesions with progressive neurological deterioration. GCS 6–8 with frontal or temporal contusions greater than 20 cm^3 with midline shift of 5 mm and/or cisternal compression. Any lesion greater than 50 cm^3.	Craniotomy with evacuation. Bifrontal decompressive craniectomy is a treatment option for diffuse, medically refractory posttraumatic cerebral edema.
Epidural hematomas	Greater than 30 cm^3 regardless of GCS. Less than 30 cm^3 and with less than a 15 mm thickness and with less than a 5 mm midline shift in patients with GCS > 8 can be managed nonoperatively.	Craniotomy and evacuation of the hematoma.
Subdural hematomas	Thickness greater than 10 mm or a midline shift greater than 5 mm regardless of GCS. All patients with GCS < 9 should undergo ICP monitoring. GCS < 9 with less than 10 mm thickness and a midline shift less than 5 mm should undergo surgical evacuation if the GCS decreased by 2 or more points and/or if the patient presents with abnormal pupils and/or ICP > 20 mmHg.	Surgical evacuation. In GCS < 9 patients, a large craniotomy with or without bone flap removal and duraplasty are recommended.
Posterior fossa mass lesions/hemorrhages	Mass effect on CT scan or with neurological deterioration referable to the lesion. No significant mass effect on CT scan and without signs of neurological dysfunction may be managed by observation.	Evacuation should be performed as soon as possible, because these patients can deteriorate rapidly, thus worsening their prognosis. Suboccipital craniectomy is the predominant method.
Depressed skull fractures	Open (compound) cranial fractures depressed greater than the thickness of the cranium should undergo operative intervention to prevent infection. Patients with open (compound) depressed cranial fractures may be treated nonoperatively if there is no clinical or radiographic evidence of dural penetration, significant intracranial hematoma, depression greater than 1 cm, frontal sinus involvement, gross cosmetic deformity, wound infection, pneumocephalus, or gross wound contamination.	Early operation is recommended to reduce the incidence of infection. Elevation and debridement is recommended as the surgical method of choice. Primary bone fragment replacement is a surgical option in the absence of wound infection at the time of surgery.
ICP monitoring	All salvageable patients (GCS 3–8) with abnormal CT scan of hematomas, contusions, swelling, herniation, or compressed basal cisterns. Also indicated in patients with severe TBI with a normal CT scan if two or more of the following features are noted at admission: age over 40 years, unilateral or bilateral motor posturing, or systolic blood pressure (BP) < 90 mmHg (level 3 recommendation).	Ventriculostomy catheter connected to an external strain gauge is the most accurate, low-cost, and reliable method. The micro strain gauge and the fiberoptic transducer are also available and reliable, but more expensive.

- Patients with Glasgow Coma Scale (GCS) scores of 6–8 (see Chapter 35, Table 35.1) with frontal or temporal contusions greater than 20 cm^3 in volume with midline shift of at least 5 mm and/or cisternal compression on CT scan may be candidates for surgery.
- Patients with any lesion greater than 50 cm^3 in volume should be treated operatively.
- Patients with parenchymal mass lesions who do not show evidence for neurological compromise, have controlled ICP, and have no significant signs of mass effect on CT scan may be managed nonoperatively with intensive monitoring and serial imaging.

Timing and method

Craniotomy with evacuation of mass lesion is recommended for those patients with focal lesions and the surgical indications listed above. Bifrontal decompressive craniectomy within 48 hours of injury is a treatment option for patients with diffuse, medically refractory posttraumatic cerebral edema, especially if bilateral, and resultant intracranial hypertension. Decompressive procedures, including subtemporal decompression, temporal lobectomy, and hemispheric decompressive craniectomy (the commonly preferred procedure), are treatment options for patients with refractory intracranial hypertension and diffuse parenchymal injury with clinical and radiographic evidence for impending transtentorial herniation (see also below, *Current opinions on decompressive craniectomy*).

Epidural hematomas[8]
Indications for surgery

- The decision to operate is based primarily on the patient's GCS score, pupillary abnormalities, and CT parameters, especially clot thickness, hematoma volume, midline shift, and the status of the basal cisterns.
- An epidural hematoma greater than 30 cm^3 should be surgically evacuated regardless of the patient's GCS score.
- An epidural hematoma less than 30 cm^3 and with less than a 15 mm thickness and with less than a 5 mm midline shift in patients with a GCS score greater than 8 without focal deficit can be managed nonoperatively with serial CT scanning and close neurological observation in a neurosurgical center.

Timing and method

It is strongly recommended that patients with an acute epidural hematoma in coma (GCS < 9) with anisocoria undergo surgical evacuation as soon as possible. There are insufficient data to support one surgical treatment method. However, craniotomy provides a more complete evacuation of the hematoma.

Epidural hematoma in the inferotemporal lobe should have a lower threshold for surgery. Hematomas in this location can cause brainstem compression at low ICP with little midline shift.[25] Additionally, one report found anisocoria, suggestive of impending herniation, to occur in patients with ICP as low as 18 mmHg.[26]

Subdural hematomas[7]
Indications for surgery

- An acute SDH with a thickness greater than 10 mm or a midline shift greater than 5 mm on CT scan should be surgically evacuated, regardless of the patient's GCS score.
- All patients with acute SDH in coma (GCS < 9) should undergo ICP monitoring.
- A comatose patient (GCS < 9) with a SDH less than 10 mm thick and a midline shift of less than 5 mm should undergo surgical evacuation of the lesion if the GCS score decreased between the time of injury and hospital admission by 2 or more points, and/or the patient presents with asymmetric or fixed and dilated pupils, and/or the ICP exceeds 20 mmHg.

Timing and method

In patients with acute SDH and indications for surgery, surgical evacuation should be performed as soon as possible. If surgical evacuation of an acute SDH in a comatose patient (GCS < 9) is indicated, it should be performed using a large craniotomy with or without bone flap removal and duraplasty.

Posterior fossa mass lesions/hemorrhages[5]
Indications for surgery

- Patients with mass effect on CT scan or with neurological dysfunction or deterioration referable to the lesion should undergo operative intervention. Mass effect on CT scan is defined as distortion, dislocation, or obliteration of the fourth ventricle, compression or loss of visualization of the basal cisterns, or the presence of obstructive hydrocephalus.
- Patients with lesions and no significant mass effect on CT scan and without signs of neurological dysfunction may be managed by close observation and serial imaging.

Timing and method

In patients with indications for surgical intervention, evacuation should be performed as soon as possible, because these patients can deteriorate rapidly, thus worsening their prognosis. Suboccipital craniectomy is the predominant method reported for evacuation of posterior fossa mass lesions, and is therefore recommended.

Depressed skull fractures[6]
Indications for surgery

- Patients with open (compound) cranial fractures depressed greater than the thickness of the cranium should undergo operative intervention to prevent infection.

- Patients with open (compound) depressed cranial fractures may be treated nonoperatively if there is no clinical or radiographic evidence of dural penetration, significant intracranial hematoma, depression greater than 1 cm, frontal sinus involvement, gross cosmetic deformity, wound infection, pneumocephalus, or gross wound contamination. Nonoperative management of closed (simple) depressed cranial fractures is a treatment option.

Timing and method

Early operation is recommended to reduce the incidence of infection. Elevation and debridement is recommended as the surgical method of choice. Primary bone fragment replacement is a surgical option in the absence of wound infection at the time of surgery. All management strategies for open (compound) depressed fractures should include antibiotics.

Current opinions on decompressive craniectomy

Decompressive craniectomy has been used to treat uncontrolled intracranial hypertension of various types of brain damage, including TBI. Patient selection, timing of surgery, type of surgery, and the clinical and radiologic severity of the brain injury are all factors that determine the outcome of this procedure. The effectiveness of very early bifrontal decompressive craniectomy was evaluated in one randomized clinical trial that included 27 children who suffered TBI. There was a reduced risk ratio for death of 0.54 (95% confidence interval [CI] 0.17–1.72) and a risk ratio of 0.54 for poor outcomes (severe disability, vegetative state, and death [SD, VS, and D] in Glasgow Outcome Score) 6–12 months after injury (95% CI 0.29–1.07).[27] Other available studies in adults are either case series or cohorts with historical controls. Their results suggest that decompressive craniectomy effectively reduces ICP in most (85%) patients who have intracranial hypertension refractory to conventional medical treatment.[28] The results of a case series of 33 patients with severe TBI who underwent decompressive craniectomy showed that the long-term (3 years) results justify the use of decompressive craniectomy, and that good clinical results are seen in up to 40% of patients who were otherwise most likely to die.[29] Further studies will be required to define the parameters of use, including the timing of surgery, the physiologic threshold, the choice of procedure, and the age limit.

More recently, the highly controversial DECRA study, whose aim was to clarify the effectiveness of bifrontal decompressive craniectomy in diffuse injury patients, was published in 2011.[30] The authors concluded that although bifrontal decompressive craniectomy improves ICP and decreases intensive care unit days, patients treated with surgery have poorer outcomes than those treated with medical management alone.[30] However, this result aroused a great deal of controversy, focusing on the patient selection criteria, randomization balance for treatment arms, methods of decompressive craniectomy, and the patient population.[31,32]

The ongoing RESCUEicp (Randomized Evaluation of Surgery with Craniectomy for Uncontrollable Elevation of ICP) study is based upon unilateral decompression, and may give us more evidence relating the effectiveness of decompressive craniectomy in TBI patients (www.rescueicp.com).

Intracranial pressure monitoring to prevent additional secondary brain injury

Methodology

ICP monitoring is a "cornerstone" of the surgical treatment, and one of the main monitoring methods to putatively decrease secondary injury processes in neurointensive care. The Brain Trauma Foundation guidelines for the management of severe TBI state that a ventriculostomy catheter connected to an external strain gauge is the most accurate, low-cost, and reliable method of monitoring ICP.[3] The catheter is ideally positioned with its tip in the frontal horn of the lateral ventricle and is coupled by fluid-filled tubing to an external pressure transducer that can be recalibrated against an external standard. The ventriculostomy ICP monitor also allows treatment of elevated ICP by intermittent drainage of cerebrospinal fluid (CSF). However, proper placement of the catheter tip in the lateral ventricle sometimes can be difficult in patients with small, compressed ventricles. Alternative devices can also be used. The micro strain gauge and the fiberoptic transducer are widely available and reliable, but more expensive. The main advantage of these monitors is their ease of insertion, especially in patients with compressed ventricles. However, subarachnoid, subdural, and epidural monitors (fluid-coupled or pneumatic) are less accurate.

The main complications of ICP monitoring are infection and hemorrhage. Infection may be confined to the skin wound, but ventriculitis occurs in 1–10% of patients. The duration of catheterization has been correlated with an increasing risk for CSF infections during the first 10 days of use. Systemic prophylactic antibiotics and routine catheter exchange are not recommended in the current TBI guidelines (level 3 recommendation).[3] The best strategies for reducing the risk of ventriculitis associated with ICP monitoring are meticulous aseptic technique during catheter insertion, use of antibiotic-impregnated catheters, and minimization of the duration of monitoring.

Although the risk of hemorrhage has been shown to be consistently low (1–2%), it is an important complication to recognize and treat. Patients with coagulopathies are at greater risk for the development of this complication, and coagulation parameters (platelet count, prothrombin time, partial thromboplastin time, INR) must be checked and treated before ICP monitor insertion.

Indications for ICP monitoring in TBI

Monitoring of ICP can result in serious complications and is therefore indicated only in patients at significant risk for the development of intracranial hypertension. Indications from the current TBI guidelines are as follows (see also Table 20.2):[3]

- ICP should be monitored in all salvageable patients with severe TBI (GCS 3–8 after resuscitation) and an abnormal CT scan of the head (e.g., hematoma, contusion, swelling, herniation, or compressed basal cisterns) (level 2 recommendation – moderate degree of clinical certainty).
- ICP monitoring is indicated in patients with severe TBI with a normal CT scan if two or more of the following features are noted at admission: age over 40 years, unilateral or bilateral motor posturing, systolic blood pressure (BP) < 90 mmHg (level 3 recommendation – degree of clinical certainty not established).

A randomized clinical trial of ICP monitoring versus "standard intensive care unit (ICU) care" has recently been performed in Bolivia and Ecuador, with no difference in outcome found.[33]

There is clear evidence that patients who do not have intracranial hypertension or who respond to ICP reduction therapies have a lower mortality than those who have intractable intracranial hypertension. This evidence thus supports the use of ICP monitoring in severe TBI patients at risk for intracranial hypertension.[34,35]

ICP threshold for TBI management

Different authors have recommended different treatment thresholds for ICP management. However, there is still no strong evidence concerning this issue, which is still controversial. The current TBI guidelines recommend treating ICP above 20 mmHg (level 2 recommendation) or using clinical and CT characteristics in addition to the ICP value to determine the need for treatment (level 3 recommendation).[3] Ratanalert et al. compared the 6-month clinical outcomes of two different thresholds (20 mmHg and 25 mmHg), and concluded

that these ICP thresholds did not differ significantly, and that ICP threshold did not influence outcome.[36]

Treatment for intracranial hypertension

For patients with sustained ICP higher than 20–25 mmHg despite the general measures described above, specific measures are added in a stepwise fashion until the ICP is controlled (Fig. 20.3).

Once hypercapnia ($PaCO_2$ > 36 mmHg) and excessive end-tidal airway pressures (e.g., "fighting the ventilator") have been excluded, then the first stage of management for raised ICP is to exclude a new mass lesion or enlargement of a preexisting cerebral contusion. A CT scan must be performed without delay. When a significant mass lesion is present, then the optimal form of management is usually surgical excision, if this is feasible.

Sedation/paralysis

ICP elevation with agitation, posturing, or "fighting the ventilator" should be prevented by analgesics and sedatives with neuromuscular blockade, if necessary. The Brain Trauma Foundation guidelines mention doses of analgesics and sedatives as follows:[3]

- Morphine sulfate
  - 4mg/h continuous infusion
  - titrate as needed
  - reverse with naloxone
- Midazolam
  - 2 mg test dose
  - 2–4 mg/h continuous infusion
  - reverse with flumazenil

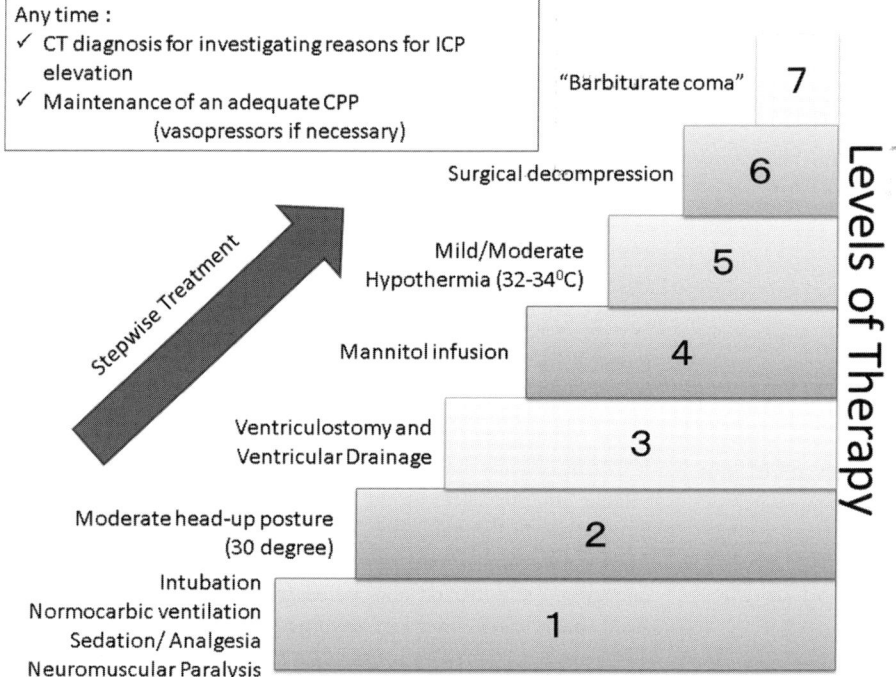

Figure 20.3 Example of a stepwise algorithm for the management of elevated intracranial pressure (ICP) at Virginia Commonwealth University and University of Miami. CPP, cerebral perfusion pressure; CT, computed tomography.

Any time :
- ✓ CT diagnosis for investigating reasons for ICP elevation
- ✓ Maintenance of an adequate CPP (vasopressors if necessary)

Stepwise Treatment

"Barbiturate coma" — 7

Surgical decompression — 6

Mild/Moderate Hypothermia (32-34°C) — 5

Mannitol infusion — 4

Ventriculostomy and Ventricular Drainage — 3

Moderate head-up posture (30 degree) — 2

Intubation / Normocarbic ventilation / Sedation/Analgesia / Neuromuscular Paralysis — 1

Levels of Therapy

- Fentanyl
  - 2 μg/kg test dose
  - 2–5 μg/kg/h continuous infusion
- Sufentanil
  - 10–30 μg test dose
  - 0.05–2 μg/kg continuous infusion
- Propofol
  - 0.5 mg/kg test bolus
  - 25–75 μg/kg/min continuous infusion (not to exceed 5 mg/kg/h)

However, there is still no strong evidence to support the efficacy of sedatives for ICP control. Only one study fulfilling the predetermined inclusion criteria for this topic exists. Kelly et al. compared the effectiveness of ICP control and patient outcome of morphine sulfate versus propofol in a double-blinded randomized controlled trial.[37] Despite a higher incidence of poor prognostic indicators in the propofol group, ICP therapy was less intensive, ICP was lower on therapy day 3, and long-term outcome was similar to that of the morphine group. According to these data, propofol is now recommended for the control of ICP as the "best" treatment option (level 3 recommendation).[3]

Ventriculostomy/ventricular drainage

Although removal of 1 mL of CSF normally does not change ICP, in patients with elevated ICP, drainage of 1–2 mL of CSF through the ventriculostomy catheter can temporarily lower ICP. The Monro–Kellie intracranial compliance curve explains this phenomenon well (Fig. 20.4). CSF drainage is an important adjunctive therapy for lowering ICP. However, as the brain

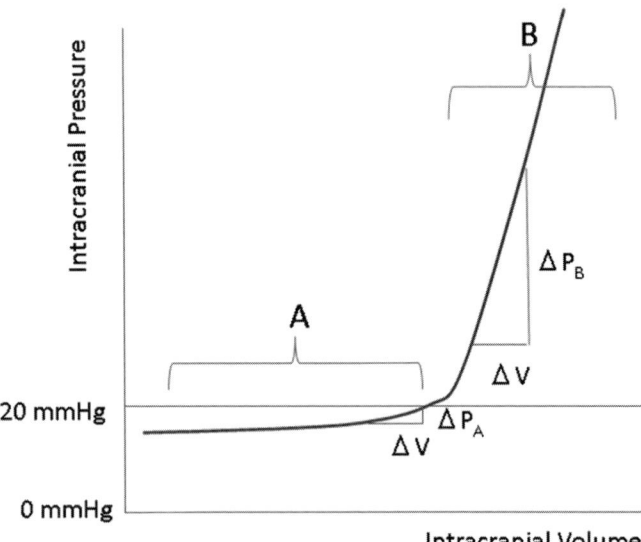

Figure 20.4 The Monro–Kellie intracranial compliance curve. (**A**) Normal ICP status: changes in intracranial volume (ΔV) are compensated without significant change in ICP (ΔP_A). (**B**) Intracranial hypertension with disruption of pressure compensatory mechanisms: when all compensatory mechanisms have been exhausted, small changes in intracranial volume (ΔV) lead to large changes in ICP (ΔP_B).

becomes more swollen, the ventricles collapse, less CSF is available for drainage, and the effectiveness of this modality is reduced.

Hyperosmolar therapy

Mannitol is widely used for the control of intracranial hypertension in TBI patients. However, there is little evidence to recommend repeated, regular administration of mannitol over several days. Mannitol is usually given as a bolus of 0.25–1 g/kg body weight (level 2 recommendation in Brain Trauma Foundation guidelines[3]). Serum osmolarity seems to be optimal when increased to 320 mOsm/L and should be kept at less than 320 mOsm/L to avoid side effects such as hypovolemia, hyperosmolarity, and renal failure.

Hypertonic saline has been also used for ICP control. Adverse effects of hypertonic saline injection include coagulopathy, hypokalemia, and acidosis.

Hypothermia therapy (see also Chapter 14)

Posttraumatic hypothermia has been shown to improve histopathological and behavioral consequences of TBI in the research setting. Hypothermia is also used to manage intracranial hypertension in the ICU in some trauma centers. The scientific literature, however, has failed to consistently support its positive influence on mortality and morbidity. Therefore, hypothermia treatment for diffuse TBI is still limited to an optional recommendation (level 3 in Brain Trauma Foundation guideline[3]). In a recent multicenter trial of hypothermia for neuroprotection, 392 patients with acute brain injury were randomized to normothermia or surface-induced hypothermia; in this study, hypothermia did not improve outcome.[38] However, there was some evidence of improved outcomes in patients who were initially hypothermic on admission and treated with continued hypothermia for 24 hours. This same study group then tried to confirm the efficacy of very early hypothermia in patients with severe TBI: the National Acute Brain Injury Study: Hypothermia II (NABISH-II).[39] In NABISH-II, early induced hypothermia did not improve outcome. In a subgroup analysis dividing the patients into those with diffuse brain injury and those with surgical hematoma evacuation, early induced hypothermia was beneficial for the latter group.[39] The authors postulated that the different pathophysiology between diffuse brain injury and hematoma may have accounted for these findings. Further clinical studies are needed for this topic.

Barbiturate therapy

Barbiturate infusion has also been used as a treatment for intracranial hypertension. Both cerebral-protective and ICP-lowering effects have been attributed to barbiturates. Other effects include alterations in vascular tone and resistance, suppression of metabolism, inhibition of free-radical-mediated lipid peroxidation, and inhibition of excitotoxicity.

Some randomized controlled trials of barbiturate therapy have been performed in severe TBI. These trials did not confirm the effectiveness of prophylactic barbiturate administration for outcome improvement after severe head injury.[40,41] On the other hand, a randomized multicenter trial demonstrated that instituting barbiturate coma in patients with refractory intracranial hypertension resulted in a twofold greater chance of controlling ICP.[35] Barbiturate therapy might be an effective agent for acutely reducing ICP in selected patients. With these data, prophylactic administration of barbiturates to induce EEG burst suppression is not recommended in the Brain Trauma Foundation guidelines (level 2).[3] However, high-dose barbiturate administration is recommended to control elevated ICP refractory to maximum standard medical and surgical treatment (level 2 recommendation).[3]

Conclusions

The pathobiology of severe TBI allows us to classify most patients as primary and secondary, focal or diffuse brain injury. Their mechanisms are heterogeneous, complex, synergistic, and still inadequately understood. Moreover, regeneration and repair are even more poorly understood. To prevent additional secondary brain injury and to optimize appropriate timing of surgical treatment versus intensive care versus natural recovery, careful monitoring and observation are needed. For anesthesiologists, understanding the concept of ICP management and the surgical indications are important as a basis for discussions of the treatment strategy with neurosurgeons.

Questions

(1) A 50-year-old female is brought to the emergency department after colliding with a tree while skiing. She had no loss of consciousness, but was a little dazed after hitting the tree. However, she seemed to improve after a short time. Twenty minutes ago, she began complaining of a mild headache and dizziness, and she has vomited once. Her GCS score is 10. On examination, the patient is sleepy and her pupils are equal bilaterally. A CT scan of the head shows an epidural hematoma of about 30 cm^3, with thickness less than 15mm and with less than a 5 mm midline shift. Which of the following is the most appropriate first step in the patient's care?
   a. Admit to ICU with serial CT scanning
   b. Emergent craniotomy and evacuation
   c. Stat MRI of brain
   d. Give mannitol

(2) A 37-year-old male is brought to the emergency room after a motor vehicle collision. He is unconscious. His blood pressure is 90/50 mmHg, pulse is 100 bpm, and respirations are 18/min. He does not follow commands and makes inappropriate sounds. On examination pupils are 2 mm and reactive bilaterally. A CT scan of the head shows a 6 mm punctate hemorrhage in the corpus callosum, and another in the parasagittal white matter, with blurring of the gray–white matter interface. Which is the most likely diagnosis?
   a. Subdural hematoma
   b. Diffuse axonal injury
   c. Epidural hematoma
   d. Subarachnoid hemorrhage
   e. Concussion

(3) A 30-year-old man is brought to the trauma center by ambulance after falling in his bathroom, while drunk. He is unarousable to voice but grimaces on sternal rub and withdraws to pain. On examination he has bruising to his head and injuries to his right arm. His right pupil is fixed and dilated. His vital signs are stable. Noncontrast CT of head shows a curved hyperdense hemorrhagic lesion, visible on 12 cuts, over his right temporal, and parietal lobe. What is the next step in management?
   a. MRI of brain
   b. Emergent craniotomy
   c. Repeat CT in 24 hours
   d. Cerebral angiogram

Questions 4–6 are based on the following case: A 46-year-old male suffers a severe TBI after falling off his motorcycle and hitting his head on the ground. He is unconscious. He has no medical problems, except a prior concussion when he was 20 playing college football. BP is 84/60 mmHg and pulse is 98 bpm. Examination shows a small bruise on his forehead but no bony abnormalities. A noncontrast CT of the head does not show any mass effect.

(4) Which of the situations below would be an indication for initiating intracranial pressure (ICP) monitoring?
   a. GCS 12 and normal CT scan of head
   b. Vomiting and headache
   c. Normal CT and BP < 90 mmHg
   d. His history of previous head trauma

(5) According to current guidelines, what is the most appropriate initial drug for controlling ICP in the ICU in the above patient?
   a. Morphine sulfate
   b. Fentanyl
   c. Phenytoin
   d. Propofol

(6) Which is the single most accurate site for ICP monitor catheter placement, in the current guidelines for ICP monitoring?
   a. Parenchymal
   b. Subdural
   c. Subarachnoid
   d. Epidural
   e. Intraventricular

(7) Which of the following is *not* a strategy in the ICU to reduce ventriculitis from ICP monitoring?
   a. The use of antibiotic-impregnated catheters
   b. Aseptic technique during catheter insertion
   c. Minimization of the duration of monitoring
   d. Routine catheter replacement after day 7

Questions 8–9 refer to the following case: A 40-year-old man is brought to the emergency department (ED) after sustaining a closed head injury and being found confused, smelling of alcohol. GCS 14 (E4 V4 M6), 36.8 °C, BP 126/80 mmHg, pulse 108 bpm, respirations 16/min. A head CT scan reveals a small hematoma in his frontal lobe. While in the ED, his GCS decreases to 7. BP is 200/120 mmHg, pulse 50 bpm and spontaneous respirations 6 breaths/min. The patient then worsens to deep coma (GCS 3) with irregular breathing.

(8) What is the most likely primary pathophysiologic abnormality?

    a. Hypoxia

    b. Delirium tremens

    c. Increased intracranial pressure (ICP)

    d. Alcohol induced encephalopathy

(9) The patient is now sedated and intubated, is in a head-up posture, and is being ventilated to a $PaCO_2$ of 35 mmHg. ICP monitoring was instituted, and ICP is over 30 mmHg. Repeat CT showed worsening of bifrontal intracranial hemorrhagic contusions which were greater than 50 cm^3 in total volume, and the CT showed compressed basal cisterns, with diffuse anteroposterior mass effect. The most appropriate *first* treatment for this situation is:

    a. Give mannitol bolus of 0.5–1 g/kg body weight

    b. Hyperventilate to $PaCO_2$ 25 mmHg

    c. Perform a craniotomy for removal of hematoma

    d. Induce mild/moderate hypothermia at 32–34 °C

(10) An 18-year-old woman involved in a motor vehicle collision is diagnosed with an acute subdural hematoma and undergoes a craniotomy. She is admitted to the ICU and has established ICP monitoring. The next day, despite the administration of mannitol and a decompressive craniectomy, the patient's ICP continues to be > 25 mmHg. The best next step in this patient's care is:

    a. Decrease blood pressure with a calcium antagonist

    b. Perform another head CT

    c. Induce hypothermia 34 °C

    d. Hyperventilate, to $PaCO_2$ of 25 mmHg

Answers

(1) b
(2) b
(3) b
(4) c
(5) d
(6) e
(7) d
(8) c
(9) c
(10) b

References

1. Binder S, Corrigan JD, Langlois JA. The public health approach to traumatic brain injury: an overview of CDC's research and programs. *J Head Trauma Rehabil* 2005; **20**: 189–95.

2. Cole TB. Global road safety crisis remedy sought: 1.2 million killed, 50 million injured annually. *JAMA* 2004; **291**: 2531–2.

3. Brain Trauma Foundation. Guidelines for the management of severe traumatic brain injury. *J Neurotrauma* 2007; **24** (Suppl 1): S1–106.

4. Bullock MR, Chesnut R, Ghajar J, *et al.* Surgical management of traumatic parenchymal lesions. *Neurosurgery* 2006; **58** (3 Suppl): S25–46.

5. Bullock MR, Chesnut R, Ghajar J, *et al.* Surgical management of posterior fossa mass lesions. *Neurosurgery* 2006; **58** (3 Suppl): S47–55.

6. Bullock MR, Chesnut R, Ghajar J, *et al.* Surgical management of depressed cranial fractures. *Neurosurgery* 2006; **58** (3 Suppl): S56–60.

7. Bullock MR, Chesnut R, Ghajar J, *et al.* Surgical management of acute subdural hematomas. *Neurosurgery* 2006; **58** (3 Suppl): S16–24.

8. Bullock MR, Chesnut R, Ghajar J, *et al.* Surgical management of acute epidural hematomas. *Neurosurgery* 2006; **58** (3 Suppl): S7–15.

9. Pettus EH, Christman CW, Giebel ML, Povlishock JT. Traumatically induced altered membrane permeability: its relationship to traumatically induced reactive axonal change. *J Neurotrauma* 1994; **11**: 507–22.

10. Buki A, Okonkwo DO, Wang KK, Povlishock JT. Cytochrome c release and caspase activation in traumatic axonal injury. *J Neurosci* 2000; **20**: 2825–34.

11. Raghupathi R. Cell death mechanisms following traumatic brain injury. *Brain Pathol* 2004; **14**: 215–22.

12. Miller JD, Butterworth JF, Gudeman SK, *et al.* Further experience in the management of severe head injury. *J Neurosurg* 1981; **54**: 289–99.

13. Bullock R, Butcher S, McCulloch J. Changes in extracellular glutamate concentration after acute subdural haematoma in the rat–evidence for an "excitotoxic" mechanism? *Acta Neurochir Suppl (Wien)* 1990; **51**: 274–6.

14. Lang DA, Hadley DM, Teasdale GM, Macpherson P, Teasdale E. Gadolinium DTPA enhanced magnetic resonance imaging in acute head injury. *Acta Neurochir (Wien)* 1991; **109**: 5–11.

15. Todd NV, Graham DI. Blood-brain barrier damage in traumatic brain contusions. *Acta Neurochir Suppl (Wien)* 1990; **51**: 296–9.

16. Sganzerla EP, Tomei G, Rampini P, *et al.* A peculiar intracerebral hemorrhage: the gliding contusion, its relationship to diffuse brain damage. *Neurosurg Rev* 1989; **12** (Suppl 1): 215–18.

17. Yokota H, Naoe Y, Nakabayashi M, *et al.* Cerebral endothelial injury in severe head injury: the significance of measurements of serum thrombomodulin and the von Willebrand factor. *J Neurotrauma* 2002; **19**: 1007–15.

18. Jamieson KG, Yelland JD. Extradural hematoma. Report of 167 cases. *J Neurosurg* 1968; **29**: 13–23.

19. Seelig JM, Becker DP, Miller JD, *et al.* Traumatic acute subdural hematoma: major mortality reduction in comatose patients treated within four hours. *N Engl J Med* 1981; **304**: 1511–18.

20. Miller JD, Bullock R, Graham DI, Chen MH, Teasdale GM. Ischemic brain damage in a model of acute subdural hematoma. *Neurosurgery* 1990; **27**: 433–9.

21. Kuroda Y, Bullock R. Local cerebral blood flow mapping before and after removal of acute subdural hematoma in the rat. *Neurosurgery* 1992; **30**: 687–91.

22. Burger R, Bendszus M, Vince GH, Solymosi L, Roosen K. Neurophysiological monitoring, magnetic resonance imaging, and histological assays confirm the beneficial effects of moderate hypothermia after epidural focal mass lesion development in rodents. *Neurosurgery.* 2004; **54**: 701–11.

23. Kuroda Y, Fujisawa H, Strebel S, Graham DI, Bullock R. Effect of neuroprotective *N*-methyl-D-aspartate antagonists on increased intracranial pressure: studies in the rat acute subdural hematoma model. *Neurosurgery.* 1994; **35**: 106–12.

24. Yokobori S, Gajavelli S, Mondello S, *et al.* Neuroprotective effect of preoperatively induced mild hypothermia as determined by biomarkers and histopathological estimation in a rat subdural hematoma decompression model. *J Neurosurg* 2013; **118**: 370–80.

25. Andrews BT, Chiles BW, Olsen WL, Pitts LH. The effect of intracerebral hematoma location on the risk of brain-stem compression and on clinical outcome. *J Neurosurg* 1988; **69**: 518–22.

26. Marshall LF, Barba D, Toole BM, Bowers SA. The oval pupil: clinical significance and relationship to intracranial hypertension. *J Neurosurg* 1983; **58**: 566–8.

27. Taylor A, Butt W, Rosenfeld J, *et al.* A randomized trial of very early decompressive craniectomy in children with traumatic brain injury and sustained intracranial hypertension. *Childs Nerv Syst* 2001; **17**: 154–62.

28. Aarabi B, Hesdorffer DC, Ahn ES, *et al.* Outcome following decompressive craniectomy for malignant swelling due to severe head injury. *J Neurosurg* 2006; **104**: 469–79.

29. Morgalla MH, Will BE, Roser F, Tatagiba M. Do long-term results justify decompressive craniectomy after severe traumatic brain injury? *J Neurosurg* 2008; **109**: 685–90.

30. Cooper DJ, Rosenfeld JV, Murray L, *et al.* Decompressive craniectomy in diffuse traumatic brain injury. *N Engl J Med* 2011; **364**: 1493–502.

31. Honeybul S, Ho KM, Lind CR, Gillett GR. The future of decompressive craniectomy for diffuse traumatic brain injury. *J Neurotrauma* 2011; **28**: 2199–200.

32. Kitagawa RS, Bullock MR. Lessons from the DECRA study. *World Neurosurg* 2013; **79**: 82–4.

33. Chesnut RM, Temkin N, Carney N, *et al.*; Global Neurotrauma Research Group. A trial of intracranial-pressure monitoring in traumatic brain injury. *N Engl J Med* 2012; **367**: 2471–81.

34. Palmer S, Bader MK, Qureshi A, *et al.* The impact on outcomes in a community hospital setting of using the AANS traumatic brain injury guidelines. *J Trauma* 2001; **50**: 657–64.

35. Eisenberg HM, Frankowski RF, Contant CF, Marshall LF, Walker MD. High-dose barbiturate control of elevated intracranial pressure in patients with severe head injury. *J Neurosurg* 1988; **69**: 15–23.

36. Ratanalert S, Phuenpathom N, Saeheng S, *et al.* ICP threshold in CPP management of severe head injury patients. *Surg Neurol* 2004; **61**: 429–34.

37. Kelly DF, Goodale DB, Williams J, *et al.* Propofol in the treatment of moderate and severe head injury: a randomized, prospective double-blinded pilot trial. *J Neurosurg* 1999; **90**: 1042–52.

38. Clifton GL, Miller ER, Choi SC, *et al.* Lack of effect of induction of hypothermia after acute brain injury. *N Engl J Med* 2001; **344**: 556–63.

39. Clifton GL, Valadka A, Zygun D, *et al.* Very early hypothermia induction in patients with severe brain injury (the National Acute Brain Injury Study: Hypothermia II): a randomised trial. *Lancet Neurol* 2011; **10**: 131–9.

40. Schwartz ML, Tator CH, Rowed DW, *et al.* The University of Toronto head injury treatment study: a prospective, randomized comparison of pentobarbital and mannitol. *Can J Neurol Sci* 1984; **11**: 434–40.

41. Ward JD, Becker DP, Miller JD, *et al.* Failure of prophylactic barbiturate coma in the treatment of severe head injury. *J Neurosurg* 1985; **62**: 383–8.

Chapter

21

Head trauma: anesthetic considerations and management

Armagan Dagal and Arthur M. Lam

Objectives

(1) Review the pathophysiology of traumatic brain injury (TBI).
(2) Summarize the systemic manifestations of acute TBI.
(3) Review the current guidelines regarding management of TBI.
(4) Discuss the anesthetic management of TBI and the potential complications.

Introduction

Traumatic brain injury (TBI) is common. Its outcome may be poor and it creates a significant burden for society. It is estimated that 1.7 million people suffer from TBI in the USA annually. Approximately 290,000 of these patients require hospital admission, 50,000–70,000 die, and 80,000 (11,000 of whom are children) require long-term rehabilitation. Currently 5.3 million people live with TBI in the USA and their overall annual healthcare costs mount up to $80–100 billion.[1]

Children aged 0–4 years, older adolescents aged 15–19 years, and adults aged 65 years and older are the most likely age groups to sustain a TBI. Falls are the leading cause of TBI-related injuries, especially in children under 4 and adults 75 and older. Car crashes, on the other hand, are the leading cause of TBI-related deaths.

The number of people inflicted with TBI amongst military personnel has been reported to be 295,200 from 2000 to 2013. The Department of Defense reported in 2013 a total of 27,324 TBI cases of varying severity: 83.6% mild, 6.8% moderate, 0.6% penetrating, 0.6% severe, and 8.4% not classifiable. There has been a steady increase in the number of military personnel with TBI over the last 13 years.[2]

Sports and recreational activities contribute to about 21% of all TBI among children and adolescents. In 2009 there were 248,418 patients with sports-related non-fatal head injuries treated at emergency departments (EDs) in the USA.[3]

A report published by the Centers for Disease Control and Prevention for the period 2001–2009 indicates that the number of sports- and recreation-related ED visits for TBI amongst persons aged ≤ 19 years increased by 62%.[3] This increase in ED visits might be explained by an increasing popularity of sports and recreational activities, a higher incidence of TBI among participants, and/or an increased awareness of the importance of early diagnosis of TBI. The number of ED visits for TBIs that resulted in hospitalization did not show a significant upward trend, so an increased awareness is more likely the explanation. Moreover, current evidence suggests that just a single episode of TBI may be associated with the later onset of depression and neurodegenerative disorders, including Alzheimer's disease (AD).[4,5]

In 2011 the Department of Health and Human Services (HHS) allocated a budget of $400 million to develop programs to understand, prevent, and reduce the incidence of TBI. The Traumatic Brain Injury Act of 1996 authorized state surveillance systems to obtain information on the number of people affected by TBI, the causes of these injuries, and their severity.

Despite enormous efforts to prevent TBI (see also Chapter 41), it continues to impose a significant burden on society, as it is the primary determinant of the quality of outcome following trauma.

State-of-the-art care of patients with TBI has evolved as progress has been made in our understanding of its underlying pathophysiology, as well as in prehospital medicine, neuroimaging, neuromonitoring, intraoperative and critical care areas, and access to multidisciplinary neurotrauma units.

Anesthesiologists are frequently involved in the care of these patients at every step of the treatment continuum. These areas are covered in this chapter.

Pathophysiology

TBI is defined as an alteration in brain function, or other evidence of brain pathology, caused by an external force.[6]

Alteration in brain function is defined as one of the following clinical signs:

- evidence of loss/decreased consciousness or mental state
- prospective/retrospective memory loss following injury
- neurologic deficits (weakness, loss of balance, change in vision, dyspraxia paresis/plegia, paralysis, sensory loss, aphasia, etc.)

Trauma Anesthesia, 2nd Edition, ed. Charles E. Smith. Published by Cambridge University Press. © Charles E. Smith, 2015.

- radiologic or laboratory evidence of brain pathology (e.g., computed tomography [CT], magnetic resonance imaging [MRI])

The evolution of TBI can be divided into two major clinical stages.

The primary injury immediately follows the head trauma. It is generally untreatable and irreversible. Although it is not treatable it is certainly preventable through education and protective measures (e.g., seatbelts, bicycle helmets: see Chapter 41).

There are two main categories of primary brain damage due to trauma: focal and diffuse injury (see Chapter 20).[7] Focal injury includes cortical or subcortical contusions and lacerations, as well as intracranial bleeding such as subarachnoid hemorrhage (SAH) and subdural hematoma (SDH) due to severe direct biomechanical energy transfer to the brain tissue.

Diffuse injury is caused by stretching and tearing of the brain tissue. It does not need any skull fracture or direct impact or crush injury to the brain surface and is therefore also seen in cases with mild TBI. The main form of diffuse injury is called diffuse axonal injury (DAI), which is due to acceleration/deceleration forces that lead to shearing of axons. The axonal tissue is more vulnerable to TBI than the vascular tissue. Thus, focal injuries are usually superimposed upon more diffuse neuronal injury. The consequences of the initial TBI include physical disruption of cell membranes and infrastructure, and disturbance of ionic homeostasis secondary to increased membrane permeability. This in turn may lead to astrocytic and neuronal swelling, relative hypoperfusion, perturbation of cellular calcium homeostasis, increased free radical generation and lipid peroxidation, mitochondrial dysfunction, inflammation, apoptosis, and DAI; these mechanisms are not preventable at this point.[8]

The brain is a metabolically active organ that requires constant delivery of oxygen and nutrients via adequate cerebral blood flow (CBF), which is usually maintained despite variations in cerebral perfusion pressure (CPP). It receives 15% of the cardiac output, and consumes 20% of total body oxygen and 25% of total body glucose. Disruption of this high metabolic demand and supply can result in irreversible damage. Secondary injury is the progression of the pathologic insults, such as ischemia, reperfusion, and hypoxia, starting immediately after the initial injury. Potentially treatable causes include hypotension (systolic BP < 90 mmHg), hypoxemia (PaO_2 < 60 mmHg), hypo/hyperglycemia, and hypo/hypercarbia. Although delayed brain ischemia appears to be the major common pathway of secondary brain injury, reperfusion hyperemia may also occur, and its prevention should be part of the treatment paradigm.

Primary injury

TBI is generally classified into three clinical categories (mild, moderate, and severe) based on the Glasgow Coma Scale (GCS: see Table 21.4, below). This classification system lacks heterogeneity and complexity to guide management and research, and therefore a new classification system has been developed with common data elements, and this has been validated through the TRACK-TBI study.[9]

Skull fractures

Skull fractures indicate a significant energy transmission to the brain with a high suspicion of intracranial injury.

Indications for surgical intervention for patients with skull fractures include:

- depressed fracture more than the thickness of the cranium
- open fracture with gross contamination
- resulting intracranial hemorrhage
- cranial nerve injury
- persistent cerebrospinal fluid (CSF) leak (most likely to be a basilar fracture)
- gross cosmetic deformity

CSF leakage is initially managed conservatively with lumbar subarachnoid drainage of CSF. If the leak persists, surgical treatment can be instituted with either endoscopic intranasal repair or a craniotomy approach. Despite the lack of strong evidence for the benefit of prophylactic antibiotics, some centers continue to use it routinely. Prophylactic anticonvulsant (e.g., phenytoin) therapy should be considered, but should be given only for open depressed skull fractures or fractures associated with an underlying brain injury, and even then given for only seven days.

Subdural hematoma

Subdural hematoma (SDH) is seen in approximately 25% of head injuries. They have the highest mortality rate of all TBIs due to underlying associated brain injury and the decrease in cerebral blood flow that accompanies these lesions. The hematoma creates a crescent shape between the brain and the dura (Fig. 21.1). It is usually caused by tearing of the bridging veins connecting the cerebral cortex and dural sinuses from acceleration–deceleration forces, as in motor vehicle crashes.

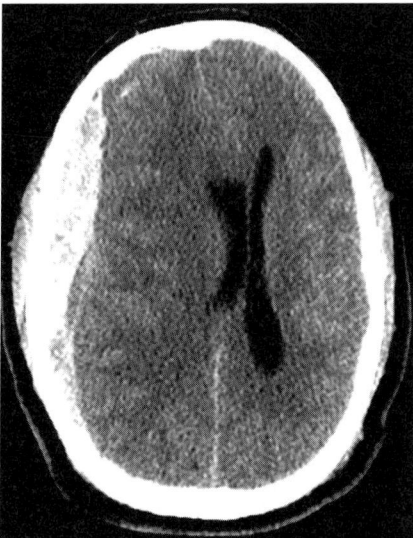

Figure 21.1 CT showing an acute subdural hematoma (SDH).

Factors affecting the outcome include hematoma thickness, magnitude of midline shift, associated contusions and edema.[10]

Immediate surgical evacuation is recommended for patients with acute SDH if:

- clot thickness > 10 mm
- midline shift > 5 mm
- GCS has decreased by ≥ 2 points from the time of injury
- asymmetric or fixed and dilated pupils
- consistently high intracranial pressure (ICP > 20 mmHg)

Epidural or extradural hematoma

Epidural hematomas are less common, accounting for 6% of head-injured patients. They generally have a better prognosis than SDH, with the main determinant of outcome being the preoperative neurologic status. Epidural hematomas are biconvex in shape on CT and are located between the dura and the skull (Fig. 21.2). The usual etiology is a torn middle meningeal artery, but the blood may also come from a skull fracture or bridging veins. The classic presentation includes a lucid interval followed by neurologic deterioration and coma.

Treatment is prompt surgical decompression (see Chapter 20) when the following criteria are met:

- supratentorial hematoma > 30 mL
- infratentorial hematoma > 10 mL
- hematoma thickness > 15 mm
- midline shift > 5 mm
- presence of other intracranial lesions

Expectant management with close observation is acceptable for small lesions.[11]

Cerebral hematoma and contusion

An intracerebral hematoma (ICH) is a collection of blood within the brain parenchyma. It can be spontaneous or traumatic. Its appearance on CT may be delayed for up to 24–48 hours following trauma. Determinants of outcome include the GCS, the presence of hypoxia, the hematoma volume, and its subsequent expansion. Surgical treatment may be necessary to control intracranial hypertension. Initially promising in limiting the growth of hematomas in patients with spontaneous intracerebral hemorrhage, the novel approach using recombinant activated factor VII (rFVIIa) did not improve outcome in a large randomized controlled study.[12] Moreover, the results of this study should not be generalized to traumatic intracranial hematomas. Contusions are areas of brain parenchyma with necrosis, hemorrhage, and infarct (Fig. 21.3). Cerebral blood flow as measured by xenon CT has been shown to be depressed in and around these lesions; it may be below ischemic thresholds. This finding has been confirmed using the newer positron emission tomography (PET) technology. Management of traumatic cerebral hematomas remains controversial, but surgical evacuation with or without decompressive craniectomy may be indicated if intracranial hypertension is refractory to medical treatment.

Surgical decision making is dependent on the location and CT imaging (see Chapter 20). Surgery for cerebral hemispheric hemorrhages is indicated if:

- hemorrhage size > 50 mL
- hemorrhage size > 20 mL with midline shift > 5 mm
- presence of basal cistern compression

For posterior fossa hemorrhages, surgery is indicated in the case of:

- significant mass effect (e.g., obliteration of fourth ventricle)[13,14]
- significant decrease in level of consciousness (LOC)

Diffuse injury

Diffuse injury is caused by sudden deceleration or rotational forces, leading to widespread cellular and axonal injury. Unlike the other lesions, the best diagnostic test for this injury is MRI

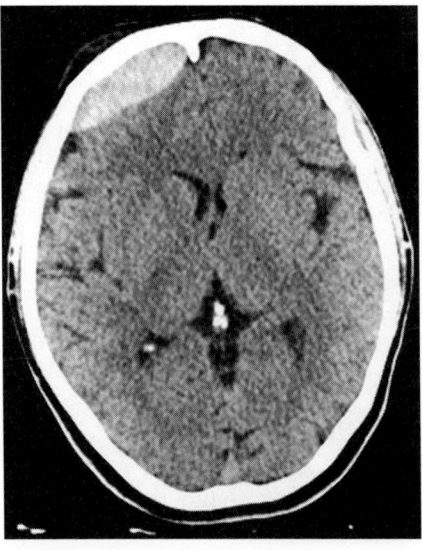

Figure 21.2 CT showing an acute epidural hematoma.

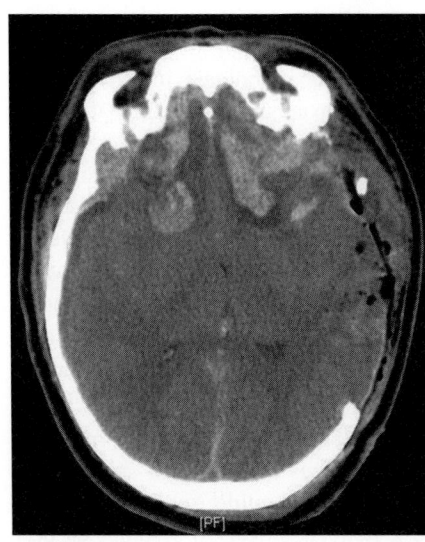

Figure 21.3 CT showing a cerebral contusion.

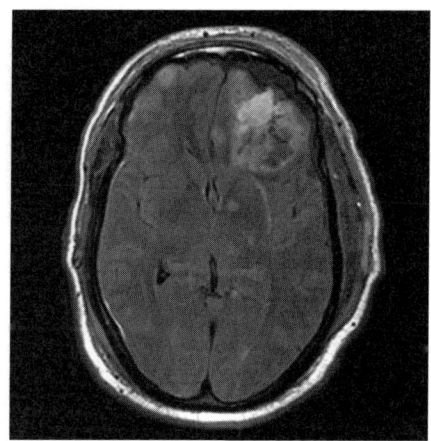

Figure 21.4 Example of shear injury on MRI.

Table 21.1 Contributing risk factors to secondary brain injury

Cerebral factors
Increased intracranial pressure
Expanding mass lesions
Hypercapnia
Hypoxemia
Venous obstruction (cervical collar, poor positioning)
Systemic hypotension (compensatory cerebral vasodilatation)
Excessive hyperventilation
Posttraumatic vasospasm (in patients with traumatic subarachnoid hemorrhage)
Seizures
Systemic factors
Hypotension
Hypoxemia
Anemia
Hypovolemia
Hyperglycemia
Hyponatremia
Hypo-osmolar state
Coagulopathy

or diffusion tensor imaging studies and not CT (Fig. 21.4). This injury is sometimes referred to as DAI, which is more accurately a pathologic diagnosis. DAI causes downstream deafferentation and disconnection in the brainstem, leading to coma. Patients with severe DAI typically present with profound coma without elevated ICP. It is classified into three categories: (1) mild DAI, coma of 6–24 hours; (2) moderate DAI, coma of more than 24 hours without decerebrate posturing; and (3) severe DAI, coma of more than 24 hours with decerebrate posturing or flaccidity. Severe DAI has a 50% mortality.[15]

Secondary injury

Secondary injury occurs after the initial injury, due to a number of events that occur as a result of or subsequent to the initial injury, which may or may not be preventable. It both represents a powerful predictor of outcome and presents an opportunity for tailored care to minimize further damage to neural tissue (Table 21.1).

It should also be remembered that head injury is a multisystem disorder. Non-neurological organ dysfunction may contribute to up to two-thirds of all deaths after severe TBI.[16] The respiratory system is affected by direct airway obstruction from reduced LOC, respiratory center dysfunction, infection, and neurogenic pulmonary edema. The cardiovascular system is affected by the elevated sympathetic activity, which may cause myocardial injury, leading to further cerebral hypoperfusion, and complicates the use of cardioactive agents. A high overall stress response results in elevated cortisol levels, subsequent hyperglycemia, and gastric stress ulcers. About one-third of patients with severe TBI develop a coagulopathy directly as a result of brain tissue injury, the presence of which is related to poor outcome.[17,18] Electrolyte imbalances frequently contribute to worsening of cerebral edema and lowering seizure thresholds. The syndrome of inappropriate antidiuretic hormone secretion (SIADH) or cerebral salt-wasting syndrome (CSWS) may occur, and both can lead to severe hyponatremia. Hypernatremia, on the other hand, may be caused iatrogenically from dehydration, or may result from

diabetes insipidus. Not infrequently, neurogenic hyperthermia can occur secondary to thermoregulatory dysfunction. The prevention and treatment of these multisystem complications plays an important part in ameliorating secondary injury and improves TBI outcomes (Table 21.2).[19]

Initial resuscitation

Immediate trauma care follows the standards of ABCDEs according to the Advanced Trauma Life Support (ATLS) principles taught by the American College of Surgeons Committee on Trauma (see Chapter 2). Rapid identification and correction of catastrophic hemorrhage is a high priority. Limitation of initial secondary brain injury depends on the prevention and treatment of hypoxia and hypotension. Therefore, initial resuscitation should aim for cardiopulmonary optimization.

The 2011 Guidelines for Field Triage of Injured Patients recommends the direct transport of patients with a field GCS of ≤ 13 or with penetrating head injuries to the Level I–II trauma center within the defined trauma system.[20] The trauma facility should have CT scan capability, immediate neurosurgical care, and the ability to monitor ICP and treat intracranial hypertension. Every effort should be made to provide the fastest mode of transport to minimize total prehospital time.[21] Despite the available evidence and recommendations, analysis of the national trauma databank showed that one-third of all

Table 21.2 Non-neurological multisystem effects of TBI

Fever		55% Neuroinflammatory (early) Infection (late) presentation
Infections	Sepsis SIRS	75% Inflammation and immunosuppression
Cardiovascular	Hypertension	Due to systemic massive catecholamine discharge
	Hypotension	Damage to brainstem in diffuse axonal injury
	Neurogenic myocardial dysfunction	Local excessive catecholamine release in the presence of normal coronary perfusion
Respiratory	Respiratory failure	41%
	Pneumonia Acute lung injury	68%
	Pulmonary edema	Could be cardiac or neurogenic origin
Hematological	Anemia	35%
	Coagulopathy	35%
Acute kidney injury		8%
Metabolic	Hyperglycemia	
	Hyponatremia	SIADH CSWS Anticonvulsants Diuretics
	Hypernatremia	Excessive mannitol use or CDI

CDI, central diabetes insipidus; CSWS, cerebral salt-wasting syndrome; SIADH, syndrome of inappropriate antidiuretic hormone secretion. % are estimates based on the literature and the authors' experience.

severe TBI incidents in the USA were first seen at another facility before transferring to a level I or II trauma center, a percentage that should be decreased.[22]

Airway and breathing

Prehospital phase

The Brain Trauma Foundation guidelines for prehospital management of severe TBI were updated in 2008.[21] According to these recommendations, indications for a definitive airway include:

- inability to maintain an adequate airway
- evidence of hypoxemia ($SpO_2 < 90\%$) despite supplemental O_2
- severe TBI with GCS ≤ 8

Minimal monitoring standards should include blood pressure, oxygenation, and end-tidal carbon dioxide ($ETCO_2$) monitoring (see Chapter 9). $ETCO_2$ should be maintained at normal range (35–40 mmHg); hyperventilation (< 35 mmHg) might only be used for a short period of time if the patient is demonstrating signs of cerebral herniation.

There are conflicting results for the effectiveness of prehospital tracheal intubation. However, a recent study on rapid sequence intubation (RSI) performed by paramedics during prehospital care has been shown to improve functional outcome at 6 months.[23] The provider's level of training and experience with advanced airway management techniques, including the appropriate use of drugs, often determines the success or failure of airway management techniques in the field. It is clear, however, that hypotension, hypoxemia, and hypercarbia must be avoided.

In-hospital phase

Indications for tracheal intubation in severe TBI in the hospital include:

- severe TBI (GCS ≤ 8)
- inability to maintain/protect an adequate airway
- increased risk of aspiration
- evidence of hypoxemia ($SpO_2 < 90\%$) despite supplemental O_2
- potential for hypercarbia due to ventilatory failure
- uncooperative, combative patients
- facilitation of further diagnostic studies

Several considerations must be kept in mind prior to intubating the trachea of patients with TBI, in addition to the skill and expertise of the physician. Patients with TBI have up to a 10% incidence of an unstable cervical spine injury. Risk factors for combined brain and spine injuries include a motor vehicle collision (MVC) and GCS ≤ 8. Therefore, manual in-line neck stabilization (MILS) is routinely done in these situations to decrease the chance of worsening a neurologic injury (see Chapter 3). MILS, however, has the potential to make laryngoscopy more difficult. The anterior portion of the cervical collar can be removed to enhance mouth opening and facilitate laryngoscopy while MILS in place. Backup plans and alternative airway devices should be available when performing an emergent intubation, including but not limited to gum elastic bougie, laryngeal mask airway, and fiberoptic or video laryngoscopy equipment (see Chapter 3). Patients with TBI should generally be intubated orally, not nasally, because of the potential risk of intracranial migration of the endotracheal tube through a basal skull fracture defect, and the long-term risk of sinus infection. A surgical airway remains a viable and appropriate option in the setting of severe facial and neck trauma with a compromised airway (see Chapters 3, 24, and 25).

There is always a risk of aspiration of gastric contents in trauma airway management. Even though inappropriately applied cricoid pressure may theoretically displace cervical fractures, and its benefit has never been proven in the trauma population, it is routinely performed during RSI.[24,25] Rice *at al.* recently defined the concept of the "cricoid pressure unit"

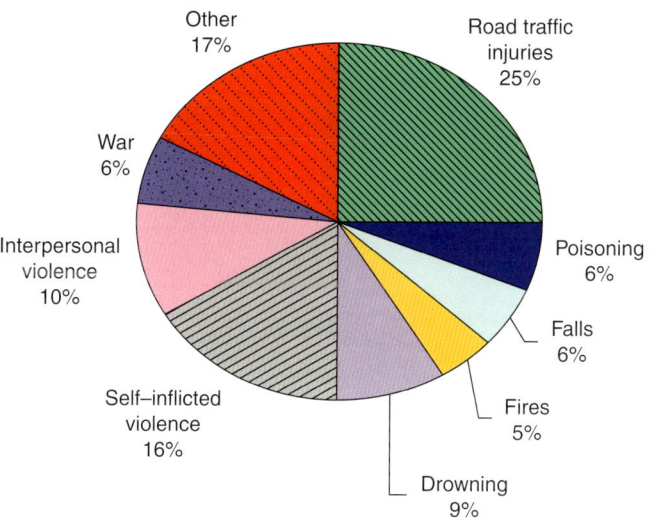

Distribution of global injury mortality by cause, 2000

- Other 17%
- Road traffic injuries 25%
- War 6%
- Poisoning 6%
- Interpersonal violence 10%
- Falls 6%
- Fires 5%
- Self–inflicted violence 16%
- Drowning 9%

Figure 1.2 Distribution of global injury mortality by cause. (From Peden M, McGee K, Sharma G. *The injury Chart Book: a Graphical Overview of the Global Burden of Injuries*. Geneva: World Health Organization, 2002.[3]).

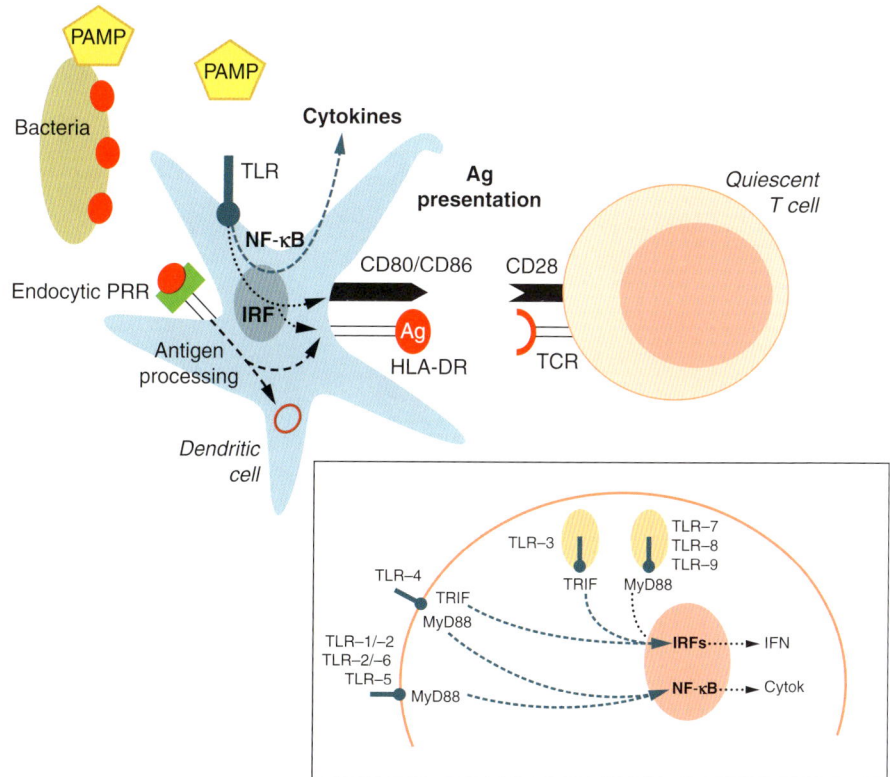

Figure 6.1 Innate immune function in trauma: functions of the dendritic cell. Pathogen-associated molecular patterns, expressed by bacteria, are recognized by toll-like receptors. Activation of the toll-like receptor signaling pathways induces expression of nuclear factor κ-dependent cytokines and interferon regulatory factor-dependent costimulatory molecules, CD80 and CD86. Pattern-recognition receptors mediate the phagocytosis of pathogens by dendritic cells. Proteins derived from the microorganisms are processed to generate antigens. The major-histocompatibility-complex class II molecules present antigens to the T-cell receptor, activating T cells. Recognition of the costimulatory molecules (CD80 and CD86) by CD28 on T cell membrane is required to fully activate T cells.

Ag, antigens; CD80, CD86, costimulatory molecules; DC, dendritic cell; HLA-DR, histocompatibility-complex class II molecules; IRF, interferon regulatory factor; NF-κB, nuclear factor κB; PAMP, pathogen-associated molecular patterns; PRR, pattern-recognition receptors; TCR, T-cell receptor; TLR, toll-like receptors. (Reproduced with permission from Asehnoune *et al.*, 2012.[17])

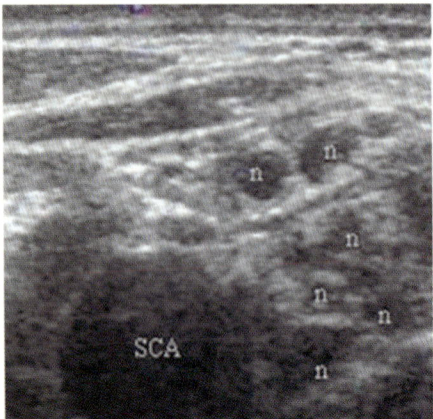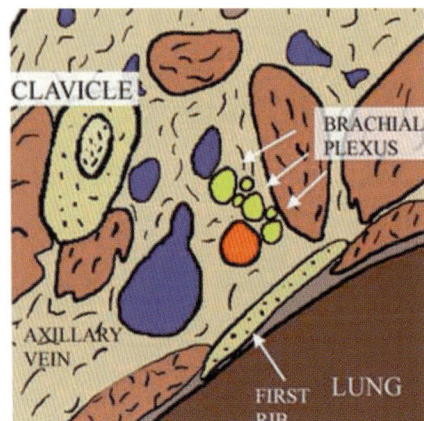

Figure 12.2 Supraclavicular sonogram of neural elements (n) adjacent to subclavian artery (SCA).

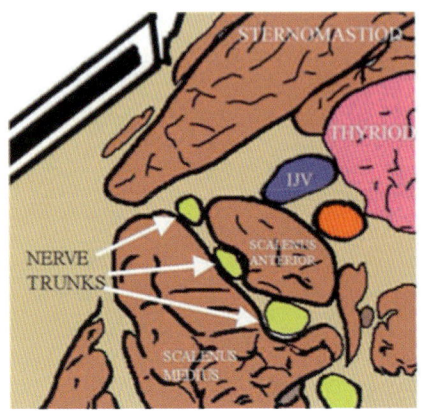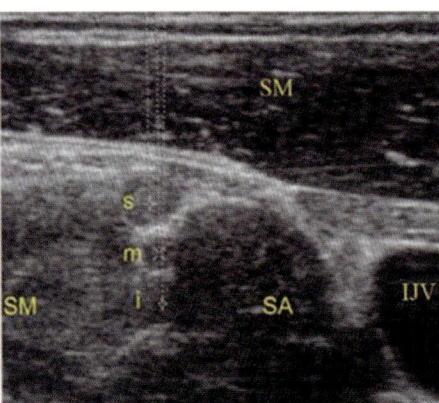

Figure 12.8 Sonographic anatomy of the brachial plexus in the interscalene region: scalenus medius (SM), scalenus anterior (SA), and sternomastoid muscle (SM); superior (s), middle (m), and inferior (i) trunks. IJV, internal jugular vein.

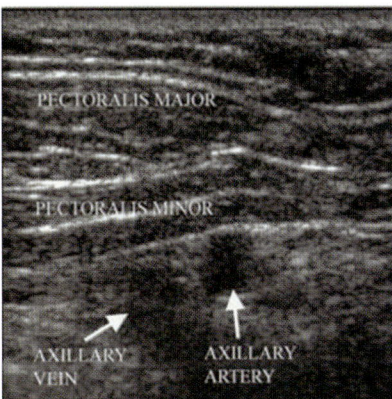 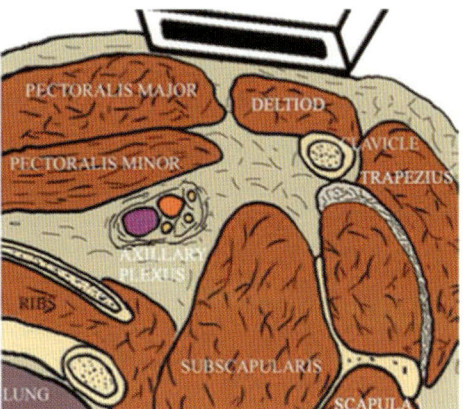

Figure 12.10 Sonographic anatomy of the brachial plexus in the infraclavicular region, medial to the coracoid.

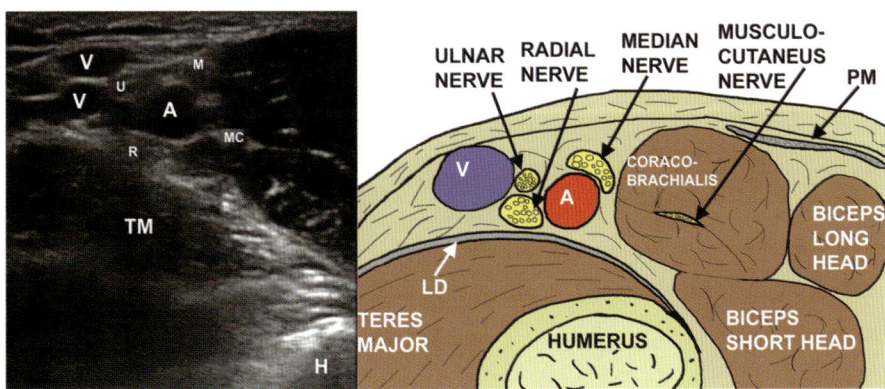

Figure 12.11 Sonographic anatomy of the brachial plexus in the axillary region: median nerve (M) ulnar nerve (U), radial nerve (R), musculocutaneous nerve (MC), axillary artery (A), axillary vein (V), humerus (H), teres major muscle (TM), pectoralis major tendon (PM), latissimus dorsi tendon (LD).

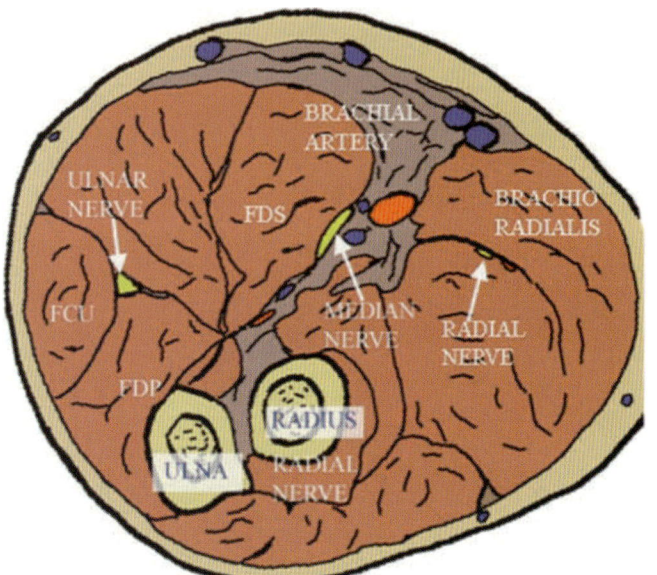

Figure 12.12 Diagram of cross-section at the cubital fossa, showing relations of radial, median, and ulnar nerves.

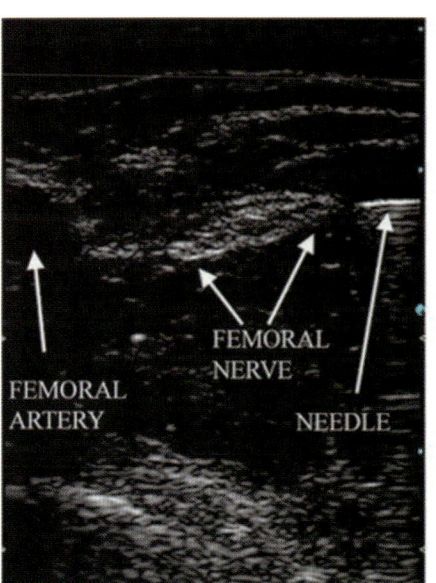
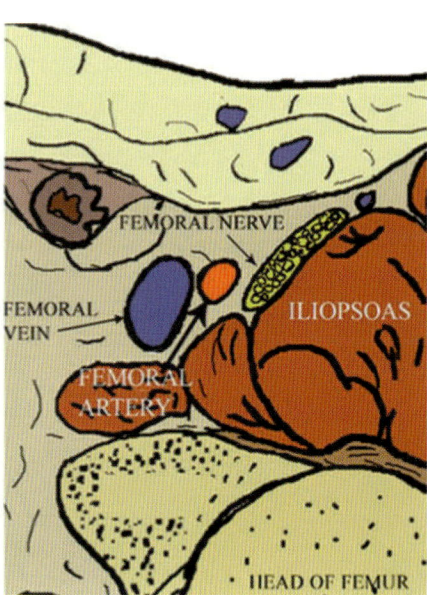

Figure 12.14 Sonographic anatomy of the femoral nerve below the inguinal ligament.

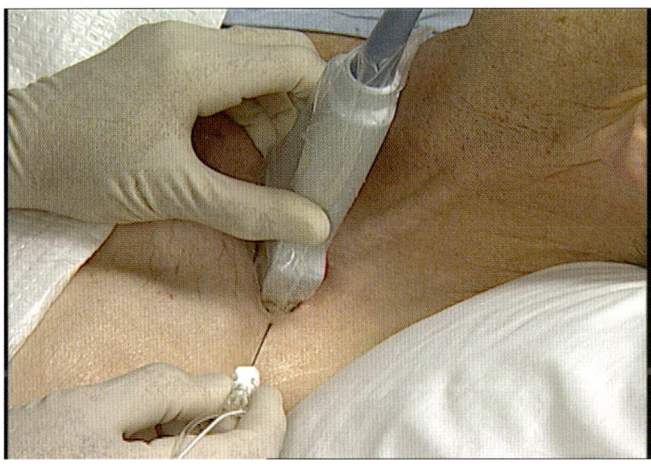

Figure 16.3 Ultrasound-guided supraclavicular block.

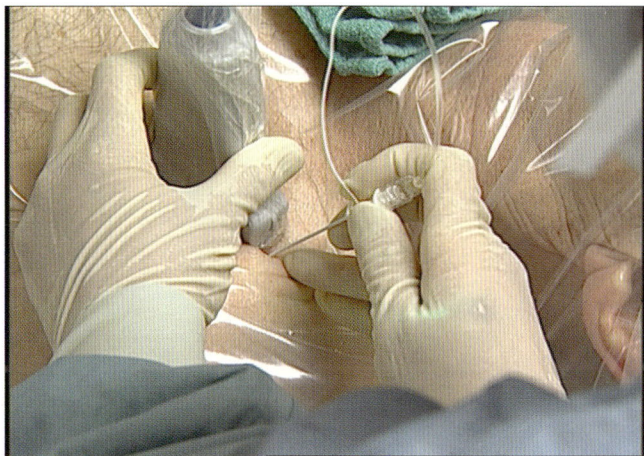

Figure 16.4 Ultrasound-guided infraclavicular block.

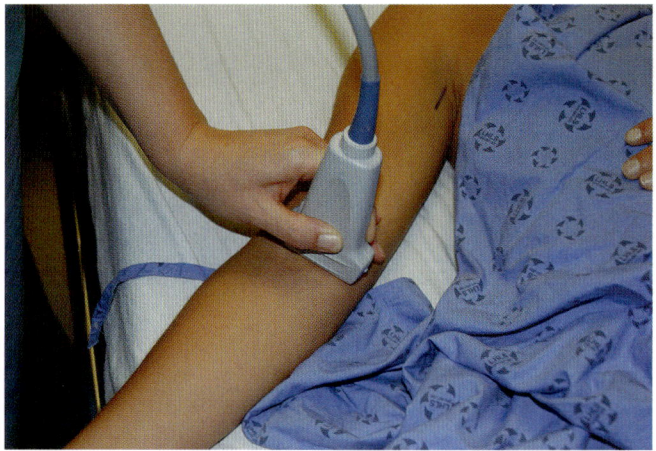

Figure 16.6 Scanning of median nerve at the elbow.

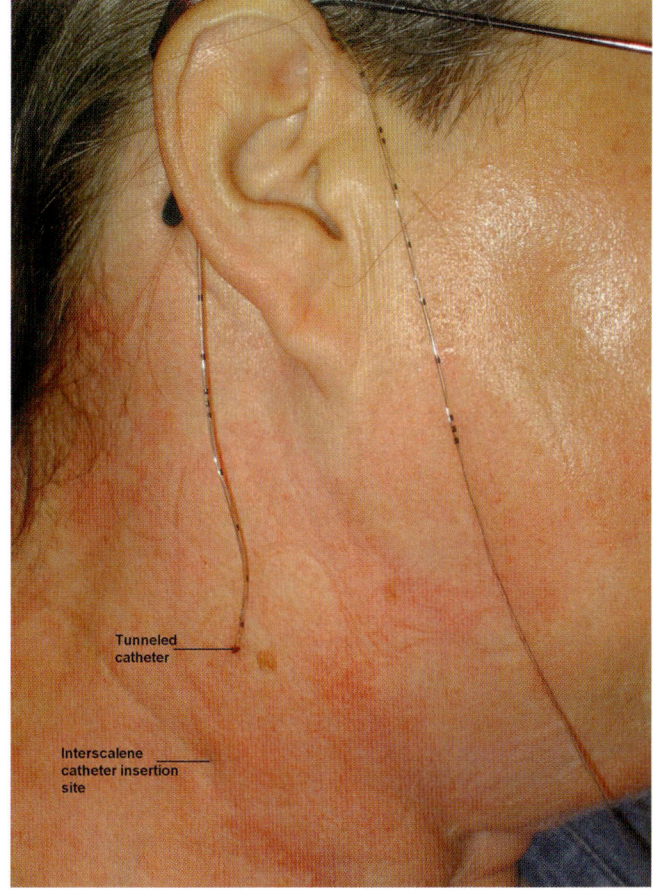

Tunneled
catheter

Interscalene
catheter insertion
site

Figure 16.13 Tunneling of catheter.

(A)

(B)

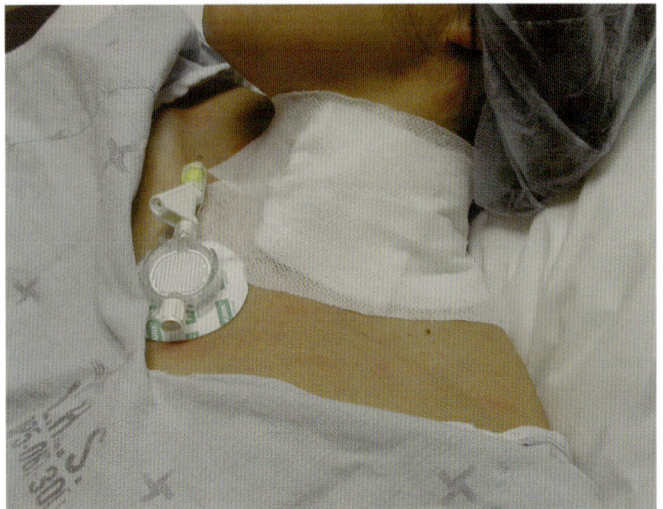
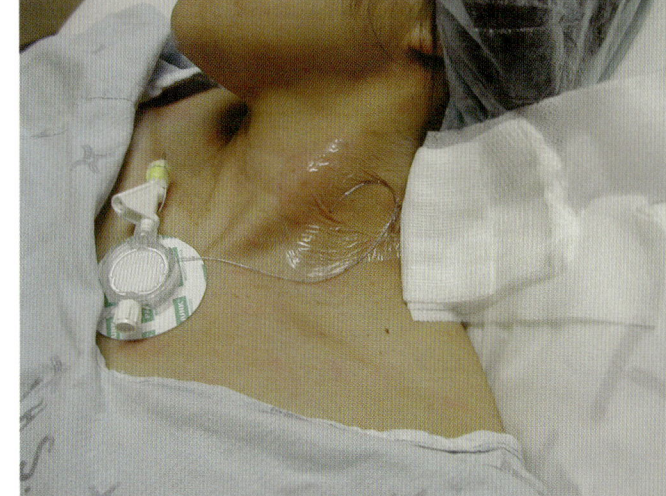

Figure 16.17 Surgeon-proof dressing.

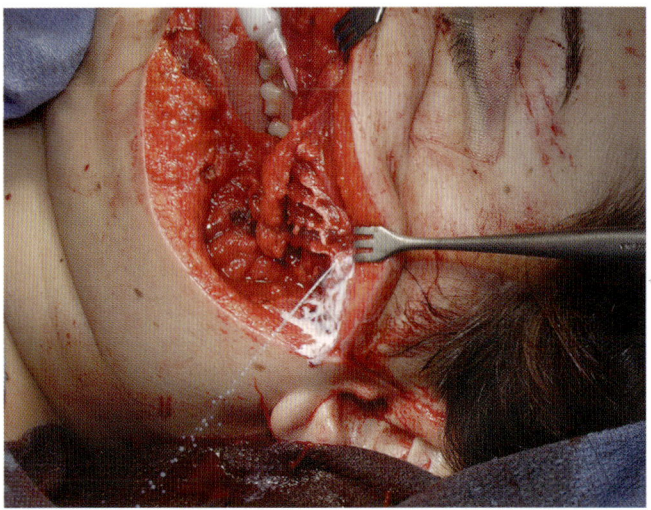

Figure 24.1 Full-thickness facial laceration through parotid duct.

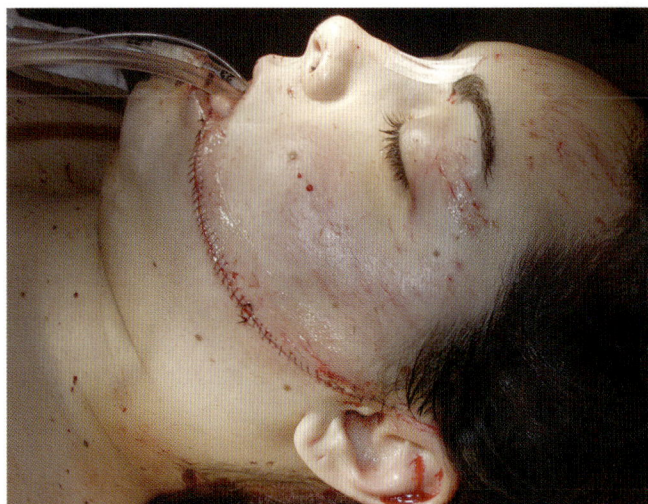

Figure 24.2 Same patient as in Figure 24.1. Propofol was used to identify the duct after cannulation.

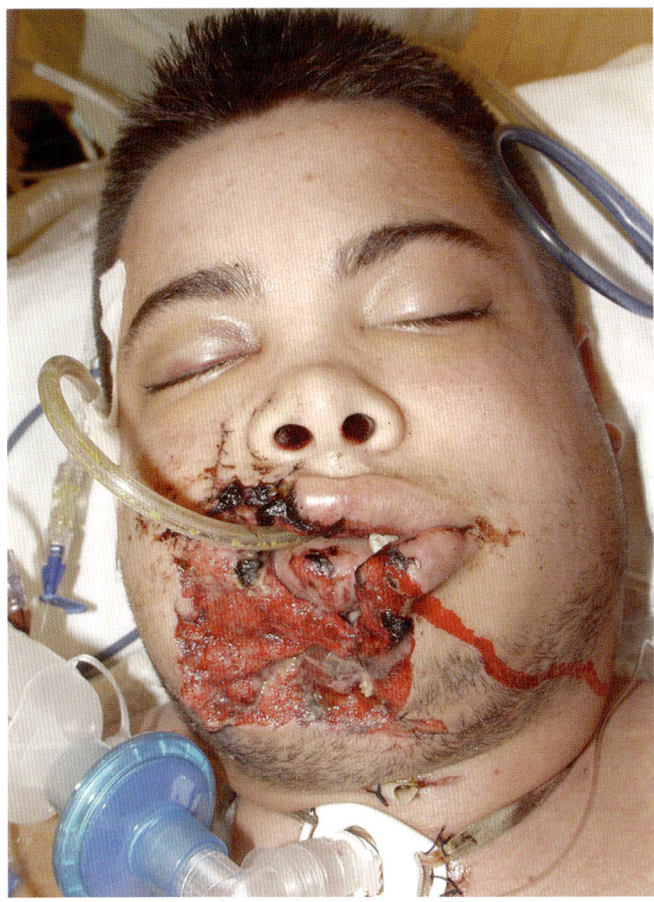

Figure 24.3 Complex lower facial soft tissue trauma after gunshot wound.

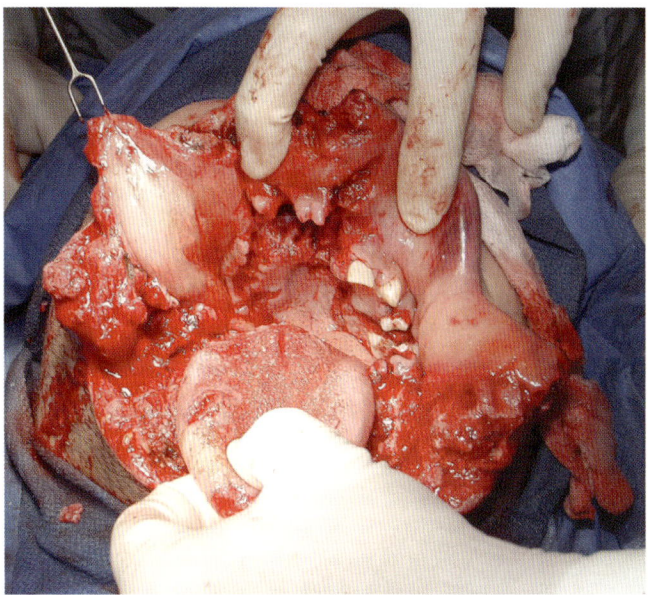

Figure 24.4 After tracheostomy and flap reflection, extensive soft tissue, hard tissue, and dentoalveolar trauma is seen.

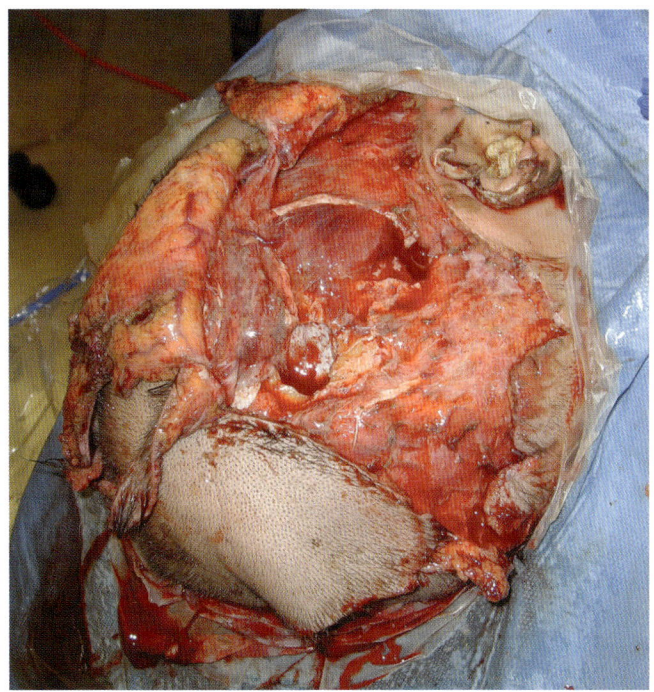

Figure 24.5 Complex scalp degloving injury in an unhelmeted motorcyclist.

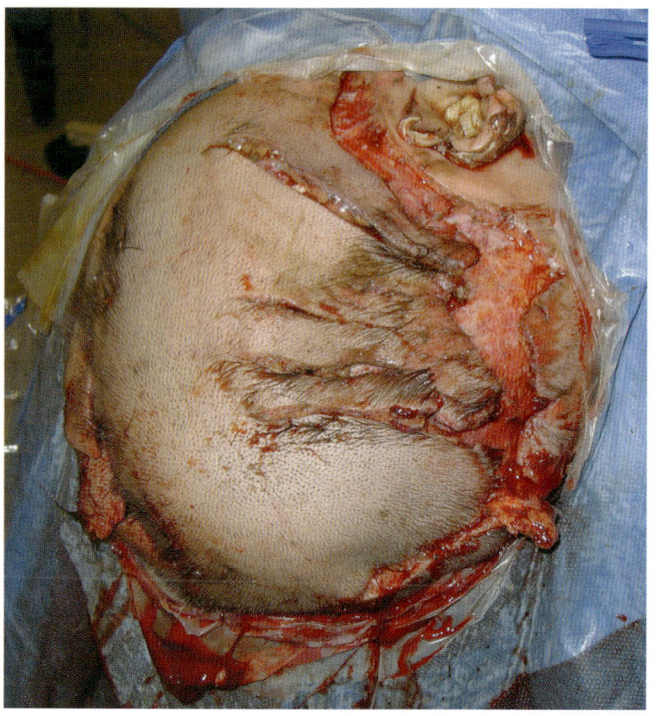

Figure 24.6 Tissue realigned, and rotational flaps utilized.

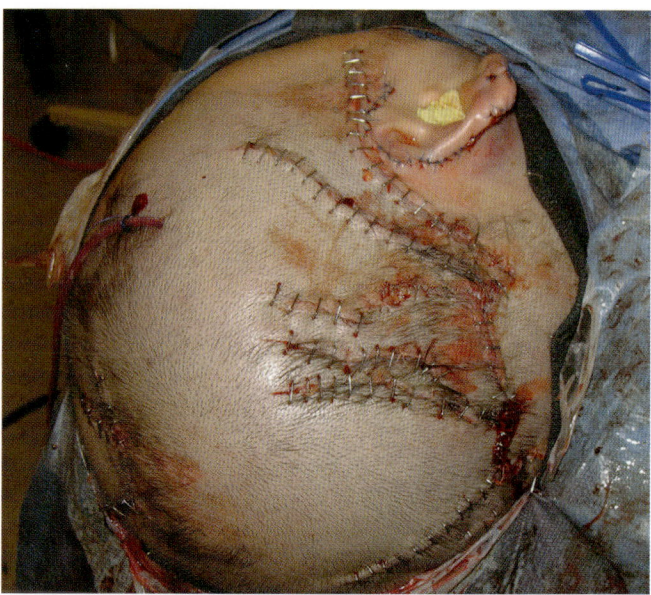

Figure 24.7 Primary repair of scalp laceration.

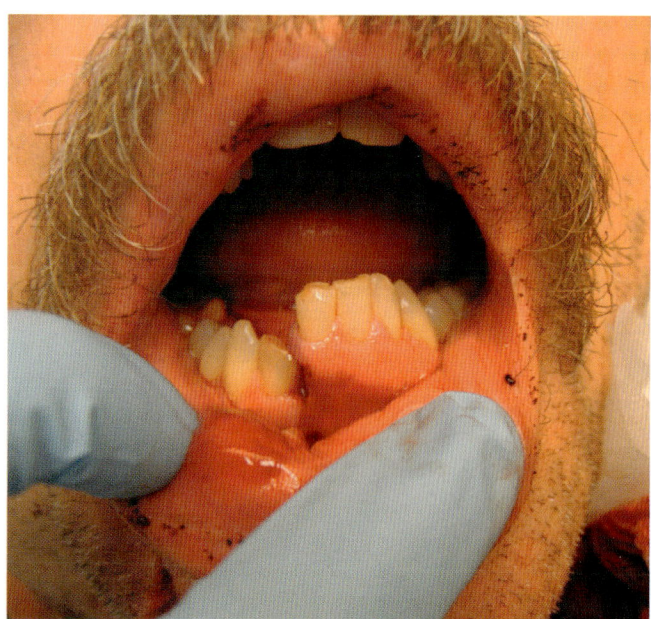

Figure 24.11 Clinic oral view of the patient in Figure 24.9 in the trauma bay.

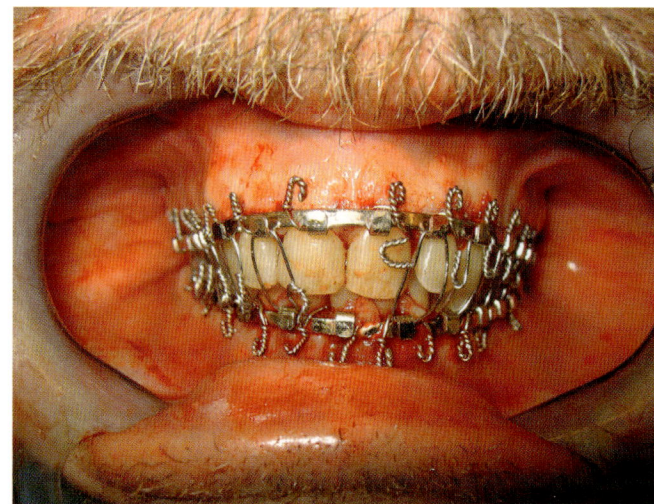

Figure 24.12 Clinical view of patient with maxillomandibular fixation (MMF) in place.

(A)

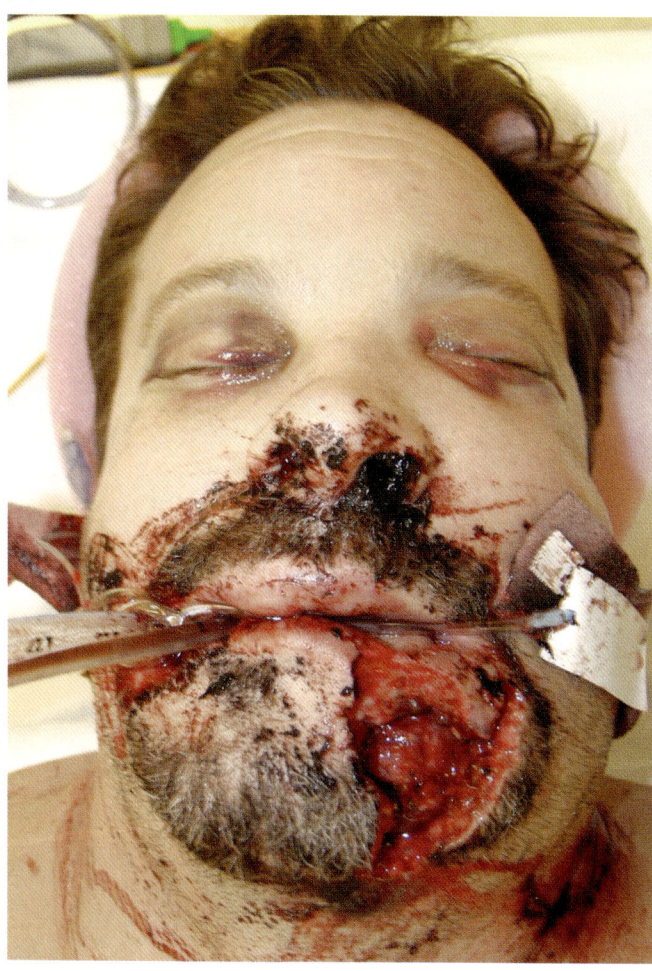

(B)

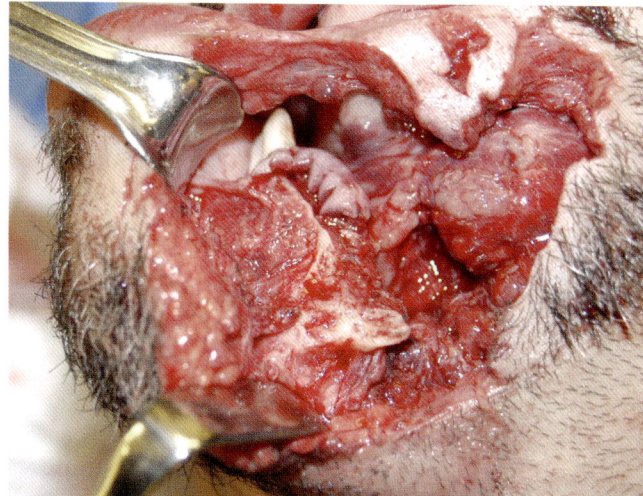

(C)

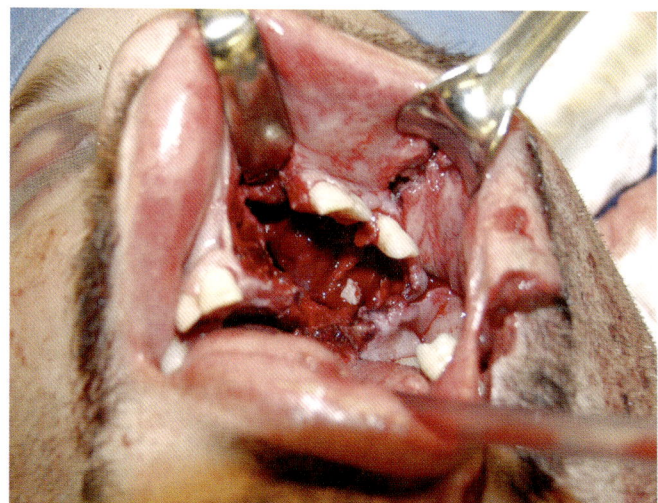

Figure 24.13 Clinical views of gunshot wound under chin with 357 handgun.

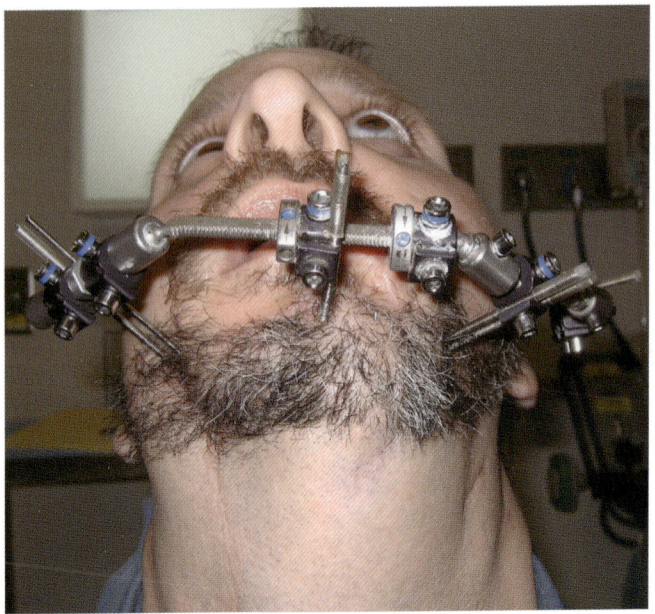

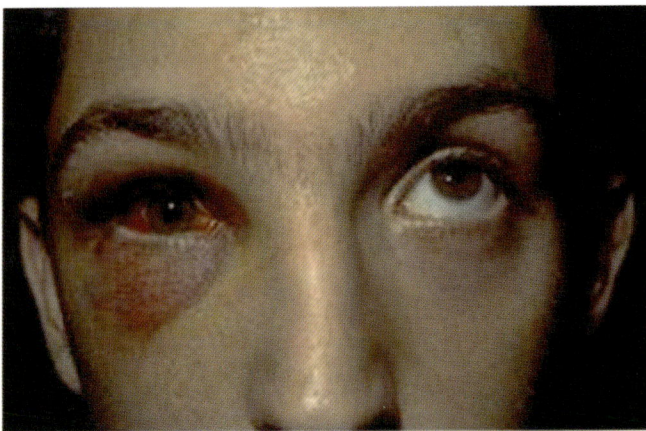

Figure 24.16 Clinical view of patient with right orbital floor fracture, with restricted superior gaze.

Figure 24.15 6 weeks postoperative view of patient with external pin fixation in place.

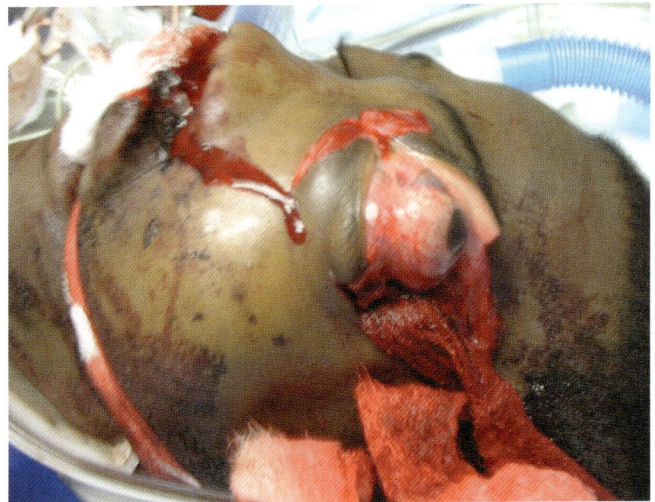

Figure 24.18 Clinical view of patient in trauma bay with extensive midface trauma.

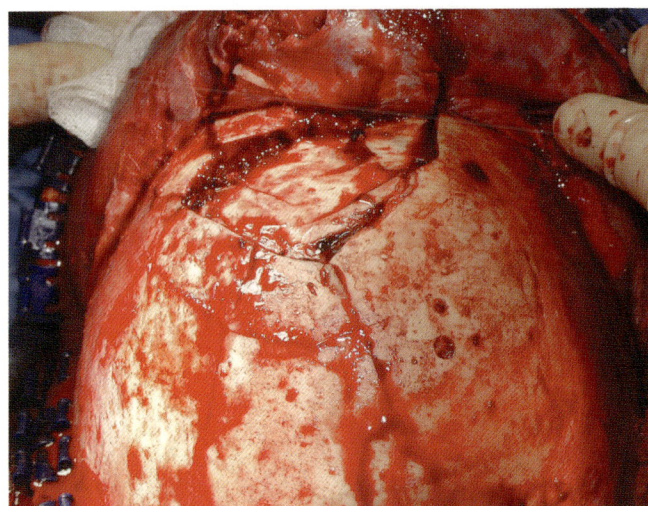

Figure 24.20 Surgical exposure of a patient with a comminuted frontal sinus fracture.

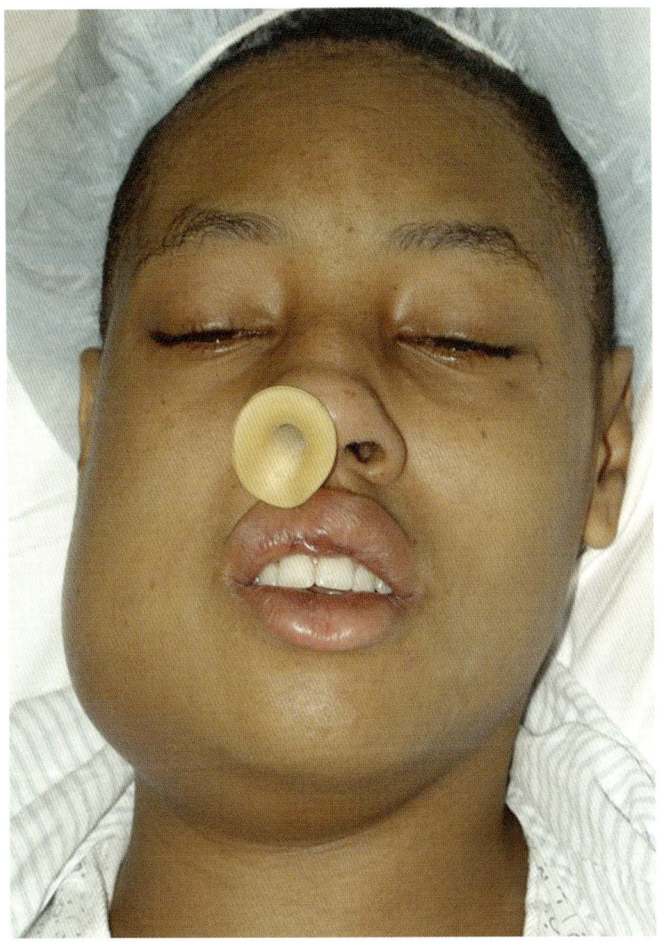

Figure 24.22 Clinical view of patient with Ludwig's angina, with nasal trumpet inserted to assist the airway temporarily.

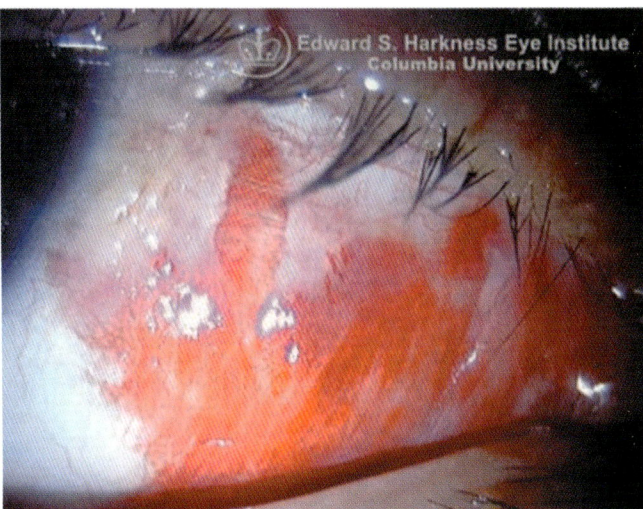

Figure 26.2 Conjunctival laceration with subconjunctival hemorrhage. This is an example of a closed-eye injury.

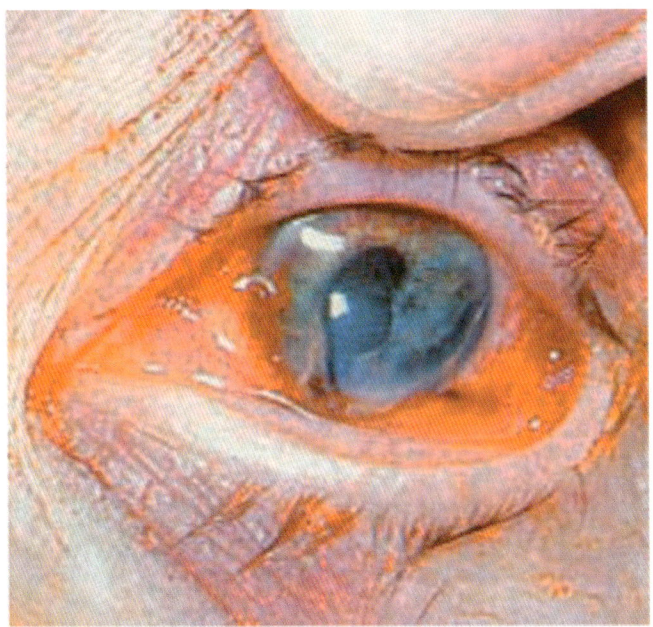

Figure 26.3 An open-eye injury resulting from trauma from a racquet.

(B)

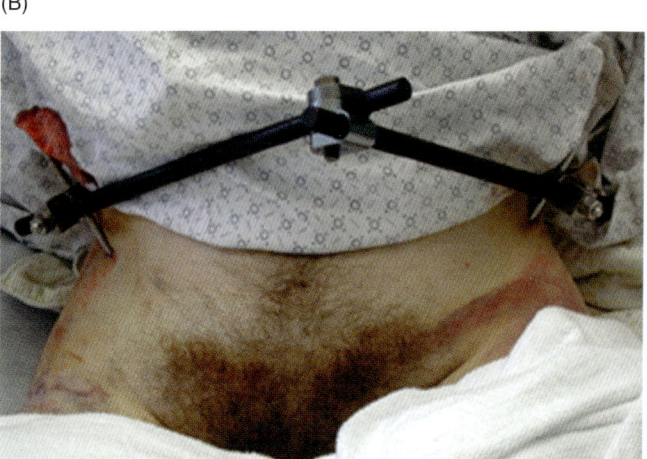

(C)

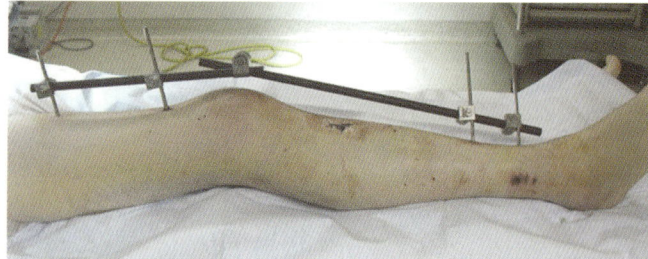

Figure 27.11 Knee dislocation. (**C**) A spanning external fixator has been placed across the knee joint to maintain the reduction of the knee.

Figure 27.8 Unstable pelvis fracture. (**B**) An anterior external fixator has been applied, as shown in the clinical photograph.

(B)

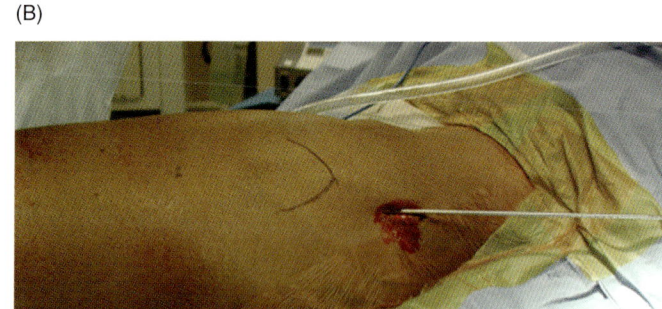

(C)

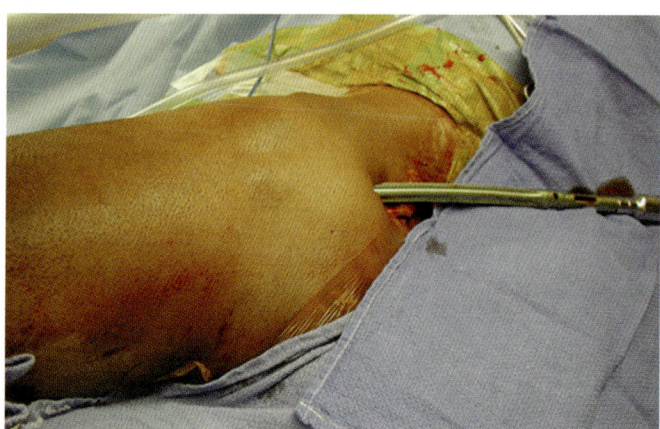

(D)

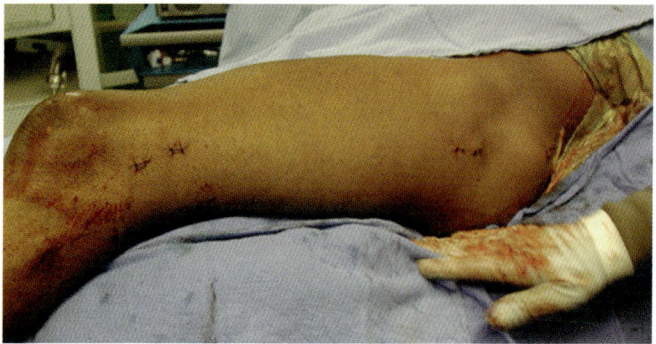

Figure 27.9 Intramedullary nailing of a femoral shaft fracture can be done percutaneously. (**B**) A wire placed with fluoroscopic assistance opens the femoral canal. (**C**) After reduction and reaming a nail is placed. Minimal surgical trauma occurs during this procedure. (**D**) This photograph demonstrates the small wounds from the nail and the locking bolts.

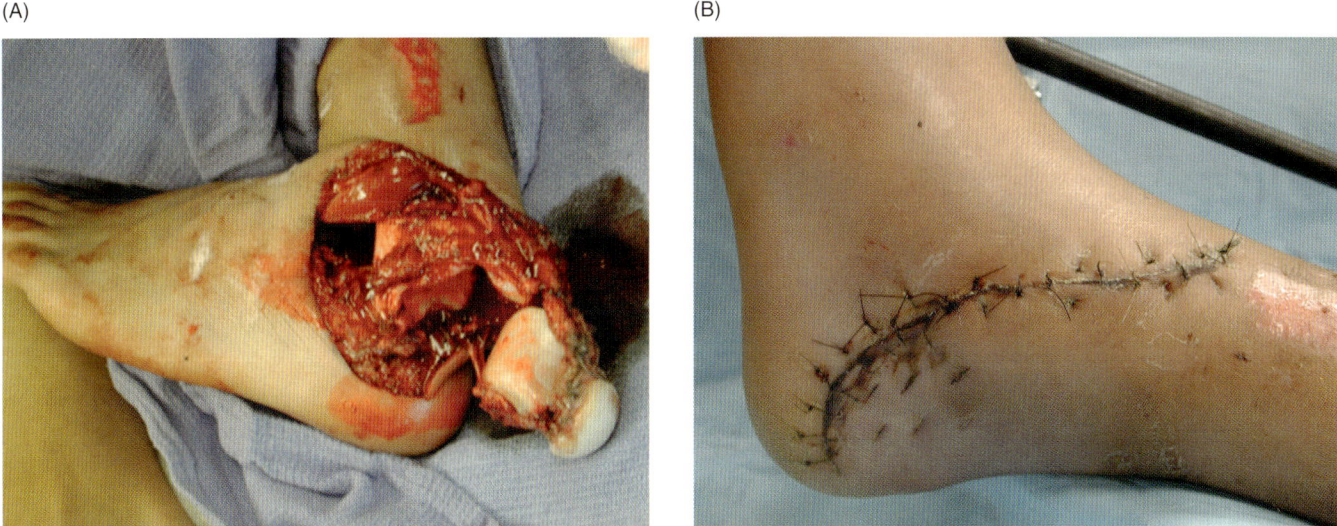

Figure 27.13 (**A**) A young man sustained injuries including an open dislocation of his talus. Emergent treatment was recommended to debride the wound and reduce the dislocation. (**B**) External fixation was used to stabilize the ankle and hindfoot.

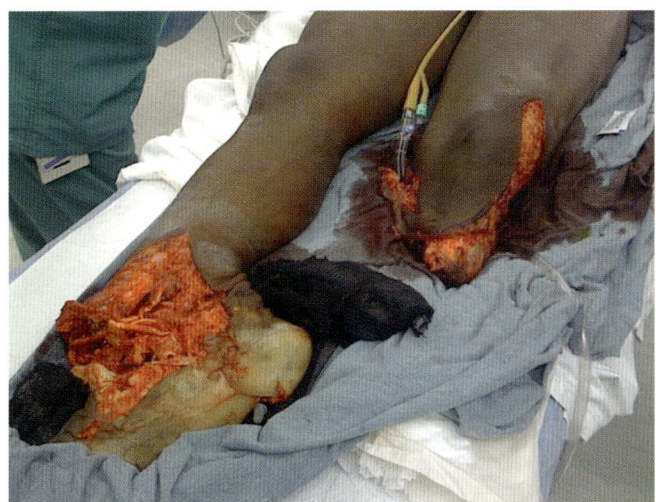

Figure 28.2 Bilateral amputations of the lower extremities.

(B)

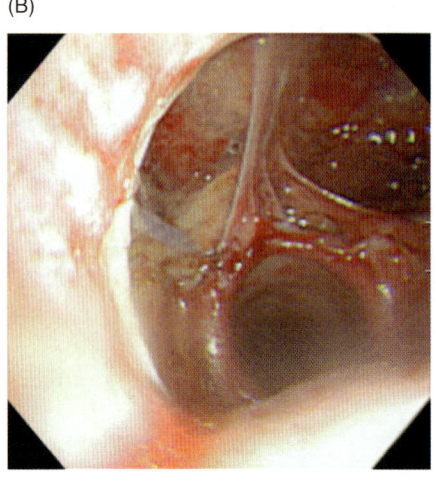

(C)

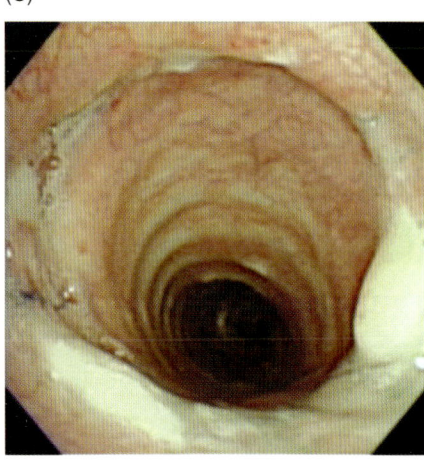

Figure 30.11 Tracheal transection secondary to blunt chest trauma. (**B**) Fiberoptic bronchoscopy through endotracheal tube reveals complete tracheal avulsion. (**C**) Trachea following surgical repair. (Used with permission from Shim *et al.* 2008.[77]).

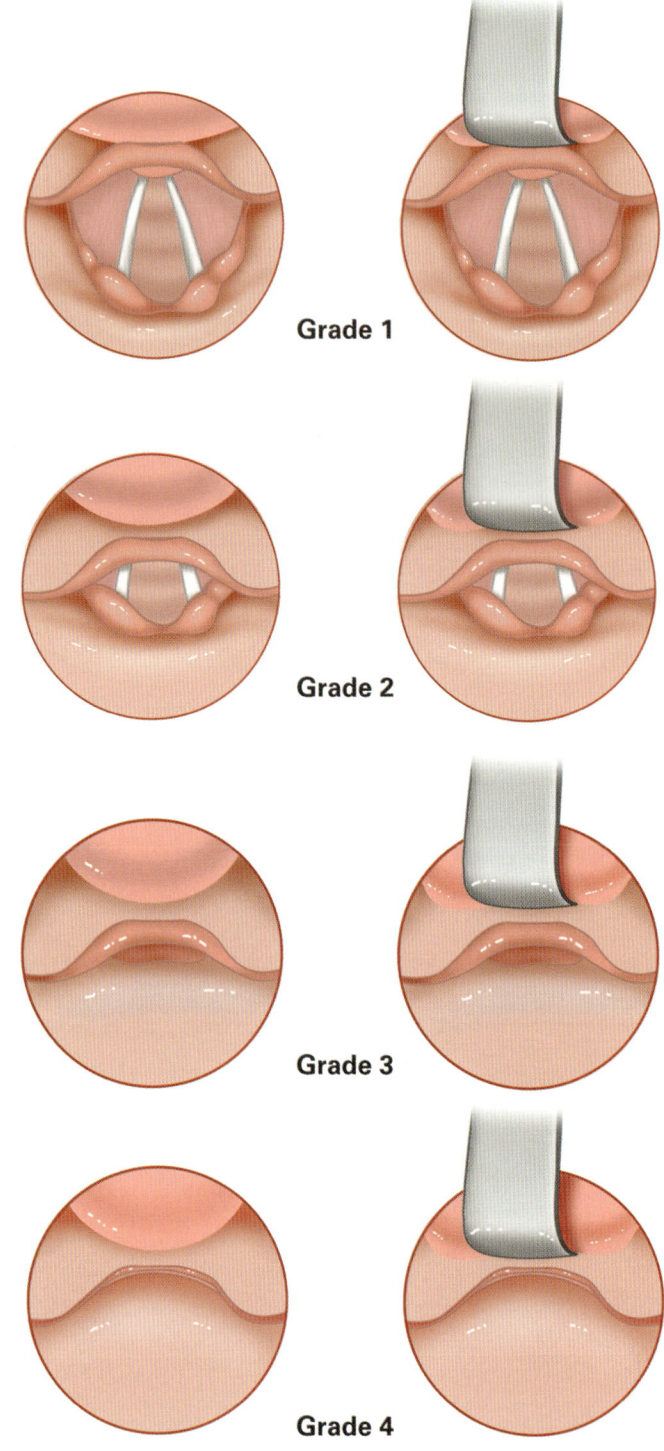

Grade 1

Grade 2

Grade 3

Grade 4

Cormack and Lehane Laryngeal Grades

Figure 34.5 Cormack and Lehane classification. Grading based on the degree of visualization of the glottic opening during direct laryngoscopy. Grade 1, entire glottis visible; grade 2, posterior portion of glottis visible; grade 3, only tip of epiglottis is visible; grade 4, only soft palate is visible. (Courtesy of medical illustrator at MetroHealth Medical Center; redrawn from Cormack and Lehane 1984.[36]).

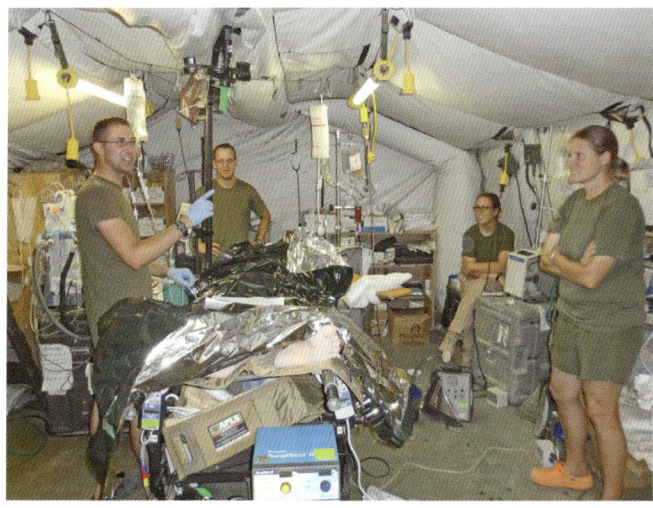

Figure 38.2 Role 2 field medical facility, Afghanistan, 2011. (Photo courtesy of C. Park.).

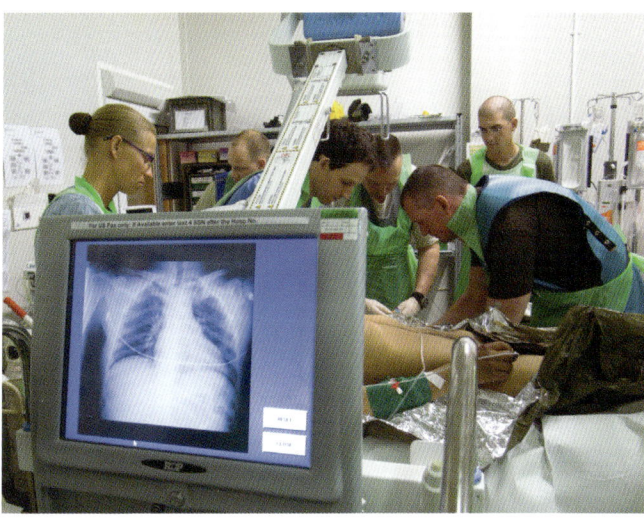

Figure 38.3 Casualty reception at the UK multinational Role 3 hospital, Afghanistan 2010. (Photo courtesy of N. Tarmey. Previously published inside the cover of *Journal of the Royal Army Medical Corps* 2010, Vol 156: reproduced with permission of the Editor.)

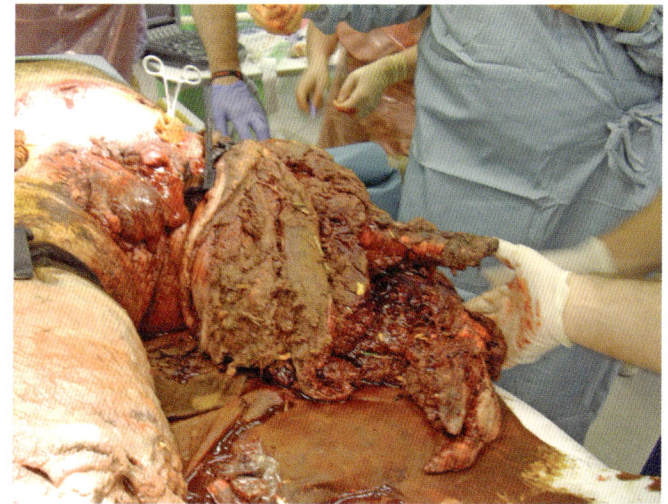

Figure 38.5 IED blast injury to the lower limbs, with proximal hemorrhage control from Combat Application Tourniquets and temporary surgical arterial ligation. (Reproduced from Parker 2011,[9] with permission of the Editor of the *Journal of the Royal Army Medical Corps*.).

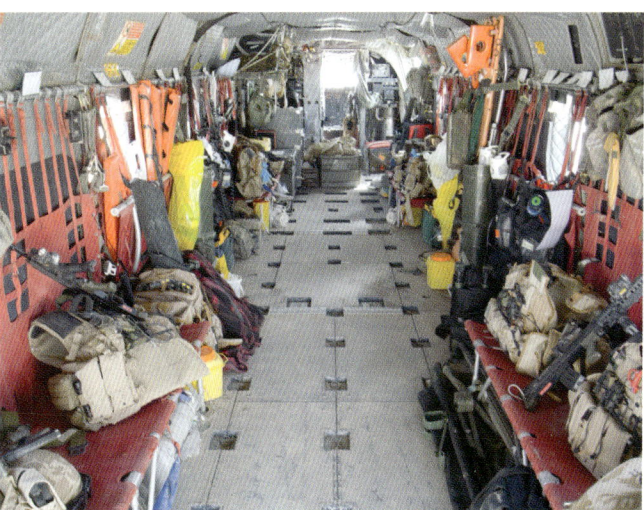

Figure 38.6 Chinook helicopter equipped for casualty evacuation by the UK Medical Emergency Response Team, Afghanistan, 2010. (Photo courtesy of N. Tarmey.).

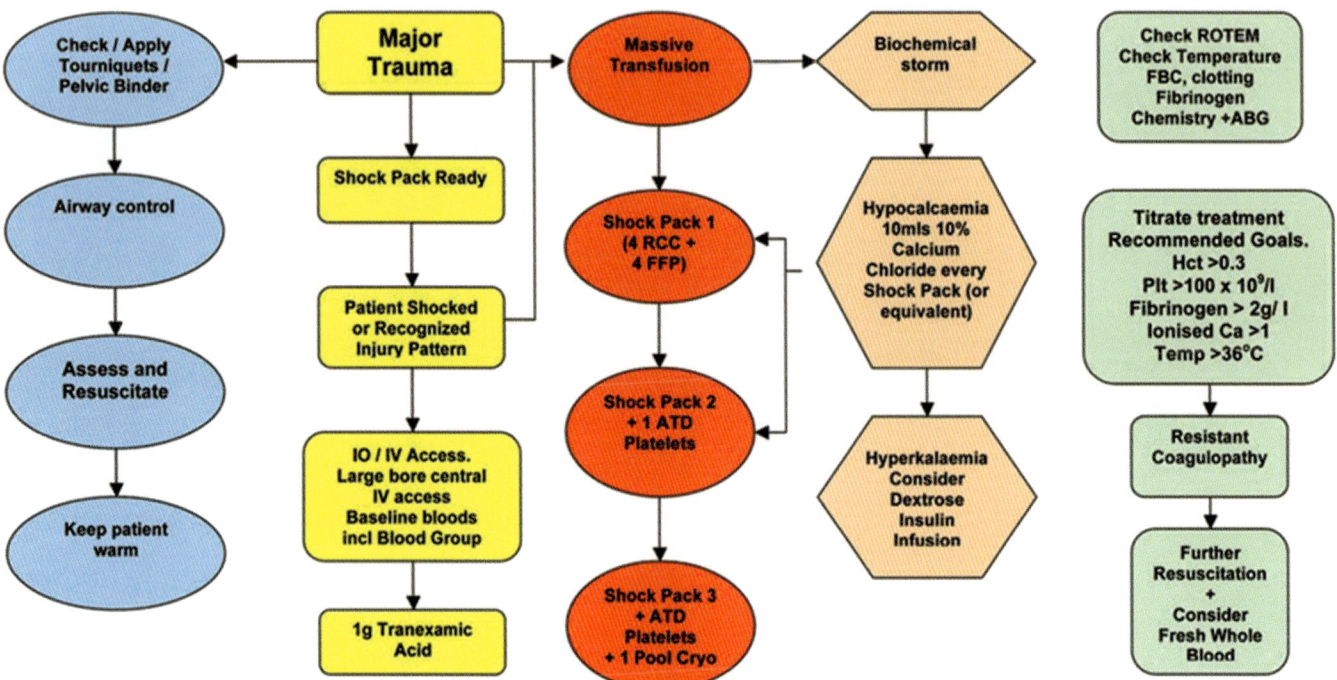

Guideline for the Transfusion Management of Major Ballistic Trauma

- Check / Apply Tourniquets / Pelvic Binder
- Airway control
- Assess and Resuscitate
- Keep patient warm

- **Major Trauma**
- Shock Pack Ready
- Patient Shocked or Recognized Injury Pattern
- IO / IV Access. Large bore central IV access Baseline bloods incl Blood Group
- 1g Tranexamic Acid

- **Massive Transfusion**
- Shock Pack 1 (4 RCC + 4 FFP)
- Shock Pack 2 + 1 ATD Platelets
- Shock Pack 3 + ATD Platelets + 1 Pool Cryo

- **Biochemical storm**
- Hypocalcaemia 10mls 10% Calcium Chloride every Shock Pack (or equivalent)
- Hyperkalaemia Consider Dextrose Insulin Infusion

- Check ROTEM Check Temperature FBC, clotting Fibrinogen Chemistry +ABG
- Titrate treatment Recommended Goals. Hct >0.3 Plt >100 x 10^9/l Fibrinogen > 2g/ l Ionised Ca >1 Temp >36°C
- Resistant Coagulopathy
- Further Resuscitation + Consider Fresh Whole Blood

Figure 38.7 UK military massive transfusion protocol. (Reproduced from Doughty et al. 2011,[18] with permission of the Editor of the *Journal of the Royal Army Medical Corps*.).

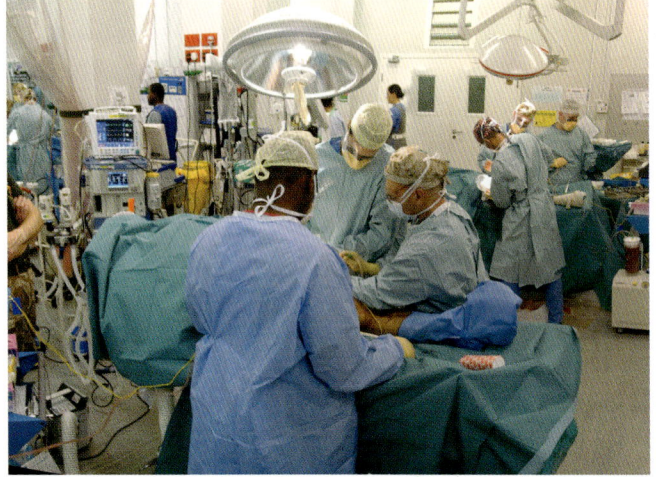

Figure 38.10 Three tables operating simultaneously at the UK Multinational Role 3 Hospital, Afghanistan, 2010. (Photo courtesy of N. Tarmey.).

and re-confirmed the effectiveness of the proper application of cricoid pressure at the post-cricoid hypopharynx.[25] In their MRI study, the hypopharynx and cricoid ring move together as a single anatomic unit, and it is this "anatomic unit" that is compressed by cricoid pressure. In addition, bimanual application of cricoid pressure may be preferable to a single-handed approach, to minimize cervical displacement.[24,25]

In terms of the induction agent of choice, one should carefully balance the importance of hemodynamic stability against the speed of onset. Hypotension is extremely detrimental to the injured brain, as discussed previously, while hypertension may increase ICP, worsening cerebral ischemia and causing cerebral herniation. It is important to emphasize that in the critically injured, the method of drug administration may be more important than the choice of anesthetic agent. Most of these patients are already severely obtunded, and they may not require full induction doses of the hypnotic agent. Since sodium thiopental is no longer available in the United States, propofol and etomidate are the only choices. Propofol decreases CBF via its effect on cerebral metabolic rate ($CMRO_2$), thereby decreasing ICP. However, it can cause severe hypotension, particularly in a hypovolemic patient (see Chapter 7).

The alternative choice is etomidate in doses of 0.2–0.3 mg/kg. This drug also decreases $CMRO_2$ and CBF but it has less effect on blood pressure. Etomidate use has been shown to inhibit adrenal hormone synthesis, with low plasma cortisol levels up to 24–48 hours after a single dose administration. This has the potential to complicate blood pressure management and may necessitate vasopressor use, and affect outcome. Care must be taken in the acutely unstable patient with the administration of any potent sedative–hypnotic drug, as it can also cause systemic hypotension. Small doses of opioids or intravenous lidocaine may be a suitable adjunct. Lidocaine, in doses of 1.0–1.5 mg/kg, decreases ICP with minimal hemodynamic effects. Neuromuscular blocking agents are routinely employed for tracheal intubation in the patient with TBI to provide excellent intubating conditions, facilitate prompt laryngoscopy, and eliminate coughing and fighting from an uncooperative patient (see Chapters 3 and 13). The main choice is between succinylcholine and rocuronium, the two agents with the fastest onset of action. It should be remembered that rocuronium, with its intermediate duration of action, may preclude neurologic examination for the next 60–90 minutes, although the availability of the reversal agent sugammadex may obviate this consideration (see Chapter 13). The main argument against the use of succinylcholine in patients with TBI is the potential increase in ICP. However, Kovarik et al. studied the effects of this drug in ventilated neurologically injured patients and observed no increase in ICP or cerebral blood flow velocity.[26] The detrimental effects of hypoxemia and hypercarbia generally outweigh any potential concern for ICP, making succinylcholine the preferred agent of choice. The initial ventilation parameters should include 100% oxygen; arterial carbon dioxide should be maintained in the low normal range (~35 mmHg). Ventilation strategy will be discussed further in the section on ventilation management, below (see also Chapter 19).

Circulation

The goal of resuscitation is to establish adequate systemic and cerebral circulation so that organ perfusion can be maintained. Blood pressure should be continuously monitored, and hypotension (systolic blood pressure < 90 mmHg) should be avoided. Isotonic intravenous fluid should be administered as necessary to restore intravascular volume and to prevent hypotension. The goal is to maintain cerebral perfusion pressure (CPP = mean arterial blood pressure – ICP) in the range 60–70 mmHg, as recommended by the Brain Trauma Foundation guidelines.[21] Hypotonic fluids should be avoided (Table 21.3). The role of colloids is controversial. According to the Saline versus Albumin Fluid Evaluation (SAFE) study, resuscitation of TBI patients with 4% albumin in the ICU is associated with a higher mortality rate and a less favorable neurologic outcome at 6 as well as at 24 months.[27] With regard to hydroxylethyl starch (HES), a further degree of caution is required, given the findings on the recent clinical trial on the administration of HES 130/0.4. The Crystalloid versus Hydroxyethyl Starch Trial (CHEST) has shown no mortality benefit but increased adverse events, including renal injury and requirement for renal replacement therapy. In the presence of significantly increased risk, and in the absence of compelling evidence of therapeutic efficacy, neither HES nor albumin should be used in patients with acute brain injury.[28,29] As for the use of hypertonic saline as a resuscitation fluid in the prehospital phase to improve neurologic outcome in patients with TBI, a multicenter randomized controlled trial was terminated early due to futility.[30] Vasopressors and inotropes may be needed after fluid resuscitation to achieve the desired CPP, but CPP > 70 mmHg should be avoided, as the use of vasopressors in this manner has been shown to increase the risk of acute respiratory distress syndrome (ARDS). In the absence of ICP monitoring, or until ICP monitoring has been established in a patient with documented TBI, mean arterial pressure (MAP) should be maintained in the 70–80 mmHg range. This recommendation is based on the assumption that ICP is between 10 and 20 mmHg.

Neurologic exam

It is important to determine the neurologic status of all patients suffering from TBI. The Glasgow Coma Scale (GCS) is a useful measure because of its simplicity and low interobserver variability. In addition, it provides important information to guide the management decisions as well as to indicate prognosis. GCS has three parameters: eye opening, vocal response, and motor response (Table 21.4). A score of 13–15 is considered mild head injury, 9–12 is a moderate head injury, and 3–8 is a severe head injury. The score should be calculated once the patient has been resuscitated and is normotensive.

Table 21.3 Intravenous fluids

Fluids	Osmolality (mOsm/kg)	Oncotic pressure (mmHg)	Na⁺ (mEq/L)	Cl⁻ (mEq/L)	K⁺ (mEq/L)	Ca²⁺/Mg²⁺ (mEq/L)	Glucose (g/L)
Plasma*	289	21	141	103	4–5	5/2	
Crystalloid							
0.9% saline	308	0	154	154			
0.45% saline	154	0	77	77			
3% saline	1030	0	515	515			
7.5% saline	2400	0	1200	1200			
LR	273	0	130	109		3/0	
D₅ LR	527	0	130	109	4	3/0	50
D₅W*	252	0					50
D₅ NS*	586	0	154	154			50
D₅ 0.45% NS*	406	0	77	77			50
Plasma-Lyte	294	0	140	98	5	0/3	
Mannitol (20%)	1098	0					
Colloid							
Hetastarch (6%)	310	31	154	154			
Albumin (5%)	290	19					

D₅W, 5% dextrose in water; LR, lactated Ringer's; Na, sodium; Cl, chloride; K, potassium; Ca, calcium; Mg, magnesium.
* Osmolality of dextrose solutions decreases as glucose enters the cells.

Table 21.4 Glasgow Coma Scale (GCS) scores

Eye opening		Verbal response		Motor response	
Spontaneous	4	Oriented	5	Obeys commands	6
To speech	3	Confused	4	Localizes to pain	5
To pain	2	Inappropriate	3	Withdraws to pain	4
None	1	Incomprehensible	2	Flexes to pain	3
		None	1	Extends to pain	2
				None	1

The status of the pupils should also be obtained. The presence of a unilateral dilated pupil suggests transtentorial herniation and is a surgical emergency, while the presence of dilated pupils bilaterally portends a dismal prognosis.

Monitoring
Computed tomography

CT has become essential in the diagnosis and management of head-injured patients (see Chapters 11 and 20). Most often patients will have serial exams in the first 24 hours after injury to document either lesion stability or extension of injury. CT scan classification of injury patterns is based on the work of

Marshall and colleagues, who classified lesions into six groups.[31] In diffuse injury I, there is no evidence of intracranial pathology. In diffuse injury II, the basal cisterns are patent and there is a midline shift of 0–5 mm. In addition there are no high- or mixed-density lesions larger than 25 mL. Diffuse injury III is characterized by a midline shift of 0–5 mm with compression of the basal cisterns and no high- or mixed-density lesions larger than 25 mL. In diffuse injury IV there is more than 5 mm of midline shift with compression or absence of the basal cisterns and no high- or mixed-density lesions larger than 25 mL. There are also categories for evacuated lesions and mass lesions of more than 25 mL. This classification scheme also provides prognostic information.

Cerebral perfusion monitors
Transcranial Doppler ultrasonography

Transcranial Doppler (TCD) ultrasonography is a noninvasive monitor used for measuring flow velocity in large cerebral vessels and assumes constant cerebral vessel diameter to estimate blood flow. It can provide information on arterial patency, ICP, pressure autoregulation, and vasoreactivity, and it can be used as a confirmatory test supporting the clinical diagnosis of brain death. Its use as an important clinical adjunct in the management of TBI patients has not been

Table 21.5 Indications for intracranial pressure (ICP) monitoring

Strong indication	Severe head injury (GCS ≤ 8) with abnormal CT scan of head Severe head injury, normal head CT, with at least two of the following: • Age ≥ 40 years • Motor posturing • Systolic blood pressure ≤90 mmHg
Possible indication	Head injury and unable to follow neurologic exam due to: • Unable to perform neuro exam (tracheal intubation and deep sedation or paralysis) • Urgent non-neurosurgical procedure

GCS, Glasgow coma scale score; CT, computed tomography.

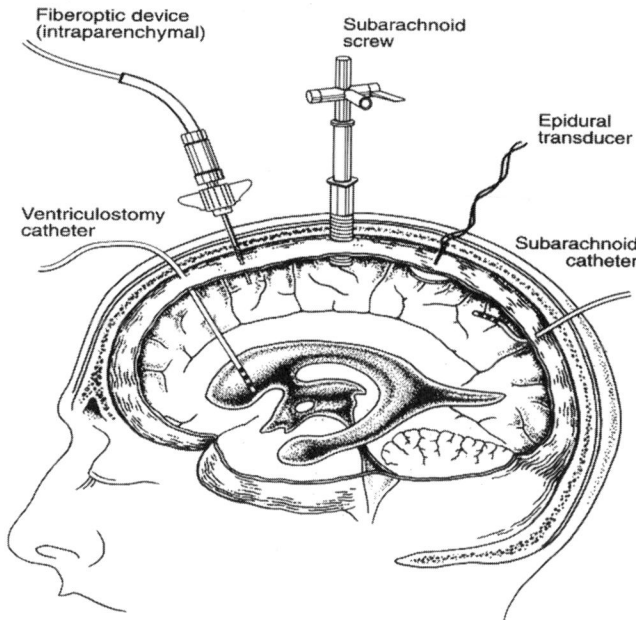

Figure 21.5 Different modalities to monitor intracranial pressure (ICP).

established. It is potentially valuable in patients with traumatic subarachnoid hemorrhage, as vasospasm can develop in 20–40% of these patients.

Laser Doppler flowmetry

Regional CBF can be measured invasively using laser Doppler flowmetry (LDF), which provides qualitative CBF information on a small volume of tissue (typically 1 mm³) and allows rapid detection of regional perfusion changes. The data are expressed in LDF units, and can be influenced by the presence of underlying major vessels, hemodilution, and various artifacts (patient movement or displacement). LDF requires a burr hole. This is an experimental tool in the management of patients with TBI.

Intracranial pressure monitoring

ICP monitoring has become standard in patients with severe TBI (see Chapter 20), even in the absence of evidence demonstrating an outcome benefit of this monitor. Treatment guidelines, including those of the Brain Trauma Foundation, base therapy on CPP, which requires monitoring of ICP.[32,33]

An ICP monitor is recommended in all patients with GCS ≤ 8 and an abnormal head CT on admission (Table 21.5). Though controversial, some studies have demonstrated that centers that use ICP monitoring less than what is indicated in Brain Trauma Foundation guidelines have a significantly higher mortality.[34] It is estimated that 53–63% of patients with severe TBI will suffer from intracranial hypertension. Earlier studies have established the value of intracranial hypertension as a negative prognostic outcome indicator. Patients with GCS ≤ 8 and exhibiting two of the following three characteristics – age more than 40 years, motor posturing, or systolic blood pressure < 90 mmHg – should also be monitored. Patients with mild or moderate head injuries can usually be managed without ICP monitoring if serial clinical examinations are feasible. A group of patients who deserve special consideration are those whose clinical conditions per se do not warrant ICP monitoring, but who have to undergo general anesthesia or sedation for a long duration (e.g., > 2 hours), negating the opportunity of serial neurologic exam. Intracranial hematomas and cerebral edema may appear or worsen after the initial CT scan for up to 48 hours after the injury; frequent neurologic examinations or continuous ICP monitoring is particularly justified during this time period. Patients with mild to moderate TBI should be individualized and discussed with the neurosurgical service prior to surgery with regard to the need for intraoperative ICP monitoring.

There are different techniques for monitoring ICP (Fig. 21.5). The gold standard is an intraventricular catheter (ventriculostomy). The catheter is inserted into the lateral ventricle through a small frontal burr hole, usually on the right side. The catheter is connected to an external pressure transducer and can be recalibrated as needed to maintain accuracy. The external auditory meatus is taken as a reference point. In addition, it allows therapeutic intervention for intracranial hypertension via drainage of CSF. Its main disadvantage is an increased risk of infection (up to 30%), as well as increased risk of hemorrhage. Less accurate but less invasive is a parenchymal catheter inserted into the brain. This system is relatively easy to insert and is associated with fewer complications (< 2%). Various transducer systems exist for the parenchymal catheter: external strain gauge (pneumatic), internal strain gauge (measures change in resistance), microchip or fiberoptic (measures change in light reflection). The preferred method of monitoring is the ventriculostomy, which allows practitioners to both monitor ICP and drain CSF. It is also the most accurate system. The fiberoptic parenchymal catheter uses a smaller burr hole, and is easier to insert but allows only the monitoring of ICP. The other methods are used less frequently. Whereas the intraventricular catheter with the external pressure transducer can be recalibrated as necessary, the parenchymal ICP monitor is calibrated prior to insertion without the possibility of recalibration. As a result, drift impairs the accuracy of this type of monitor over time (but is generally regarded as negligible). Other types of ICP monitors include epidural systems and subarachnoid bolts. These monitors are thought to be less accurate than the ventricular catheter and the parenchymal fiberoptic monitor, and are used infrequently.

The normal upper limit of ICP is 10–15 mmHg, and most authorities recommend treatment when the ICP exceeds 20–25 mmHg. Specific therapies to decrease ICP will be discussed in the *Management principles* section, below. The ICP tracing has normal variability over the course of the cardiac cycle. Prolonged elevation in ICP is known to be pathologic. However, recent evidence has shown that even a brief number of episodes are also predictive of a poor outcome, which may justify a more proactive treatment.[35]

As mentioned above, ICP monitoring had been established as a standard early on, precluding the possibility of conducting any randomized controlled trials in the developed countries. In a recent landmark multicenter randomized clinical trial conducted in South America, Chesnut *et al.* reported that ICU care focused on maintaining ICP ≤ 20 mmHg (as guidelines recommend) to avoid poor outcome was not superior to care based on serial CT and neurologic clinical examination.[36] However, there are many confounding factors in the study, including the protracted prehospital transport time. The general consensus is that the results from this trial do not invalidate the potential utility of ICP monitoring in TBI, but rather it emphasizes the importance of serial CT imaging and careful clinical examination as part of the management paradigm.

Cerebral oxygenation monitors

Jugular venous oxygenation

A jugular venous bulb catheter allows measurement of the oxygen saturation of the venous drainage from the brain ($SjvO_2$) (see Chapter 9). This catheter allows continuous monitoring of jugular venous pressure as well as intermittent withdrawal of a venous blood sample for gas and lactate analysis. Continuous monitoring of $SjvO_2$ can be achieved using a fiberoptic oximetric catheter inserted via a conduit. Confirmation of catheter placement is usually made with a lateral cervical spine film, on which the tip of the catheter should lie above the inferior border of C1. For the best representation of the metabolic state of the brain, the catheter should be placed in the dominant jugular vein, most commonly the right side. Side dominance can also be predicted using ultrasound, where the dominant vein appears larger.

To compensate for inadequate perfusion or low oxygen-carrying capacity, the brain increases oxygen extraction from hemoglobin, causing a decrease in $SjvO_2$. On the other hand, a metabolically quiescent brain extracting little oxygen will result in a high $SjvO_2$ value. An $SjvO_2$ below 50% or higher than 75%

in severe TBI has been associated with poor prognosis. Continuous $SjvO_2$ monitoring is particularly useful in TBI when a measure such as hyperventilation, which reduces global CBF without reducing cerebral metabolic rate, is used. In addition, lactate levels on blood samples drawn from this catheter can reveal anaerobic metabolism in the brain. The limitation of the jugular bulb catheter is that it only offers insight into the global balance of CBF and metabolism. A study using PET showed that 13% of the brain has to be ischemic before $SjvO_2$ falls below 50%.[37]

Brain tissue oxygenation

The brain tissue PO_2 ($PbtO_2$) monitor allows continuous direct measurement of local brain tissue oxygen supply and demand balance. The polarographic sensor-mounted catheter can be inserted into the brain parenchyma during a craniotomy in the operating room or through a burr hole at the bedside. The devices most widely used employ one of two different techniques: Clark electrode (most common) or optical technique.

An adequate CPP in TBI is encouraging, but does not guarantee an adequate blood supply to meet the metabolic needs of the brain. $PbtO_2$ complements ICP information in that it provides insight into oxygen delivery and consumption. A level below 15 mmHg is concerning for cerebral hypoxia, and warrants intervention in TBI. In nonrandomized clinical studies of patients with TBI, $PbtO_2$ has been shown to correlate well with treatment effects and outcome.[38,39] Despite these studies, the role of $PbtO_2$ monitoring in the management of TBI remains controversial. A randomized controlled trial on the utility of $PbtO_2$ in patients with TBI is under way as of 2012.

Accuracy of $PbtO_2$ will depend on the zone of insertion (normal vs. injured vs. at-risk tissue) and depth of insertion. The probe should be positioned near tissue that is at risk and potentially salvageable, and under a subdural hematoma. Eloquent locations (sensory, motor, language, visual cortex, hypothalamus and thalamus, internal capsule, brainstem) should be avoided. When structurally normal tissue is monitored, probes should be placed in the subcortical white matter of the more injured hemisphere.

Normal brain tissue oxygen tension has a wide variability and is dependent on both normal arterial PO_2, at about 90 mmHg, and venous PO_2, at about 35 mmHg. Most importantly, there is a dominant ($> 70\%$) venous microcirculation. Thus, it is assumed that $PbtO_2$ mainly reflects venous PO_2.

In practical terms, $PbtO_2$ values of 10–20 mmHg have been suggested as a threshold for initiating measures to raise brain tissue oxygenation.[40] As $PbtO_2$ typically increases with increase in PaO_2, the ratio of $PbtO_2$ to PaO_2 has also been suggested as a useful threshold, but this is much less well documented.

Interventions that increase CBF, decrease $CMRO_2$, or increase the oxygen content of blood would improve brain tissue oxygenation. Such interventions include raising CPP,

Table 21.6 Summary of Brain Trauma Foundation recommendations for severe TBI

Blood pressure (BP)	Monitor and avoid hypotension (systolic < 90 mmHg).
Hyperosmolar therapy	Mannitol is the preferred choice.
Intracranial pressure (ICP)	ICP monitoring is recommended when there is a risk of intracranial hypertension. Ventricular catheter with external pressure transducer is the preferred choice. Parenchymal catheter is the alternative when ventriculostomy cannot be performed, or if there is an obstruction in the fluid couple. Treat when ICP is > 20 mmHg.
Cerebral perfusion pressure (CPP)	Treat with fluid and vasopressors to maintain CPP 50–70 mmHg.
Brain oxygenation	Jugular venous oxygen saturation (SjO_2) and brain tissue oxygen monitoring recommended in addition to standard ICP monitors. Treat when SjO_2 < 50% or brain tissue oxygen tension < 15 mmHg.
Oxygenation	Monitor and avoid hypoxia (PaO_2 < 60 mmHg or oxygen saturation < 90%).
Arterial carbon dioxide ($PaCO_2$)	Prophylactic hyperventilation ($PaCO_2$ ≤ 25 mmHg) is not recommended. Hyperventilation is recommended as a temporizing measure for the reduction of elevated ICP.
Temperature	Prophylactic hypothermia is not significantly associated with decreased all-cause mortality. Hypothermia may have higher chances of reducing mortality when cooling is maintained for more than 48 hours.
Glucose control	Hyperglycemia is associated with worsened outcome.
Thromboprophylaxis	Intermittent pneumatic compression stockings and low-dose heparin or low molecular weight heparin recommended for deep venous thrombosis prophylaxis
Antiseizure prophylaxis	Anticonvulsants are indicated within 7 days of injury. Anticonvulsants are not recommended for late posttraumatic seizure prophylaxis.
Steroids	Steroids do not improve outcome or lower ICP, and increase complications.

using sedative drugs to suppress $CMRO_2$, or optimizing hematocrit. Because of the limited amount of oxygen that is dissolved in the blood apart from hemoglobin, increasing the PaO_2 alone would not be expected to raise $PbtPO_2$.

Paradoxically, increasing FiO_2 frequently does raise $PbtPO_2$, and is often deployed, even when the saturation of hemoglobin is already at or near 100%.

Near-infrared spectroscopy

Near-infrared spectroscopy (NIRS) is a noninvasive method of detecting cerebral tissue oxygenation. It is based on reflectance spectroscopy and measures the light reflected from chromophobes in the brain (hemoglobin) to derive the regional oxygen saturation. In this manner, it provides an indication of the balance between flow and metabolism.

Individual variations in extracranial tissue (hence contamination), arterial to venous blood volume ratio, systemic blood pressure, $PaCO_2$, hematocrit, and regional cerebral blood volume (CBV) are factors that can influence cerebral tissue oxygenation, and this creates potential difficulties when attempting to establish a consensus value for the NIRS-derived thresholds for ischemia/hypoxia. It is generally accepted that normal range varies between 60% and 75%, with a coefficient of variation of almost 10%.[41]

Management principles

Table 21.6 summarizes current recommendations concerning the management of severe TBI.

Intracranial pressure and cerebral perfusion pressure (ICP/CPP)

Intracranial hypertension predisposes patients to poor outcomes. In a study carried out by Treggiari *et al.* the rate of death in a TBI population tripled if the ICP increased from 20 to 40 mmHg.[42] The main goal for patients with TBI is to control ICP and provide an adequate CPP, defined as MAP – ICP; many techniques are available to shift this balance in a favorable direction (Table 21.7). Some controversy exists regarding what constitutes the optimal ICP and CPP. Prior recommendations were to maintain the CPP at 70 mmHg or above and to lower ICP when it exceeded 20–25 mmHg. Subsequently CPP goals were redefined to be kept between 60 and 70 mmHg, as aggressive attempts to raise CPP beyond 70 mmHg increase the incidence of ARDS.[39]

Osmotic therapy

Reduction of ICP in patients with head injuries can be accomplished effectively by using osmotic diuretics. Both mannitol and hypertonic saline are effective in the treatment of intracranial hypertension.[43] Mannitol is the most commonly used agent and is available for intravenous administration in either a 20% or a 25% solution. Common dosages range from 0.25 to 1 g/kg of body weight. Mannitol may be used on a repeated schedule, but the serum osmolarity should be monitored. Osmolarity is generally kept below 320 mOsm/L to prevent renal dysfunction, although there are no data to support this threshold. With high-dose mannitol (2 g/kg), hyperkalemia

Table 21.7 Methods for controlling intracranial pressure (ICP)

Cerebrospinal fluid (CSF)	Mannitol or other hypertonic solution (decrease production) External CSF drainage • Ventricular catheter • Lumbar drain • Ventriculoperitoneal (VP) or ventriculoatrial (VA) shunt • Serial lumbar punctures
Brain	Mannitol or hypertonic saline • ± furosemide Decompressive craniectomy Resection of contusion or other mass lesions
Blood volume	Mannitol (reflex vasoconstriction?) Hyperventilation Hypothermia Head elevation, neutral neck position Deep propofol or barbiturate sedation • ± paralysis Control of seizures

can occur and serum potassium should be monitored. The mechanism of ICP reduction by mannitol may be related to its osmotic effect in shifting fluid from the brain tissue compartment to the intravascular compartment as well as its ability to improve blood rheology by decreasing blood viscosity. The latter effect has been postulated to cause reflex vasoconstriction, which keeps blood flow constant while reducing blood volume and ICP. In addition, mannitol, like other hypertonic fluids, decreases production of CSF.

Some individuals may benefit from the use of furosemide in combination with mannitol. The duration of the ICP decrease due to simultaneous administration of both diuretics may be prolonged compared to either agent used alone.

Various concentrations of hypertonic saline, alone or in combination with dextran, have been used for the management of elevated ICP, primarily in the setting of intracranial hypertension refractory to mannitol therapy. Hypertonic saline administration results in less dehydration and electrolyte disturbance, and may have anti-inflammatory actions with reduction in leukocyte adhesion and endothelial cell edema.[44] As the blood–brain barrier is impermeable to sodium ions, hypertonic saline establishes a gradient that facilitates the movement of water from the brain into the intravascular space. In addition to efficacy, the benefit of hypertonic saline includes the lack of severe electrolyte disturbance, which is common with mannitol. The brisk diuresis seen with mannitol is absent with hypertonic saline. Hypertonic saline increases serum osmolarity directly rather than by inducing osmotic diuresis. It is used in a 3% solution (513 mmol/L) in boluses of approximately 150 mL, in a 7.5% solution (1283 mmol/L) in 75 mL boluses, in a 23.4% solution (4008 mmol/L) in 30 mL boluses, or in a 3% solution as an infusion at a rate of 20–40 mL/h. It is also available as a 2% solution that can be administered via a peripheral venous catheter. If hypertonic saline with a concentration of $\geq 3\%$ is chosen, a central venous catheter should be inserted.[45]

Required serum sodium concentration can be approximated using the following formula:

$$\text{Required Na}^{2+} = (\text{LBW} \times \% \text{BW}) \times (\text{Target Na}^{2+} - \text{Current Na}^{2+})$$

where Na^{2+} is in millimoles per liter; LBW = lean body weight in kilograms; BW = % of body weight that is water (0.5 for a woman and 0.6 for a man); target Na^{2+} is generally referred to as 150 mmol/liter.

Following prolonged infusion in the intensive care unit, hypertonic saline should be tapered off slowly to prevent subsequent hyponatremia and rebound cerebral edema. In situations where hypertonic saline causes an unacceptable hyperchloremic acidosis, a mixture of sodium chloride and sodium acetate can be used.

Ventilation

Hyperventilation may be useful in a patient who suddenly develops signs of herniation, or during surgery to provide better conditions for surgical exposure. Hyperventilation causes cerebral vasoconstriction, primarily in the small-resistance arterioles in the brain; this vasoconstriction reduces CBF, CBV, and therefore ICP. The decrease in CBV and the fall in ICP occur virtually simultaneously with initiation of hyperventilation. The reduction in CBV is achieved at the expense of CBF. Excessive and prolonged hyperventilation may therefore cause unintended vasoconstriction, which leads to cerebral ischemia.[46]

Chronic hyperventilation should generally be avoided. In situations where prolonged hyperventilation is necessary because of failure of other agents to control ICP, monitoring of PbtO_2, SjvO_2, and cerebral venous lactate is desirable, to avoid hypocapnia-induced ischemia.

Anemia and coagulopathy

Monitoring of regional and/or global cerebral oxygenation may help determine transfusion needs, and brain tissue oxygen tension and NIRS monitoring have been utilized for this purpose. Currently available evidence supports a hemoglobin threshold level of 8–9 g/dL. In the context of ongoing bleeding, lower levels (e.g., 7 g/dL) may result in brief periods of profound anemia, which may cause inadequate brain perfusion. Patients with TBI transfused with a high platelet to red blood cell ratio (e.g., 1:1) experienced improved 30-day survival. A proposed mechanism may involve improved blood–brain barrier healing with activation of oligodendrocytes and repair of demyelination.[47]

The brain is rich in tissue thromboplastin, and severe TBI initially induces a hypercoagulable state with microemboli, creating a multisystemic injury. Subsequently an overwhelmed inhibitory mechanism leads to a consumption coagulopathy and/or disseminated intravascular coagulopathy (DIC) in up to 35% of cases, which is associated with a poor prognosis. When coagulopathy is observed clinically, it must be treated vigorously as guided by the coagulation profile. Fresh frozen plasma (FFP) is indicated when the international normalized ratio (INR) exceeds 1.4. Prothrombin complex concentrates may be used instead of or in addition to plasma. Platelets should be given when the count is below 100,000/μL. Platelets should also be given if the patient is receiving aspirin therapy and there is clinical bleeding despite a normal platelet count.

Glycemic control

The development of hyperglycemia in patients with severe TBI is associated with poor prognosis. However, tight glycemic control is not recommended. Patients with neurologic injury may have poor correlation of systemic glucose with brain tissue glucose concentration, which leads to higher variability, cerebral osmotic shifts, and a higher incidence of hypoglycemia. Hyperglycolysis has been described in TBI, and metabolically disturbed brain tissue appears to be at risk for local glucose depletion even when systemic glucose levels are within the lower normal range.[48]

Intraoperative hyperglycemia is found to be common in adults undergoing urgent/emergent craniotomy for TBI, and it is predicted by the severity of TBI, the presence of subdural hematoma, preoperative hyperglycemia, and age ≥ 65 years. A target glucose of 140–180 mg/dL is generally considered a reasonable goal. Continuous closed-loop glucose control systems, consisting of pumps for the infusion of appropriate amounts of insulin and a glucose sensor for the detection and/or monitoring of glucose levels regulated by computerized algorithms, is an emerging method that could assist in the management.[49]

Electrolyte disturbance

Patients with severe TBI or other brain injury can develop diabetes insipidus, SIADH, and CSWS. The former usually leads to hypernatremia, whereas the latter two result in hyponatremia. SIADH is associated with a hypervolemic state, whereas CSWS is associated with a hypovolemic state. Determination of plasma and urine sodium as well as osmolality is generally helpful, but will not necessarily sort out the diagnosis. Careful assessment of hemodynamic and volume status, as well as intake and output, will guide institution of appropriate treatment.

Hypothermia

Moderate hypothermia has been considered a potentially useful therapeutic modality in head injury for many years. There is ample experimental evidence to support this contention. The theoretical benefits of hypothermia in preventing secondary brain injury may include;

- reduction in brain metabolic rate (6–7% for every 1 °C decrease in core temperature)
- ICP reduction
- attenuation of blood–brain barrier permeability
- reduction of the critical threshold for oxygen delivery
- calcium antagonism
- blockade of excitotoxic mechanisms
- preservation of protein synthesis
- reduction of intracellular acidosis
- modulation of the inflammatory response
- reduction in edema formation
- suppression of free radicals and antioxidants and modulation of apoptotic cell death

Despite these theoretical considerations, repeated multicenter randomized clinical trials in head-injured patients have failed to demonstrate any beneficial effects on outcome. Moreover, hypothermia increases the risk of pneumonia and wound infection and may cause electrolyte and coagulation abnormalities (see Chapter 14). The Brain Trauma Foundation guidelines cite prophylactic hypothermia as a level 3 treatment option (degree of clinical certainty not established) that may confer better outcomes when the target temperature is maintained for ≥ 48 hours. Despite the controversies surrounding the use of hypothermia in TBI, there is still evidence for some metabolic advantage, in that moderate hypothermia might have a preferential beneficial effect in "at-risk" brain tissue, and is efficacious in decreasing ICP. Consequently, mild hypothermia may be useful in the setting of intracranial hypertension refractory to other interventions.[50] Success may depend on the timing of hypothermia onset and duration, temperature targets, rate of rewarming, and avoidance of rebound increases in ICP. Currently, there are two trials still under way (Eurotherm hypothermia and POLAR).[51]

In contrast to hypothermia, the devastating effects of hyperthermia are well established, and fever in a brain-injured patient must be treated promptly and vigorously.

Cerebral metabolic therapy with electrical burst suppression

Propofol infusion may be beneficial in the management of TBI by decreasing cerebral metabolic rate, CBV, and consequently ICP. However, it can cause hypotension, and prolonged infusions are associated with the additional risk of metabolic acidosis with lactate production and myocardial dysfunction (propofol infusion syndrome). Originally described in children, propofol infusion syndrome is now recognized in young adults, and carries significant morbidity and mortality. The addition of remifentanil (or other opioid) may help to reduce the dose requirements of propofol.

Propofol can be used in a dose–response manner to provide ICP control, ranging from mild sedation to pharmacologically induced coma. Although some type of electroencephalography (EEG) monitoring, such as the Bispectral Index, has been advocated for sedation monitoring, it is not necessary at low-dose infusion rates. Continuous EEG monitoring must be employed, however, when maximal suppression of metabolic activity is required. Propofol doses required for EEG burst suppression are usually around 2–5 mg/kg. This is titrated in slowly over a 5-minute period with a background maintenance infusion of 10–15 mg/kg/h.

Corticosteroids

Steroids have profound anti-inflammatory actions and can reduce brain edema in inflammatory and neoplastic conditions. Results from the CRASH trial, however, indicated that, not only does steroid use show no benefit in TBI: the treatment group had a higher mortality and morbidity because of an increased incidence of pneumonia and infection.[52] Thus, high-dose steroids are not indicated for use in severe TBI. However, anterior pituitary and adrenal insufficiency is common in these patients, particularly in the elderly or those who have a DAI and skull base fracture. Steroids may improve hemodynamic responsiveness in these patients when used in physiologic doses under close laboratory assessment of the hypothalamic–pituitary–adrenal axis.

Decompressive craniectomy

Decompressive craniectomy is used to manage intractable intracranial hypertension after TBI. In patients who have sustained a TBI and have severe cerebral edema, it is postulated that removing a large portion of the skull will allow more room for the increased volume of brain and thus decrease ICP and improve survival. In addition, decompressive craniectomy has also been shown to improve brain tissue oxygenation, CBF, and cerebral compliance. However, the question that remains is whether this intervention improves meaningful outcome. Potential complications with this procedure include hematoma, increased cerebral edema, and infection. A retrospective cohort study by Aarabi and coworkers reported a 50% incidence of good recovery in 50 patients.[53] The Australian multicenter DECRA trial reported that, in patients with severe diffuse TBI and refractory intracranial hypertension, early bifrontotemporoparietal decompressive craniectomy lowers the ICP and the length of stay in the ICU but leads to more unfavorable outcomes.[54] Rates of death were found to be similar in both the craniectomy group (19%) and the standard-care group (18%) at 6 months. The technique, timing, and selection of patients (ICP 20 vs. 25 mmHg) for decompressive craniectomy have been criticized. The randomized evaluation of surgery with craniectomy for uncontrollable elevation of intracranial pressure (RESCUEicp) trial is a currently recruiting patients (www.rescueicp.com).

Post-TBI epilepsy

TBI is a major cause of acquired epilepsy. The incidence of seizures has been reported to be 2–30%, depending on the severity of TBI. Seizures are classified as:

- immediate, which occur < 24 h after injury
- early, which occur < 1 week after injury
- late, which occur > 1 week after injury (posttraumatic epilepsy)

Risk factors for immediate and early seizures include:

- depressed skull fracture
- intracerebral hematoma
- subdural hematoma

Patients with any of these risk factors have a 25% chance of developing immediate or early posttraumatic seizures. Immediate seizures and early seizures are risk factors for the development of later epilepsy. The definition of posttraumatic epilepsy requires the occurrence of at least one late, unprovoked seizure in a person with a structural TBI. Approximately 80% of individuals who develop posttraumatic epilepsy have their first seizure within the first 12 months after injury, and more than 90% have a seizure by the end of the second year.

Proposed risk factors for epilepsy include:

- high severity of TBI
- immediate or early seizures
- female gender
- family history of epilepsy
- contusion with subdural hematoma
- skull fracture
- loss of consciousness or amnesia > 1 day
- age > 65 years

As posttraumatic seizures may only develop a number of years after the initial injury, it may reasonably be expected that seizures could be prevented with the prophylactic use of antiepileptic medications. Phenytoin and carbamazepine have been shown to prevent early seizures with some success. However, clinical trials have shown that prophylactic conventional antiepileptic drugs do not protect or prevent late development of epilepsy.[55]

Anesthetic management

Patients sustaining TBI may require emergent and nonemergent surgery for neurosurgical and non-neurosurgical indications. Priorities remain the same in all circumstances: prevention of cerebral ischemia, optimization of CPP, and management of intracranial hypertension.

Emergent neurosurgery

These patients commonly arrive in the operating room with an endotracheal tube in place. If they are not tracheally intubated, the same principles that were discussed in the section on *Airway and breathing*, above, should be applied, and the possibility of an unstable C-spine should always be taken into consideration. Often there is little time available for the preoperative assessment; one's approach must be concise and focused to obtain the pertinent information in a brief amount of time. These patients will probably have other systemic injuries that need to be assessed and addressed. A brief neurologic exam should include GCS, review of the CT scan findings, and examination of the pupillary reflexes. Drug- and alcohol-related intoxications are common and may influence the response of the patient to anesthetic agents. Review should include all available medical, surgical, and anesthetic history, allergies, and current medications including anticoagulant use (e.g., clopidogrel, aspirin, or warfarin) and herbal supplements. Relevant laboratory data (hematocrit, hemoglobin, coagulation profile, glucose, electrolytes, arterial blood gas) and planning of the postoperative management (ICU care) should be considered.

The hemodynamic status of the patient must be evaluated. Patients may demonstrate Cushing's response, exhibiting hypertension and bradycardia, which signifies brainstem compression from raised ICP. However, these classic findings may be masked by hypovolemia, and their absence does not rule out brainstem compression. An assessment of volume status is therefore always indicated. This may be difficult to accomplish, as urine output may be augmented by the use of mannitol, and hematocrit is decreased by ongoing blood loss. Cardiac output monitoring (see Chapter 9) will allow a more rational approach to fluid replacement, particularly in those patients requiring significant doses of inotropes or vasopressors to maintain an adequate CPP. In general, whenever there is a strong index of suspicion of hypovolemia, a volume challenge of 500 mL of crystalloid should be given. In adults, isolated brain injury generally does not result in hypotension, although this can occur with significant scalp blood loss (in both adults and children). The presence of hypotension in an adult with an isolated brain injury should prompt reevaluation of all other systems to rule out other sources of blood loss, such as a ruptured spleen.

Appropriate monitoring is established, and this must also take into account the immediate need for surgical decompression. Standard monitors include electrocardiography, pulse oximetry, capnography, temperature, urine output, and non-invasive blood pressure measurement (see Chapter 9). An arterial catheter is highly desirable for continuous blood pressure monitoring and blood sampling, but its placement should not delay obtaining adequate intravenous access (see Chapter 5). Two large-bore intravenous catheters are required at a minimum. Although a central venous catheter and retrograde jugular bulb catheter may be of value, time constraints usually do not permit their insertion.

Patients undergoing emergent neurosurgery usually do not have ICP monitors in place, but one can assume the presence of intracranial hypertension in the setting of an acute space-occupying lesion because the brain is unable to accommodate sudden increases in intracranial volume. Therefore, hyperventilation can be done until the dura is opened. Another area to focus on is the management of blood pressure. Compensatory hypertension should be tolerated in the period before the cranium has been opened. Hypotension during this period should

be treated aggressively. Assuming a minimum ICP of 20 mmHg, mean arterial blood pressure should be at least 80 mmHg. A combination of fluid and vasopressors may be used to accomplish this goal. Intravenous volume loading in the early stages of the anesthetic is appropriate, particularly in patients with other injuries and significant blood loss, as the hypertensive response can mask hypovolemia. Post-decompressive hypotension should be expected. The major risk factors include a low GCS, absence of basal cisterns on CT, and bilateral dilated pupils. Preemptive management is preferred, with continued volume administration along with vasopressors as appropriate.

The choice of anesthetic agents should be based on the clinical condition of the patient. As a general rule, nondepolarizing neuromuscular blocking agents should be administered to prevent inadvertent movement or coughing while in Mayfield pins. The most important goals are smooth induction, preservation and maintenance of hemodynamic stability, maintenance of CPP, control of $CMRO_2$, CBF, and ICP, and prompt postoperative emergence to allow neurologic assessment. Intravenous anesthetics seem well suited for this goal. Propofol decreases $CMRO_2$, CBF, and ICP, has been shown to offer some degree of neuroprotection, and does not impair flow metabolism coupling or cerebral autoregulation. Volatile anesthetic agents may be used when brain swelling is not a prime concern. In low doses volatile agents are not potent vasodilators, but they do not have the vasoconstrictive properties of propofol. Their main advantage is the ease and speed of titration, especially for the newer agents, sevoflurane and desflurane. Similar to the intravenous agents, they may offer neuroprotection and reduction in $CMRO_2$. Isoflurane – and, to a much lesser extent, sevoflurane – may lead to an increase in cerebral blood flow in a dose-dependent manner, and thus may potentially increase ICP. Keeping the dose less than 1 MAC can minimize these effects. In addition, volatile agents may impair cerebral autoregulation, although sevoflurane has less of an effect than isoflurane. Consequently, with high or labile ICP, the authors' anesthetic of choice is a total intravenous anesthesia technique with propofol and remifentanil infusion. Care must be taken to avoid overdosage, and the associated hypotension and compromise of CPP. Once the dura is open, decisions on anesthetic management can be based on the appearance of the brain. When an ICP monitor is in place and the ICP is controlled, it is reasonable to choose a volatile agent and switch to propofol should the ICP increase. Nitrous oxide increases $CMRO_2$, CBF, and ICP in head-injured patients and should be avoided. Opioids can be used safely in these patients as long as blood pressure is not compromised and the patient is mechanically ventilated.

Other surgery
Emergent

TBI patients require emergent surgical management of non-cranial injuries, which may be complex and challenging. Life-threatening conditions (e.g., major hemorrhage) take priority, and there might be not enough time to investigate the neurological injuries. The anesthesiologist therefore needs to employ a high index of suspicion based on history, mechanism of injury, level of consciousness, and pupillary status. If pupillary asymmetry exists or the history suggests a high likelihood of intracranial injury, consultation with the neurosurgeon should be obtained and ICP monitoring may be initiated. The presence of dilated pupils bilaterally may suggest brain death or a nonsalvageable patient. This can be confirmed intraoperatively with the use of TCD ultrasonography. TCD may also be useful as a semiquantitative noninvasive assessment of ICP if the presence of coagulopathy precludes placement of an ICP monitor. TCD evidence of oscillating flow signifies the onset of cerebral circulatory arrest. If the patient is stabilized, surgery can be followed by a CT scan of the head and a possible return to the OR for definitive neurosurgical management. If an ICP monitor is placed and demonstrates intracranial hypertension, appropriate immediate intervention may include head elevation, neutral neck position, to prevent any obstruction to venous drainage, elevation of MAP, administration of mannitol, and conversion to total intravenous anesthesia.

Nonemergent

Patients who have sustained TBI frequently have other injuries, especially orthopedic injuries requiring operative fixation. The timing of surgery in these patients remains a controversial issue. One must balance the need for operative fixation of fractures to decrease the incidence of complications related to immobility, such as atelectasis, pneumonia, and venous thromboembolism, against the risks of performing surgery in patients with unstable ICP and CPP. These patients have altered physiologic mechanisms such as cerebral autoregulation and are extremely susceptible to secondary brain insults, especially hypotension.

In the absence of good evidence, the following recommendations provide a conservative approach to the management of nonemergent, non-neurosurgical procedures:

(1) Uncontrolled intracranial hypertension should preclude all but emergent surgery.
(2) Patients with an abnormal head CT scan should have ICP monitoring in the operating room, in particular for long-duration surgeries in the first 48 hours after injury.
(3) Consideration should be given to advanced neuromonitoring, including TCD, jugular bulb oximetry, and brain tissue oxygenation.
(4) If ICP becomes unstable, surgery should be terminated and a head CT should be obtained.

Summary and conclusions

Traumatic brain injury is common, and it is a major public health problem. Physicians following guidelines and protocols should take into account individual patient variability and disease-specific factors. Along with the development of such guidelines, recent advances in prehospital medicine,

neuroimaging, neuromonitoring, intraoperative and critical care areas, and access to multidisciplinary neurotrauma units, have made significant contributions to some substantial improvements in the care of the TBI patient.

Government agencies have made extensive efforts to develop programs to understand, prevent, and reduce the incidence of TBI. In-hospital trauma management continues to focus on the prevention of secondary injuries. Despite a progressive reduction in mortality, no single treatment has been shown to improve outcome. TBI is a multisystem disorder. Non-neurological organ dysfunction makes a significant contribution to the overall mortality.

Interventions that increase CBF, improve brain oxygenation, and prevent further neuronal cell death are the main areas of focus. Multimodal neuromonitoring modalities are rapidly progressing and guiding decision making. Understanding these technologies and their limitations is paramount for appropriate patient care.

Anesthesiologists are frequently involved in the care of the TBI patient, at every step of the treatment continuum.

Questions

(1) **Which of the following is correct with regard to traumatic brain injury (TBI)?**
   a. Injury occurring at the scene is termed primary injury
   b. Secondary injuries due to hypoxia and hypotension are not preventable
   c. Open fractures do not usually require surgery
   d. Skull fractures are always associated with intracranial lesions
(2) **With regard to primary TBI, which of the following is correct?**
   a. Diffuse axonal injury is best diagnosed using CT
   b. Cerebral hematoma may require decompressive craniectomy for refractory intracranial hypertension
   c. Epidural hematoma has a worse prognosis than intracerebral hematoma
   d. Subdural hematoma is the least frequent injury
(3) **Considering the initial resuscitation of the patient with TBI after blunt trauma, which of the following is correct?**
   a. Neck stabilization is rarely done for rapid sequence intubation in the prehospital setting
   b. Tracheal intubation should ideally be accomplished via the nasal route
   c. Succinylcholine is contraindicated in head injury patients
   d. Propofol may cause severe hypotension in hypovolemic brain-injured patients
(4) **Concerning fluid and drug administration in hypotensive TBI patients, which of the following is correct?**
   a. Patients should be run dry in order to minimize cerebral edema

b. Hypotonic fluids should be avoided

c. Vasopressors and inotropes should be avoided

d. Mean arterial pressure (MAP) should be maintained in the 100–110 mmHg range

(5) Regarding intracranial pressure (ICP) monitoring of the TBI patient, which of the following is correct?

a. Cerebral perfusion pressure (CPP) is not affected by ICP

b. Intraventricular catheters cannot measure ICP accurately

c. The upper limit of normal for ICP is 25 mmHg

d. ICP monitoring is recommended for patients with an abnormal head CT and GCS < 8

(6) Concerning acute TBI:

a. Both primary injury and secondary injury can be treated effectively

b. Secondary injury, some of which can be prevented, occurs after the primary event

c. Hypoxia and hypotension do not contribute to secondary injury with TBI

d. Patients with TBI do not suffer spinal cord injury

(7) Identify the correct statement regarding airway management in TBI:

a. Patients with TBI generally do not have ventilation problems

b. Patients who are obtunded and unable to protect their airway should have their tracheas intubated immediately to prevent aspiration

c. After tracheal intubation, all patients with TBI should be hyperventilated to $PaCO_2$ of 25 mmHg

d. To improve cerebral blood flow, $PaCO_2$ should be maintained at 50 mmHg or above

Questions 8–11 are based on the following case: A patient with TBI and GCS of 7 is admitted to the emergency department. CT scan showed a large subdural hematoma with midline shift. The patient is scheduled for emergent craniotomy.

(8) The next step in this patient's management should be:

a. Peritoneal lavage to rule out other injuries

b. Placement of a pulmonary artery catheter to facilitate hemodynamic monitoring

c. Perform tracheal intubation to protect the airway and ensure adequate oxygenation and ventilation

d. CT survey to rule out orthopedic injuries

(9) Before induction of anesthesia, essential laboratory assessments should include:

a. Thyroid function testing

b. Transthoracic echocardiography

c. MRI of the brain

d. Hematocrit and coagulation profile

(10) Potential intraoperative complications include:

a. Coagulopathy

b. Hypernatremia

c. Hyperglycemia

d. All of the above may occur

(11) After opening of dura and decompression, blood pressure suddenly decreases to 60 mmHg systolic. This can be secondary to all of the causes listed below, *except*:

a. Large and ongoing blood loss from coagulopathy

b. Sudden loss of sympathetic tone from release of intracranial hypertension

c. Concealed systemic bleeding, for instance, an undetected ruptured spleen

d. Surgical damage to the medulla

Answers

(1) a
(2) c
(3) d
(4) b
(5) d
(6) b
(7) b
(8) c
(9) d
(10) d
(11) d

References

1. Coronado VG, Xu L, Basavaraju SV, et al. Surveillance for traumatic brain injury-related deaths: United States, 1997–2007. *MMWR Surveill Summ* 2011; **60** (5): 1–32.

2. US Department of Defense. TBI worldwide numbers 2013. http://dvbic.dcoe.mil/sites/default/files/uploads/Worldwide-Totals-2013.pdf (accessed September 2014).

3. Centers for Disease Control and Prevention. Nonfatal traumatic brain injuries related to sports and recreation activities among persons aged ≤19 years: United States, 2001–2009. *MMWR Morb Mortal Wkly Rep* 2011; **60**: 1337–42.

4. Fleminger S, Oliver DL, Williams WH, Evans J. The neuropsychiatry of depression after brain injury. *Neuropsychol Rehabil* 2003; **13**: 65–87.

5. Fleminger S, Oliver DL, Lovestone S, Rabe-Hesketh S, Giora A. Head injury as a risk factor for Alzheimer's disease: the evidence 10 years on; a partial replication. *J Neurol Neurosurg Psychiatry* 2003; **74**: 857–62.

6. Menon DK, Schwab K, Wright DW, Maas AI. Position statement: definition of traumatic brain injury. *Arch Phys Med Rehabil* 2010; **91**: 1637–40.

7. Werner C, Engelhard K. Pathophysiology of traumatic brain injury. *Br J Anaesth* 2007; **99**: 4–9.

8. Chesnut RM. Care of central nervous system injuries. *Surg Clin North Am* 2007; **87**: 119–56, vii.

9. Yue JK, Vassar MJ, Lingsma H, et al. Transforming Research and Clinical Knowledge in Traumatic Brain Injury (TRACK-TBI) pilot: multicenter

implementation of the common data elements for traumatic brain injury. *J Neurotrauma* 2013; **13**: 1831–44.

10. Bullock MR, Chesnut R, Ghajar J, *et al*. Surgical management of acute subdural hematomas. *Neurosurgery* 2006; **58** (3 Suppl): S16–24.

11. Bullock MR, Chesnut R, Ghajar J, *et al*. Surgical management of acute epidural hematomas. *Neurosurgery* 2006; **58** (3 Suppl): S7–15.

12. Mayer SA, Brun NC, Begtrup K, *et al*. Efficacy and safety of recombinant activated factor VII for acute intracerebral hemorrhage. *N Engl J Med* 2008; **358**: 2127–37.

13. Bullock MR, Chesnut R, Ghajar J, *et al*. Surgical management of traumatic parenchymal lesions. *Neurosurgery* 2006; **58** (3 Suppl): S25–46.

14. Bullock MR, Chesnut R, Ghajar J, *et al*. Surgical management of posterior fossa mass lesions. *Neurosurgery* 2006; **58** (3 Suppl): S47–55.

15. Johnson VE, Stewart W, Smith DH. Axonal pathology in traumatic brain injury. *Exp Neurol* 2013; 24635–43.

16. Kemp CD, Johnson JC, Riordan WP, Cotton BA. How we die: the impact of nonneurologic organ dysfunction after severe traumatic brain injury. *Am Surg* 2008; **74**: 866–72.

17. Allard CB, Scarpelini S, Rhind SG, *et al*. Abnormal coagulation tests are associated with progression of traumatic intracranial hemorrhage. *J Trauma* 2009; **67**: 959–67.

18. Wafaisade A, Lefering R, Tjardes T, *et al*. Acute coagulopathy in isolated blunt traumatic brain injury. *Neurocrit Care* 2010; **12**: 211–19.

19. Lim HB, Smith M. Systemic complications after head injury: a clinical review. *Anaesthesia* 2007; **62**: 474–82.

20. Sasser SM, Hunt RC, Faul M, *et al*. Guidelines for field triage of injured patients: recommendations of the National Expert Panel on Field Triage, 2011. *MMWR Recomm Rep* 2012; **61** (RR-1): 1–20.

21. Badjatia N, Carney N, Crocco TJ, *et al*.; Brain Trauma Foundation. Guidelines for prehospital management of traumatic brain injury, 2nd edition. *Prehosp Emerg Care* 2008; **12** (Suppl 1): S1–52.

22. Sugerman DE, Xu L, Pearson WS, Faul M. Patients with severe traumatic brain injury transferred to a Level I or II trauma center: United States, 2007 to 2009. *J Trauma Acute Care Surg* 2012; **73**: 1489–97.

23. Bernard SA, Nguyen V, Cameron P, *et al*. Prehospital rapid sequence intubation improves functional outcome for patients with severe traumatic brain injury: a randomized controlled trial. *Ann Surg* 2010; **252**: 959–65.

24. Sultan P. Is cricoid pressure needed during rapid sequence induction? *Br J Hosp Med (Lond)* 2008; **69**: 177.

25. Rice MJ, Mancuso AA, Morey TE, Gravenstein N, Deitte L. The anatomical correction of cricoid pressure. *Minerva Anestesiol* 2010; **76**: 304.

26. Kovarik WD, Mayberg TS, Lam AM, Mathisen TL, Winn HR. Succinylcholine does not change intracranial pressure, cerebral blood flow velocity, or the electroencephalogram in patients with neurologic injury. *Anesth Analg* 1994; **78**: 469–73.

27. Cooper DJ, Myburgh J, Finfer S, *et al*. Albumin resuscitation for traumatic brain injury: is intracranial hypertension the cause of increased mortality? *J Neurotrauma* 2013; **30**: 512–18.

28. Reinhart K, Perner A, Sprung CL, *et al*. Consensus statement of the ESICM task force on colloid volume therapy in critically ill patients. *Intensive Care Med* 2012; **38**: 368–83.

29. Murkin JM. "Primum non nocere": the role of hydroxyethyl starch 130/0.4 in cerebral resuscitation. *Can J Anaesth* 2012; **59**: 1089–94.

30. Bulger EM, May S, Kerby JD, *et al*. Out-of-hospital hypertonic resuscitation after traumatic hypovolemic shock: a randomized, placebo controlled trial. *Ann Surg* 2011; **253**: 431–41.

31. Marshall LF, Marshall SB, Klauber MR, *et al*. The diagnosis of head injury requires a classification based on computed axial tomography. *J Neurotrauma* 1992; **9** (Suppl 1): S287–92.

32. Bratton SL, Chestnut RM, Ghajar J, *et al*. Guidelines for the management of severe traumatic brain injury. VIII. Intracranial pressure thresholds. *J Neurotrauma* 2007; **24** (Suppl 1): S55–8.

33. Bratton SL, Chestnut RM, Ghajar J, *et al*. Guidelines for the management of severe traumatic brain injury. VII. Intracranial pressure monitoring technology. *J Neurotrauma* 2007; **24** (Suppl 1): S45–54.

34. Barmparas G, Singer M, Ley E, *et al*. Decreased intracranial pressure monitor use at level II trauma centers is associated with increased mortality. *Am Surg* 2012; **78**: 1166–71.

35. Stein DM, Hu PF, Brenner M, *et al*. Brief episodes of intracranial hypertension and cerebral hypoperfusion are associated with poor functional outcome after severe traumatic brain injury. *J Trauma* 2011; **71**: 364–73.

36. Chesnut RM, Temkin N, Carney N, *et al*.; Global Neurotrauma Research Group. A trial of intracranial-pressure monitoring in traumatic brain injury. *N Engl J Med* 2012; **367**: 2471–81.

37. Coles JP, Fryer TD, Smielewski P, *et al*. Incidence and mechanisms of cerebral ischemia in early clinical head injury. *J Cereb Blood Flow Metab* 2004; **24**: 202–11.

38. Maloney-Wilensky E, Gracias V, Itkin A, *et al*. Brain tissue oxygen and outcome after severe traumatic brain injury: a systematic review. *Crit Care Med* 2009; **37**: 2057–63.

39. Spiotta AM, Stiefel MF, Gracias VH, *et al*. Brain tissue oxygen-directed management and outcome in patients with severe traumatic brain injury. *J Neurosurg* 2010; **113**: 571–80.

40. McCarthy MC, Moncrief H, Sands JM, *et al*. Neurologic outcomes with cerebral oxygen monitoring in traumatic brain injury. *Surgery* 2009; **146**: 585–90.

41. Highton D, Elwell C, Smith M. Noninvasive cerebral oximetry: is there light at the end of the tunnel? *Curr Opin Anaesthesiol* 2010; **23**: 576–81.

42. Treggiari MM, Schutz N, Yanez ND, Romand JA. Role of intracranial pressure values and patterns in predicting outcome in traumatic brain injury: a systematic review. *Neurocrit Care* 2007; **6**: 104–12.

43. Oddo M, Levine JM, Frangos S, *et al*. Effect of mannitol and hypertonic saline on cerebral oxygenation in patients with severe traumatic brain injury and refractory intracranial

hypertension. *J Neurol Neurosurg Psychiatry* 2009; **80**: 916–20.

44. Rizoli SB, Rhind SG, Shek PN, *et al.* The immunomodulatory effects of hypertonic saline resuscitation in patients sustaining traumatic hemorrhagic shock: a randomized, controlled, double-blinded trial. *Ann Surg* 2006; **243**: 47–57.

45. Ropper AH. Hyperosmolar therapy for raised intracranial pressure. *N Engl J Med* 2012; **367**: 746–52.

46. Bratton SL, Chestnut RM, Ghajar J, *et al.* Guidelines for the management of severe traumatic brain injury. XIV. Hyperventilation. *J Neurotrauma* 2007; **24** (Suppl 1): S87–90.

47. Brasel KJ, Vercruysse G, Spinella PC, *et al.* The association of blood component use ratios with the survival of massively transfused trauma patients with and without severe brain

injury. *J Trauma* 2011; **71** (2 Suppl 3): S343–52.

48. Magnoni S, Tedesco C, Carbonara M, *et al.* Relationship between systemic glucose and cerebral glucose is preserved in patients with severe traumatic brain injury, but glucose delivery to the brain may become limited when oxidative metabolism is impaired: implications for glycemic control. *Crit Care Med* 2012; **40**: 1785–91.

49. Oddo M, Schmidt JM, Mayer SA, Chiolero RL. Glucose control after severe brain injury. *Curr Opin Clin Nutr Metab Care* 2008; **11**: 134–9.

50. Wang Q, Li AL, Zhi DS, Huang HL. Effect of mild hypothermia on glucose metabolism and glycerol of brain tissue in patients with severe traumatic brain injury. *Chin J Traumatol* 2007; **10**: 246–9.

51. Rosenfeld JV, Maas AI, Bragge P, *et al.* Early management of severe traumatic brain injury. *Lancet* 2012; **380**: 1088–98.

52. Edwards P, Arango M, Balica L, *et al.* Final results of MRC CRASH, a randomised placebo-controlled trial of intravenous corticosteroid in adults with head injury-outcomes at 6 months. *Lancet* 2005; **365**: 1957–9.

53. Aarabi B, Hesdorffer DC, Ahn ES, *et al.* Outcome following decompressive craniectomy for malignant swelling due to severe head injury. *J Neurosurg* 2006; **104**: 469–79.

54. Cooper DJ, Rosenfeld JV, Murray L, *et al.* Decompressive craniectomy in diffuse traumatic brain injury. *N Engl J Med* 2011; **364**: 1493–502.

55. Christensen J. Traumatic brain injury: risks of epilepsy and implications for medicolegal assessment. *Epilepsia* 2012; **53** (Suppl 4): 43–7.

Surgical considerations for spinal cord trauma

Cynthia Nguyen and Timothy Moore

Objectives

(1) Differentiate between a *complete* and an *incomplete* spinal cord injury.
(2) Describe the clinical presentation of complete and incomplete spinal cord syndromes.
(3) Review the two major considerations for surgical treatment of spinal cord injuries.
(4) Recognize unique surgical considerations in high cervical spinal cord injuries and unstable thoracic injuries.

Introduction

Spinal cord injury (SCI) is a devastating event for the patient, and for society. There are approximately 200,000 Americans with SCI. There are almost 12,000 new cases of spinal cord injuries per year. A large percentage of these injuries are in males ages 20–40. The cost to society in maintaining care and quality of life is difficult to calculate.

Surgical intervention has made a significant impact on outcome with these injuries. The development of improved spinal instrumentation has allowed surgeons to approach the spine from 360 degrees. Varied approaches allow decompression of the neurologic elements and the ability to impart a stable spinal segment that improves mobilization and rehabilitation.

The role of surgery in spinal cord injury continues to evolve. A multidisciplinary approach is necessary to optimize outcomes in spinal cord injuries. The orthopedic or neurologic surgeon remains a key component in the treatment of the patient with an acute traumatic event. These patients are best served by a center that provides optimal care from the day of injury to the final day of spinal cord rehabilitation. Access to spinal cord injury centers has been shown to decrease the proportion of complete injuries and mortality.

Patterns of neurologic injury

Spinal cord injuries usually result from a high-energy mechanism. Most of these injuries involve a motor vehicle crash, fall from height, penetrating trauma, or sports injuries. In the

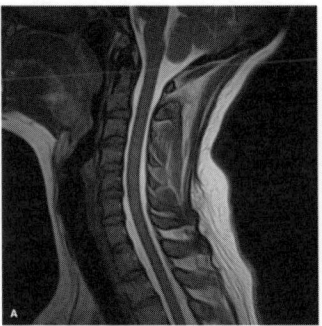
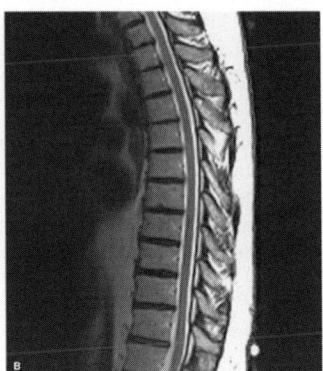
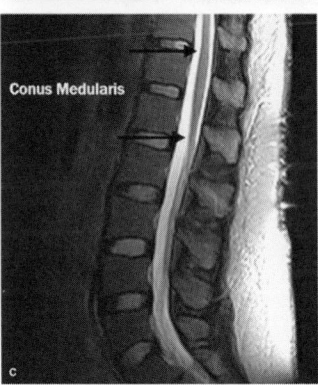

Conus Medularis

Figure 22.1 (**A**) Midsagittal T2 MRI of normal cervical spine and spinal cord. Injuries to the cervical spine can produce every type of neurological injury, from complete spinal cord injury to nerve root compression producing radicular deficit. (**B**) Midsagittal T2 MRI of normal thoracic spine and spinal cord. Injuries to the thoracic spine tend either to cause devastating spinal cord injury or to leave the patient neurologically normal. (**C**) Midsagittal T2 MRI of normal lumbar spine, spinal cord, conus medularis, and cauda equina. Injuries involving these levels can produce the full spectrum of neurological injuries, from complete spinal cord injury to conus medularis syndrome to cauda equina syndrome to radicular nerve injury.

experience of a large urban Level I trauma center, over one-fifth of patients with spine trauma suffer spinal cord injuries.[1] Anatomically, spinal cord injuries can occur from the occiput to the level of the conus medularis (Fig. 22.1). The majority of spinal cord injury happens in the cervical spine.[2] In the cervical spine, the most common level of injury is C5, followed by C4 then C6. The next most commonly involved level is T12. Neurologic findings with injuries at T12 are often mixed with

Trauma Anesthesia, 2nd Edition, ed. Charles E. Smith. Published by Cambridge University Press. © Charles E. Smith, 2015.

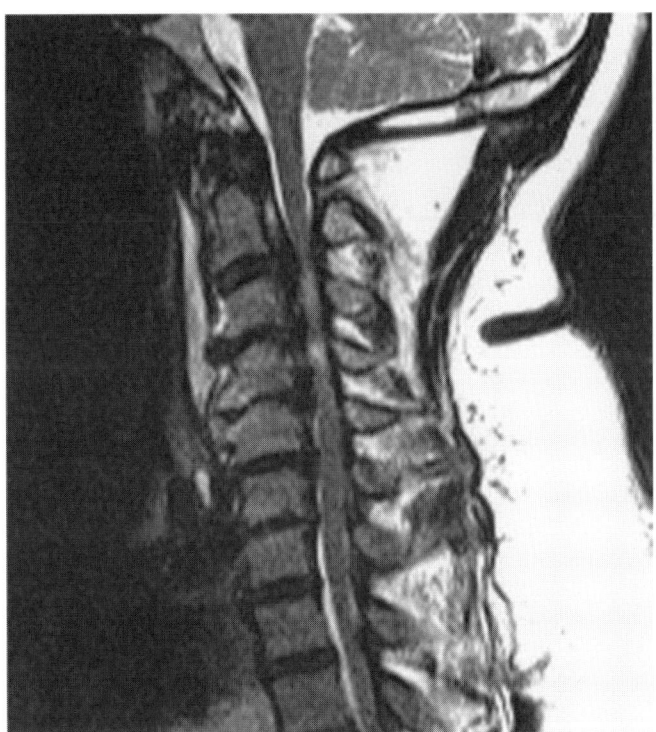

Figure 22.2 Midsagittal T2 MRI of a 62-year-old male who fell from standing height in his home. He was immediately unable to move his extremities and lost control of his bladder. The patient has significant ossification of the posterior longitudinal ligament, causing baseline severe stenosis of his cervical spinal cord.

upper and lower motor neuron symptoms termed conus medullaris syndrome. Injuries below the conus most often result in cauda equina syndrome or lower extremity peripheral nerve injuries. These injuries cause lower motor neuron symptoms with or without bowel and bladder dysfunction.

Specific anatomic variants make certain patients prone to more devastating neurologic injury. Elderly patients are at higher risk of spinal cord injury after low-energy trauma due to degenerative changes causing spinal stenosis and their inability to protect their head and spine from ground-level falls. Congenital cervical stenosis from ossification of the posterior longitudinal ligament can decrease the space available for the neurologic elements. Minor traumatic events in this setting can have devastating consequences. The patient in Figure 22.2 fell from standing, striking his head on a wall. He was unable to move his extremities and lost control of his bladder. He presented to our trauma center about 3 hours after the fall with labored respirations and no motor function below his trapezius (cranial nerve 11). This is an example of minimal trauma causing a devastating complete spinal cord injury in the setting of severe cervical stenosis.

The pathophysiology of SCI involves the primary injury from the initial insult, then secondary injury from the body's response. The primary injury to the cord is usually from the direct force of the precipitating event, leading to cord compression, distraction, or laceration. Secondary mechanisms,

including vascular changes, electrolyte changes, and initiation of neurotransmitter cascades, predictably add insult to the primary injury. These mechanisms are summarized in Figure 22.3. The majority of SCI research is devoted to minimizing these secondary mechanisms.

It is important to clarify the type of neurologic injury upon presentation. The accurate diagnosis of a neurologic injury is best conveyed to the patient and family as soon as possible. *Spinal shock* is a controversial scenario characterized by loss of bulbocavernosus reflex lasting up to 48 hours after an acute injury. It refers to the loss of reflexes and flaccidity seen after SCI, due to the immediate massive depolarization of neuronal axons caused by the physical disruption of neural elements from the injury. Some authors feel complete spinal cord injury cannot be diagnosed until resolution of spinal shock after the uninjured neural tissue has been given time to repolarize. A patient may present with what appears to be a complete spinal cord injury only to have return of bulbocavernosus reflex after spinal shock has resolved. *Neurogenic shock* is characterized by hypotension with bradycardia. The paradoxical bradycardic response to hypotension is caused by the interruption of the normal sympathetic response. Neurogenic shock must be differentiated from other types of shock, particularly hypovolemic (see Chapter 4). The incidence of neurogenic shock in patients with cervical SCI is 19.3%, compared with 7% in patients with thoracic SCI, and 3% in patients with lumbar SCI.[3] Timely restoration of the patient's blood pressure is crucial to prevent ischemia to end organs, including preventing added insult to the spinal cord after injury (see also Chapter 23). After other causes of shock are ruled out, management of neurogenic shock includes adequate fluid resuscitation as well as judicious use of pressors. Crystalloid fluids should be given to maintain a mean arterial blood pressure above 70 mmHg. Excessive fluid administration should be avoided. Hemodynamic and echocardiographic monitoring are useful in this regard (see Chapters 9 and 10). If fluid resuscitation is inadequate to ensure organ perfusion, inotropic agents such as dopamine may be added to improve perfusion pressure (see also Chapter 23). Severe bradycardia may need to be treated with atropine, glycopyrolate, or a pacemaker. Table 22.1 shows some of the differences between the different types of clinical shock.

The American Spinal Injury Association (ASIA) has formulated a comprehensive evaluation of spinal cord function (Fig. 22.4). *Complete spinal cord injury* is defined as an injury with no motor or sensory function below a certain level. The motor level is defined as the lowest level at which there is at least three-fifths strength on both sides of the body. An *incomplete spinal cord injury* exists if any motor or sensory function remains or if there is sacral sparing. Sacral sparing is evidenced by preservation of some function of the sacral nerves, including perianal sensation, rectal tone, or the ability to flex the great toe.

Neurologic injury can be classified in many ways. Surgeons tend to look at neurologic injury from a strictly anatomic

Table 22.1 Neurogenic versus other types of shock in trauma (see also Chapter 4). Spinal shock refers to loss of reflexes and flaccidity after spinal cord injury and should not be confused with neurogenic and other forms of shock.

	Neurogenic	Hypovolemic	Cardiogenic	Tension pneumothorax	Septic
Etiology	Spinal cord injury	Hemorrhage	Pump failure, tamponade	Decreased blood return to the heart, hypoxemia	Varied
Heart rate	Decrease	Increase	Increase	Increase	Increase
Peripheral blood vessels	Vasodilatation	Vasoconstriction	Vasoconstriction	Vasoconstriction	Vasodilatation

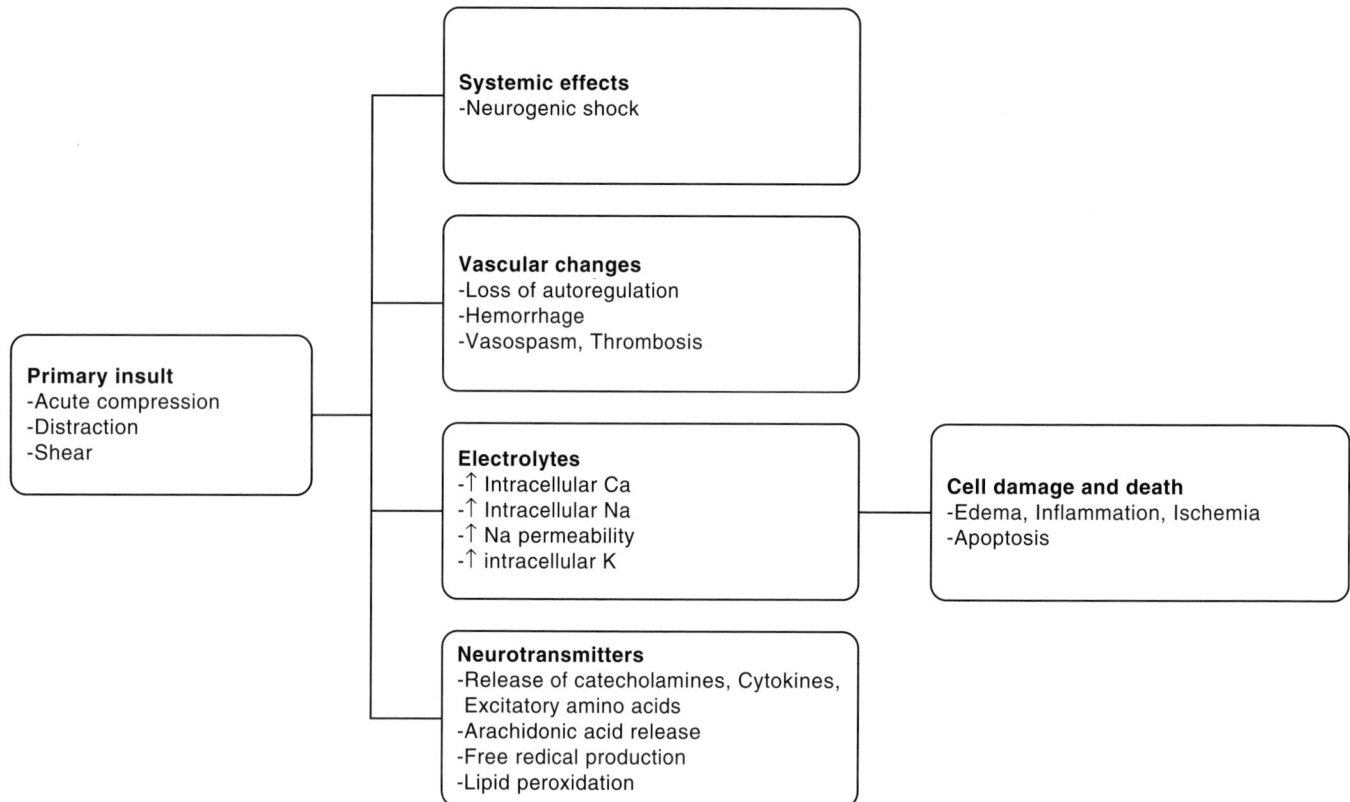

Figure 22.3 Primary and secondary mechanisms of acute spinal cord injury.

standpoint. Injuries can be viewed as a spectrum from a neurologically intact state to complete spinal cord injury (as defined above). Deficits can be further characterized as lower motor versus upper motor neuron injuries.

Lower motor neuron injuries tend to present with unilateral extremity findings. Sensory deficits tend to follow a dermatomal pattern that is suggestive of the level of injury. Motor deficits involve the extremity musculature supplied by the injured nerve root. Investigations often find compression of a specific nerve root by fracture anatomy, hematoma, or some other type of extrinsic compression. A superior articular facet fracture with displacement is a common injury that often involves radicular symptoms from compression of the nerve root by the displaced fracture fragment (Fig. 22.5).

Upper motor neuron injuries often involve a lesion of the spinal cord above the level of the conus. These injuries are

characterized as complete or incomplete injuries. Complete injuries carry a poorer prognosis for recovery than do incomplete injuries. Complete injuries can result from multiple etiologies. Spinal cord infarcts can result from vascular insufficiency (Fig. 22.6). Spinal cord transection can result from direct trauma to the supporting bony and ligamentous structures (Fig. 22.7).

A traumatic injury to the conus medullaris can create a pattern characterized by both upper and lower motor neuron findings. These injuries often involve both hyper- and flaccid reflexes, mixed bowel and bladder findings, with peripheral nerve root involvement to a varying degree.

Incomplete injuries to the cervical spine often involve syndromes of neurologic findings. *Central cord syndrome* usually occurs in a cervical spine with significant spondylosis (arthritis) and stenosis. It is often caused from a hyperextension mechanism

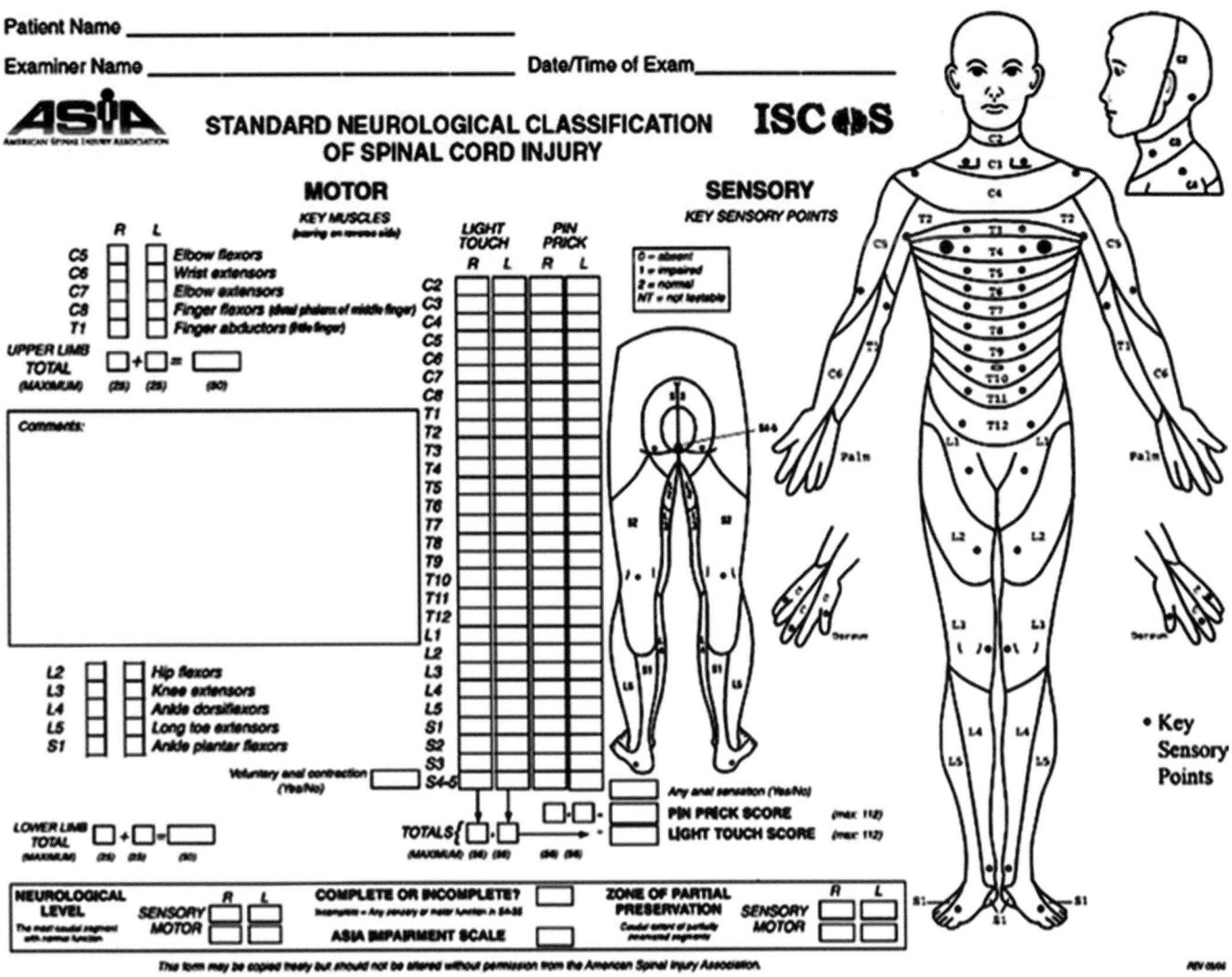

Figure 22.4 American Spinal Injury Association (ASIA) neurological classification of spinal cord injury.

causing a "pinching" of the spinal cord and damage to the central fibers. This syndrome involves relative sparing of lower extremity function with disproportionately greater upper extremity impairment, especially motor. Patients with this type of injury will have neurologic improvement 50% of the time. Patients can have transient quadriplegia but soon evolve to upper extremity loss of motor and sensation, while the lower extremity symptoms tend to resolve.

Brown-Séquard syndrome involves damage to one side of the spinal cord. This most often occurs from penetrating trauma, such as a gunshot wound or stab wound. The syndrome is characterized by ipsilateral motor and position sense loss and contralateral pain and temperature loss below the level of injury. This incomplete syndrome carries the best prognosis for recovery in that up to 90% of patients will have some form of neurologic recovery.

Anterior cord syndrome involves damage to the anterior spinal cord, often from a vascular insult to the anterior spinal

artery. The mechanism most often responsible is a flexion–compression force to the cervical spine. Patients often lose motor function below the level of the injury. The hallmark of this injury is preservation of deep pressure and vibratory sensation. This syndrome carries the poorest prognosis for recovery, with under 20% of patients gaining any neurologic recovery.

Posterior cord syndrome is extremely rare and involves damage to the posterior columns resulting in loss of deep pressure and vibration. These patients cannot ambulate without visual feedback.

The American Spinal Injury Association has adopted a modification of the Frankel classification that has allowed providers effective communication, prognosis, and treatment direction in dealing with neurologic injuries (Fig. 22.8). The ASIA score is designated once spinal shock has resolved. This assessment allows for rehabilitation protocols to be established and instituted in a timely manner.

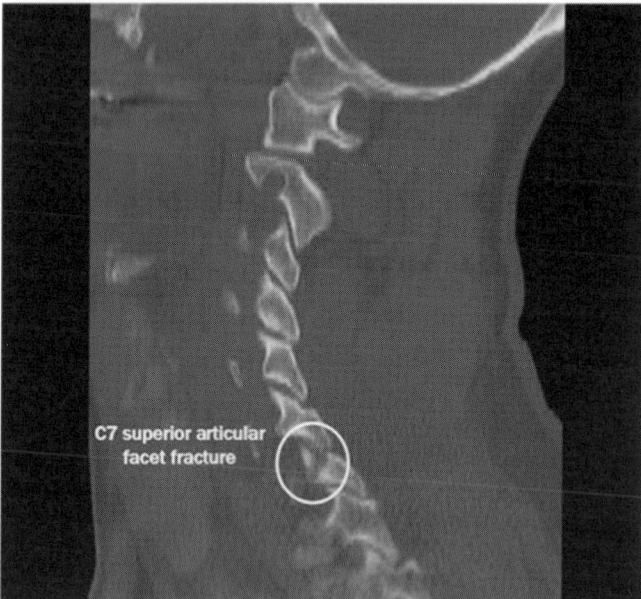

Figure 22.5 Sagittal CT scan through the facet joints showing a superior articular facet fracture of C7. The patient presented after a motor vehicle crash with unilateral triceps weakness and dysesthesias in the C7 dermatome. The patient was treated with Gardner–Wells traction to reduce the subluxated facet and then taken to the operating room for an anterior cervical diskectomy and fusion at C6–C7, with complete resolution of his radicular symptoms.

Surgery

Surgery has always played a controversial role in the care of spinal cord injuries. Spinal cord injuries have historically been considered injuries without the likelihood of functional improvement. Due to the efficiency of first responders, establishment of trauma centers, and advances in surgical techniques, surgery can have a profound effect in the functional recovery of spinal cord injured patients. Surgical intervention should be considered if there is any extrinsic compression of the neurologic elements or if the spine is considered unstable.

Surgery for SCI is a highly specialized field. Orthopedic surgeons who have completed a spine fellowship with trauma exposure are qualified to care for traumatic SCI. Neurologic surgeons get exposure to traumatic spinal injuries during their residency but often choose a fellowship that provides more exposure to these injuries. Orthopedic or neurosurgical providers who care for these injuries tend to work in tertiary care centers, often affiliated with university programs involved in teaching residents and ancillary care givers. Most providers feel a patient's outcome is optimized by early intervention of a center with the resources to care for these highly specialized injuries. The role of the trauma team at such a center is to identify patients with potential spine injuries. Until these are ruled out, the patient must remain in full spinal immobilization, including a cervical collar. If an injury is identified on radiography, or if the patient has a neurologic deficit, a consult should be obtained from either the neurosurgical or orthopedic service.

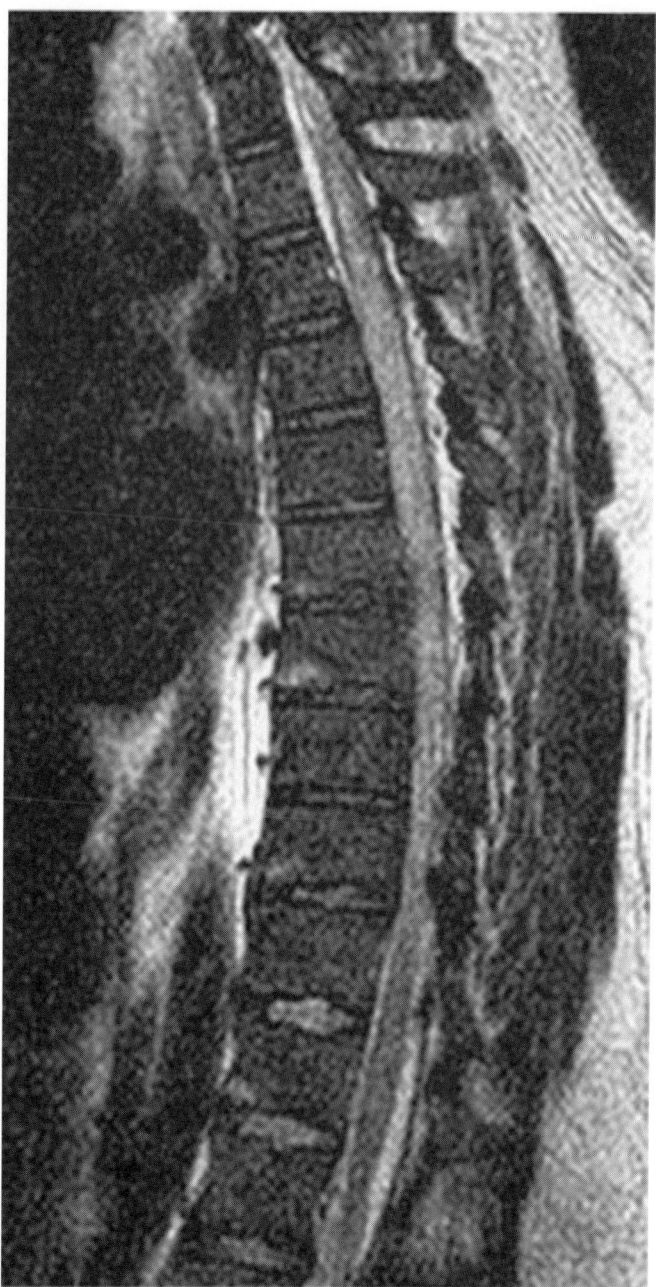

Figure 22.6 Midsagittal T2 MRI of the thoracic spine showing multiple-level spinal cord edema resulting from spinal cord infarct in a polytrauma patient.

There are two considerations in the surgical treatment of patients with SCI: stabilization and decompression. There are many scenarios to consider. Spinal cord injury without radiographic abnormality (SCIWORA) is uncommon but can be followed without surgical intervention. More common is extrinsic compression of the neural elements, creating the neurologic injury. This scenario often involves some element of spinal instability. A surgeon must consider both decompression and stabilization when evaluating the patient.

While most providers agree that surgery plays an important role, controversy exists concerning administration of

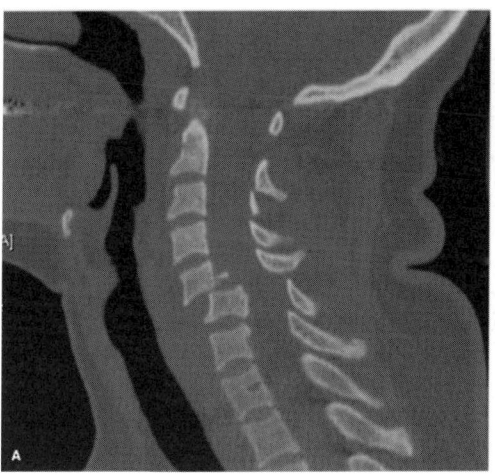
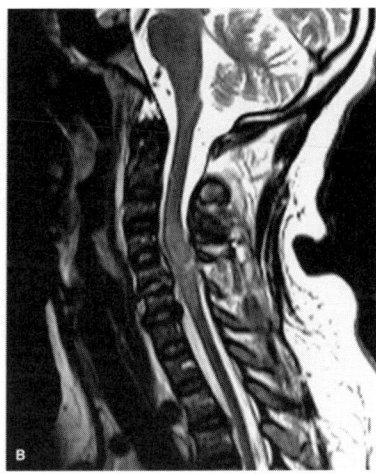

Figure 22.7 (**A**) Midsagittal CT scan of bilateral facet fracture–dislocation of C5–C6. (**B**) Midsagittal T2 MRI after emergent reduction, showing near-transection of the cervical spinal cord with edema extending up to the level of the C3–C4 disk space. This patient underwent surgical stabilization without any neurologic return.

ASIA IMPAIRMENT SCALE

☐ **A** = **Complete:** No motor or sensory function is preserved in the sacral segments S4-S5.

☐ **B** = **Incomplete:** Sensory but not motor function is preserved below the neurological level and includes the sacral segments S4-S5.

☐ **C** = **Incomplete:** Motor function is preserved below the neurological level, and more than half of key muscles below the neurological level have a muscle grade less than 3.

☐ **D** = **Incomplete:** Motor function is preserved below the neurological level, and at least half of key muscles below the neurological level have a muscle grade of 3 or more.

☐ **E** = **Normal:** Motor and sensory function are normal.

CLINICAL SYNDROMES (OPTIONAL)

☐ Central Cord
☐ Brown-Sequard
☐ Anterior Cord
☐ Conus Medullaris
☐ Cauda Equina

Figure 22.8 American Spinal Injury Association (ASIA) impairment scale.

Administration of steroids

Administration of high-dose steroids is felt by many to limit the secondary effects of spinal cord injuries. There has been a large amount of research involving the efficacy, timing, dosage, duration, and morbidity of this treatment. The National Acute Spinal Cord Injury Study has been established to make recommendations concerning the role of methyl-prednisolone in spinal cord injuries. Despite three summits, controversy still exists concerning the benefit of steroid treatment.[4–6]

The use of steroids is ultimately the decision of the treating physician and treatment protocols established by their institution. In a study of 305 providers, 90% routinely implemented steroids in acute spinal cord injuries but only 20% felt it improved clinical outcome.[4] Many providers and institutions feel there may be legal ramifications if steroids are not utilized. However, there are significant side effects and morbidity associated with this treatment. Multiple organ systems are affected by the administration of high-dose steroids, and complications include higher rates of sepsis and pneumonia and prolonged ICU stays.

Most providers feel that the use of steroids is at best controversial. The authors conclude that the use of steroids should be utilized on a case-by-case basis. A fracture dislocation in the midthoracic spine with complete spinal cord injury is different from a unilateral facet dislocation at C6–C7 with an incomplete spinal cord injury. In midthoracic injuries, the risks of the treatment outweigh the benefits, and minimal functional improvement can be expected. Motor improvement in the cervical spine can have a huge effect on rehabilitation, ability to transfer, and independence in activities of daily living. The level of injury plays a major factor in steroid utilization. In a review of the literature, Sayer *et al.* concluded there was insufficient evidence to support the use of methylprednisolone in acute spinal cord injuries.[5] Steroids are not indicated for SCI secondary to penetrating trauma.

steroids, timing of surgery, and techniques of stabilization. Because of the devastating nature of spinal cord injuries, it has been difficult to complete randomized, prospective studies looking at the efficacy of surgical intervention. Most providers make decisions based on their experience and the protocols established by the institution in which they provide care.

Timing of surgery

Even more controversial than steroid administration is the timing of surgery in SCI. There are many factors that play a role in the timing of surgery. Patients involved in high-energy mechanisms may not be medically optimized for early surgical intervention. Strict adherence to the Advanced Trauma Life Support (ATLS) protocol with respect to injury diagnosis and resuscitation is paramount in decreasing mortality and prioritizing care. Complete evaluation of the patient's spine may be safely deferred, especially in the presence of hemodynamic instability, as long as the spine is immobilized properly.

Studies have shown that recovery in SCI depends on degree of extrinsic spinal cord compression, initial severity of neurologic injury, and duration of neurologic compression. Animal models have shown improvement in motor function with early decompression.[7,8] Previously, these results had not been shown in humans,[9,10] though multiple studies have shown decreased morbidity, shorter length of acute hospital stay, and safety of early surgery.[10–14] Results of the Surgical Timing in Acute Spinal Cord Injury Study (STASCIS) indicate an improvement in ASIA scale in cervical SCI patients with early decompression (defined as < 24 hours from injury) compared to patients with late decompression.[15]

Anderson and Bohlman have shown neurologic improvement in complete and incomplete quadriplegics with late decompression.[16,17] These decompressive operations were performed, on average, 15 months in the complete injuries and 13 months in the incomplete injuries after the trauma. Late decompression, up to 4.5 years out, has also been shown to improve dysesthetic pain in thoracolumbar injuries.[18]

Most surgeons feel that decompression of the neurologic elements can benefit patients with traumatic injuries, although the optimal time for the decompressive surgery remains controversial. Incomplete injuries are usually decompressed in an emergent or urgent manner. The prognosis for complete injuries remains poor, and urgent decompression does not appear to affect functional recovery.

Unique surgical considerations

Spinal cord injuries can create unique scenarios that the surgical team must consider when preparing for surgery. The surgeon's goal is for the patient to come through the operation with a stable spine and decompressed neurologic elements. These operations often involve the use of spinal cord monitoring and specialized intubation and positioning techniques.

Positioning a patient with an unstable spine can be a challenge. A patient with an unstable cervical fracture–dislocation and incomplete neurologic injury often requires awake fiberoptic oral or nasotracheal intubation without manipulation of the head and neck (see Chapter 3). Spinal cord monitoring can be obtained at baseline and checked during and after positioning of the patient. Unstable thoracic injuries that are treated posteriorly often necessitate awake supine tracheal intubation on a table capable of atraumatic prone positioning. The following case illustrates some of these surgical principles. A 52-year-old man sustained the injury in Figure 22.9A from a fall from 25 feet (7.6 m). Physical exam revealed an incomplete SCI with decreased sensation below the level of the fracture dislocation. This injury is unstable in that it involves all three columns of the spine, and the spinal cord is in jeopardy of sustaining further injury if reduction and stabilization of the fracture–dislocation is not accomplished. Surgical considerations include both decompression and stabilization. The patient was taken to the operating room and placed supine on a flat Jackson table. Awake tracheal intubation was accomplished without any change in neurologic status. Spinal cord monitoring was accomplished in the supine position and baseline potentials were obtained. The

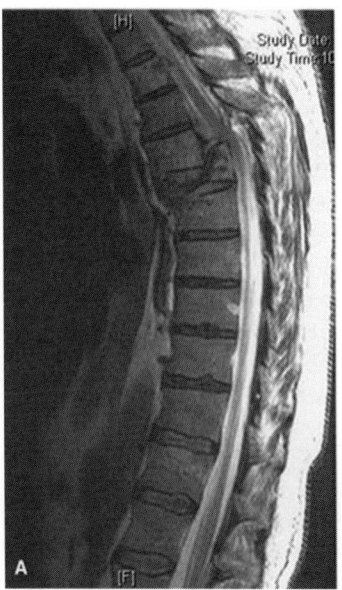
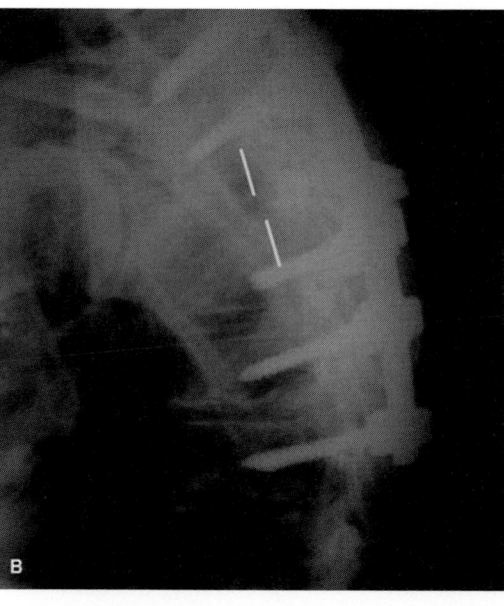

Figure 22.9 (**A**) Midsagittal T2 MRI showing T4–T5 fracture–dislocation and "tenting" of spinal cord over T5 vertebral body. (**B**) Lateral thoracic radiograph after posterior pedicle screw stabilization, showing near-anatomic reduction of the T4–T5 fracture–dislocation. The reduction was achieved by simply positioning the patient in the prone position and reducing the upper screws into the lower thoracic screws with a straight bar.

prone Jackson board with posts was placed on top of the patient. The patient was "flipped" to the prone position, asked to move his feet while the spinal cord monitoring was evaluated for any changes. General anesthesia was then induced by the anesthesia team. The patient underwent posterior stabilization with pedicle screw instrumentation (Fig. 22.9B) and woke up neurologically intact. The act of rolling the patient to the prone position reduced the fracture–dislocation enough to decompress the spinal cord. The spinal cord monitoring potentials actually improved from the supine to the prone position. The patient remains neurologically intact over a year from his injury.

Many patients with high cervical spinal cord injuries will require long-term ventilatory support. If decompression and/or stabilization are required, the timing of tracheostomy must be considered. If a stabilization procedure is required, this might be accomplished through a posterior approach. Percutaneous tracheostomy can be performed safely without increasing surgical site infections if done 6–10 days after the spinal procedure.[19] Early tracheostomy in SCI patients has been associated with shorter duration of mechanical ventilation and shorter ICU stays.[20]

Decompression of the neurological elements

As mentioned above, there are two surgical considerations in traumatic spinal cord injuries: decompression and stabilization. Often there is some element of extrinsic compression causing or contributing to the neurologic deficit. This compression can be caused by bone, disk herniation, hematoma, or foreign bodies, as in gunshot injuries. Magnetic resonance imaging (MRI) plays a major role in determining the nature of neurologic compression. Many providers feel that patients with acute traumatic SCI should be transported to an institution with 24-hour MRI capability.

Dislocations in the cervical spine are common and often present with varying degrees of neurological injury. The anatomy of the facet joints renders them susceptible to dislocation with and without fractures. Facet dislocations impart instability through the facet and anterior column. These dislocations can be reduced with skeletal traction upon presentation to the trauma center. Accurate assessment of spinal cord function upon presentation has been discussed previously. A lateral cervical spine x-ray (Fig. 22.10A), computed tomography (CT) scan (Fig. 22.10B), and MRI (Fig. 22.10C) are important studies to obtain. Once the diagnosis of cervical facet dislocation with neurologic injury is made, urgent reduction should be undertaken. Reduction can be accomplished by skeletal traction with serial neurologic assessments in a cooperative patient (Fig. 22.10D).

Decompression of the neurological elements is the most important factor in determining the approach utilized in traumatic spinal surgery. In the cervical spine, decompression is usually accomplished by the anterior approach. Decompression can involve single-level diskectomies to multiple-level corpectomies. Rarely does the injury pattern necessitate a posterior approach. This is illustrated by a lamina fracture with displacement ventrally causing compression of the spinal cord (Fig. 22.11).

The thoracic spine is relatively stiff. Thoracic injuries tend to be stable without neurologic injury or grossly unstable with devastating injury to the spinal cord. Most of these injuries either do not require decompression or can be effectively decompressed by rolling the patient to the prone position. Decompressing the spinal cord posteriorly can be accomplished by a transpedicular approach in which the pedicles are removed to the level of the posterior vertebral body. This allows access to the ventral surface of the spinal cord through the posterior approach.

Decompression of the thoracolumbar (T10–L2) spine remains controversial among providers. A reproducible, validated classification system that provides an algorithm for treatment and prognosis does not exist. Vaccaro et al. presented a classification system based on fracture morphology, neurologic injury, and the integrity of the posterior osteoligamentous complex.[21] This system reproducibly characterizes these injuries while directing the surgeon in the surgical approach for decompression and stabilization. In a summit attended by 21 of the worlds' leading neurologic and orthopedic trauma spinal surgeons, there was fairly high agreement in surgical decision making when presented with different types of injuries.[22] Presently, most providers feel the anterior approach affords a more thorough decompression of the spinal cord, conus medullaris, and cauda equina. This approach is often utilized for incomplete spinal cord injuries. Surgery usually involves a retroperitoneal approach, corpectomy of the fractured vertebrae, strut graft or structural cage placement, and instrumentation of the vertebrae above and below the injury. If the posterior osteoligamentous complex is involved, the anterior procedure is often augmented by posterior stabilization. If the neurologic injury is purely radicular, this can be effectively decompressed from a standard midline posterior approach.

Stabilization

Usually surgery in traumatic spinal cord injuries involves both decompression and stabilization. However, operative stabilization of an injured vertebral segment often needs to be performed in neurologically intact patients. This procedure usually involves fusion of at least one motion segment. A surgeon cannot make the patient any better than "neurologically intact." The risk of iatrogenic neurologic injury always exists with surgery, but it is a more important consideration when operating on a patient with an unstable injury without a neurologic deficit.

In the cervical spine, stabilization can be accomplished by either an anterior or a posterior approach. The anterior approach involves diskectomy and/or corpectomy with bone graft (auto- or allograft) reconstruction and fusion with or without hardware. Posterior approaches involve stabilization

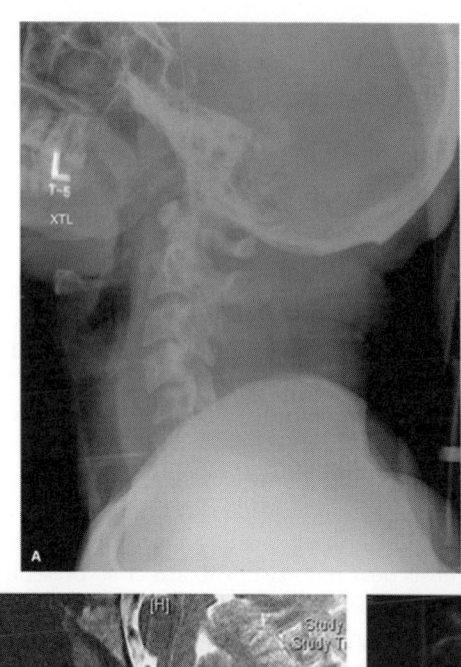

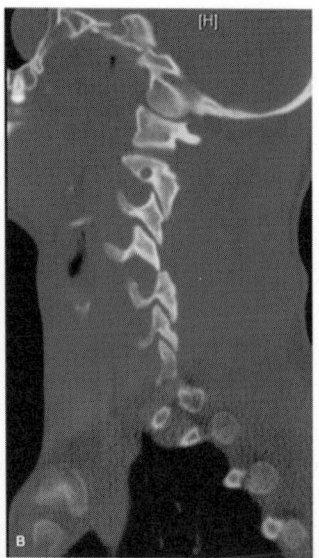

Figure 22.10 (**A**) Lateral cervical spine radiograph showing traumatic subluxation of C4–C5. (**B**) Sagittal CT through facet joints showing C4–C5 facet dislocation. (**C**) Midsagittal T2 MRI showing C4–C5 subluxation and large disk fragment causing spinal cord compression. (**D**) Lateral cervical spine radiograph taken after the patient was placed in Gardner–Wells traction and reduced. The patient underwent anterior cervical diskectomy and fusion with resolution of his central cord syndrome about 3 months after the injury.

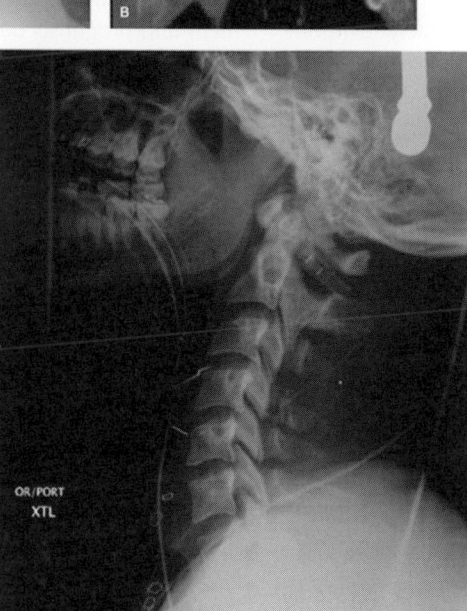

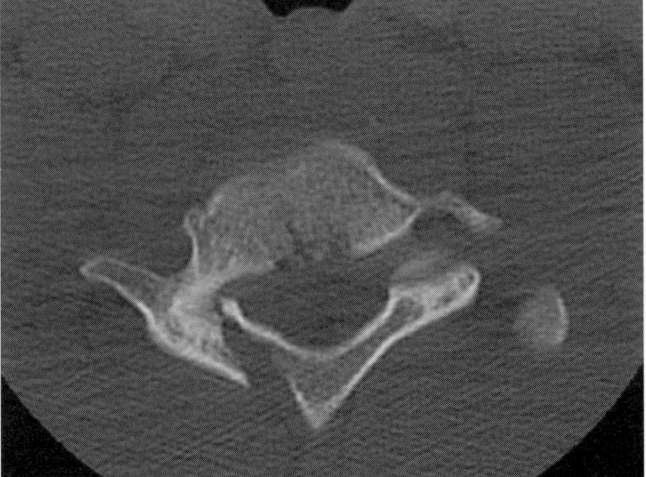

Figure 22.11 Axial CT scan through C7 showing displaced lamina and lateral mass fractures, necessitating a posterior approach for decompression.

with lateral mass instrumentation with bone grafting. In general, the anterior approach is better tolerated than the posterior. The surgical stabilization approach can be performed based on the surgeon's preference. The surgeon must critically analyze each injury and assess which approach will provide stability for the patient with the fewest motion segments being fused. Many times the injury warrants a combined approach with extensive anterior and posterior reconstructions. Brodke *et al.* studied 52 consecutive patients with traumatic spinal injuries, and found no difference in outcomes when comparing the anterior to the posterior approach.[23]

Stabilization procedures for the thoracic and lumbar spines are usually performed through a posterior approach. The use of pedicle screws has allowed the spine surgeon predictable and safe instrumentation for most unstable injuries. As mentioned above, anterior decompression procedures often need posterior augmentation. These procedures can be performed under one anesthetic or staged, based on the condition of the patient.

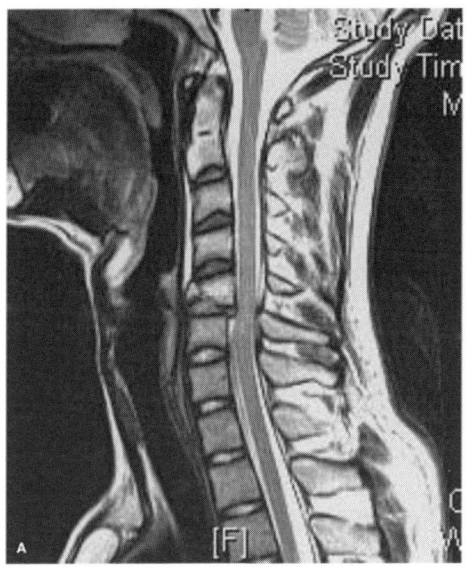 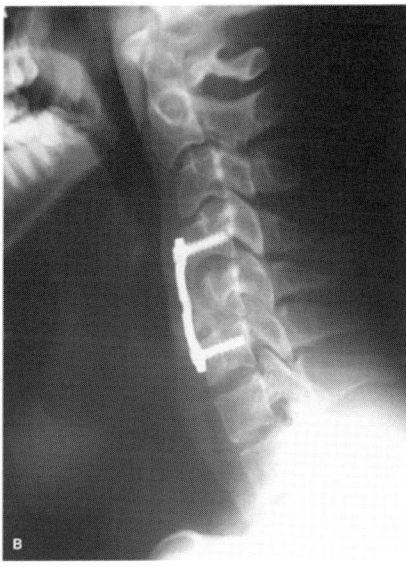

Figure 22.12 (**A**) Midsagittal T2 MRI showing C5 fracture with retrolisthesis causing spinal cord compression. (**B**) Lateral cervical spine radiograph postoperatively after C5 corpectomy C4–C6 cervical fusion with iliac crest bone graft and anterior instrumentation.

The stability of a motion segment is not always apparent to the surgeon. Posttraumatic instability can evolve at the time of injury or years after the injury. Most surgeons tend to brace traumatic injuries and follow them with sequential radiographs. Certain injuries are prone to instability and therefore are often treated with surgical stabilization. Cervical injuries that cause neurologic deficits usually require decompression of the neurologic elements. The decompression renders the motion segment(s) unstable, necessitating a stabilization procedure (Fig. 22.12).

Conclusions

Surgery is an important aspect in the multidisciplinary approach to improving function of spinal cord injury patients. Surgery involves decompression and stabilization to impart a stable motion segment while protecting the neurologic elements from further injury. The optimal timing, pharmacologic benefit, and surgical approach continue to evolve. Only through continued basic science research, improvement in spinal instrumentation, and the development of classification systems and treatment protocols will surgeons be able to maximize their contribution to the care of these highly specialized patients.

Questions

(1) The majority of spinal cord injuries occur in which part of the spine?
 a. Cervical
 b. Thoracic
 c. Lumbar
 d. Sacral
 e. Thoracolumbar junction

(2) All of the following are secondary causes of injury to the spinal cord, *except*:
 a. Vascular changes
 b. Electrolyte changes

 c. Initiation of neurotransmitter cascades
 d. Free radical production
 e. Suppression of immune responses

(3) A 27-year-old male presents to the ED after a motor vehicle accident. Imaging reveals liver lacerations, splenic lacerations and a C4/5 fracture–dislocation. The patient starts to become hypotensive and bradycardic en route to the OR. Which type(s) of shock should you be concerned about?
 a. Neurogenic
 b. Septic
 c. Hypovolemic
 d. Hypovolemic and neurogenic
 e. Neurogenic and septic

(4) What are the two main goals of surgery for patients with spinal cord injury?
 a. Stabilization of motion segment and restoring neurologic function
 b. Stabilization and decompression of neurologic elements
 c. Decompression of neurologic elements and early motion
 d. Restoring neurologic function and pain relief
 e. Pain relief and prevention of infection

(5) Which statement is true regarding timing of interventions for spinal cord injuries?
 a. Immediate administration of steroids has been shown to definitively improve neurologic function
 b. Percutaneous tracheostomies in ventilator dependent patients should be delayed for 1–2 weeks due to risk of infection
 c. The timing of surgery is controversial, but most surgeons address incomplete injuries in an urgent manner
 d. Complete spinal cord injuries should be prioritized over incomplete injuries for surgical intervention

e. Early surgery leads to prolonged ICU stays and increased hospital costs

(6) **What determines the surgical approach (anterior vs. posterior) in spinal cord injury patients?**
   a. Prognosis for neurologic recovery
   b. Decompression of neurologic elements
   c. Incomplete versus complete injuries
   d. Respiratory function
   e. Timing of surgery

(7) **Concerning surgery for injuries of the cervical spine:**
   a. Both anterior and posterior approaches may be needed
   b. Posterior approaches are better tolerated than anterior approaches.
   c. Anterior approaches to the cervical spine lead to longer hospital stays
   d. Intubation is prolonged to protect the patient's airway
   e. Anterior cervical approaches are preferred to prevent swelling

(8) **Which of the following is *not* a factor in assessing thoracolumbar (T10–L2) injuries?**
   a. Neurologic function
   b. Fracture pattern
   c. Presence of cauda equina syndrome
   d. Integrity of posterior osteoligamentous complex
   e. Central cord syndrome

(9) **Which of these statements regarding the necessity for surgical intervention in spinal cord injuries is correct?**
   a. Neurologically intact patients do not usually need surgical stabilization
   b. Patients with complete spinal cord injuries do not benefit from surgery
   c. Surgical decompression is warranted for injuries with extrinsic spinal cord compression
   d. Late decompression has been shown to have no benefit in patients with neurologic deficits
   e. Surgical stabilization is needed for the majority of thoracic injuries

(10) **Posttraumatic instability:**
   a. Can be predicted based on the amount of neurologic deficit
   b. May evolve years after the injury
   c. Is more common with a posterior surgical approach
   d. Is an indication for administration of steroids
   e. Can be treated by bracing exclusively

Answers

(1) a
(2) e
(3) d
(4) b
(5) c
(6) b
(7) a
(8) e
(9) c
(10) b

References

1. Oliver M, Inaba K, Tang A, *et al.* The changing epidemiology of spinal trauma: a 13-year review from a Level I trauma centre. *Injury* 2012; **43**: 1296–300.

2. Grossman RG, Frankowski RF, Burau KD, *et al.* Incidence and severity of acute complications after spinal cord injury. *J Neurosurg Spine* 2012; **17** (1 Suppl): 119–28.

3. Guly HR, Bouamra O, Lecky FE; Trauma Audit and Research Network. The incidence of neurogenic shock in patients with isolated spinal cord injury in the emergency department. *Resuscitation* 2008; **76**: 57–62.

4. Eck JC, Nachtigall D, Humphreys SC, Hodges SD. Questionnaire survey of spine surgeons on the use of methylprednisolone for acute spinal cord injury. *Spine (Phila Pa 1976)* 2006; **31**: E250–3.

5. Sayer FT, Kronvall E, Nilsson OG. Methylprednisolone treatment in acute spinal cord injury: the myth challenged through a structured analysis of published literature. *Spine J* 2006; **6**: 335–43.

6. Kubeck JP, Merola A, Mathur S, *et al.* End organ effects of high-dose human equivalent methylprednisolone in a spinal cord injury rat model. *Spine (Phila Pa 1976)* 2006; **31**: 257–61.

7. Shields CB, Zhang YP, Shields LB, *et al.* The therapeutic window for spinal cord decompression in a rat spinal cord injury model. *J Neurosurg Spine* 2005; **3**: 302–7.

8. Carlson GD, Minato Y, Okada A, *et al.* Early time-dependent decompression for spinal cord injury: vascular mechanisms of recovery. *J Neurotrauma* 1997; **14**: 951–62.

9. Vaccaro AR, Daugherty RJ, Sheehan TP, *et al.* Neurologic outcome of early versus late surgery for cervical spinal cord injury. *Spine (Phila Pa 1976)* 1997; **22**: 2609–13.

10. McKinley W, Meade MA, Kirshblum S, Barnard B. Outcomes of early surgical management versus late or no surgical intervention after acute spinal cord injury. *Arch Phys Med Rehabil* 2004; **85**: 1818–25.

11. Ball JR, Sekhon LH. Timing of decompression and fixation after spinal cord injury–when is surgery optimal? *Crit Care Resus* 2006; **8**: 56–63.

12. Fehlings MG, Perrin RG. The role and timing of early decompression for cervical spinal cord injury: update with a review of recent clinical evidence. *Injury* 2005; **36** (Suppl 2): B13–26.

13. Guest J, Eleraky MA, Apostolides PJ, Dickman CA, Sonntag VK. Traumatic central cord syndrome: results of surgical management. *J Neurosurg* 2002; **97** (1 Suppl): 25–32.

14. Kishan S, Vives MJ, Reiter MF. Timing of surgery following spinal cord injury. *J Spinal Cord Med* 2005; **28**: 11–19.

15. Fehlings MG, Vaccaro A, Wilson JR, *et al.* Early versus delayed decompression for traumatic cervical spinal cord injury: results of the

Surgical Timing in Acute Spinal Cord Injury Study (STASCIS). *PLoS One* 2012; **7** (2): e32037.

16. Bohlman HH, Anderson PA. Anterior decompression and arthrodesis of the cervical spine: long-term motor improvement. Part I: improvement in incomplete traumatic quadriparesis. *J Bone Joint Surg Am* 1992; **74**: 671–82.

17. Anderson PA, Bohlman HH. Anterior decompression and arthrodesis of the cervical spine: long-term motor improvement. Part II: improvement in complete traumatic quadriplegia. *J Bone Joint Surg Am* 1992; **74**: 683–92.

18. Bohlman HH, Kirkpatrick JS, Delamarter RB, Leventhal M. Anterior decompression for late pain and paralysis after fractures of the thoracolumbar spine. *Clin Orthop Relat Res* 1994; (300): 24–9.

19. O'Keeffe T, Goldman RK, Mayberry JC, Rehm CG, Hart RA. Tracheostomy after anterior cervical spine fixation. *J Trauma Injury Infection Crit Care* 2004; **57**: 855–60.

20. Ganuza JR, Garcia Forcada A, Gambarrutta C, *et al*. Effect of technique and timing of tracheostomy in patients with acute traumatic spinal cord injury undergoing mechanical ventilation. *J Spinal Cord Med* 2011; **34**: 76–84.

21. Vaccaro AR, Lehman RA, Hurlbert RJ, *et al*. A new classification of thoracolumbar injuries: the importance of injury morphology, the integrity of the posterior ligamentous complex, and neurologic status. *Spine (Phila Pa 1976)* 2005; **30**: 2325–33.

22. Vaccaro AR, Lim MR, Hurlbert RJ, *et al*. Surgical decision making for unstable thoracolumbar spine injuries: results of a consensus panel review by the Spine Trauma Study Group. *J Spinal Disord Tech* 2006; **19**: 1–10.

23. Brodke DS, Anderson PA, Newell DW, Grady MS, Chapman JR. Comparison of anterior and posterior approaches in cervical spinal cord injuries. *J Spinal Disord Tech* 2003; **16**: 229–35.

Anesthesia for spinal cord trauma

Armagan Dagal and Arthur M. Lam

Objectives

(1) Review the prevalence and types of spinal cord injuries.
(2) Evaluate airway management choices in patients with spinal cord injuries.
(3) Review the implications of spinal cord injuries for intraoperative anesthetic management.
(4) Discuss the anesthetic implications of neuromonitoring in patients with spinal cord injuries.
(5) Develop an understanding of perioperative and posttraumatic medical complications after spinal cord injuries.

Introduction

Spinal cord injury (SCI) is a common disease. It occurs when biomechanical forces applied to the spinal column exceed the strength of the spinal column unit (see Chapter 22). Management of the SCI is complex. Specialty centers providing multidisciplinary care and intensive care units with sophisticated monitoring capabilities play an integral role in the care of SCI patients and have been shown to improve outcomes. Anesthesiologists are frequently involved in many aspects of the care of the patient with SCI, including airway management, initial resuscitation, intraoperative and intensive care, as well as acute pain management. An in-depth understanding of this devastating disease therefore is required for optimal outcomes.

Prevalence and etiology of spinal cord injury

SCI encompasses a wide range of pathologies, from a minor sprain to a life-threatening tetraplegia. The bony structure of the spine encloses, protects, and supports the delicate spinal cord. A cord injury may occur anywhere from the articulation of the cervical spine with the occiput to the sacrum. Spinal fractures or ligamentous injury may or may not have associated spinal cord damage, the presence of which would define the SCI. Insult to the cord comprises a spectrum of disease states depending on the location of the injury and the nature of the deficit (see Chapter 22).

The annual incidence of spinal fracture is reported to be 19–88 per 100,000 in the USA. Approximately 6% of the spinal column fractures will have an underlying spinal cord injury, accounting for up to 11–53 per million persons. This would translate to approximately 12,400 new cases in 2012.[1]

Men are four times more likely than women to sustain an SCI. The average age is around 41 years. Most SCIs are associated with an injury to the vertebral column as well as a coexisting traumatic injury to other regions. About 40% of the injuries occur because of motor vehicle collisions (MVCs), followed by falls and acts of violence. Acts of violence and sports-related injuries tend to decline with advancing age, while falls increase with advancing age, becoming the leading cause of SCI among victims who are at least 50 years of age.[1,2]

Some 250,000 Americans are currently living with the debilitating consequences of SCI, and its related healthcare costs are estimated to be $9.7 billion annually.

Spine precautions are important in the initial management of trauma patients. About 50% of patients with cord injury arrive at the emergency department without a diagnosis of severe SCI from prehospital settings (see Chapter 2). This highlights the critical importance of employing full spine precautions during transfer of these patients. The risk of SCI is higher in patients who have sustained serious injuries by specific mechanisms (falls > 2 meters, high-speed MVC, penetrating injuries), and who have decreased level of consciousness or chest injuries.

About 10% of spinal column injuries occur at more than one vertebral level.

Anatomy of the spinal cord

The spinal column is the bony structure made up of seven cervical, twelve thoracic, and five lumbar vertebrae, as well as the sacrum. The spinal cord exits the skull through the foramen magnum and enters the canal formed by the vertebral bodies. In the adult, the cord terminates at approximately the lower aspect of the first lumbar vertebral body. The vertebral bony column protects the cord while supporting the body and allowing movement through articulation of each vertebral body with adjacent bodies.

Adequate blood supply to the entire cord is essential. The spinal cord is supplied by two vascular systems that function independently from each other. The central system, which supplies the anterior two-thirds of the spinal cord, is derived from the single anterior spinal artery (ASA), and its blood flow is centrifugal. The peripheral system mainly supplies the peripheral and posterior parts of the spinal cord, and its blood flow is directed towards the center of the cord via the two posterior spinal arteries (PSA) and the pial arterial plexus.[3]

The ASA runs caudad along the length of the spinal cord and receives contributories from the radicular arteries via the intercostal vessels. The artery of Adamkiewicz is the most important radicular vessel, typically joining the ASA in the lower thoracic region and providing blood supply to the thoracolumbar cord. The PSA arises from the posterior branches of the vertebral arteries and receives contributions from the radicular arteries (Fig. 23.1).

Recent data from animal models concerning the collateral network blood supply of the cord indicate that there are extensive longitudinal interconnections between the spinal cord and the paravertebral tissues, including the muscles along the vertebral column which also receive contributions from the subclavian, hypogastric, and iliac arteries. This rich collateral blood supply may help to explain preservation of spinal cord perfusion when segmental vessels are interrupted. Again, in animal studies it has been shown that the muscular arterial component dominates the anatomy of the network when compared to the small arteries feeding the spinal cord directly. The anatomic imbalance between the vascular input to muscle and spinal cord may result in a "steal phenomenon" diverting the blood from the spinal cord to the paravertebral muscles when they are in high metabolic activity. This might explain the improvements in the spinal cord ischemic tolerance through reduction in muscle and spinal cord metabolism with the application of moderate hypothermia and neuromuscular blockade.[4,5]

Classification of vertebral column injuries

The nature of the bony injury is important, as it will guide further management of the patient regardless of the neurological injury (see Chapter 22). An unstable injury puts the neural elements at risk and will necessitate some intervention to provide stability, which may be nonsurgical, with an application of a thoracolumbosacral orthosis (TLSO) or halo-vest traction, or surgical. Determining the stability of the injury is therefore essential for surgical and anesthetic decision making.

Traumatic spinal dislocations, vertebral fractures, and fracture–dislocations are classified by the Orthopedic Trauma Association classification system.[6] In brief, the anatomic regions cervical, thoracic, and lumbar spine are assigned an A, B, or C type for the mechanism of the injury and are numbered 1, 2, or 3 for the injury severity. A-type fractures occur because of axial loading to the anterior spinal column and are frequently stable. The A3 subtype of burst fractures

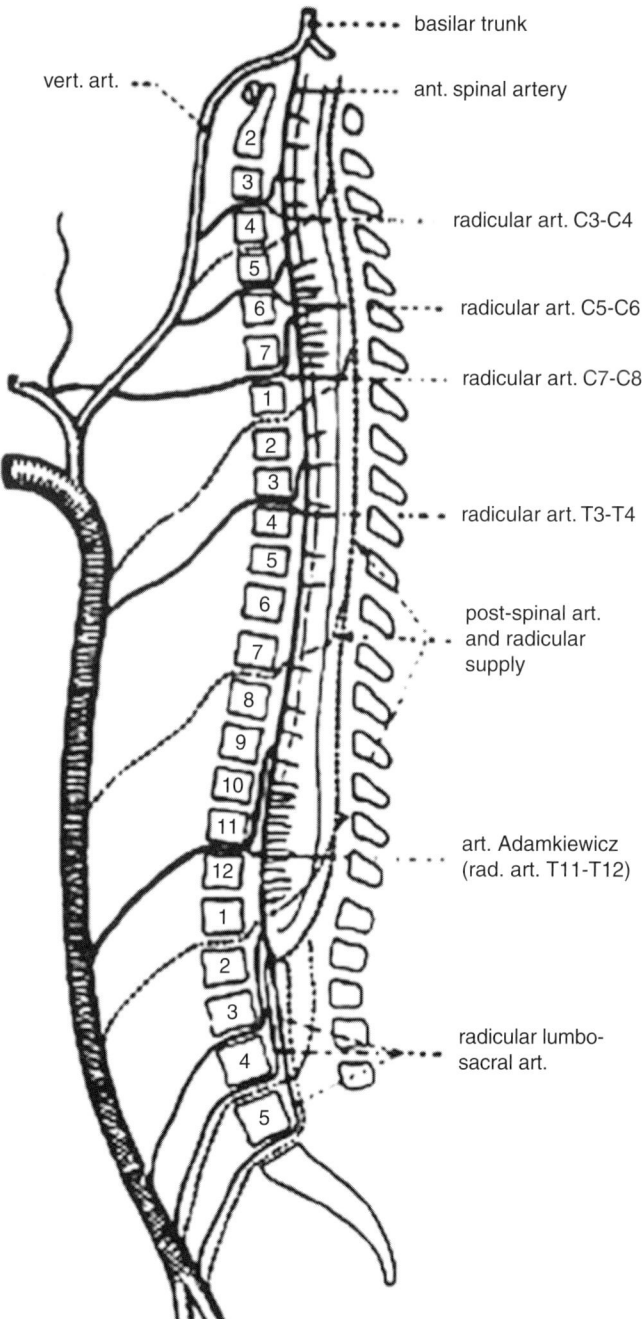

Figure 23.1 Vascular supply of the spinal cord.

may be associated with acute SCI in the case of fragment dislocation into the spinal canal, leading to spinal cord compression. The entity of B-type injuries represents unstable three-column injuries secondary to flexion–distraction (B1/B2) or hyperextension (B3) mechanisms. C-type fractures represent rotationally unstable fracture dislocations and carry the highest severity. The incidence of associated neurologic SCI can be graded from minimum in C1-type to maximum in C3-type injury (Table 23.1).[7]

Table 23.1 The Orthopedic Trauma Association classification system

Fracture type	Axial compression			Flexion/distraction or hyperextension			A or B type with rotation		
	A1	A2	A3	B1	B2	B3	C1	C2	C3
Mechanism	Impaction/ compression	Split	Burst	Flexion/ distraction ligamentous	Flexion/ distraction osseous	Hyperextension	Rotational wedge	Rotational flexion/ extension	Rotational shear
Stability	Stable	Stable	Stable/ unstable	Unstable	Unstable	Unstable	Unstable	Unstable	Unstable
Management	Nonoperative	Nonoperative	Nonoperative/ operative	Operative	Operative	Operative	Operative	Operative	Operative

Previously, the most common system used for classification was Denis's three-column approach,[4] which was developed for the thoracolumbar spine. In this system, the anterior column contains the anterior longitudinal ligament, as well as the anterior half of the vertebral body and disk. The middle column contains the posterior half of the vertebral body and disk, as well as the posterior longitudinal ligament. The posterior column contains the facets, pedicles, spinous processes, and interspinous ligaments. Instability occurs when a fracture disrupts two or more columns. As a result, injuries such as compression fractures, which affect the anterior column, are stable. Burst fractures, affecting the anterior and middle column, and flexion–distraction injuries, affecting the anterior and posterior columns, are both unstable.

Types of spinal cord injury
Primary injury

Injury to the spinal cord typically involves bony and/or ligamentous injury to the vertebral column. Fractures and ligamentous damage can cause primary injury to the cord through various mechanisms, including canal compromise with a direct injury followed by disruption of the blood flow to the cord. In 19–34% of cases there may be a spinal cord injury without radiographic abnormality (SCIWORA).[7] SCIWORA is generally seen in children and is uncommon in the adult population (see also Chapter 34). The term is sometimes used inappropriately to diagnose patients who have spinal cord injury without computed tomography (CT) evidence of trauma (SCIWOCTET). SCIWOCTET refers to the patients with CT scans showing canal stenosis and significant degenerative changes in the cervical spine. These degenerative changes may cause moderate or severe canal stenosis. Trauma to the cervical spine, with its disk osteophyte complexes, bony spurring, and thickened ligamentum flavum, causes cord contusion and subsequent neurologic deficit. It is more commonly seen in men beyond 50 years of age. A ground-level fall is the usual mechanism, with subsequent negative CT scan of the head, and it is exclusively seen in those with moderate to severe degenerative changes noted on the CT of the cervical spine.[8]

The cord can be completely transected, but this rarely occurs. Instead, the nature of the initial damage is likely mediated through a combination of insults, including compression, contusion, or stretch, leading to loss of spinal cord microcirculation, loss of autoregulation, hemorrhage, and vasospasm, all of which result in cord ischemia and infarction in this immediate area, called the central zone. This primary injury cannot be modified by treatment.

Examples of common spine injuries are shown in Figures 23.2–23.6.

Secondary injury

The goal of care in SCI patients is to prevent secondary injury, thereby maintaining the viability of the penumbra. Penumbra is defined as the immediate area surrounding the central zone. Penumbra defines the zone of decreased blood flow that can progress either to severe ischemia and necrosis or to reperfusion and tissue survival. Preservation or reduction in the size of this zone leads to substantial clinical benefits.

Neuronal injury triggers a cascade of deleterious events initiated by a robust immune response leading to neuroinflammation, neurodegradation, and cytotoxicity within the injured spinal cord tissue. These mediators include proinflammatory cytokines, chemokines, and complement activation products. This is followed by an infiltration of neutrophils, macrophages, and lymphocytes into the injured neuronal tissue. These leukocytes play a role in the local release of neurotoxic molecules, including reactive oxygen species, nitrogen-derived free radicals, proteases, and other neurotoxic enzymes, which eventually lead to breakdown of the blood–spinal cord barrier (BSCB). When the protective effect of the BSCB is lost, systemic toxic molecules leak into the subarachnoid space in the injured spinal cord. This self-perpetuating exacerbated neuroinflammation leads to spinal cord edema, delayed neuronal cell death, and exacerbation of the secondary injury.[9,10]

Hypotension due to hemorrhage or loss of systemic vasomotor tone due to neurogenic shock further exacerbates the secondary injury by worsening the ischemia.

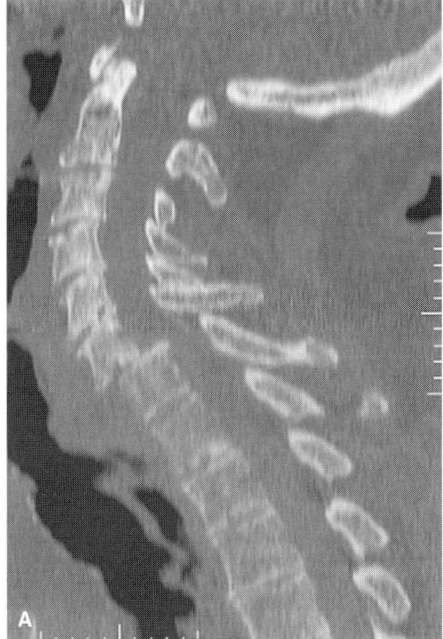
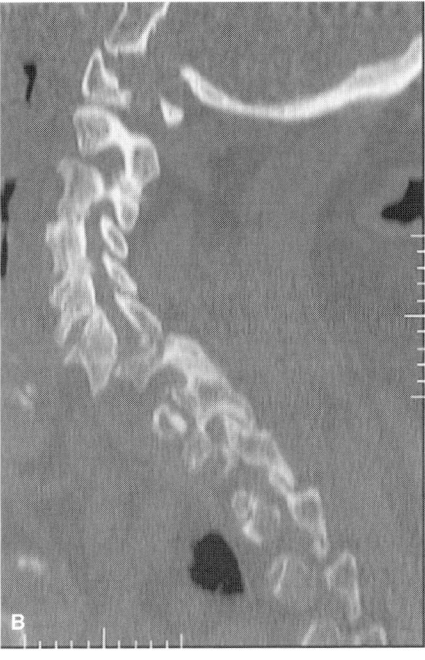

Figure 23.2 (A) Two images of a patient's cervical spine with a traumatic unilateral jumped facet.

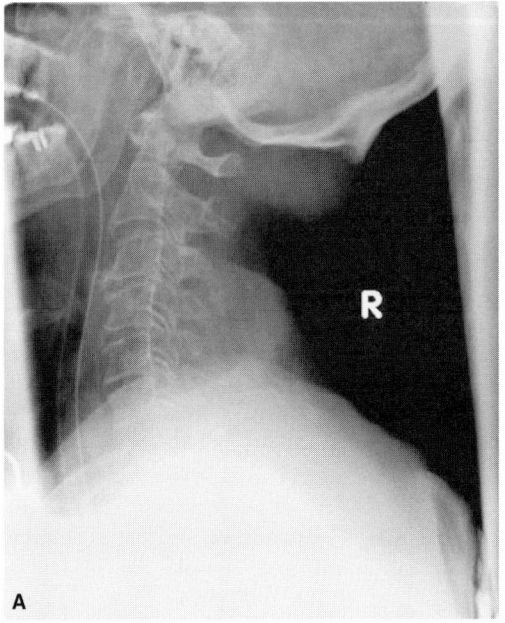
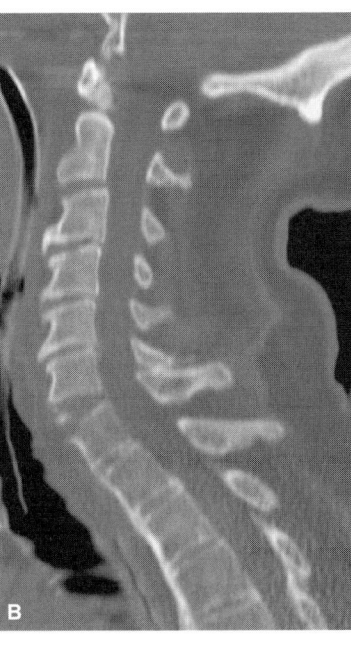

Figure 23.3 (A) A lateral plain film of the cervical spine demonstrating anterior-extension injury. (B) Also seen in the sagittal CT reconstruction.

American Spinal Injury Association (ASIA) classification

In an effort to categorize the sensory and motor impairments following SCI, and to improve functional prognostication, the ASIA classification was developed (Table 23.2). This system rates cord injuries by using a neurologic impairment scale (letters A through E). ASIA A is a complete cord lesion in which no motor or sensory function is preserved in the sacral segments S4–S5. ASIA B is incomplete, with only sensory function spared below the lesion, including S4–S5. ASIA C indicates an incomplete injury where more than half the important muscle groups below the injury have motor scores of less than 3. ASIA D is an incomplete injury where more than half of the muscle groups have motor scores of 3 or better. ASIA E indicates a neurologically intact individual.

Central, anterior, posterior, and Brown-Séquard injuries

Injury to the spinal cord will present with a different clinical picture depending on the location and severity of the injury (Table 23.3, Fig. 23.7). Complete and incomplete injury is differentiated by the presence or by the absence of the sensory

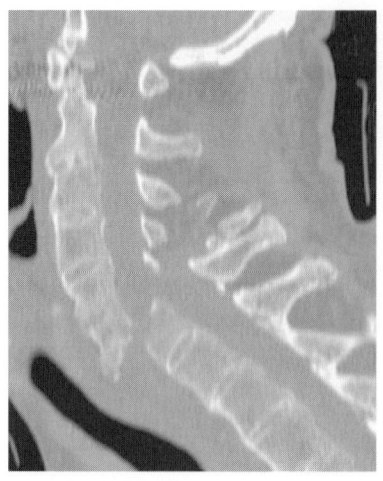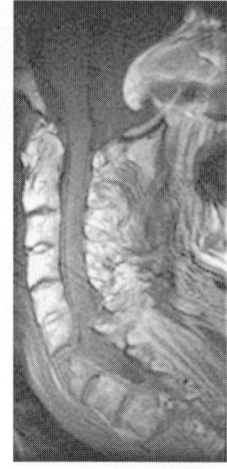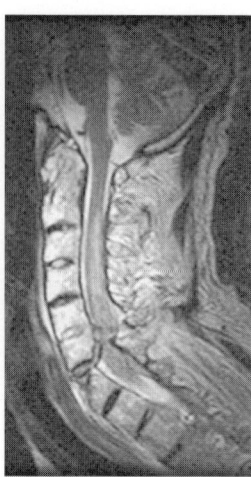

Figure 23.4 Images of the cervical spine in a patient with ankylosing spondylitis who suffered an extension–distraction injury, with obvious canal compromise.

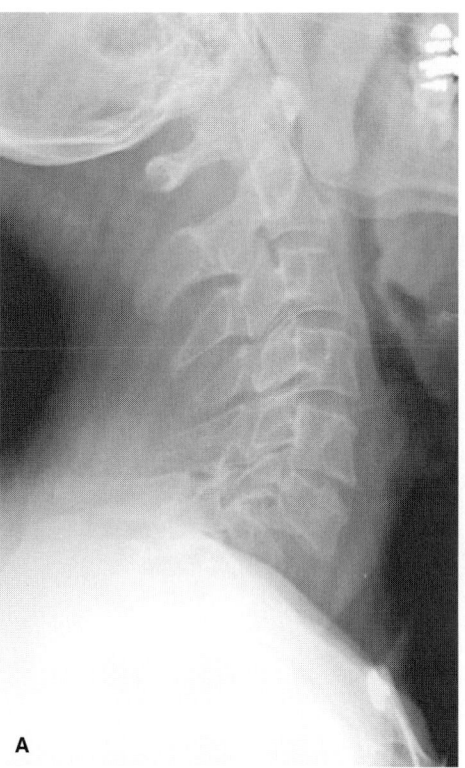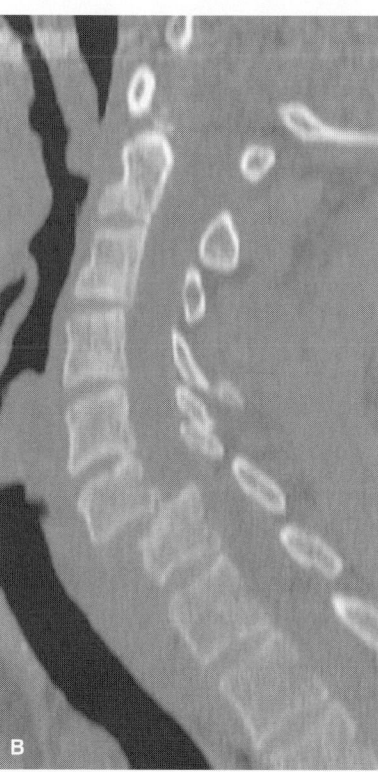

A   B

Figure 23.5 (**A**) Radiograph and (**B**) CT image showing bilateral facet override.

or motor function in the S4–S5 (perineal, specifically anal sensation) region.

Complete

About 30% of SCI patients present with a complete cord lesion and have no afferent and efferent signal transmission below the level of the injury.[2]

Incomplete

Central cord syndrome is a cervical lesion probably caused by hemorrhage into the cord following trauma. It is characterized by greater severity of paresis in the upper extremities than in the lower, bladder dysfunction, and variable loss of sensory function below the lesion. It is typically seen in the elderly population with a preexisting arthropathy following a hyperextension injury.

Anterior cord syndrome is generally due to a disruption of blood flow through the ASA at the level of the injury, either from a bone fragment or from a herniated disk. The resultant ischemic injury to the anterior portion of the cord disrupts motor function below the level, but has a variable effect on sensory function. Pain and temperature tracts are typically interrupted as well, but proprioception remains intact.

Posterior cord injury is a rare entity in which the dorsal column, carrying touch, vibration, and proprioception, is compromised.

Table 23.2 American Spinal Injury Association (ASIA) classification of spinal cord injury

ASIA A	Complete	No motor or sensory in sacral segments S4–S5
ASIA B	Incomplete	Sensory spared below lesion, including S4–S5
ASIA C	Incomplete	Motor score ≤ 3 for > 50% of major muscle groups
ASIA D	Incomplete	Motor score > 3 for > 50% of major muscle groups
ASIA E	Intact	No motor or sensory deficit

Table 23.3 Cord syndromes

Syndrome	Description
Central cord	Cervical lesion with upper-greater than lower-extremity paresis
Anterior cord	Anterior spinal artery disruption with loss of motor below lesion
Posterior cord	Rare, with loss of touch, vibration, and proprioception below lesion
Brown-Séquard	Interruption of lateral half of cord, with loss of ipsilateral motor and touch, and loss of contralateral pain and temperature
Cauda equina	Compression of nerve roots below conus, with saddle anesthesia, urinary retention, and fecal incontinence

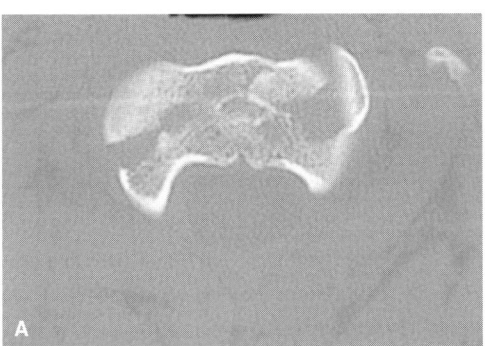

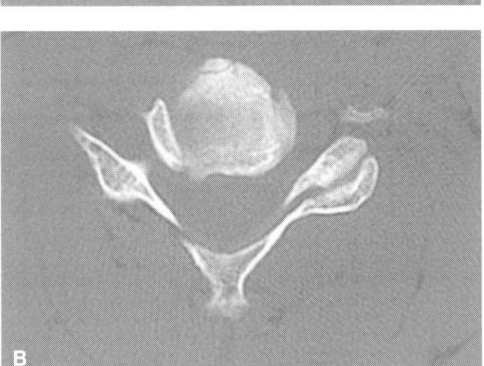

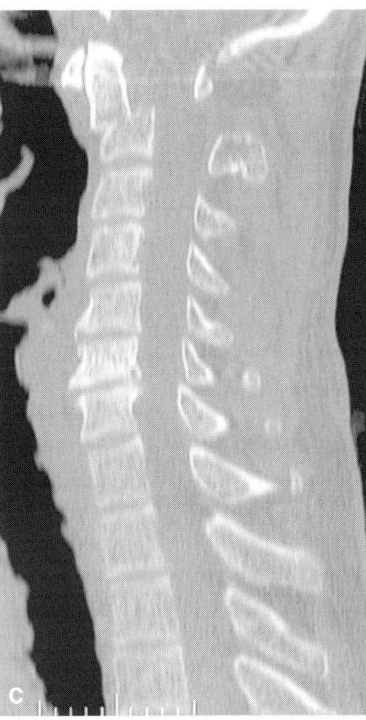

Figure 23.6 (**A, B**) Axial and (**C**) sagittal CT images demonstrating multiple cervical spine fractures.

Brown-Séquard syndrome is characterized by the interruption of the lateral half of the spinal cord, typically through penetrating trauma. It is rare to see a patient with the full spectrum of findings in Brown-Séquard. These would include loss of motor, touch, and vibration sensation ipsilateral to the lesion, with pain and temperature sensation lost contralateral to the lesion.

Cauda equina syndrome is the result of injury below the level of the conus, or caudal end of the cord, typically below L2. The cauda equina is compressed, typically resulting in perineal or "saddle" anesthesia, urinary retention, fecal incontinence, and a varying degree of lower-extremity weakness.

Common comorbid injuries

SCI from trauma does not always occur in isolation. Approximately 50% of patients with a spine injury have concomitant trauma. Injury to the cervical spine is often associated with blunt cerebrovascular injury, traumatic brain injury (TBI), and facial fractures (see Chapters 20, 21, 24, 25). About 20–60% of patients with SCI have concurrent TBI. Also, 24% of patients with SCI have associated thoracic trauma, which is inherently associated with vascular injury (see Chapters 29 and 30); in addition, one must consider the possibility of pneumothorax, blunt cardiac injury, and pulmonary contusion. Lumbar spine fractures may also be associated with both hollow viscus and solid organ

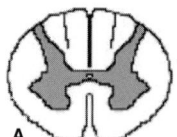 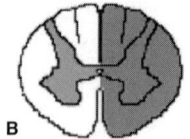 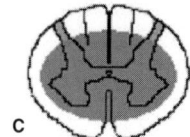 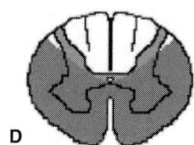

Figure 23.7 Several types of spinal cord injuries. (**A**) Cross-sectional representation of the uninjured spinal cord. (**B**) Brown-Séquard, with unilateral injury to gray and white matter. (**C**) Central cord syndrome, with sparing of the tracts near the surface of the cord. (**D**) Anterior cord syndrome due to disruption of the anterior spinal artery.

injuries (see Chapters 31 and 32). Furthermore, many of the associated injuries, including long-bone fractures (23%), may involve significant hemorrhage (see Chapters 27 and 28).[11–16]

In addition to concomitant trauma, we can expect an increasing trend in the prevalence of preexisting comorbidity for the SCI population as the mean age increases. Coronary artery disease, hypertension, chronic obstructive pulmonary disease, diabetes, and chronic kidney disease and their related pharmacotherapy (antihypertensives, antiplatelets, anticoagulants, hypoglycemics) all complicate the anesthetic management of a patient with an SCI.

Clinical manifestations of injury

Two possible presentations exist:

(1) isolated SCI
(2) polytrauma that includes SCI

In both cases, acute management priorities include the maintenance of oxygenation, blood pressure optimization, and spinal stabilization according to Advanced Trauma Life Support (ATLS) principles. The clinical picture is complicated by sensory and/or motor deficits, cardiorespiratory disturbances, multiorgan dysfunction, and the need for surgical interventions.

In addition to varying degrees of motor and sensory deficits below the level of the SCI, hypotension is also common. Hypotension could be related to hemorrhage, cardiac dysfunction, and neurogenic shock, or to a combination of causes (see Chapters 4 and 22). Hypotensive, low-volume resuscitation is contraindicated in hemorrhaging trauma patients with coexisting brain and spinal cord injuries. At the authors' institutions, a mean arterial pressure (MAP) of > 80 mmHg is recommended in the first 48–72 hours or for 24 hours post decompression/stabilization (whichever is longer) to provide adequate perfusion pressure to optimize tissue oxygenation for the injured central nervous system.[17,18]

Neurogenic shock refers to the combination of hypotension and bradycardia following SCI. Systemic hypotension develops because of a loss of sympathetic autonomic activity, with a decreased vascular tone. Bradycardia following high thoracic or cervical spine injuries results in unopposed parasympathetic activity at the heart due to the disruption of the cardiac accelerator fibers. The incidence of neurogenic shock may be as high as 19%.[19–21] In addition to the baseline hypotension, these patients are at particular risk for orthostatic hypotension, as they cannot compensate for dependent venous pooling.

Interestingly, neurogenic shock may not be evident in the early phase of SCI. The bradycardic component of neurogenic shock takes about 2 hours to develop and is often preceded by an initial tachycardia, which along with hypotension may mimic hemorrhagic shock. It is important to realize that permissive hypotensive management in this situation may exacerbate secondary injury.[21]

Spinal shock indicates loss of sensory, reflex, and motor functions after trauma (see also Chapter 22). The loss of spinal cord reflexes is not permanent. The initial areflexic, flaccid phase transitions to a hyperreflexic phase in 1–6 weeks. In the flaccid paralysis phase failure of the respiratory muscles, including the diaphragm and the intercostals below the level of the injury, can lead to acute respiratory failure and death.

Initial management
Urgent airway management

The initial management of the patient with spine trauma should follow the standard practices of care for trauma patients in general, with initial emphasis on airway, breathing, and circulation as outlined in ATLS (see Chapter 2). Tracheal intubation can be particularly challenging in the patient with SCI, especially if the lesion is in the cervical spine (see Chapter 3). In addition, tracheal intubation frequently needs to be accomplished before the presence or location of an injury can be confirmed. As a result, many acute trauma patients who require urgent or emergency endotracheal intubation are treated as if they had a C-spine injury. The goal of intubation is to secure the airway with as little movement of the cervical spine as possible. Early assessment of a patient and diagnosis of SCI at the site of injury by experienced providers therefore is an important step to determine the need for spinal immobilization. Patients who are alert, awake, not intoxicated, with no associated distracting injury, who are free from neck pain and tenderness, and who have a normal motor and sensory exam can be cleared without further radiologic investigation.

Immobilization

Airway management in patients suffering from a C-spine injury is challenging, because airway maneuvers will cause movement of the neck and increase the risk of further deterioration of SCI. C-spine immobilization is established by positioning the patient's neck in neutral alignment using a rigid cervical collar, sandbags, tape, and a backboard (Fig. 23.8).[22] An exception to this may be the penetrating trauma patient, in whom spine immobilization may result in delayed resuscitation and is not recommended.[23]

The standard urgent or emergent tracheal intubation technique for a patient with a presumed or known C-spine injury is rapid sequence induction (RSI) with cricoid pressure and manual in-line stabilization (MILS) (see Chapters 3 and 13). Because a hard collar places a significant restriction on mouth opening and laryngoscopy, the anterior part of the cervical collar is usually removed while MILS is being applied.[24] The goal of MILS is to minimize any neck movement during airway management.[25] The benefit of MILS has been questioned, however, since it may impair glottic visualization during conventional direct laryngoscopy, and cause the laryngoscopist to apply more lifting force, which could be transmitted to the spine.[26] Nonetheless, MILS is routinely done, either from the head of the bed or from the side of the bed while facing the patient (Fig. 23.9). The assistant's hands should cover the mastoid processes and the occiput to provide adequate stabilization and opposing force to the laryngoscopy.

Regarding the choice of muscle relaxant, succinylcholine remains the gold standard for rapid sequence intubation in the early stages of SCI management (see Chapter 13). Succinylcholine should be avoided from day 3 up to 9 months following SCI, because of the risk of succinylcholine-induced hyperkalemia caused by denervation hypersensitivity. Rocuronium should be considered as an alternative.

Hemodynamic stabilization

Neurogenic shock with loss of sympathetic tone results in reduced spinal cord perfusion pressure (SCPP) and exacerbates secondary injury. Up to 80% of cervical SCI patients develop volume-resistant hypotension, and 90% of complete and 53% of incomplete SCI patients require vasopressors for blood pressure support for up to 7 days post injury.[27–29] Isotonic crystalloid resuscitation is appropriate. In addition, other concomitant injuries may cause significant blood loss, which will also necessitate aggressive resuscitation with crystalloid and possibly blood products. Excessive volume resuscitation, particularly in combination with a poorly functioning heart, can be deleterious with its contribution to systemic and airway edema, cardiac failure, and electrolyte and coagulation abnormalities. Ongoing assessment of volume status is essential. Not all hypotension should be treated with more volume, particularly if normovolemia has been achieved. Further volume infusion at this point may worsen cardiac and pulmonary function. Goal-directed treatment using cardiac output monitoring devices should be considered to help achieve acceptable resuscitation targets. Echocardiography is valuable for monitoring heart function and quantifying the hemodynamic state (see also Chapters 9 and 10).

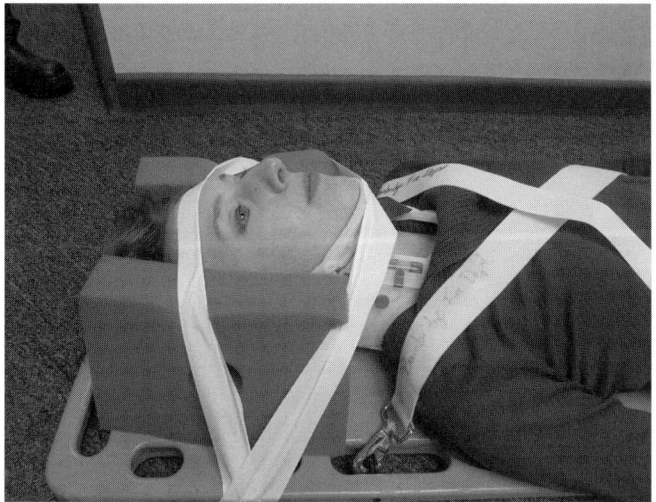

Figure 23.8 C-spine immobilization.

(A)

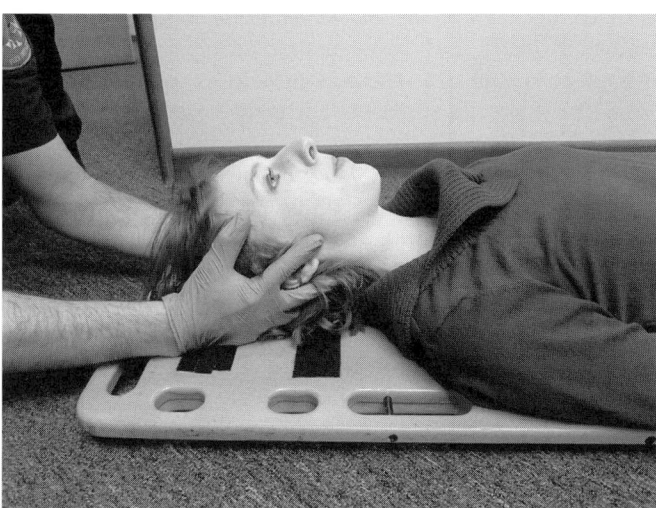

(B)

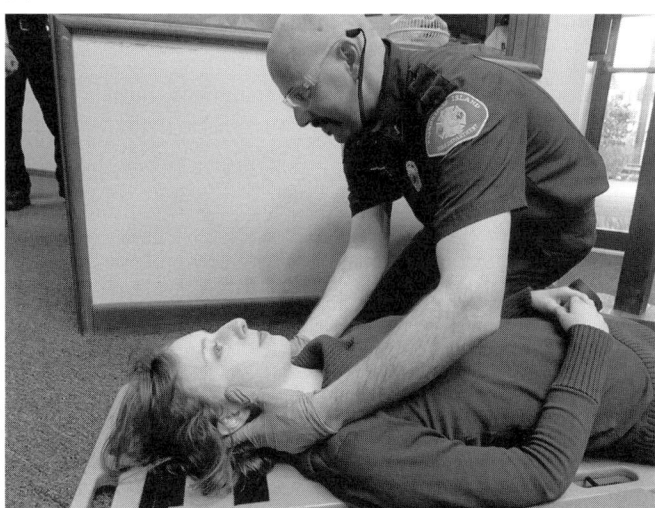

Figure 23.9 Manual in-line stabilization. Approach from (**A**) the top or (**B**) the front of the patient.

Maintaining MAP between 85 and 90 mmHg for the first 7 days following acute SCI to improve spinal cord perfusion is the current recommendation of the American Association of Neurological Surgeons (AANS) and the Congress of Neurological Surgeons (CNS).[30]

Inotropic agents or vasopressors should be considered in addition to adequate volume resuscitation when the targeted perfusion pressure cannot be maintained by fluid infusion alone. Care should be taken to avoid masking hypovolemia or ongoing blood loss. The choice of inotrope or pressor must be based on the clinical picture and individualized to the patient and his or her comorbidities. Patients with isolated injuries to the lower spinal cord frequently do not require such agents to maintain an adequate systemic blood pressure. Higher cord lesions result in greater sympathectomy, more extensive vasodilatation, and thus increased vascular capacitance. Although volume is beneficial in this setting, a pure α agonist such as phenylephrine is a reasonable choice to restore vascular tone. Patients with higher lesions, in the upper thoracic or cervical spine, with concomitant hypotension and bradycardia are not well served by phenylephrine. Dopamine or norepinephrine is the preferable choice to restore cardiac inotropy, chronotropy, and peripheral vascular tone. Vasopressin has a vasoconstrictive and catecholamine-sparing effect, and may be useful in patients with persistent hypotension. However, its antidiuretic effects may lead to increased water retention and hyponatremia, with potential exacerbation of intracellular edema after injury. Thus, its role in SCI is not well defined, and it should be used with some caution.

Bradycardia leading to cardiovascular instability requires attention and treatment with atropine or glycopyrrolate. Persistent bradycardia is usually seen with high-level cord lesions (C1–C5), which may require infusion of isoprenaline or pacemaker (temporary) application.

Radiologic evaluation and cervical spine clearance

In trauma, as part of the secondary survey, the radiologic evaluation of the cervical spine is frequently initiated with CT scans. When an awake and asymptomatic patient demonstrates the following, no further radiological examination and immobilization is required:

- no neck pain or tenderness
- no focal neurological deficit
- no painful distracting injury
- able to complete a functional range of motion on examination

As most major trauma patients do not meet these criteria, further evaluation is usually necessary, following the Eastern Association for the Surgery of Trauma (EAST) 2009, American College of Radiology 2012, and the AANS and CNS recommendations.[31–33]

Awake symptomatic, and obtunded and unevaluable

- A thin-section multi-detector-row CT with sagittal and coronal reconstructions is the recommended screening procedure.
- Once a decision is made to scan the patient, the entire spine should be examined, owing to the high incidence of noncontiguous multiple injuries.
- Thoracic, lumbar, and pelvic CT examinations may be used instead of primary spine imaging.
- Conventional radiography is the preferred choice in children age 14 years or under. In the cervical region, recommended views are anteroosterior (AP), lateral, and open-mouth; in the thoracic and lumbar regions, AP and lateral only.
- Three-view radiography has limited use in adults and should be used only when CT is not available and for help to resolve nondiagnostic CT studies due to motion artifacts.
- Flexion–extension radiography is not useful in the acute injury period because of muscle spasm.
- Magnetic resonance imaging (MRI) is the procedure of choice for evaluating patients with a suspected SCI or for cord compression, as well as for determining the integrity of the spinal ligaments, particularly in obtunded patients.
- CT, however, has been shown in the literature to be as effective as MRI for determining spinal stability. Spine surgeons may prefer to use MRI.
- Dynamic fluoroscopy should not be used to evaluate for ligamentous injury in obtunded patients.
- CT angiography (CTA) is recommended to assess for vertebral artery injury in selected patients who meet the modified Denver Screening Criteria after blunt cervical trauma (focal neurological deficit, arterial hemorrhage, cervical bruit in a patient less than 50 years of age, expanding neck hematoma, neurological exam inconsistent with head CT scan, cerebrovascular accident on follow-up head CT not seen on initial head CT).

While CT scans are most sensitive for bony injury, MRI is well suited to detect soft tissue injury, including SCI (see also Chapters 11 and 22). The role of MRI in evaluation of the spine in the acute period is currently unclear. Its utility is somewhat limited by the length of time to acquire an image. It is clearly useful in several situations. The presence of a neurologic deficit that is inconsistent with the injury found on plain films and CT should prompt an MRI evaluation. In addition, patients without radiographic evidence of injury who have neurologic deficit may have SCIWORA and should certainly undergo MRI evaluation.

AANS/CNS recommends that in an awake and symptomatic patient with normal CT findings, C-spine immobilization should continue until the patient is asymptomatic, or it can be discontinued following normal and adequate dynamic flexion/extension films or normal MRI results within the first 48 hours or at the discretion of the treating physician.

In an obtunded or otherwise unevaluable patient with normal CT findings, C-spine immobilization should continue until the patient is asymptomatic, or following normal MRI results within the first 48 hours, or at the discretion of the treating physician who has expertise in the management of SCI patients.

Role for steroids

Steroid use for SCI was ushered in by the NASCIS (National Spinal Cord Injury Study) II and III studies from the 1990s, which showed clinically significant improvement in the motor function of SCI patients. Although these improvements in motor function appear to be modest, one to two levels of improvement of motor level can be quite significant if the injury is in the cervical spine. The results of these studies confirming the benefit of methylprednisolone have been criticized and disputed.[34] There are numerous reasons why avoidance of systemic steroids might be desirable if they are not indicated, such as their association with hyperglycemia, infection, and polyneuropathy of critical illness. In addition, because the SCI patient population has a high incidence of associated head injury, it is worthwhile to consider the large randomized study of methylprednisolone therapy on head-injury patients, which found an increased risk of death in patients receiving methylprednisolone both at 2 weeks and at 6 months.[35]

In their recent revision, the CNS/AANS no longer recommends routine administration of methylprednisolone for the treatment of acute SCI. The US Food and Drug Administration (FDA) does not approve methylprednisolone application in this clinical setting. In fact, high-dose steroids are associated with harmful side effects including infection, respiratory compromise, gastrointestinal hemorrhage, and death.[36]

Timing of surgical intervention

The purpose of surgical intervention is to decompress the neural structures and stabilize the spinal column to prevent further injury to the cord (see Chapter 22). Management of the patient with SCI frequently requires intervention for associated life-threatening trauma, such as TBI or abdominal or pelvic hemorrhage (see Chapters 20, 27, and 32). Surgical decompression of the spinal cord with fixation of the spinal column must wait until the patient is clinically appropriate for the procedure. If the patient remains hemodynamically unstable or develops acute respiratory distress syndrome (ARDS), then the delay may be significant, from days to weeks. There are both preclinical and clinical data that exist to suggest that early operative fixation of isolated SCI improves neurologic outcome and decreases complication rate and length of stay in the intensive care unit (ICU) compared with delayed surgery or conservative treatment.[37–40]

The Surgical Timing in Acute Spinal Cord Injury Study (STASCIS) revealed that decompressive surgery prior to 24 hours after SCI was safe and was associated with improved neurologic outcome (defined as at least two-grade ASIA Impairment Scale improvement at 6 months follow-up). This was true even after multivariate regression analysis, adjusted for preoperative neurological status and steroid administration.[40] It is recognized that current evidence favoring "early" spinal surgery lacks strength and is subject to publication bias. However, what evidence there is clearly supports early intervention.[41]

Intraoperative management
Airway management and anesthesia (see also Chapter 3)

If a patient with SCI does not require tracheal intubation in the prehospital or emergency department setting, then he or she will need further airway management upon presentation to the operating room. Given the less urgent nature of tracheal intubation in this setting, options in addition to RSI with in-line stabilization may be considered by the anesthesiologist.

Prehospital and intrahospital transfers require that the patient is immobilized in the neutral position using a rigid cervical collar, sandbags, tape, and a backboard. This combination has been shown to produce the greatest stabilization of the neck.[23] Later on, nonsurgical stabilization techniques may be employed, including adjuncts such as neck collars, halo-vest devices, or neck traction.

For some patients, by the time they arrive in the operating room for surgery they may have been cleared of C-spine injury both radiologically and clinically. The technique for induction of anesthesia and tracheal intubation should therefore be determined by their other injuries, comorbidities, and airway exam.

Patients with presumed or confirmed C-spine injury require careful planning, however. RSI remains a viable option, particularly in trauma with someone who is unable to cooperate with an awake procedure. If the patient has fasted, a standard induction followed by intubation with in-line stabilization may be a reasonable option as well. In most trauma patients, however, some consideration must be given to the risk of aspiration. Even if sufficient time has passed since the last meal, the stomach may not have emptied adequately for a standard induction. The stress of trauma, narcotics, and ileus due to SCI may all put the patient at risk for regurgitation and aspiration.

It has been clinically shown that, in the normal spine, direct laryngoscopy leads to the extension of the C-spine, predominantly at the atlantooccipital junction, and to a lesser extent at the C1/C2 joint. The subaxial cervical segments (C4–C7) are minimally displaced but additional flexion occurs at the cervicothoracic junction. Instability of the occiput–atlas–axis complex may lead to anterior movement of the atlas during direct laryngoscopy, thereby reducing the space available for the spinal cord. Because the cervical collar significantly restricts mouth opening during laryngoscopy, the anterior part of the

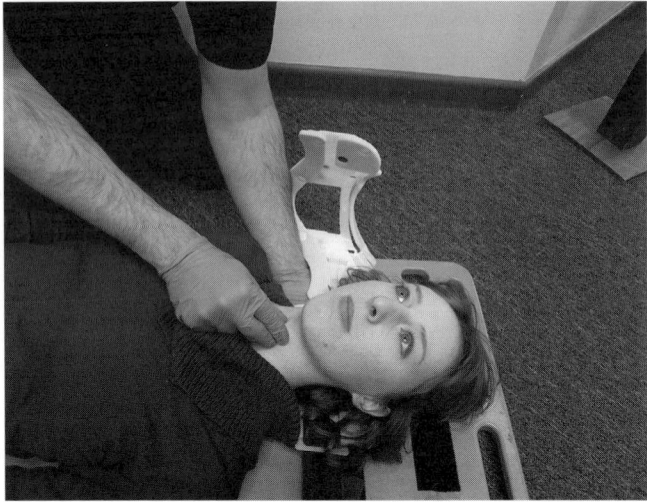

Figure 23.10 Bimanual application of cricoid pressure.

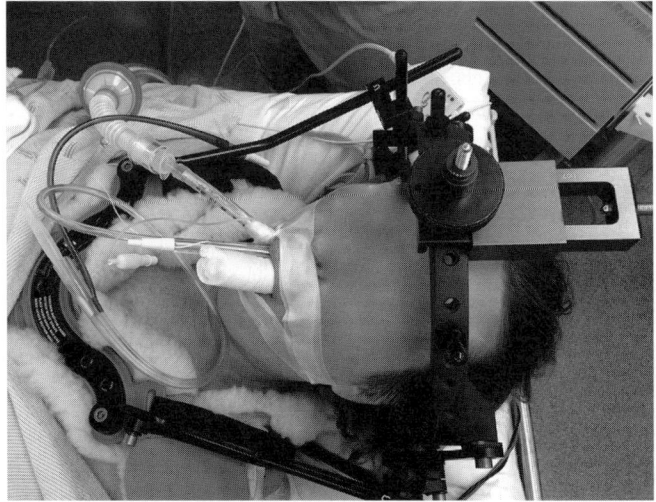

Figure 23.11 Spine stabilization with a halo device.

cervical collar can be removed while in-line stabilization is applied. The gum elastic bougie, now included in the ATLS airway algorithm, facilitates tracheal intubation in this situation (see Chapter 3). Carefully applied basic airway maneuvers such as chin lift, jaw thrust, and mask ventilation have been shown to produce some degree of cervical flexion, but this is comparable to direct laryngoscopy. Use of oral and nasal airway adjuncts may improve the ventilation and reduce the manual manipulation required. Even supraglottic devices can produce posterior soft tissue pressure and cervical flexion. When cricoid pressure is required, the authors prefer bimanual application (rather than the traditional single-handed approach) because of the theoretical advantage of less spine movement. With bimanual application, the operator's one hand is compressing the cricoid ring while the other hand supports the neck from behind to minimize downward displacement (Fig. 23.10).

The most conservative approach to airway management in this setting is awake intubation with flexible fiberoptic bronchoscopy (FOB) via the oral or nasal route (see Chapter 3).

In trauma, a major limitation to FOB is the lack of visibility in the presence of blood and secretions. If blood is present, it is best to avoid FOB. Topicalization of an airway requires time and may result in patient discomfort and coughing. It is difficult to accomplish this in some patients who are particularly anxious or uncooperative while immobilized in a supine position. If such a patient is an appropriate candidate for bag-mask ventilation, then FOB may be accomplished after induction of anesthesia. It may be more suitable to use in cases where the patient is stabilized with external fixators (halo-vest) (Fig. 23.11), or has fixed flexion deformities such as a previous cervical spine fusion, ankylosing spondylosis, or severe rheumatoid arthritis with limited mouth opening. While FOB may expose the C-spine to the least amount of movement, this procedure requires significant skill and a cooperative patient (if it is to be performed in an awake

patient). For the anesthetized patient, this procedure may require jaw thrust or tongue pull, which can theoretically expose the patient to some movement.

Video laryngoscopy has been shown to improve the intubation success rate when cervical in-line stabilization is applied. In terms of cervical motion, there is no consistent evidence to favor these devices. Video laryngoscopes promise a more steep learning curve and skill retention than flexible fiberoptic intubation and offer significant improvement in terms of ease of visualization of the vocal cords compared with direct laryngoscopy.[42]

Each airway maneuver has its inherent weaknesses and advantages. There is no conclusive evidence that an optimal airway management strategy in patients with cervical instability affects outcome. The most appropriate choice will often depend on the practitioner's experience with a particular technique and the specifics of the clinical situation.[43]

Reintubation rates following extubation are reported to be as high as 5% after anterior cervical spine procedures. This rate is probably even higher in anteroposterior cervical spine procedures. The decision whether or not to extubate the trachea at the end of the surgical procedure is influenced by many factors. These include the ease of intubation, extent and duration of surgery, surgical complications (e.g., recurrent laryngeal nerve injury), prone positioning, blood loss, subsequent fluid balance, and other coexisting medical conditions and injuries. The absence of a cuff leak in the spontaneously breathing patient has not consistently been shown to predict subsequent airway obstruction, but the presence of a cuff leak generally indicates a patent airway after extubation. When in doubt, extubating the patient's trachea with an airway exchange catheter in situ can facilitate immediate emergent reintubation if necessary. It is important to note that progressive airway swelling may continue to occur up to several days following surgery. Therefore keeping the patient intubated for a prolonged period is not a practical approach but highlights the importance of close monitoring in an appropriate post-operative care unit. Good clinical judgment is paramount, and if there is a concern, it is prudent to delay extubation.

Intraoperative management and monitoring technique

The American Society of Anesthesiologists' minimum monitoring standards are required for all surgical patients (see Chapter 9).

Most surgery for spine trauma carries a significant risk of blood loss. Two large-bore peripheral intravenous catheters are therefore required for volume and blood-product administration. In large thoracic or lumbar spine surgeries, particularly in the prone position, central venous access may be warranted. Advantages of central venous catheters are: easy access to venous circulation when arms are positioned out of direct reach, appropriate access for inotropes and vasopressors (if required), secure large-bore access for volume resuscitation. Central venous catheters may help guide goal-directed treatment by allowing measurement of mixed venous oxygen saturation and lactate levels as well as the calculation of the ocular perfusion pressure (OPP = MAP – central venous pressure [CVP]). Although there are currently no data to support the notion that an adequate ocular perfusion pressure decreases the incidence of postoperative visual loss, maintaining an ocular perfusion pressure of 60 mmHg is reasonable. CVP is neither a good indicator of preload nor a predictor of cardiac function in response to volume administration when used alone.

An arterial catheter is essential, as it allows serial measurements of hematocrit, glucose, electrolytes, and arterial blood gases, as well as continuous blood pressure monitoring. In addition, respiratory variation of the blood pressure waveform from the arterial line is an extremely useful indicator of volume responsiveness in the mechanically ventilated patient (see Chapter 9: systolic pressure variability, pulse pressure variability).

Today, various devices are available to measure or estimate cardiac output using different methods. These minimally invasive devices track stroke volume continuously, provide dynamic indices of fluid responsiveness, and allow assessment of the volumetric preload variables. All these variables, together with calibrated or noncalibrated (trending) cardiac output monitoring, may improve patient outcome when they are coupled with appropriate hemodynamic management strategies and clinical judgment.

Neuromonitoring

The goal of surgery in the setting of SCI is not only to stabilize the spinal column, but also to prevent further injury to the cord. Unfortunately, the surgery itself, such as achieving fracture reduction or placing hardware, has potential for causing further injury. Intraoperative neuromonitoring is frequently performed in order to minimize further risk to the cord (see Chapter 9). Several modalities are commonly used, and each has specific anesthetic implications. Neuromonitoring during spine procedures is done with evoked potential monitoring. In brief a small stimulus (electrical impulse) is applied to the patient; it is transmitted through a specific pathway in the nervous system, and subsequently measured at its termination, where the continued presence of signal indicates an intact pathway.

Patients with complete SCIs or nearly complete SCIs will have no transmission of signal through the lesion, and neuromonitoring is therefore not possible. It is, however, reasonable to perform some baseline measurements in patients who are thought to have incomplete injuries. If some signal persists, then it may be worth the effort to monitor and attempt to preserve it.

There is a high level of evidence that, when used in combination, intraoperative multimodal neuromonitoring is sensitive and specific enough to detect neuronal injury. However, the evidence is not strong to suggest that intraoperative monitoring reduces the risk of new or worsened perioperative neurological deficit. Successful neuromonitoring requires a high level of communication between the surgeon, the anesthesiologist, and the neurophysiologist/monitoring personnel.[44,45]

Neurophysiologic monitoring modalities

Somatosensory evoked potentials

Somatosensory evoked potentials (SSEPs) are the most common type of intraoperative neuromonitoring modality for spine surgery. An electrical stimulus is applied peripherally, and the signal is measured by using scalp electrodes over the sensory cortex. The most common sites for stimulation are the posterior tibial and peroneal nerves for the lower extremities, and the median and ulnar nerves for the upper extremities. In the context of spine surgery, SSEP monitoring is useful for confirming the integrity of the posterior column, where afferent pathways predominate. A 50% decrease in the amplitude of the signal and a 10% increase in signal latency are considered clinically significant and should prompt the surgeon to revise the ongoing surgical plan. Volatile anesthetics and nitrous oxide decrease the amplitude and increase the latency in a dose-dependent manner. If only SSEP monitoring is performed, then a low-dose volatile anesthetic combined with a generous opioid supplementation would be a reasonable anesthetic choice. SSEP is generally well preserved with intravenous anesthetics, even in the setting of EEG burst suppression. Total intravenous anesthesia (TIVA) is therefore a preferred alternative to a volatile anesthetic for the purpose of neuromonitoring.

Because SSEP only detects injury to the sensory pathways of the spinal cord, isolated injury to the descending pathways could potentially be missed, such as a nerve root injury during a pedicle screw insertion. Because of the need for signal averaging (usually 256–512 sweeps) of the EEG, SSEP generally lags behind the real-time clinical picture. Therefore, one major concern is that by the time monitoring changes become apparent, irreversible neurological damages may have already occurred. The addition of motor evoked potential (MEP) monitoring – which, due to its large amplitude, does not require signal averaging – would increase the accuracy in this high-risk clinical circumstance.

Motor evoked potentials

Motor evoked potentials (MEPs) have become an increasingly standard technique for detecting injury to efferent motor tracts all the way from the cortex to the peripheral nerve, and thereby complement SSEP for spinal cord monitoring. This technique involves depolarization of the motor cortex via transcranial electrical stimulation. Electromyographic potentials are then recorded over muscles via compound muscle action potentials in both upper and lower extremities or by epidural electrodes placed caudal to the region at risk (D-wave).

The compound muscle action potential is much more sensitive to the effects of anesthetics than SSEP. TIVA is essential for adequate signal quality. A continuous infusion of propofol with remifentanil, sufentanil, or fentanyl in combination with ketamine and/or dexmedetomidine is an appropriate technique. Neuromuscular relaxants must be avoided. MEPs are only assessed in intervals when there is a high risk of nerve injury, whereas SSEP tends to be a continual measurement. Therefore, if the injury does not correspond to the time of measurement there might be a delay before it is recognized. An 80% reduction in the signal amplitude or more than 100 V increase in minimum stimulus threshold are considered clinically significant changes. Transcranial electrical stimulation has a theoretical risk of seizure generation, and this should be taken into consideration. A soft bite-block is mandatory to prevent teeth injury or tongue lacerations during depolarization of the motor cortex.

D-wave MEPs are fairly resistant to the effects of anesthetics and allow the use of intraoperative muscle relaxants. A 20% reduction in D-wave amplitude is considered as a warning, while a 50% reduction indicates a significant neuronal injury. D-wave MEP has higher false-positive rates and misses the signals from the nerve roots and cauda equina. This modality therefore is more suited for intramedullary spine surgery monitoring.

Visual evoked potentials

Visual evoked potential (VEP) monitoring is accomplished through stimulation of the retina with light from light-emitting diodes in goggles worn by the patient, with subsequent measurement of cortical electrical activity. Recent concern over postoperative visual loss (POVL) has prompted exploration of its application to prone spine surgery. Abnormal readings mostly result from ischemic optic neuropathy and cortical blindness. However, VEPs are exquisitely sensitive to the influence of anesthetics, which thus far has precluded the potential utility of this modality to monitor visual function during spine surgery.

Spontaneous electromyography

Although it is not an evoked potential, spontaneous electromyography (EMG) can be monitored simultaneously with SSEP and MEP to provide an additional continual monitor. This technique relies on the strong motor activity in a preselected muscle group that occurs when a relevant nerve root is "irritated" by the surgeon. EMG in an adequately anesthetized patient should be minimal, but surgical contact with a large peripheral nerve should stimulate activity. This monitoring modality is particularly useful in either cervical or lumbar spine surgery, when the surgeon is working around nerve roots that form either the brachial plexus or the lumbar sacral plexus. The deltoid and biceps are the most commonly monitored muscles. Anesthetic considerations include the avoidance of neuromuscular relaxants. Hypothermia and electrocautery can create interference and generate false-positive readings.

Management of significant intraoperative neuromonitoring changes indicative of impending neurologic impairment

- Rule out surgical and equipment related factors: communicate with the surgeon and the neuromonitoring team.
- Rule out physiologic causes: correct hypotension, hypothermia (and avoid hyperthermia), and metabolic abnormalities.
- Correct severe anemia.
- Raise MAP > 85 mmHg to increase spinal cord perfusion.
- Turn off inhalational agents and start TIVA if not already utilized.
- Consider steroid infusion (methylprednisolone 30 mg/kg IV load then 5.4 mg/kg/h IV).

Effects of anesthetic agents

Halogenated anesthetic agents and nitrous oxide have dose-related depressant effects more than TIVA. When only SSEP signals are monitored, keeping the anesthetic concentration to < 1 MAC (preferably 0.5 MAC) of an agent is compatible with satisfactory recording. However, in the event of a potential signal loss it might become difficult to exclude the effect of the inhaled agent, and this aspect must be taken into consideration. Inhaled agents should generally be avoided when MEP monitoring is undertaken.

Propofol and thiopental attenuate the amplitude of virtually all modalities of evoked potentials but do not obliterate them. SSEP and MEP can be monitored even during burst suppression induced by these agents.

Ketamine and etomidate may enhance the amplitude of MEP, while dexmedetomidine may have either negligible or some depressant effects in higher doses.

Neuromuscular relaxants must be avoided during MEP and spontaneous EMG monitoring. However, relaxants may be used to facilitate tracheal intubation provided their effects have worn off or are reversed prior to the time neuromonitoring commences. Alternatively, the trachea may be intubated without the use of relaxants if early baseline measurements are desired. An induction dose of remifentanil is an alternative method and obviates the need of neuromuscular blockade. Remifentanil does not affect SSEPs or MEPs.

Opioids and benzodiazepines have negligible effects on recording of evoked potentials.

Patient positioning

Patient positioning for spine surgery requires the same careful attention to pressure-point padding and neutral extremity positioning as with any surgery. It is somewhat more difficult to achieve satisfactory padding in the prone position. Whether using the Mayfield device to hold the head in pins, foam prone pillow, or ProneView adjustable mirror, it is essential to be certain that there is no pressure on the globes or nose. The head support may move over time, and the eyes and nose should be checked periodically and recorded. In addition, slight reverse Trendelenburg may facilitate venous drainage from the head and reduce congestion and intraocular pressure. Padding on the chest must not creep up or down and compress the neck or liver and other intraabdominal organs. The ulnar nerve is particularly exposed at the ulnar groove and the brachial plexus at the axilla, and both have the potential to receive direct pressure from positioning, especially when the arms are placed in the swimmer's position. Other areas of concern include the breasts, which may suffer from pressure necrosis, and the male genitalia, which should not be compressed. The knees and toes also are at risk for pressure sores.

Temperature regulation and therapeutic hypothermia

Due to the loss of cutaneous vasomotor tone below the level of injury, patients with SCI have difficulty with thermoregulation and are therefore at risk of developing accidental hypothermia in the acute injury period. Measures to prevent hypothermia should therefore be employed (see Chapter 14).

There is evidence that modest hypothermia in the setting of a central nervous system injury may decrease secondary injury through a variety of mechanisms such as reduction in the level of excitotoxic metabolite glutamate in the cerebrospinal fluid (CSF), reduced vasogenic edema at the site of injury, decreased neutrophil invasion, preservation of blood flow, and reduced tissue metabolism, energy requirements, oxidative stress, apoptosis, and tissue hemorrhage.

Important determinants of a successful technique are the cooling method (local, surface, or intravascular), therapeutic time window, rate, duration, and degree of temperature depression, and importantly rewarming and prevention of

associated complications such as infection.[46] Modest systemic hypothermia (32–34 °C) when initiated early (< 8 hours) has the potential to provide neuroprotection without incurring the complications associated with deep hypothermia. A prospective multicenter randomized trial of hypothermia for acute SCI is at the planning stage, and may provide more conclusive evidence.[47]

Despite emerging potential for temperature modulation for spinal function preservation and recovery, the American Association of Neurological Surgeons and the Congress of Neurological Surgeons published a statement in November 2007, updated November 2013, concluding that there was insufficient scientific evidence to support or oppose systemic or local hypothermia for traumatic spine injury.[48]

Glucose management

Many patients with SCI become hyperglycemic either from the stress of the injury or from the subsequent effects of methylprednisolone. Appropriate glucose management therefore is imperative both in the operating room and in the ICU.

Hypoglycemia, hyperglycemia, and increased variability in blood glucose concentrations are associated with worse outcomes. According to the findings of the NICE-SUGAR (Normoglycemia in Intensive Care Evaluation-Survival Using Glucose Algorithm Regulation) trial, the use of intensive insulin therapy to achieve strict glucose control (80–110 mg/dL) is associated with higher 90-day mortality due to a higher incidence of severe hypoglycemic episodes. Neuronal tissue is particularly vulnerable to a diminished energy supply. Both anesthesia and SCI potentially mask the signs of hypoglycemia and make the clinical diagnosis more difficult. Frequent measurements of glucose are routinely done in anesthetized patients on insulin drips. Closed loop glucose control systems with computerized mathematical algorithms can help guide appropriate management. A glucose level of 140–180 mg/dL is generally targeted in most patients.[49]

Complications of anesthesia for spine surgery
Postoperative visual loss

Although there are many potential complications of spine surgery, including massive hemorrhage, venous air embolism, myocardial infarction, pulmonary edema, nerve injury, and pressure necrosis, the complication of postoperative visual loss (POVL) is a particular concern in prone spine surgery. POVL is a significant concern because it has no proven treatment strategies and is associated with poor outcomes (see Chapter 26).

Its overall incidence is reported to be up to 0.2% in spine surgery. The four recognized causes of POVL are ischemic optic neuropathy (ION) (approximately 89%), central retinal artery occlusion (CRAO) (approximately 11%), cortical infarction, and external ocular injury. Most of the ION cases are due to posterior ischemic optic neuropathy (PION), which is characterized by afferent papillary defect, normal funduscopy, and visual field loss. With time, optical nerve atrophy occurs, at which point PION is indistinguishable from anterior ischemic optic neuropathy (AION).

Recently published results from the POVL Registry report that the incidence of ION is in the range of 0.017–0.1%. Risk factors in major spinal fusion surgery in the prone position include obesity, male sex, use of the Wilson frame, longer anesthetic/surgical duration, greater blood loss, and lesser use of colloid in volume replacement.[50]

While the majority of ION cases result in bilateral visual loss, all CRAO cases present with unilateral visual loss. The unilateral nature of CRAO can be explained by direct compression of the eye from inadvertent malpositioning on a headrest. Use of Mayfield pins is the best way to avoid pressure to the eyes and nose to prevent this type of ischemic visual loss.

Cortical blindness is typically associated with states of profound hypotension such as cardiac arrest or cardiac bypass procedures, where a thromboembolic event leads to visual cortex ischemia. Of the four causes of visual loss, cortical infarction has the best chance for recovery.

External ocular injury can be prevented by avoiding direct injury to the cornea and maintaining its natural moisture with properly closed eyelids or aqueous eye ointment.

The following recommendations are included in the updated ASA practice advisory on POVL:[51]

- elevation of the head of the bed
- keeping the head in a neutral position
- using colloids along with crystalloids for volume replacement
- consideration for staging long procedures in high-risk patients
- continuous systemic blood pressure monitoring
- periodical check on hemoglobin or hematocrit values
- avoidance of direct pressure on the globe

Given the devastating consequences of POVL, increased recognition, and the possibility of subsequent litigation, a properly conducted informed consent becomes an important part of the preoperative discussion for patients scheduled for complex spine surgery. Trauma may hinder this process, but if possible the patient's vision should be documented immediately before and after the surgery. A high index of suspicion for vision impairment and frequent documentation to indicate that the eyes are free from pressure should be part of the perioperative anesthesia practice. Visual complaints warrant an immediate ophthalmology consult,[51,52] although as yet no effective treatment is available.

Denervation hyperkalemia from succinylcholine

Muscle denervation via SCI results in rapid upregulation of acetylcholine receptor isoforms across the muscle belly, not just localized to the neuromuscular junction, which are stimulated by acetylcholine, succinylcholine, and choline. The profound hyperkalemia that can result from the use of succinylcholine in these circumstances becomes potentially lethal. Although it is unclear at what point succinylcholine use becomes unsafe, it is probably appropriate to avoid it after 48 hours post injury (see Chapter 9).

Autonomic hyperreflexia

Although the return of spinal cord reflexes following SCI might mitigate the problems of hypotension and orthostasis, the return may also signify the onset of autonomic hyperreflexia. It is characterized by episodes of profound hypertension accompanied by cutaneous vasoconstriction below the site of the lesion and compensatory vasodilatation with flushing above. This generally occurs as a result of stimulation to an area below the site of the lesion, e.g., from catheterization of the bladder. The mechanism is an intense reflex sympathetic arc completed in the spinal cord below the lesion, unmodulated by influence from medullary centers above. It may be accompanied by baroreflex-mediated bradycardia. It can arise intraoperatively, during urinary catheterization, or as a result of surgical stimulation. The primary treatment for this phenomenon is preventive by "deafferentation" using regional anesthetic techniques when appropriate, and secondarily by "deepening" the anesthetic when this occurs. Autonomic hyperreflexia is most commonly observed in persons with SCI above T6, as at this level there are inadequate vascular beds above to compensate for the vasoconstriction below.

Later issues with spinal cord injury

The incidence of acute medical complications following SCI is reported to be 58%. Approximately 78% of these complications appear to present in the first 14 days. The rates of medical complications are higher in more severe SCI ASIA grades. Respiratory failure, pneumonia, pleural effusion, anemia, cardiac dysrhythmia, and severe bradycardia appear to be the most commonly observed complications. The observed mortality rate is reported to be 3.5% and associated with increased age and preexisting morbidity.

Conclusions

It is challenging for the anesthesiologist to deal with the many complicating medical issues during the perioperative management of patients with spinal cord injury. Recognition of the presence and knowledge of the impact and the severity of specific complications after SCI can help to tailor an optimal anesthetic plan.[53]

Questions

(1) Concerning spinal cord injuries:
  a. They are more common in women than in men
  b. They are most commonly seen in the elderly population

c. Motor vehicle collisions are the leading cause in adults

d. Around 30% of spinal column injuries occur at more than one level

(2) **Identify the correct statement regarding the anatomy of the spinal cord:**

a. It is made up of 8 cervical, 11 thoracic, 5 lumbar and sacral segments

b. The anterior one-third of the spinal cord is supplied via the anterior spinal artery, which arises from the intercostal arteries

c. The artery of Adamkiewicz is an important radicular artery providing blood to the thoracolumbar cord

d. The cord terminates at approximately L4 in adults

(3) **Regarding neuromonitoring:**

a. SSEP monitoring assesses the integrity of the posterior column

b. A 50% decrease in SSEP signal amplitude and latency is considered clinically significant

c. A 50% reduction in MEP signal amplitude is considered clinically significant

d. Nitrous oxide does not affect the evoked potential signals

(4) **For C-spine clearance:**

a. Three-view radiography is generally adequate to clear the C-spine

b. Flexion extension radiography is recommended after acute injury

c. Dynamic fluoroscopy is recommended for evaluation of ligamentous injury in the obtunded patient

d. MRI is the imaging study of choice when there is negative CT findings in a patient with neurologic deficit

(5) **Which of the following criteria is *not* required to be met in order to clear awake and asymptomatic patients without radiological evaluation?**

a. Absence of neck pain

b. Free from focal neurological deficit

c. Isolated spinal injury

d. Absence of pain with passive neck movement

(6) **Which of the following statements is true concerning immobilization for spine protection?**

a. Rigid cervical collar, sandbags and tape are adequate for C-spine immobilization

b. Penetrating trauma patients do not require spine immobilization for transportation

c. The C-spine cannot never be cleared without imaging

d. All trauma patients must be immobilized during prehospital care until their spine is cleared by a physician

(7) **Regarding injury classification systems:**

a. In the Orthopedic Trauma Association classification letter A refers to axial compression

b. In the Orthopedic Trauma Association classification B3 refers to stable injury

c. ASIA B refers to intact sensory and motor score ≤ 3 for > 50% of major muscle groups

d. ASIA E refers to complete injury

(8) **ASA practice advisory on perioperative visual loss does *not* state:**

a. The head of the bed should be kept above the heart

b. Hemoglobin should be kept above 9 g/dL

c. Colloids should be used for volume replacement

d. Staging should be considered for high-risk patients having long surgery

For questions 9–12, match each of the statements (9–12) with the best answer (a–d).

(9) **Associated with worsening of original injury (secondary injury)**

(10) **Spinal cord injury without radiographic abnormality**

(11) **Central cord syndrome**

(12) **Brown-Séquard syndrome**

a. Occurs more commonly in children than adults

b. Hypotension due to hemorrhage or loss of systemic vasomotor tone

c. Increased upper- versus lower-extremity weakness, associated with bladder dysfunction, and variable loss of sensory function below the lesion

d. Loss of motor and touch sensation ipsilateral to the lesion, with pain and temperature sensation lost contralateral to the lesion

Answers

(1) c
(2) c
(3) a
(4) d
(5) d
(6) b
(7) a
(8) b
(9) b
(10) a
(11) c
(12) d

References

1. Devivo MJ. Epidemiology of traumatic spinal cord injury: trends and future implications. *Spinal Cord* 2012; **50**: 365–72.

2. National Spinal Cord Injury Statistical Center (NSCISC). Spinal Cord Injury Facts and Figures at a Glance, 2013. https://www.nscisc.uab.edu (accessed September 2014).

3. Martirosyan NL, Feuerstein JS, Theodore N, *et al*. Blood supply and vascular reactivity of the spinal cord under normal and pathological conditions. *J Neurosurg Spine* 2011; **15**: 238–51.

4. Etz CD, Kari FA, Mueller CS, *et al*. The collateral network concept: a reassessment of the anatomy of spinal cord perfusion. *J Thoracic Cardiovascular Surg* 2011; **141**: 1020–8.

5. Etz CD, Kari FA, Mueller CS, *et al*. The collateral network concept: remodeling of the arterial collateral network after experimental segmental artery sacrifice. *J Thoracic Cardiovascular Surg* 2011; **141**: 1029–36.

6. Marsh JL, Slongo TF, Agel J, *et al*. Fracture and dislocation classification compendium – 2007: Orthopaedic Trauma Association classification, database and outcomes committee. *J Orthop Trauma* 2007; **21** (10 Suppl): S1–133.

7. Launay F, Leet AI, Sponseller PD. Pediatric spinal cord injury without radiographic abnormality: a meta-analysis. *Clin Orthop Relat Res* 2005; **433**: 166–70.

8. Como JJ, Samia H, Nemunaitis GA, *et al*. The misapplication of the term spinal cord injury without radiographic abnormality (SCIWORA) in adults. *J Trauma Acute Care Surg* 2012; **73**: 1261–6.

9. Stahel PF, VanderHeiden T, Finn MA. Management strategies for acute spinal cord injury: current options and future perspectives. *Curr Opin Crit Care* 2012; **18**: 651–60.

10. Borgens RB, Liu-Snyder P. Understanding secondary injury. *Q Rev Biol* 2012; **87**: 89–127.

11. Saboe LA, Reid DC, Davis LA, Warren SA, Grace MG. Spine trauma and associated injuries. *J Trauma* 1991; **31**: 43–8.

12. Holly LT, Kelly DF, Counelis GJ, *et al*. Cervical spine trauma associated with moderate and severe head injury: incidence, risk factors, and injury characteristics. *J Neurosurg* 2002; **96** (3 Suppl): 285–91.

13. Hackl W, Hausberger K, Sailer R, Ulmer H, Gassner R. Prevalence of cervical spine injuries in patients with facial trauma. *Oral Surg Oral Med Oral Pathol Oral Radiol Endod* 2001; **92**: 370–6.

14. Rabinovici R, Ovadia P, Mathiak G, Abdullah F. Abdominal injuries associated with lumbar spine fractures in blunt trauma. *Injury* 1999; **30**: 471–4.

15. Chen Y, DeVivo M. Epidemiology of extraspinal fractures in acute spinal cord injury: data from the Model Spinal Cord Injury Care Systems, 1973–1999. *Topics Spinal Cord Injury Rehabil* 2005; **11**: 18–29.

16. Raw RM. Could the open door crack on perioperative visual loss be even bigger? *Anesthesiology* 2012; **117**: 432–3.

17. Spahn DR, Bouillon B, Cerny V, *et al*. Management of bleeding and coagulopathy following major trauma: an updated European guideline. *Crit Care* 2013; **17**: R76.

18. Brenner M, Stein DM, Hu PF, *et al*. Traditional systolic blood pressure targets underestimate hypotension-induced secondary brain injury. *J Trauma Acute Care Surg* 2012; **72**: 1135–9.

19. Mallek JT, Inaba K, Branco BC, *et al*. The incidence of neurogenic shock after spinal cord injury in patients admitted to a high-volume level I trauma center. *Am Surg* 2012; **78**: 623–6.

20. Summers RL, Baker SD, Sterling SA, Porter JM, Jones AE. Characterization of the spectrum of hemodynamic profiles in trauma patients with acute neurogenic shock. *J Crit Care* 2013; **28**: 531 e1–5.

21. Guly HR, Bouamra O, Lecky FE, Trauma A, Research N. The incidence of neurogenic shock in patients with isolated spinal cord injury in the emergency department. *Resuscitation* 2008; **76**: 57–62.

22. Podolsky S, Baraff LJ, Simon RR, *et al*. Efficacy of cervical spine immobilization methods. *J Trauma* 1983; **23**: 461–5.

23. Theodore N, Hadley MN, Aarabi B, *et al*. Prehospital cervical spinal immobilization after trauma. *Neurosurgery* 2013; **72** (Suppl 2): 22–34.

24. Manoach S, Paladino L. Laryngoscopy force, visualization, and intubation failure in acute trauma: should we modify the practice of manual in-line stabilization? *Anesthesiology* 2009; **110**: 6–7.

25. Crosby ET. Airway management in adults after cervical spine trauma. *Anesthesiology* 2006; **104**: 1293–318.

26. Santoni BG, Hindman BJ, Puttlitz CM, *et al*. Manual in-line stabilization increases pressures applied by the laryngoscope blade during direct laryngoscopy and orotracheal intubation. *Anesthesiology* 2009; **110**: 24–31.

27. Vale FL, Burns J, Jackson AB, Hadley MN. Combined medical and surgical treatment after acute spinal cord injury: results of a prospective pilot study to assess the merits of aggressive medical resuscitation and blood pressure management. *J Neurosurgery* 1997; **87**: 239–46.

28. Levi L, Wolf A, Belzberg H. Hemodynamic parameters in patients with acute cervical cord trauma: description, intervention, and prediction of outcome. *Neurosurgery* 1993; **33**: 1007–16.

29. Tuli S, Tuli J, Coleman WP, Geisler FH, Krassioukov A. Hemodynamic parameters and timing of surgical decompression in acute cervical spinal cord injury. *J Spinal Cord Med* 2007; **30**: 482–90.

30. Ryken TC, Hurlbert RJ, Hadley MN, *et al*. The acute cardiopulmonary management of patients with cervical spinal cord injuries. *Neurosurgery* 2013; **72** (Suppl 2): 84–92.

31. Como JJ, Diaz JJ, Dunham CM, *et al*. Practice management guidelines for identification of cervical spine injuries following trauma: update from the Eastern Association for the Surgery of Trauma Practice Management Guidelines Committee. *J Trauma* 2009; **67**: 651–9.

32. American College of Radiology. ACR appropriateness criteria: suspected spine trauma, 2012. http://www.acr.org/~/media/ACR/Documents/AppCriteria/Diagnostic/SuspectedSpineTrauma.pdf (accessed September 2014).

33. Ryken TC, Hadley MN, Walters BC, *et al*. Radiographic assessment. *Neurosurgery* 2013; **72** (Suppl 2): 54–72.

34. Sayer FT, Kronvall E, Nilsson OG. Methylprednisolone treatment in acute spinal cord injury: the myth challenged through a structured analysis of published literature. *Spine J* 2006; **6**: 335–43.

35. Edwards P, Arango M, Balica L, *et al*. Final results of MRC CRASH, a randomised placebo-controlled trial of intravenous corticosteroid in adults with head injury-outcomes at 6 months. *Lancet* 2005; **365**: 1957–9.

36. Hurlbert RJ, Hadley MN, Walters BC, *et al.* Pharmacological therapy for acute spinal cord injury. *Neurosurgery* 2013; **72** (Suppl 2): 93–105.

37. La Rosa G, Conti A, Cardali S, Cacciola F, Tomasello F. Does early decompression improve neurological outcome of spinal cord injured patients? Appraisal of the literature using a meta-analytical approach. *Spinal Cord* 2004; **42**: 503–12.

38. Furlan JC, Noonan V, Cadotte DW, Fehlings MG. Timing of decompressive surgery of spinal cord after traumatic spinal cord injury: an evidence-based examination of pre-clinical and clinical studies. *J Neurotrauma* 2011; **28**: 1371–99.

39. Carreon LY, Dimar JR. Early versus late stabilization of spine injuries: a systematic review. *Spine (Phila Pa 1976)* 2011; **36**: E727–33.

40. Fehlings MG, Vaccaro A, Wilson JR, *et al.* Early versus delayed decompression for traumatic cervical spinal cord injury: results of the Surgical Timing in Acute Spinal Cord Injury Study (STASCIS). *PLoS One* 2012; **7** (2): e32037.

41. van Middendorp JJ, Hosman A, Doi SA. The effects of the timing of spinal surgery after traumatic spinal cord injury: a systematic review and meta-analysis. *J Neurotrauma* 2013; **30**: 1781–94.

42. Aziz M. Airway management in neuroanesthesiology. *Anesthesiol Clin* 2012; **30**: 229–40.

43. Robitaille A. Airway management in the patient with potential cervical spine instability: continuing professional development. *Can J Anaesth* 2011; **58**: 1125–39.

44. Fehlings MG, Brodke DS, Norvell DC, Dettori JR. The evidence for intraoperative neurophysiological monitoring in spine surgery: does it make a difference? *Spine (Phila Pa 1976)* 2010; **35** (9 Suppl): S37–46.

45. Lall RR, Lall RR, Hauptman JS, *et al.* Intraoperative neurophysiological monitoring in spine surgery: indications, efficacy, and role of the preoperative checklist. *Neurosurg Focus* 2012; **33** (5): E10.

46. Levi AD, Casella G, Green BA, *et al.* Clinical outcomes using modest intravascular hypothermia after acute cervical spinal cord injury. *Neurosurgery* 2010; **66**: 670–7.

47. Ahmad F, Wang MY, Levi AD. Hypothermia for acute spinal cord injury: a review. *World Neurosurg* 2014; **82**: 207–14.

48. O'Toole JE, Wang MC, Kaiser MG. Hypothermia and human spinal cord injury: updated position statement and evidence based recommendations from the AANS/CNS Joint Section on Disorders of the Spine Peripheral Nerves. http://www.spinesection.org/files/pdfs/Hypothermia%20Position%20Statement%20Oct%202013.pdf (accessed October 2014).

49. NICE-SUGAR Study Investigators, Finfer S, Chittock DR, Su SY, *et al.* Intensive versus conventional glucose control in critically ill patients. *N Engl J Med* 2009; **360**: 1283–97.

50. Postoperative Visual Loss Study Group. Risk factors associated with ischemic optic neuropathy after spinal fusion surgery. *Anesthesiology* 2012; **116**: 15–24.

51. American Society of Anesthesiologists Task Force on Perioperative Visual Loss. Practice advisory for perioperative visual loss associated with spine surgery. *Anesthesiology* 2012; **116**: 274–85.

52. Lee LA. Perioperative visual loss and anesthetic management. *Curr Opin Anaesth* 2013; **26**: 375–81.

53. Grossman RG, Frankowski RF, Burau KD, *et al.* Incidence and severity of acute complications after spinal cord injury. *J Neurosurg Spine* 2012; **17** (1 Suppl): 119–28.

Chapter

24

Oral and maxillofacial trauma: surgical considerations

Marcello Guglielmi, Rishad Shaikh, Ketan P. Parekh, and Cecil S. Ash

Objectives

(1) Review the role of the maxillofacial surgeon in patients with oral and maxillofacial trauma.

(2) Discuss the surgical considerations for patients with oral and maxillofacial facial trauma, including fractures of the upper and lower jaws, orbital fractures, midface fractures, and facial lacerations.

(3) Review the implications of head and neck infections, including Ludwig's angina.

Introduction

Maxillofacial surgery is the specialty of the dental and medical profession and is the only surgical specialty in the United States that receives at least 5–6 months of anesthesia training during residency. Therefore, maxillofacial surgeons are experienced in managing the airway both surgically and nonsurgically, and work closely with anesthesiologists to ensure optimal airway management. The training in anesthesia permits the maxillofacial surgeon to perform surgical procedures in an office setting using intravenous sedation or general anesthesia.

Injuries to the oral and maxillofacial region impart a high degree of emotional, as well as physical, trauma to patients. There are a number of causes of facial trauma including motor vehicle collisions (MVCs), falls, sports injuries, interpersonal violence, and work-related injuries (see Chapter 1). The type of injuries can range from minor (e.g., avulsion of a tooth) to extremely severe injuries of the skin and bones of the face (Figs. 24.1–24.7). Typically, injuries are classified as either simple or complex soft tissue injuries (skin and gums), bony injuries (fractures), or injuries to special regions such as the eyes, nerves, or salivary glands.

Dentoalveolar injuries

Dentoalveolar injuries are relatively common. In the adult population these injuries may be caused by MVCs, bicycles, falls, assaults, sports injuries, and industrial accidents. These injuries may be also iatrogenic: from dentists and physicians

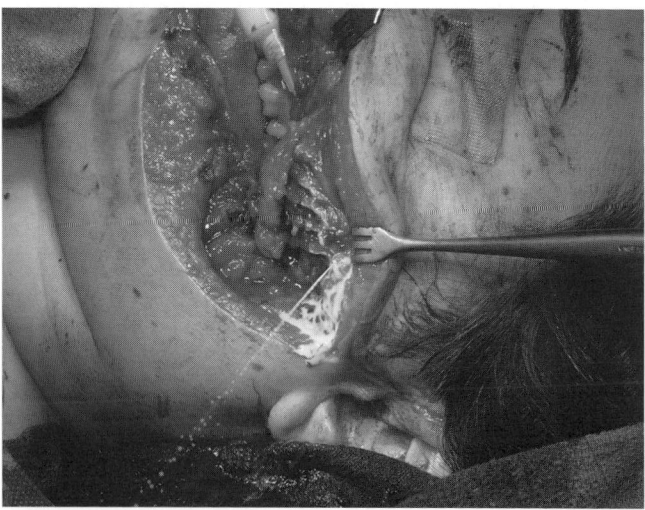

Figure 24.1 Full-thickness facial laceration through parotid duct. *A black and white version of this figure will appear in some formats. For the color version, please refer to the plate section.*

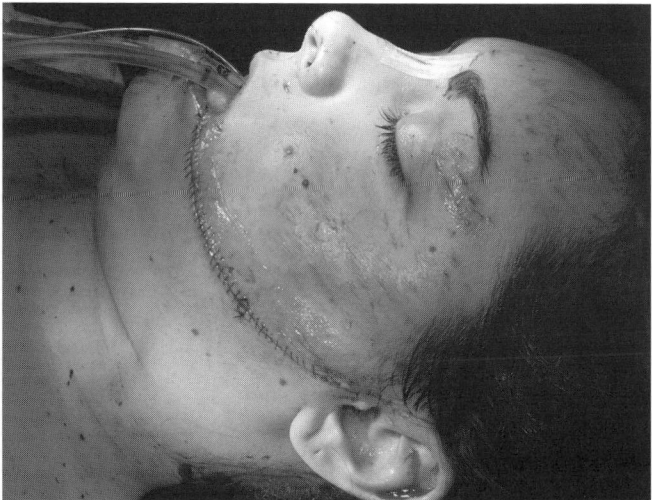

Figure 24.2 Same patient as in Figure 24.1. Propofol was used to identify the duct after cannulation. *A black and white version of this figure will appear in some formats. For the color version, please refer to the plate section.*

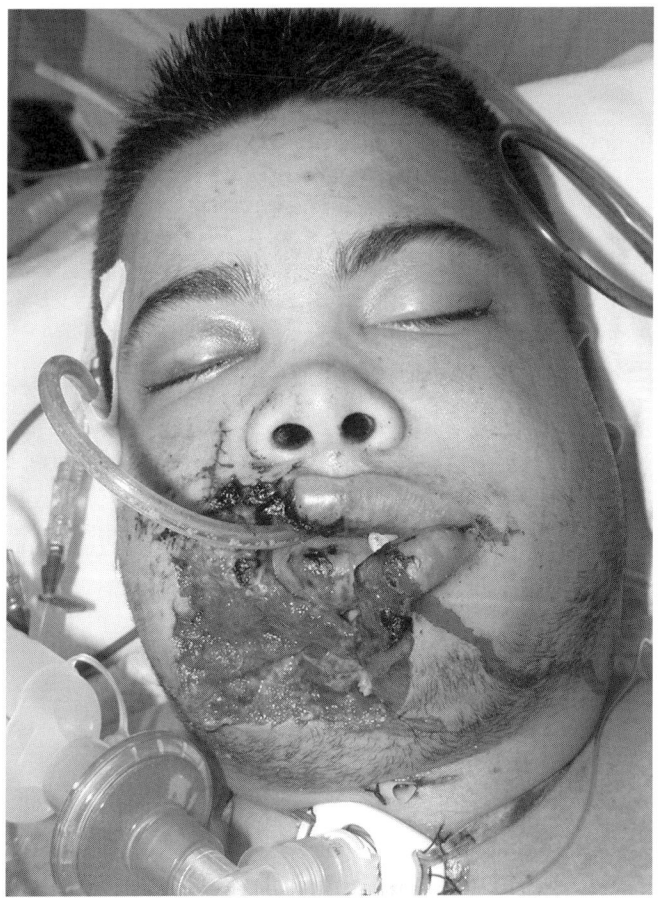

Figure 24.3 Complex lower facial soft tissue trauma after gunshot wound. *A black and white version of this figure will appear in some formats. For the color version, please refer to the plate section.*

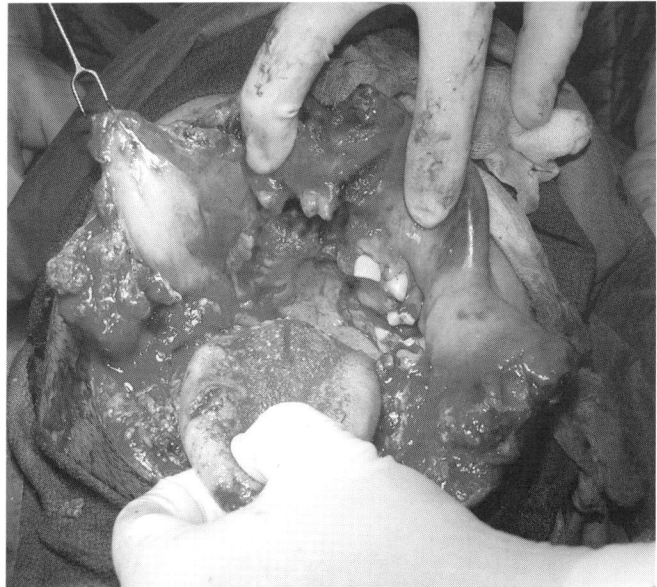

Figure 24.4 After tracheostomy and flap reflection, extensive soft tissue, hard tissue, and dentoalveolar trauma is seen. *A black and white version of this figure will appear in some formats. For the color version, please refer to the plate section.*

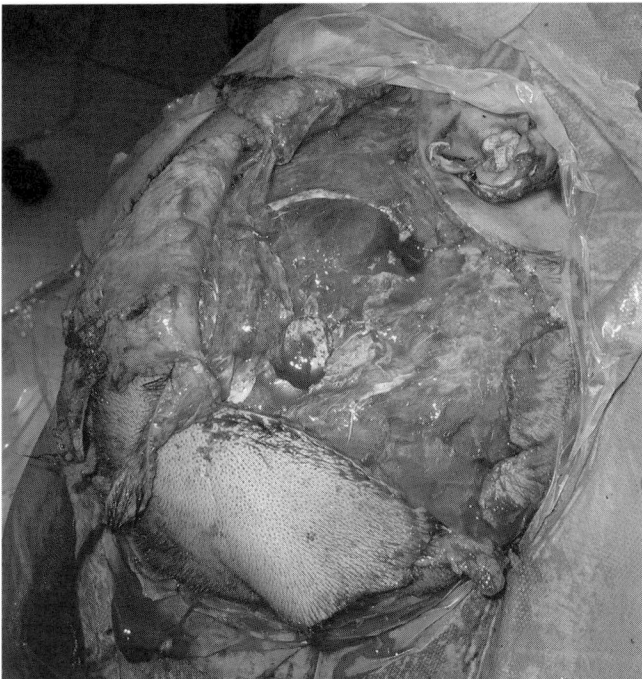

Figure 24.5 Complex scalp degloving injury in an unhelmeted motorcyclist. *A black and white version of this figure will appear in some formats. For the color version, please refer to the plate section.*

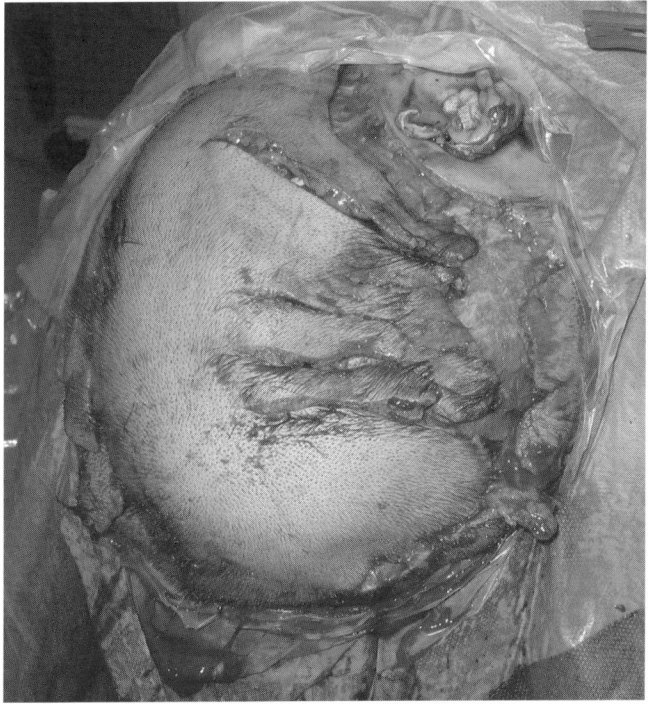

Figure 24.6 Tissue realigned, and rotational flaps utilized. *A black and white version of this figure will appear in some formats. For the color version, please refer to the plate section.*

during oral procedures or by anesthesia providers during endotracheal intubation.

Maxillofacial surgeons are usually involved in treating fractures in the supporting bone or in replanting teeth which have been displaced or avulsed. These types of injuries are treated by

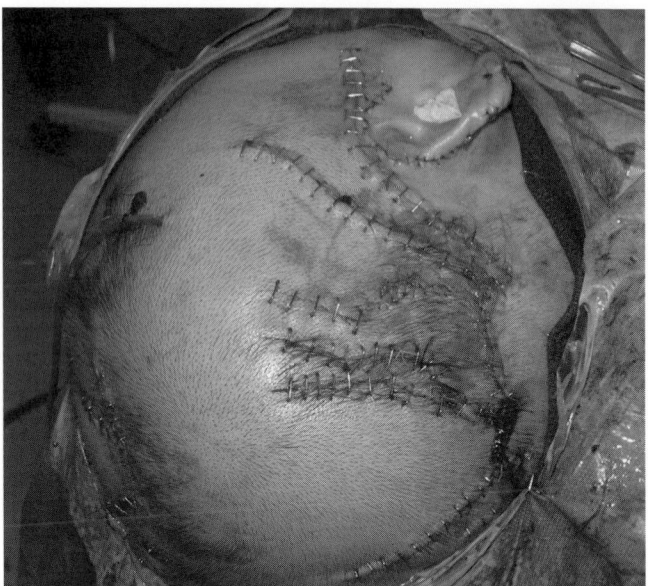

Figure 24.7 Primary repair of scalp laceration. *A black and white version of this figure will appear in some formats. For the color version, please refer to the plate section.*

one of a number of forms of "splinting" (stabilizing by wiring or bonding teeth together). If a tooth is avulsed, it should be kept inside the mouth by the patient or placed in salt water, milk, or Hank's balanced solution when available. As a general rule, the sooner the tooth is re-inserted into the dental socket the better the prognosis. Dentoalveolar trauma may be classified as: dental avulsion, dental luxation and extrusion, enamel and crown fracture, dental intrusion, dental concussion and subluxation, root fracture, and alveolar bone fracture. Injuries to the teeth and alveolar bone process should be considered emergency conditions, because a successful outcome depends on prompt attention to the injury. Therefore, the patient should be evaluated as soon as possible. It is imperative that each tooth the patient had before the accident is accounted for. If during clinical examination a tooth or crown is found missing and no history suggests that it was lost at the scene, radiographic examination of the oral soft tissues, chest, and abdominal region is necessary to rule out the presence of the missing piece within the tissues or other areas of the body, such as the tracheobronchial tree or gastrointestinal tract.[1]

Injuries to children's teeth require special attention: the peak period for trauma to the primary teeth is 18–40 months of age, because this is a time of increased mobility for the relatively uncoordinated toddler. Injuries to primary teeth usually result from falls and collisions as the child learns to walk and run. Dental trauma also may occur as a result of an altercation, child abuse, or other causes. Again, prompt treatment is essential for the long-term health of an injured tooth. Obtaining dental care within 30 minutes can make the difference between saving or losing a child's tooth.

With permanent teeth, school-aged boys suffer oral trauma almost twice as frequently as school-aged girls. Sports accidents and fights are the most common causes of dental trauma in teenagers. The upper (maxillary) central incisors are the most commonly injured teeth. Maxillary teeth protruding more than 4 mm are 2–3 times more likely to suffer dental trauma in comparison to normally aligned teeth.

One of the most common causes of complaints against anesthesiologists is dental trauma during intubation. Warner *et al.* found that the frequency of tooth contact with a regular Macintosh blade is significantly increased with nonreassuring signs of difficult intubation on airway examination such as poor visualization of the uvula (e.g., Mallampati class III/IV), inability to prognath the jaw, incomplete range of motion of the head and neck, decreased interincisor gap, and protruding maxillary incisors with prominent overbite.[1] The risk of dental trauma should be discussed with the patient preoperatively, especially in patients with anatomic predictors of difficult intubation (see Chapter 3). Teeth traumatized during intubation necessitate an immediate dental consultation for evaluation and treatment. The goal in the treatment of any dentoalveolar injury is reestablishing normal form and function of the masticatory apparatus, in addition to aesthetics.

Mandible fractures

History

The history of mandible fractures dates as far back as 1600 BC in the writings of the Edwin Smith Papyrus, the world's earliest known medical document. Hippocrates was quoted describing the bandaging of fractures as a means of stabilization in 400 BC. Today the principles first described for immobilization by Hippocrates are combined with the more modern advances of open reduction and internal fixation to treat a variety of mandibular fractures.

Incidence and pathophysiology

The mandible is the second most frequently fractured bone of the face, after the paired nasal bones. Of these fractures the angle is the most commonly fractured site, followed by the body, condyle, symphysis, ramus, coronoid, and alveolus. The ratio of mandible to zygomatic to maxillary fractures is reported as 6:2:1. In a study of 4711 patients treated with facial fractures, 45% had a fracture of the mandible.[2,3] Assault was the most common mechanism, followed by MVCs, falls, and sporting injuries. Males are 3–6 times more likely to have a mandible fracture than females, and 40–60% of mandible fractures are associated with other injuries. Ten percent of these are lethal. The most commonly associated injury is to the chest. Cervical spine injury is associated in 2.6% of mandible fractures. Although this incidence is low, missing a cervical spine injury may be catastrophic. Condylar fractures at times can be displaced superiorly, with the fragment herniating through the roof of the glenoid fossa into the floor of the middle cranial fossa, which can be associated with a dural tear.

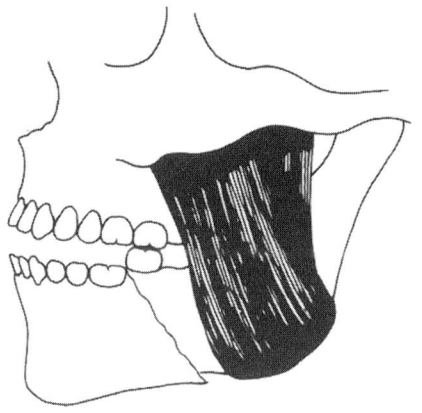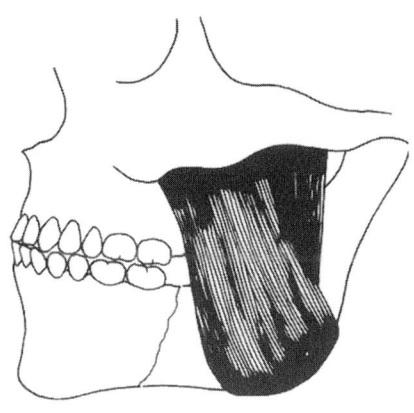

Figure 24.8 Lateral view of skull showing masseter muscle pull on an unfavorable fracture pattern (left) and a favorable fracture pattern (right).

Mandibular fractures usually occur in two or more locations because of the bone's unique U or V shape. When treating mandibular fractures, the rule is to suspect a second fracture until proven otherwise. The fracture may occur at a site separate from the initial site of the direct trauma. Fractures of the mandible are often classified as favorable or unfavorable, depending on the angulation of the fracture and force of the muscle pull proximal and distal to the fracture (Fig. 24.8). The masticatory muscles – masseter, medial pterygoid, lateral pterygoid, and temporalis – insert into different areas of the mandible to provide mobility, support, and function. The directional pull of these muscles will determine the stability of certain fracture patterns. The masseter and temporalis muscles exert an upward pull on the angle of the mandible, which will distract horizontally unfavorable fractures from each other in a vertical direction. The medial and lateral pterygoid muscles exert a medial pull on the ramus of the mandible and will distract vertically unfavorable fractures medially. Because of the strength of these muscles, displaced fractures often cannot be reduced without the use of a neuromuscular blocking agent (NMBA).

The mandible may also be simply dislocated without an associated fracture. Dislocation of the mandible can be spontaneous in a patient with laxity of the temporomandibular joint (TMJ) ligaments, especially in females. The dislocation usually occurs after a large yawn or after a prolonged dental procedure. Patients usually present in considerable pain. Due to spasms of the masseter and pterygoid muscles, the condyles are directed up the anterior aspect of the articular eminence, preventing normal mouth closure. Treatment of this problem is based on the frequency and/or ability of the patient to self-reduce, versus the need for surgical reduction of the dislocation. Reduction of the mandible can be accomplished under local anesthesia or intravenous sedation, or, in rare circumstances, under general anesthesia with the use of a NMBA (see Chapter 13). The Dawson maneuver is a well-described method to reduce the dislocation. In this maneuver, the thumbs are placed over the molar teeth of the patient and the dislocated jaw is pushed downward and backward. In severe cases, open joint surgery is indicated (often bilaterally). With

surgery, the TMJ ligaments can be tightened and the joint reshaped to decrease future dislocations.

Dislocation of the mandible can also occur during tracheal intubation. Prompt recognition and immediate intervention should take place in the operating room prior to emergence from anesthesia.

Evaluation and treatment

Evaluation of facial fractures is usually part of the Advanced Trauma Life Support (ATLS) secondary survey (see Chapter 2) unless there are issues with the airway. For example, patients with severely displaced bilateral mandibular injuries in which the tongue is displaced back into the airway may require urgent tracheotomy. If no airway issues are noted, mandibular fractures are evaluated after more serious life-threatening injuries have been addressed.

During the secondary survey, a complete examination is carried out, including palpation for step-off deformities, malocclusion, open bite deformities, floor of mouth hematomas or ecchymosis, crepitus, and chin and lower lip numbness. Missing teeth may prompt a chest x-ray and lateral neck film to inspect the airway or cervical esophagus for a foreign body.[4,5]

Radiographic evaluation with a panorex x-ray (Fig. 24.9) allows for bidimensional evaluation of fractures of the entire mandible. In addition, the stability and health of the teeth can be evaluated. A submental vertex radiograph can be used for evaluation of the condyles and subcondylar regions.[6,7] Computed tomography (CT) scan of the face without contrast is done when multiple facial fractures are suspected (Figs. 24.10, 24.11). The 3D reconstruction can also be very useful, especially in cases of panfacial fracture.

Treatment of mandible fractures initially entails a tetanus toxoid booster as indicated by immunization records. Almost all fractures can be considered open, as they usually communicate with either the skin or the oral cavity.[8] Bacteria involved in associated infections of mandibular fractures include the normal oral flora of aerobic Gram-positive cocci, anaerobic Gram-positive cocci, and anaerobic Gram-negative rods. Oral care should be instituted with 0.12% chlorhexidine solution to help remove superficial bacteria.

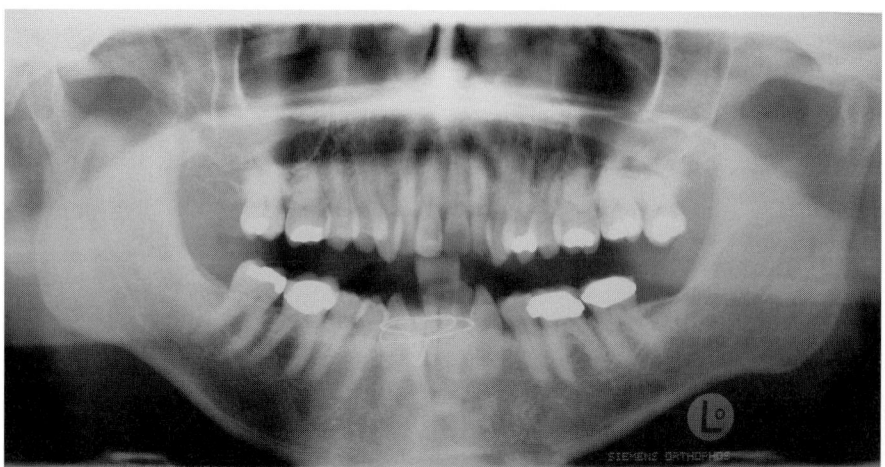

Figure 24.9 Panoramic radiograph, or panorex, of a mandible fracture.

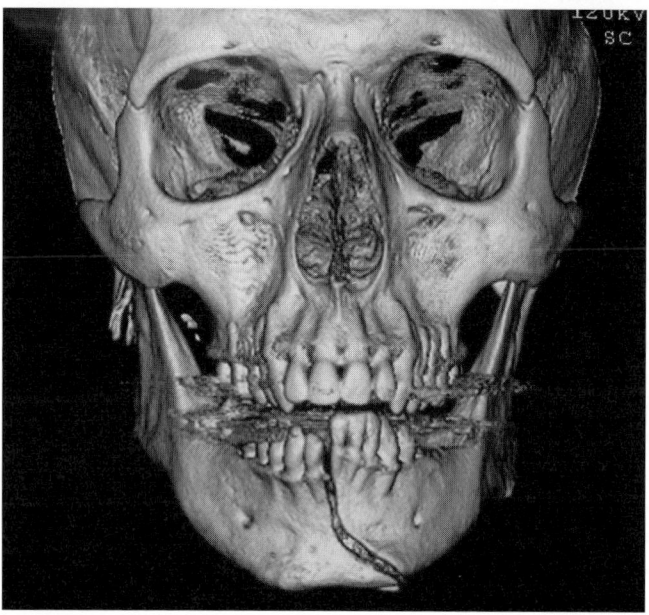

Figure 24.10 CT of the same patient as in Figure 24.9, showing mandibular symphysis fracture.

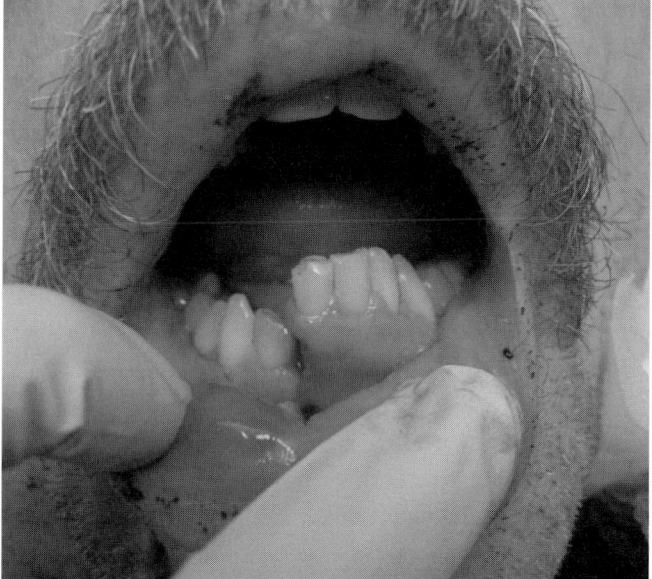

Figure 24.11 Clinic oral view of the patient in Figure 24.9 in the trauma bay. *A black and white version of this figure will appear in some formats. For the color version, please refer to the plate section.*

Basic principles of orthopedic surgery also apply to treatment of mandibular fractures, including reduction, fixation, immobilization, and supportive therapies.[9] Union of fracture segments will only take place in the absence of mobility. The stability of fracture segments is key for proper healing.[10] Goals of treatment are to restore occlusion and function by ensuring union of fracture segments.[11,12]

Treatment options for mandible fractures include: rigid fixation, semi-rigid fixation, nonrigid (closed reduction), or observation. A restricted soft diet may be the only treatment necessary for a unilateral nondisplaced fracture of the condyle when normal occlusion exists. If the patient develops malocclusion and/or pain, he or she may need to be managed with maxillomandibular fixation (MMF) or wiring of teeth together for 6 weeks (Fig. 24.12).[13] MMF or closed reduction

is also used for severely comminuted fractures, which heal better with the periosteum intact, avoiding surgical exposure of the fracture that could impair vascularization of the area.[14] Condylar fractures treated with open reduction may also lead to damage of the TMJ structure and facial nerve function.[15] These fractures are also classically treated with MMF.[16] However, a history of asthma, psychiatric disorder, seizures, malnutrition, or gastrointestinal disorders with severe nausea and vomiting may lead the surgeon away from MMF, because the patient may not tolerate having his or her jaws wired closed. At times, emergent reduction and fixation is undertaken in the emergency department to help with pain management and fracture stabilization until definitive treatment is completed. The mandible must be immobilized for 2–6 weeks for most

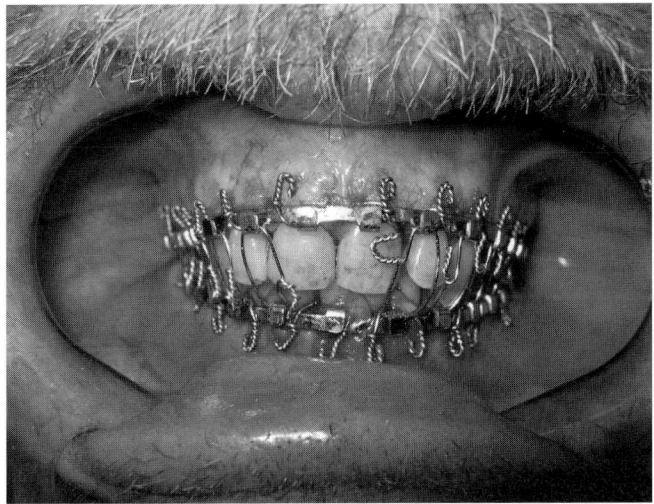

Figure 24.12 Clinical view of patient with maxillomandibular fixation (MMF) in place. *A black and white version of this figure will appear in some formats. For the color version, please refer to the plate section.*

fractures. Liquid diet supplemented with boost is always advised. The average weight loss is 10–15 pounds (4.5–7 kg).

MMF involves the placement of arch bars onto the gingiva of the maxilla and mandible. These bars are fixed into place with a 24 gauge wire to the interdental spaces of the teeth from the left to the right first molars. Once the arch bars are secure and the fracture is reduced with the patient in normal occlusion, fish loops made out of 26 gauge wire are placed to wire the mandible to the maxilla with the desired occlusion. The fish loops are used in selectively bringing the correct opposing pairs of teeth together.

MMF can be achieved also with the use of maxillomandibular titanium screws applied between the alveolar bone of adjacent roots, usually between upper and lower cuspid and bicuspid bilaterally. Fish loops made out of 24 gauge wire are passed through those screws to stabilize the mandible and maxilla into the patient's occlusion.

In true rigid fixation, healing occurs primarily without callus formation, allowing early return of function. Classical indications for open reduction include malocclusion despite MMF. Rigid fixation methods include the lag screw technique, compression plating, reconstruction plates, and external pin fixation. Open reduction with nonrigid fixation is more forgiving and easier to place; it still requires MMF and is useful in angle and parasymphyseal fractures. External pin fixation is usually necessary in comminuted fractures such as those seen with gunshot wound (GSW) injuries (Figs. 24.13–24.15).

Many complications may arise following the treatment of mandible fractures, including nonunion, malunion, infections, and ankylosis. Contributory factors include: the nature of the injury, comorbidities (e.g., diabetes mellitus, immunocompromised status), and noncompliance with the postoperative care (i.e., smoking, alcohol, or eating solid food during the healing period).[17] The potential for developing ankylosis is dependent on several factors, including the location and extension of the condylar injury, age, and the posttreatment immobilization period.

Midface fractures

Etiology and pathophysiology

Fractures of the midface are most often associated with facial trauma. The most common cause of these injuries is MVCs, followed by physical assaults, falls, sports injuries, industrial accidents, and GSWs. The diagnosis and treatment of facial fractures are important. Fractures of the facial skeleton alter the patient's physical appearance and possibly may disrupt the function of the masticatory system, ocular system, olfactory system, and nasal airway. Precise anatomic reduction and fixation of such fractures leads to superior functional and cosmetic outcomes.

Though facial trauma does represent a serious injury, the workup and treatment of facial fractures is part of the secondary survey when adhering to the ATLS protocol. Life-threatening problems, such as a threatened airway, should be addressed first.

In a patient with extensive facial trauma with the possibility of skull base injury, endotracheal intubation may not be possible and a surgical airway may be necessary (see Chapter 3). Fortunately only a small number of patients with extensive facial trauma require a cricothyroidotomy or tracheostomy for initial airway management. Submental intubation (intubation through the floor of the mouth) may be considered as temporary airway management, especially in a patient with nasal and nasoethmoid complex fractures (see Chapter 25 for a more in-depth description of submental intubation).

The patient who has sustained a force severe enough to cause significant facial injury must be assumed to have a cervical spine injury until proven otherwise. Epistaxis may be problematic and hemodynamically important. Hypovolemic shock or airway compromise can result secondary to profuse bleeding. Although epistaxis can have an anterior or posterior source, it most often originates in the anterior nasal cavity. Nasal bleeding usually responds to first-aid measures such as compression. When epistaxis does not respond to simple measures, the source of the bleeding needs to be identified and treated appropriately. Treatments to be considered include topical vasoconstriction, chemical cautery, electrocautery, anterior nasal packing (nasal tampon or gauze impregnated with petroleum jelly), posterior gauze packing, use of a balloon system (including a modified Foley catheter), and arterial ligation or angioembolization

Once the patient is stabilized per ATLS protocol, secondary evaluation with an accurate history and physical can take place. On physical examination one should document the presence and location of lacerations, ecchymosis, asymmetries, crepitus, tenderness, bony stepoffs, and canthal tendon disruption. Ophthalmologic examination deserves special mention in the diagnosis and treatment of facial trauma (see Chapter 26).

(A)

(B)

(C)

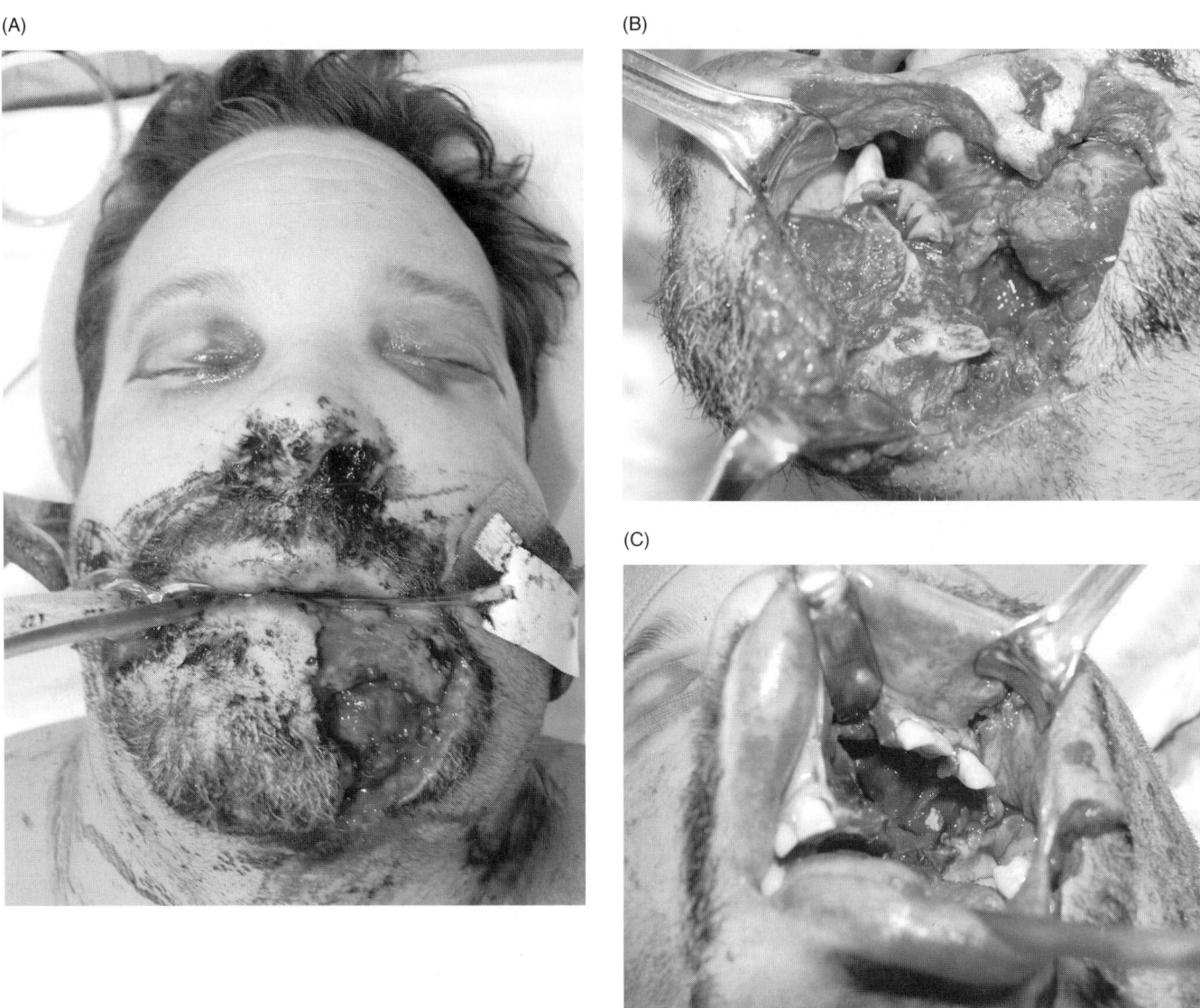

Figure 24.13 Clinical views of gunshot wound under chin with 357 handgun. *A black and white version of this figure will appear in some formats. For the color version, please refer to the plate section.*

Testing of visual acuity is the most important component of the ophthalmologic exam and should be performed immediately. Traumatic optic neuropathy, open globe injuries, and retrobulbar hematoma are ophthalmologic emergencies. Monocular diplopia is an indicator of possible unilateral globe or retinal injury and requires immediate ophthalmologic consultation. Retrobulbar hematoma is an emergent condition that needs to be addressed with lateral canthotomy as soon as possible to avoid blindness of the affected eye.

It is important to document visual acuity, pupillary function, and ocular mobility, and to inspect the anterior chamber for blood (hyphema) and the fundus for gross disruption. Evaluation of extraocular movements (EOM) may be difficult or restricted by edema of the soft tissues. At times a forced duction testing is required if the possibility of orbital entrapment exists. This is done by grasping the sclera in the fornix

and mechanically moving the globe. Inhibition of the globe moving would be indicative of entrapment and possible need for exploration (Figs. 24.16, 24.17).

After ophthalmologic evaluation, the face, ears, nose, mouth, and mandible should be systematically examined. The face should be assessed for asymmetry, facial shortening, a mobile midface, palpable step-offs, Battle's sign (ecchymosis behind the ear), raccoon eyes (periorbital bruising/ecchymosis), paresthesia, rhinorrhea, otorrhea, traumatic blindness, hemotympanum, restricted extraocular movements, septal hematoma, trismus, and dental malocclusion.

Even with the most thorough physical exam, radiological imaging remains an important adjunct in the evaluation of the facial trauma patient (see Chapter 11). If facial fractures are suspected, a high-resolution CT and 3D reconstruction is the procedure of choice. A CT of the face without contrast is

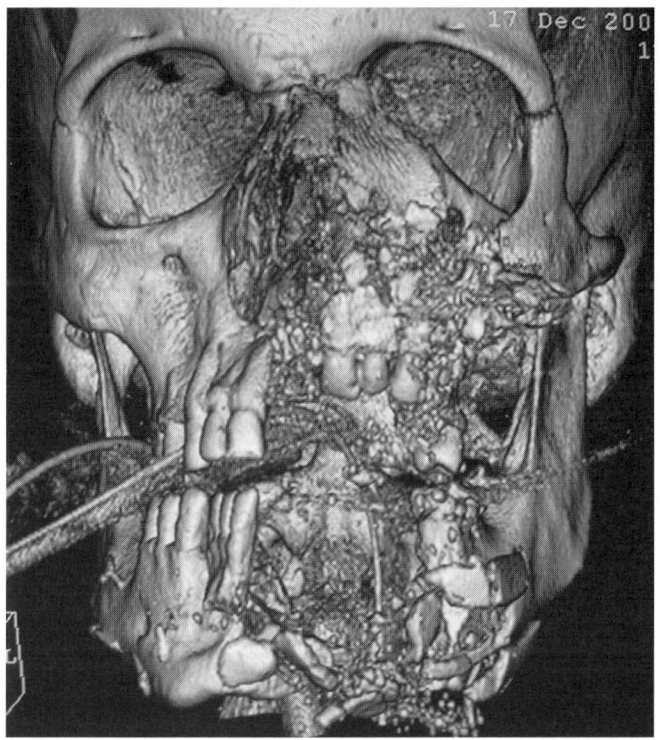

Figure 24.14 3D CT showing extensive hard tissue and dentoalveolar damage.

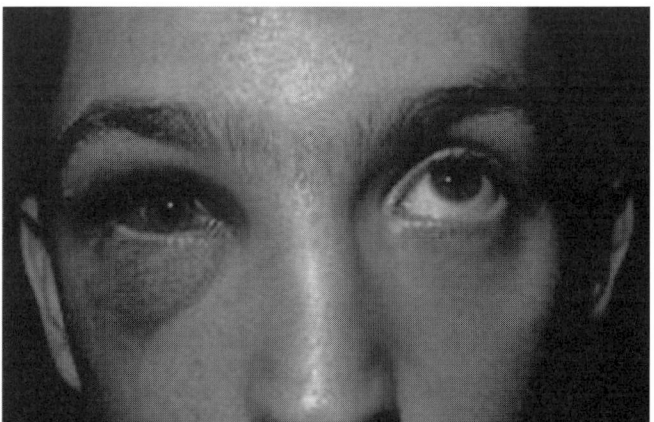

Figure 24.16 Clinical view of patient with right orbital floor fracture, with restricted superior gaze. *A black and white version of this figure will appear in some formats. For the color version, please refer to the plate section.*

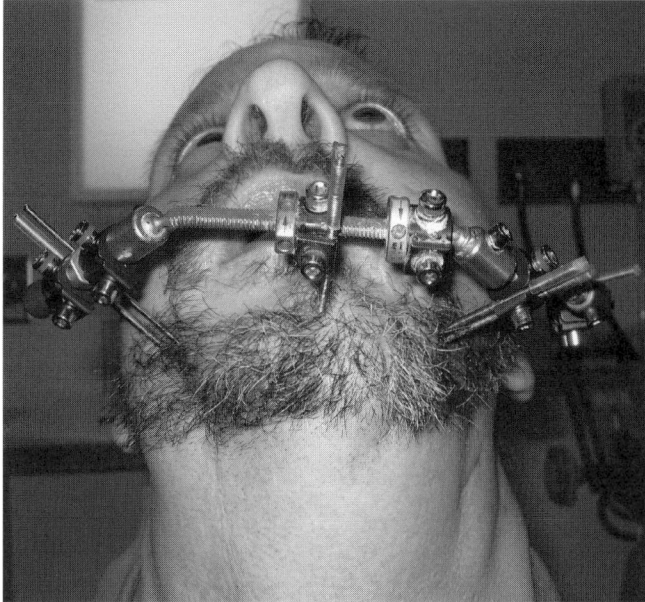

Figure 24.15 6 weeks postoperative view of patient with external pin fixation in place. *A black and white version of this figure will appear in some formats. For the color version, please refer to the plate section.*

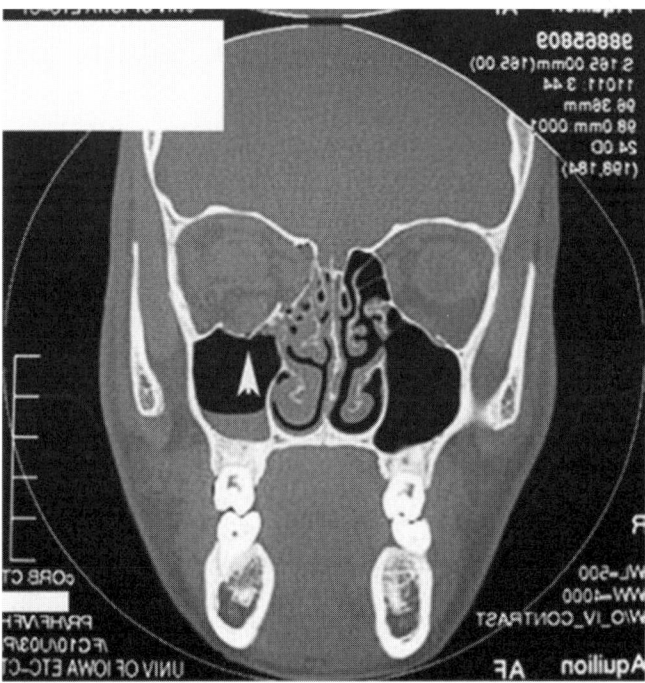

Figure 24.17 Coronal CT of same patient as in Figure 24.16, with a right orbital floor fracture.

standard care. The bones of the skull and face collectively make up the most complex area of skeletal anatomy in the human body. This complex anatomy is shown with great detail by CT, as are fractures of the facial bones, and soft tissue complications can be evaluated to a far greater degree with CT (Figs. 24.18, 24.19). Three-dimensional CT reconstruction is useful when treatment planning, or when communicating the degree of the trauma with the patient or the family.

Facial fractures most often occur in young males. The male to female incidence of these fractures is 4:1. The most common midface fracture is the nasal fracture, followed by the zygomaticomaxillary complex fracture (tripod fracture), and the Le Fort I–II–III fractures. Facial fractures are uncommon in the pediatric population (less than 10%), due to the increased resilience of a child's facial skeleton or the smaller relative dimensions of the midface compared to the cranium.[18]

In 1901, René Le Fort, a Frenchman, described his now famous classification of facial fractures. Le Fort's work described the lines of weakness in the facial skeleton through which most fractures occur. These lines where the facial bones break after trauma have become known as the Le Fort I, II, and III fractures. This work served as the stepping stone for the development of the specialty of maxillofacial surgery.[19] In

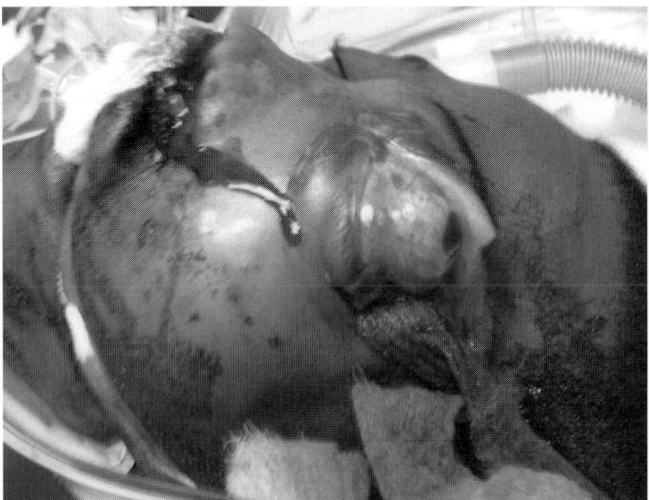

Figure 24.18 Clinical view of patient in trauma bay with extensive midface trauma. *A black and white version of this figure will appear in some formats. For the color version, please refer to the plate section.*

addition, these fracture lines have served as a guide for facial osteotomies used to correct posttraumatic and congenital facial anomalies.

The Le Fort I fracture essentially separates the lower maxilla, including the alveolar ridge and teeth, from the rest of the midface. The fracture classically travels through the inferior portion of the piriform aperture. It separates the maxilla from the pterygoid plates and from the nasal and zygomatic structures. The characteristic finding is an anterior open bite due to the medial and inferior traction of the medial and lateral pterygoids on the mobile maxillary fragment. The maxilla may be mobile but is often mildly impacted.

The Le Fort II fracture is sometimes called a pyramidal fracture because of its shape. This type of fracture includes the entire piriform aperture in the distracted midface. Le Fort II fractures are most often a result of forces applied near the level of the nasal bones.

The Le Fort III fracture, also referred to as a craniofacial disassociation fracture, consists of a fracture line that passes through the lateral orbit superior to the zygoma which is attached to the maxilla. The bones of the midface are essentially disarticulated from the cranium, giving a characteristic dish face appearance.

Most of the time midfacial fractures are combinations of the previously mentioned injuries, such as a mixture of Le Fort II and Le Fort III complex fractures.

(A)

(B)

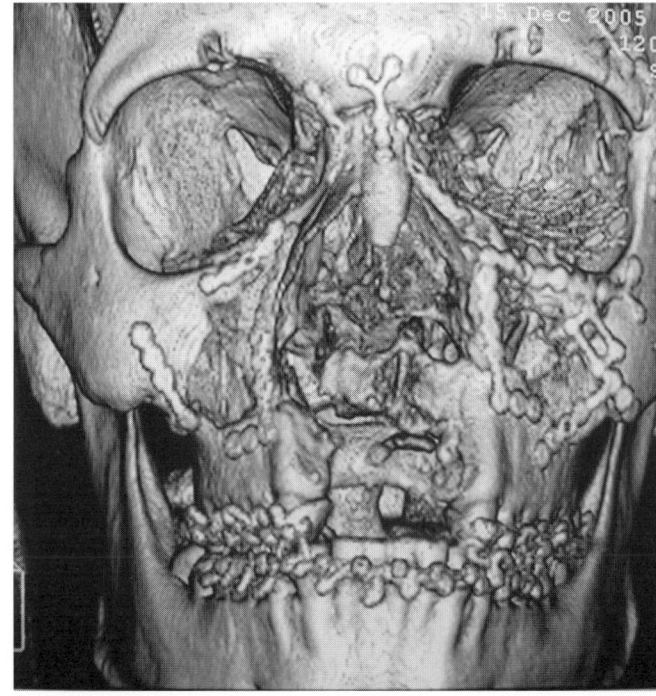

Figure 24.19 3D CT of same patient (**A**) before and (**B**) after repair.

The nose is the most frequently injured facial structure, undeniably because of its prominent position on the face. The physical exam is most accurate when performed prior to post-traumatic edema. Palpation of the nasal bones may reveal mobility or crepitus, indicating a nasal fracture. Any clots at this time should be gently suctioned, and minor bleeding can be controlled with topical preparations. Visual inspection of the septum must be performed to rule out a septal hematoma. Septal hematomas require immediate evacuation and drainage when discovered. If left untreated, septal hematomas can cause fibrosis and narrowing of the nasal passages, distortion of the septum, and/or formation of an abscess. They can also cause pressure necrosis of the septum, leading to septal perforation and eventually to complete necrosis with formation of a saddle-nose deformity. The majority of nasal injuries are identified after significant edema resolves in the multitrauma patient. Therefore, with the exception of grossly displaced fractures, open fractures, and septal hematomas, treatment of most nasal fractures is delayed 3–10 days to allow swelling to resolve.

The zygoma is a relatively strong bone, and serves as a buttress of the facial skeleton. A fracture of the zygoma itself is quite rare, and most fractures are associated with weaker suture lines associated with the zygomatic arch. Fractures of the zygoma are more associated with lateral trauma, as opposed to Le Fort fractures, which result more from anterior facial trauma. Because of the zygomatic articulation with the maxilla and the frontal and temporal bones, fracture patterns in this area are sometimes referred to as zygomaticomaxillary complex (ZMC) or tripod fractures. Because of the zygoma's association with the orbit, fractures of the zygoma may cause orbital fractures. Isolated orbital fractures do also occur, the most common type being an orbital floor fracture or "blow-out" fracture. This type of fracture is most often from an object that bypasses the bony prominences of the zygoma and orbital rims, and transmits its force directly to the globe. This then causes increased orbital pressure, which in turn fractures either the orbital floor or the medial wall, which represents the thinnest bony portion of the orbital cavity. Less common are fractures of the lateral and superior walls of the orbit, where the bone is thicker.

Naso-orbital-ethmoid (NOE) fractures are most often associated with trauma to the central midface. The NOE complex consists of a complex skeletal framework including bones of the nose, orbits, maxilla, and cranium. Fractures in this area are some of the most difficult and challenging of all facial fractures to treat. NOE fractures may be isolated but are most often found in combination with Le Fort or panfacial fractures. Fractures in this area cause a collapse and telescoping of the nasal bones and ethmoids and may lead to fracture of the cribriform plate. In cases in which disruption of the cribriform plate is a possibility, a nasogastric tube insertion is contraindicated because of the risk of inserting the tube intracranially.[20] This complication of nasogastric tubes has been reported.[20,21] In most cases, the nasotracheal tube is too wide to penetrate

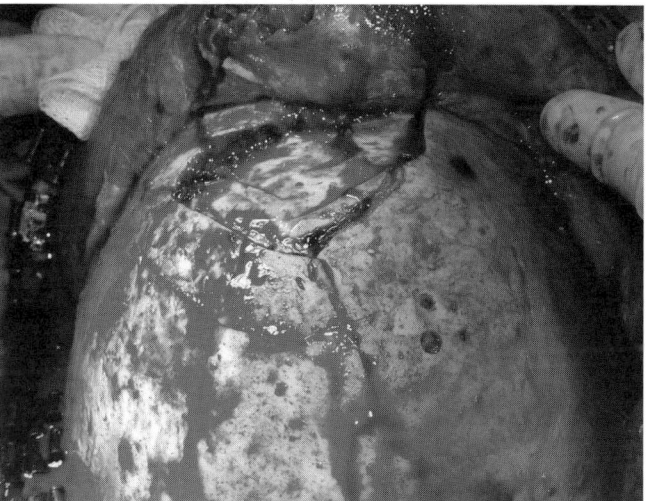

Figure 24.20 Surgical exposure of a patient with a comminuted frontal sinus fracture. *A black and white version of this figure will appear in some formats. For the color version, please refer to the plate section.*

the cribriform plate. The suspicion level should also be high for cerebrospinal fluid (CSF) rhinorrhea in all NOE fractures. A common finding associated with comminuted NOE fractures is traumatic telecanthus due to the disruption of the medial canthal tendon. Inadequate treatment and reduction will often lead to permanent telecanthus, flattened nasal bridge, and rounding of the palpebral fissure.

Frontal sinus fractures represent some of the least common injuries that affect the facial skeleton. The incidence is 5–15% of all facial fractures. However, because the frontal sinus makes up part of the brain, the potential for fatality from these injuries is much greater than with other facial fractures (Figs. 24.20, 24.21). During patient evaluation all frontal sinus fractures should be regarded as head injuries. Significant intracranial injury occurs more commonly with injury to the frontal sinus (12–17% of the time) than with injury to the mandible or midface. A thorough neurological examination is extremely important. Neurosurgical consultation should be obtained promptly in the presence of abnormal neurological radiologic studies or if there is a change in mental status. Isolated anterior table fractures of the frontal bone need repair if there is an aesthetic concern for the patient. Fractures of the posterior table of the frontal bone require close surveillance for signs and symptoms of CSF leakage such as double ring signs of nasal drainage (blood surrounded by clear ring onto paper filter), salty taste of patient's nasofrontal secretions, or a positive β_2 isotransferrin test. In this case obliteration and cranialization is the surgical treatment of choice.

Treatment

The goal of surgical treatment is to reestablish skeletal relationships while restoring and preserving function of vital structures. Most important are the restoration of dental occlusion, masticatory function, nasal function, ocular position,

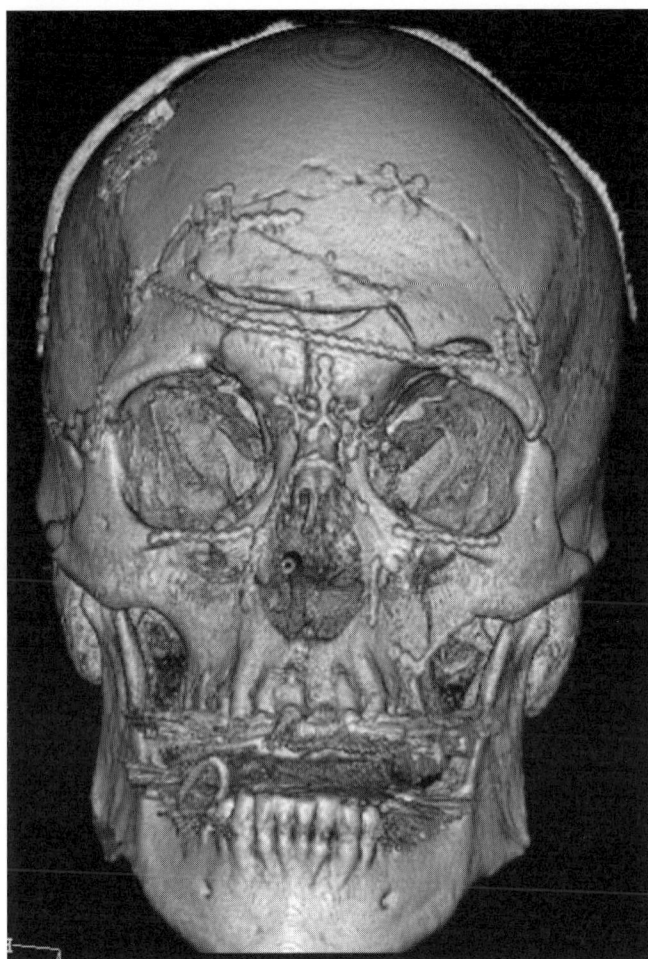

Figure 24.21 Postoperative 3D CT after repair of frontal sinus fracture.

ocular mobility, and orbital volume. Aesthetics are important but secondary to function. Whenever facial structures are injured, treatment must be directed toward maximal rehabilitation of the patient.

The timing of repair for facial fractures is a subject of debate and varies between surgeons. At times, immediate repair is completed in the stable patient, but a delay of 7–10 days may allow edema to decrease and provide easier manipulation of bones and soft tissue during surgical repair. Waiting longer than 14 days is not recommended, because of possible formation of fibrous unions in the fractured segments, making extended delayed repair more difficult if not impossible. Conditions that may warrant delayed repair are hemodynamic instability, increased intracranial pressure (ICP), CSF leaks, Glasgow Coma Scale (GCS) score ≤ 5, evidence of intracranial hemorrhage, midline intracranial shift, and basal cistern effacement on CT.

Surgical reconstruction of the face is based on the concept of the facial skeleton buttress. Facial skeleton buttresses are rigid bony frameworks that absorb and transmit forces applied to the facial skeleton. They prevent the disruption of the facial skeleton until a critical level of stress is reached. Facial buttresses are divided into vertical and horizontal.

- Vertical facial buttresses absorb and transmit the masticatory forceps to the skull; they include lateral piriform, the nasofrontal area, and the zygomaticomaxillary complex.
- Horizontal buttresses include greater palatine bones and frontal bone.

Multiple surgical approaches are often required to achieve the necessary exposure in cases where open reduction and internal fixation is required. Obvious methods of direct access through facial wounds are used whenever possible. Other common routes are coronal, hemicoronal, transconjunctival, subciliary, nasoantral window, labiobuccal, Gillies, and lateral brow incisions. Descriptive details of these approaches are beyond the scope of this chapter. Regardless of the type of facial fracture or the surgical approach used, the initial procedure should be to place the teeth in the proper occlusion and then appropriately reduce the bony fractures.

Although the timing of fracture repair may differ, the goals in the treatment of facial fractures remain the same: function and cosmetic restoration and prevention of early and late complications including malunions, CSF leaks, globe injuries, extraocular muscle entrapment, epiphora, lacrimal injuries, mucocele formation, brain abscess, osteomyelitis, and acute and chronic sinusitis.

Head and neck infections

Head and neck infections are some of the most difficult problems to manage. They may present in conjunction with facial trauma due to contamination, especially with delayed treatment. Infections may range from low-grade, well-localized infections that require only minimal treatment to severe, life-threatening fascial space infections. Maxillofacial surgeons are usually consulted to manage head and neck infections of dental origin. Even with the advent of antibiotics and improved dental health, serious odontogenic infections still sometimes result in death. These deaths occur when the infection reaches areas distant from the dentoalveolar process.

Head and neck infections of odontogenic origin are most commonly part of the indigenous bacteria that are part of the normal oral flora. They are primarily aerobic Gram-positive cocci, anaerobic Gram-positive cocci and anaerobic Gram-negative rods. The majority of these infections are polymicrobial in nature. Antibiotics are used in an adjunctive role in treating patients with odontogenic infections. Surgical treatment remains the primary method of treatment in most patients.

When the infection spreads from the affected teeth it erodes through the cortical plate of the alveolar process. A general rule is that the infection will erode through the thinnest bone. Most odontogenic infections penetrate the bone to become a vestibular (localized) abscess; on occasion they may erode into fascial spaces. Primary fascial spaces include the canine/maxillary, buccal, submandibular, and sublingual spaces.[22] Maxillary odontogentic infections that

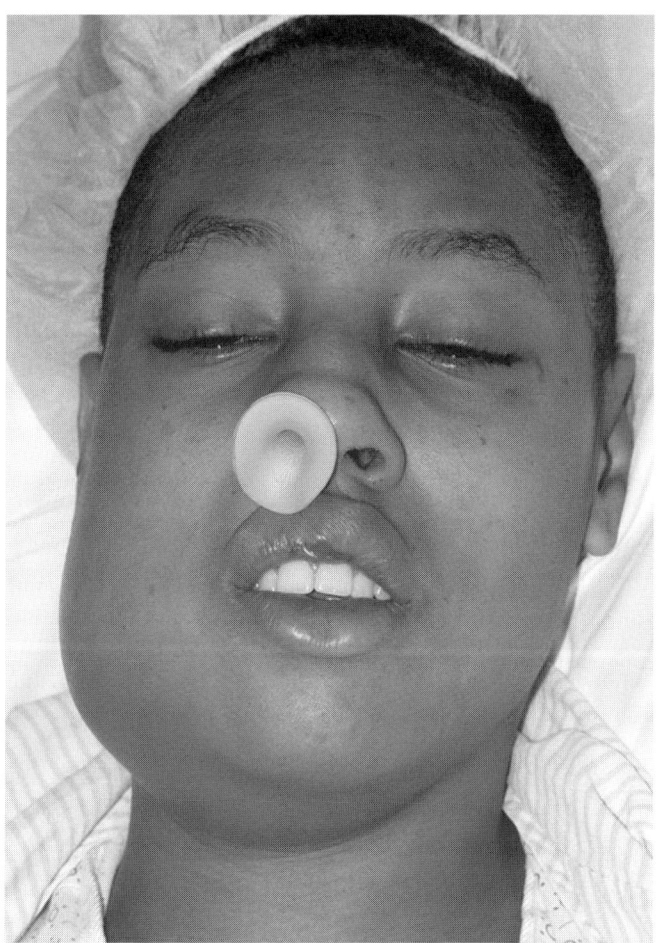

Figure 24.22 Clinical view of patient with Ludwig's angina, with nasal trumpet inserted to assist the airway temporarily. *A black and white version of this figure will appear in some formats. For the color version, please refer to the plate section.*

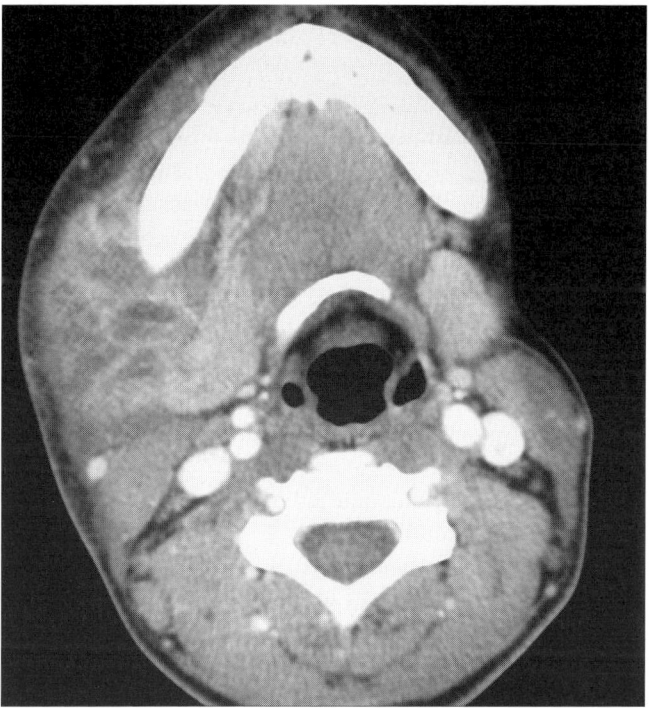

Figure 24.23 Axial CT view of same patient with Ludwig's angina.

spread superiorly can lead to orbital cellulitis or cavernous sinus thrombosis. When bilateral submandibular, sublingual and submental spaces are involved, this is known as *Ludwig's angina*, a life-threatening infection (Figs. 24.22, 24.23). If proper treatment is not received for infections of the primary spaces, the infections may extend posteriorly to involve the secondary fascial spaces. At this point the infections become more severe, causing greater complications and greater morbidity. Infections involving these spaces are very difficult to treat without surgical intervention.[23] Secondary fascial spaces include the masseteric space, pterygomandibular space, and temporal space. Extension beyond the secondary fascial space is rare. However, extension from here leads into the deep cervical spaces. Deep cervical space infections are serious life-threatening infections and require immediate surgical consultation and possible endotracheal intubation. The deep cervical spaces include the lateral pharyngeal space and the retropharyngeal space. Infections in these areas pose the greatest potential complications such as skull-base/brain abscess, upper airway obstruction, aspiration of pus into the lungs and subsequent asphyxiation, and severe infection in the thorax.

The management of infections, whether mild or severe, always has five standard goals: (1) medical support of the patient, (2) treatment with proper antibiotics, (3) surgical removal of the source, (4) surgical drainage with drain placement, and (5) close reevaluation.[24] However, fascial space infections require more extensive and aggressive management. Initial imaging (CT of the face with contrast) will demonstrate the exact extent of the swelling and potential airway compromise, and is invaluable to both the surgeon and the anesthesiologist. However, patients with potential or actual airway compromise should be taken directly to the operating room for definitive airway management rather than wait for imaging. The anesthesiologist must be prepared for emergency airway management. Awake fiberoptic nasotracheal intubation may be urgently required (see Chapter 3). An emergency tracheostomy or cricothyroidotomy set should be available in the operating room, and the surgeon should be present and ready to obtain a surgical airway, if necessary. One review reported that 67% of patients with Ludwig's angina required either anticipatory or emergent intubation.[23]

Summary

Injuries to the oral and maxillofacial region can be complex. These injuries are usually evaluated during the secondary survey unless there are airway difficulties, in which case a surgical airway may be necessary. The oral and maxillofacial surgeon, with expertise in diagnosis and treatment of facial trauma, including fractures of the upper and lower jaws and orbits, facial lacerations, and Le Fort midface fractures, as well as in airway management, has a vital role in trauma management. A multidisciplinary team approach is important for optimal patient outcome following oral and maxillofacial trauma.

Acknowledgments

Clinical photographs courtesy of Dr. Jon P. Bradrick, former Director/Associate Professor of Oral and Maxillofacial Surgery, MetroHealth Medical Center – CASE School of Medicine, Cleveland, Ohio; and Dr. Ketan Parekh, former Chief Resident, Oral and Maxillofacial Surgery, MetroHealth Medical Center – CASE School of Medicine, Cleveland, Ohio.

Questions

(1) What is the best imaging modality for assessing mandible fractures?
   a. Plain film panoramic radiography (panorex or dental orthopantomogram)
   b. Computed tomography
   c. Magnetic resonance imaging
   d. Bone scan

(2) What is the best radiographic imaging modality for assessing maxillary (midface) fractures?
   a. Plain film panoramic radiography (panorex or dental orthopantomogram)
   b. Computed tomography
   c. Magnetic resonance imaging
   d. Bone scan

(3) Which of the following are considered to be ophthalmologic emergencies in association with midface trauma?
   a. Traumatic optic neuropathy
   b. Open globe injury
   c. Retrobulbar hematoma with optic nerve compression
   d. All the above

(4) A 28-year-old female presents with significant facial swelling after dental extractions. You suspect Ludwig's angina. What is the best radiographic imaging modality to assess if there is airway compromise?
   a. Plain film panoramic radiography
   b. Computed tomography with contrast agent
   c. Computed tomography without contrast agent
   d. Magnetic resonance imaging

(5) What sensory nerve distribution deficit would you expect in a Le Fort II fracture?
   a. Maxillary division of the trigeminal (V)
   b. Mandibular division of the trigeminal (V)
   c. Ophthalmic division of the trigeminal (V)
   d. Facial nerve (VII)

(6) What is the incidence of cervical spine injuries associated with facial trauma?
   a. 2.6%
   b. 10%
   c. 26%
   d. 42%

(7) A patient has an uncomplicated mandible fracture with no other injuries, and the maxillofacial surgeon plans to treat this by closed reduction (wire maxilla and mandible closed – MMF). Which of the following would be the preferred route of tracheal intubation?
   a. Oral
   b. Nasal
   c. Emergent cricothyroidotomy
   d. Tracheostomy

(8) What is the most common cause of midface fractures associated with facial trauma in the United States?
   a. Physical assaults
   b. Motor vehicle collisions
   c. Falls
   d. Sports injury

(9) How soon must an avulsed tooth be re-inserted into the dental socket following dental trauma for the best prognosis?
   a. 30 minutes
   b. 45 minutes
   c. 60 minutes
   d. Time is not a factor, a tooth may always be re-inserted

(10) Severe epistaxis may be treated by which of the following?
   a. Nasal packing
   b. Surgical ligation
   c. Embolization
   d. All the above

Answers

(1) a
(2) b
(3) c
(4) b
(5) a
(6) a
(7) b
(8) b
(9) c
(10) d

References

1. Warner ME, Benenfeld SM, Warner MA, Schroeder DR, Maxson PM. Perianesthetic dental injuries: frequency, outcomes, and risk factors. *Anesthesiology* 1999; **90**: 1302–5.

2. Ellis E. Treatment methods for fractures of the mandibular angle. *Int J Oral Maxillofac Surg* 1999; **28**: 243–52.

3. Ellis E, Ghali GE. Lag screw fixation of mandibular angle fractures. *J Oral Maxillofac Surg* 1991; **49**: 234–43.

4. Fonseca RJ, Walker RV. *Oral and Maxillofacial Trauma*. Philadelphia, PA: Saunders, 1991, pp. 359–405.

5. Fonseca RJ, Walker RV. *Oral and Maxillofacial Trauma*. Philadelphia, PA: Saunders, 1991, pp. 576–99.

6. Dolan KD, Jacoby CG. Facial fractures. *Semin Roentgenol* 1978; **13**: 37–51.

7. Dolan KD, Jacoby CG, Smoker WR. The radiology of facial fractures. *Radiographics* 1984; **4**: 575–663.

8. Marciani RD, Anderson GE, Gonty AA. Treatment of mandibular angle fractures: transoral internal wire fixation. *J Oral Maxillofac Surg* 1994; **52**: 752–6.

9. Choung R, Donoff RB, Guralnick WC. A retrospective analysis of 327 mandibular fractures. *J Oral Maxillofac Surg* 1983; **41**: 305–9.

10. Bailey BJ, Prater M. Mandible fractures. *Online Textbook of Otolaryngology*, November 27, 1996.

11. Bailey BJ. *Head and Neck Surgery: Otolaryngology, Mandible Fractures.* Philadelphia, PA; Lippincott, 1998, pp. 977–88.

12. Banks P, Brown A. *Fractures of the Facial Skeleton.* London: Butterworth-Heinemann, 2001, pp. 152–7.

13. Gates GA. *Current Therapy in Otolaryngology: Head and Neck Surgery, Mandible Fracture*, 6th edition. Philadelphia, PA: Mosby, 1998, pp. 150–2.

14. Hoffman WY. Rigid internal fixation vs. traditional techniques for the treatment of mandible fractures. *J Trauma* 1990; **30**: 1032–5.

15. Hall MB. Condylar fractures: surgical management. *J Oral Maxillofac Surg* 1994; **52**: 1189–92.

16. Walker R. Condylar fractures: nonsurgical management. *J Oral Maxillofac Surg* 1994; **52**: 1185–8.

17. James RB, Fredrickson C, Kent JN. Prospective study of mandibular fractures. *J Oral Surg* 1981; **39**: 275–81.

18. Peterson LJ, Ellis E, Hupp JR, Tucker MR. *Contemporary Oral and Maxillofacial Surgery*, 4th edition, St Louis, MO: Mosby. 2003, pp. 343, 509–27.

19. Mathog RH. *Atlas of Craniofacial Trauma.* Philadelphia, PA: Saunders, 1992, pp. 25–119.

20. Muzzi DA. Losasso TJ. Cucchiara RF. Complication from a nasopharyngeal airway in a patient with a basilar skull fracture. *Anesthesiology* 1991; **74**: 366–8.

21. Marlow TJ, Goltra DD, Schabel SI. Intracranial placement of a nasotracheal tube after facial fracture: a rare complication. *J Emerg Med* 1997; **15**: 243–4.

22. Hiatt JL, Gartner LP. *Textbook of Head and Neck Anatomy*, 2nd edition. Baltimore, MD: Williams & Wilkins, 1987, pp. 103–5.

23. Har-El G, Aroesty JH, Shaha A, Lucente FE. Changing trends in deep neck abscesses: a retrospective study of 110 patients. *Oral Surg Oral Med Oral Pathol* 1994; **77**: 446–50.

24. Haug RH, Buchbinder D. Incisions for access to craniomaxillofacial fractures. *Atlas Oral Maxillofac Surg Clin North Am* 1993; **1** (2): 1–29.

Chapter 25

Anesthesia for oral and maxillofacial trauma

Olga Kaslow and Elena J. Holak

Objectives

(1) Comprehend the unique anesthetic challenges related to specific anatomic locations of oral and maxillofacial injury.

(2) Understand acute airway management in patients with maxillofacial trauma.

(3) Describe the Le Fort classification and associated anesthetic implications.

(4) Appreciate the challenges of blunt versus penetrating trauma to the face.

(5) Discuss concomitant injuries associated with maxillofacial trauma occurring as a result of proximity to the traumatized area.

Introduction

Care of the patient with oral and maxillofacial (OMF) injuries presents a unique challenge for the anesthesiologist, as trauma-related anatomic distortions directly involve the airway. Aspiration, hemorrhage, and foreign bodies in the airway may be life-threatening. We will discuss unique challenges facing the practitioner in treating oral and maxillofacial trauma.

Anesthetic challenges related to specific anatomic locations of OMF injury

Facial fractures are frequently associated with damage to the **soft tissues** (skin and gums), and also to the structures and organs within the face (eyes, nerves, salivary glands). **Facial lacerations** need timely surgical repair to achieve good cosmetic results, and this is usually performed under local anesthesia or nerve blocks in the emergency department (ED) (see Chapter 2). **Isolated injury to the teeth and alveolar processes** should be urgently treated by the dentist or oral surgeon, and this may be carried out in an office setting. These interventions do not require an anesthesiologist's expertise.[1]

Missing teeth, crowns, dentures and their parts should be accounted for in a patient with maxillofacial trauma as early as possible to rule out foreign-body aspiration. Advanced Trauma Life Support (ATLS) protocol calls for a detailed assessment of facial injuries only during the secondary survey – a late stage in the evaluation process (see Chapter 2).[2] This delay, in addition to restrictive conditions in the trauma bay, may compromise the value of this evaluation. Although the prevalence of aspiration of teeth and dental prosthesis in patients with maxillofacial trauma is low (0.5% in 10 years), the consequences, especially when misdiagnosed or diagnosed too late, may be grave.[3]

To prevent aspiration, all patients with maxillofacial trauma, both intubated and spontaneously breathing, must be thoroughly examined for the presence of a foreign body: the mouth must be inspected for oral injury, including avulsed or loosely attached teeth, empty alveolar sockets, and missing dental appliances. High vacuum suction followed by thorough oral examination must be performed. Should tracheal intubation be indicated, all dentures and other removable oral devices or loosely attached teeth, crowns, and bridges must be removed prior to direct laryngoscopy.

Foreign bodies in the oral cavity may be either swallowed or lodged, and subsequently pushed into the upper airway and tracheobronchial tree during intubation. While swallowing may be asymptomatic, aspiration produces signs and symptoms that vary according to foreign body size and the level of obstruction.

Laryngeal obstruction with a large foreign body may manifest as choking and gagging, and if the foreign body is not retrieved it may progress to severe hypoxemia with cyanosis. After the object has passed through the vocal cords and into the trachea, an inspiratory stridor and cough is produced. Further advancement of the foreign body into the bronchial tree may lead to development of cough, wheezing, and decreased breath sounds – the most common symptoms of aspiration.

If evidence exists that teeth and dentures have been lost at the scene, a radiographic exam of the oral cavity, chest, and abdomen should be done promptly. Most aspirated foreign bodies can be retrieved from the upper airway using Magill or DeBakey forceps. A foreign body in the lower airway may require the use of a rigid or flexible bronchoscope.[3]

Mandible fractures usually occur in two or more places due to the bone's unique U shape; a second fracture should be suspected until proven otherwise. The stability of the fragments is determined by the directional pool of the muscles of

---

mastication. The strength of the pull is often too strong to be reduced without neuromuscular blockade (need for general anesthesia). Bilateral ("bucket handle") or comminuted fractures of the anterior mandible carry the risk of airway obstruction. Loss of tongue support causes posterior displacement and partial or complete blockage of the airway.

Most mandible fractures are considered open because of damage to the skin or oral mucosa. Antibiotics are therefore required. Current methods of mandible fracture fixation call for mandibular immobilization, typically associated with wiring the jaws for several weeks. Patients may experience significant weight loss without appropriate nutritional support.[1] **Zygomatic arch** and condylar neck fractures may significantly limit jaw opening, leading to difficult or failed intubation using conventional or video laryngoscopy (see Chapter 3). The fragment of the condylar fracture might be superiorly displaced, causing herniation through the roof of the glenoid fossa to the middle cranial fossa, potentially resulting in a dural tear. These injuries are often associated with trauma to the chest and cervical spine (C-spine).[1]

Midface fractures often result in a compromised airway and may necessitate emergent surgical intervention with tracheostomy placement.[4] Epistaxis may be significant and can affect hemodynamic stability. A substantial amount of blood may be swallowed and fill the stomach, inducing vomiting. **Midface fractures** follow specific lines of weakness and have been characterized according to their anatomic location and displacement pattern by René Le Fort in the early twentieth century as follows (see also Chapter 24):

- Le Fort I: horizontal fracture that separates the tooth-bearing part of the maxilla from the rest of the maxilla; does not complicate intubation.
- Le Fort II: pyramidal-shaped fracture separating the maxilla and the nose from the upper lateral midface and zygoma; a high index of suspicion exists for a concomitant fracture of the skull base.
- Le Fort III: midface is separated and frequently displaced posteriorly; it is often associated with fractures of the skull base.

Naso-orbital-ethmoid (NOE) fractures, either isolated or in combination with Le Fort or panfacial fractures, may damage the cribriform plate and sphenoid sinus. In this case, nasal insertion of the endotracheal or gastric tube carries a risk of intracranial penetration. Nasal fiberoptic intubation with oxygen flow through the suction port (sometimes done to improve visualization and oxygenation) might introduce air and contaminated secretions into the fractured skull base.[1] A strong association exists between midface fractures and head and cervical spine injuries.

Anesthetic challenges related to the mechanism of OMF trauma

Understanding the mechanisms of maxillofacial trauma provides insight into appropriate treatment plans, therapy, and expectation of outcome. For example, the mechanism of

trauma, the velocity of the projectile, and tissue penetration all factor into the equation for treatment. These parameters are explored in more detail below.

Blunt trauma occurs most commonly in civilian settings secondary to motor vehicle accidents, falls, and battery. It generally results in less soft tissue damage than penetrating trauma, although frequently associated with C-spine and head injuries. Blunt trauma causes predictable linear fracture patterns in the maxilla and mandible, often with damage to the associated dentition.[5] Facial fractures from blunt trauma result in airway compromise due to posterior displacement of midface structures into the oropharynx, occlusion with the tongue and soft tissue with loss of bony support, and obstruction due to severe swelling and hemorrhage.[6]

Penetrating trauma to the face from projectiles leads to devastating outcomes. Victims may develop rapid airway obstruction and neurovascular compromise, and require complex reconstruction of bone and soft tissue defects (Fig. 25.1).

The extent of damage from ballistic missiles varies depending upon weapon caliber, mass, and velocity. Other factors that influence injury include tissue resistance, range,

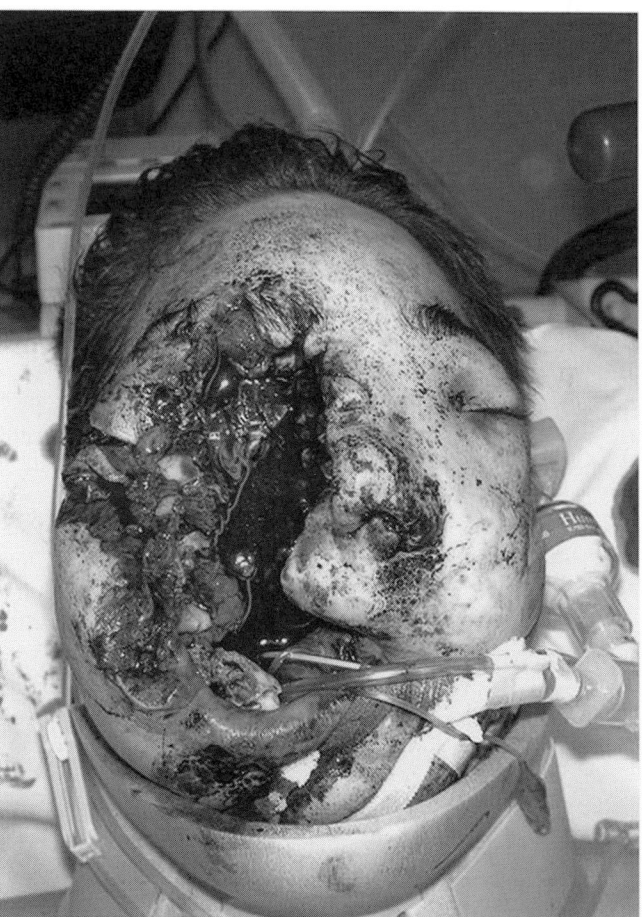

Figure 25.1 Complex panfacial trauma following a self-inflicted gunshot wound to the face with extensive bony and soft tissue injury including orbital and deep sinus cavity involvement. Airway management was quickly and safely initiated by direct laryngoscopy and intubation despite the massive facial wounds. (Courtesy of Jonathan M. Bock, MD, Medical College of Wisconsin.)

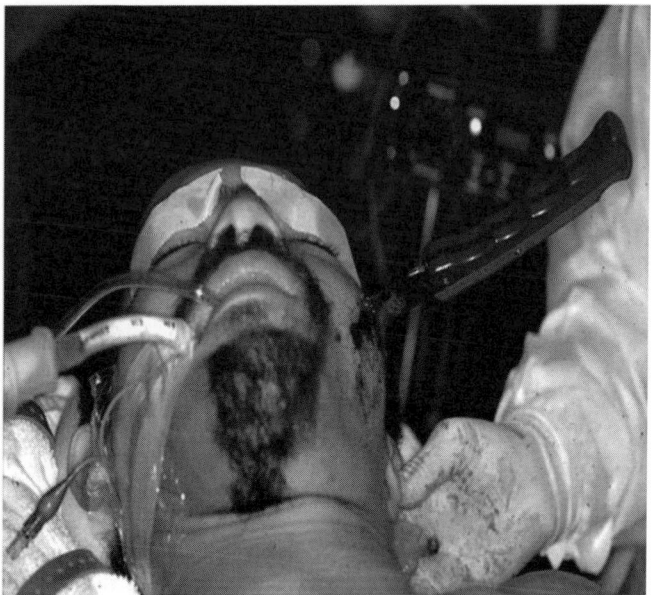

Figure 25.2 Deeply penetrating knife wound to the face with high likelihood of associated great vessel injury. Airway management should minimize manipulation of the penetrating object to prevent massive hemorrhage and possible neurovascular compromise. (Courtesy of Jonathan M. Bock, MD, Medical College of Wisconsin.)

and the specific missile type with its associated ability to fragment, yaw, and tumble.[7]

Velocity is a key determinant of the missile's wounding capability. A twofold increase in velocity means a fourfold increase in energy, with devastating consequences.[8]

The principal mechanisms of injury of low-velocity missiles are laceration and crushing of tissues associated with missile penetration (Fig. 25.2). Additionally, high-velocity missiles produce cavitation and stress effects. Their ability to tumble or yaw creates extensive damage to the surrounding tissues. When traversing the trunk or limb, their high energy is partially absorbed by thick body tissues; however, when such missiles strike the face, with a small muscle mass, significant damage occurs with comminution of the bone and formation of a large explosive exit wound. Thus, airway disruption is significantly more likely after high-velocity injury.

Civilian gunshot injuries to the face are usually of low velocity, and are most often managed at specialized trauma centers in a timely manner. Conversely, **unique characteristics of war injuries** occur due to specific high-velocity missile types, resulting in massive damage to bone and soft tissue. Additionally, delays often occur in the patient's evacuation and medical care (see Chapter 38).[8,9]

Blast injuries may result in unique and complex injury patterns (see Chapter 38). Three mechanisms of injuries due to explosions are described: **primary** blast injuries are caued by the mass movement of air, also known as blast wind. Air-filled structures typically damaged in the maxillofacial area are the ear and paranasal sinuses. **Secondary** blast injury is caused by flying debris, which is responsible for most of the casualties during explosions. **Tertiary** blast injury occurs when victims

are thrown into the air and strike the ground, incurring multiple injuries complicated by gross contamination.[5,8]

Chemical, electrical, or flame burns cause severe obliteration of the airway secondary to tissue edema and soft tissue friability. Immediate airway management is imperative, as the airway will become compromised secondary to ongoing tissue injury and edema.

Anesthetic challenges related to concomitant injuries and multiple trauma

Maxillofacial fractures are associated with a significant number of concomitant injuries occurring as a result of proximity of vital structures to the traumatized area. For example, the brain, cranial nerves, complex bone structure, airway, C-spine, major blood vessels, and salivary glands may also be injured. The force applied to the facial skeleton during trauma disperses and transmits to the cranial vault and C-spine in predictable patterns, causing distinct combinations of head and neck injuries. These injuries must be suspected and investigated in all patients with multiple trauma and associated craniofacial injuries. Knowledge of these concomitant injuries allows the anesthesiologist to develop an appropriate patient care plan and prevent further complications. C-spine injury must be assumed until proven otherwise by clinical examination and radiological studies (see Chapter 3). The anesthetic goals should include C-spine protection during the patient's transfer and airway management, as well as maintaining adequate spinal cord perfusion (see Chapter 23). This is done in an effort to avoid the disastrous sequelae of unrecognized spine injuries.

In order to review the incidence and to establish the association among facial fractures, C-spine injuries, and head injuries, Mulligan *et al.* analyzed the National Trauma Data Bank data on more than 2.7 million reported traumas between 2002 and 2006, and reported that 6.7% of the patients with facial fractures had associated cervical spine injuries, and 67.9% incurred head injury.[10] Of the patients with a facial fracture, 1.5% underwent spinal surgery, and 10.8% required a neurosurgical procedure. In a study of facial fractures and concomitant injuries in trauma patients, cerebral hematoma (e.g., subdural hematoma) was the most frequently observed (43.7%), and pulmonary injury (e.g., lung contusion) was the second most commonly associated injury (31.1%).[11]

The following relationships have been demonstrated between the anatomical location of the facial fracture and both C-spine and intracranial injuries:

- Fractures to the upper face (supraorbital rim, orbital roof, frontal bone, and frontal sinus) are transmitted directly to the intracranial contents, resulting in severe intracranial injuries. A high likelihood of mid- and lower C-spine trauma (C3–C7) occurs, with associated high mortality.
- Bilateral fractures of both the mandible and the midface (nose, maxilla, zygoma, and ethmoids) often results in

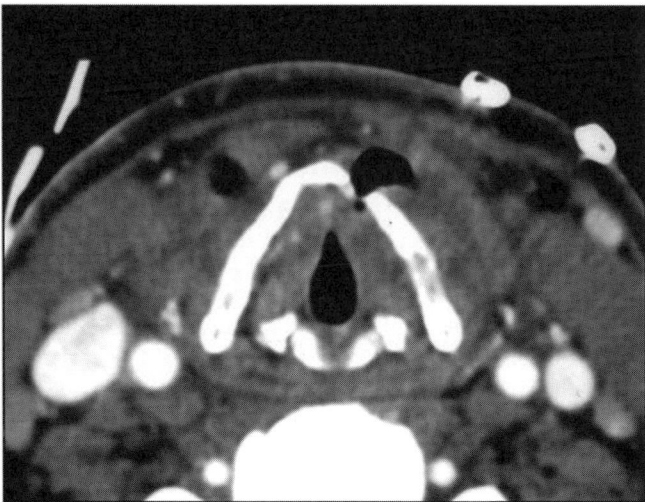

Figure 25.3 Comminuted laryngeal fracture. While rare, direct laryngeal impact can cause fractures and instability of the laryngeal cartilage framework, leading to complications in airway management. Signs of deep cervical emphysema are present, suggesting an open communication or laceration into the endolarynx. Treatment generally proceeds with awake tracheotomy followed by direct microlaryngoscopy for documentation of endolaryngeal injury, followed by laryngeal cartilage framework reconstruction as needed and possible endolaryngeal stent placement. (Courtesy of Jonathan M. Bock, MD, Medical College of Wisconsin.)

dissipation of the applied force, although high-energy impact may result in death.

- Unilateral injuries of the midface are transmitted to the skull base, whereas unilateral mandible trauma is transmitted to the upper C-spine (C1–C2), causing concomitant injuries.[12]

Maxillofacial trauma may also present in combination with **laryngotracheal injuries**. The most common mechanism is blunt trauma due to motor vehicle collisions or sports accidents, and penetrating wounds from gunshots and stabbings. This type of trauma may result in fractures of the hyoid bones and thyroid and cricoid cartilages, with separation of cricoid cartilage from the larynx and the trachea (Fig. 25.3). Laryngeal and tracheal injuries may be underrecognized; therefore, it is imperative for all members of a trauma team to be vigilant for signs and symptoms of these injuries in order to perform rapid airway intervention. Common signs of laryngotracheal trauma include stridor, subcutaneous emphysema, neck hematoma and ecchymosis, hemoptysis, laryngeal tenderness, and voice changes. Laryngotracheal trauma may also be associated with C-spine, esophageal, and vascular injuries.[13]

Preoperative assessment

Assessment and manipulation of the damaged airway with severe distortion of anatomical landmarks, complicated by hemorrhage and tissue edema, presents a serious challenge for the anesthesiologist. In an airway emergency occurring in a patient with facial trauma, airway evaluation should be performed promptly, often simultaneously with the salvage maneuvers. However, if time allows, airway assessment should be thorough and include all available pertinent information and data (see Chapter 3).

The mechanism of injury is usually obtained from first responders, and occasionally from a responsive patient. Results of the primary and secondary surveys allow estimation of the complete burden of injury and whether there are changes in a patient's condition. For example, if neurological assessment reveals an altered level of consciousness, lateralizing neurologic symptoms, paralysis, asymmetric pupillary size, irregular breathing pattern, and clinical signs of raised intracranial pressure (ICP), immediate establishment of a definitive airway is warranted, utilizing agents and techniques that are safe for both maintaining hemodynamic stability and decreasing the ICP (see Chapter 21).

Thorough airway assessment should be performed without delay, since the rapid development of facial edema may quickly obstruct the upper airway. The need to protect the C-spine during airway assessment may interfere with the examination: the rigid C-collar restricts mouth opening and reduces visualization of both the oral cavity and the patient's neck. Eliciting an appropriate verbal response from the patient assures preserved level of conscience and intact vocal cords. Direct examination of the airway is absolutely necessary and should include inspection of the mouth and pharynx for foreign bodies and bleeding. Airway assessment should include evaluation of facial and neck deformity, swelling, neck motion; dental injury, nasal patency, mouth opening, and a Mallampati score (see Chapter 3).

Preliminary or finalized radiological results, including chest x-ray, spine evaluation, and head computed tomography (CT), are of paramount importance to the anesthesiologist in predicting the level of airway difficulty and helping to develop an appropriate plan.[14,15]

Airway obstruction in a patient with maxillofacial trauma results from multiple factors, with the most common materials being blood, secretions, and vomitus (Table 25.1). An awake patient may swallow blood and secretions; however, the swallowing process may be painful and difficult in a patient with a midface or mandible fracture. Swallowing may be impossible in a patient who is intoxicated or unconscious. Swallowed blood accumulates in the stomach, predisposing to nausea and vomiting. Suctioning the mouth should be done with caution to avoid gagging and vomiting.

Comminuted anterior mandible fractures create significant soft tissue swelling and bleeding, with bilateral ("bucket handle") fractures resulting in loss of tongue support. High-impact midface fractures may lead to crumpling displacement of the bony fragments backwards and downwards, causing gross soft tissue swelling extending into the pharynx. Posterior pharyngeal hematoma secondary to C-spine fracture may precipitate airway obstruction as well. Tissue swelling and hematoma with airway compromise may also occur after seemingly minor trauma in the anticoagulated patient (e.g., warfarin).

Trauma to the anterior neck may present with bruising, swelling, and subcutaneous emphysema. These physical findings are suggestive of laryngeal and tracheal injury. Stridor, coarse voice and hemoptysis are ominous signs for impending airway obstruction.[14,16]

Close attention must be paid to the patient's request or attempt to sit up. This may indicate an early sign of airway compromise due to partial obstruction from swelling, bleeding, or loss of tongue support. Sitting and leaning forward allows passive drainage of oral and nasal secretions and blood and relieves the posterior tongue's displacement following a comminuted mandible fracture. Potential spinal injury should be ruled out before allowing the patient to sit; a hard cervical collar should be worn and the head carefully supported to reduce axial load. When the sitting position is contraindicated because of head, spine, pelvic, or extensive extremity trauma, tracheal intubation may be necessary.[17,18]

A high index of suspicion for **impending airway compromise should be maintained**. Frequent reassessment is mandatory in order to detect changes such as declining level of consciousness, vomiting, or development of shock.

Table 25.1 Factors contributing to airway obstruction in maxillofacial trauma.

Foreign bodies	Blood and secretions accumulated in the pharynx of a supine patient who is unable to swallow Teeth, dentures, loose crowns Vomitus, food particles
Displaced facial bone fragments	Posterior displacement of midface structures into the oropharynx Bilateral mandibular fracture with loss of tongue support
Soft tissue swelling	Face, tongue, and neck tissue swelling develop within a few hours after injury
Cervical spine injury	Retropharyngeal hematoma due to cervical spine fracture contributes to airway collapse and complicates visualization of the larynx during intubation Hard collar and manual in-line stabilization make airway evaluation difficult and limit visualization during laryngoscopy
Neck trauma	Hyoid bone fractures, trauma to laryngeal cartilages and trachea lead to significant swelling and airway distortion Injury to the jugular vein and carotid artery leads to formation of expanding hematoma
Inability to swallow and clear secretions	Due to pain, swelling, and impaired level of consciousness
Impaired level of consciousness	Traumatic brain injury, shock, and/or intoxication cause loss of protective airway reflexes

Symptoms such as cyanosis, dysphonia, agitation, dyspnea, and accessory muscle recruitment usually indicate urgent or emergent requirement for a definitive airway.

Acute airway management in a patient with maxillofacial trauma (see also Chapters 2 and 3)

Initial evaluation and management of the trauma patients follows the ABCDE sequence of the Advanced Trauma Life Support (ATLS) protocol:[2]

- Airway maintenance with C-spine protection
- Breathing and ventilation
- Circulation with hemorrhage control
- Disability: neurologic status
- Exposure/environmental control

The airway in the patient with maxillofacial trauma is of primary concern and often presents as a true emergency (Fig. 25.4).

Absolute indications for immediate airway control include apnea, respiratory distress due to unrelieved airway obstruction, altered consciousness, and pronounced neurologic deficit. **Urgent indications** include penetrating neck trauma, chest injury with respiratory compromise, persistent hypotension, nonresponsive to resuscitation, and altered mental status. **Relative indications** include impending respiratory failure,

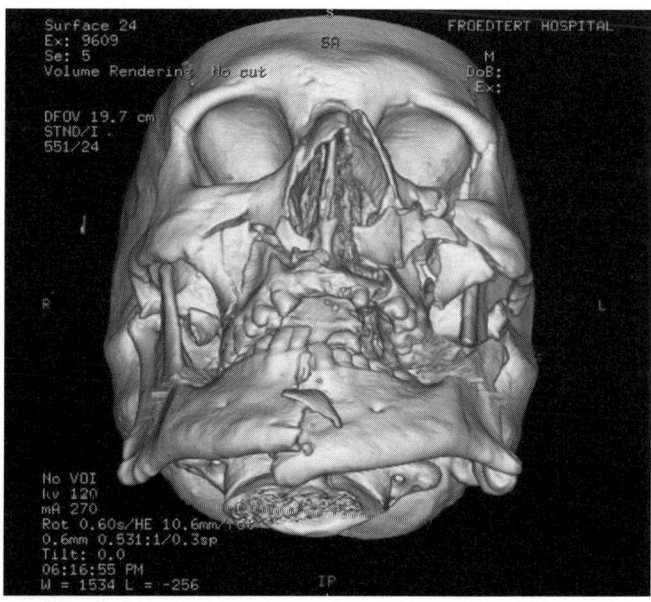

Figure 25.4 Three-dimensional CT reconstruction of complex panfacial bony trauma, demonstrating comminuted zygomatic, naso-orbital, and maxillary fractures on the left as well as an unstable anterior mandible fracture. Airway management for patients with unstable mandible fractures often requires awake tracheotomy, as mandible instability may not allow for appropriate laryngeal exposure on laryngoscopy, and endotracheal tube presence can interfere with rigid fixation techniques such as maxillomandibular fixation (MMF). (Courtesy of Jonathan M. Bock, MD, Medical College of Wisconsin.)

risk of airway deterioration with diagnostic procedures and sedation and analgesia.[6]

The anesthesiologist must have a clear plan of action before attempting to intubate the trachea in the patient with facial trauma (see Chapter 3). **Preparation** to deal with the "difficult airway" and **a backup plan**, including the ability to rapidly perform a surgical airway, are of paramount importance.

One must ensure immediate **availability of adequate equipment and experienced assistance**. High-flow oxygen must be provided with pulse oximeter monitoring. High-volume suction should be in working condition. A bag-mask and a ventilator should be prepared. Both intubating equipment (laryngoscopes, different types of blades, video-assisted intubating devices (e.g., GlideScope), and the airway maintenance adjuncts (oral airway, bougie, laryngeal mask airways [LMA], laryngeal tube airway [LTA]) must be ready to use. A cricothyroidotomy kit should be available in the event of failure to intubate.

C-spine precautions: after high-velocity craniofacial trauma, C-spine injury must be assumed until proven otherwise. C-spine protection is provided by applying a fitted hard collar and immobilizing the patient on a backboard. The C-collar limits an optimal access to the airway, face, and neck. An incorrectly applied collar may aggravate airway compromise and elevate ICP by decreasing venous return from the head and neck.

Airway maintenance maneuvers

Maintaining an open airway can often be achieved with simple methods: clearing the mouth of secretions and debris and applying traction to the mandible by performing a **chin lift and jaw thrust.** Bilateral mandibular ("bucket handle") fractures may cause the tongue to lose support and fall back, thus occluding the airway. Manual reduction of a posteriorly displaced mandibular fragment may be performed by grasping and pulling the mandible along with the tongue in a forward motion to relieve airway obstruction. These maneuvers should be performed with caution, to prevent any movement of the C-spine.

Oral airways are not tolerated by awake patients as they provoke gagging and precipitate vomiting. **Nasal airways** are better tolerated, although epistaxis may result, presenting a potential problem in midface trauma with suspected anterior skull base fracture.

Adequate **preoxygenation is difficult** to achieve in an unconscious patient. **Bag-mask ventilation** may be attempted, but difficulties may arise. Extreme caution must be exercised to prevent harming the patient with facial injuries, as an adequate mask seal is difficult to attain. The pressure applied by the face mask may further displace the facial bone fragments, therefore worsening the airway obstruction, potentially forcing the air into subdural space.

Methods of tracheal intubation depend on several factors including the patient's overall condition, the degree of urgency, and the extent of maxillofacial damage. A choice must be made between **awake and asleep intubation techniques.** Conscious patients are usually able to control their airway, but this is not the case with uncooperative and unresponsive patients. If difficult laryngoscopy is anticipated in a cooperative spontaneously breathing patient, an awake intubation should be planned.[5,15–20]

For awake intubation, the airway mucosa is topically anesthetized with local anesthetic agents. The authors prefer 4% lidocaine (maximum dose of 3–4 mg/kg) administered via nebulizer or atomizer. Although glossopharyngeal and superior laryngeal nerve blocks may provide excellent conditions for an awake intubation, they are impractical in a patient with maxillofacial trauma because good mouth opening and neck movement are required to perform these blocks. Sedation may be achieved with dexmedetomidine infusion (0.2–0.7 µg/kg/h), remifentanyl, or small boluses of ketamine, midazolam, or alfentanil. Intubation is generally accomplished with laryngoscopy (conventional, video-assisted) or fiberoptic bronchoscopy depending on skills, judgment, and experience of the clinician and availability of equipment.

Route of intubation: nasal versus oral versus surgical airway

The role and safety of nasotracheal intubation in a patient with oral and maxillofacial trauma has been debated in anesthesiology literature for many years. Controversial points include: management of patients with a skull base fracture; emergent intubation when no radiologic studies are available to evaluate the extent of maxillofacial and cranial injury; and the risks of a blind intubation technique.

Current literature reports a few anecdotal cases of inadvertent intracranial placement of a nasal endotracheal tube (ETT). At the same time, intracranial placement of a nasogastric tube (NGT) has been reported more often, perhaps because of the smaller diameter of the NGT and a lack of control in directing its insertion compared to the ETT. Thirty-eight cases of intracranial placement of NGT are reported in the literature.[21] The most common entry site was the cribriform plate, and less commonly the sphenoid sinus. Both of these anatomic structures lie within the midline of the central anterior skull base. Fractures located in this area are very serious in nature, as brain penetration commonly occurs. Conversely, skull base fractures located laterally and posteriorly are not considered hazardous for intracranial penetration.

When placement of the gastric tube is indicated, an oral route is the preferred choice in a patient with maxillofacial trauma. The consequences of inadvertent intracranial NGT placement are catastrophic, with a high mortality rate. If a gastric tube needs to be placed nasally, the integrity of the skull base should be confirmed both clinically and radiographically.[22]

Goodison *et al.* proposed a guideline for airway management in patients with maxillofacial trauma complicated by skull base fracture in both acute and elective settings.[23] For definitive repair, a head CT scan with slices 3 mm or less should be performed. If CT is diagnostic of anterior central skull base fracture, then awake or asleep fiberoptic nasal intubation may be safely attempted, allowing clear visualization of the nasopharynx and the vocal cords.

In situations of emergent tracheal intubation or in patients not stable enough to undergo CT, the presence of common symptoms and signs consistent with basilar skull fracture should be considered: periorbital ecchymosis or "raccoon eyes," retroauricular ecchymosis or "Battle's sign," cerebrospinal fluid leak, and facial nerve palsy; however, the absence of these signs does not rule out skull base fracture.

Nasal fiberoptic intubation in an emergent setting commonly does not provide for controlled and well-prepared conditions compared to an elective setting. For example, deteriorating mental status and inability to cooperate may preclude the use of sedation and adequate topical anesthesia. Blind nasal intubation may lead to contamination of intracranial contents, with devastating consequences, and is not recommended.

Definitive airway management
Endotracheal intubation

Rapid sequence induction (RSI) with cricoid pressure and manual in-line cervical immobilization is the technique of choice in patients with adequate mouth opening. However, direct laryngoscopy may fail in a patient with extensive maxillofacial trauma. Visualization of the vocal cords may be limited by accumulation of blood, secretion, edema, and anatomic distortion. Attempts to open the mouth to insert the blade may fail as well. Awake patients with bilateral temporomandibular joint (TMJ) fractures present with restricted mouth opening due to pain or trismus. However, it should not be assumed that limited mouth opening will improve after induction of anesthesia and neuromuscular blockade.

Choice of instrumentation

Various video-laryngoscopes (e.g., Glidescope, C-MAC), fiberoptic bronchoscope (FOB), Bullard laryngoscope, or lighted stylet may be utilized, depending upon availability of equipment and the expertise of the anesthesiologist (see Chapter 3).

The FOB is a useful instrument in experienced hands for awake intubation in cooperative, spontaneously breathing patients with topically anesthetized airways. However, it has limited use for emergent intubation. Poor visualization of both the oral and nasal airways obscured with blood, secretions, swelling, and tissue disruption may cause the fiberoptic approach to be difficult or impossible.

An **intubating lighted stylet (light wand)** is another useful tool in the hands of skilled providers. A lighted oral approach is utilized to secure the airway when direct visualization is not possible and mouth opening is limited.

Supraglottic airway devices

The laryngeal mask airway (**LMA**) is a helpful adjunct, especially when direct laryngoscopy fails. Rapid insertion of an LMA can provide sufficient oxygenation and ventilation to the patient. However, it is not a definitive airway and does not provide protection from aspiration of gastric contents (see Chapter 3). The LMA can also be used as a conduit for tracheal intubation over a fiberoptic bronchoscope. LMAs should be avoided in the presence of an implanted oral foreign body or distorted intraoral anatomy. The LMA will be difficult to place in patients with limited mouth opening.

Surgical airway (cricothyroidotomy and tracheotomy) is usually the last step in the difficult airway algorithm for securing an airway with maxillofacial trauma (see Chapter 3). It is needed when intubation and ventilation by other means prove difficult or impossible, as in the case of upper airway obstruction, extensive facial edema and deformity, and failed nasal or orotracheal intubation. It is prudent to have an experienced surgeon immediately available during airway management, since both **cricothyroidotomy** and **tracheotomy** may pose problems in patients with severe edema and anatomic distortions of the face and neck.[14,20]

Cricothyroidotomy is less time-consuming, is associated with fewer complications, and can be later converted to a definitive tracheotomy once the patient is stabilized. Tracheal cannulation through the cricothyroid membrane followed by jet ventilation may be life-saving during difficult airway situations. Care should be taken to avoid barotrauma.

An awake tracheostomy under local anesthesia may be indicated in an otherwise cooperative patient who is not in respiratory distress. Awake tracheostomy is also preferred for patients with existing or suspected laryngeal injuries, since conventional laryngoscopy and orotracheal intubation may disrupt laryngeal structures, create a "false passage," or facilitate laryngotracheal separation. In stable patients, flexible fiberoptic nasolaryngoscopy may be performed to examine the extent of injury.[12]

Bleeding from maxillofacial injuries

Maxillofacial injuries alone are unlikely to be the cause of hemorrhagic shock. Most injuries result in minor slow venous bleeding from the nose or mouth which can be controlled with conventional measures. The incidence of life-threatening hemorrhage from facial fractures occurs in approximately 1.2% of cases.[24] Profuse bleeding from panfacial fractures is often difficult to stop, because of the complex vascularization of the OMF region. Control of bleeding improves airway patency and may be achieved with "damage control" maneuvers such as:

- rapid manual reduction and stabilization of displaced bone fragments
- tight packing of the oral cavity with abdominal swabs; in certain circumstances nasal packing may also be necessary
- occlusion with nasal balloons or Foley catheters

When packing and fracture reduction is ineffective in controlling hemorrhage, angiographic embolization in the interventional radiology suite may become necessary (see Chapter 11). Angiography should also be considered when clinical diagnosis is unreliable and surgical access is technically difficult. Other techniques to consider are emergent intermaxillary fixation, transcatheter arterial embolization, and surgical ligation of the external carotid and its branches.[24,25]

Bleeding may not be apparent if a patient is unable to clear oral secretions due to pain or altered sensorium. Blood and saliva that accumulate in the oropharynx may cause airway obstruction, obscuring visualization of the vocal cords during intubation. Additionally, aspiration may occur in an unconscious patient, as blood is often swallowed in a supine position, thus predisposing to vomiting and subsequent aspiration.

Anesthetic management of elective OMF repair

The timing of surgical repair of maxillofacial trauma depends upon the extent and severity of associated injuries (see Chapter 24). In patients with multiple trauma, life-, sight-, and limb-threatening injuries are addressed first. In stable patients with contaminated facial wounds, surgery is required within a few hours.

Surgical management of facial gunshot wounds consists of three phases and often requires multiple operations:

(1) debridement, fracture stabilization, and primary closure
(2) hard tissue reconstruction if soft tissue coverage is adequate
(3) rehabilitation of the oral vestibule and alveolar ridge, and secondary correction of residual deformities[7]

Current practice advocates treating ballistic wounds to the face in otherwise stable patients early and in one stage. The surgery includes exposure of the displaced bony fragments with immediate stabilization by rigid fixation, and bone grafting is performed if necessary. Soft tissue injuries are repaired simultaneously and with primary closure.[9]

Definitive repair of maxillofacial injuries in a severely injured patient may be deferred until the patient's overall condition is stable, pertinent clinical evaluations and imaging studies are completed, and the facial edema is resolved, allowing easier manipulation of bone fragments and soft tissue (see Chapter 24). Mandibular fractures are usually repaired within 24–48 hours, other facial fractures within 7–14 days. After 10–14 days, fractures are more difficult to reduce correctly. Reestablishing proper dental occlusion is usually achieved first, followed by reduction of the other bony fractures. The ultimate goal of surgical repair is to restore nasal function, mastication, orbital integrity, and ocular position and mobility.

Since the airway is shared between the surgeon and the anesthesiologist, the decision on appropriate placement of the ETT should be made and agreed upon by both clinicians. The type of airway management for elective maxillofacial repair depends on many factors including neurologic injuries, hemodynamic and respiratory status, and the need for prolonged mechanical ventilation.

Oral intubation, commonly used for obtaining emergent airway access, is undesirable for elective cases for several reasons. Firstly, an orally placed ETT interferes with surgical access to the oral cavity and precludes occlusion of the teeth, an essential requirement for intramaxillary and maxillomandibular fixation. Secondly, oral intubation may be complicated by residual airway swelling and deformity, as well as limited mouth opening.[26]

The nasal route for **intubation** would interfere neither with the surgical approach to the oral cavity nor with achieving dental occlusion. It is advocated for patients with limited mouth opening and for those who do not require nasal surgery. It is contraindicated in patients with nasal trauma and bleeding disorders. Side effects of nasotracheal intubation include infection, epistaxis, sinusitis, otitis media, and nasal injury.[26]

Tracheostomy is frequently performed for facilitation of elective maxillofacial repair, and in patients with comminuted spine and head injuries requiring multiple surgeries. Tracheostomy allows repeated and safe airway access. Compared with endotracheal intubation, tracheostomy is more comfortable for the patient, and allows for suctioning of secretions and easy re-insertion in the case of accidental decannulation. Tracheostomy requires a qualified surgeon, and the procedure may be time-consuming, especially in patients with unfavorable anatomy. Tracheostomy necessitates special care postoperatively, is expensive, and may cause complications. Early complications include bleeding, pneumothorax, subcutaneous emphysema, and laryngeal nerve injury. Delayed complications include wound and respiratory infection, scarring, subglottic tracheal stenosis, tracheomalacia, and the formation of tracheoesophageal, trachoinnominate, and tracheocutaneous fistulas.[4,26]

Retromolar intubation was first documented by Bonfils in 1983.[27] After performing a standard oral intubation, the ETT is moved to the space between the back of the last molar and the anterior portion of the ascending mandibular ramus, or the missing tooth space. The surgeon then secures the tube with sutures to the molar. If coexisting tooth loss exists, the tube may be sutured to the selected tooth on the maxillary side. This intubation method has been advocated for patients who need simultaneous nasal surgery and restoration of dental occlusion (e.g., fractures of zygoma and maxilla as well as Le Fort II fractures).[28] This technique is noninvasive, fast, and easy to perform. The trachea of patients with difficult airway anatomy and limited mouth opening may be intubated through their retromolar space with the fiberoptic bronchoscope. The limiting factor is the size of the retromolar space. Because the retromolar space becomes smaller with age and eruption of molars, it may be inadequate to accommodate the ETT in some adults. Smaller ETTs (6.5 Fr and 7.0 Fr) have been recommended for female and male patients, respectively.[28]

The retromolar space can be enlarged by osteotomy, although this procedure might result in permanent bone damage. The patency of this space should be confirmed preoperatively by placing the patient's index finger in the space, followed by occlusion of the teeth. Intraoperatively, it is essential to monitor airway pressures and tidal volume during the period of dental occlusion, which can occlude the ETT. Complications associated with retromolar intubation include oral mucosal trauma and long buccal nerve palsy.[26]

Submental intubation (intubation through the floor of the mouth in the submental area) may be done in patients with complex craniofacial, nasal, and maxillary injuries, especially when oral and nasal intubation are inappropriate.[29,30] This method of securing the airway is advocated for patients who do not require prolonged ventilation and airway protection, and it permits avoidance of tracheostomy. The procedure is done after induction of general anesthesia and orotracheal intubation. The proximal end of the ETT (regular or reinforced tube) is passed through a surgical incision in the floor of the mouth and secured to the skin with sutures. There is a risk of accidental extubation during tube advancement through the submental region. If proximal tube retrieval and its connection to the breathing circuit are delayed, life-threatening hypoxia may ensue.

Although submental intubation is technically simple and fast, and allows for dental occlusion and better cosmesis, it should not be considered for patients with laryngotracheal disruption, gunshot facial trauma, and for those who need prolonged mechanical ventilation. Contraindications include local tissue infection, bleeding disorders, and predisposition to keloid formation. The anesthesiologist needs to be aware that surgical maneuvers resulting in compression or kinking of the submentally positioned ETT result in increased airway pressure and decreased tidal volume. Suctioning of the oral cavity and insertion of an orogastric tube might present some difficulties. Postoperatively, submental intubation may be complicated by airway edema, hematoma, infection, and injury to the submandibular and sublingual glands.[26]

Summary

Maxillofacial trauma presents a variety of unique challenges in airway management, as airway structures are frequently compromised, with distortion of anatomical landmarks. This requires immediate assessment of damaged structures and securing a pathway for alveolar ventilation. Blunt versus penetrating trauma, as well as soft tissue injury, must be taken into account. Concomitant injuries occurring as a result of proximity to traumatized maxillofacial structures have to be evaluated. A clear plan of action must be in place for tracheal intubation, with a back-up plan which may include a surgical airway. Maxillofacial injuries can indeed create the most difficult airway scenarios faced by the clinician. The successful management of these complex patients requires appropriate skills, quick decision making, and efficient communication.

Acknowledgments

The authors are grateful to Dr. Jonathan M. Bock, Assistant Professor, Division of Laryngology & Professional Voice, Department of Otolaryngology & Communication Sciences, Medical College of Wisconsin, for providing figures and figure legends.

Questions

(1) **An inebriated patient presents to the trauma bay with facial injuries, swelling, and bruising. He requests to sit up. The appropriate response is to:**
   a. Deny the request: the patient should be sedated and restrained
   b. Deny the request: the patient is drunk and incapable of making decisions
   c. Administer IV sedation and allow the patient to sit up
   d. Place a rigid cervical collar and allow the patient to sit up with the head and neck carefully supported. Attempt to rule out a spinal cord injury

(2) **Concerning bag-mask ventilation (BMV) in an unconscious but breathing patient with facial trauma:**
   a. BMV should always be performed to adequately preoxygenate before intubation
   b. Obtaining an adequate mask seal is relatively easy in patients with facial trauma.
   c. BMV may displace facial bone fragments, worsen airway obstruction, and introduce air into the subdural space
   d. BMV is always contraindicated, because of the risk of a full stomach

(3) **Which maxillofacial trauma patient has a reasonable indication for submental intubation?**
   a. The patient requiring emergent intubation for airway obstruction
   b. The patient presenting for elective repair of Le Fort II/III fractures without a need for prolonged mechanical ventilation
   c. The patient scheduled for elective repair of multiple facial fractures requiring prolonged mechanical ventilation
   d. The patient with laryngotracheal disruption

(4) **An unconscious patient with facial trauma presents with multiple loose and broken teeth. At what point during the patient's care should loose and broken teeth be accounted for and retrieved?**
   a. After the primary and secondary ATLS survey and after complete stabilization of the patient's vital signs
   b. Never
   c. After full recovery from life-threatening injuries
   d. Loosely attached and broken teeth should be removed if intubation is indicated, followed by thorough oral examination and vacuum suction

(5) Fiberoptic bronchoscopic intubation in a patient with maxillofacial trauma:

    a. Is best used for awake cooperative patients after topicalization of the airway

    b. Is best utilized for emergent intubation

    c. Is a valuable intubation tool for nasal intubation in patients with epistaxis

    d. Is safer than a surgical airway for patients with massive facial trauma with soft tissue disruption

(6) Regarding the nasal approach to intubation in a patient with maxillofacial trauma:

    a. It is best performed using a blind technique

    b. It should never be performed in the presence of Le Fort fractures

    c. Nasotracheal intubation is acceptable when performed with fiberoptic bronchoscopy in patients with Le Fort II/III fractures, provided that the cribriform plate is intact and the fractures do not cross the midline

    d. Only a gastric tube should be placed nasally; oral placement of the endotracheal tube is preferred

(7) True or false? Midface fractures are associated with neck and C-spine injuries.

(8) The extent of damage from ballistic missiles varies depending on all of the following, *except*:

    a. weapon caliber

    b. mass

    c. bone density

    d. velocity

(9) Which of the following is an absolute indication for airway control in a trauma patient?

    a. Severe neurologic deficit with impaired ventilation

    b. Mild stridor

    c. Moderate shortness of breath

    d. Wheezing

(10) A supraglottic airway (e.g., LMA) provides:

    a. A definitive airway

    b. Sufficient oxygenation but inadequate ventilation

    c. A protected airway

    d. A conduit for tracheal intubation utilizing a fiberoptic bronchoscope

Answers

(1) d
(2) c
(3) b
(4) d
(5) a
(6) c
(7) True
(8) c
(9) a
(10) d

References

1. Parekh K, Ash C. Oral and maxillofacial trauma. In Smith C, ed., *Trauma Anesthesia*. Cambridge: Cambridge University Press, 2008; pp. 417–30.

2. American College of Surgeons Committee on Trauma. *ATLS: Advanced Trauma Life Support For Doctors*, 8th edition. Chicago, IL: ACS, 2008.

3. Casap N, Alterman M, Lieberman S, Zeltser R. Enigma of missing teeth in maxillofacial trauma. *J Oral Maxillofac Surg* 2011; **69**: 1421–9.

4. Holmgren E, Bagheri S, Bell RB, Bobek S, Dierks EJ. Utilization of tracheostomy in craniomaxillofacial trauma at a level-1 trauma center. *J Oral Maxillofac Surg* 2007; **65**: 2005–10.

5. Gibbons AJ, Patton DW. Ballistic injuries of the face and mouth in war and civil conflict. *Dent Update* 2003; **30**: 272–8.

6. Mohan R, Iyer R, Thaller S. Airway management in patients with facial trauma. *J Craniofacial Surg* 2009; **20**: 21–3.

7. Glapa M, Kourie J, Doll D, Degiannis E. Early management of gunshot injuries to the face in civilian practice. *World J Surg* 2007; **31**: 2104–10.

8. Kummoona R, Muna AM. Evaluation of immediate phase of management of missile injuries affecting maxillofacial region in Iraq. *J Craniofacial Surg* 2006; **17**: 217–23.

9. Motamedi MH. Primary treatment of penetrating injuries to the face. *J Oral Maxillofac Surg* 2007; **65**: 1215–18.

10. Mulligan RP, Friedman JA, Mahabir RC. A nationwide review of the associations among cervical spine injuries, head injuries, and facial fractures. *J Trauma* 2010; **68**: 587–92.

11. Alvi A, Dogherty T, Lewen G. Facial fractures and concomitant injuries in trauma patients. *Laryngoscope* 2003; **113**: 102–6.

12. Mithani SK, St.-Hilaire HM, Brooke BS, *et al.* Predictable patterns of intracranial and cervical spine injury in craniomaxillofacial trauma: analysis of 4786 patients. *Plast Reconstr Surg* 2009; **123**: 1293–301.

13. Verschueren DS, Bell RB, Bagheri SC, Dierks EJ, Potter BE. Management of laryngo-tracheal injuries associated with craniomaxillofacial trauma. *J Oral Maxillofac Surg* 2006; **64**: 203–14.

14. Kaslow O, Gollapudy S. Anesthetic considerations for ocular and maxillofacial trauma. In Varon AJ, Smith C, eds., *Essentials of Trauma Anesthesia*. Cambridge: Cambridge University Press, 2012, pp. 198–208.

15. Perry M. Maxillofacial trauma: developments, innovations and controversies. *Injury* 2009; **49**: 1252–9.

16. Chesshire NJ, Knight D. The anaesthetic management of facial trauma and fractures. *BJA CEPD Rev* 2001; **1**: 108–12.

17. Perry M, Dancey A, Mireskandari K, *et al.* Emergency care in facial trauma-a maxillofacial and ophthalmic perspective. *Injury* 2005; **36**: 875–96.

18. Perry M, Morris C. Advanced trauma life support (ATLS) and facial trauma: can one size fit all? Part 2: ATLS, maxillofacial injuries and airway management dilemmas. *Int J Oral Maxillofac Surg* 2008; **37**: 309–20.

19. Bramhall J. Anesthesia for maxillofacial trauma. [lecture online] 2004. http://faculty.washington.edu/bramhall/lectures/trauma/max.html (accessed September 2014).

20. Curran JE. Anaesthesia for facial trauma. *Anaesth Intensive Care Med* 2008; **9**: 338–43.

21. Psarras K, Lalountas MA, Symeonidis NG, *et al*. Inadvertent insertion of a nasogastric tube into the brain: case report and review of literature. *Clin imaging* 2012; **36**: 587–90.

22. Genu PR, de Oliveira DM, Vasconcellos RJ, Nogueira RV, Vasconcelos BC. Inadvertent intracranial placement of a nasogastric tube in a patient with severe craniofacial trauma: a case report. *J Oral Maxillofac Surg* 2005; **62**: 1435–8.

23. Goodisson DW, Shaw GM, Snape L. Intracranial intubation in patients with maxillofacial injuries associated with base of skull fractures? *J Trauma* 2001; **50**: 363–6.

24. Bynoe RP, Kerwin AJ, Parker HH, *et al*. Maxillofacial injuries and life threatening hemorrhage: treatment with transcatheter arterial embolization. *J Trauma* 2003; **55**: 74–9.

25. Cogbill TH, Cothren CC, Ahearn MK, *et al*. Management of maxillofacial injuries with severe oronasal hemorrhage: a multicenter perspective. *J Trauma* 2008; **65**: 994–9.

26. Das S, Das TP, Ghosh PS. Submental intubation: a journey over the last 25 years. *J Anaesthesiol Clin Pharmacol* 2012; **28**: 291–303.

27. Bonfils P. Difficult intubation in Pierre-Robin children, a new method: the retromolar route. *Anaesthetist* 1983; **32**: 363–7.

28. Lee SS, Huang SH, Wu SH, *et al*. A review of intraoperative airway management for midface facial bone fracture patients. *Ann Plast Surg* 2009; **63**: 162–6.

29. Lima SM, Asprino L, Moreira R, deMorales M. A retrospective analysis of submental intubation in maxillofacial trauma patients. *J Oral Maxillofac Surg* 2011; **69**: 2001–5.

30. Gadre KS, Waknis PP. Transmylohyoid/submental intubation: review, analysis, and refinements. *J Craniofac Surg* 2010; **21**: 516–19.

Chapter

26

Eye trauma and anesthesia

Martin Dauber and Steven Roth

Objectives

(1) Define the basic anatomic and physiologic concepts of ocular trauma.

(2) Review the anesthetic implications of eye injuries, including blindness following major surgery.

(3) Evaluate the use of succinylcholine in patients with open-globe injuries and consider pharmacologic alternatives.

Introduction

Trauma to the eyes and resulting blindness can have a life-altering impact. This chapter will present the implications for the anesthesiologist of trauma to the eye. Ocular trauma and basic ophthalmic anatomy and physiologic concepts will be defined, and the incidence of these potentially devastating injuries will be reviewed. Anesthetic implications, including the timing of surgery, anesthetic drug selection, and other perianesthetic concerns, will be addressed. The use of succinylcholine in patients with open-globe injuries is a long-standing controversy which will be addressed. Blindness following major trauma and resuscitation has significant implications for physicians caring for trauma patients.

Definitions

A standard terminology for eye injury that has been adopted in the United States and internationally is known as the Birmingham Eye Trauma Terminology (BETT; Fig. 26.1). The entire globe is considered, and the BETT is unambiguous, consistent, and simple to use. It provides a nomenclature with low interobserver variation and allows for easy communication between healthcare providers, analogous to the Glasgow Coma Scale (GCS) for brain injuries. The definitions it provides will be utilized in this chapter. The BETT system clearly defines all injuries and places each type of injury within a comprehensive system of the whole eyeball.[1]

The eye wall is defined as the cornea and the sclera. A full-thickness wound of these layers is an *open-globe* injury, whereas a *closed-globe* injury does not involve a full-thickness wound (Fig. 26.2). Mechanisms of injury include contusion, laceration, and rupture. Contusions can occur by direct delivery of energy (e.g., choroidal rupture) or through changes in the shape of the globe (e.g., angle recession).[2] Because the eye

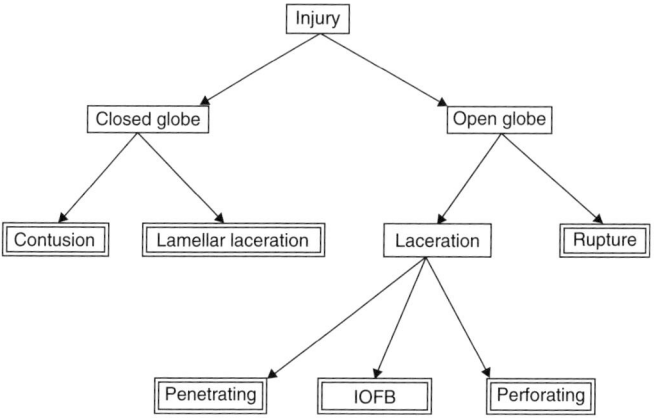

Figure 26.1 The Birmingham Eye Trauma Terminology (BETT) system. The double-framed boxes show the diagnoses employed in clinical practice. IOFB, intraocular foreign body.

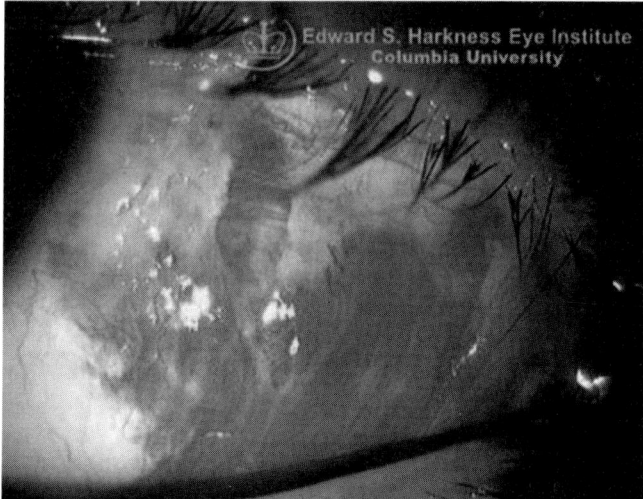

Figure 26.2 Conjunctival laceration with subconjunctival hemorrhage. This is an example of a closed-eye injury. *A black and white version of this figure will appear in some formats. For the color version, please refer to the plate section.*

Trauma Anesthesia, 2nd Edition, ed. Charles E. Smith. Published by Cambridge University Press. © Charles E. Smith, 2015.

is filled with vitreous, an incompressible liquid, a direct impact will increase the intraocular pressure (IOP), assuming the globe is intact. If vitreous or anterior chamber contents extrude (i.e., leak out) the eye is decompressed. The eye wall will rupture at its weakest point, such as at the point of impact or dehiscence of a previously surgically sutured site. The actual wound, therefore, is produced by an inside-out mechanism, whereas, in lacerations of the full thickness of the eye wall caused by sharp objects, the result is an outside-in mechanism of injury.

Incidence and epidemiology

Eye trauma is a significant and disabling health problem in the United States, where approximately 2.5 million injuries occur annually at a cost of more than $4 billion.[2] The National Institute for Occupational Safety and Health indicates that between 600,000 and 700,000 work-related eye injuries occur annually, with the construction industry at the highest risk.[3] An ocular foreign body is the most common type of injury, accounting for one-third of cases. Open wounds and contusions make up one-fourth of all work-related ocular injuries. Chemical, thermal, and radiation burns constitute the remaining eye injuries. This chapter will deal primarily with mechanical trauma to the eye, as the other injuries rarely present to the operating room.

In a 2012 investigation of the incidence of eye injuries in Canada, 2% of adults (including 3% of men and 1% of women) reported sustaining an eye injury that required medical attention during the previous year. Approximately one-third of these occurred at home, and one-third occurred at work. Sports accounted for 9%, sharp objects 23%, dirt/debris 12%, and blunt objects 7%. One-quarter of eye injuries resulted in the need to take time off from work.[4] No equivalent recent data are available for the United States.

There are approximately 40,000 eye injuries related to sports annually in the United States, most occurring in children and young adults (Fig. 26.3). Prevention of almost all of these injuries and the resultant blindness would be possible if proper eye protection were employed. Masks and eye guards are available for baseball, football, basketball, soccer, racquetball, and other sports, and are required by certain sports agencies.[5] These lenses are made from polycarbonates and should bear the approval of the American Society for Testing and Materials (ASTM).

Associated injuries

The location of the eye within the bony orbit results in frequent associated injuries to the head and neck. These other injuries include traumatic brain injuries, as well as cervical spine trauma with and without neurologic compromise (see Chapters 20–23). Because these associated injuries potentially have profound physiologic and prognostic implications, as well as a great impact on anesthetic plans, they must be addressed prior to ophthalmologic intervention. Nonetheless,

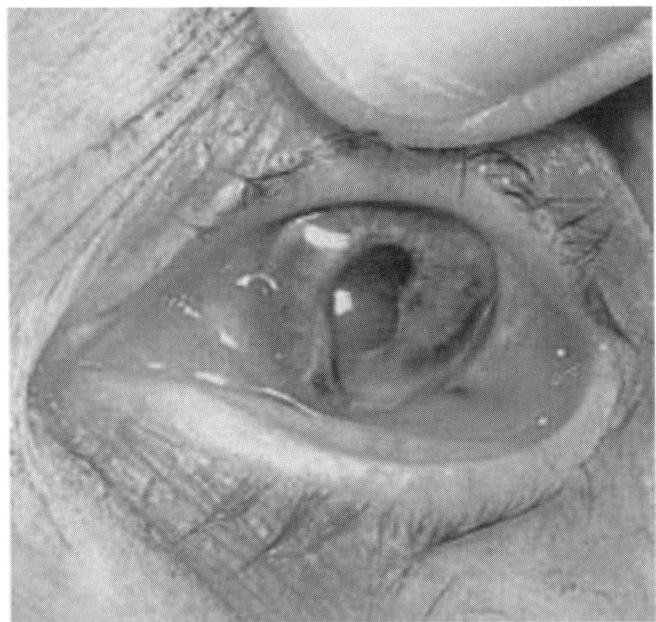

Figure 26.3 An open-eye injury resulting from trauma from a racquet. *A black and white version of this figure will appear in some formats. For the color version, please refer to the plate section.*

early and thorough examination of the eyes should be accomplished to the greatest extent possible, preferably by an ophthalmologist skilled in ocular trauma care.

Ophthalmologic evaluation

Patients who are suspected of having sustained orbital or periorbital/facial trauma must undergo a complete ophthalmologic evaluation after initial stabilization and trauma evaluation. The extent of soft tissue and intraocular injury and bony disruption must be assessed. Acute or progressive loss of the visual axis from corneal opacification, cataract formation, or intraocular bleeding can inhibit complete ophthalmologic examination within a short time and may prevent appropriate diagnosis. The exam by the ophthalmologist will include assessment of visual acuity, pupillary condition and function, motility of the eye, and intraocular pressure (IOP). Anterior segment evaluation with a slit lamp or handheld lens and funduscopic inspection of the posterior segment will be performed on the trauma patient as well.

If penetrating injury to the globe is present, further examination will be limited so the globe can be shielded to prevent further extrusion of intraocular contents. If necessary, antiemetics such as metoclopramide, serotonin antagonists (e.g., ondansetron), and/or promethazine can be administered early to prevent vomiting-induced elevations in IOP. Transdermal scopolamine ought to be avoided, as it may blur vision by causing mydriasis and thereby confuse ophthalmologic diagnosis. In many reviews, prediction of a favorable visual outcome from ruptured globes included visual acuity of 20/200 on admission, rupture anterior to the insertion of the rectus muscles, length less than 1.0 cm, and a penetrating mechanism of injury.[6,7] Predictors of poor visual outcome include visual acuity no better than light perception, wounds extending posterior to the recti muscles or longer than 1.0 cm, or a blunt mechanism of injury. Aggressive surgical management may, nonetheless, be undertaken in these high-risk patients to prevent visual loss.

IOP is the ophthalmic issue most important to the anesthesiologist, after the possibility of visual salvage has been ascertained. In trauma patients, the IOP is important at either high or low values. Extremely low pressures may indicate occult globe penetration, although this is by no means pathognomonic, as the IOP may be low, high, or normal in the case of a ruptured globe. Extremely high pressure may indicate retrobulbar hemorrhage, which may be a harbinger of central retinal arterial occlusion or optic nerve damage. Either elevated or depressed IOP may cause pain and nausea.

Pediatric considerations

Most of the considerations regarding adult ocular trauma patients are the same in children, but there are recognizable differences regarding epidemiology, timing of repair of fractures, and the impact these repairs may have on the growth of the child. Craniofacial anatomical differences in children under 7 years of age make them more susceptible to orbital roof fractures. These fractures rarely require surgical intervention, in contrast to other orbital and midface fractures.[8] The difference in incidence may be due to the increased craniofacial ratio in infants, lower facial bone density and thickness, and underdeveloped paranasal sinuses. Children are thus less likely to present for emergency anesthesia for orbital fractures.

Timing of surgery

The ophthalmologist's evaluation will presumably lead to a rational surgical or nonsurgical plan based both on the eye findings and on the overall condition of the patient. In polytrauma patients, ocular interventions are typically postponed unless other injuries are not severe and visual salvage is possible. In unstable patients, regardless of the ophthalmologic imperative or likely visual prognosis, delay of eye surgery is necessarily indicated. In patients with isolated eye injuries or those without life-threatening or other major trauma, the timing of ophthalmologic surgery needs to be determined by the need for urgent versus delayed surgery. Delay of surgery is preferred if the risk of visual loss is not thereby increased. Further medical evaluation of both trauma-related issues (e.g., central nervous system and cervical spine injuries) and coexisting medical disease can occur during the interval between the trauma and the surgery. Also, in the situation of delayed ophthalmologic intervention, "full-stomach" status may be improved, or, at the very least, antacid and antireflux prophylactic medications can be administered so that they can begin to exert their pharmacologic effects, in order to decrease the risk from aspiration of gastric contents.

The determination by the ophthalmologist of the possibility of vision salvage or the certainty of full visual loss must enter into the consideration of the need for emergency anesthesia. In the absence of other injuries that require immediate induction of general anesthesia, the risks of emergency anesthesia in the unprepared patient must be balanced against the potential benefit of ophthalmologic intervention. Additionally, many injuries to the eye, especially those to the external tissues (eyelid, conjunctiva, cornea, and iris) may be treated medically or under local or topical anesthesia in the emergency department rather than in the operating room. If the patient is anesthetized for treatment of other injuries in any case, however, the ophthalmologist may choose to treat the eye injuries under the same general anesthetic.

Intraocular pressure

A thorough discussion of IOP is beyond the scope of this chapter, although some basic concepts will be reviewed. A comprehensive review of this topic for anesthesiologists is available in a chapter by McGoldrick and Gayer.[9] In many ways the principles of IOP are similar to those of intracranial pressure (ICP), a subject more familiar to most anesthesiologists.

The balance between production and elimination of the aqueous humor maintains IOP (Fig. 26.4). Two-thirds of this liquid humor is produced by the ciliary bodies through the mechanism of active secretion. This process is modulated by both the carbonic anhydrase and cytochrome oxidase systems. The remaining third is produced by passive filtration in the anterior surface of the iris. Drainage occurs via the trabecular network, the canal of Schlemm, and the episcleral vessels.[10] Maintenance of IOP within the normal range of 10–20 mmHg is important for ocular homeostasis. Pressures greater than 22 mmHg are considered abnormal, and prolonged elevations of IOP can lead to permanent visual loss. The IOP may be 1–6 mmHg higher while the patient is supine rather than sitting upright, which is the typical position for patients during ophthalmologic examination. As in any semi-closed system, the factors that may influence and alter IOP include external, internal, and wall tension. In trauma patients, the condition of the extraocular muscles, bony injuries around the orbit, retching or vomiting, and iatrogenic manipulations all may affect external compression. Rupture of the globe causing extrusion of contents or hemorrhage into the globe as a result of blunt trauma can influence the internal contribution to IOP.

Succinylcholine and the eye

Succinylcholine remains the only depolarizing neuromuscular blocker available for clinical use. Its rapid onset, short duration, and long history of clinical experience make it a preferred drug for rapid sequence intubation in the trauma patient (see Chapter 13). Despite some undesirable adverse effects, succinylcholine remains an integral option in the anesthetic plan of many emergency patients. It exerts presynaptic,

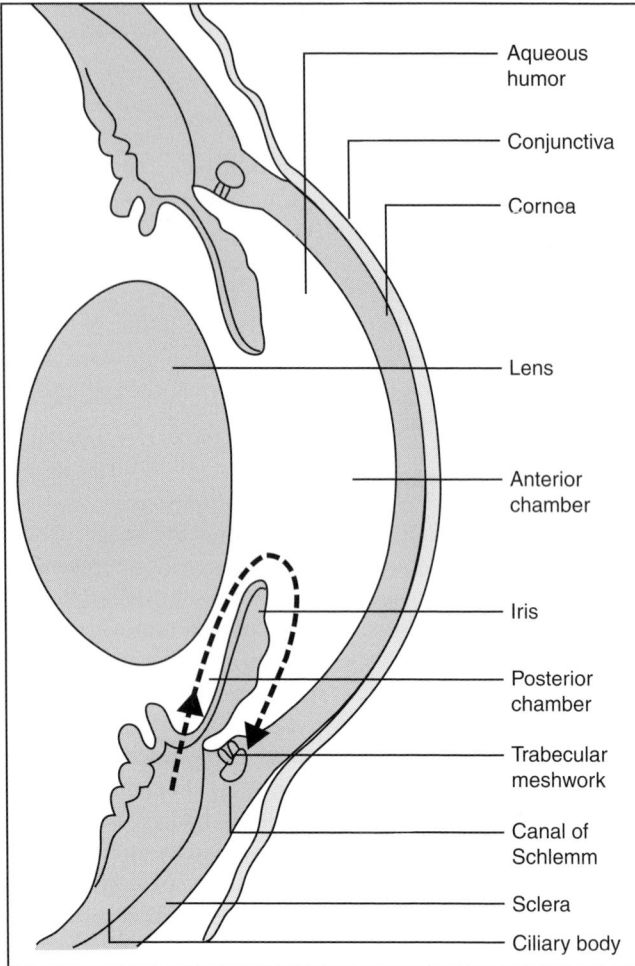

Figure 26.4 Diagram of the flow of aqueous humor in the eye.

postsynaptic, and extrajunctional effects. Clinically, succinylcholine depresses the height of a single twitch and facilitates tracheal intubation.

The publication in the general medical literature of the potential role that succinylcholine could play in anesthesia practice occurred in 1952.[11] The following year it was reported in Europe that succinylcholine measurably increased IOP.[12] The American literature then followed, with the publication of several anecdotes from ophthalmologists that exudation of vitreous occurred after patients received succinylcholine.[13] It was suggested in the anesthesia literature that this loss of vitreous occurred when succinylcholine was given under "light anesthesia" conditions. It was stated that the use of succinylcholine in intraocular surgery was "hazardous."[14] This reputation has persisted in many forms since that time.

In a 1986 retrospective review of the experience at the Wills Eye Hospital of open-eye trauma patients, 81% of patients underwent general anesthesia. Eighty-eight percent of those underwent an intravenous induction, 90% of whom received succinylcholine. The remainder, all of whom were children, had an inhalation induction. Operative reports were reviewed

in detail, as were progress notes from the postoperative period. No extrusion of vitreous was noted in any patient who had received succinylcholine. In addition, the authors noted in their discussion that they were not aware of any anecdotal reports from Wills Eye Hospital of loss of eye contents in eye trauma patients over the prior decade.[15] Case reports of succinylcholine-induced vitreous extrusion followed, as did other institutional anecdotes of the reported ocular safety of succinylcholine.[16,17]

Scientific study of the effects of succinylcholine on the open globe followed these reports. Intraocular pressure increases in humans 1 minute after succinylcholine administration, and peaks at an elevation of 9 mmHg within 6 minutes. Many mechanisms have been proposed for this increase, including the contraction of extraocular muscles in response to succinylcholine forcing globe contents out of the orbit. A cat model, however, did not substantiate this theory.[18] An elegant study in humans undergoing enucleation under general anesthesia demonstrated that the increase in IOP after succinylcholine occurs even after detachment of all of the extraocular muscles.[19] The current theory for the succinylcholine-induced elevation in IOP is related to a vascular mechanism, whereby either choroidal vascular dilatation or decrease in vitreous drainage as a result of elevated central venous pressure (causing an increase in resistance to outflow) decreases drainage of vitreous through the canal of Schlemm.[20]

Several techniques have been advocated for the blunting of the elevation in IOP from succinylcholine. Included among them are "self-taming," defasciculating with nondepolarizing relaxants, and other pharmacologic pretreatment. Self-taming implies the administration of a small, subclinical dose of succinylcholine (0.2 mg/kg in this study) 1 minute prior to the rapid sequence intubating dose. This has been shown to be ineffective and, in fact, the IOP rises in response to the small dose.[21] Lidocaine (intravenous dose of 1 mg/kg) blunts the increase caused by succinylcholine and further blunts the rise in IOP seen with endotracheal intubation, though *d*-tubocurare and diazepam provide neither benefit.[22] All of the opioids commonly used in clinical anesthesia, including fentanyl, alfentanil, sufentanil, and remifentanil, have been shown to blunt the IOP elevation following succinylcholine and intubation.[23–25] Nifidipine, nitroglycerin, propranolol, and clonidine all exert protective effects on IOP, but may be contraindicated in the polytrauma patient.[26–28] A major limitation to these studies is that they were done in elective surgical patients without eye injuries and with intact globes.

The use of nondepolarizing muscle relaxants in high doses is an alternative to succinylcholine for rapid sequence induction and intubation (see Chapter 13). Currently the duration of paralysis provided by these agents (e.g., rocuronium 1.2 mg/kg) may be excessive for the anticipated duration of eye trauma surgery. Sugammadex (Org 25969, trade name, Bridion) is an agent for the early reversal of deep neuromuscular blockade by the modified steroid agent rocuronium, and has some efficacy against vecuronium and pancuronium. It is the first selective relaxant binding agent. Although not yet available in the US and Canada, it is available in Europe, Australia, and New Zealand. The main advantage of sugammadex is rapid and complete reversal of neuromuscular blockade without relying on inhibition of acetylcholinesterase. As such, its administration is associated with much greater cardiovascular and autonomic stability than the traditional reversal agents.[29]

It is clear that succinylcholine does indeed increase IOP. However, during the period surrounding the induction of anesthesia, there are many factors that also change IOP. These include supine positioning, coughing, retching, Valsalva maneuvers, or crying. In addition, mask ventilation with compression of the orbit while awaiting paralysis from the slower-onset nondepolarizing neuromuscular relaxants will directly elevate IOP. Coughing during intubation from any cause will also adversely affect IOP and is to be avoided. Airway assessment combined with ophthalmologic impressions need to be discussed by the anesthesia and ophthalmology teams. Maintenance of ventilation is essential to all plans, independent of ocular implications. If rapid sequence induction and intubation is deemed appropriate, propofol, thiopental, opioids, and other drugs have been shown to minimize the effect of succinylcholine on IOP. If difficult tracheal intubation is anticipated, a determination of the viability of the eye is critical. If vision is not to be preserved, awake intubation can be selected (see Chapter 3). If the possibility of restoration or salvage of vision exists, IOP elevation will need to be avoided prior to any intubation sequence.

In light of the benefits and safety of succinylcholine for facilitating intubation as part of the standard rapid sequence induction of anesthesia in the full-stomach patient, its clinical use should not be limited. The main point is that, in the situation of an open-eye injury, the patient needs to be deeply anesthetized and immobile. How to do that is a matter of individual preference and should be tailored according to the patient's needs and the anesthesiologist's preferences.

Ischemic optic neuropathy (ION)

Ischemic optic neuropathy, the leading cause of sudden visual loss in patients 50 years of age or older, primarily occurs spontaneously without warning signs, and rarely is found in the setting of nonocular surgery. There are two types of ION: anterior (AION) and posterior (PION). Of the two, AION is far more common in the overall population and has been more extensively studied than PION. ION has been found after a wide variety of surgical procedures, with the majority having followed cardiothoracic surgery,[30–32] instrumented spinal fusion operations,[33,34] head and neck surgery,[35] and surgery on the nose or sinuses.[36,37] However, cases have also been described after vascular surgery, general surgical, and urologic procedures, cesarean delivery, gynecologic surgery, and liposuction.[38–43] With advances in trauma resuscitation, patients who would have died before are surviving, and the incidence of ION and the resultant blindness is likely to increase in these patients.

Current knowledge and controversies

Perioperative ION appears to be a multifactorial disease, and, unlike spontaneously occurring ION, it can occur in younger patients. Because there are few case–control studies and no prospective studies, the risk factors have not yet been well defined.[44,45] Another puzzling feature of this dreaded complication is that it is unclear why some patients develop AION and others develop PION. Some possible factors involved in the etiology of perioperative ION are common in multiple trauma patients, including decreased systemic blood pressure, large blood loss, increased intraocular or orbital venous pressure, abnormal autoregulation of the optic nerve circulation and/or anatomic variation in the blood supply to the optic nerve, emboli, use of vasopressors, the presence of systemic diseases such as hypertension, diabetes, and atherosclerosis, and retrobulbar hemorrhage. It seems that one or more of these factors are often involved in an individual patient, and in an unpredictable fashion.

Intraoperative hypotension has been cited as an important risk factor by a number of authors of case reports,[39,46,47] but it is not always present, suggesting that hypotension itself might not be responsible. Hypotension can potentially lead to decreases in perfusion pressure in the optic nerve. The anterior optic nerve would be susceptible to damage from hypotension, leading to AION either because of anatomical variation in the circulation or because of abnormal autoregulation and inability to adequately compensate for a decrease in perfusion pressure. The posterior optic nerve would be at potential risk, leading to PION, because of the relatively limited blood supply reaching this area, which might be potentiated by hypotension. It is difficult to precisely define the degree of hypotension that is potentially harmful, as actual pre- and intraoperative blood pressures were not available in many of the reported cases of ION in the literature, and hence the safe "lower limits" of blood pressure are not known.

From case reports of perioperative ION, it is apparent that, on average, patients sustained considerable blood loss and had decreased hemoglobin concentration intraoperatively. Routine clinical practice based on the National Institutes of Health (NIH) Consensus Panel on Blood Transfusion and the American Society of Anesthesiologists (ASA) practice guidelines indicate that transfusion is generally not required for hemoglobin values greater than 8.0 g/dL (see Chapter 8).[48,49] A number of authors have suggested that allowing hemoglobin to decrease to such low values may be putting patients at increased risk for ION;[39,50] however, whether practice should be changed in surgical procedures for major trauma surgery remains controversial. In the setting of uncontrolled hemorrhage, where blood volume is not maintained, decreased oxygen delivery to the optic nerve could result in either AION or PION.[51,52] Just how low or for how long hemoglobin concentration must decrease to lead to this complication is not known. However, the presence of recurrent and profound hemorrhage has been described in many reports. The effects of combined hypotension and hemodilution on hemodynamics and O_2 delivery in the optic nerve have not been studied but remain a concern.

Intraocular pressure changes and venous hemodynamics in the eye

AION and PION have been reported in the setting of massive fluid replacement, and many reports include patients who were operated on in the prone position. This raises the possibility that either external pressure on the globe or a build-up of pressure internally within the eye could be related to ION. It is unlikely that PION is related to external pressure, because the retrolaminar optic nerve is not exposed to the IOP. In addition, an increase in IOP would not be likely to produce an isolated ION without also causing retinal damage, because sustained increases in IOP significantly decrease both retinal and choroidal blood flows.[53]

The theory that massive fluid resuscitation could be a pathogenic factor in perioperative ION remains speculative, but does have some merit. Conceivably, fluid therapy could result in increased IOP, and/or accumulation of fluid in the optic nerve. Because the vessels in the optic nerve are small and relatively easily compressed, especially in the posterior optic nerve, large-volume replacement might lead to decreased arterial supply, or increased orbital venous pressure and the risk of venous stasis. Because the central retinal vein and draining veins exit out of the optic nerve, it is possible that an "internal compartment syndrome" may occur in the optic nerve. In a remarkable report, Cullinane et al. found that 2.6% of trauma patients who were resuscitated successfully by using more than 20 L of crystalloid in a 24-hour period developed ION.[54] Patients were said, in this publication, to have sustained AION, but from the ocular findings reported it appears the diagnosis was in fact PION. These patients received massive blood replacement and were acidotic, most had abdominal compartment syndrome, and the lowest hematocrit ranged from 7.5% to 28%. Also, very high levels of positive end-expiratory pressure (PEEP) (average 29 cmH_2O) were used to ventilate these patients. Although there are many complicating factors in these patients, massive fluid and blood replacement seem likely as possible etiologic factors for ION.

Vasopressors

Hayreh theorized that AION is related to excessive secretion of vasoconstrictors, which could in turn lower optic nerve perfusion to dangerously low levels.[52,54] Clinicians often use vasopressors to maintain blood pressure, especially after cardiac surgery. Shapira et al. showed an association between prolonged use of epinephrine or long bypass time and ION in patients undergoing open heart surgery.[30] Lee and Lam reported a case of ION in a patient after lumbar spine fusion during which a phenylephrine infusion was used to maintain blood pressure.[55] However, these reports cannot distinguish whether vasopressors altered hemodynamics in the optic nerve

or if the use of vasopressors represents a marker for patients with profound systemic abnormalities.

Prognosis and treatment

Unfortunately, there is no proven treatment for ION. Williams et al. have reviewed the attempted treatments.[50] Acetazolamide lowers IOP and may improve flow to the optic nerve and retina.[56,57] Diuretics such as mannitol or furosemide reduce edema. In the acute phase, corticosteroids may reduce axonal swelling, but in the postoperative period they increase the risk of wound infection. Because steroids are of unproven benefit, their use must be carefully weighed. Increasing ocular perfusion pressure or hemoglobin concentration may be appropriate when ION occurs in conjunction with significant decreases in blood pressure and hemoglobin concentration. Maintaining head-up position could be valuable if increased ocular venous pressure is suspected. Similarly, IOP should be lowered if an increase is documented. Optic nerve decompression is an operative procedure that could restore circulation in the optic nerve. However, in a multicenter trial sponsored by the National Eye Institute, this operation was found to be ineffective and possibly harmful; because of the adverse findings, this study was terminated prematurely.[58] Despite the devastating nature of ION, our limited understanding of the pathogenesis of this disorder, at this time, does not yet enable us to make rational recommendations that are likely to completely prevent its occurrence.

Conclusions

Although typically not life-threatening in the terms that anesthesiologists usually consider, ocular trauma can have devastating consequences that alter lifestyle. Current evidence favors the judicious use of succinylcholine in trauma patients to facilitate rapid and excellent tracheal intubation conditions when appropriate, and when maneuvers to prevent acute elevations in IOP are instituted. Ophthalmologic evaluation, treatment, and prognostication allow anesthetic management of these patients that can optimize the visual outcome while exerting the minimum necessary effects on the overall physiology of the trauma patient. Ischemic optic neuropathy is a devastating complication that may be found in the perioperative period in patients who have been successfully resuscitated from massive trauma. The etiology remains unclear, but patients with visual deficit should be examined immediately by an ophthalmologist to determine cause and provide any possible treatment.

Questions

For questions 1–3, match each of the statements (1–3) with the best answer (a–e).
(1) **Ischemic optic neuropathy**
(2) **Ocular foreign body**
(3) **Open-globe injury**
  a. Laceration of the globe from penetrating trauma

b. Always associated with loss of vitreous and anterior eye chamber contents

c. Full-thickness injury of the eye wall including cornea and sclera

d. Leading cause of blindness in patients more than 50 years old

e. Most common type of eye injury

(4) Which of the following is associated with increased intraocular pressure?

a. Retching

b. Coughing

c. Crying

d. Valsalva maneuver

e. All of the above

(5) Concerning succinylcholine and intraocular pressure (IOP), which of the following statements is true?

a. IOP to 50 mmHg within 5 minutes after administration of succinylcholine

b. Succinylcholine causes contraction of extraocular muscles and extrusion of vitreous in cats

c. Increased IOP may be due to choroidal vascular dilatation or decrease in vitreous drainage

d. A small dose of succinylcholine (self-taming) is effective in blunting the rise in IOP

e. The combination of high-dose rocuronium and suggamadex has been shown to be safe for eye trauma patients.

(6) Potential methods for dealing with duration of nondepolarizing neuromuscular blockade (NDNMB) in excess of surgery time include:

a. Early antagonism with larger than typical doses of acetylcholinesterase

b. Tracheal extubation while patient somewhat weak to decrease risk of coughing and elevation of IOP

c. Utilization of suggamadex if the NDNMB was not a modified steroid

d. Prolonged sedation and ventilation until clinical signs of reversal are satisfactory

(7) Anesthesia-related causes of postoperative visual loss include all of the following except:

a. Anterior ischemic optic neuropathy

b. Posterior ischemic optic neuropathy

c. Retinal detachment

d. Central retinal artery occlusion

e. Cortical blindness

(8) In approaching the polytrauma patient with ocular trauma, the anesthesia evaluation of potential for preservation of vision should take precedence over:

a. Duration of proposed operations

b. Thoracic injuries

c. Abdominal injuries

d. Elevation in intracranial pressure

e. Full-stomach considerations

(9) Concerning decreasing the IOP response to succinylcholine:

a. Prevention of fasciculations with NDNMB prevents the increase in IOP

b. Self-taming doses of succinylcholine (e.g., 0.2 mg/kg) prevent the increase in IOP

c. Lidocaine is effective in blunting the increase in IOP

d. Nifidipine, nitroglycerin, propranolol, and clonidine all exert protective effects on IOP, and are therefore ideal in the polytrauma patient

(10) Understanding all of the following is important to anesthetic management of ocular trauma patients to help optimize the visual outcome while exerting the minimum necessary effects on the overall physiology, except:

a. The ophthalmologic evaluation

b. Planned ophthalmologic treatment

c. Visual prognostication

d. Ophthalmologic need for intraoperative diuresis

Answers

(1) d

(2) e

(3) c

(4) e

(5) c

(6) d

(7) c

(8) a

(9) d

(10) d

References

1. Kuhn F, Morris R, Witherspoon CD. Birmingham Eye Trauma Terminology (BETT): terminology and classification of mechanical eye injuries. *Ophthalmol Clin N Am* 2002; **15**: 139–43.

2. National Society to Prevent Blindness. *Vision Problems in the U.S. – Data Analysis, National Society to Prevent Blindness.* Chicago, IL: NSPB, 2002.

3. United States Consumer Product Safety Commission, Directorate for Epidemiology; National Injury Information Clearinghouse. *National Electronic Injury Surveillance System. Product Summary Report.* Bethesda, MD, US Consumer Product Safety Commission, 2003.

4. Gordon, KD. The incidence of eye injuries in Canada. *Can J Opthalmol* 2012; **47**: 351–3.

5. USA Racquetball Association. Official Rules of Racquetball, September 2004. http://usra.org/Rulebook/tabid/839/ Default.aspx (accessed September 2014).

6. Grove AS. Computerized tomography in management of orbital trauma. *Ophthalmology* 1982; **89**: 433–40.

7. Harlan JB, Pieramici DJ. Evaluation of patients with ocular trauma. *Ophthalmol Clin N Am* 2002; **15**: 153–61.

8. Koltai PJ, Amjad I, Meyer D, Feustel PJ. Orbital fractures in children. *Arch Otolaryngol Head Neck Surg* 1995; **121**: 1375–9.

9. McGoldrick KE, Gayer S. Anesthesia and the eye. In Barash P, Cullen B, Stoelting R, eds., *Clinical Anesthesia*, 5th edition. Philadelphia PA: Lippincott, Williams and Wilkins, 2006, pp. 974–96.

10. Forrester JV, Dick AD, *et al. The Eye: Basic Sciences in Practice*. Philadelphia, PA: Saunders, 2002.

11. Foldes FF, Menall PG, Borrego-Hinojosa JM. Succinylcholine: a new approach to muscular relaxation in anesthesiology. *N Engl J Med* 1952; **247**: 596–600.

12. Hofman H, Holzer H, Bock J, *et al.* The effect of muscle relaxants on intraocular pressure. *Klin Monatsbl Augenheilk* 1953; **123**: 1–15.

13. Lincoff HA, Breinin GM, Devoe AG. The effect of succinylcholine on the extraocular muscles. *Am J Ophthalmol* 1957; **43**: 440–4.

14. Dillon JB, Sabawala P, Taylor DB, *et al.* Action of succinylcholine on eye muscles and intraocular pressure. *Anesthesiology* 1957; **18**: 44–9.

15. Libonati MM, Leahy JJ, Ellison N. The use of succinylcholine in open eye surgery. *Anesthesiology* 1986; **62**: 637–40.

16. Rich AL, Witherspoon CD, Morris RE, *et al.* Use of nondepolarizing anesthetic agents in penetrating ocular injuries. *Anesthesiology* 1986; **65**: 108–9.

17. Donlon JV. Succinylcholine and open eye injuries. *Anesthesiology* 1986; **65**: 526–7.

18. Moreno RJ, Kloess P, Carlson DW. Effect of succinylcholine on the intraocular contents of open globes. *Ophthalmology* 1991; **98**: 636–8.

19. Kelly RE, Dinner M, Turner LS, *et al.* Succinylcholine increases intraocular pressure in the human eye with the extraocular muscles detached. *Anesthesiology* 1993; **79**: 948–52.

20. Metz HS, Venkatesh B. Succinylcholine and intraocular pressure. *J Pediatr Ophthalmol Strabismus* 1981; **18**: 12–14.

21. Verma RS. "Self-Taming" of succinylcholine-induced fasciculations and intraocular pressure. *Anesthesiology* 1979; **50**: 245.

22. Mahajan RP, Grover VK, Munjal VP, *et al.* Double blind comparison of lidocaine, tubocurarine and diazepam pretreatment in modifying intraocular pressure increases. *Can J Anaesth* 1987; **34**: 41–5.

23. Alexander R, Hill R, Lipham WJ, *et al.* Remifentanil prevents an increase in intraocular pressure after succinylcholine and tracheal intubation. *Br J Anaesth* 1998; **81**: 606–7.

24. Georgiou M, Parlapani A, Argiriadou H, *et al.* Sufentanil or clonidine for blunting the increase in intraocular pressure during rapid-sequence induction. *Eur J Anaesthesiol* 2002; **19**; 819–22.

25. Sweeney J, Underhill S, Dowd T, *et al.* Modification by fentanyl and alfentanil of the intraocular pressure response to suxamethonium and tracheal intubation. *Br J Anaesth* 1989; **63**: 688–91.

26. Indu B, Batra YK, Puri GD, *et al.* Nifidipine attenuates the intraocular pressure response to intubation following succinylcholine. *Can J Anaesth* 1989; **36**: 269–72.

27. Mahajan RP, Grover VK, Sharma SL, *et al.* Intranasal nitroglycerine and intraocular pressure during general anesthesia. *Anesth Analg* 1988; **67**: 631–6.

28. Cook JH, Feneck RO, Smith MB. Effect of pre-treatment with propranolol on intra-ocular pressure changes during induction of anesthesia. *Eur J Anaesthesiol* 1986; **3**: 449–57.

29. Naguib M. Sugammadex: another milestone in clinical neuromuscular pharmacology. *Anesth Analg* 2007; **104**: 575–81.

30. Shapira OM, Kimmel WA, Lindsey PS, *et al.* Anterior ischemic optic neuropathy after open heart operations. *Ann Thorac Surg* 1996; **61**: 660–6.

31. Shahian DM, Speert PK. Symptomatic visual deficits after open heart operations. *Ann Thorac Surg* 1989; **48**: 275–9.

32. Sweeney PJ, Breuer AC, Selhorst JB, *et al.* Ischemic optic neuropathy: a complication of cardiopulmonary bypass surgery. *Neurology* 1982; **32**: 560–2.

33. Roth S, Thisted RA, Erickson JP, *et al.* Eye injuries after non ocular surgery: a study of 60,965 anesthetics from 1988 to 1992. *Anesthesiology* 1996; **85**: 1020–7.

34. Roth S, Nunez R, Schreider BD. Visual loss after lumbar spine fusion. *J Neurosurg Anesthesiol* 1997; **9**: 346–8.

35. Chutkow JG, Sharbrough FW, Riley FC. Blindness following simultaneous bilateral neck dissection. *Mayo Clin Proc* 1973; **48**: 713–17.

36. Buus DR, Tse DT, Farris BK. Ophthalmic complications of sinus surgery. *Ophthalmology* 1990; **97**: 612–19.

37. Maniglia AJ. Fatal and major complications secondary to nasal and sinus surgery. *Laryngoscope* 1989; **99**: 276–83.

38. Warner ME, Warner MA, Garrity JA, *et al.* The frequency of perioperative vision loss. *Anesth Analg* 2001; **93**: 1417–21.

39. Brown RH, Schauble JF, Miller NR. Anemia and hypotension as contributors to perioperative loss of vision. *Anesthesiology* 1994; **80**: 222–6.

40. Chun DB, Levin DK. Ischemic optic neuropathy after hemorrhage from a cornual ectopic gestation. *Am J Obstetr Gynecol* 1997; **177**: 1550–2.

41. Gupta M, Puri P, Rennie IG. Anterior ischemic optic neuropathy after emergency caesarean section under epidural anesthesia. *Acta Anaesthesiol Scand* 2002; **46**: 751–2.

42. Williams GC, Lee AG, Adler HL, *et al.* Bilateral anterior ischemic optic neuropathy and branch retinal artery occlusion after radical prostatectomy. *J Urol* 1999; **162**: 1384–5.

43. Minagar A, Schatz NJ, Glaser JS. Liposuction and ischemic optic neuropathy: case report and review of literature. *J Neurol Sci* 2000; **181**: 132–6.

44. Roth S. The effects of isovolumic hemodilution on ocular blood flow. *Exp Eye Res* 1992; **55**: 59–63.

45. Roth S, Barach P. Post-operative visual loss: still no answers – yet. *Anesthesiology* 2001; **95**: 575–6.

46. Katz DM, Trobe JD, Cornblath WT, *et al.* Ischemic optic neuropathy after lumbar spine surgery. *Arch Ophthalmol* 1994; **112**: 925–31.

47. Lee AG. Ischemic optic neuropathy following lumbar spine surgery. *J Neurosurg* 1995; **83**: 348–9.

48. Consensus conference: perioperative red blood cell transfusion. *JAMA* 1988; **260**: 2700–3.

49. American Society of Anesthesiologists. Practice guidelines for blood component therapy: a report by the American Society of Anesthesiologists Task Force on Blood Component Therapy. *Anesthesiology* 1996; **84**: 732–47.

50. Williams EL, Hart WM, Tempelhoff R. Postoperative ischemic optic neuropathy. *Anesth Analg* 1995; **80**: 1018–29.

51. Roth S, Gillesberg I. Injuries to the visual system and other sense organs. In Benumof JL, Saidman LJ, eds., *Anesthesia and Perioperative Complications*, 2nd edition. St. Louis, MO: Mosby, 1999, pp. 377–408.

52. Hayreh SS. Anterior ischemic optic neuropathy. VIII. Clinical features and pathogenesis of post-hemorrhagic amaurosis. *Ophthalmology* 1987; **94**: 1488–502.

53. Roth S, Pietrzyk Z. Blood flow after retinal ischemia in cats. *Invest Ophthalmol Vis Sci* 1994; **35**: 3209–17.

54. Cullinane DC, Jenkins JM, Reddy S, *et al.* Anterior ischemic optic neuropathy: a complication after systemic inflammatory response syndrome. *J Trauma* 2000; **48**: 381–7.

55. Lee LA, Lam AM. Unilateral blindness after prone lumbar surgery. *Anesthesiology* 2001; **95**: 793–5.

56. Rassam SM, Patel V, Kohner EM. The effect of acetazolamide on the retinal circulation. *Eye* 1993; **7**: 697–702.

57. Hayreh SS. Anterior ischaemic optic neuropathy. III. Treatment, prophylaxis, and differential diagnosis. *Br J Ophthalmol* 1974; **58**: 981–9.

58. Ischemic Optic Neuropathy Decompression Trial Research Group. Optic nerve decompression surgery for non-arteritic anterior ischemic optic neuropathy is not effective and may be harmful. *JAMA* 1995; **273**: 625–32.

Objectives

(1) To define priorities and goals in the management of musculoskeletal trauma.

(2) To discuss the potential advantages and disadvantages of early fracture fixation.

(3) To describe patient and injury characteristics necessary to formulate a treatment plan.

(4) To develop treatment strategies for urgent and emergent musculoskeletal problems.

Introduction

Trauma is the leading cause of death and disability in the United States in people under the age of 45 years, accounting for more than 100,000 deaths each year and annual medical expenses of over $280 billion.[1-3] Most trauma-related deaths are associated with closed head injuries or rapid exsanguination soon after the injury. Survivors of the initial traumatic event are at risk for various life-threatening complications, many of which are directly related to their musculoskeletal injuries. Trauma care has evolved to address the immediate musculoskeletal insult and to mitigate secondary complications. Essential goals of treatment include resuscitation, pain relief, improved alignment and stability, enhanced mobility, and ultimately restoration of function. The long-term ramifications for musculoskeletal function are profound, affecting most activities of daily living as well as vocational and recreational pursuits.

Goals of treatment

Resuscitation

The American College of Surgeons Committee on Trauma has developed Advanced Trauma Life Support (ATLS) algorithms for initial evaluation and resuscitation of the trauma patient.[4] These validated protocols are practiced at trauma centers throughout the United States and involve primary, secondary, and tertiary surveys of the patient (see Chapter 2). The primary survey is a stepwise evaluation of airway, breathing, circulation, disability, and exposure. This primary survey is followed by a secondary survey in which a detailed history and physical examination is completed. The tertiary survey involves serial evaluations of the patient's status throughout the hospital course.

The primary survey will identify the location and severity of most injuries and will determine the patient's physiological status, including the presence of shock. There are multiple causes of shock in the trauma patient such as hypovolemic, cardiogenic, tension pneumothorax, neurogenic, and sepsis (see Chapter 4). Musculoskeletal injuries are associated with hemorrhage. Hypovolemic shock is most frequently encountered in trauma patients, especially those with pelvis and long-bone fractures. Shock results in tissue hypoperfusion, hypoxemia, activation of the inflammatory cascade, and immune dysfunction.[5-7] Reduction and fixation of fractures will generally promote control of hemorrhage and the pathophysiology of shock, aiding in the resuscitation of the patient.

Pain relief

Pain indicates to the patient that an injury has occurred. It is an invaluable tool to identify injuries in a multiply injured patient, especially during the secondary and tertiary ATLS surveys. Painful stimuli from an injury aid in diagnosis of the problem and initiation of treatment, so that further damage of the surrounding structures can be avoided. Despite these beneficial aspects of pain, pain induces sympathetic discharge, which can contribute to a hyperinflammatory response, increasing the risk of morbidity and mortality in severely injured patients (see Chapter 15).[7] Pain also leads to splinting and impaired ventilation, which causes atelectasis. Atelectasis may result in hypoxemia or pneumonia. Additionally, pain can adversely affect the outcome of an injury, by becoming the primary focus of the patient and his or her family. Chronic pain is associated with poor physical and mental functional outcome scores after orthopedic trauma (see Chapter 17). Uncontrolled and constant pain also contributes to continued immobility, which can lead to thromboembolic events, decreased motion, pulmonary complications, and even death.

Trauma Anesthesia, 2nd Edition, ed. Charles E. Smith. Published by Cambridge University Press. © Charles E. Smith, 2015.

Prompt yet judicious pain control is critical in the care of the multiply injured patient. Pain control can be achieved by several different methods. Fracture stabilization, whether provisional or definitive, will provide some pain relief. Reduction of dislocated joints significantly decreases pain. Early fracture fixation has been associated with reduced narcotic medication usage, potentially resulting in less respiratory depression and fewer other adverse effects.[8] Fracture stabilization combined with various medications, including nonsteroidal anti-inflammatory drugs, opioids, analgesics, antidepressants, and anticonvulsants, can be used effectively to maximize patient comfort and recovery.

Alignment and stability

Early stabilization and restoration of alignment of fractures is an essential step in the resuscitation and pain relief of trauma patients. Unstable pelvis, acetabulum, and femur fractures are often definitively managed within the first 24 hours.[9–16] The urgency and type of stabilization varies among different types of injuries and will depend on the overall status of the patient. Strategies to stabilize a fracture range from a simple splint placed outside the hospital providing axial stability, to early appropriate surgical care restoring fracture alignment, and placing complex implants. General principles of management for fractures of long bones, such as the tibia and femur, include correction of longitudinal, angular, and rotational deformities. Definitive treatment is frequently with intramedullary nails, but plates and external fixators can also be used to accomplish these goals. Articular fractures, involving joint surfaces, demand strict attention to accurate reduction and rigid internal fixation, commonly with plates and screws. These procedures are often undertaken on a delayed basis, several days or even weeks after injury, to allow for swelling around the fracture to decrease, reducing risks of wound healing problems and infections.[17,18] Provisional external fixation spanning the injured joint is frequently done within 48 hours after injury to control fracture alignment and to provide pain relief for complex intraarticular lower extremity fractures.

Enhanced mobility

Once fractures are stabilized, a patient's mobility will improve. Improved mobility of the multiply injured patient has positive effects and can start in the field when traction and splints are applied. Even crude initial splints facilitate nursing care and decrease secondary soft tissue injury during transport. Definitive stabilization of individual fractures permits a patient to initiate early range of motion of the associated joints and to optimize flexibility. The benefits of enhanced mobility go beyond the pain relief and obvious functional and psychological gains. A patient with restored mobility is at decreased risk of venous stasis, deep venous thrombosis, and pulmonary emboli, which can be fatal. Improved mobility decreases the need for continued nursing care, minimizes hospital stay, and ultimately facilitates return to pre-injury level of function.

Restoration of function

The ultimate goal of trauma care and intervention is to return the patient to his or her pre-injury status. This could be as simple as a nonoperative treatment plan, or it could involve multiple different procedures and possibly staged reconstruction that can take many months. It is expected that orthopedic patients with multiple injuries, particularly those with injuries to lower extremity joints, will not reach a level of maximal function for up to 24 months. Treatment of musculoskeletal injury thus has a dramatic impact on the patient, and on society, given the demographics of trauma patients. The typical trauma patient is a young male laborer, contributing significantly to the workforce. In addition to the direct costs of medical treatment and rehabilitation, indirect costs of lost productivity due to premature morbidity and mortality are substantial.[1,3] Optimization of all aspects of trauma care will restore function and minimize costs to society.

Timing of musculoskeletal care
Prioritization of musculoskeletal injuries

The type of treatment and the timing thereof in a patient with multiple system trauma and fractures are controversial. Decisions should be undertaken in a collaborative fashion with all members of the team providing care. Life-threatening and limb-threatening musculoskeletal injuries are addressed *emergently*. These include patients with massive hemorrhage from pelvic fractures or multiple long-bone fractures, arterial injury in an extremity, and compartment syndrome. In these situations, orthopedic management contributes to resuscitation and promotes viability of life and limb. Other musculoskeletal injuries are recommended to be treated on an *urgent* basis. These include open fractures, as well as mechanically unstable pelvis, acetabulum, or femur fractures, hip fractures, and dislocated joints.

Definitive management for most other articular fractures, and isolated extremity injuries can be on a *subacute* basis. This ensures that the systemic resuscitation for the trauma has been completed, nutrition has been addressed, and underlying medical conditions have been evaluated and optimized. Furthermore, many articular injuries have severe soft tissue swelling, which precludes open reduction and internal fixation in the first several days. Extensile surgical approaches (larger incisions allowing open reductions with direct visualization and manipulation of the fracture fragments) for some of these fractures, including the tibial plateau, tibial plafond, and calcaneus, can result in disastrous soft tissue complications and deep infections when undertaken too soon after injury – not allowing for the initial soft tissue swelling to subside.[17,18]

Benefits of early fixation

The majority of multiply injured patients have musculoskeletal injuries. Orthopedic injuries place the patient at risk for complications such as fat embolism, acute respiratory distress syndrome (ARDS), and sepsis. Many studies have documented the positive effects of early fracture management in reducing morbidity and mortality.[9–11,13–16,19–24] Reduction and stabilization of fractures stop bleeding and provide pain relief.[8] Early fixation prevents prolonged recumbency and enhances mobilization from bed, both of which are key factors in reducing atelectasis, pneumonia, and organ failure.[22,23,25,26] In addition to better pulmonary function, some of the benefits of early fracture fixation are improved wound care, fewer wound complications, and lower risk of thrombotic complications. These effects are even more profound in patients with multiple system injury versus those with an isolated fracture (Table 27.1).

In terms of timing, the concept of early fixation has evolved from weeks to hours. In 1982, Goris et al. published a report that supported fixation within the first 24 hours to reduce morbidity, ARDS, and sepsis rates.[19] Johnson et al. completed a retrospective review of 132 multiple trauma patients with two major fractures and an Injury Severity Score (ISS) of 18 or greater.[13] They noted an increased incidence of ARDS when fixation was delayed beyond 24 hours. The overall ARDS incidence was 7% in the early fixation group versus 39% in the group with fixation beyond 24 hours. Early definitive long-bone fixation and external fixation methods have continued to evolve and are now considered to be an integral part of the initial care. Recent attention has been placed on adequately resuscitating patients prior to undergoing definitive fixation. In resuscitated patients, early definitive fracture care is associated with low rates of pulmonary complications, and hospital and ICU stays are minimized.[22,23,25,30,31,33,34]

Two-hit model of organ dysfunction

An important consideration in the development of a treatment plan for patients with multiple system injuries and unstable fractures is whether the physiological state of the patient has been optimized to tolerate surgery. Trauma constitutes a burden to the patient, much of which is related to associated hemorrhage. The injury itself may be considered the "first hit." Surgery to stabilize fractures will provide control of bony bleeding and provide pain relief and pulmonary benefits; however, the surgery also causes further hemorrhage, a so-called "second hit." When the second hit exceeds a theoretical threshold level, severe systemic inflammation may occur. In this model, severely injured patients with massive hemorrhage enter a state called systemic inflammatory response syndrome (SIRS), which has been associated with multiple organ failure and death.[5–7,35–38] (see also Chapters 4 and 6). Fracture fixation will contribute to this secondary response, and, depending on the amount of blood loss generated by surgery, can result in SIRS in underresuscitated patients. An adequate level of resuscitation is crucial in minimizing the impact of the second hit and its adverse consequences.[30,33]

Damage control orthopedics

Damage control orthopedics is a concept to provide early fracture stabilization, while minimizing the second hit caused by prolonged surgical procedures.[27,28,37,39] This tactic generally involves avoiding longer definitive procedures with large blood loss, in favor of shorter surgical procedures (see Chapter 18). An example would be stabilization of a femur fracture with provisional external fixation instead of definitive fixation with an intramedullary nail. Although some studies have suggested decreased initial operative times and less bleeding with a damage control strategy,[28,32,34,37,39] many unstable pelvis fractures cannot be provisionally stabilized with external fixation.[40] Acetabulum fractures and spine fractures also cannot be stabilized with external fixation, limiting the applicability of the damage control concept.[41] Furthermore, the need for additional (definitive) surgery on a delayed basis, e.g., conversion of a femoral external fixator to an intramedullary nail, and the potential for more complications and costs, makes this practice controversial.[42,43] Currently, it is unclear exactly which patients benefit from a damage control strategy.[23,34] Recent studies suggest that definitive fixation of femoral shaft, pelvis, and acetabulum fractures is well tolerated in most patients, with no damage control tactics, as long as adequate resuscitation has occurred.[16,22,23,25,30,31,33]

Decision-making process

The majority of current data supports early fracture stabilization (Table 27.1). The exact timing of surgical intervention will depend on the magnitude and duration of acidosis, and the response to resuscitation. Injury complexity and underlying factors, including patient age and cardiac function, are also important considerations. The orthopedic surgeon, trauma critical care team, and anesthesiologist must work together to decide the appropriate timing of surgical intervention and fracture fixation.

Primary parameters of trauma management
Physiologic

Many different physiologic parameters are used in the evaluation of the multiply injured patients. Early and accurate assessment of the cardiovascular system is critical in the care of the trauma patient. Identification and characterization of shock promotes immediate, appropriate intervention (see Chapter 4). Basic physiologic parameters assessed include the heart rate, blood pressure, temperature, respiratory rate, urine output, and mental status (Table 27.2). Assessment of these values can be used to estimate fluid and blood loss. Other more advanced parameters can be obtained such as systolic pressure and pulse pressure variability, stroke volume, cardiac output, systemic vascular resistance, and cardiac filling pressures (see Chapters 9 and 10). These values can be used to differentiate types of shock and to make fine adjustments during volume replacement.

Table 27.1 Selected studies regarding timing of fixation for unstable orthopedic injuries. The level of evidence in most studies is poor. The majority of published information to date supports early fixation, although in recent years some authors have questioned this as a routine strategy.

Author, year	Study type	Comparison	# patients	Results
Lozman et al. 1986[20]	Randomized, prospective	Femur and tibia treatment immediate, versus nonop	Not specified	Mean cardiac index higher and mean shunt lower with immediate fixation. **Supports early fixation.**
Bone et al. 1989[9]	Randomized, prospective	Femur fixation <24 hours versus >24 hours	178	Fixation after 24 hours associated with more pulmonary complications, greater length of stay, more ICU days, greater costs of care. **Supports early fixation.**
Pape et al. 2007[27]	Randomized, prospective	Femur fixation with IM nail versus damage control (external fixation)	121	Stable patients treated with early IM nail had shorter ventilation times. Borderline patients treated with early DCO had less acute lung injury. No differences in pneumonia, ARDS, MOF for IM nail versus DCO.
Seibel et al. 1985[24]	Retrospective cohort	Group 1 = immediate fixation femur or acetabulum and mobilization Group 2 = 10 days of traction postop Group 3 = 30 days of traction postop	56	More pulmonary failure, sepsis, fracture complications, and narcotic usage when mobilization delayed. **Supports early fixation.**
Pape et al. 1993[28]	Retrospective cohort	Femur fixation < 24 hours versus > 24 hours	106	Patients without concurrent thoracic trauma had shorter intubation time and shorter ICU stay when treated early. Patients with severe chest trauma had more ARDS and mortality with early fixation.
Poole et al. 1992[29]	Retrospective cohort	Femur fixation < 24 hours versus > 24 hours versus nonop in patients with head injury	114	Risk of pulmonary complications not related to timing of fixation. No difference in neurological outcomes among the three groups.
Morshed et al. 2009[30]	Retrospective cohort of National Trauma Databank	Definitive fixation of femur < 12 hours, 12–24 hours, 24–48 hours, 48–120 hours, > 120 hours	1759	Definitive treatment within 12–24 hours after injury associated with lower mortality.
O'Toole et al. 2009[31]	Retrospective review	Resuscitation (lactate < 2.5) before early IM nail	227	78% of patients treated with early IM nail. DCO used for severe head injury or underresuscitated patients. ARDS occurred in < 2% overall. **Supports early fixation in resuscitated patients.**
Tuttle et al. 2009[32]	Retrospective cohort	Femur fixation with IM nail versus damage control (external fixation)	97	Shorter OR times and EBL with DCO. No differences for pneumonia, ARDS, MOF, length of stay for IM nail versus damage control
Lefaivre et al. 2010[33]	Retrospective cohort	Definitive fixation of femur < 8 hours, 8–24 hours, > 24 hours	1958	Definitive treatment within 8–24 hours after injury associated with lower mortality.
Nahm et al. 2011[22]	Retrospective cohort	Femur fixation < 24 hours versus > 24 hours	750	Fixation after 24 hours associated with more pulmonary complications, other complications, greater length of stay, more ICU days. **Supports early fixation.**
Harvin et al. 2012[25]	Retrospective cohort	Femur fixation < 24 hours versus > 24 hours	1376	Fixation after 24 hours associated with more pulmonary complications, greater length of stay, more hospital charges. **Supports early fixation.**
Rixen et al. 2005[34]	Review of retrospective studies	Femur fixation < 24 hours versus > 24 hours	1465	The use of provisional or definitive external fixation in these patients increased over this time period, and was associated with an increased Injury Severity Score (ISS), a lower Glasgow Coma Scale (GCS), thoracic trauma, a base deficit > 6.0, or an elevated prothrombin time. However, **no advantage to external fixation versus primary femoral stabilization with a nail or plate was seen.**

ARDS, acute respiratory distress syndrome; DCO, damage control orthopedics (external fixator); EBL, estimated blood loss; ICU, intensive care unit; IM, intramedullary; MOF, multiorgan failure; nonop, nonoperative; OR, operating room; postop, postoperative.

Table 27.2 Classification for hemorrhagic shock

	Class I	Class II	Class III	Class IV
Blood loss (mL)	Up to 750	750–1500	1500–2000	> 2000
Blood loss (% of volume)	Up to 15%	15–30%	30–40%	> 40%
Heart rate	< 100	> 100	> 120	> 140
Blood pressure	Normal	Normal	Decreased	Decreased
Pulse pressure (mmHg)	Normal	Decreased	Decreased	Decreased
Respiratory rate	14–20	20–30	30–40	> 35
Urine output (mL/h)	> 30	20–30	5–15	Negligible
Mental status	Slightly anxious	Mildly anxious	Confused	Lethargic

Laboratory

Several laboratory parameters routinely obtained during care of the multiply injured patient are crucial for appropriate management. In combination with physiologic parameters and physical exam, these are usually sufficient for resuscitation. Severe musculoskeletal trauma and associated hemorrhage result in tissue hypoperfusion, which leads to acidosis. The extent of acidosis can be assessed by determining the pH, base excess/deficit, or lactate. Normalization of these values within 24 hours of injury is predictive of survival.[44–48] The pH and base excess are less specific than lactate, and they are more easily regulated by the body's compensatory mechanisms. pH and base excess are also more subject to confounders such as alcohol ingestion or renal disease; thus, lactate is considered the most reliable indicator of resuscitation. This value can be used as a guide in the volume repletion of the trauma patient.[45,47,48] Improvement in lactate over time is one of the most accurate and specific indicators of a patient's volume repletion and tissue oxygenation.

Guidelines for adequacy of resuscitation have been proposed to provide an objective level to guide the timing of definitive fracture fixation. Early results suggest that a patient with improving acidosis, as measured by pH $\geq$ 7.25, base excess $\geq$ –5.5 mmol/L, or lactate < 4.0 mmol/L will benefit from definitive fracture care, as long as severe head injury or other medical pathology do not preclude it. These parameters have been termed "early appropriate care" (EAC), and surgical stabilization of spine, pelvis, acetabulum, and femur fractures is recommended within 36 hours of injury.[22]

Secondary parameters of trauma management

Soft tissue: swelling, wounds

Many high-energy musculoskeletal injuries are associated with severe soft tissue damage or destruction. Although open fractures and unstable femoral and pelvic fractures are managed urgently, many fractures of the extremities are managed provisionally with splinting or external fixation until the soft tissues have healed sufficiently to tolerate additional surgical incisions.[17,18] Articular fractures, involving joint surfaces, demand strict attention to anatomic reduction and rigid internal fixation, commonly with plates and screws. Many of these fractures are definitively treated on a delayed basis, several days or even weeks after injury, to allow for swelling around the fracture to decrease. This reduces risks of wound healing problems and infections. In some cases definitive management is with external fixation, depending on the injury and patient characteristics.

Nutrition

Adequate nutrition is essential for healing of wounds and fractures. Trauma increases caloric needs, making it difficult to maintain body weight and protein stores during the healing period. The burden of multiple trauma and the inability to take food by mouth, possibly due to associated injuries which may necessitate ventilatory support, lead to a catabolic state after injury. Inadequate nutrition is associated with increased risks of infection, wound and fracture healing problems, and decubitus ulcers. Trauma also produces stress, which leads to more gastric acid production and increased intestinal translocation of bacteria. Early enteral nutrition will mitigate these issues in trauma patients. Sometimes it is prudent to delay reconstructive procedures associated with fractures until nutrition has been optimized.

Musculoskeletal emergencies

Major orthopedic trauma occurs in approximately 80% of multiply injured patients. The incidence of orthopedic trauma in these patients is approximately equal to the incidence of head injury, twice that of thoracic injury, and four times that of abdominal injury.[49–51] The following discussion will provide a basic approach to musculoskeletal trauma, including the pelvis and extremities. It will describe mechanisms of injury and resultant pathology and will outline initial treatment measures. Emergent and urgent injuries will be reviewed and treatment guidelines will be discussed.

Life-threatening injuries

Musculoskeletal injuries can be life-threatening when they are associated with massive hemorrhage. Bleeding can be due to an isolated fracture or the combination of multiple fractures and blood loss from other body systems. Pelvic fractures and bilateral femur fractures are the two most frequent injuries that can cause bleeding of this magnitude. Usually this bleeding will be into a closed space – not immediately obvious to the examiner. Open fractures with extensive soft tissue destruction and/or arterial injury, in addition to being limb-threatening, are also life-threatening because of the amount of associated hemorrhage.

Pelvic ring injuries

Certain pelvic fractures can be associated with blood loss of several liters. Very large forces are required to disrupt the stability of the pelvis. Unstable pelvic fractures have mortality rates of 10–21%.[52–58] Urgent resuscitation and early stabilization can minimize morbidity and mortality in these patients. A basic understanding of the fracture pattern, anatomy, and biomechanics is therefore essential for treatment.

The pelvis is a bony ring composed of two innominate bones and the sacrum (Fig. 27.1). Pelvic stability comes primarily from the posterior sacroiliac complex, providing about 60% of the ring stiffness.[56,57] The pelvic floor and the symphysis pubis also contribute to pelvic stability. Because of its ring structure, if the pelvis is fractured in one location, another fracture or dislocation is very likely to be present. Injuries to the pelvic ring may be classified based on the direction of initial impact. Progressive force in a given direction will generate instability of pelvic structures in a predictable fashion. Associated injuries and blood loss are associated with the pattern of pelvic fractures based on the direction of impact.[49,52,54,56,58,59]

Anteroposterior injuries occur with direct force to the anterior pelvis or external rotation force to the hemipelvis

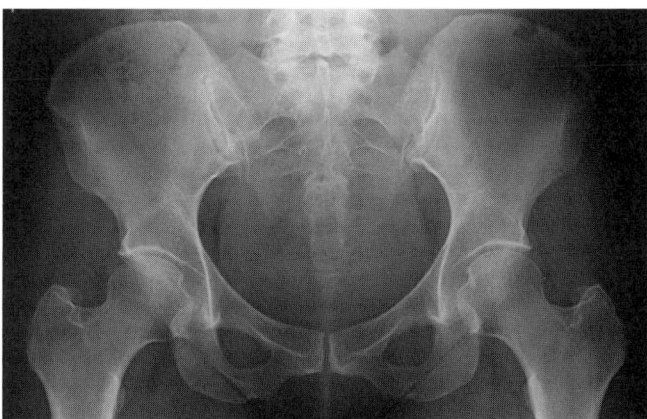

Figure 27.1 The pelvis is a bony ring consisting of the two innominate bones and the sacrum. Sacroiliac ligaments, sacrospinous ligaments, sacrotuberous ligaments, and the symphysis pubis are important stabilizing elements depicted on this anteroposterior pelvis radiograph.

through the femur. These commonly occur in head-on motor vehicle collisions or in crush injuries. Forces "open" the anterior pelvic ring by externally rotating the innominate bones. The pubic symphysis may fracture and widen – the so-called open-book pelvis fracture – and/or the pubic rami may fracture (Fig. 27.2). Continued forces produce fractures and dislocations to the posterior pelvic ring, ultimately resulting in displacement of one or both hemipelves. The amount of bleeding associated with a pelvic fracture is related to the magnitude of displacement of the posterior pelvic ring.[49,52,58] Because a single pelvis radiograph depicts only one point in time, it does not necessarily demonstrate the degree of displacement that occurred at the time of the injury. A high index of suspicion for significant bleeding is essential when the diagnosis of an open-book pelvic fracture is made. Prompt physiological assessment for hemodynamic instability is imperative.

Lateral compression injuries are due to lateral impact to the pelvis. Most often this happens in a motor vehicle collision or a fall onto the side. Impaction of the sacrum on the side of the forces is usually seen, along with pubic ramus fractures, as the affected hemipelvis internally rotates (Fig. 27.3). This is the most common pelvic fracture pattern. Progressive force can completely destabilize the affected hemipelvis, producing a sacroiliac dislocation or fracture–dislocation. Lastly, the contralateral hemipelvis can become unstable, rotating externally. Blood loss and neurological injuries are generally related to the magnitude of displacement of the posterior pelvic ring, although massive hemorrhage is much less likely with this injury pattern than with an open-book fracture.[49,52,57,60,61]

So-called vertical shear injuries are caused by axial force to the pelvis. Vertical shear injuries are often the result of a fall from a height or a motorcycle crash. The affected hemipelvis will be displaced superiorly, creating instability of the posterior pelvic ring (Fig. 27.4). Concomitant stretching of the lumbosacral plexus and vascular structures are frequent with this fracture pattern. Associated hemorrhage can be extremely severe, depending on the magnitude of posterior pelvic displacement.

Other musculoskeletal injuries occur with 60–80% of pelvic ring fractures.[49,51,52] Severe open-book pelvic fractures and vertical shear fracture patterns are often associated with other injuries. Vertical shear fractures frequently occur with multiple other fractures in the same lower extremity. Open-book fractures often occur with severe abdominal and chest trauma. With each of these types of pelvic fracture, the pelvic fracture has a high propensity to cause massive hemorrhage. In contrast, lateral compression pelvic ring fractures are not associated with as much bleeding, and thus associated head injuries and abdominal injuries are potentially more problematic than the pelvic fracture. Whitbeck et al. described 43 patients with complete disruption of the sacroiliac joint and a mortality rate of 21%.[58] Half of those who died succumbed to massive hemorrhage, while 25% of the fatalities were secondary to traumatic brain injury, and the other 25% were due to multiple organ failure over the first several days.

(A)

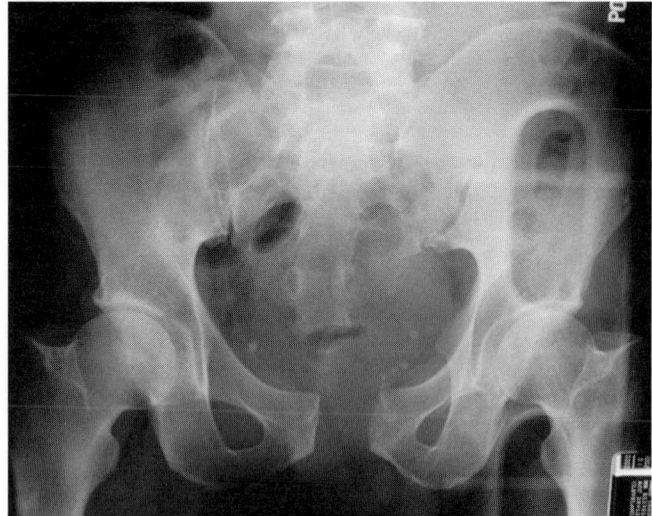

(B)

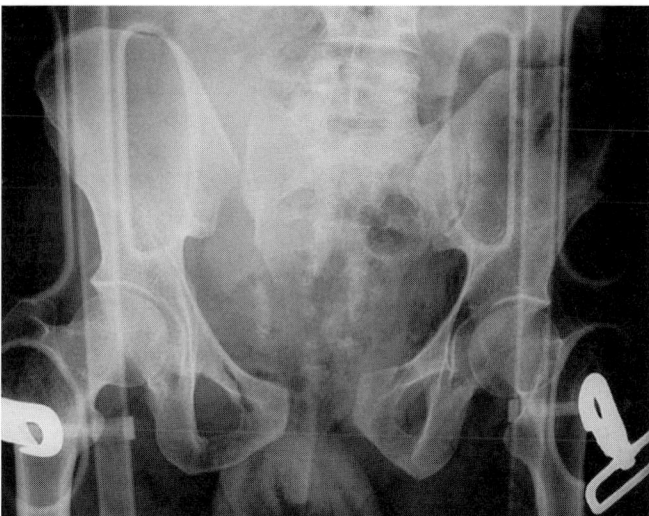

(C)

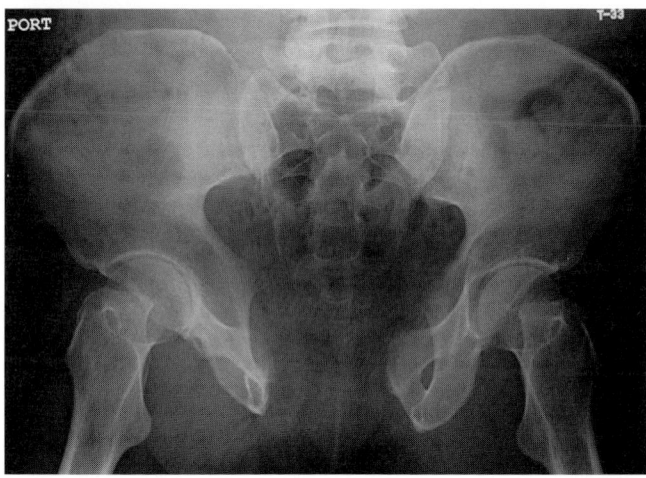

Figure 27.2 Progression of injury to the pelvic ring seen with an anteriorly directed force. This is called an anteroposterior compression (APC) or open-book injury. (**A**) Diastasis of the pubis symphysis occurs. Further force causes external rotation of each hemipelvis, disrupting the posterior pelvic ring. The sacroiliac joints may be dislocated (**B**) on one side or (**C**) bilaterally. With increased displacement of the posterior pelvic ring, more bleeding will occur.

In order to minimize mortality, acute management of unstable pelvic fractures must first address bleeding. Open fractures, urogenital trauma, and gastrointestinal injury in conjunction with pelvic fractures are infrequent, and are also considered surgical emergencies.[50,53,62]

Bleeding is the most frequent initial problem associated with pelvic fractures. Three sources of bleeding may be seen: bony, venous, and arterial. Blood loss secondary to the fractured bone surfaces is usually insignificant. However, the proximity of major branches of the iliac vessels to the sacroiliac joints results in bleeding when the posterior pelvic ring is displaced. Bleeding from the sacral venous plexus can be extensive, with blood loss up to 3–10 liters. The retroperitoneum of the intact pelvis can hold 4 L of blood before tamponade occurs. Since the pelvis is shaped like a cone, the volume available for blood to accumulate is proportionate to the radius cubed. Initial management should consist of provisional reduction of open-book patterns (reducing the size of the pelvis radius), by manually closing the pelvic ring with a sheet or binder.[63] This decreases the pelvic volume and will rapidly tamponade bleeding from the sacral plexus (Fig. 27.5).

Very rarely there is major arterial injury associated with fracture of the pelvic ring. This occurs in about 6–8% of unstable pelvic fractures.[59,64] Angiography and embolization or pelvic packing are life-saving measures in patients with an arterial injury.[53,65–67] If the patient is unresponsive and severely hypotensive, despite aggressive fluid replacement and pelvic reduction, emergent angiography should be performed to stop arterial bleeding (Figs. 27.6, 27.7).

Urgent surgical interventions in patients with unstable pelvic fractures are aimed at provisional or definitive reduction and stabilization of the pelvic ring, which promotes tamponade by reducing the bleeding from bone surfaces and decreasing the pelvic volume to a normal level. Fortunately, modern techniques of surgical stabilization for sacroiliac dislocations and fracture–dislocations are usually performed percutaneously with fluoroscopic assistance in the supine position.[68]

(A)

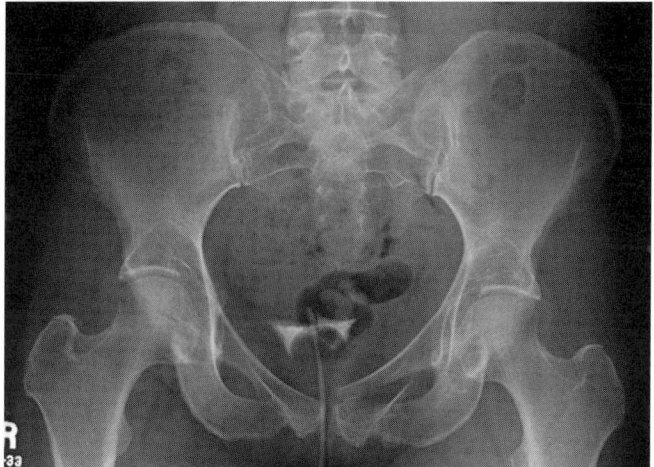

(B)

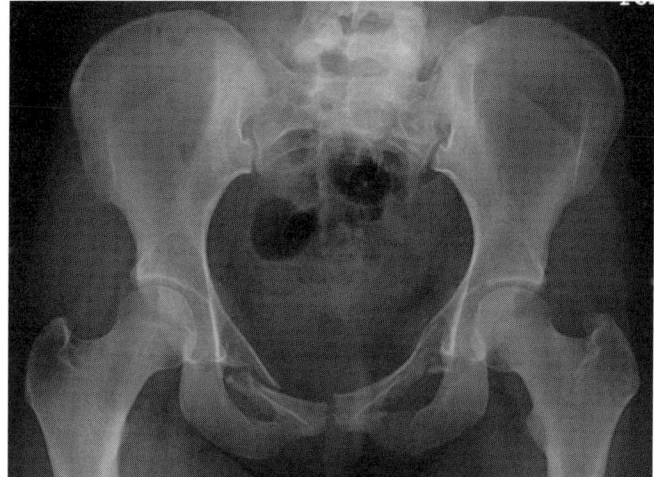

(C)

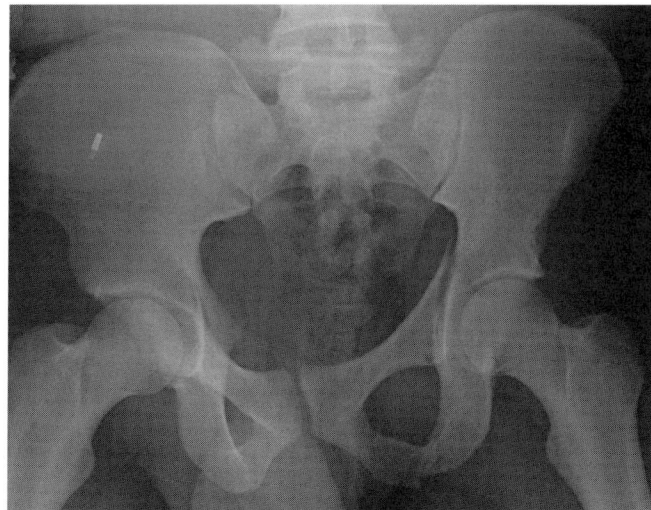

Figure 27.3 Progression of injury to the pelvic ring seen with a laterally directed force. This is called a lateral compression injury (LC) and is the most common pattern of pelvic fracture. This force causes disruption of the ipsilateral posterior pelvic ring, in the form of (**A**) an anterior sacral fracture and pubic ramus fractures. With continued force, (**B**) the posterior pelvic ring will dislocate, and eventually (**C**) the contralateral hemipelvis will experience an external rotation deformity.

This minimizes surgical time and blood loss. Reduction and stabilization of the anterior pelvic ring are often performed during the same surgical procedure (Fig. 27.8). Whenever possible, expeditious definitive management is undertaken.[14,16,49,63,69] This may consist of open reduction and internal fixation of a symphyseal disruption or anterior pelvic external fixation.[40]

Special mention should be made of open pelvic fractures. In addition to the pelvic ring injury and associated hemorrhage and neurological insult, visceral injuries are more common, and a high rate of infection is seen. Mortality of open pelvic fractures historically approached 50%.[53,54,62] Control of bleeding is the most important initial measure, followed by debridement and packing of open wounds. Diverting colostomy should be considered in patients with posterior or perineal wounds or rectal trauma.[70,71] Extraperitoneal bladder tears are repaired in patients with surgically treated anterior pelvic fractures. This reduces the risk of

pelvis osteomyelitis. A team approach, including anesthesiology, general surgery, orthopedics, urology, and gynecology, is essential in the management of these complex, often critically ill patients.[59]

Long-bone fractures

Life-threatening hemorrhage can occur with bilateral femoral shaft fractures or multiple long-bone fractures, with mortality rates of up to 25%.[72–75] Although this group of patients is likely to have major injuries to other systems, which would increase mortality risk, the hemorrhage associated with multiple long-bone fractures is impressive. Mean blood loss associated with a femoral shaft fracture is 1500 mL, and for a humeral or tibial shaft fracture it is 750 mL. This does *not* include additional bleeding generated by surgery. Frequently the fracture hematoma is within a closed space, not immediately obvious to the examiner, which can result in a

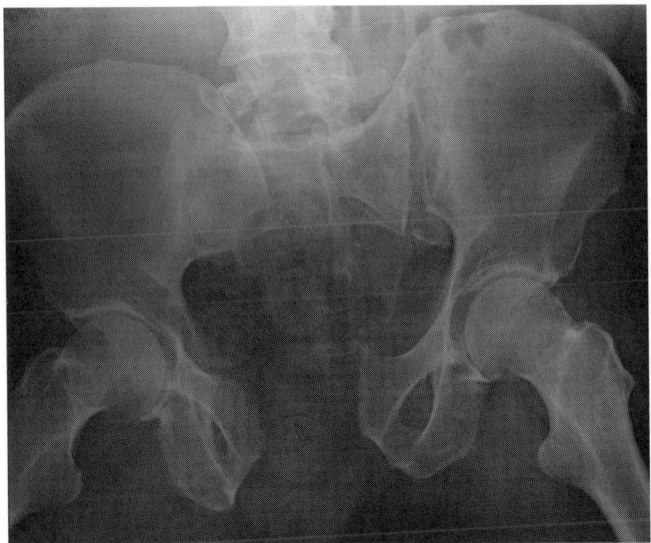

Figure 27.4 An axial force to the pelvis through one of the legs causes significant instability of the pelvic ring due to injuries of the pubic symphysis or rami as well as the entire posterior ligamentous complex. The affected hemipelvis displaces superiorly, which is called a vertical shear injury. The magnitude of posterior pelvic ring injury correlates with the amount of bleeding.

(A)

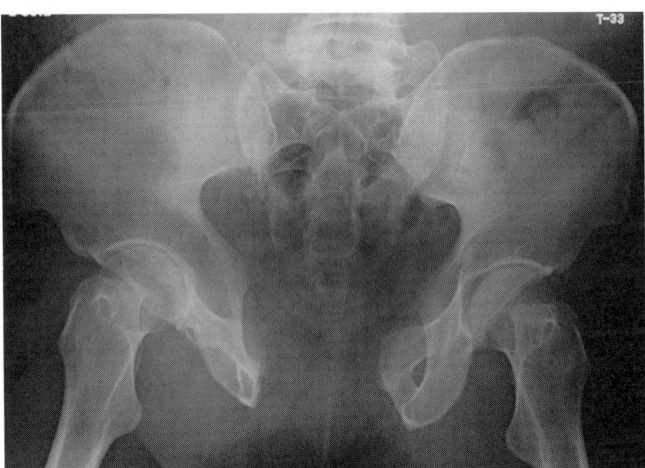

(C)

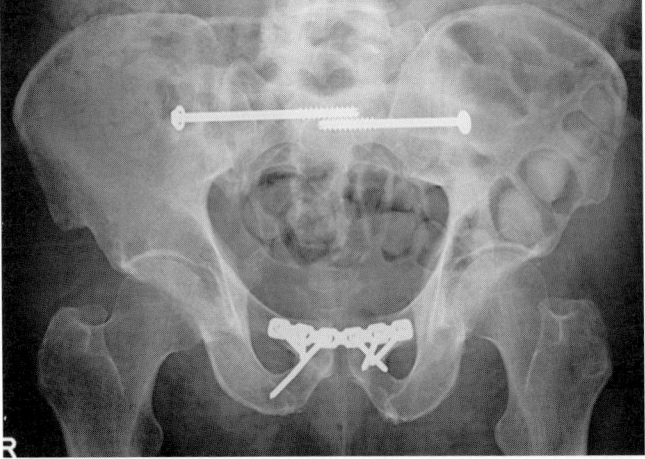

dangerous delay in resuscitation. Immediate treatment measures should be undertaken when bilateral femur fractures or multiple long-bone fractures are identified. Central access or two large-bore intravenous lines is recommended (see Chapter 5).

Most femoral and tibial shaft fractures in adults are definitively treated with reamed intramedullary nailing. Unstable femoral fractures are usually fixed within 24 hours of injury to reduce the risk of pulmonary complications.[9,22,23,33] Fixation eliminates the need for skeletal traction and recumbency. It also provides control of bleeding from the fracture, and thus it is considered part of the resuscitation. During surgery, careful monitoring by the anesthesia team is crucial. Adjunctive volume replacement will depend on the pattern and number of fractures, as well as other injuries contributing to bleeding.

Isolated femoral shaft fractures may be treated on a fracture table in a lateral or supine position, depending on surgeon preference. However, most patients with multiple long-bone fractures are treated in a supine position on a flat radiolucent operating table, which will facilitate surgical access and

(B)

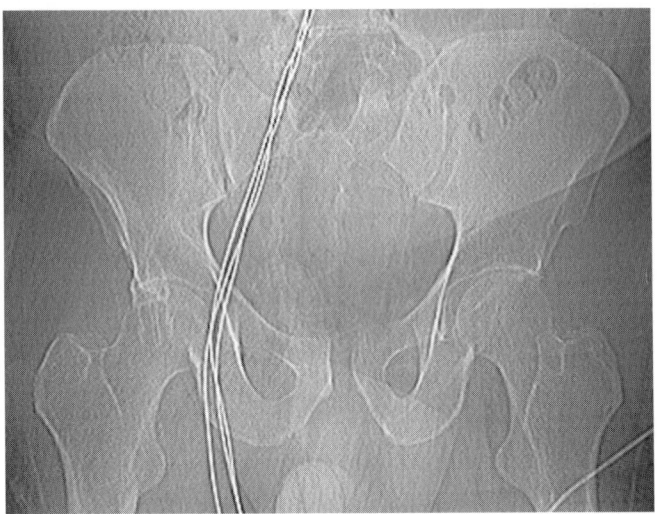

Figure 27.5 (**A**) An open-book pelvic fracture with bilateral sacroiliac dislocations will result in massive, possibly life-threatening hemorrhage. (**B**) Prompt identification and manual reduction of the injury by binding the pelvic ring with a sheet or commercial binder decreases pelvic volume. This also results in improved alignment, comfort, and control of venous bleeding by promoting tamponade. (**C**) Hours later definitive fixation may be undertaken, consisting of percutaneous reduction and fixation of the posterior ring and open reduction and internal fixation of the anterior ring.

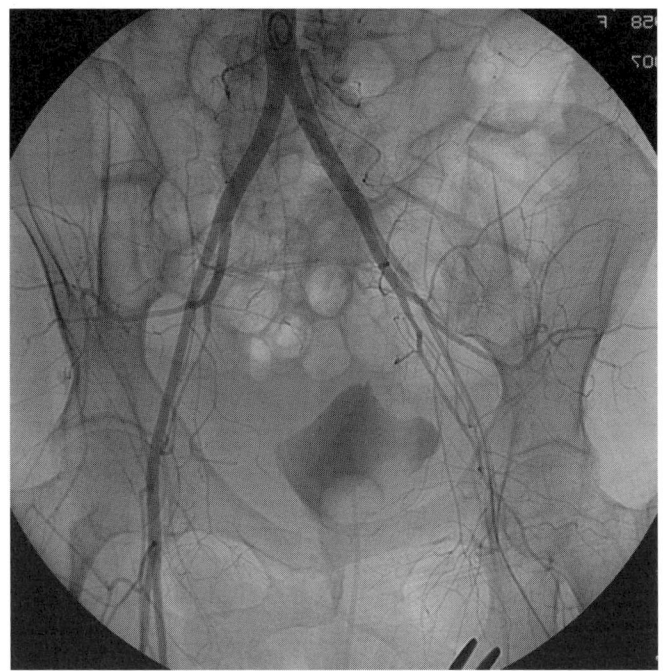

Figure 27.6 Pelvic angiography of a hemodynamically unstable patient with an open-book injury. Initial sheeting and fluid resuscitation did not improve his hypotension, and emergent angiography revealed injury to the external iliac artery.

radiographic imaging for all the injuries. Neuromuscular blockade (full paralysis) assists the surgeon in reducing fractures. Intramedullary nailing is often a percutaneous procedure (Fig. 27.9). The surgery itself is not likely to generate substantial bleeding; however, blood loss from long-bone fractures should not be underestimated. Occasionally, in a critically ill patient, provisional external fixation (damage control orthopedics) is used to stabilize long-bone fractures, as this can be accomplished in several minutes with minimal bleeding (Fig. 27.10). This strategy is employed only in those patients who cannot tolerate early definitive fixation, most often secondary to severe head injury or cardiac dysfunction.[27,31,39]

Limb-threatening injuries

Traumatic amputation

Traumatic amputation and near-amputation are severe open fractures. Direct pressure to control bleeding is imperative, as is expeditious antibiotic and tetanus prophylaxis for any open fracture. Reimplantation, especially with certain hand injuries, and salvage of near-amputation may be possible, if this can be completed within the first several hours of injury. Crush injuries, prolonged ischemia time, severe trauma elsewhere in the limb, serious systemic injury, advanced age, and underlying

Figure 27.7 An algorithm for evaluation and treatment of unstable pelvic ring injury.

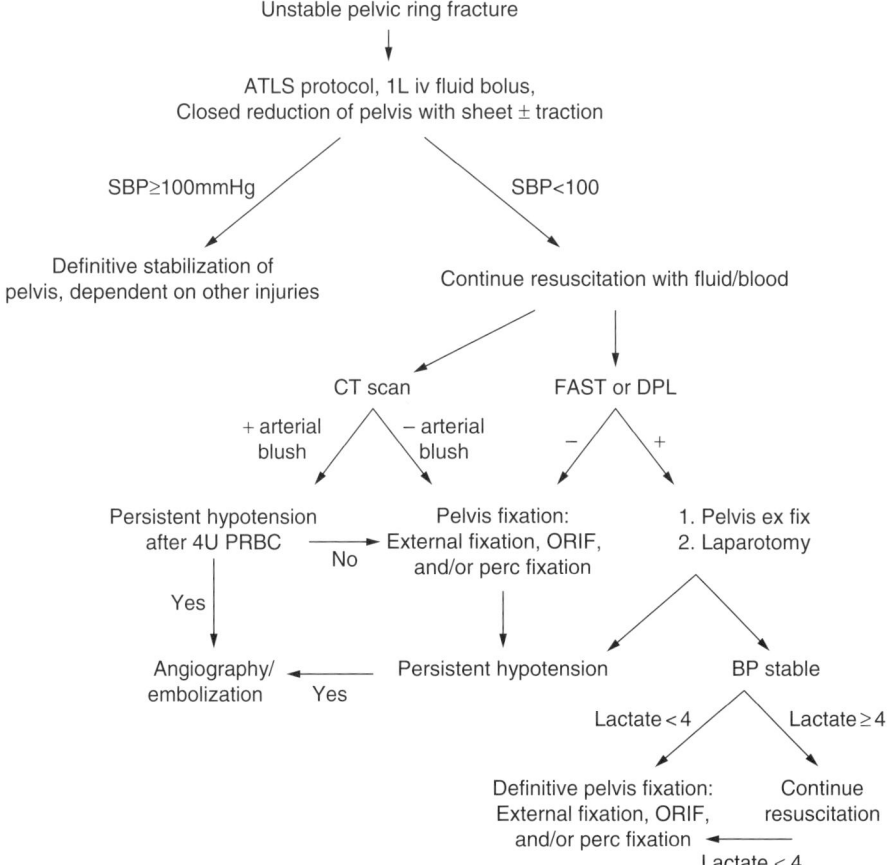

(A)

(B)

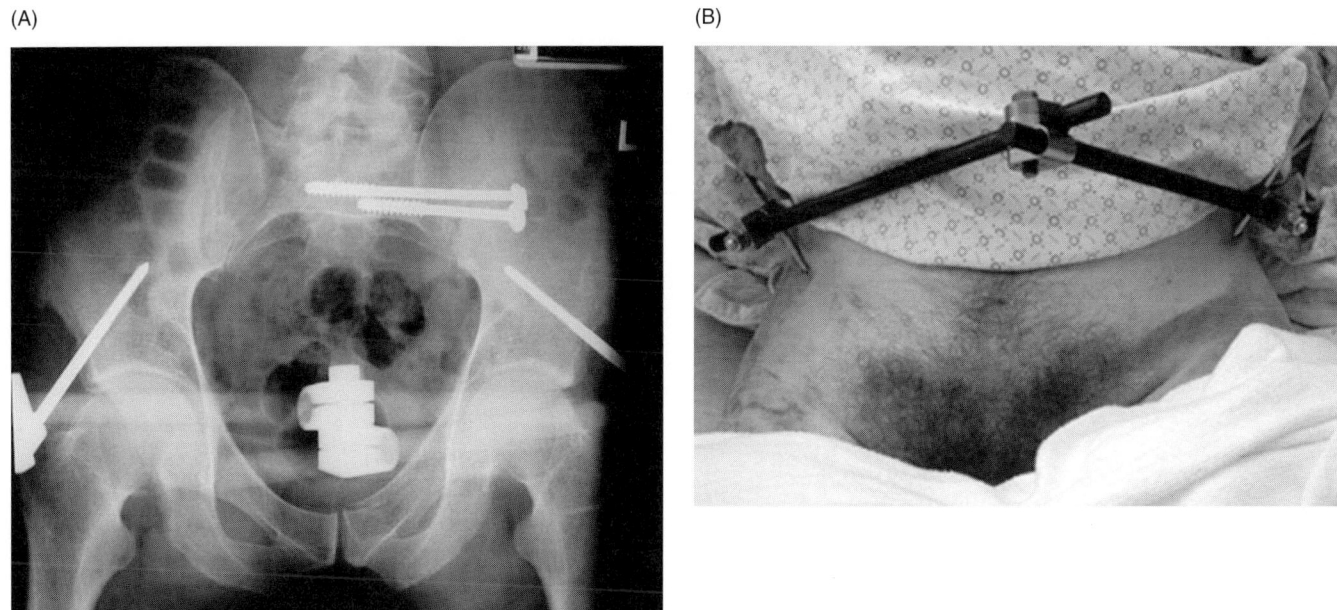

Figure 27.8 (**A**) Anteroposterior pelvis radiograph after reduction and fixation of an unstable pelvis fracture. The alignment of the pelvic ring has been restored and screws stabilize the left sacroiliac joint. (**B**) An anterior external fixator has been applied, as shown in the clinical photograph. *A black and white version of this figure will appear in some formats. For the color version, please refer to the plate section.*

(A)

(B)

(C)

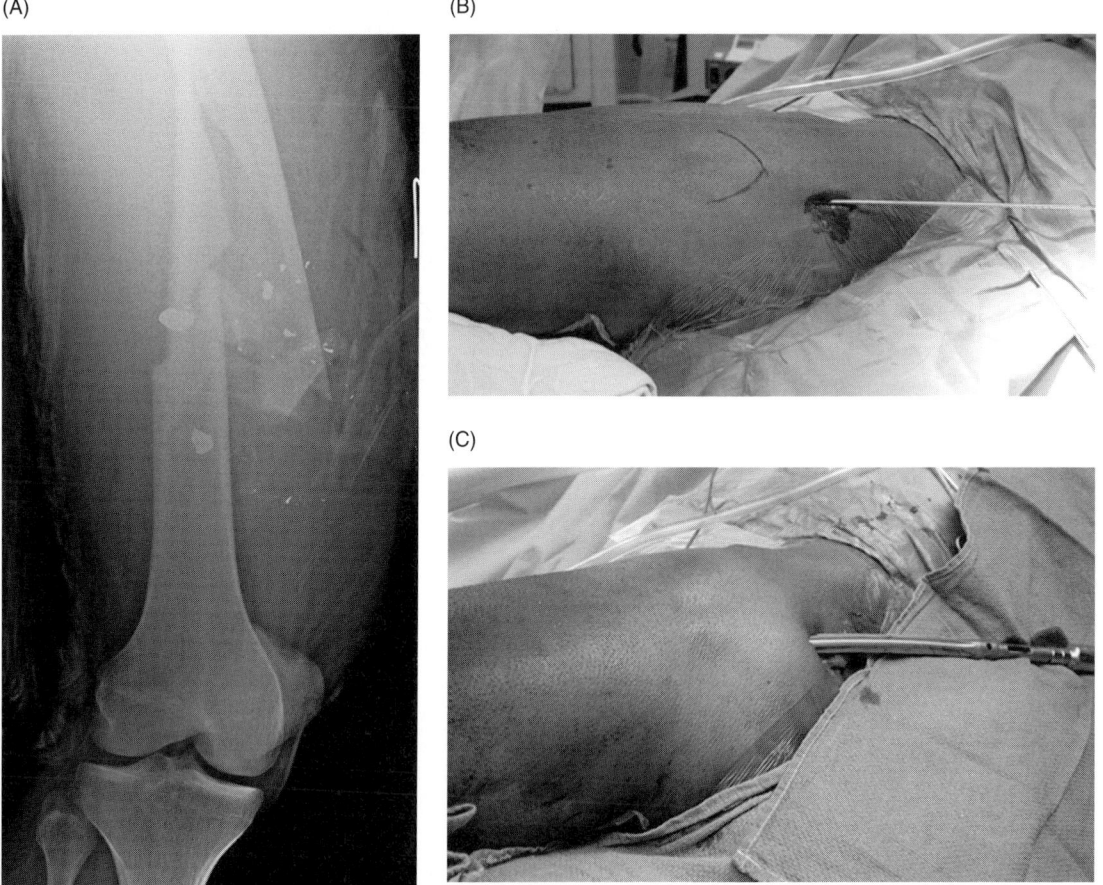

Figure 27.9 (**A**) Intramedullary nailing of a femoral shaft fracture can be done percutaneously. (**B**) A wire placed with fluoroscopic assistance opens the femoral canal. (**C**) After reduction and reaming a nail is placed. Minimal surgical trauma occurs during this procedure. (**D**) This photograph demonstrates the small wounds from the nail and the locking bolts. (**E**) Anteroposterior radiograph of the healed femur fracture 4 months after intramedullary nail. *A black and white version of this figure will appear in some formats. For the color version, please refer to the plate section.*

(D)

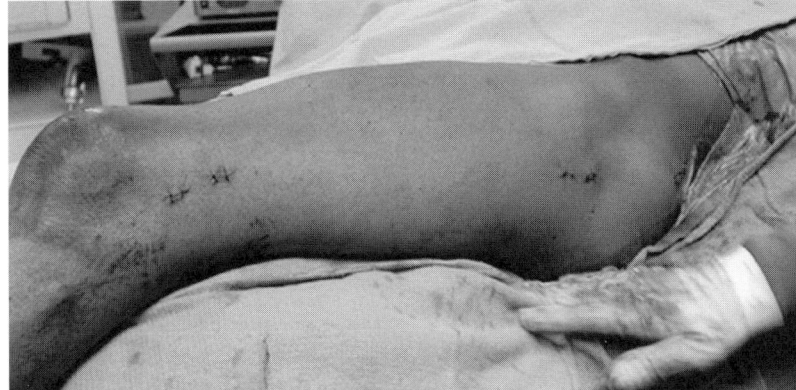

(E)

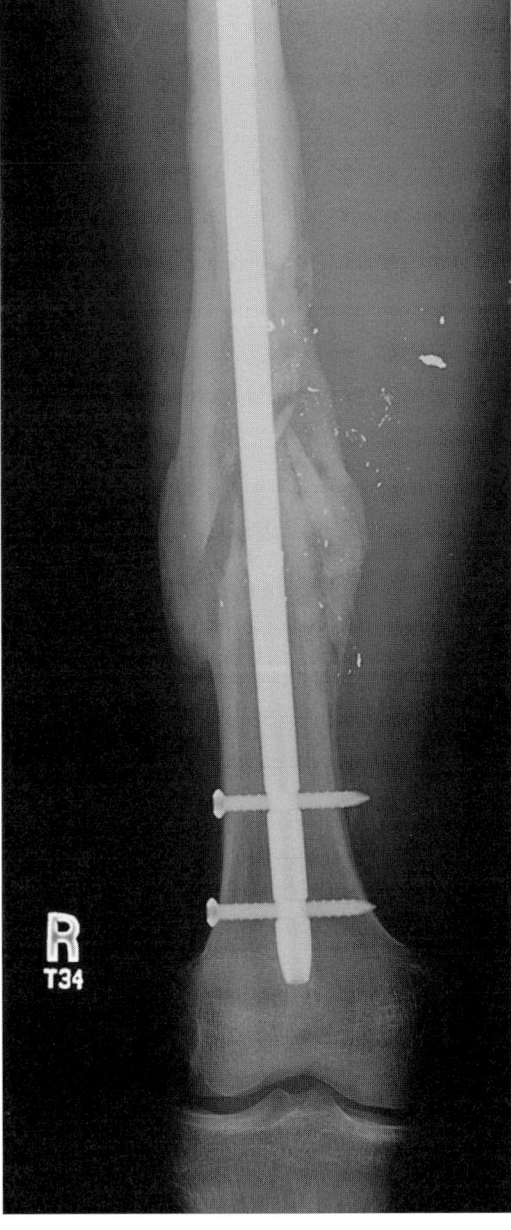

Figure 27.9 *(cont.)*

medical conditions are factors decreasing the likelihood of successful salvage.[76–78] Emergent surgery is recommended to examine the affected area, perform surgical debridement, and control hemorrhage.

In rare cases, amputation is undertaken to stop bleeding in a severely mangled extremity with multiple fractures and severe soft tissue destruction. This can be life-saving and can reduce the wound and injury burden in a multiply injured person. More commonly salvage is attempted with provisional or definitive stabilization of fractures. External fixation is a rapid means of stabilizing fractures in patients who are

critically ill and underresuscitated. External fixation can generally be performed in several minutes with minimal surgical trauma. Serial debridement and later definitive fixation (versus amputation) can be done after discussions with the patient and other subspecialists.

Vascular injury

Injury to the major arterial flow to a limb is a surgical emergency. More than 75% of such injuries occur from penetrating trauma, while blunt trauma causing fractures and dislocations is a less common etiology for vascular injury.

(A)

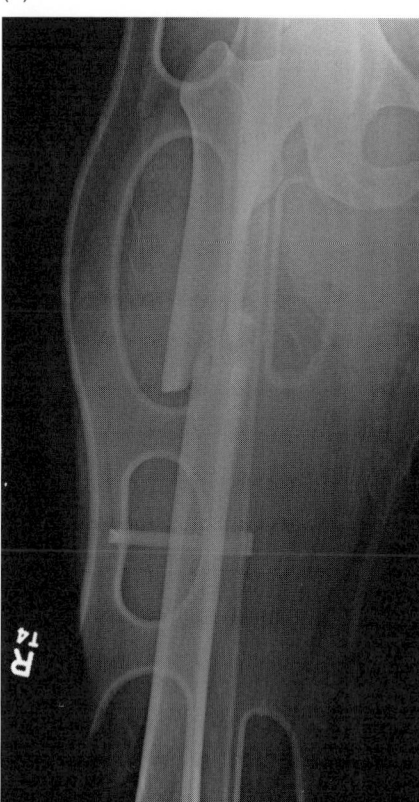

(B)

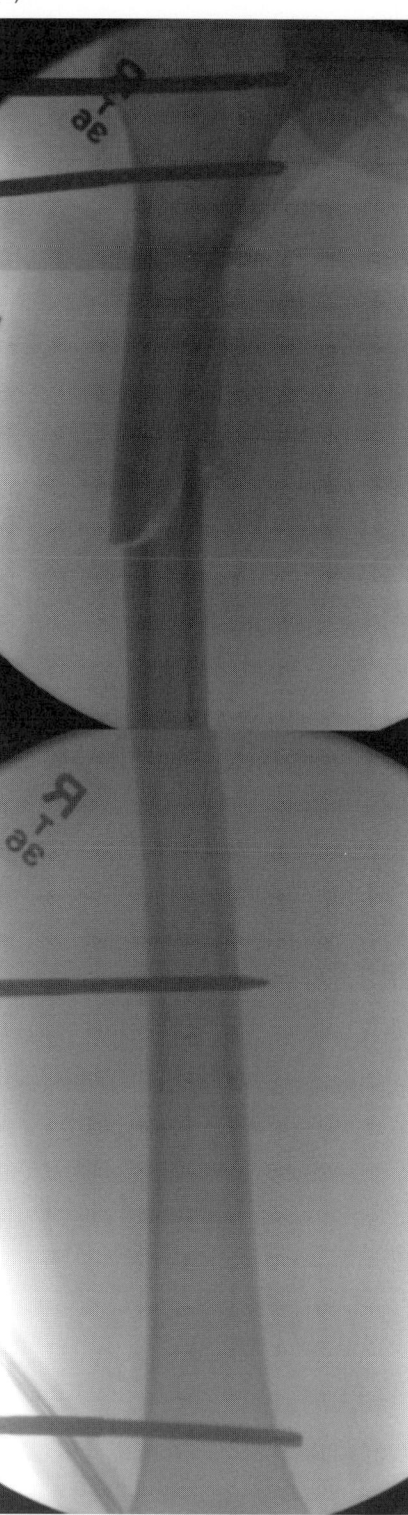

Figure 27.10 (A) A displaced femoral shaft fracture was treated with damage control due to severe subarachnoid hemorrhage with persistently elevated intracranial pressures, which precluded definitive fixation of the fracture. (B) An external fixator can be placed within approximately 20 minutes with minimal blood loss, providing adequate temporary stability for the fracture without ongoing skeletal traction.

Traumatic knee dislocations are an exception to this rule, as the incidence of arterial injury is 16–25% (Fig. 27.11).[79–81] Patients with a major arterial injury present with pallor, coolness, and decreased pulses in an extremity. Massive bleeding or an expanding hematoma may be present. Fracture malalignment, constrictive dressings, and hypotension can cause or contribute to these findings. Dressings should be loosened and fractures should be reduced, followed by rapid reassessment of limb perfusion. When a pulse is palpable or Dopplerable but asymmetrical, a vascular injury is suspected.

(A)

(B)

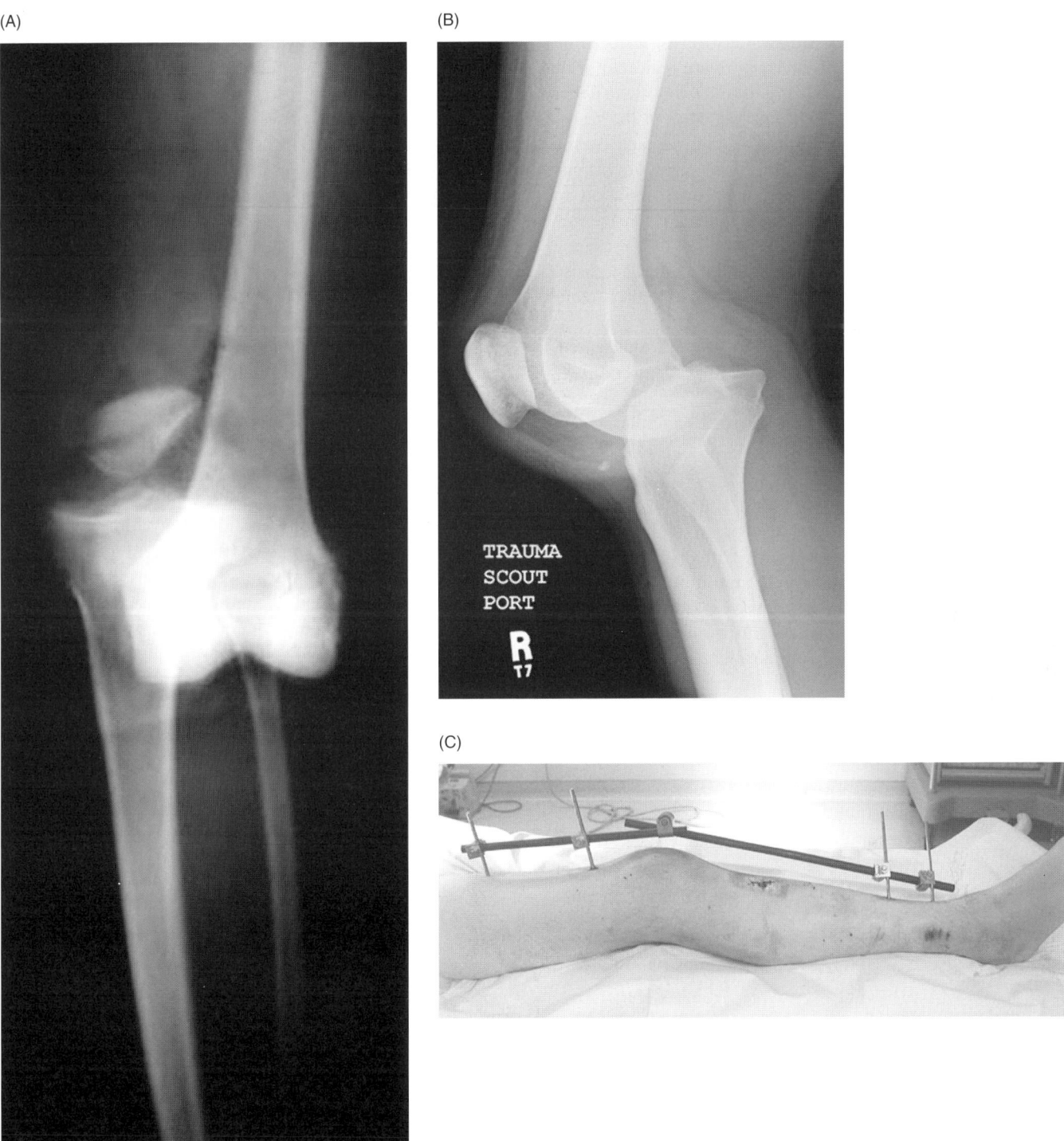

TRAUMA
SCOUT
PORT

R
T7

(C)

Figure 27.11 (A, B) Anteroposterior and lateral radiographs of a knee dislocation. The incidence of arterial injury with a knee dislocation is up to 25%, due to tethering of the popliteal artery at the trifurcation. (C) A spanning external fixator has been placed across the knee joint to maintain the reduction of the knee. *A black and white version of this figure will appear in some formats. For the color version, please refer to the plate section.*

Ankle–brachial indices (ABI) should be obtained in these patients in the emergency room. The ABI is measured by placing a blood pressure cuff on the upper arm and inflating it to obtain a measurement of the systolic pressure. The procedure is then repeated at the ankle of the affected leg. The ABI is the ratio of the systolic pressure of the ankle over the systolic pressure of the arm. If an ABI is less than 0.9, assessment for vascular injury is indicated.[82,83] When an extremity is pulseless despite reduction and splinting, emergent surgical exploration is essential to preserve the limb. Within 6 hours of ischemia, myonecrosis and loss of neurological function will ensue.

When a patient has a major arterial injury requiring revascularization in conjunction with a fracture or dislocation, reduction and stabilization of the fracture are indicated prior to the vascular procedure. Stabilizing the bone first (with either provisional or definitive methods) ensures safety of the vascular repair, thereby avoiding further arterial damage during fracture reduction and fixation. In some cases provisional external fixation may be the most appropriate method in maintaining limb alignment, without requiring extensive surgical time and dissection. Rarely, if several hours of ischemia have transpired, a temporary vascular shunt should be placed to provide flow to the limb before undertaking fracture stabilization. Subsequently, definitive revascularization is performed. Notably, once a limb has been revascularized, distal fasciotomy should be considered to prevent compartment syndrome after the reperfusion occurs. Ongoing resuscitation with blood and fluid replacement by the anesthesia team is an integral part of this process.

Compartment syndrome

Extremity trauma can also lead to compartment syndrome. When the interstitial pressure in a closed osteofascial compartment rises and causes capillary compromise, local tissue becomes ischemic and necrosis begins. Closed or open fractures, severe soft tissue trauma or crush injury, and arterial injury are potential causes of compartment syndrome. Hemorrhage in a closed space, arterial spasm, and reperfusion of an ischemic area are part of the sequential pathophysiology. Compartment syndrome will often develop over a period of hours after injury; thus, careful serial monitoring of patients at risk is extremely important. Compartment syndrome develops from a reduced gradient between diastolic blood pressure and compartment pressure (Fig. 27.12). Compartment ischemia can occur with elevated compartment pressure with normal diastolic pressure, or, in a patient with hypotension, with slightly elevated compartment pressure

Therefore, it is crucial to diligently monitor those severely injured patients who may have prolonged hypotension from bleeding and/or head injury. These patients are at particularly high risk for ischemic damage. Irreversible muscle fiber changes are seen after 6 hours of ischemia, and irreversible nerve damage is seen after 12 hours of ischemia.[84]

The most common locations of compartment syndrome are the lower leg and the volar forearm. Important early signs and symptoms are pain out of proportion to that expected and tense swelling of the affected region. Pain will usually be severe at rest and will increase dramatically with passive motion of the involved muscles. Decreased distal sensation will follow, with a loss of proprioception seen before other types of sensory loss. Complete anesthesia and weakness are late findings, which are not likely to be present until irreversible loss of function has occurred. A high index of suspicion must be maintained in patients with altered states of consciousness or in patients on large doses of pain medication, so that a

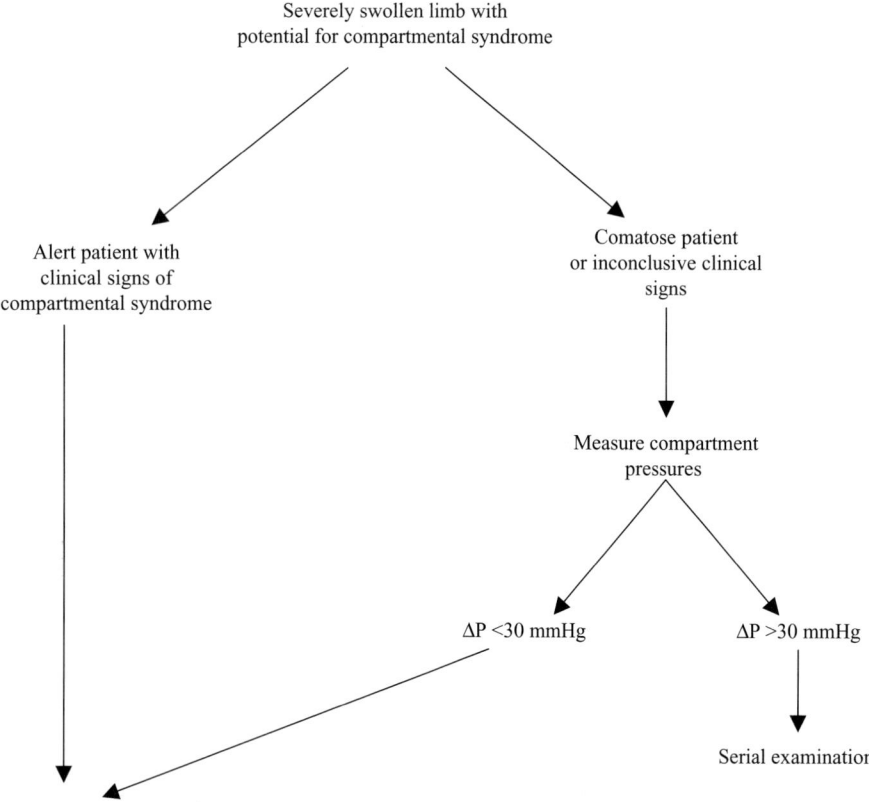

Figure 27.12 An algorithm for evaluation and treatment of compartment syndrome. ΔP indicates the difference in pressure between the diastolic blood pressure and the compartment pressure.[84]

Severely swollen limb with
potential for compartmental syndrome

Alert patient with
clinical signs of
compartmental syndrome

Comatose patient
or inconclusive clinical
signs

Measure compartment
pressures

ΔP <30 mmHg

ΔP >30 mmHg

Serial examination

Fasciotomy

diagnosis of compartment syndrome is not missed. Furthermore, spinal and epidural anesthesia as well as peripheral nerve blocks are contraindicated in patients at risk for compartment syndrome, because clinical findings could be missed – the most important of which is pain out of proportion to what is expected.

If compartment syndrome is diagnosed, the *only* effective treatment is surgical fasciotomy. Without emergent fasciotomy, muscle and nerve damage are imminent, and necrosis will ensue. Fasciotomy is performed by incising the skin over the affected compartments and incising each fascial compartment. This can be completed within minutes. When compartment syndrome is present in association with a fracture, additional treatment to stabilize the fracture is indicated to prevent further insult to the soft tissues. This could include external fixation, but may be definitive internal fixation, depending on the fracture pattern and the overall status of the patient.

Urgent musculoskeletal problems
Surgery recommended within 6–8 hours
Open fracture

Open fractures are classified by their associated soft tissue injury and level of contamination (Table 27.3).[85,86] As the severity increases, so does the risk of infection and other complications. Intravenous antibiotics are administered expeditiously and tetanus immunization is updated. All adult patients with an open fracture should receive a first-generation cephalosporin, such as cefazolin (2 g IV), followed by repeated dosing at a minimum of every 8 hours. With a known cephalosporin allergy, clindamycin is a good alternative (900 mg IV). High-energy open fractures, or cases with gross contamination, should receive Gram-negative coverage as well. Gentamicin (4–5 mg/kg IV every 24 hours) is effective.[87] In an elderly patient or in patients with renal insufficiency,

levofloxacin 500 mg may be given instead of gentamicin. Fractures with soil contamination should also be treated with penicillin, 4 million units IV every 4 hours, in order to treat anaerobes, especially *Clostridia*.[85,86]

Open fractures are surgical emergencies. After a delay of 6–8 hours from the time of injury, infection rates begin to rise, particularly for high-energy fractures.[85,86,88] Debridement and irrigation in the operating room are recommended. These are generally combined with provisional or definitive fixation, as soon as is safely possible. Stabilization of an open fracture provides support to the surrounding soft tissues and decreases the risk of infection.[89,90] Occasionally, provisional external fixation is preferred, because of massive contamination, surgical delay, or instability of the patient due to hemorrhage or head injury. Muscular relaxation during the procedure facilitates reduction of the fracture.

Traumatic arthrotomy

Some injuries will produce a wound that communicates with an underlying joint. When a traumatic arthrotomy is present, intravenous antibiotics and tetanus are administered, similar to an open fracture. Urgent surgical debridement and irrigation of the joint are recommended to decrease the risk of infection. This should be undertaken within the first several hours of injury.

Dislocations

Dislocated joints cause significant pain and deformity, along with impairment of motion. Some dislocations are associated with neurological or vascular injuries (Table 27.4).[79–81,91,92] A dislocated joint should be anatomically reduced as soon as possible, and stabilized as indicated to prevent recurrence. Neuromuscular paralysis is necessary for reductions to be performed safely. Closed reductions, in which the dislocation is manually manipulated without surgery, are possible in most cases. Some dislocations are most safely undertaken in the operating room under general anesthesia. This permits

Table 27.3 Classification of open fractures[85,86]

Type 1	Wound 1 cm or less in length, clean, low-energy injury with minimal soft tissue damage and simple fracture pattern.
Type 2	Wound more than 1 cm in length. More extensive soft tissue damage with flaps, avulsion, or crush components.
Type 3A	Severe soft tissue damage and high-energy wound of variable size, but adequately covering bone. Includes some gunshot injuries.
Type 3B	Type 3 injuries with extensive bone exposure and necessitating flap coverage. Also includes less complex wounds with gross contamination and shotgun blasts.
Type 3C	Type 3 injuries with vascular lesion requiring repair to preserve limb viability.

Table 27.4 Fractures and dislocations associated with neurological or vascular injury

Fracture or dislocation	Structure injured
Clavicle or first rib fracture	Subclavian artery
Shoulder dislocation	Axillary artery or nerve
Humeral shaft fracture	Radial nerve
Supracondylar humerus fracture	Brachial artery
Hip dislocation	Sciatic nerve
Femoral shaft fracture	Superficial femoral artery
Supracondylar femur fracture	Popliteal artery
Knee dislocation	Popliteal artery, common peroneal nerve
Proximal tibia or fibula fracture	Common peroneal nerve

(A)

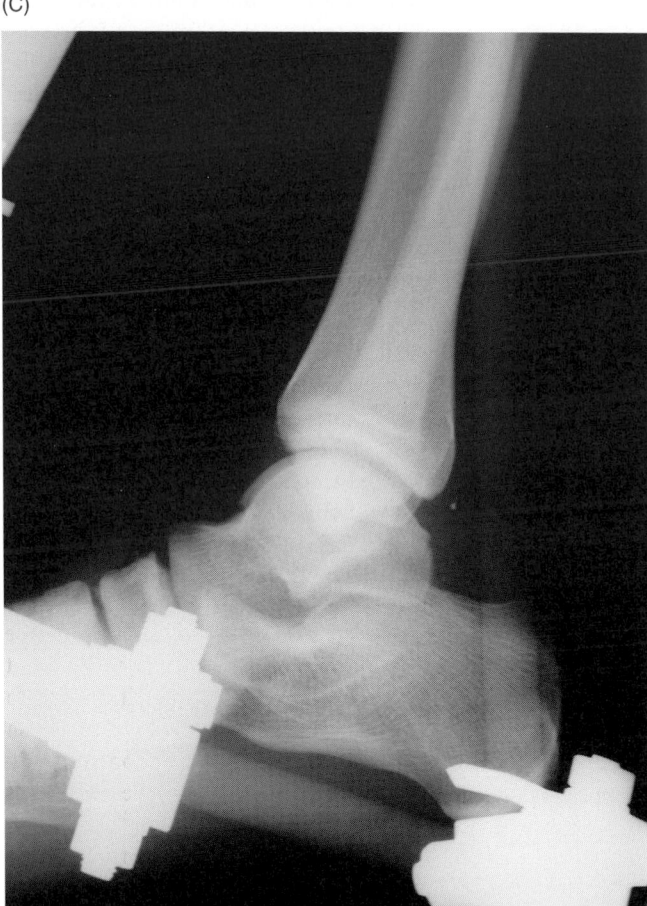

(B)

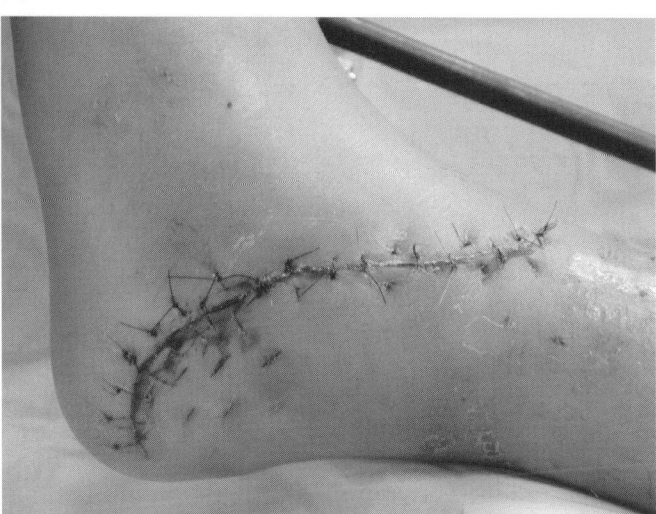

(C)

Figure 27.13 (**A**) A young man sustained injuries including an open dislocation of his talus. Emergent treatment was recommended to debride the wound and reduce the dislocation. (**B,C**) External fixation was used to stabilize the ankle and hindfoot. *A black and white version of this figure will appear in some formats. For the color version, please refer to the plate section.*

optimal neuromuscular blockade (see Chapter 13) and promotes safe airway management. Orthopedic complications such as nerve damage and iatrogenic fracture are kept to a minimum when general anesthesia is used. Dislocations of the subtalar joint and the native hip joint are two examples of

reductions that are often performed in the operating room (Figs. 27.13, 27.14).[92] Rarely a dislocated joint cannot be reduced through closed means, and surgery is required to perform an open reduction. Urgent management of all dislocations is an important goal. Of particular concern are

(A)

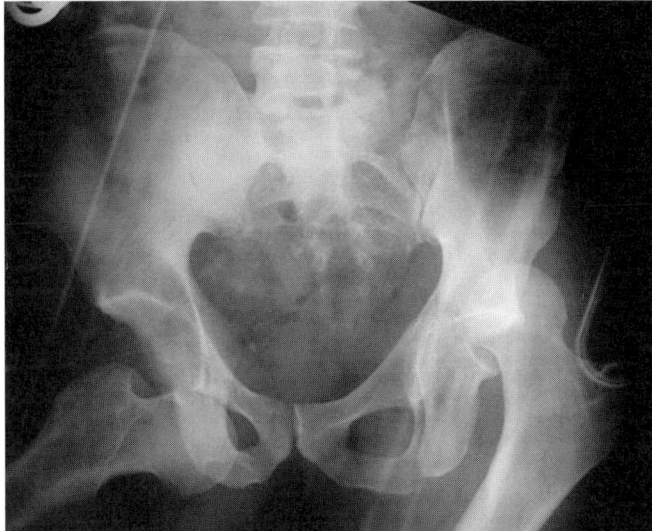

(B)

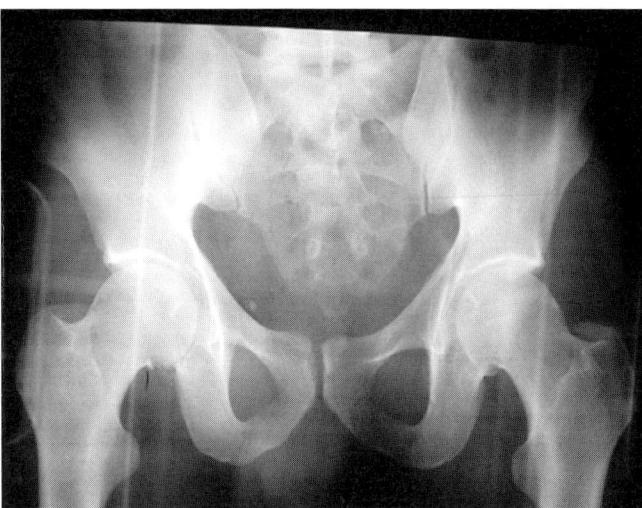

Figure 27.14 (**A**) A young man sustained bilateral hip dislocations in a rollover motor vehicle collision as showed by this anteroposterior radiograph of the pelvis. The right hip has an obturator dislocation, and the left hip has a posterior dislocation. (**B**) Closed reductions were performed under general anesthesia.

dislocations of the talus and of the femoral head, where the duration of the dislocation likely correlates with the development of osteonecrosis, due to stretching of the arteries to these areas.[93–95]

Displaced femoral neck fracture in young adult

Hip fractures occur commonly in general orthopedic practice. Most are low-energy events in elderly people. These are not typically treated as emergencies. On the other hand, young adults may sustain these fractures as the result of high energy-trauma. Reduction and stabilization of the fracture are recommended to reestablish femoral alignment and stability and to promote mobilization from bed. Femoral neck fractures in young adults are considered to be orthopedic emergencies. These should be treated urgently to minimize the potential for osteonecrosis of the femoral head. Osteonecrosis is a devastating complication leading to advanced arthrosis, which may be treated with hip arthrodesis or arthroplasty, neither of which is desirable for a young adult. It is believed that ongoing insult to the arterial supply of the femoral head, caused by displaced intracapsular hip fractures, may be alleviated by open reduction of the fracture. Rigid internal fixation likely optimizes the potential for fracture healing and regeneration of the blood supply to the femoral head.[96,97]

General anesthesia is preferred when performing open reduction of high-energy displaced femoral neck fractures. Some surgeons prefer to perform this procedure on a fracture table with traction against a perineal post. This is done in a supine position. Others prefer supine positioning using manual traction. In all cases, neuromuscular blockade facilitates anatomic reduction of the fracture (Fig. 27.15).

Surgery recommended within 24 hours
Unstable pelvis/acetabulum or femur fracture

Early stabilization of femoral shaft fractures and unstable fractures of the pelvis, acetabulum, or spine reduces complication rates, especially those related to pulmonary compromise and sepsis.[9–16,19–25,32,98] This has been attributed to elimination of prolonged skeletal traction and recumbency.[24] Either definitive or provisional fracture fixation (with external fixation) could serve this purpose. Fixation of long-bone fractures also helps decrease the incidence of fat embolism syndrome.[99,100] Initial traction is a first step in preventing this process; however, definitive stabilization is more efficacious. In most cases this is done with intramedullary nails. The benefits of early stabilization are greater in multiply injured patients than in those with isolated orthopedic injury.[9,16]

Confounding factors such as associated injuries to the head, chest, or abdomen, and the severity of injury, have not been accounted for in most of the published literature to date.[10,12,50,55,98] Treatment of unstable skeletal injury in patients with concomitant head injury is also controversial. Delay in femoral stabilization in this group of patients appears to increase the risk of pulmonary complications.[26] Although the presence of any head injury is not a contraindication to femoral or pelvic stabilization, the question whether early stabilization increases the risk of central nervous system complications has not been answered.[12,23,26,29,101] Optimal treatment timing in this subgroup of patients most likely depends on maintenance of adequate cerebral perfusion pressure (CPP), which is defined as the mean arterial pressure (MAP) minus the intracranial pressure (ICP). Cerebral perfusion pressure of 60–70 mmHg is recommended with a goal ICP less than 20 mmHg (see Chapter 21).[12,26,101] When these

(A) (B) (C)

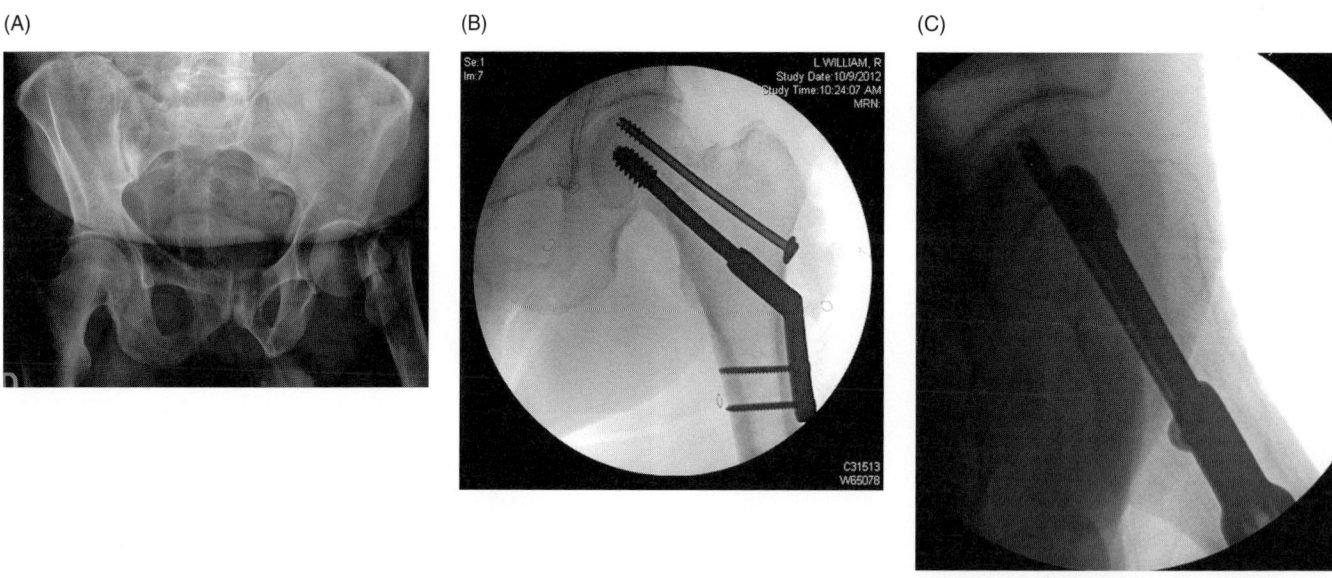

Figure 27.15 (**A**) A young man fell two stories and sustained multiple injuries including a displaced left femoral neck fracture, seen on this anteroposterior radiograph. (**B, C**) Open reduction and internal fixation were performed.

parameters are not met, a damage control tactic using external fixation should be considered.

Concern has also been raised about the optimal treatment for patients with long-bone fractures and chest injury. Intramedullary nailing is the standard of care for most femoral and tibial shaft fractures. Reaming is the mechanical enlargement of the intramedullary canal to provide improved fit of the nail and to permit placement of a larger-diameter nail. Reaming has been speculated to contribute to pulmonary problems in patients with chest injury by producing fat emboli and increasing inflammation. Bosse *et al.* have addressed some of these questions. In a large, retrospective study using carefully matched patients, they compared groups with femoral shaft fracture, femoral shaft fracture and chest injury, and chest injury alone.[10] Femoral shaft fractures were treated within 24 hours of injury with reamed intramedullary nailing or plating (which avoids the potential pulmonary insults from reaming and intramedullary nailing). The incidence of ARDS was 2% overall. There were no differences in the rates of ARDS, pneumonia, multiple organ failure, or death in any of the patient groups after treatment with a plate versus a nail. It is likely that the initial injury burden and associated hemorrhage contribute to an increased risk of complications. Patients who sustain severe chest trauma are more likely to have pulmonary problems. Current practice supports stabilizing femoral fractures within 24 hours of injury with reamed intramedullary nails, even when chest injury is present, in order to minimize adverse pulmonary sequelae.[9,10,13,22,23,102]

Proximal femoral fracture in the elderly (see also Chapter 36)

Hip fractures are among the most common fractures treated by orthopedic surgeons in community practice. Usually they result from a fall from standing height in an elderly person.

In almost all cases, surgical treatment is recommended to repair the fracture or to perform a hip arthroplasty. This provides pain relief and promotes mobility from bed. Mortality associated with hip fractures in the elderly population is substantial, which is primarily a reflection of declining overall health. Mortality approximately doubles when surgery is performed more than 48 hours after injury.[103] Overall, men have mortality rates of 30% within 1 year and 40% within 2 years, and women have mortality rates of approximately 15% within 1 year and 23% within 2 years. Mortality is generally related to underlying functional, mental, and medical status.[104–108] The risk of death increases dramatically with nonoperative management. For this reason, surgery is recommended for nearly all patients with any ambulatory ability. Expeditious medical assessment to provide cardiac risk stratification and to correct any fluid or electrolyte problems is imperative, to prepare them for surgery within 24 hours of the injury.[109] The type of surgical treatment depends on the fracture location and pattern as well as the overall status of the patient.

Femoral neck fractures

Nondisplaced or impacted femoral neck fractures can be treated with screw fixation. These patients are generally placed in a supine position on a fracture table. Neuromuscular relaxation is not required, since the fracture does not need to be reduced. Percutaneous screws may be placed through an incision measuring approximately 5 cm. This procedure does not usually cause much blood loss, and the actual surgical time ranges between 15 and 30 minutes (Fig. 27.16).

Displaced femoral neck fractures in elderly patients are treated with hemiarthroplasty. Surgery is performed in the

(A)

(B)

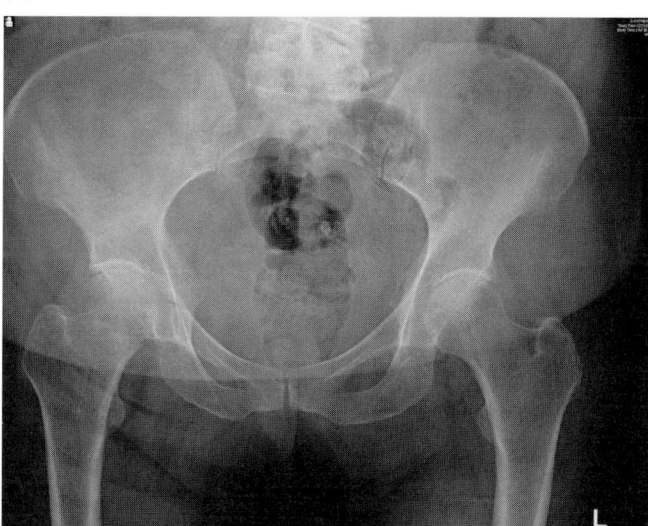
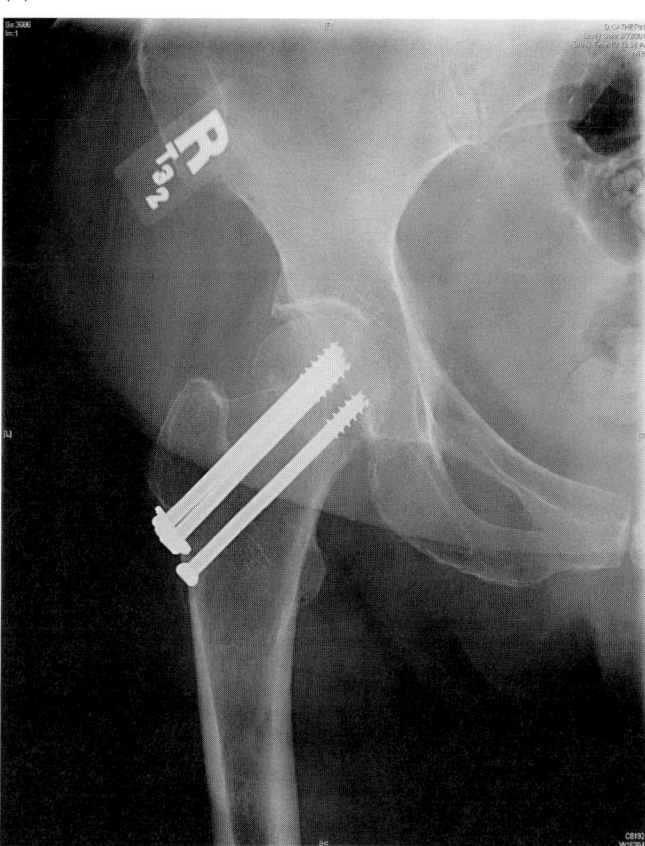

Figure 27.16 (**A**) An elderly woman fell from standing height, sustaining a minimally displaced, impacted right femoral neck fracture. (**B**) Closed reduction and percutaneous pinning was performed.

lateral position. Cement is used to stabilize the prosthesis in most patients with poor bone quality and advanced age. Cementation increases the surgical time and can predispose to hypotension during the pressurization of the cement. Blood loss is substantially increased when comparing hemiarthroplasty with screw fixation, and surgical times range from 30 to 75 minutes (Fig. 27.17).

Intertrochanteric fractures

Intertrochanteric fractures occur in the transitional zone between the femoral neck and the femoral shaft. These fractures usually do not disrupt the blood supply to the femoral head. Generally, patients are physiologically older, with more osteoporosis and dependent functional status, when compared to femoral neck fracture patients.[110] For surgery, they are usually placed in a supine position on a fracture table. A closed reduction is performed before the sterile preparation and drape. Subsequently, the fracture is stabilized with either a plate and screw device or an intramedullary hip screw device, at the discretion of the surgeon. In general, the surgical time and blood loss are slightly less than with a hemiarthroplasty procedure.

Complicating factors

Spine protection

Trauma patients who have been tracheally intubated prior to surgery or who have altered mental status will be unable to complain of neck or back pain. Neurological examination in these patients will not be reliable. Furthermore, patients with major fractures or dislocations have a "distracting injury": that is, the severity of pain and deformity in that area could distract them from complaining of the pain related to a spine injury. Imaging of the spine may be incomplete. Thus, spinal precautions should be used in *all* of these patients. Cervical collars are kept in place and patients should lie flat in bed. A backboard is used for transport, but patients should not be maintained on a backboard for a prolonged period of time. This is painful and can cause skin irritation.

In the operating room, the team should protect the spine by using a log-rolling technique for transfer of the patient to the table. If the cervical collar is to be removed for tracheal intubation, in-line stabilization of the neck should be maintained until the collar is replaced (see Chapters 3 and 23). Care should be taken to ensure that cervical collars are the

(A)

(B)

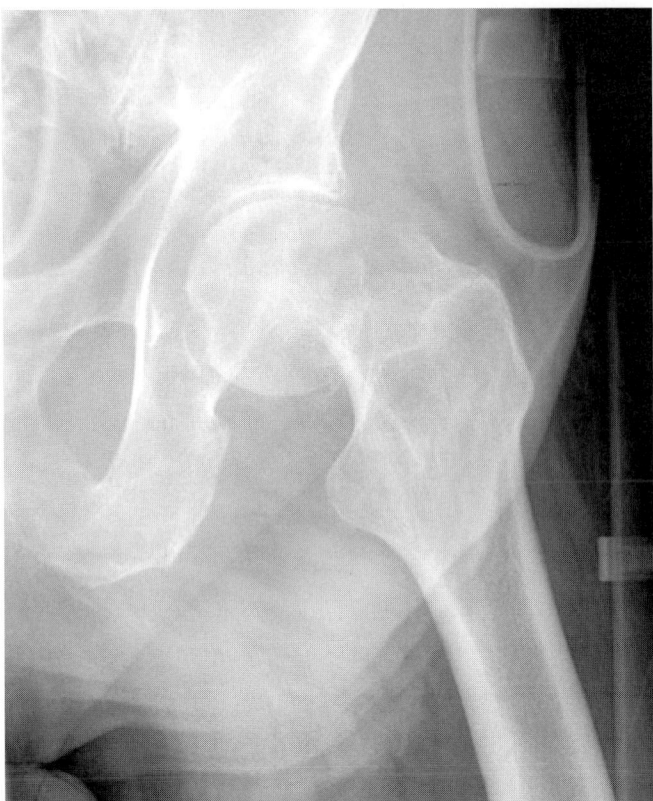
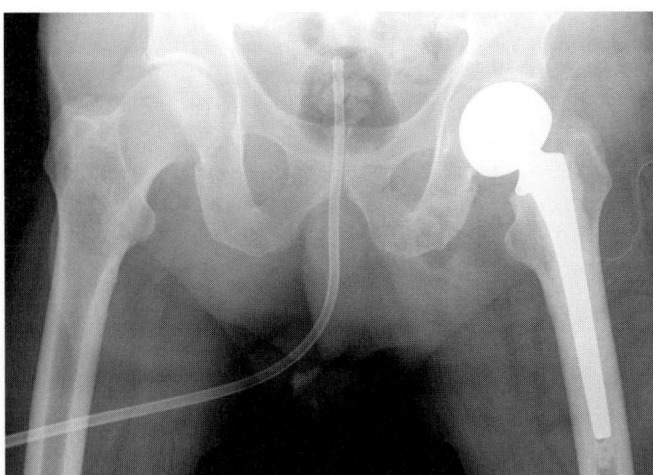

Figure 27.17 (**A**) An elderly man fell, sustaining a displaced femoral neck fracture. (**B**) Hip hemiarthroplasty was performed.

appropriate size and are positioned safely. This is particularly important when positioning a patient prone, which is frequently done to approach an acetabulum or spine fracture.

NPO status

Urgent and emergent procedures are often necessary in patients who have a full stomach or whose history is unknown. Communication between the surgeon and the anesthesiologist regarding rationale for surgery and plan of treatment is important to optimize patient safety and expedite the procedure.

Summary

Musculoskeletal trauma care has evolved to a high level. Treatment goals include resuscitation, pain relief, improved stability and alignment, enhanced mobility, and ultimately restoration of function. History, physical examination, radiographs, and careful assessment of the physiological status of the patient will provide information to determine the timing, type, and sequence of care. A team strategy employing the expertise of critical care specialists, trauma surgeons, orthopedic surgeons, and anesthesiologists is essential in optimizing the management of these patients, who are often critically ill. Some musculoskeletal injuries are life-threatening or limb-threatening. These are treated emergently. Examples include massive

hemorrhage from some pelvic fractures, multiple long-bone fractures, arterial injury in an extremity, and compartment syndrome. Various injuries should be treated on an urgent basis. These include open fractures, where the risk of infection increases after surgical delay. Unstable fractures of the pelvis, acetabulum, or femur, hip fractures, and dislocated joints are also addressed with urgent surgical care. Early fixation of major orthopedic injuries, which would otherwise require bedrest, with or without traction, has been shown to reduce pulmonary complications and hospital stay, both of which are associated with lower hospital costs. It is essential that patients are adequately resuscitated before proceeding with definitive fracture care. The role of damage control orthopedics with provisional external fixation has not been clearly defined; thus communication and collaboration among providers and sound clinical judgment in these cases will optimize outcomes.

Questions

(1) **Potential life-threatening orthopedic injuries include:**
   a. Traumatic amputation of lower leg
   b. Bilateral closed femur fractures
   c. Open-book pelvic fracture
   d. All of the above

(2) **The best initial measure to control bleeding from a pelvic fracture is:**

a. Open reduction and internal fixation of the acetabulum within the first 12 hours after injury
b. Angiography
c. Splenectomy and pelvic packing
d. Reduction of the pelvis with a circumferential sheet or binder

(3) **True or false? In a patient with severe chest trauma, definitive fixation of femur fractures should be delayed for at least 48 hours to minimize the risk of ARDS.**

(4) **The most reliable laboratory parameter to measure the adequacy of resuscitation is:**
a. pH
b. Hematocrit
c. Lactate
d. INR

(5) **True or false? In the first 24 hours after injury, third-generation cephalosporins and fluoroquinolone antibiotics are an acceptable alternative to surgical debridement to minimize infection of open fractures.**

(6) **Which of the following statements about compartment syndrome is correct?**
a. Compartment syndrome develops from a reduced gradient between systolic pressure and compartmental pressure
b. Compartment syndrome should be carefully observed for 6–8 hours before proceeding with fasciotomy
c. Compartment syndrome is seen when the gradient between cerebral perfusion pressure and MAP decreases
d. Compartment syndrome results from increased interstitial pressure in a closed osteofascial compartment, causing ischemia and necrosis of muscle and nerve
e. All of the above

(7) **Damage control orthopedics refers to:**
a. Procedures performed concurrently with the primary and secondary surveys in the emergency room

b. Plating of rib fractures
c. Application of splints or slings for fractures of the femur, pelvis, and acetabulum
d. Provisional application of external fixation for fractures of the femur or pelvis
e. Early stabilization of the spine once the exploratory laparotomy has been completed

(8) **Arterial injury is seen in 16–25% of patients who sustain a:**
a. Knee dislocation
b. Hip fracture–dislocation
c. Pelvic fracture
d. Humerus fracture

(9) **True or false? Patients have mortality of 30–40% in the first year after hip fracture when they are managed nonoperatively.**

(10) **Systemic inflammatory response syndrome (SIRS) may be minimized by:**
a. Judicious resuscitation in patients with multiple system trauma
b. Performing genetic testing upon arrival to the trauma bay
c. Incorporating a spinal rehabilitation protocol
d. Ensuring all spinal, pelvis, and femur fractures are stabilized within 12 hours of injury

Answers

(1) d
(2) d
(3) False
(4) c
(5) False
(6) d
(7) d
(8) a
(9) False
(10) a

References

1. Finkelstein EA, Fiebelkorn IC, Corso PS, Binder SC. Medical expenditures attributable to injuries: United States, 2000. *MMWR Morb Mortal Wkly Rep* 2004; **53**: 1–4.

2. Centers for Disease Control and Prevention. Injury prevention and control: trauma care. www.cdc.gov/TraumaCare (accessed September 2014).

3. National Safety Council. Estimating the costs of unintentional injuries. http://www.nsc.org/news_resources/injury_and_death_statistics/Pages/EstimatingtheCostsof UnintentionalInjuries.aspx (accessed September 2014).

4. American College of Surgeons. *Advanced Trauma Life Support*, 9th edition. Chicago, IL: ACS, 2012.

5. Pape HC, van Griensven M, Rice J, *et al.* Major secondary surgery in blunt trauma patients and perioperative cytokine liberation: determination of the relevance of biochemical markers. *J Trauma* 2001; **50**: 989–1000.

6. Pape HC, van Griensven MV, Hildebrand FF, *et al.* Systemic inflammatory response after extremity or truncal fracture operations. *J Trauma* 2008; **65**: 1379–84.

7. Waydhas C, Nast-Kolb D, Trupka A, *et al.* Posttraumatic inflammatory response, secondary operations, and late multiple organ failure. *J Trauma* 1996; **40**: 624–30.

8. Barei DP, Shafer BL, Beingessner DM, *et al.* The impact of open reduction and internal fixation on acute pain management in unstable pelvic ring injuries. *J Trauma* 2010; **68**: 949–53.

9. Bone LB, Johnson KD, Weigelt J, Scheinberg R. Early versus delayed stabilization of femoral fractures: a prospective randomized study. *J Bone Joint Surg Am* 1989; **71A**: 336–40.

10. Bosse MJ, MacKenzie EJ, Riemer BL, et al. Adult respiratory distress syndrome, pneumonia, and mortality following thoracic injury and a femoral fracture treated either with intramedullary nailing with reaming or with a plate: a comparative study. *J Bone Joint Surg Am* 1997; **79A**: 799–809.

11. Charash WE, Fabian TC, Croce MA. Delayed surgical fixation of femur fractures is a risk factor for pulmonary failure independent of thoracic trauma. *J Trauma* 1994; **37**: 667–72.

12. Dunham CM, Bosse MJ, Clancy TV, et al. Practice management guidelines for the optimal timing of long-bone fractures stabilization in polytrauma patients: the EAST Practice Management Guidelines work group. *J Trauma* 2001; **50**: 958–67.

13. Johnson KD, Cadambi A, Seibert GB. Incidence of adult respiratory distress syndrome in patients with multiple musculoskeletal injuries: effect of early operative stabilization of fractures. *J Trauma* 1985; **25**: 375–84.

14. Latenser BA, Gentilello LM, Tarver AA, Thalgott JS, Batdorf JW. Improved outcome with early fixation of skeletally unstable pelvic fractures. *J Trauma* 1991; **31**: 28–31.

15. Plasier BR, Meldon SW, Super DM, Malangoni MA. Improved outcome after early fixation of acetabular fractures. *Injury* 2000; **31**: 81–4.

16. Vallier HA, Cureton BA, Eckstein C, Oldenburg FP, Wilber JH. Early definitive stabilization of unstable pelvis and acetabulum fractures reduces morbidity. *J Trauma* 2010; **69**: 677–84.

17. Barei DP, Nork SE, Mills WJ, Henley MB, Benirschke SK. Complications associated with internal fixation of high-energy bicondylar tibial plateau fractures utilizing a two-incision technique. *J Orthop Trauma* 2004; **18**: 649–57.

18. Sirkin M, Sanders R, DiPasquale T, Herscovici DJ. A staged protocol for soft tissue management in the treatment of complex pilon fractures. *J Orthop Trauma* 1999; **13**: 78–84.

19. Goris RJ, Gimbrere JS, van Niekerk JL, Schoots FJ, Booy LH. Early osteosynthesis and prophylactic mechanical ventilation in the multitrauma patient. *J Trauma* 1982; **22**: 895–903.

20. Lozman J. Deno DC, Feustel PJ, et al. Pulmonary and cardiovascular consequences of immediate fixation or conservative management of long-bone fractures. *Arch Surg* 1986; **21**: 992–9.

21. McHenry TP, Mirza SK, Wang J, et al. Risk factors for respiratory failure following operative stabilization of thoracic and lumbar spine fractures. *J Bone Joint Surg Am* 2006; **88A**: 997–1005.

22. Nahm NJ, Como JJ, Wilber JH, Vallier HA. Early appropriate care: definitive stabilization of femoral fractures within 24 hours of injury is safe in most patients with multiple injuries. *J Trauma* 2011; **71**: 175–85.

23. Nahm NJ, Vallier HA. Timing of definitive treatment for femoral shaft fractures in patients with multiple injuries: a systematic review of randomized and nonrandomized trials. *J Trauma* 2012; **73**: 1046–63.

24. Seibel R, LaDura J, Hassett JM, et al. Blunt multiple trauma (ISS 36), femur traction, and the pulmonary failure-septic state. *Ann Surg* 1985; **202**: 283–95.

25. Harvin JA, Harvin WH, Camp EC, et al. Early femur fracture fixation is associated with a reduction in pulmonary complications and hospital charges: a decade of experience with 1376 diaphyseal femur fractures. *J Trauma* 2012; **73**: 1440–2.

26. Starr AJ, Hunt JL, Chason DP, Reinert CM, Walker J. Treatment of femur fracture with associated head injury. *J Orthop Trauma* 1998; **12**: 38–45.

27. Pape HC, Rixen D, Morley J, et al. Impact of the method of initial stabilization for femoral shaft fractures in patients with multiple injuries at risk for complications (borderline patients). *Ann Surg* 2007; **246**: 491–9.

28. Pape HC, Hildebrand F, Pertschy S, et al. Changes in the management of femoral fractures in polytrauma patients: from early total care to damage control orthopedic surgery. *J Trauma* 2002; **53**: 452–61.

29. Poole GV, Miller JD, Agnew SG, Griswold JA. Lower extremity fracture fixation in head-injured patients. *J Trauma* 1992; **32**: 654–9.

30. Morshed S, Miclau T, Bembom O, et al. Delayed internal fixation of femoral shaft fracture reduces mortality among patients with multisystem trauma. *J Bone Joint Surg Am* 2009; **91A**: 3–13.

31. O'Toole RV, O'Brien M, Scalea TM, et al. Resuscitation before stabilization of femoral fractures limits acute respiratory distress syndrome in patients with multiple traumatic injuries despite low use of damage control orthopaedics. *J Trauma* 2009; **67**: 1013–21.

32. Tuttle MS, Smith WR, Williams AE, et al. Safety and efficacy of damage control external fixation versus early definitive stabilization for femoral shaft fractures in the multiple-injured patient. *J Trauma* 2009; **67**: 602–5.

33. Lefaivre KA, Starr AJ, Stahel PF, Elliott AC, Smith WR. Prediction of pulmonary morbidity and mortality in patients with femur fracture. *J Trauma* 2010; **69**: 1527–36.

34. Rixen D, Grass G, Sauerland S, et al. Evaluation of criteria for temporary external fixation in risk-adapted damage control orthopedic surgery of femur shaft fractures in multiple trauma patients: "evidence-based medicine" versus "reality" in the trauma registry of the German Trauma Society. *J Trauma* 2005; **59**: 1375–95.

35. Harwood PJ, Giannoudis PV, van Griensven M, Krettek C, Pape HC. Alterations in the systemic inflammatory response after early total care and damage control procedures for femoral shaft fracture in severely injured patients. *J Trauma* 2005; **58**: 446–52.

36. Nast-Kolb D, Waydhas C, Gippner-Steppart C, et al. Indicators of the posttraumatic inflammatory response correlate with organ failure in patients with multiple injuries. *J Trauma* 1997; **42**: 446–54.

37. Pape HC, van Griensven M, Sott AH, et al. Impact of intramedullary instrumentation versus damage control for femoral fractures on immunoinflammatory parameters: prospective randomized analysis buy the EPOFF study group. *J Trauma* 2004; **55**: 7–13.

38. Pape HC, Schmidt RE, Rice J, et al. Biochemical changes after trauma and skeletal surgery of the lower extremity: quantification of the operative burden. *J Orthop Trauma* 2004; **18**: S24–31.

39. Scalea TM, Boswell SA, Scott JD, et al. External fixation as a bridge to intramedullary nailing for patients with multiple injuries and with femur fractures: damage control orthopedics. *J Trauma* 2000; **48**: 613–23.

40. Tucker MC, Nork SE, Simonian PT, Routt ML. Simple anterior pelvic

external fixation. *J Trauma* 2000; **49**: 989–94.

41. Stahel PF, VanderHeiden T, Flierl MA, *et al.* The impact of a standardized "spine damage control" protocol for unstable thoracic and lumbar spine fractures in severely injured patients. *J Trauma* 2013; **74**: 590–6.

42. Bhandari M, Zlowodzki M, Tornetta P, Schmidt A, Templeman DC. Intramedullary nailing following external fixation in femoral and tibial shaft fractures. *J Orthop Trauma* 2005; **19**: 140–4.

43. Harwood PJ, Giannoudis PV, Probst C, Krettek C, Pape HC. The risk of local infective complications after damage control procedures for femoral shaft fracture. *J Orthop Trauma* 2006; **20**: 181–9.

44. Davis JW, Shackford SR, Mackersie RC, Hoyt DB. Base deficit as a guide to volume resuscitation. *J Trauma* 1988; **28**: 1464–7.

45. Guyette F, Suffoletto B, Castillo J, *et al.* Prehospital serum lactate as a predictor of outcomes in trauma patients: a retrospective observational study. *J Trauma* 2011; **70**: 782–6.

46. Husain FA, Martin MJ, Mullenix PS, Steele SR, Elliott DC. Serum lactate and base deficit as predictors of mortality and morbidity. *Am J Surg* 2003; **185**: 485–91.

47. Ouellet JF, Roberts DJ, Tiruta C, *et al.* Admission base deficit and lactate levels in Canadian patients with blunt trauma: are they useful markers of injury? *J Trauma* 2012; **72**: 1532–5.

48. Paladineo L, Sinert R, Wallace D, *et al.* The utility of base deficit and arterial lactate in differentiating major from minor injury in trauma patients with normal vital signs. *Resuscitation* 2008; **77**: 363–8.

49. Burgess AR, Eastridge BJ, Young JW, *et al.* Pelvic ring disruptions: effective classification system and treatment protocols. *J Trauma* 1990; **30**: 848–56.

50. Nahm NJ, Como JJ, Vallier HA. The impact of major operative fractures in blunt abdominal injury. *J Trauma* 2013; **74**: 1307–14.

51. Riska EB, vonBonsdorff H, Hakkinen S, *et al.* Primary operative fixation of long bone fractures in patients with multiple injuries. *J Trauma* 1977; **17**: 111–21.

52. Dalal SA, Burgess AR, Siegel JH, *et al.* Pelvic fracture in multiple trauma: classification by mechanism is key to pattern of organ injury, resuscitative requirements, and outcome. *J Trauma* 1989; **29**: 981–1000.

53. Holstein JH, Culemann U, Pohlemann T; Working Group Mortality in Pelvic Fracture Patients. What are predictors of mortality in patients with pelvis fractures? *Clin Orthop Relat Res* 2012; **470**: 2090–7.

54. Smith W, Willams A, Agudelo J, *et al.* Early predictors of mortality in hemodynamically unstable pelvis fractures. *J Orthop Trauma* 2007; **21**: 31–7.

55. Starr AJ, Griffen DR, Reinert CM, *et al.* Pelvic ring disruptions: prediction of associated injuries, transfusion requirement, pelvic angiography, complications, and mortality. *J Orthop Trauma* 2002; **16**: 553–61.

56. Tile M. Acute pelvic fractures: I. Causation and classification. *J Am Acad Orthop Surg* 1996; **4**: 143–51.

57. Tile M. Pelvic ring fractures: should they be fixed? *J Bone Joint Surg Br* 1988; **70B**: 1–12.

58. Whitbeck MG, Zwally HJ, Burgess AR. Innominosacral dissociation: mechanism of injury as a predictor of resuscitation requirements, morbidity, and mortality. *J Orthop Trauma* 2006; **20**: S57–63.

59. Routt ML, Simonian PT, Ballmer F. A rational approach to pelvic trauma: resuscitation and early definitive stabilization. *Clin Orthop Relat Res* 1995; **318**: 61–74.

60. Denis F, Davis S, Comfort T. Sacral fractures: an important problem. Retrospective analysis of 236 cases. *Clin Orthop Relat Res* 1988; **227**: 67–81.

61. Gibbons KJ, Soloniuk DS, Razack N. Neurologic injury and patterns of sacral fractures. *J Neurosurg* 1990; **72**: 889–93.

62. Jones AL, Powell JN, Kellam JF, *et al.* Open pelvic fractures: a multicenter retrospective analysis. *Orthop Clin North Am* 1997; **28**: 345–50.

63. Routt ML, Falicov A, Woodhouse E, Schildhauer T. Circumferential pelvic antishock sheeting: a temporary resuscitation aid. *J Orthop Trauma* 2006; **20**: S3–6.

64. O'Neill PA, Rinna J, Sclafani S. Tornetta P. Angiographic findings in pelvic fractures. *Clin Orthop Relat Res* 1996; **329**: 60–7.

65. Osborn PM, Smith WR, Moore EE, *et al.* Direct retroperitoneal pelvic packing versus pelvic angiography: a comparison of two management protocols for haemodynamically unstable pelvic fractures. *Injury* 2009; **40**: 54–60.

66. Smith WR, Moore EE, Osborn P, *et al.* Retroperitoneal packing as a resuscitation technique for hemodynamically unstable patients with pelvic fractures: report of two representative cases and a description of the technique. *J Trauma* 2005; **5**: 1510–14.

67. Tai DK, Li WH, Lee KY, *et al.* Retroperitoneal pelvic packing in the management of hemodynamically unstable pelvic fractures: a level 1 trauma center experience. *J Trauma* 2011; **71**: E79–86.

68. Routt ML, Kregor PJ, Simonian PT, Mayo KA. Early results of percutaneous iliosacral screws placed with the patient in the supine position. *J Orthop Trauma* 1995; **9**: 207–14.

69. Probst C, Probst T, Gaensslen A, *et al.* Timing and duration of the initial pelvic stabilization after multiple trauma in patients from German Trauma Registry: is there an influence on outcome? *J Trauma* 2007; **62**: 370–7.

70. Pell M, Flynn WJ, Seibel RW. Is colostomy always necessary in the treatment of open pelvic fractures? *J Trauma* 1998; **45**: 371–3.

71. Woods RK, O'Keefe G, Rhee P, Routt ML, Maier RV. Open pelvic fracture and fecal diversion. *Arch Surg* 1998; **133**: 281–6.

72. Copeland CE, Mitchell KA, Brumback RJ, Gens DR, Burgess AR. Mortality in patients with bilateral femoral fractures. *J Orthop Trauma* 1998; **12**: 315–19.

73. Kobbe P, Vodovotz Y, Kaczorowski DJ, Billiar TR, Pape HC. The role of fracture-associated soft tissue injury in the induction of systemic inflammation and remote organ dysfunction after bilateral femur fractures. *J Orthop Trauma* 2008; **22**: 385–90.

74. Nork SE, Agel J, Russell GV, *et al.* Mortality after reamed intramedullary nailing of bilateral femur fractures. *Clin Orthop Relat Res* 2003; **415**: 272–8.

75. Willett K, Al-Khateeb H, Kotnis R, Bouamra O, Lecky F. Risk of mortality: the relationship with associated injuries and fracture treatment methods in

469

patients with bilateral femoral shaft fractures. *J Trauma* 2010; **69**: 405–10.

76. Bosse MJ, MacKenzie EJ, Kellam JF, *et al.* A prospective evaluation of the clinical utility of the lower-extremity injury-severity scores. *J Bone Joint Surg Am* 2001; **83A**: 3–14.

77. Johansen K, Daines M, Howey T, Helfet D, Hansen ST. Objective criteria accurately predict amputation following lower extremity trauma. *J Trauma* 1990; **30**: 568–72.

78. Lange RH, Bach AW, Hansen ST, Johansen KH. Open tibial fractures with associated vascular injuries: prognosis for limb salvage. *J Trauma* 1985; **25**: 203–8.

79. Green NE, Allen BL. Vascular injuries associated with dislocation of the knee. *J Bone Joint Surg Am* 1977; **59A**: 236–9.

80. Treiman GS, Yellin AE, Weaver FA, *et al.* Examination of the patient with a knee dislocation. The case for selective arteriography. *Arch Surg* 1992; **127**: 1056–62.

81. Wascher DC, Dvirnak PC, DeCoster TA. Knee dislocation: initial assessment and implications for treatment. *J Orthop Trauma* 1997; **11**: 525–9.

82. Johansen K, Lynch K, Paun M. Copass M. Non-invasive vascular tests reliably exclude occult arterial trauma in injured extremities. *J Trauma* 1991; **31**: 515–19.

83. Mills WJ, Barei DP, McNair P. The value of the ankle-brachial index for diagnosing arterial injury after knee dislocation: a prospective study. *J Trauma* 2004; **56**: 1261–5.

84. McQueen MM, Court-Brown CM. Compartment monitoring in tibial fractures: the pressure threshold for decompression. *J Bone Joint Surg Br* 1996; **78B**: 99–104.

85. Gustilo RB, Anderson JT. Prevention of infection in the treatment of one thousand and twenty-five open fractures of long bones: retrospective and prospective analyses. *J Bone Joint Surg Am* 1976; **58A**: 453–8.

86. Gustilo RB, Mendoza RM, Williams DN. Problems in the management of type III (severe) open fractures: a new classification of type III open fractures. *J Trauma* 1984; **24**: 742–6.

87. Sorger JI, Kirk PG, Ruhnke CJ, *et al.* Once daily, high dose versus divided, low dose gentamicin for open fractures. *Clin Orthop Relat Res* 1999; **366**: 197–204.

88. Patzakis MJ. Management of open fracture wounds. *Instr Course Lect* 1987; **36**: 367–9.

89. Franklin JL, Johnson KD, Hansen ST. Immediate internal fixation of open ankle fractures: report of thirty-eight cases treated with a standard protocol. *J Bone Joint Surg Am* 1984; **66A**: 1349–56.

90. Moed BR, Kellam FJ, Foster RJ, Tile M, Hansen ST. Immediate internal fixation of open fractures of the diaphysis of the forearm. *J Bone Joint Surg Am* 1986; **68A**: 1008–17.

91. Fassler PR, Swiontkowski MF, Kilroy AW, Routt ML. Injury of the sciatic nerve associated with acetabular fracture. *J Bone Joint Surg Am* 1993; **75A**: 1157–66.

92. Tornetta P, Mostafavi HR. Hip dislocation: current treatment regimens. *J Am Acad Orthop Surg* 1997; **5**: 27–36.

93. Hawkins LG. Fractures of the neck of the talus. *J Bone Joint Surg Am.* 1970; **52A**: 991–1002.

94. Stuart JM, Milford LW. Fracture-dislocation of the hip: An end result study. *J Bone Joint Surg Am* 1954; **36A**: 315–42.

95. Yue JJ, Wilber JH, Lipuma PJ, *et al.* Posterior hip dislocations: a cadaveric angiographic study. *J Orthop Trauma* 1996; **10**: 447–54.

96. Jain R, Koo M, Kreder HJ, *et al.* Comparisons of early and delayed fixation of subcapital hip fractures in patients sixty years of age or less. *J Bone Joint Surg Am* 2002; **84A**: 605–12.

97. Swiontkowski MF, Winquist RA, Hansen ST. Fractures of the femoral neck in patients between the ages of twelve and forty-nine years. *J Bone Joint Surg Am* 1984; **66A**: 837–46.

98. Carlson DW, Rodman GH, Kaehr D. Hage J, Misinski M. Femur fractures in chest-injured patients: is reaming contraindicated? *J Orthop Trauma* 1998; **12**: 164–8.

99. Gurd AR, Wilson RI. The fat embolism syndrome. *J Bone Joint Surg Br* 1974; **56B**: 408–16.

100. Lindeque BG, Schoeman HS, Dommisse GF, Boeyens MC, Vlok AL. Fat embolism and the fat embolism syndrome: a double-blind therapeutic study. *J Bone Joint Surg Br* 1987; **69B**: 128–31.

101. Bhandari M, Guyatt GH, Kjera V, *et al.* Operative management of lower extremity fractures in patients with head injuries. *Clin Orthop Rel Res* 2003; **407**: 187–98.

102. Reynolds MA, Richardson JD, Spain DA, *et al.* Is the timing of fracture fixation important for the patient with multiple trauma? *Ann Surg* 1995; **222**: 470–8.

103. Zuckerman JD, Skovron ML, Koval KJ, Aharonoff GB, Frankel VH. Postoperative complications and mortality associated with operative delay in older patients who have a fracture of the hip. *J Bone Joint Surg Am* 1995; **77A**: 1551–6.

104. Aharanoff GB, Koval KJ, Skovron ML, Zuckerman JD. Hip fractures in the elderly: predictors of one ear mortality. *J Orthop Trauma* 1997; **11**: 162–5.

105. Cornwall R, Gilbert MS, Koval KJ, Strauss E, Siu AL. Functional outcomes and mortality vary among different types of hip fractures: a function of patient characteristics. *Clin Orthop Relat Res* 2004; **425**: 64–71.

106. Daugaard CL, Jorgensen HL, Riis T, *et al.* Is mortality after hip fracture associated with surgical delay or admission during weekends and public holidays? A retrospective study of 38,020 patients. *Acta Orthop* 2012; **81**: 609–13.

107. Endo Y, Aharonoff GB, Zuckerman JD, Egol KA, Koval KJ. Gender differences in patients with hip fracture: a greater risk of morbidity and mortality in men. *J Orthop Trauma* 2005; **19**: 29–35.

108. Richmond J. Aharonoff GB, Zuckerman JD, Koval KJ. Mortality risk after hip fracture. *J Orthop Trauma* 2003; **17**: 53–6.

109. McLaughlin MA, Orosz GM, Magaziner J, *et al.* Preoperative status and risk of complications in patients with hip fracture. *J Gen Intern Med* 2006; **21**: 219–25.

110. Koval KJ, Shovron ML, Aharonoff GB, Zuckerman JD. Predictors of functional recovery after hip fracture. Effect of general versus regional anesthesia. *Clin Orthop Rel Res* 1998; **348**: 37–41.

Chapter

28

Anesthesia considerations for musculoskeletal trauma

Jeff Gadsden

Objectives

(1) Review the anesthetic considerations for complex musculoskeletal injuries including pelvic and long-bone fractures, traumatic amputations, and crush syndrome.

(2) Discuss issues related to the timing of surgical fixation of specific fractures.

(3) Discuss the impact of anesthetic management on morbidity and mortality following hip fracture.

(4) Review the pathophysiology and anesthetic concerns relating to acute compartment syndrome, fat embolism, and complex regional pain syndrome.

(5) Summarize the postoperative concerns following musculoskeletal trauma, specifically pain and delirium.

Introduction

Musculoskeletal injury is common in the trauma patient. While bony fractures and muscular injuries can occur anywhere on the body, the extremities are disproportionately affected. Approximately 60% of multiple trauma patients with an Injury Severity Score (ISS) of $\geq$ 16 have extremity injury of some type, and 18% have both lower and upper extremity injuries.[1] Over 30% of the same population will have two or more extremity fractures. Mechanism of injury is an important epidemiologic factor – for example, those in motor vehicle collisions (MVCs) have a significantly higher prevalence of extremity injury; similarly, due to improvements in battlefield medicine and body armor, modern military combatants have a dramatically reduced rate of fatal torso injury, meaning that while more survive, they have much higher rates of serious extremity injury. While patients with isolated extremity injuries typically go on to have very good outcomes, it has been shown that orthopedic and general health outcomes become significantly poorer if the same injury is present in a polytrauma patient.[2]

It is often easy to assign musculoskeletal injuries a secondary level of importance, and certainly initial measures such as life-saving resuscitation and control of life-threatening injuries take priority in the severely injured patient. However, management of the patient with musculoskeletal trauma is more than just fixing broken bones. There are frequently multiple considerations that impact the anesthetic plan and carry potential for complications. In addition, the trauma anesthesiologist has the potential to significantly improve the quality of recovery, morbidity, and, in some cases, mortality of the patient with careful application of trauma care principles. In this chapter, several broad considerations will be discussed: complex musculoskeletal injuries, timing of fracture repair, the specific management of anesthesia for hip fracture, complications associated with musculoskeletal trauma, and, finally, postoperative concerns.

Complex musculoskeletal injuries

While minor, non-life-threatening bony and soft tissue injuries are extremely common in most trauma patients, serious musculoskeletal injuries are not infrequent, especially in the multiply injured population.

Pelvic fractures

Disruption of the bony ring of the pelvis occurs at a rate of about 100,000 per year in the US, and accounts for approximately 3% of skeletal trauma. The main mechanism of injury is blunt trauma, typically from side-impact vehicle collisions, pedestrian-struck injuries, motorcycle crashes, and falls. There are several classification systems in use that are based on the anatomical nature of the fracture(s); most simply, a stable fracture has one break point and minimal disruption to the pelvic ring, as well as minimal bleeding; unstable fractures have two or more break points and are associated with a higher bleeding risk (see Chapter 27). One specific type of unstable pelvic fracture is the "open-book" fracture (Fig. 28.1); this is commonly seen when anterior–posterior forces on the pelvis result in a separation or fracture of the pubic rami and the subsequent rotation of the hemipelves outwards, with associated disruption of the posterior pelvis. While not as common as long-bone fractures, pelvic fractures are frequently life-threatening and mandate careful attention to pre-anesthetic evaluation.

The pelvic ring can withstand a large amount of force before fracturing, and as a result these injuries are markers

Trauma Anesthesia, 2nd Edition, ed. Charles E. Smith. Published by Cambridge University Press. © Charles E. Smith, 2015.

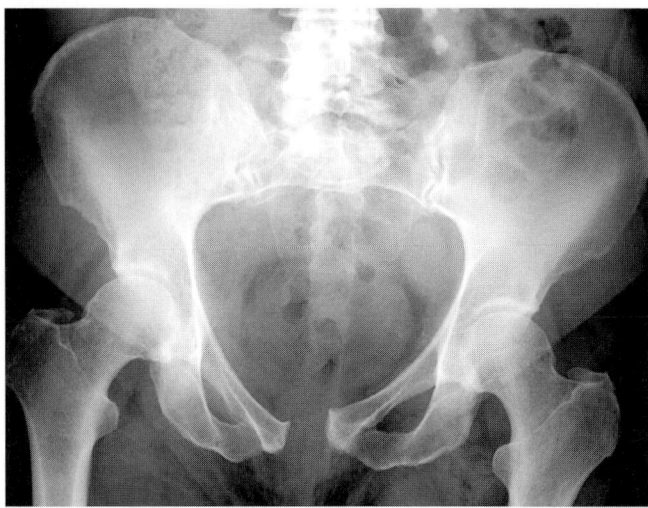

Figure 28.1 Anteroposterior x-ray of the pelvis showing an open-book fracture.

of injury severity. Because of the high amount of energy transfer associated with pelvic fractures, injuries to the abdominal and pelvic viscera are common, and correlation of injury pattern between bony structure and underlying soft tissue is high. For example, fracture of the anterior aspect of the pelvic ring (i.e., the pubis) is associated with bladder and urethral injury; patients with suspected urethral injuries should undergo retrograde urethrogram prior to bladder catheter insertion to avoid further injury. Similarly, sacral fractures commonly coincide with injuries to the rectum. Female patients require special attention to rule out injury to the uterus, ovaries, and vagina; clearly the risk to the fetus in the case of pelvic trauma in the pregnant patient is high.

Hemorrhage remains the principal cause of death in these patients. The overall mortality rate is typically 5–10%, but may be as high as 40% when pelvic fracture is associated with hemodynamic instability.[3] The internal and external iliac arteries and veins (as well as their branches) traverse the pelvic brim, and may be injured in the course of mechanical disruption of the pelvis. The large veins are much more likely to be torn than arteries, and while these low-pressure vessels occasionally stop bleeding spontaneously, prompt therapy is frequently required, especially in unstable fractures. External pelvic stabilization is a maneuver aimed at reducing the pelvic volume (thereby accelerating pelvic tamponade) while preventing further shearing of vascular structures. Several methods have shown mixed success in reducing transfusion requirements and/or blood loss – these include pneumatic antishock garments, external pelvic fixation, and the pelvic C-clamp. In contrast, temporary pelvic binders are inexpensive and easy to use, and can be rapidly applied in order to provide mechanical stability by prehospital or emergency department personnel (e.g., SAM pelvic sling). Patients may present to the operating room with a binder in place; in order to minimize disruption of the clot and prevent deterioration, the binder should ideally

be left in place until the patient is fully resuscitated and coagulopathy treated.

Since the majority (85–90%) of bleeding sources in pelvic fracture are venous, most patients will not benefit from angiographic embolization techniques. Indications for angiography include continued instability in the absence of nonpelvic causes of bleeding, extravasation of contrast material on CT scan, or major pelvic fracture in patients > 60 years of age, regardless of hemodynamic status (due to a high correlation with positive angiography).[4] Once performed, embolization is usually successful in halting bleeding. For instances where angiography is unavailable, or where it would unnecessarily delay treatment, preperitoneal packing of the pelvis can be done to control hemorrhage.

Clearly one of the main considerations for the anesthesiologist caring for a patient with pelvic fracture is predicting the need for, and managing transfusion of, blood components. Massive transfusion protocols (MTPs) are frequently required to mitigate the profound hemodynamic instability that can accompany these injuries (see Chapter 6).

Traumatic amputations

Management of patients with traumatic amputations, whether complete or incomplete, poses several challenges for the anesthesiologist. The energy required to sever a limb is often high, and multiple other life- or limb-threatening injuries may coexist. Traumatic amputations are rarely simple, and much of the affected limb can be crushed and/or mangled (Fig. 28.2). A decision must be made by the surgeon as to how much of the limb to salvage and/or amputate in order to achieve the best functional result. Hemorrhage is the foremost concern, and patients often present to the trauma bay or the operating room profoundly hypovolemic. The principles of damage control resuscitation should be employed in order to prevent hemodilution, acidosis, and hydrostatic disruption of any clot that may have already formed at the site of injury. These include permissive hypotension pending surgical control of the hemorrhage, maintenance of normothermia, aggressive warming of the patient, prevention of worsening acidosis, and the early use of blood component therapy with high ratios of plasma to packed red blood cells (see Chapter 6). A more in-depth discussion of damage control resuscitation is presented in Chapter 18.

Amputation is associated with severe acute pain that can develop into long-term pain syndromes. These are generally categorized as stump pain, which is localized to the site of amputation, and phantom limb pain, which is defined as a noxious sensory phenomenon in the missing limb. The latter pathologic pain syndrome occurs in 30–85% of patients after limb amputation. Phantom sensation is defined as the sensory perception of a missing body part without pain.

The ability of any one anesthetic technique or medication to alter the progression from acute to chronic pain in amputees is unclear, and the evidence is somewhat contradictory.

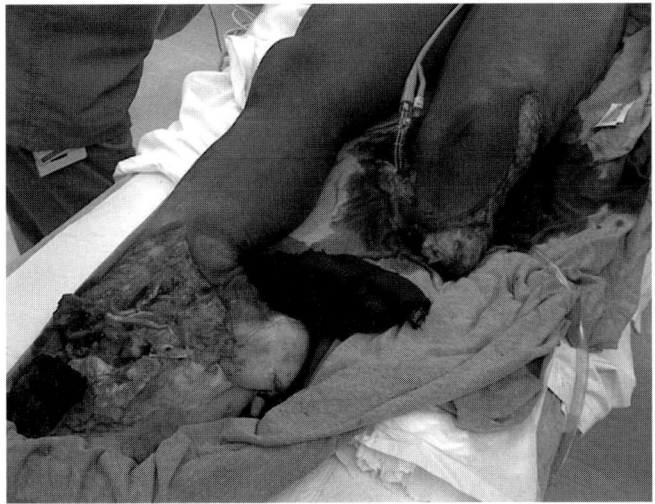

Figure 28.2 Bilateral amputations of the lower extremities. *A black and white version of this figure will appear in some formats. For the color version, please refer to the plate section.*

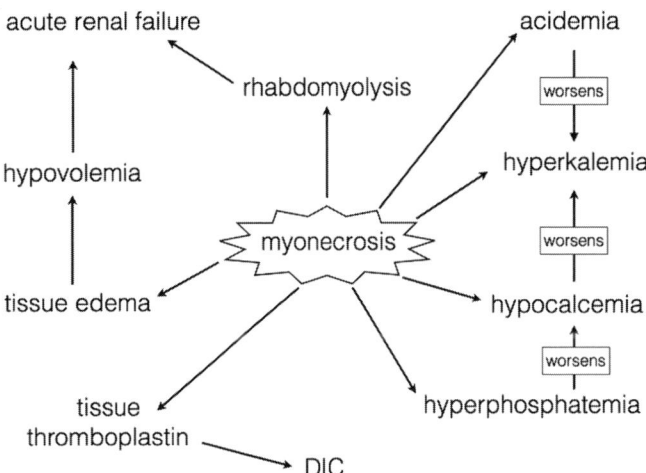

Figure 28.3 Pathophysiology of crush syndrome. DIC, disseminated intravascular coagulation.

Part of this may be related to study design and the lack of continued analgesia into the postoperative period. However, patients undergoing elective amputation for critical limb ischemia appear to have a reduced incidence of chronic pain syndromes when effective analgesia is instituted prior to and continued after the surgical procedure. This may be independent of the type of analgesia (e.g., regional versus intravenous opioids).[5] While it may be difficult to translate these data to traumatic amputations, there is little downside to excellent analgesia, and once the initial goals of resuscitation and hemodynamic stability are achieved, pain control should be high on the list of priorities for traumatic amputations (see Chapters 15–17).

Crush syndrome

Crush injuries are not typical of everyday trauma, but are important in the setting of disasters, either natural or otherwise, such as earthquakes, landslides, hurricanes, or bombings. External mechanical pressure acting continually on muscle tissue disrupts the permeability of the sarcolemma, and leads to tissue edema and eventual ischemia. Muscle is capable of surviving ischemia for up to 2–4 hours, but muscle necrosis usually occurs by 6 hours. Upon relief of the pressure (e.g., when a victim is extricated) blood flow is re-established and a reperfusion injury occurs, leading to further edema and myofascial compartment syndrome. With myocyte necrosis, intracellular contents are released, resulting in the characteristic findings in *crush syndrome*, the systemic manifestations of local muscle injury (Fig. 28.3).

Hypovolemic shock from massive third-spacing and hyperkalemic cardiac arrest are the leading causes of early death in crush syndrome.[6] Aggressive intravenous volume replacement addresses both of these issues simultaneously, and is the mainstay of early treatment. The earlier that volume resuscitation

can begin, the higher the likelihood of avoiding permanent renal injury; ideally this is initiated at the scene of an MVC, prior to extrication of the victim. Alkalinization of the urine should also begin as soon as possible, in order to prevent acute kidney injury from myoglobinemia.[6] Forced diuresis of at least 200 mL/h with a urine pH of > 6.5 has been advocated by some, which can be achieved by the addition of approximately 50 mEq bicarbonate to each liter of normal saline. In order to prevent alkalemia, patients often require treatment with acetazolamide. Intravenous infusion rates of > 500 mL/h are not unusual in this setting in order to maintain adequate fluid and renal homeostasis, and volume overload is a concern, especially in those with poor ventricular function. Potassium-containing solutions (e.g., lactated Ringer's) should be avoided. Other specific therapies for hyperkalemia include insulin and glucose, calcium, β_2 agonists, potassium binding resins (e.g., Kayexalate), and, if refractory, hemodialysis. Mannitol is a common adjunct during treatment of crush syndrome, as it promotes a forced diuresis, increases intravascular volume, is a free-radical scavenger, and may reduce intracompartmental pressures during compartment syndrome. Throughout the perioperative period, careful and repeated assessments of volume status and calculation of the fluid requirements are critical, as is frequent monitoring of electrolyte balance and osmolarity.

Hypocalcemia results from the intracellular sequestration of calcium in affected muscle tissue, and is particularly dangerous as it enhances the potential for hyperkalemic arrhythmias by decreasing the cardiac myocyte threshold potential. Hyperphosphatemia occurs due to muscle breakdown, and further worsens hypocalemia by precipitating calcium and decreasing vitamin D production. Tissue factor levels are typically elevated following crush injury, which can lead to disseminated intravascular coagulopathy (DIC).

In addition to addressing concerns relating to hypovolemia and myonecrosis, the preoperative assessment of the patient with crush syndrome must also include a thorough clinical evaluation of the airway and respiratory system, as inhalation injury due to dust and/or smoke is common. Early tracheal intubation and control of the airway is often a prudent course if there is any suspicion of airway or respiratory impairment. Especially in the setting of potential thermal injury to the airway from superheated air (e.g., bombings), the dynamics of the airway exam can change as the mucosal tissues become edematous.

Long-bone fracture

Fractures of the femur, tibia, or humerus typically require a moderate to high amount of energy transfer, especially in young patients, and a careful search for associated injuries should be performed. Hemorrhage is a major concern, especially with femoral shaft fractures, and the average blood loss associated with an isolated femoral shaft fracture has been estimated to exceed 1200 mL.[7] The soft tissues surrounding the long bone can accommodate much of the extravasated volume, leading to potential delays in effective resuscitation. Reduction and stabilization of the fracture are early goals, and have been shown to reduce ongoing blood loss, pulmonary complications, and pain (see Chapter 27). In patients who are hemodynamically unstable or require other urgent therapy or investigations (e.g., angiography, head computed tomography), external fixation devices can be quickly applied and definitive fixation delayed until the patient is deemed fit enough. Another consideration in long-bone fracture is the risk of fat embolism syndrome, discussed in detail later in this chapter.

Timing of fracture repair

Anesthesiologists are frequently involved in weighing priorities in times of competing surgical urgency, especially at night and on weekends when nursing staff and resources are not at full capacity. Both open fractures and hip fractures are examples of common injuries that have specific constraints with respect to timing of surgery, and knowledge of these issues is important for the trauma anesthesiologist.

Open fractures

Open fractures are considered an urgent surgical problem, and must be irrigated and debrided within 6–8 hours in order to prevent infection, although the human data supporting this are scant. Several studies have in fact failed to show a relationship between timing of open fracture repair and risk for infection or nonunion, although early debridement has nonetheless remained the standard of care. Other factors that may influence the risk of infection include the time from injury to arrival at hospital, and timing of initial antibiotic treatment.[8] Gunshot wounds in civilian medicine typically occur from handguns, and represent a low-energy mechanism. In such cases where the fracture is stable, extensive exploration of the wound may lead to a higher risk of infection. In contrast,

high-velocity gunshot wounds (e.g., from rifles) are always treated as open fractures because of the extensive tissue damage that occurs. In addition, the velocity with which the bullet travels through the soft tissue creates a vacuum, drawing bacteria and other foreign debris into the wound.

The decision regarding the timing of definitive closure is related to the character of the wound itself: clean wounds that can be closed atraumatically can often undergo primary closure at the time of debridement, whereas delayed closure may be the best course in cases where tissue quality is a concern.

Hip fractures (see also Chapter 36)

Patients with hip fracture frequently have multiple comorbid conditions that influence their pre- and perioperative care, and although the correction of any and all abnormalities is optimal, delay in the surgical management of these patients leads to pain and distress, and is associated with an increase in complication rates.[9] Patients should be fully evaluated, and particular attention should be paid to restoration of circulatory volume and optimization of any conditions such as electrolyte abnormalities, poorly controlled diabetes, congestive heart failure, or significant anemia. However, delaying surgery in an attempt to achieve unrealistic medical goals should be discouraged. For example, further workup and treatment of a pneumonia prior to surgery may not result in an improved outcome, as the patient's overall condition will likely continue to deteriorate in the presence of continued immobility and pain. Similarly, routine preoperative cardiac testing in hip fracture patients appears to make no difference to management plans, and adds an average delay of 3.3 days to surgery.[10] In contrast, clinical evaluation of cardiac disease appears to be as reliable as noninvasive cardiac testing.[10] Guidelines of preoperative testing from the American College of Cardiology and the American Heart Association do not support the use of additional cardiac investigations in most patients, and tests such as echocardiography should be individualized to patients with specific clinical findings (e.g., a murmur and/or history suggestive of aortic stenosis).[11]

Routine "medical clearance" in patients with fractures is an outdated concept that is both economically wasteful and a contributor to further delays. Solicitation of medical consultations should be done judiciously and with a specific question in mind. Even when problems are identified preoperatively, there is often little to do. An audit of over 5400 Scottish hip fracture patients demonstrated that, of patients that were delayed due to a major abnormality, only 47% had the problem corrected prior to eventual presentation to the operating room, thereby unnecessarily exposing the patient to further risk while awaiting optimization.[9]

While older studies appeared to show a mixed effect of a surgical delay on outcomes, more recent data have pointed toward a survival benefit to early (e.g., < 24–48 hours) surgical treatment of hip fractures (Table 28.1). Recognition of the importance of this effect has prompted many institutions and

Table 28.1 Selected studies on the timing of hip fracture and mortality

Reference	Design	Outcome
Daugaard et al. 2012[12]	Retrospective review of prospective database (n = 38,020)	In-hospital mortality ↑ with delay (OR 1.32 for each 24 h)
Smeets et al. 2012[13]	Retrospective (n = 388)	48 hour delay ↑ in-hospital mortality (RR 3.4) and 1-month mortality (RR 2.7) each 24 h
Uzoigwe et al. 2013[14]	Retrospective review of prospective database (n = 2056)	In-hospital mortality ↑ with delay (OR 1.98 > 24 h vs. < 24 h, and OR 3.8 > 12 h vs. < 12 h)
Moja et al. 2012[15]	Meta-analysis (n = 191,873)	Early hip surgery (< 48 h) ↓ in-hospital mortality (OR 0.74)

OR, odds ratio; RR, relative risk.

health advocacy bodies such as the UK National Institute for Health and Care Excellence (NICE) to adopt recommendations and clinical pathways with the goal of early surgical therapy for this population. In addition to mortality benefits, a reduction in the lag time between presentation to the emergency room and surgery in hip fracture patients has been shown to decrease the incidence of postoperative delirium, a common problem in this older group of patients.[16]

Management of anesthesia for hip fracture

It is widely recognized that geriatric hip fracture patients are at high risk for in-hospital morbidity and mortality (see Chapter 36). Editorials and pro–con debates abound regarding the optimal anesthetic technique for various surgical procedures, and in many cases the data are insufficient to sway clinicians to one side. Until fairly recently, this had been the case with hip fracture, but this is changing. The main problems facing readers of the literature were heterogeneity in study design, patient population, and procedure type, which often precludes a meaningful overall conclusion. The number of randomized controlled trials performed in the last 20 years that examine the effect of anesthetic technique on outcome for hip fracture surgery is small. Moreover, despite data from these studies showing good outcomes such as reductions in post-anesthesia care unit (PACU) discharge time, hypotension, and myocardial ischemia with neuraxial techniques, these results should be interpreted with caution as they tend to be from small studies.

More recently, however, two studies were published that looked at very large numbers of patients in order to answer the question. Luger and colleagues conducted a meta-analysis of 34 randomized controlled trials, 14 observational studies, and 8 reviews/meta-analysis publications (n = 18,715) and demonstrated that neuraxial anesthesia was associated with significantly reduced early mortality, fewer incidents of deep venous thrombosis, less postoperative confusion, and fewer overall pulmonary complications, including postoperative hypoxia, pneumonia, and fatal pulmonary embolism.[17] There were no differences between groups in the rates of arrhythmias, myocardial events, congestive heart failure, intraoperative blood loss, renal failure, or stroke. Hypotension also seemed to occur independently of anesthetic technique, although a careful look at the individual studies reveals that continuous spinal has an advantage over single-injection spinal in this regard. This is an attractive technique for this population – it is reliable, it is easy to perform, and it allows for a slow level to be built up in a patient who may have decreased cerebrospinal fluid (CSF) levels and spinal canal volumes. In addition, geriatric patients are typically low-risk for post-dural puncture headache, and the placement of a spinal catheter is usually free of side effects.

In 2012, Neuman and colleagues published a retrospective analysis of a prospectively collected database collected over 2 years from 126 New York State hospitals.[18] Over 18,000 patients admitted for hip fracture were identified and the association between type of anesthesia and patient outcomes tested. Regional anesthesia was found to reduce the risk of in-hospital mortality relative to general anesthesia by 29%, and the risk of pulmonary complications by 25%. At the same time, cardiovascular morbidity was no different between groups. These are difficult data to ignore, and this landmark study has tilted what in the past was often considered a balance of anesthesiologist preference. While not yet a standard of care, the burden of proof is increasingly on the anesthesia provider to show why it is more appropriate to proceed with a general anesthetic in this group of patients.

One common reason that influences the decision to administer general anesthesia in hip fracture patients is coagulopathy. Patients presenting for hip fracture are frequently on anticoagulant or antiplatelet drugs for a variety of reasons, such as atrial fibrillation, cerebrovascular disease, or the presence of coronary stents. While the incidence of spinal hematoma following instrumentation of the neuraxis in such patients is very difficult to quantify, it can safely be assumed to be somewhat above baseline. Various organizations such as the American Society of Regional Anesthesia and Pain Medicine (ASRA) have put forth recommendations to guide decision making in these cases, but since evidence is limited, the guidelines are largely based on pharmacologic data. For example, a factor VII activity level of 40% is generally associated with adequate hemostasis. Since factor VII is the vitamin-K-dependent clotting factor with the shortest half-life, and an international normalized ratio (INR) of 1.5 reflects an activity level of > 40%, ASRA states that it should be safe to administer neuraxial anesthesia if the INR is < 1.5.[19] Similarly, various European societies advocate for acceptable thresholds of < 1.4 or < 1.5.[20,21]

A difficulty with these statements is that they fail to account for individual patient characteristics. For example, what is the obligation of the anesthesiologist to avoid spinal anesthesia for hip fracture (and therefore confer a 25–30% reduction in mortality and pulmonary complications), if the INR is slightly elevated (e.g., 1.6)? The Scandinavian Society of Anaesthesiology and Intensive Care Medicine has issued a thoughtful document on this issue that stratifies the recommended INR threshold based on the expected benefit: if a spinal is being considered for analgesia reasons only, the recommended maximum INR should be ≤ 1.4.[22] However, if it is being used in a situation where it has been shown to decrease morbidity, that threshold may be increased to < 1.8; if expected to reduce mortality, it increases again to < 2.2. Because the incidence of spinal hematoma is larger with epidural and combined spinal–epidural, the respective thresholds are ≤ 1.2, < 1.6, and < 1.8. Clearly, every decision of this sort must be individualized to the patient, and a careful risk–benefit analysis applied considering all of the competing care priorities.

Complications of musculoskeletal trauma

Acute compartment syndrome

A potentially devastating complication of musculoskeletal trauma is acute compartment syndrome, which occurs when the pressure within a closed anatomic compartment rises above a capillary perfusion pressure, compromising the circulation and tissue function within that space (see also Chapter 27). When the capillaries collapse, flow through the tissue beds and into the venous system ceases, leading to tissue hypoxia and the release of mediators increasing vascular permeability. The resultant leakage of fluid through capillary and muscle membranes increases edema, leading to further worsening of the intracompartmental pressure, and eventual muscle necrosis and rhabdomyolysis.

Tibial fracture is the leading cause of acute compartment syndrome, particularly the proximal and middle thirds of the diaphysis (due to the bulkier muscle mass compared with the distal leg).[23] Other common fracture sites leading to acute compartment syndrome include diaphyseal fractures of the forearm and distal radius fractures, although blunt soft tissue injury is a relatively common cause. Younger age (< 35) is a risk factor, increasing the incidence of acute compartment syndrome following tibial fracture by 30-fold, and males outnumber females by approximately 10 to 1.[24] There appears to be no difference in compartment syndrome rates following open versus closed fractures.

The diagnosis of acute compartment syndrome has traditionally been based on the presence of clinical symptoms and signs, especially pain out of proportion. However, clinical signs are often unreliable and can be late indicators of injury. The few studies that have investigated the utility of clinical signs and symptoms have shown a sensitivity and positive predictive value of only 11–15%,[25] prompting some major trauma intensive care units to abandon physical examination as part of the screening process for compartment syndrome, and instead rely solely on objective measurements of compartmental pressures or tissue ischemia such as direct compartmental pressure monitoring or near-infrared spectroscopy (NIRS). This latter technique is based on the principle that chromophores such as oxyhemoglobin and deoxyhemoglobin absorb near-infrared light to varying degrees, and the reflected pattern can be quantified to give a picture of oxygen uptake and extraction in tissues. NIRS is noninvasive and appears to correlate well to tissue perfusion pressures.[26] However, its use may be limited in the deep posterior compartment of the leg due to interference from more shallow tissues. Despite the availability of objective monitors, many clinicians still rely on the presence or absence of pain as a diagnostic tool for acute compartment syndrome, and fear of missing the diagnosis has led many surgeons and anesthesiologists to advocate against the use of neuraxial and peripheral nerve blocks in the trauma population. Indeed, epidural analgesia has been implicated in the delayed diagnosis of compartment syndrome in at least three patients, all of whom had *dense* bilateral motor blocks for more than 18 hours after their operations.[24] A common finding in these three cases was a lack of breakthrough pain because of their profound sensory and motor blockade. In contrast, the remaining literature suggests that neuraxial analgesia may in fact facilitate the diagnosis due to increasing severity of breakthrough pain, provided a low-concentration solution is used (e.g., 0.1–0.2% ropivacaine). The ischemic pain of compartment syndrome is difficult to mask with dilute analgesic solutions of local anesthetic, and requires surgical anesthetic concentrations to control. To date there are no convincing reports of peripheral nerve blocks delaying the diagnosis of acute compartment syndrome. Similarly, there is no literature to support the view that opioids are inherently safer than regional anesthesia in this setting, and there have been multiple reports of delayed diagnosis of compartment syndrome attributable to opioid analgesia.[24]

This controversial issue is often framed in the context of patient safety *versus* quality analgesia; these two are not, however, mutually exclusive. Ignoring the ethical obligation to treat pain following injury, it is nonsensical to rely on such an insensitive and subjective means of diagnosing a potentially catastrophic complication as the clinical exam. Some anesthesiologists have therefore called for the mandated use of objective monitoring in patients deemed high-risk, which would then permit the rational use of whatever analgesic modality is most appropriate.[27]

Continuous peripheral nerve catheter techniques can be advantageous, as the concentration of the local anesthetic can be altered throughout the perioperative and postoperative course to match the intervention (surgical procedure vs. post-operative pain) or to stop the infusion entirely if required (see Chapter 16). Catheters can be placed at any time during the hospital course and left "dry" (or with a small infusion of saline to prevent clotting), and then bolused when appropriate. When possible, dilute solutions of local anesthetics (e.g., ropivacaine 0.2%) should be used.

Fat embolism syndrome

Fat embolism syndrome (FES) is a constellation of signs and symptoms that are related to the presence of fat droplets in the peripheral and lung microcirculation.[28] Long-bone fracture is the principal etiology, and risk factors include both the movement of unstable bone fragments and the reaming of medullary cavities. Femoral shaft fractures are particularly prone to developing FES (incidence of 7.6%), compared with 0.3–1.3% for all fractures combined.[29] The risk increases with the number of bones fractured – for example, FES occurs in up to 33% of patients with bilateral femoral fractures.[30] Soft tissue blunt trauma may be a frequently overlooked cause of FES; in one report of 53 fatalities following extensive soft tissue trauma, over half were found to have died from FES, despite the absence of long-bone fracture.[31] The authors hypothesized that mechanical disintegration of adipose tissue was the etiology in those cases.

The classic presentation of FES includes respiratory distress and hypoxemia, central nervous system derangements, pulmonary hypertension and system hypotension, and petechial rash of the upper torso and conjunctiva. Other findings include retinopathy (including retinal fat globules), thrombocytopenia, arrhythmias, oliguria, and myocardial ischemia. There are two principal explanations for the varying pathologic and clinical manifestations of FES. The mechanical hypothesis argues that fat from disrupted bone marrow accumulates in the microcirculation, acting as a mechanical obstruction to blood flow, both in the pulmonary system (causing pulmonary hypertension) and in the systemic circulation (due to passage via a patent foramen ovale or other shunt), which accounts for the CNS, skin, and other organ changes. Detractors from this theory point out the failure of it to explain the 24- to 72-hour interval between injury and onset of the syndrome that is frequently seen. The alternative hypothesis states that fat in the blood is degraded to toxic intermediaries, including free fatty acids, which then go on to cause injury to the multiple organ systems. This biochemical theory explains the delay in symptoms, as it takes some time for fat to be degraded in the plasma. It is probable that both mechanisms play a role in the variable picture seen in FES.

Blood gas analysis will frequently show marked hypoxemia, as well as respiratory alkalosis from tachypnea. Fat globules may be seen in the urine, blood, or sputum, but these are unreliable tests and should not be relied upon. Chest x-ray findings typically occur in 30–50% of cases, but often present 12–24 hours after the initial event; these include bilateral

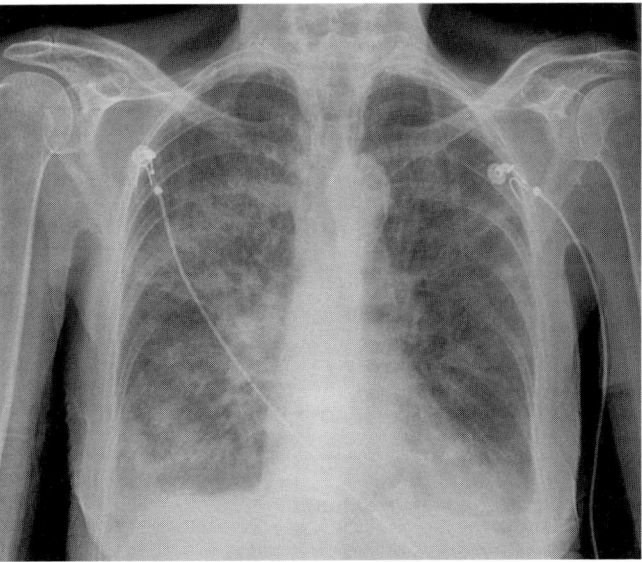

Figure 28.4 Chest x-ray findings in fat embolism syndrome, demonstrating widespread bilateral alveolar infiltrates.

diffuse interstitial and alveolar densities (Fig. 28.4).[32] Patients with FES frequently show hypointense lesions on cerebral T1W magnetic resonance imaging.[33]

Treatment of FES is supportive, and should include oxygen therapy, ventilatory and hemodynamic support and intravenous fluids. Corticosteroids have been shown in some cases to benefit patients, but there is an absence of rigorous studies supporting this.[34] Despite the need for advanced resuscitation, the overall mortality is low and most patients recover fully. Probably the single most important intervention in reducing the morbidity and incidence of FES is early immobilization of fractures.[35] The longer the period of time that the broken ends of the long bone are displaced and prone to mechanical disruption, the higher the risk of fat emboli.

Complex regional pain syndrome

Complex regional pain syndrome (CRPS) is a relatively common disorder following limb trauma that is characterized by continuing regional pain disproportionate to what would be expected for the inciting injury (see Chapter 17). Severity can vary from very mild to incapacitating, and can last for decades. In CRPS I (formerly reflex sympathetic dystrophy) there is typically minor soft tissue trauma or bone fracture, but no overt nerve lesion. In contrast, CRPS II (formerly causalgia) must be associated with a peripheral nerve injury for diagnosis. The exact pathophysiology is unclear, but likely involves both a central mechanism that promotes maladaptive sensory and autonomic responses to injury, and local factors such as tissue acidosis and neurogenic inflammation. The constellation of findings can include abnormal sensory, motor, sudomotor, vasomotor, and trophic changes, localized to the affected area (Table 28.2).

Table 28.2 Clinical features of complex regional pain syndrome (CRPS) type I

Abnormality	Specific features
Sensory	Hyperalgesia, allodynia
Vasomotor	Vasoconstriction (decreased skin temperature, pale skin color) or vasodilatation (increased skin temperature, red/dark skin color)
Sudomotor	Edema, hypo/hyperhydrosis
Motor	Decreased range of motion, weakness, tremor, dystonia
Trophic	Atrophy of the skin, hair, and nails; osteoporosis

Fractures are often reported as the most common precipitating event, especially of the distal forearm and leg (i.e., wrist and ankle). In Colles' fracture, for example, the incidence of CRPS is up to 37%.[36] Other risk factors appear to be female sex and injury to a motor nerve.[37] Identification of these high-risk patients in the trauma population provides a potential opportunity to offer preventive therapy. For example, the *N*-methyl-D-aspartate (NMDA) receptor antagonist ketamine has received increasing attention as a means to prevent the central sensitization that leads to amplification of noxious pain signals in CRPS. Ketamine is thought to reverse the chronic depolarized state in neuropathic pain such as CRPS by occupying the NMDA receptors in the spinal cord, thereby preventing glutamate from exerting its excitatory effect. A recent systematic review found only a few controlled trials and several observational studies, although the results appear to be generally in favor of its use.[38] The optimal dosing schedule is unclear: single perioperative doses, as well as long-term high-dose infusions of ketamine, have been reported as successful.

One simple and effective preventive measure against CRPS for patients with wrist and ankle fractures is the administration of vitamin C. A dose of 500–1000 mg PO daily for 45–50 days following injury has been shown to reduce the risk of developing CRPS by 80%, and therefore unless contraindicated should be part of the clinical pathway for this subset of trauma patients.[39]

Regional anesthetic blocks have the theoretical advantage of halting the sympathetic efferent flow to the extremity, which has been implicated in CRPS I. Observational studies suggest that patients with latent CRPS may have a reduced risk of having their disease "rekindled" when regional blocks are performed for extremity surgery, compared with general anesthesia alone.[40] However, while this is an attractive theory, large-scale randomized controlled studies are lacking.

Postoperative concerns

Pain management

Pain is a substantial burden to the injured patient, and the provision of quality postoperative analgesia must be a high priority. One of the principles that guides modern acute pain practice is the aggressive use of multimodal analgesia, in an effort to reduce the side-effect profile of any one class of drugs, but in particular opioids (see Chapter 15). Opioid-related adverse events range from those that can be considered a nuisance (e.g., pruritis), to those that have an effect on patient comfort, satisfaction, and hospital length of stay (e.g., nausea and vomiting, ileus, constipation, confusion), and finally to those that are life-threatening (e.g., respiratory depression). The American Society of Anesthesiologists (ASA) task force, amongst others, has recommended that whenever possible, all patients receive around-the-clock nonsteroidal anti-inflammatory drugs (NSAIDs), COX-2 inhibitors, and/or acetaminophen, unless contraindicated.[41]

Pain has consequences beyond the obvious emotional and physical discomfort. For example, pain associated with an isolated rib fracture confers a 20% chance of respiratory failure due to splinting, hypoventilation, atelectasis, and pneumonia; this number jumps to approximately 50% if there is underlying pulmonary contusion.[42] This type of case highlights the need to individualize the choice of pain management strategy to the patient and the type of injury. Simply administering opioids may provide good pain control, but may also result in further hypoventilation and overall worsening of the patient's condition.

Muscle spasm is an occasional contributor to acute pain following bony fracture, and is caused by an increase in the firing rate of a spinal cord reflex arc; motor fibers supplying the muscles overlying the fracture are activated and contract at an abnormal rate, producing the spasm or cramping. This type of contraction is particularly painful in a fracture that has not yet been repaired, when the two mobile ends of the broken shaft come in contact. Ice is the mainstay of first-line treatment. Muscle-relaxant medications such as cyclobenzaprine or benzodiazepines are mildly effective for this type of spasm. For unremitting spasm, treatment can be aimed at interrupting the spinal reflex arc by anesthetizing the culprit nerve – for example, spasm associated with a femoral fracture might require any combination of femoral, obturator, and/or sciatic nerve blocks depending on the involved muscle group. This is generally very effective, but requires a team approach to the care of the patient and an appreciation for other considerations relating to a nerve block such as compartment syndrome.

The traumatized patient is at risk for the development of chronic pain (see Chapter 17). Acute and chronic pain were at one time thought to be separate entities (e.g., physiologic versus neuropathic), but increasingly it is being realized that they are two ends of a spectrum and injured patients are at risk for transformation to longstanding pain and suffering. The incidence of chronic pain following severe trauma is dependent on several factors such as the type of injury and psychological health, but in general almost half of patients report accident-related pain 3 years after the injury.[43] Those with chronic pain tend to demonstrate significantly more symptoms of posttraumatic stress disorder, depression, and anxiety, more disability, and more days off work.

Posttraumatic pain can occur with any injury, but common chronic pain syndromes include headache following traumatic brain injury, CRPS following injury to a distal extremity, posttraumatic abdominal or thoracic pain, and pain related to spinal injury such as nerve root or cord compression, or vertebral fracture.

One group of patients at particular risk for chronic pain following trauma are amputees, as noted earlier in this chapter. Phantom limb pain is present in up to 85% of amputees, and is often severe enough to interfere with a patient's employment and social life. There are several postulated factors that predict the incidence and severity of phantom limb pain, but one that is potentially modifiable by anesthesiologists is the presence or absence of good preoperative pain control. In one randomized controlled study of 65 patients undergoing amputation, high-quality analgesia with either epidural or intravenous opioids for 48 hours prior to and 48 hours following surgery led to decreased incidence and intensity of phantom limb pain at 6 months.[5] While the literature is somewhat equivocal on the efficacy of peripheral nerve blocks, including continuous catheters, in preventing chronic pain following amputation, several observational studies have reported good results, especially if the infusion of local anesthetic is started at the time of surgery and continued for several days after the procedure.

Delirium

The geriatric trauma patient is at high risk for perioperative delirium, particularly if he/she has preexisting dementia, is male, or undergoes a hip fracture procedure lasting longer than 2 hours (see Chapter 36).[16] Because of the multifactorial nature of delirium, including baseline mental and behavioral capacity, metabolic disturbances, the effect of drugs (particularly sedatives and opioid analgesics), the presence of pain, and an unfamiliar environment, it is difficult to expect a single intervention to reduce the incidence of this complication.

Avoidance of traditional opioid analgesics may be one of the most promising strategies for reducing delirium in trauma patients. Many trauma critical care units have shifted to the use of dexmedetomidine rather than benzodiazepines and/or opioids for sedation, to provide a more rapid and clearer neurologic recovery with fewer episodes of delirium.[44] Regional anesthetic techniques may also be beneficial. A randomized controlled trial found that hip fracture patients deemed to be at risk for delirium who received daily fascia iliaca blocks pre- and postoperatively had a significantly reduced incidence of delirium compared with those randomized to sham fascia iliaca block, likely a result of reduced pain and opioid requirements, both known contributors to delirium.[45] This supports the notion that regional analgesia should be initiated as soon as possible (i.e., in the emergency department if possible) for these high-risk patients, and continued until the intensity of pain is low enough to justify halting the block.

Summary

Injuries to the musculoskeletal system are usually assigned a secondary level of importance compared to injuries to the airway, central nervous system, or visceral organs. However appropriate during the early stages of resuscitation and initial management, this triage strategy should not lead to an underestimation of the importance of these types of injuries. Fractures and soft tissue trauma carry the potential to be life-threatening, and frequently lead to life-long disability and/or a reduction in the functional quality of life. Quality anesthetic care of the patient with musculoskeletal trauma demands recognition of the potential complications associated with these injuries; more importantly, the trauma anesthesiologist must be aware of the opportunities to intervene in order to reduce long-term morbidity and mortality, including appropriate use of regional anesthesia during hip fracture repair.

Questions

(1) **The most common cause of death following pelvic fracture is:**
   a. Abdominal compartment syndrome
   b. Hemorrhage
   c. Thromboembolism
   d. Septic shock
   e. None of the above

(2) **Early treatment priorities in the setting of significant crush injury should include:**
   a. Aggressive volume replacement
   b. Alkalinization of the urine
   c. Treatment with mannitol
   d. Intravenous calcium
   e. All of the above

(3) **Routine preoperative cardiac testing in hip fracture patients leads to an average delay of surgical fixation of:**
   a. 6 hours
   b. 24 hours
   c. 48 hours
   d. 80 hours
   e. 1 week

(4) **The use of regional anesthesia compared with general anesthesia for hip fracture repair is associated with a significant reduction in:**
   a. Cardiac complications
   b. Incidence of acute kidney injury
   c. Risk of stroke
   d. In-hospital mortality
   e. Hospital length of stay

(5) **Fracture of which bone is the leading cause of acute compartment syndrome?**
   a. Tibia
   b. Fibula
   c. Radius
   d. Ulna
   e. Humerus

(6) The sensitivity and positive predictive value of clinical signs in the diagnosis of acute compartment syndrome is approximately:
   a. 1–2%
   b. 11–15%
   c. 25–30%
   d. 75–80%
   e. 92–95%

(7) Which of the following is *not* a feature of fat embolism syndrome (FES)?
   a. Hypoxemia
   b. Thrombocytopenia
   c. Bronchospasm
   d. Retinopathy
   e. Oliguria

(8) The risk of complex regional pain syndrome following wrist and ankle fracture can be reduced with the use of:
   a. Vitamin A
   b. Vitamin B_{12}
   c. Vitamin C
   d. Vitamin E
   e. None of the above

(9) An isolated rib fracture leads to what approximate risk of respiratory failure due to splinting, atelectasis, and pneumonia?
   a. 10%
   b. 20%
   c. 30%
   d. 50%
   e. 75%

(10) Which of the following are risk factors for postoperative delirium in patients undergoing hip fracture repair?
   a. Preexisting dementia
   b. Male sex
   c. Surgical repair lasting longer than 2 hours
   d. Opioid analgesia
   e. All of the above

Answers

(1) b
(2) e
(3) d
(4) d
(5) a
(6) b
(7) c
(8) c
(9) b
(10) e

References

1. Banerjee M, Bouillon B, Shafizadeh S, *et al.* Epidemiology of extremity injuries in multiple trauma patients. *Injury* 2012; **44**: 1015–21.

2. Gallay SH, Hupel TM, Beaton DE, Schemitsch EH, McKee MD. Functional outcome of acromioclavicular joint injury in polytrauma patients. *J Orthop Trauma* 1998; **12**: 159–63.

3. White CE, Hsu JR, Holcomb JB. Haemodynamically unstable pelvic fractures. *Injury* 2009; **40**: 1023–30.

4. Cullinane DC, Schiller HJ, Zielinski MD, *et al.* Eastern Association for the Surgery of Trauma practice management guidelines for hemorrhage in pelvic fracture: update and systematic review. *J Trauma* 2011; **71**: 1850–68.

5. Karanikolas M, Aretha D, Tsolakis I, *et al.* Optimized perioperative analgesia reduces chronic phantom limb pain intensity, prevalence, and frequency: a prospective, randomized, clinical trial. *Anesthesiology* 2011; **114**: 1144–54.

6. Malinoski DJ, Slater MS, Mullins RJ. Crush injury and rhabdomyolysis. *Crit Care Clin* 2004; **20**: 171–92.

7. Lieurance R, Benjamin JB, Rappaport WD. Blood loss and transfusion in patients with isolated femur fractures. *J Orthop Trauma* 1992; **6**: 175–9.

8. Fulkerson EW, Egol KA. Timing issues in fracture management: a review of current concepts. *Bull NYU Hosp Jt Dis* 2009; **67**: 58–67.

9. Gadsden J. Blocks in anesthetized patients. *Reg Anesth Pain Med* 2009; **34**: 604.

10. Ricci WM, Della Rocca GJ, Combs C, Borrelli J. The medical and economic impact of preoperative cardiac testing in elderly patients with hip fractures. *Injury* 2007; **38** (Suppl 3): S49–52.

11. Fleisher LA, Beckman JA, Brown KA, *et al.* ACC/AHA 2007 guidelines on perioperative cardiovascular evaluation and care for noncardiac surgery. *J Am Coll Cardiol* 2007; **50**: e159–241.

12. Daugaard CL, Jørgensen HL, Riis T, *et al.* Is mortality after hip fracture associated with surgical delay or admission during weekends and public holidays? A retrospective study of 38,020 patients. *Acta Orthop* 2012; **83**: 609–13.

13. Smeets SJM, Poeze M, Verbruggen JPAM. Preoperative cardiac evaluation of geriatric patients with hip fracture. *Injury* 2012; **43**: 2146–51.

14. Uzoigwe CE, Burnand HGF, Cheesman CL, *et al.* Early and ultra-early surgery in hip fracture patients improves survival. *Injury* 2013; **44**: 726–9.

15. Moja L, Piatti A, Pecoraro V, *et al.* Timing matters in hip fracture surgery: patients operated within 48 hours have better outcomes. A meta-analysis and meta-regression of over 190,000 patients. *PLoS ONE* 2012; **7** (10): e46175.

16. Lee HB, Mears SC, Rosenberg PB, *et al.* Predisposing factors for postoperative delirium after hip fracture repair in individuals with and without dementia. *J Am Geriatr Soc* 2011; **59**: 2306–13.

17. Luger TJ, Kammerlander C, Gosch M, *et al.* Neuroaxial versus general anaesthesia in geriatric patients for hip fracture surgery: does it matter? *Osteoporos Int* 2010; **21** (Suppl 4): S555–72.

18. Neuman MD, Silber JH, Elkassabany NM, Ludwig JM, Fleisher LA. Comparative effectiveness of regional

versus general anesthesia for hip fracture surgery in adults. *Anesthesiology* 2012; **117**: 72–92.

19. Horlocker TT, Wedel DJ, Rowlingson JC, *et al.* Regional anesthesia in the patient receiving antithrombotic or thrombolytic therapy: American Society of Regional Anesthesia and Pain Medicine evidence-based guidelines (third edition). *Reg Anesth Pain Med* 2010; **35**: 64–101.

20. Vandermeulen D, SIngelyn F, Vercauteren M, *et al.* Belgian guidelines concerning central neuraxial blockade in patients with drug-induced alteration of coagulation: an update. *Acta Anaesthesiol Belg* 2005; **56**: 139–46.

21. Gogarten W, Vandermeulen E, Van Aken H, *et al.* Regional anesthesia and antithrombotic agents: recommendations of the European Society of Anaesthesiology. *Eur J Anaesthesiol* 2010; **27**: 999–1015.

22. Breivik H, Bang U, Jalonen J, *et al.* Nordic guidelines for neuraxial blocks in disturbed haemostasis from the Scandinavian Society of Anaesthesiology and Intensive Care Medicine. *Acta Anaesthesiol Scand* 2010; **54**: 16–41.

23. McQueen MM, Gaston P, Court-Brown CM. Acute compartment syndrome. Who is at risk? *J Bone Joint Surg Br* 2000; **82**: 200–3.

24. Mar GJ, Barrington MJ, McGuirk BR. Acute compartment syndrome of the lower limb and the effect of postoperative analgesia on diagnosis. *Br J Anaesth* 2009; **102**: 3–11.

25. Ulmer T. The clinical diagnosis of compartment syndrome of the lower leg: are clinical findings predictive of the disorder? *J Orthop Trauma* 2002; **16**: 572–7.

26. Reisman WM, Shuler MS, Kinsey TL, *et al.* Relationship between near infrared spectroscopy and

intra-compartmental pressures. *J Emerg Med* 2013; **44**: 292–8.

27. Hocking G. Re: The use of regional anaesthesia in patients at risk of acute compartment syndrome. *Injury* 2007; **38**: 872–3.

28. Akhtar S. Fat embolism. *Anesthesiol Clin* 2009; **27**: 533–50.

29. Stein PD, Yaekoub AY, Matta F, Kleerekoper M. Fat embolism syndrome. *Am J Med Sci* 2008; **336**: 472–7.

30. Johnson MJ, Lucas GL. Fat embolism syndrome. *Orthopedics* 1996; **19**: 41–8.

31. Hiss J, Kahana T, Kugel C. Beaten to death: why do they die? *J Trauma* 1996; **40**: 27–30.

32. Greenberg HB. Roentgenographic signs of posttraumatic fat embolism. *JAMA* 1968; **204**: 540–1.

33. Satoh H, Kurisu K, Ohtani M, *et al.* Cerebral fat embolism studied by magnetic resonance imaging, transcranial Doppler sonography, and single photon emission computed tomography: case report. *J Trauma* 1997; **43**: 345–8.

34. Babalis GA, Yiannakopoulos CK, Karliaftis K, Antonogiannakis E. Prevention of posttraumatic hypoxaemia in isolated lower limb long bone fractures with a minimal prophylactic dose of corticosteroids. *Injury* 2004; **35**: 309–17.

35. Riska EB, Myllynen P. Fat embolism in patients with multiple injuries. *J Trauma* 1982; **22**: 891–4.

36. Dijkstra PU, Groothoff JW, ten Duis HJ, Geertzen JHB. Incidence of complex regional pain syndrome type I after fractures of the distal radius. *Eur J Pain* 2003; **7**: 457–62.

37. Demir SE, Ozaras N, Karamehmetoğlu SS, Karacan I, Aytekin E. Risk factors for complex regional pain syndrome in

patients with traumatic extremity injury. *Ulus Travma Acil Cerrahi Derg* 2010; **16**: 144–8.

38. Azari P, Lindsay DR, Briones D, *et al.* Efficacy and safety of ketamine in patients with complex regional pain syndrome: a systematic review. *CNS Drugs* 2012; **26**: 215–28.

39. Shibuya N, Humphers JM, Agarwal MR, Jupiter DC. Efficacy and safety of high-dose vitamin C on complex regional pain syndrome in extremity trauma and surgery: systematic review and meta-analysis. *J Foot Ankle Surg* 2013; **52**: 62–6.

40. Rocco AG. Sympathetically maintained pain may be rekindled by surgery under general anesthesia. *Anesthesiology* 1993; **79**: 865.

41. Apfelbaum JL, Ashburn MA, Connis RT, Gan TJ, Nickinovich DG. Practice guidelines for acute pain management in the perioperative setting: an updated report by the American Society of Anesthesiologists Task Force on Acute Pain Management. *Anesthesiology* 2012; **116**: 248–73.

42. Livingston DH, Shogan B, John P, Lavery RF. CT diagnosis of Rib fractures and the prediction of acute respiratory failure. *J Trauma* 2008; **64**: 905–11.

43. Jenewein J, Moergeli H, Wittmann L, *et al.* Development of chronic pain following severe accidental injury. Results of a 3-year follow-up study. *J Psychosom Res* 2009; **66**: 119–26.

44. Riker RR, Fraser GL. Altering intensive care sedation paradigms to improve patient outcomes. *Anesthesiol Clin* 2011; **29**: 663–74.

45. Mouzopoulos G, Vasiliadis G, Lasanianos N, *et al.* Fascia iliaca block prophylaxis for hip fracture patients at risk for delirium: a randomized placebo-controlled study. *J Orthop Traumatol* 2009; **10**: 127–33.

Cardiac and great vessel trauma

Leonardo Canale, Inderjit Gill, and Christopher Smith

Objectives

(1) Review the etiologies and consequences of cardiac and great vessel trauma.

(2) Discuss the clinical presentation of cardiac and great vessel trauma.

(3) Evaluate diagnostic strategies for cardiac and great vessel trauma.

(4) Become familiar with decision making and techniques for emergency thoracotomy, a potentially life-saving procedure.

(5) Identify hemorrhage control methods for cardiac and great vessel trauma which a emergency physician should be proficient with until a cardiovascular surgeon arrives.

(6) Discuss the definitive treatment of cardiac and great vessel trauma.

(7) Become familiar with endovascular stenting techniques in aortic trauma.

Introduction

Blunt and penetrating cardiac and great vessel trauma are associated with potentially life-threatening injuries requiring a high index of suspicion. Cardiac tamponade is often associated with injury to the heart and may quickly lead to hemodynamic compromise, necessitating prompt diagnosis and intervention. The aorta and great vessels are most commonly injured in a blunt manner associated with multisystem trauma, often the result of rapid deceleration. The majority of patients succumb to this type of injury and do not survive to present to a hospital. A high index of suspicion for cardiac and aortic injury should be present in any patient involved in trauma to the chest, and appropriate diagnostic measures taken once stabilized.

Cardiac trauma

The heart lies in the mediastinum between the two lungs and is enclosed within the pericardium. The surface of the heart exposed to the anterior chest wall is formed 55% from the right ventricular wall, 20% from the left ventricular wall, 10% from the right atrial wall, 10% from the ascending aorta and pulmonary artery, and 5% from the venae cavae.

Although the heart appears to be well protected by the bony structures, in reality it is highly vulnerable to injury. Missiles and knives entering the thoracic cavity from any side have the potential to injure the heart. Similarly, any decelerating or compressive injury may result in trauma to the heart. The incidence of traumatic injury to the heart is difficult to establish. Many patients with cardiac injury succumb at the scene of the injury. Aggressive resuscitation and rapid transport by trained personnel enable more patients with potentially lethal cardiac trauma to reach the hospital alive. The survival of these patients is directly related to rapidity of diagnosis, which requires a high index of suspicion and treatment of their injury.

Etiologies of cardiac trauma

Categorization of traumatic heart disease is based on the mechanism of injury (Table 29.1). We will discuss the pathophysiologic mechanisms, clinical features, diagnostic strategies, and management of the most common patterns below.

Penetrating cardiac trauma

Penetrating trauma is the most common cause of significant cardiac injury seen in hospital settings, with the predominant injury being from guns and knives.[1,2] Its high lethality has not improved over several decades. A population-based study of trauma admissions has determined its incidence as 1 per 210 admissions, with a general survival of 19.3%, 9.7% for gunshots, and 32.6% for stab wounds.[3] In the United States, gunshot wounds outnumber stab wounds by almost 2 to 1,[4] while in other parts of the world, such as China, stabbings compromise most of the penetrating cardiac injuries.

Anatomy and pathophysiology

Penetrating wounds of the heart are most frequently associated with penetrating wounds to the "cardiac box" (inferior to the clavicles, superior to the costal margin, and medial to the midclavicular line). However, they may also occur in patients

Trauma Anesthesia, 2nd Edition, ed. Charles E. Smith. Published by Cambridge University Press. © Charles E. Smith, 2015.

Table 29.1 Etiology of traumatic heart diseases

I. Penetrating
A. Stab wounds: knives, swords, ice picks, fence posts, wire, sporting objects
B. Gunshot wounds: low/high-caliber, handgun, rifles, nail guns, lawnmower projectiles
C. Shotgun wounds: close range, distant

II. Blunt
A. Motor vehicle accident: seatbelt, airbag
B. Vehicular: pedestrian accident
C. Falls from height
D. Crushing: industrial accident
E. Blasts: explosives, grenades
F. Assault (aggravated)
G. Sternal or rib fractures
H. Recreational: sporting events (bull goring), baseball

III. Iatrogenic
A. Catheter induced
B. Pericardiocentesis induced

IV. Metabolic
A. Traumatic response to injury
B. "Stunning"
C. Systemic inflammatory response syndrome (SIRS)

V. Others
A. Burn
B. Electrical
C. Factitious: needles, foreign bodies
D. Embolic: missiles

Modified from: Mattox KL, Estrera AL, Wall MJ. Traumatic heart disease. In Zipes DP, Libby P, Bonow RO, Braunwald E, eds., *Braunwald's Heart Disease*, 7th edition. Philadelphia, PA: Elsevier Saunders; 2005, pp.1781–8.

with wounds to the remainder of thorax, lower neck, and upper abdomen. These wounds may produce a variety of lesions, including: (1) penetrating wounds of the pericardium; (2) penetrating wounds of the cardiac wall; (3) penetrating wounds of the interventricular septum; (4) perforating or lacerating wounds of the cardiac valves, chordae tendineae, or papillary muscles; and (5) perforating or lacerating wounds of the coronary vessels.

The right ventricle is the most frequently injured heart chamber owing to its anterior anatomic location, followed closely by the left ventricle.[1]

Victims of gunshot wounds usually have more severe physiologic impairment than those with stab wounds. Gunshot wounds cause larger defects in the myocardium and pericardium, through-and-through wounds, and a larger number of injuries to other vital organs, leading to hemorrhage and exsanguination. Stab wounds are more likely to produce small injuries that seal off during systole, leading to cardiac tamponade.

Cardiac tamponade

Cardiac tamponade results when sufficient pressure is exerted upon the heart by blood, fluid, or air accumulated in the pericardial sac that interferes with its diastolic filling and systolic output. As pericardial fluid accumulates, a decrease in ventricular filling occurs, leading to a decrease in stroke volume. A compensatory rise in catecholamines leads to tachycardia and increased right-sided heart filling pressures. The limits of distensibility are reached, and the septum shifts toward the left side, further compromising left ventricular function. If this cycle persists, ventricular function can continue to deteriorate, leading to irreversible shock. As little as 60–100 mL of blood in the pericardial sac can produce the clinical picture of tamponade.

Clinical features

The clinical presentation of penetrating injuries may vary according to the rate of bleeding and the size of defect the injury creates in the pericardium. If the pericardium remains sealed, the clinical presentation may be acute cardiac tamponade.

The clinical manifestations of acute cardiac tamponade may vary with the rate and volume of accumulation of blood in the pericardial sac. Massive and rapid accumulation of blood within the pericardium usually results in severe tamponade, cardiac arrest, and sudden death. Patients with less rapid and massive accumulation of blood may be restless, complaining of air hunger, or in shock. The skin may be cold and moist, and the lips may be mildly cyanotic. The visible superficial neck veins are distended and may have paradoxical filling during inspiration (Kussmaul's sign). The systolic blood pressure is usually below normal and may decrease during inspiration, 10 mmHg or more, with no significant decrease in heart sounds (pulsus paradoxus). The pulse pressure is narrow, and the pulse is rapid and hypodynamic. The venous pressure is elevated, the heart sounds may be distant and muffled, and there may or may not be a pericardial friction rub.

However, many of these clinical manifestations may not be present in patients with acute traumatic cardiac tamponade. In fact the classic Beck's triad of decreased arterial pressure, muffled heart sounds, and elevated central venous pressure has been observed in only about one-third to two-thirds of patients with traumatic cardiac tamponade, although over 90% of them have one of these signs. Pulsus paradoxus, distension of the superficial neck veins, and elevation of the central venous pressure can also be caused by other conditions, such as tension pneumothorax, pulmonary emphysema, or cardiac failure. If the pericardial defect caused by penetrating trauma is large and remains open, the blood drains into the pleural space and produces hemothorax and hemorrhagic shock.

Another clinical picture with which the patient may present following a penetrating cardiac trauma is that of an intermittently decompressing tamponade. In this case, intermittent hemorrhage from the intrapericardial space occurs, decompressing and partially relieving tamponade. The clinical picture may wax and wane depending on the intrapericardial pressure and volume and total blood loss. In general, this condition is more compatible with a longer survival than are the first two clinical presentations.

Diagnostic strategies

Owing to the absence and/or lack of specificity of some of the clinical manifestations of acute cardiac tamponade, its diagnosis may be overlooked unless a high index of suspicion is maintained.

Chest radiography is nonspecific, but it can identify hemothorax or pneumothorax. A normal cardiac silhouette may be seen even in the presence of tamponade, since in acute situations small amounts of fluid may be enough to cause this syndrome. Other possibly indicated examinations include ultrasonography, central venous measurements, subxiphoid pericardial window, thoracoscopy, and pericardiocentesis.

Ultrasonography (see also Chapter 10)

Surgeons are increasingly performing ultrasonography for thoracic trauma, paralleling the use of ultrasonography for abdominal trauma. Focused assessment with sonography for trauma (FAST) evaluates four anatomical windows for the presence of intraabdominal or pericardial fluid.[5] FAST examination, if performed by a trained surgeon, has a sensitivity of nearly 100% and a specificity of 97.3%.[5] Echocardiographic features of tamponade include collapse of the thin, flexible right atrial free wall for greater than one-third of systole, diastolic collapse of the right ventricle, inferior vena cava plethora, and respiratory variations of left and right ventricular diastolic filling (see Chapter 10). Echocardiography may be useful in identifying and characterizing valvular abnormalities and septal defects. A false-negative result may occur if there is a pericardial rupture draining blood from the pericardial sac to the pleura, avoiding the accumulation of blood around the heart.

Subxiphoid pericardial window

Subxiphoid pericardial window has been performed both in the emergency department and in the operating room with the patient receiving either local or general anesthesia. Via subxiphoid vertical incision, a small hole is made in the pericardium to determine the presence of blood. Maintaining adequate preload is necessary to prevent further hemodynamic deterioration. If general anesthesia is required, induction of anesthesia and initiation of positive-pressure ventilation decreases preload and may lead to cardiac arrest (see Chapters 7 and 30). The disadvantage of a subxiphoid pericardial window is that it is an invasive procedure, and if a major injury is found a second thoracic incision is required for definitive repair. Ultrasonographic evaluation has almost eliminated the role of subxiphoid pericardial window in the evaluation of cardiac trauma (see Chapter 10).

Pericardiocentesis

In the setting of trauma, cardiac tamponade is acute and caused by hemorrhage. Clot forms quickly and is not amenable to needle drainage. Currently, many trauma surgeons discourage pericardiocentesis for acute trauma. Recurrence of tamponade and subsequent increase in mortality, as well as a significant incidence of false-negative results and potential for iatrogenic injury, makes pericardiocentesis a less than optimal diagnostic tool.

Central venous pressure measurements

In the absence of immediate availability of ultrasonography, the determination of central venous pressure (CVP) is the best test for reinforcing the suspected diagnosis of acute traumatic cardiac tamponade. The combination of shock and an elevated CVP in a patient with cardiac trauma should immediately suggest cardiac tamponade. Other differential considerations for these signs include tension pneumothorax, right ventricular myocardial contusion, superior vena cava obstruction, ruptured tricuspid valve, or preexisting severe pulmonary disease.

Management

Only a small subset of patients with significant cardiac injury will reach the emergency department, and expeditious transport to a designated trauma facility is essential for survival. Transport times of less than 5 minutes and successful endotracheal intubation are positive factors for survival.

Initial management in the emergency department

On initial presentation to the emergency department, airway, breathing, and circulation (ABCs) under Advanced Trauma Life Support (ATLS) protocol are evaluated and established (see Chapter 2).[6] Two large-bore intravenous catheters are inserted, and blood is typed and crossmatched. The patient is examined for signs and symptoms of cardiac tamponade. A pneumothorax or hemothorax, which are often associated with penetrating cardiac trauma, must be treated expeditiously with tube thoracostomy. Bedside echocardiography should be performed as quickly as possible to establish the diagnosis of pericardial effusion with tamponade physiology (see Chapter 10), which then mandates urgent surgical repair. Patients with penetrating cardiac injury invariably require surgical repair. The location (operating room versus emergency department) and timing (immediate versus urgent) depend on the patient's clinical status.

Decision making for emergency department thoracotomy

Emergency department thoracotomy is a drastic, dramatic, and potentially life-saving procedure in which trauma surgeons and emergency physicians should be proficient. With thoracotomy, the goal is (1) to relieve any cardiac tamponade, (2) to support cardiac function with direct cardiac compression and/or crossclamping of the aorta to improve coronary perfusion, and (3) to perform internal defibrillation when

Table 29.2 Outcome of emergency department thoracotomy

Condition	Survival (%)
Cardiac arrest in field	0
Cardiac arrest in emergency department	30
Agonal in emergency department	40
Unresponsive shock in emergency department	50

Modified from Brown J, Grover FL. Trauma to the heart. *Chest Surg Clin N Am* 1997; **7**: 325.

indicated. The decision should be based on a realistic judgment that the patient has a chance of survival but will not tolerate any delay in operative intervention. It is also important to consider not performing thoracotomy for cases in which there is virtually no chance of salvaging a neurologically uncompromised patient.

Important information in formulating a decision to perform emergency department thoracotomy includes time of injury, transport time to the emergency department, the time of vital signs or cardiac electrical activity or both ceased. Consequently, guidelines have been established for performing thoracotomy, to restrict the procedure to patients with some chance of achieving a neurologically functional outcome (Table 29.2). Patients with penetrating trauma with signs of life in the field, even if only electrical activity on cardiac monitor or agonal respirations, are candidates for emergency department thoracotomy if transport time is less than 10 minutes.[7]

For patients in cardiac arrest, tracheal intubation and duration of cardiopulmonary resuscitation (CPR) correlate with survival following thoracotomy. The value of field intubation has been shown to be dramatic: the average time of CPR tolerated by intubated survivors is double that of nonintubated survivors.

Airway control and anesthesia for emergency department thoracotomy

Prior to beginning thoracotomy, the patient's trachea should be intubated and the lungs manually ventilated. Selective one-lung ventilation is an established technique in thoracic surgery and may facilitate emergency department thoracotomy. Common approaches to one-lung ventilation and lung isolation include the use of a double-lumen tube or a bronchial blocker placed through an endotracheal tube (see Chapter 33, Table 33.3). It is acknowledged, however, that availability of and experience with lung isolation techniques is often limited in the emergency department setting. The right lung can be selectively intubated by blindly advancing a single-lumen endotracheal tube to a depth of 30 cm (measured at the corner of mouth) in adult patients. Comatose patients undergoing resuscitation may regain consciousness during successful thoracotomy, but the use of paralyzing agents may mask the return of awareness. The clinician must be cognizant of this

phenomenon and administer adequate analgesic and amnesic agents together with neuromuscular blocking drugs. Ideally, agents with minimal effects on cardiovascular performance should be used.

Surgical techniques for emergency department thoracotomy

A left anterolateral thoracotomy incision over the fifth rib with dissection into the fourth intercostal space provides best access to the heart and great vessels. An incision just beneath the nipple in the male or along the inframammary fold in the female will approximate the fourth intercostal space. Just before opening the pleura, ventilation should be stopped momentarily to prevent injury to the lung. Once the left pleural space is entered, the lung is retracted to expose the descending aorta and pericardium. The pericardium should be opened anterior and parallel to the left phrenic nerve. When the site of the injury cannot be reached, a transsternal extension into the right chest is performed with a Liebsche knife or osteotome. This usually requires ligation of both internal thoracic arteries.

Hemorrhage control and surgical management

Definitive treatment involves surgical exposure through a thoracotomy or median sternotomy. Control of bleeding via suturing heart muscle and heart wall (cardiorrhaphy) may be required. Poor cardiorrhaphy technique can result in enlargement of the lacerations or injury to the coronary arteries. If the initial treating physician is uncomfortable with the suturing technique, digital pressure can be applied until a more experienced surgeon arrives. Other techniques that have been described include the use of a Foley balloon catheter[8] and a skin stapler.[9] Alternatively, with large wounds that cannot be palpably controlled, an incomplete horizontal mattress suture should be placed on either side of the wound.[10] The free ends are then crossed to stop the bleeding.

Wounds of the atria are initially managed with partial occlusion. Because of the thin structure and instability of the atrial wall, digital pressure will not effectively stop bleeding. Suture techniques for penetrating cardiac injuries range from simple 3–0 Prolene interrupted sutures, with or without Teflon felt pledgets, to simple running or mattress sutures. A needle with larger curve may make it easier to enter the muscle tissue at a right angle, and also to drive the needle following its curve, thus avoiding tear of the muscle. The bite on the myocardium should be large, as it will ensure a more secure repair. Small bites increase the risk of tearing. Injuries close to coronary arteries need special care: avoid pledget sutures and take bites deep to the coronary itself.

Although the right ventricle is a lower-pressure chamber than the left ventricle, the right ventricle muscle wall is much thinner than the left, and is therefore more prone to tearing if deep and inadequate bites are taken.

On a beating heart, cardiorrhaphy may be quite challenging to perform. Cardiopulmonary bypass with cardioplegic arrest can be used, especially for multichamber injuries.

Elective cardiac arrest using temporary ventricular fibrillation should be a last resort for repair of difficult wounds.

We have reported the use of intravenous administration of adenosine to cause temporary asystole to allow easy and accurate placement of sutures for a left ventricular laceration.[11] The usual dose of 6–12 mg of adenosine is sufficient to achieve temporary asystole within 30 seconds of injection and gives the surgeon the time to do the repair on a motionless heart. Owing to adenosine's ultra-short half-life, the asystolic period lasts for only a few seconds (15–20 seconds in our patient). Cardiac stabilization devices have been reported to successfully immobilize the site of injury in penetrating cardiac wounds and for traumatic coronary injuries.

Management of the wounded heart that has spontaneously arrested is controversial. Some clinicians have recommended a rapid repair of ventricular wounds while the heart is arrested. Others consider immediate cardiac massage and reversal of cardiac arrest to be more important. Immediate cardiac massage to maintain blood flow is probably the best approach. When cardiac arrest occurs, physiologic reserves have been depleted, and a delay for repair during arrest would only diminish the chance of a successful resuscitation.

Wounds of the septa, valves, and coronary arteries require definitive repair in the operating room. Hemorrhage from a coronary artery can generally be controlled with digital pressure. If the artery is a small branch or if it is lacerated in the distal third, ligation might be used. On the other hand, in proximal lesions, especially of the left anterior descending artery, a bypass graft with or without cardiopulmonary bypass and cardioplegic arrest will need to be constructed. A dramatic special circumstance is the inability, after proper cardiac repair, to close the chest without hemodynamic compromise. The effect of cardiac distension, muscle edema, and volume overload may preclude chest or sternal closure. The use of modified vacuum-assisted closure during the first 2 days may allow a later return to the operating room for definitive closure.

Blunt cardiac trauma
Anatomy and pathophysiology

Nonpenetrating or *blunt cardiac injury* has replaced the term "cardiac contusion" and describes injury ranging from minor bruises of the myocardium to cardiac rupture. It can be caused by direct energy transfer to the heart or compression of the heart between the sternum and vertebral column at the time of the accident. Blunt cardiac injury includes injuries sustained during external cardiac massage as a part of cardiopulmonary resuscitation, such as cardiac contusion and cardiac rupture.

Although myocardial blunt trauma may be mistaken for myocardial infarction (MI), there are several pathological differences between the two. With MI, the transition between infarcted and normal tissue is gradual, muscle damage is confined to a defined artery territory, and generalized coagulation necrosis is the final pathway of the lesion. In myocardial blunt trauma, normal and contused tissues show a defined boundary. The healing process eventually leads to patchy and irregular fibrosis.

Blunt cardiac injury usually results from high-speed motor vehicle collisions (MVCs), in which the chest wall strikes against the steering wheel. Other causes, such as falls from heights, crushing injuries, blast injuries, and direct blows, are less common.

Within this spectrum, blunt cardiac injuries can manifest as free septal rupture, free wall rupture, coronary artery thrombosis, cardiac failure, complex arrhythmia, simple arrhythmia, and/or rupture of chordae tendineae or papillary muscles.[12]

Several mechanisms have been postulated by which the heart may be injured in cases of nonpenetrating trauma. The heart has a relatively free movement in an anteroposterior direction within the chest; in cases of sudden deceleration, the heart continues to move forward because of its momentum, striking the sternum with considerable force. The biomechanics of cardiac rupture include direct transmission of increased intrathoracic pressure to the chambers of the heart; hydraulic effect from a large force applied to the abdominal or extremity veins, causing a force to be transmitted to the right atrium, resulting in rupture; or a decelerating force between fixed and mobile areas, which explains for example the atrio-caval tears.[13] Blunt rupture of the cardiac septum occurs most frequently in late diastole or early systole near the apex of the heart.[13] Multiple ruptures and disruption of the conduction system have been reported. From autopsy data, blunt cardiac injury with ventricular rupture most often involves the left ventricle.[13]

Following blunt trauma acute thrombus formation may occur, especially in diseased, atheromatous vessels, and result in coronary artery occlusion and MI. Blunt pericardial rupture results from pericardial tears secondary to intraabdominal pressure or lateral deceleration forces. The heart can be displaced into either pleural cavity or even into the peritoneum. Cardiac herniation with cardiac dysfunction may occur in conjunction with these tears.

The most common cause of myocardial rupture due to blunt trauma is a high-speed MVC (72%), followed by pedestrian injuries (16%).[14] Myocardial ruptures due to blunt cardiac trauma are usually immediately fatal. It is estimated that from all blunt trauma admissions, blunt cardiac rupture is present in 0.045%.[14] Even in those that arrive alive in the hospital overall mortality approaches 90%. Delayed rupture of the heart also may occur weeks after blunt trauma, probably as a result of necrosis of a contused or infarcted area of myocardium. Another possible complication from cardiac trauma is the development of a pseudoaneurysm, from the pericardial sealing of a localized rupture. A defect on the ventricular wall with a narrow neck between the ventricle and the lesion is suggestive of a pseudoaneurysm. Usually it is suspected by a echocardiography, but ideally magnetic resonance imaging (MRI) should be used to define anatomy and diagnosis. Ventricular pseudoaneurysm carries a high risk of spontaneous rupture followed by tamponade and death. Therefore, surgery should always be considered.

The immediate ability of the patient to survive cardiac rupture depends on the integrity of the pericardium. An intact pericardium or a tear in the pericardium which is small enough to seal itself may protect from immediate exsanguination. These patients may survive for variable periods but eventually develop significant hemopericardium and pericardial tamponade.

Clinical features

Blunt cardiac trauma presents clinically as a spectrum of injuries of varying severity. Although most patients with blunt cardiac injury have external signs of thoracic trauma (e.g., contusion, abrasions, palpable crepitus, rib or sternum fractures, visible flail segments), absence of visible thoracic lesions decreases the suspicion but does not exclude cardiac injury. Other associated injuries may include pulmonary contusion, pneumothorax, hemothorax, external fracture, and great vessel injury.

In cases of blunt cardiac injury, conduction disturbances and arrhythmias are common (Table 29.3). Impaired perfusion status, and conduction abnormalities by damaged myocytes or vagal sympathetic reflexes, may result in a variety of supraventricular or ventricular arrhythmias. Of special concern is the condition called commotio cordis, in which sudden ventricular fibrillation (VF) or asystole follows even moderate cardiac contusion. It is believed that when a kinetic impact over the precordial area occurs near the T-wave period of the cardiac cycle, sudden VF may develop, requiring prompt assessment if mortality is to be avoided. If the impact occurs near the R wave, asystole may occur.

The clinical presentation of a patient who has sustained a myocardial rupture is usually that of cardiac tamponade or severe intrathoracic hemorrhage. Signs and symptoms of cardiac tamponade are similar to those with penetrating cardiac injuries, as discussed previously. Initial inspection may reveal little more than a bruised area over the sternum or no external

physical evidence at all. The following findings are suggestive of a possible myocardial rupture:

(1) hypotension disproportionate to the suspected injury
(2) hypotension unresponsive to rapid fluid resuscitation
(3) massive hemothorax unresponsive to thoracostomy and fluid resuscitation
(4) persistent metabolic acidosis
(5) presence of pericardial effusion on FAST or echocardiography, elevation of central venous pressure, and prominent neck veins, with continued hypotension despite fluid resuscitation

Diagnostic strategies

Significant controversy exists regarding the importance of establishing the diagnosis of blunt cardiac injury in otherwise hemodynamically stable patients. Most blunt myocardial injuries probably do not cause significant complications. The relative risk of a life-threatening dysrhythmia is far too low to warrant routine admission for all patients with blunt chest trauma. Yet no reliable diagnostic test exists to identify those patients at greatest risk. Along with a high suspicion, utilizing a combination of electrocardiogram, troponin, and echocardiography for appropriate patients may improve the diagnosis, risk stratification, and disposition of patients sustaining blunt cardiac injury.

Electrocardiogram

In cases of blunt cardiac injury, conduction disturbances (Table 29.3) are common, and thus a screening 12-lead ECG could be helpful for evaluation. The most sensitive but least specific sign of blunt myocardial injury is sinus tachycardia.[13] Other possible disturbances include T-wave and ST-segment changes, as seen with myocardial bruising.[13] The presence of ECG abnormalities is neither specific enough to confirm the diagnosis of myocardial trauma nor reliable enough to predict subsequent complications.

Cardiac enzymes

Because myocardial contusion is characterized histologically by intramyocardial hemorrhage and necrosis of myocardial muscle cells, cardiac enzymes were the first screening tools used to detect myocardial injury. Creatine kinase (CK) is nonspecifically increased in trauma patients as a result of associated skeletal muscle injury, and CK-MB levels have been found to be falsely elevated, and to be a nonspecific finding in multiple-trauma patients. CK-MB levels are of limited utility to screen for myocardial contusion and are no longer recommended.

Serum cardiac troponins, troponin I and troponin T, are highly specific for myocardial injury. If troponin I or T concentrations are within normal ranges on initial evaluation, a secondary measurement after 4–6 hours should be performed to reliably exclude myocardial injury.

Table 29.3 Arrhythmias associated with blunt cardiac injury

Sinus tachycardia

Sinus bradycardia

First-degree atrioventricular block

Right bundle branch block with hemiblock

Third-degree block

Atrial fibrillation

Premature ventricular contractions

Ventricular tachycardia

Ventricular fibrillation

Echocardiography (see also Chapter 10)

Two-dimensional echocardiography is useful in diagnosing myocardial blunt injury by evaluating wall motion abnormalities and identifying associated lesions such as thrombi, pericardial effusion with or without concomitant tamponade, left ventricular ejection fraction, and valvular disruption.[15] Echocardiographic signs of cardiac tamponade include cardiac chamber compression (mainly right-sided), inferior vena cava (IVC) distension, Doppler flow velocity paradoxus and paradoxical motion of the interventricular septum.[2] Echocardiography should be considered in patients with positive ECG findings, elevated troponin level, or unexplained hypotension.[16]

Cardiac magnetic resonance imaging

Cardiac magnetic resonance imaging (CMRI) is helpful in assessing the extent of myocardial damage, areas of infarct, wall motion abnormalities, and valvular dysfunction.[17] It has inherent limitations in the emergency setting, such as the need for long imaging times and the time needed to screen for contraindications to MRI. In cardiac trauma the main role for CMRI is in the post-admission period. Myocardial blunt trauma can be differentiated from myocardial infarction. CMRI is ideal for confirmation of a pseudoaneurysm.

Multidetector computed tomography

Multidetector computed tomography (MCT) has great value in assessing patients with both blunt and penetrating heart trauma. In addition to evaluating general thoracic trauma (pneumothorax, pulmonary contusion, hemothorax) and great vessel trauma (ascending or descending thoracic aorta dissection or rupture), CT has a high sensitivity for pneumopericardium, pericardial effusion, pericardial rupture, myocardial rupture, and cardiac luxation. MCT coronary angiography can be performed at the same time as cardiac CT if there is suspicion of coronary artery dissection or thrombosis secondary to the blunt trauma. Pericardial rupture followed by cardiac herniation into the pleural space or abdomen can lead to left ventricle strangulation, which is easily demonstrated by MCT. This diagnosis would prompt surgical correction. Before the advent of MCT, pericardial tears were very difficult to detect and were mainly diagnosed during surgery or autopsy studies. Pneumopericardium can also develop after pericardial tear and is a known cause of tamponade. Chest x-ray and CT of the chest may be diagnostic. If concomitant tamponade physiology is present, a subxiphoid window is mandatory.

Management

Since blunt cardiac trauma may present with a variety of clinical syndromes, management depends on the specific case. Most complications of myocardial blunt trauma manifest within 12 hours of admission.

On admission, treatment of suspected myocardial contusion should be similar to that of an MI: intravenous line, cardiac monitoring, and administration of oxygen and analgesic agents. Arrhythmias should be treated with appropriate medications as per current advanced cardiac life support guidelines.

No data exist to support prophylactic pharmacologic agents for arrhythmia prophylaxis. Measures should be taken to treat and prevent conditions which increase myocardial irritability, such as metabolic acidosis and electrolyte imbalances. Although general anesthesia is avoided in the setting of acute MI, no complications have been reported in patients with suspected myocardial contusions receiving general anesthesia for necessary operations.[18] In the setting of depressed cardiac output caused by blunt cardiac injury, careful fluid administration by monitoring filling pressures closely is advised. Inotropic support may be required after optimal preload is ensured. Intraaortic balloon counter-pulsation may be considered in cases of refractory cardiogenic shock.

Treatment of patients with a myocardial rupture is very similar to the treatment of penetrating cardiac injuries and is directed toward immediate decompression of cardiac tamponade and control of hemorrhage. Emergency thoracotomy and pericardiotomy may be required prior to transport to the operating room. After emergency thoracotomy and pericardiotomy, the myocardial rupture should be controlled until the patient can be transferred to the operating room for definitive repair. Temporary hemorrhage control techniques such as digital pressure, vascular clamp, Foley insertion, sutures, and definitive repair are similar to those for penetrating cardiac trauma.

Valvular injuries are relatively uncommon complications after blunt cardiac trauma. Left-sided valves are more commonly affected, because of the higher pressures on the left side compared to the right. A rapid increase in intracardiac chamber pressure against a closed valve can lead to leaflet or papillary muscle tear and consequent valve insufficiency.[19] Injury to a cardiac valve should be suspected in the setting of pulmonary edema or congestive heart failure after blunt chest trauma or if a murmur in auscultation suggests this. The aortic valve is the most common valve to be damaged, especially the noncoronary cusp. The mitral valve can become insufficient through injury to the papillary muscles, chordae tendineae, or leaflets. Presentation of this mitral valve injury varies from immediately post trauma to several weeks later when an initially small mitral regurgitation progress to a severe one. Tricuspid regurgitation, the least common valve lesion, is usually secondary to chordae tendineae rupture, and can either develop immediately after trauma or manifest years after. The decision to operate on any of the valves, and the timing of any surgery, will depend on the degree of regurgitation, associated symptoms, and concurrent traumatic lesions of other systems.

Coronary injury secondary to blunt trauma is a rare event, occurring in less than 2% of blunt chest trauma cases.[20] Dissection and intimal tearing are the mode of lesion in most cases, arising from deceleration injury, compression of the artery between heart and sternal bone, and even coronary spasm. The most common site involved is the left anterior descending artery. Dissection usually leads to acute MI. If suspicion is high, coronary angiogram is the gold standard for diagnosis. Treatment options include percutaneous coronary artery intervention and coronary artery bypass surgery.

Iatrogenic cardiac injury

Iatrogenic cardiac injury can occur with central venous line insertion, cardiac catheterization procedures, and pericardiocentesis. Common sites of injury include the superior atrial-caval junction and the superior vena cava-innominate junction. These small perforations often lead to a compensated cardiac tamponade. Drainage by pericardiocentesis is often unsuccessful, and evacuation via subxiphoid pericardial window or full median sternotomy is required. The site of injury may be sealed and difficult to find. Complications from coronary artery catheterization including perforation or dissection of the coronary arteries, cardiac perforation, and aortic dissection can be catastrophic and require emergent operation. Other potential iatrogenic causes of cardiac injury include external and internal cardiac massage, pericardiocentesis, and intracardiac injections.

Metabolic cardiac injury

Metabolic cardiac injury refers to cardiac dysfunction in response to trauma and may be associated with injuries caused by burns, electrical injury, sepsis, the systemic inflammatory response syndrome, and multisystem trauma.[21] The exact mechanism responsible for this dysfunction is unclear, but responses to trauma induce a mediator storm, which is a release of cytokines that may affect the myocardium and clinically manifest as conduction disturbances or decreased contractility leading to decreased cardiac output. Treatment of metabolic cardiac injury has been supportive, with correction of initiating insults.

Electrical injury

Cardiac complications are most often the cause of death after electrical injury, including lighting strikes. The cardiac complications after electrical injury include immediate cardiac arrest, acute myocardial necrosis with or without ventricular failure, pseudoinfarction, myocardial ischemia, arrhythmias, conduction abnormalities, acute hypertension with peripheral vasospasm, and asymptomatic, nonspecific abnormalities evident on an electrocardiogram. Damage from electrical injury may be due to:

(1) direct effects on the excitable tissues
(2) heat generated from the current
(3) accompanying associated injuries such as those due to falls, explosions, or fire

Intracardiac missiles

Intracardiac missiles are foreign bodies that are embedded in the myocardium, retained in the trabeculations of the endocardial surface, or free in a cardiac chamber or pericardium. These may be the result of direct penetrating chest injury or injury to a peripheral vascular structure with embolization to the heart. Location and other considerations determine the type of complications that can occur and the treatment required. Observation might be considered when the missile is (1) right-sided, (2) embedded completely in the wall, (3) contained within a fibrous covering, (4) not contaminated, or (5) producing no symptoms. Right-sided missiles can embolize to the lung, at which point they can be removed, or in rare cases they embolize "paradoxically" through a patent foramen ovale or atrial septal defect. Left-sided missiles can manifest as systemic embolization shortly after the initial injury. Diagnosis may be done with radiographs in two projections, fluoroscopy, echocardiography, or angiography.[13] Removal is recommended for missiles that are left-sided, larger than 1–2 cm, rough in shape, or produce symptoms.

Although surgery with or without cardiopulmonary bypass has been advocated in the past, a large percentage of right-sided foreign bodies are currently removed by interventional radiological methods.

Great vessel trauma

Blunt aortic injury, either aortic transection or acute rupture, is one of the leading causes of posttraumatic death, with the majority of the patients dying before presenting to hospital. Patients who survive to present at the hospital remain with a poor prognosis, with mortality rates at 6 hours and 24 hours of 30% and 50% respectively.[22] As a result, these patients have traditionally been managed with rapid open surgical intervention once the diagnosis of aortic injury has been confirmed.[23] More recently, it has been recommended to delay surgical intervention to permit the management and stabilization of any associated injuries with the goal of reducing the mortality rate associated with emergent repair of an aortic injury.[22] Other recent important changes in dealing with aortic injury are the advent of MCT, clinical management with aggressive blood pressure and cardiac contractility control, and the more widespread use of aortic endovascular repair techniques.

Anatomy and pathophysiology

The classic mechanism of aortic injury in trauma is associated with a rapid deceleration and stress located at the aortic isthmus, which is the junction between the relatively fixed descending aorta and relatively mobile aortic arch. The most common site of injury is the aortic isthmus (36–54%), followed by the aortic arch (8–18%) and the descending thoracic aorta (11–21%).[24] The injury to the aorta most commonly involves all three layers of the aorta, with complete disruption between the edges.[24] Incomplete or partial disruption of the aorta may also occur, and in some cases may result in focal dissection or the development of an intramural hematoma.[24] The high mortality associated with this injury is a result of frank exsanguination associated with complete aortic disruption,[22] but the

Table 29.4 Physical signs and symptoms of aortic injury

Physical signs
Hemodynamic instability
Fractures • Sternum • First rib, multiple rib fractures • Clavicular
Unequal upper limb blood pressures
Paraplegia and paraparesis
Symptoms
Dyspnea
Back pain
Voice hoarseness

Table 29.5 TRAINS: Traumatic Aortic Injury Score

Finding	Score
Widened mediastinum	4
Hypotension	2
Long-bone fracture	2
Hemothorax	1
Lung contusion	1
Left scapula fracture	1
Pelvic fracture deformity	1

Score $\geq$ 4 indicates high risk of traumatic aortic injury. Modified from Mosquera *et al.* 2012.[27]

strength of the adventitia may permit those patients with incomplete transection to survive to hospital. It should also be noted that in addition to aortic disruption, blunt trauma may result in trauma to the brachiocephalic vessels, most commonly involving the base of the innominate artery.[25] In addition to aortic injury, patients often suffer other multiple associated injuries that contribute to their morbidity and mortality, and complicate their surgical management. Spinal cord perfusion is a critical aspect, due to the incidence of paraplegia following both open and endovascular management.

Clinical features

Aortic rupture is an entity that requires a high index of suspicion in any trauma patient, and the incidence increases in the presence of multitrauma injuries. Unfortunately, less than half of the cases present with specific signs or symptoms of an aortic injury, and the presentation may be insidious. Thus, identifying the mechanism and severity of the trauma is critical in making the diagnosis of aortic injury, and in any case of high-speed injury, rapid deceleration, falls, or blast injuries one should suspect the possibility of aortic rupture. Classical signs and symptoms that should raise the suspicion of an aortic injury include hemodynamic instability, fractures involving the upper thorax, unequal upper limb blood pressure, paraplegia or paraparesis, dyspnea, and hoarseness (Table 29.4).

The classical trauma risk scores such as Injury Severity Score, Revised Trauma Score, and Trauma Injury Severity Score show no relationship between the overall severity of trauma and the degree of aortic injury.[26] Based on this assumption, Mosquera and colleagues developed and validated a simple score (TRAINS: Traumatic Aortic Injury Score) to detect patients at high risk of having an aortic traumatic injury.[27] The score is based on radiologic and physical findings (Table 29.5). Patients with a score $\geq$ 4 would be at high risk of traumatic aortic injury and should be managed with IV β-blocker control of blood pressure and heart rate; and should undergo a three-phase vascular MCT for definitive diagnosis

of aortic injury, and transesophageal echocardiography (TEE) if the patient was tracheally intubated. This diagnostic approach had a sensitivity of 93% and specificity of 85%.

Injuries to the brachiocephalic vessels, unlike aortic disruption, are usually less commonly associated with frank bleeding and hemorrhagic shock, as the hematoma is usually contained within the upper mediastinum. Clinical suspicion of a brachiocephalic injury should be considered in patients with widening of the upper mediastinum and discrepancies in upper limb blood pressures, both which are also seen in the setting of aortic disruption.

Diagnostic strategies

In the initial diagnostic assessment of a trauma patient, CT is often performed to rule out suspected head injuries and intraabdominal pathology (see Chapter 11). However, a decision to examine the thoracic aorta should be guided by a detailed clinical history and initial assessment of the chest radiograph. Although the chest radiograph is not a reliable screening test for aortic injury, radiographic abnormalities are noted in the majority of chest radiographs in the setting of aortic injury (Table 29.6). In any patient suspected of having an aortic injury, CT scanning of the chest should be obtained, often in conjunction with CT scanning of other regions of the body. The diagnosis of acute thoracic aortic pathology is now most commonly made with CT.[28] Continued improvements in CT technology with helical and multirow detector CT, and multiplanar reformation and volume rendering techniques, have resulted in CT being the definitive screening test for major thoracic vascular injury.[28] It is important to examine both the contrast-enhanced and non-contrast-enhanced CT scans to maximize the ability to identify the aortic pathology, including aortic dissection and intramural hematoma.[29] Findings suggestive of aortic disruption include wall thickening, filling defects, aortic hematoma (paraaortic and intramural), intimal flaps, and extravasation of contrast.[28]

A recent grading system of blunt aortic injury with CT angiography (CTA) aims to discriminate patients with varying degrees of aortic injury, from minimal intimal tear to aortic

Table 29.6 Radiographic evidence suggestive of aortic injury

Widened mediastinum > 8.0 cm
Mediastinum:chest ratio > 0.25
Opacification of aorto-pulmonary window
Irregular aortic knob
Blurred aortic contour
Deviation of nasogastric tube
Tracheal deviation to patient's right
Pulmonary contusion
Widened left paraspinal line
Left apical cap
Other rib fractures
Thoracic spine fracture
Depressed left main bronchus
First rib fracture
Clavicular fracture

Table 29.7 Vancouver simplified grading system with CT angiography for blunt aortic injury

Grade	Finding
I	Intimal flap, thrombus, or intramural hematoma < 1 cm
II	Intimal flap, thrombus, or intramural hematoma > 1 cm
III	Pseudoaneurysm (simple or complex, no extravasation)
IV	Contrast extravasation (with or without pseudoaneurysm)

Modified from Lamarche et al. 2012.[30]

Table 29.8 Sensitivity and specificity of various modalities in diagnosing aortic transection

	Sensitivity	Specificity
Contrast-enhanced CT	100%	100%
Transesophageal echocardiography	63–100%	84–100%
Aortography	100%	100%

transection,[30] and to create a common language for radiologists, trauma specialists, and surgeons (Table 29.7). In this study the degree of aortic injury correlated to overall mortality and the need for aortic intervention. In addition to identifying the aortic pathology, CT imaging is crucial in determining the suitability of an endovascular repair, in procedural planning (examining proximal and distal landing zones and access vessels), and for device sizing. Injuries to the brachiocephalic vessels will also be identified with CT imaging, although some authors recommend angiography as a means of ruling out great vessel injury.[25]

Aortography is less commonly performed, because of the advances in and the less invasive nature of CT imaging, although historically it was considered the gold standard in identifying aortic pathology, and with experienced operators it can yield sensitivity and specificity rates approaching 100%. The role of TEE in the diagnosis of traumatic aortic rupture has been established (see Chapter 10).[31] However, theoretical concerns do exist with this semi-invasive procedure, which can cause changes in blood pressure and potentially exacerbate a clinical condition most commonly lethal due to exsanguination. Table 29.8 shows the sensitivity and specificity of diagnostic modalities for aortic injury.

Management

Initial management

The majority of patients presenting with aortic trauma have associated trauma-related injuries, and appropriate ATLS-guided assessment is mandatory in all patients (see Chapter 2).[23] As in the management of standard trauma patients, focus should be made on hemodynamic stabilization and controlled ventilation. The rapid identification of life-threatening conditions mandating intervention with a definitive airway, chest tube thoracostomy, and in some cases thoracotomy or laparotomy to deal with life-threatening injuries, precedes the ordering of time-consuming diagnostic tests.

Preoperative management should include a head CT in any patient suspected of a head injury to rule out any intracranial injury requiring surgical relief in patients who are clearly not exsanguinating (see Chapters 20 and 21). In hemodynamically unstable patients, prompt institution of surgical intervention to control exsanguination is recommended. Intraoperative TEE may be used to facilitate the identification of aortic injury (see Chapter 10).

Open surgery

Open surgery is considered the traditional management for blunt thoracic aortic injury. Surgical management is aimed at correcting the aortic disruption, and is either performed with or without ("clamp and sew") the use of lower body perfusion. Proponents of adjunctive perfusion techniques cite added spinal cord and visceral perfusion during the period the aorta is crossclamped. Irrespective of the technique used, rates of paraplegia range between 0% and 10%.[22] The ability to selectively ventilate the right lung (when uninjured) either via selective right bronchial intubation or with a double-lumen tube will facilitate surgical exposure (see Chapter 33). Surgical access is gained with the patient positioned in the right lateral decubitus position, ensuring access to the left groin for possible access to the femoral vessels for the use of partial left heart bypass. A standard fourth interspace posterolateral thoracotomy is done. The incision should be large enough to facilitate exposure of the thoracic aorta below the level of disruption, and of the aortic arch between the left common carotid and left subclavian arteries. Manipulation or dissection of the isthmus or tear must be avoided until vascular access proximal and distal to the aorta is established. Depending on the stability of the patient, the decision may be made to establish partial left heart bypass prior to exposure. Once the injured aorta is identified, an interposition graft is sutured into place, thus restoring aortic continuity. Published series of emergent surgical repair of blunt aortic injury report mortality rates in the 15–30% range.[22,23] Complicating the surgical repair of this traumatic injury is the frequently associated pulmonary injury, as well as potential injury involving the abdominal organs and brain. Postoperative morbidity after successful surgical repair is further complicated by the associated injuries, which often prolong the intensive care unit stay and delay convalescence.

Surgical management of an injury involving the brachiocephalic vessels is best managed via a standard median sternotomy, allowing access to the ascending aorta and arch vessels. Standard vascular techniques of obtaining proximal and distal vascular control prior to entry into the injured area apply. The incision may be extended into the right neck to provide additional exposure to the innominate artery, with appropriate adjunctive supportive measures or monitoring techniques, including cardiopulmonary bypass, cerebral protection, and selective carotid shunting.[25] Healthy young individuals may tolerate standard clamping and sewing of an interposition graft without any adverse sequelae. Long-term patency rates of these interposition grafts, such as an aorto-innominate artery bypass, approach 96% at 10 years.

Surgical approach to blunt thoracic aortic injury

Clamp and sew

This repair technique has the advantage of being the simplest method, and it does not require knowledge or experience with extracorporeal perfusion, or cannulation of the heart or great vessels. Also, in hemodynamically unstable patients who are not candidates for vascular cannulation for partial bypass due to instability, crossclamping of the aorta may be necessary to avoid rapid exsanguination. Repair of an aortic transection may be performed in this setting with low rates of paraplegia when associated with aortic crossclamp times of less than 30 minutes.[25] The average duration of crossclamping has, however, been reported to be as high as 41 minutes. Factors contributing to prolonged periods of aortic crossclamping include fragility and friability of the aorta, and extensive hematoma complicating identification of anatomic structures. In patients with aortic tears involving the distal arch or subclavian artery, clamping proximal to the subclavian artery may be associated with an increased incidence of spinal cord ischemia in the absence of a distal perfusion strategy.

Lower body perfusion

The goal of lower body perfusion is to provide perfusion at a mean pressure of 60–70 mmHg to the body distal to the aortic clamp, minimizing the risk of spinal cord and visceral ischemia. Blood may be shunted either from the left heart or from the right heart, oxygenated or deoxygenated respectively. Concerns of lower body perfusion are based on the need for extracorporeal circuits and the need for anticoagulation, which may be contraindicated in cases of closed head or lung injury. The decision to use systemic heparinization will influence the method of lower body perfusion. The use of heparin-bonded tubing and a Bio-Medicus pump (Medtronic, Minneapolis, MN) may allow the avoidance of systemic heparinization. Partial left heart bypass involves actively shunting oxygenated blood from the left atrium to the lower body, with return through either the distal thoracic aorta or the femoral artery. It permits control of blood pressure proximal to the aortic clamp during clamping, and facilitates volume manipulation. Although this technique does not aid in oxygenation, as there is no oxygenator in the circuit, it does permit lower levels of heparinization to be used.

Right atrial to femoral artery bypass shunts deoxygenated blood from the right atrium to the femoral artery. This type of circuit may involve the use of an oxygenator, heat exchanger, and systemic heparinization, and may provide complete cardiopulmonary support if required. This technique becomes useful if the proximal anastomoses must be performed under deep hypothermic circulatory arrest owing to involvement of the aortic arch.

Thoracic endovascular aortic repair (TEVAR)

Over the last two decades there has been a revolution in the management of vascular pathology with endovascular techniques utilizing catheter-based devices. Initially, this occurred primarily in the arenas of peripheral arterial disease, carotid artery disease, and abdominal aortic aneurysm. It has now evolved to include the thoracic aorta. Although procedure-related morbidity and mortality may often favor endovascular techniques, clinical equipoise has not routinely been demonstrated when compared to standard open surgical techniques. Guidelines for the endovascular management of vascular pathology remain in flux. Although technical success rates are typically quite high, in some vascular territories there remain limitations in long-term efficacy and durability. This is most notable in endovascular treatment of arterial occlusive disease. Long-term data are not yet available for some endovascular procedures. Less than perfect technical success, the need for re-intervention, and the ongoing debates regarding endovascular procedures versus open surgical procedures, all continue to catalyze ongoing advances in catheter-based technology. However, at least in the case of endovascular treatment of aortic pathology, the benefits of reduced procedure-related complications, as well as reduced early and intermediate morbidity and mortality, appear to outweigh the disadvantages associated with the higher re-intervention rate for endovascular procedures. As will be discussed, this is especially true in the endovascular management of blunt traumatic injury of the thoracic aorta, the majority of which involves the proximal descending thoracic aorta, just distal to the origin of the left subclavian artery.

Endovascular aneurysm repair (EVAR) of the abdominal aorta was born out of the cardiopulmonary complications associated with open surgical repair of abdominal aortic aneurysms and is now established as a low-mortality and low-morbidity alternative to open aneurysm repair. Although long-term mortality rates may converge in these patients, early and intermediate-term mortality favors EVAR.[32] The same coaxial, over-the-wire techniques applied to other vascular territories have been broadly applied to the pathologies of the thoracic aorta, with the same pattern of lower early and intermediate-term morbidity and mortality. These pathologies primarily include those of the descending thoracic aorta: degenerative aneurysm disease, dissection, intramural hematoma, and penetrating ulcers. There are presently many FDA-approved commercially available devices specific to the descending thoracic aorta.

Readily available access to imaging with intravenous contrasted CT makes the diagnosis of traumatic aortic injury incidental in many patients who survive to the hospital (Fig. 29.1; see also Chapter 11). Contemporary MCT scanners provide high-resolution axial imaging rendered in 1–3 mm thickness slices that can be reformatted into sagittal, coronal, and 3D images. Optimally, axial imaging is obtained from the base of the skull to the femoral heads. This allows for scrutiny of the circle of Willis, the vertebral arteries, the arch branch vessels, the extent and severity of the thoracic aortic injury, the relationship of the injury to the left subclavian artery origin, the diameter of the thoracic aorta, and the adequacy of the access vessels.

Because there were no thoracic stents available, early experiences with endovascular repair of blunt thoracic aortic injury were obtained utilizing devices intended for treatment of the abdominal aorta. The thoracic aorta has unique technical considerations. The thoracic aorta has a larger diameter than the abdominal aorta, there is significant angulation in the transition from the transverse arch to the descending aorta, and it is a greater distance from the femoral artery. Despite the inherent limitations of abdominal aortic devices, early outcomes were still quite favorable, and there was a significant trend in shifting practice patterns toward endovascular treatment of blunt aortic injury, with reduced morbidity and mortality.[33,34] With advances in stent grafts designed specifically for the thoracic aorta, clinical outcomes have remained excellent.[35,36] Devices designed for the treatment of thoracic aneurysmal disease were targeted toward larger-diameter aortas. The trauma patient is typically younger in age and

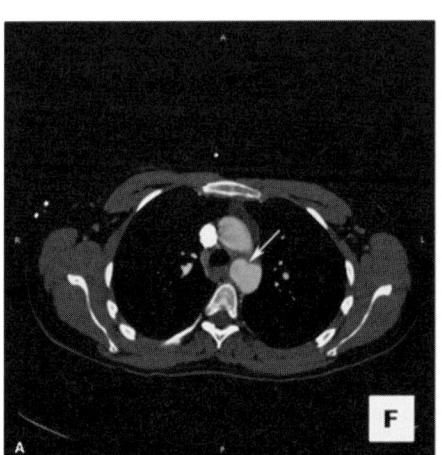
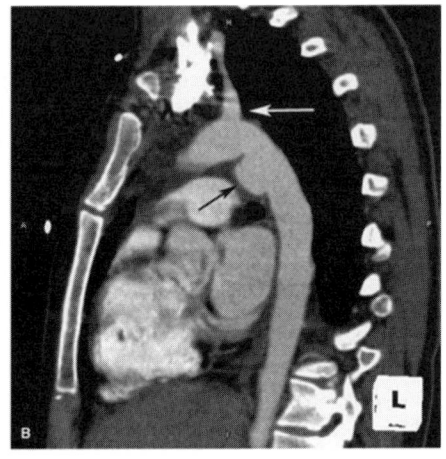
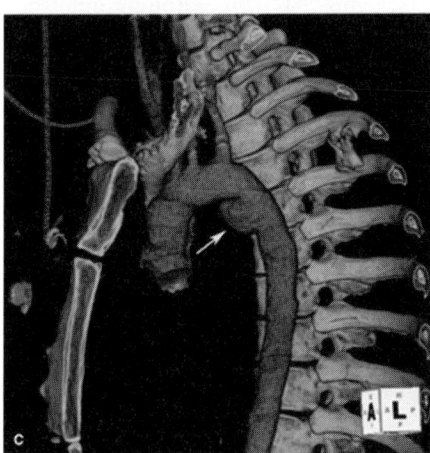

Figure 29.1 Traumatic disruption of the aorta. (**A**) Axial image of a chest CT that demonstrates posttraumatic aortic wall disruption (arrow) in a young patient with a normal aorta. (**B**) Multiplanar reconstruction view in the same patient demonstrates the bulging of the aorta (black arrow) just distal to the left subclavian artery (white arrow). (**C**) Volumetric 3D reconstruction of the same CT scan demonstrates the aortic transection just distal to the origin of the left subclavian artery. The heart and pulmonary artery have been removed to facilitate visualization of the aortic arch and descending thoracic aorta.

unlikely to have aneurysmal disease; thus, the diameter of the thoracic aorta is smaller than that encountered in the aneurysm patient. Some contemporary devices have been tailored in design, trialed and approved for use in the treatment of blunt injury to the thoracic aorta.

As noted earlier, the patient with blunt thoracic aortic injury typically has multiple other injuries including brain injury, spine injury, long-bone injury, pelvic fracture, and intraabdominal solid organ and hollow viscus injury. Theoretically, this makes endovascular repair all the more appealing. Until the patient arrives in the operating room, in an effort to control shear stress on the injured aorta and prevent delayed rupture, blood pressure and heart rate are controlled as aggressively as possible. This is done in the context of the patient's other injuries, not forsaking end-organ perfusion. This is largely achieved by the administration of short-acting intravenous β-blocker therapy.

During endovascular repair of the thoracic aorta, the patient is placed in the supine position. Open surgical exposure of one femoral artery is performed to accommodate the introduction of the large-caliber stent delivery system. Percutaneous sheath access to the contralateral femoral artery or the left brachial artery for introduction of the angiographic imaging catheter is also obtained. This eliminates the need to place the patient in the lateral decubitus position required for open repair. Hence, patient positioning in the setting of concomitant spine, pelvic, and long-bone injury is simplified. In the absence of a thoracotomy, single-lung ventilation is no longer required, mitigating some of the challenges associated with ventilating the typically contused lungs. The procedure can be performed under local anesthesia at the femoral access sites, which minimizes the hemodynamic lability often encountered in these multiply injured patients during open repair. Occasionally, access across the iliac and femoral arteries is not possible owing to small vessel diameter, native arterial disease, or a combination of the two. In these circumstances, it may be necessary to obtain access to the more proximal vasculature through transperitoneal or retroperitoneal exposure of the abdominal aorta or iliac arteries. Certainly in this circumstance, general anesthesia is preferred. Therapeutic systemic anticoagulation is not mandatory during endovascular repair, but can be used to prevent peri-catheter thrombus formation and its potential complications. However, expedient endovascular repair can be performed quite safely in the absence of any anticoagulation whatsoever. Surgical blood loss is typically insignificant during endovascular repair and large-volume fluid resuscitation is not required, except as indicated for the patient's other injuries. Contrast media is required for intraoperative imaging, and consideration is given to patients with renal dysfunction.

In taking care of the patient undergoing endovascular repair of thoracic aortic injuries, it is important to understand that all endovascular techniques are performed with some common principles. These include obtaining remote vessel access, guidewire traversal of the target lesion, delivery of the therapeutic device to the target lesion, and adequate imaging.

Intraoperative fluoroscopy is used to guide all wire, catheter, and device manipulations. Standard radiation safety should be exercised. Digital subtraction angiography is an essential adjunct in performing endovascular surgery. This can be done with either fixed unit imaging systems or portable C-arm imaging with digital subtraction capability. With the patient in the supine position, the C-arm gantry is typically angled at 40–45 degrees left of midline, allowing for maximum display of the transverse aortic arch and its transition into the descending thoracic aorta. ECG leads are kept out of the field of imaging over the chest as much as possible to avoid any visual interference in device positioning and deployment. Intraoperative TEE has been described, but is not widely used. Successful exclusion of the injury with the endograft can require device deployment with partial or complete coverage of the left subclavian artery origin. Therefore, intraarterial pressure monitoring should be performed through right upper extremity access when at all possible. The working wire over which the device is positioned and deployed is typically reflected off the aortic valve, with the potential to traverse the valve into the left ventricle. Therefore, attention is given to intraoperative cardiac arrhythmias, which are communicated to the operating surgeon. Technical success is predicated upon obtaining adequate seal of the endograft against the aortic wall proximal and distal to the injury. These are termed the "landing zones." The adequacy of the seal in the landing zones is dependent upon proper device selection according to preoperative imaging analysis. The device is selected according to the diameter of the aorta and the desired treatment length in order to cover sufficient aorta in the proximal and distal landing zones. In patients with degenerative diseases of the aorta, the required length of the landing zone is 2 cm. In patients with traumatic aortic injury, the length of normal aorta proximal to the injury, but distal to the subclavian artery, is typically much shorter than 2 cm. This can influence the decision to partially or completely cover the origin of the left subclavian artery with the endograft. Coverage of the left subclavian artery can be performed safely in the overwhelming majority of patients, reserving revascularization for patients with symptomatic arm ischemia.[37–39] This can be accomplished by endovascular means in selected patients, or by surgical revascularization with left carotid to subclavian artery bypass or subclavian artery to carotid artery transposition. Regardless of the management of the subclavian artery, technical success remains quite high and endoleaks are not typically encountered after repair of thoracic aortic injuries.

Results of endovascular repair of thoracic aortic injury are excellent and compare quite favorably to open repair, such that endovascular repair has all but completely replaced open repair (Fig. 29.2).[33,34] In comparison to open repair, the incidences of spinal cord ischemia, stroke, and death are all significantly lower for endovascular repair. Composite mortality rates less than 8%, stroke rates less than 1%, and paraplegia rates less

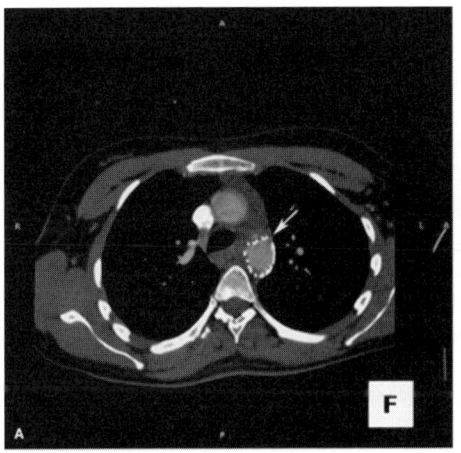

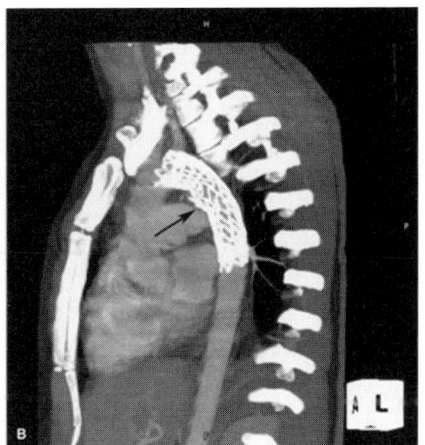

Figure 29.2 (A) Axial CT scan in the same patient as in Figure 29.1 following endovascular stent graft placement (arrow), demonstrating exclusion of the transected portion of the thoracic aorta with no evidence of extravasation of contrast. (B) Multiplanar reconstruction in the same patient showing the stent graft placed in the proximal descending thoracic aorta just distal to the origin of the left subclavian artery. Note contrast filling of the left subclavian artery demonstrating patency. (C) Volumetric 3D reconstruction of the postprocedure CT scan, demonstrating a thoracic stent graft in situ with successful exclusion of the aortic transection.

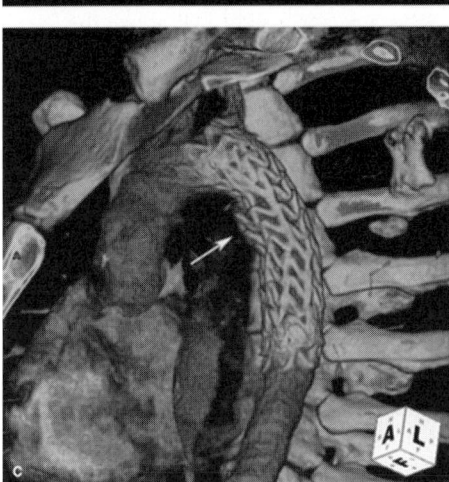

than 1% have all been reported.[35,36] Postulated reasons for the difference in the incidence of spinal cord ischemia may be the avoidance of aortic clamping and decreased variations in spinal cord perfusion pressure. The role of reperfusion injury to the spinal cord after hemodynamic compromise associated with open repair also appears to be mitigated with endovascular repair. Although the incidence of spinal cord ischemia after endovascular repair approaches zero, it is not zero. Factors that appear to increase risk of spinal cord ischemia are those that may affect collateral flow to the cord: hypotension, long length of aorta covered by the stent, coverage of the left subclavian artery, distal thoracic aortic coverage, previous infrarenal aortic replacement, and significant occlusive disease involving the internal iliac arteries. Treatment of spinal cord ischemia is targeted at manipulating spinal perfusion pressure: elevating mean arterial pressure with pressors and decreasing intrathecal pressure with lumbar spinal drainage.[40] Intraoperative monitoring with somatosensory evoked potentials or motor evoked potentials can identify patients with spinal cord ischemia in real time. However, this type of monitoring is not easily implemented in trauma patients, nor is it necessary during TEVAR of traumatic injuries, as the risk of spinal ischemia is exceedingly low.

Long-term follow-up data are lacking, as is a consensus for definitive guidelines regarding postoperative device surveillance after TEVARs.

In our institution, we have performed 13 endovascular repairs of blunt thoracic aortic injuries over the last 3 years. Twelve involved the proximal descending thoracic aorta and one involved the distal descending thoracic aorta. There have been no deaths, spinal cord ischemia, or strokes. Two patients have had partial or complete coverage of the left subclavian artery without the need for revascularization of the left upper extremity, early or late. All patients have been treated with a single device component. All patients were discharged from the hospital. There have been no endoleaks, pseudoaneurysms, or dissections present at follow-up ranging from 1 to 40 months. Over this same time interval, we have not utilized open repair in any patient with blunt thoracic aortic injury.

It is safe to conclude that endovascular repair of blunt thoracic aortic injury has become the preferred treatment for these patients. The technical expertise and knowledge required to successfully treat this entity in an endovascular manner requires a comprehensive operating room team that possesses the appropriate knowledge and endovascular skills. At our institution, we utilize collaboration between cardiothoracic surgery and peripheral vascular surgery to conduct the operative treatment of these injuries. Other centers may use a different model. Additionally, the care that these severely injured patients require adds more complexity to the management of this life-threatening condition. It also demands an institutional commitment to the care of these complex patients. Still, long-term follow-up data are required for this treatment modality.

Questions

(1) Which cardiac chamber is more exposed to the anterior chest wall?
a. Right ventricle
b. Left ventricle
c. Right atrium
d. Left atrium
e. Aorta

(2) Which of the following cardiac structures may be injured in penetrating cardiac trauma?
a. Pericardium
b. Coronary arteries
c. Cardiac valves
d. Interventricular septum
e. All of the above

(3) Which of the following clinical signs is *not* seen in cardiac tamponade?
a. Normal or low blood pressure
b. Elevation of central venous pressure
c. Pulse pressure may be narrow
d. The visible superficial neck veins may be distended and have paradoxical filling during inspiration
e. All of the above may be clinical signs of cardiac tamponade

(4) Goals of emergency department thoracotomy include:
a. Relieve cardiac tamponade
b. Potential crossclamping of the aorta to improve coronary perfusion
c. Permit direct cardiac massage
d. Internal cardiac defibrillation
e. All of the above

(5) Which of the following therapeutic measures should be performed first when considering an emergency department thoractomy?
a. Rapid infusion of packed red blood cells
b. Chest compressions
c. Stabilization of the airway
d. Skin incision
e. Insertion of two large-bore intravenous lines

(6) Which of the following signs is *not* suggestive of blunt cardiac injury?
a. Hypotension disproportionate to the suspected injury
b. Massive hemothorax unresponsive to thoracostomy and fluid resuscitation
c. Persistent metabolic acidosis
d. Presence of pericardial effusion on FAST or echocardiography, elevation of central venous pressure, and prominent neck veins with continuing hypotension despite fluid resuscitation
e. All of the above may be suggestive of a blunt cardiac injury

(7) What region of the aorta is most commonly involved in blunt aortic injury?
a. Ascending aorta
b. Aortic arch
c. Isthmus of the aorta
d. Abdominal aorta
e. Descending thoracic aorta right just above the diaphragm

(8) Open surgical repair of a blunt aortic injury is most commonly performed via which of the following incisions?
a. Midline laparotomy
b. Sternotomy
c. Right thoracotomy
d. Left thoracotomy
e. Clam-shell incision

(9) Thoracic endovascular aortic repair is a therapeutic option for the management of a blunt aortic injury. Which of the following is a contraindication to this technique?
a. Adequate vascular access
b. Insufficient landing zones to deploy the stent graft
c. Associated organ injury
d. Hypotension
e. None of the above is a contraindication

(10) Which of the following is the most sensitive and specific method for diagnosis of cardiac tamponade in acute cardiac trauma?
a. Central venous pressure measurements
b. Ultrasonography
c. Subxiphoid pericardial window
d. Pericardiocentesis
e. None of the above

Answers

(1) a
(2) e
(3) e
(4) e
(5) c
(6) e
(7) c
(8) d
(9) b
(10) b

References

1. Asensio JA, Soto SN, Forno W, *et al.* Penetrating cardiac injuries: a complex challenge. *Surg Today* 2001; **31**: 1041–53.

2. Asensio JA, Berne JD, Demetriades D, *et al.* One hundred five penetrating cardiac injuries: a 2-year prospective evaluation. *J Trauma* 1998; **44**: 1073–82.

3. Rhee PM, Foy H, Kaufmann C, *et al.* Penetrating cardiac injuries: a population-based study. *J Trauma* 1998; **45**: 366–70.

4. Asensio JÁ, Garcia-Nunez LM, Petrone P, *et al.* Penetrating cardiac injuries in America: predictors of outcome in 2016 patients from the National Trauma Data Bank; in preparation. As quoted by Asensio JÁ, Garcia-Nunez LM, Petrone P. Trauma to the heart. In Feliciano DV, Mattox KL Moore EE, eds., *Trauma*, 6th edition. New York, NY: McGraw Hill, 2008, pp. 569–88.

5. Rozycki GS, Feliciano DV, Schmidt JA, *et al.* The role of surgeon-performed ultrasound in patients with possible cardiac wounds. *Ann Surg* 1996; **223**: 737–44.

6. American College of Surgeons. *Advanced Trauma Life Support*, 9th edition. Chicago, IL: ACS, 2012.

7. Stratton SJ, Brickett K, Crammer T. Prehospital pulseless, unconscious penetrating trauma victims: field assessments associated with survival. *J Trauma* 1998; **45**: 96–100.

8. Wilson SM, Au FC. In extremis use of a Foley catheter in a cardiac stab wound. *J Trauma* 1986; **26**: 400–2.

9. Macho JR, Markison RE, Schecter WP. Cardiac stapling in the management of penetrating injuries of the heart: rapid control of hemorrhage and decreased risk of personal contamination. *J Trauma* 1993; **34**: 711–15.

10. Roberts JR, Hedges JR, Chanmugam AS. *Clinical Procedures in Emergency Medicine*, 4th edition. Philadelphia, PA: Saunders, 2004.

11. Lim R, Gill IS, Temes RT, Smith CE. The use of adenosine for repair of penetrating cardiac injuries: a novel method. *Ann Thorac Surg* 2001; **71**: 1714–15.

12. Lin JC, Ott RA. Acute traumatic mitral valve insufficiency. *J Trauma* 1999; **47**: 165–8.

13. Mattox KL, Estrera AL, Wall MJ. Traumatic heart disease. In Zipes DP, Braunwald E, eds., *Braunwald's Heart Disease a Textbook of Cardiovascular Medicine.* Philadelphia, PA: Saunders, 2005, pp. 1781–8.

14. Teixeira PG, Inaba K, Oncel D, *et al.* Blunt cardiac rupture: a 5-year NTDB analysis. *J Trauma* 2009; **67**: 788–91.

15. Hiatt JR, Yeatman LA, Child JS. The value of echocardiography in blunt chest trauma. *J Trauma* 1988; **28**: 914–22.

16. Brooks SW, Young JC, Cmolik B, *et al.* The use of transesophageal echocardiography in the evaluation of chest trauma. *J Trauma* 1992; **32**: 761–5.

17. Co SJ, Yong-Hing CJ, Galea-Soler S, *et al.* Role of imaging in penetrating and blunt traumatic injury to the heart. *Radiographics* 2011; **31**: E101–15.

18. Pevec WC, Udekwu AO, Peitzman AB. Blunt rupture of the myocardium. *Ann Thorac Surg* 1989; **48**: 139–42.

19. Banning AP, Pillai R. Non-penetrating cardiac and aortic trauma. *Heart* 1997; **78**: 226–9.

20. Prêtre R, Chilcott M. Blunt trauma to the heart and great vessels. *N Engl J Med* 1997; **336**: 626–32.

21. Sharkey SW, Shear W, Hodges M, *et al.* Reversible myocardial contraction abnormalities in patients with an acute noncardiac illness. *Chest* 1998; **114**: 98–105.

22. Merrill WH, Lee RB, Hammon JW, *et al.* Surgical treatment of acute traumatic tear of the thoracic aorta. *Ann Surg* 1988; **207**: 699–706.

23. Hunt JP, Baker CC, Lentz CW, *et al.* Thoracic aorta injuries: management and outcome of 144 patients. *J Trauma* 1996; **40**: 547–55.

24. Feczko JD, Lynch L, Pless JE, *et al.* An autopsy case review of 142 nonpenetrating (blunt) injuries of the aorta. *J Trauma* 1992; **33**: 846–9.

25. Hirose H, Moore E. Delayed presentation and rupture of a posttraumatic innominate artery aneurysm: case report and review of the literature. *J Trauma* 1997; **42**: 1187–95.

26. Malhotra AK, Fabian TC, Croce MA, *et al.* Minimal aortic injury: a lesion associated with advancing diagnostic techniques. *J Trauma* 2001; **51**: 1042–8.

27. Mosquera VX, Marini M, Muñiz J, *et al.* Traumatic aortic injury score (TRAINS): an easy and simple score for early detection of traumatic aortic injuries in major trauma patients with associated blunt chest trauma. *Intensive Care Med* 2012; **38**: 1487–96.

28. Novelline RA, Rhea JT, Rao PM, *et al.* Helical CT in emergency radiology. *Radiology* 1999; **213**: 321–39.

29. Yoshida S, Akiba H, Tamakawa M, *et al.* Thoracic involvement of type A aortic dissection and intramural hematoma: diagnostic accuracy–comparison of emergency helical CT and surgical findings. *Radiology* 2003; **228**: 430–5.

30. Lamarche Y, Berger FH, Nicolaou S, *et al.* Vancouver simplified grading system with computed tomographic angiography for blunt aortic injury. *J Thorac Cardiovasc Surg* 2012; **144**: 347–354.e1.

31. Cinnella G, Dambrosio M, Brienza N, *et al.* Transesophageal echocardiography for diagnosis of traumatic aortic injury: an appraisal of the evidence. *J Trauma* 2004; **57**: 1246–55.

32. Lederle FA, Freischlag JA, Kyriakides TC, *et al.*; Open Versus Endovascular Repair (OVER) Veterans Affairs Cooperative Study Group. Outcomes following endovascular vs open repair of abdominal aortic aneurysm: a randomized trial. *JAMA* 2009; **302**: 1535–42.

33. Demetriades D, Velmahos GC, Scalea TM, *et al.* Operative repair or endovascular stent graft in blunt traumatic thoracic aortic injuries: results of an American Association for the Surgery of Trauma multicenter study. *J Trauma* 2008; **64**: 561–71.

34. Demetriades D, Velmahos GC, Scalea TM, *et al.* Diagnosis and treatment of blunt thoracic aortic injuries: changing perspectives. *J Trauma* 2008; **64**: 1415–19.

35. Celis RI, Park SC, Shukla AJ, *et al.* Evolution of treatment for traumatic thoracic aortic injuries. *J Vasc Surg* 2012; **56**: 74–80.

36. Patel HJ, Hemmila MR, Williams DM, *et al.* Late outcomes following open and endovascular repair of blunt thoracic aortic injury. *J Vasc Surg* 2011; **53**: 615–21.

37. Maldonado TS, Dester D, Rockman CB, *et al.* Left subclavian artery coverage during thoracic endovascular aneurysm repair does not mandate revascularization. *J Vasc Surg* 2013; **57**: 116–24.

38. Antonello M, Menegolo M, Maturi C, *et al.* Intentional coverage of the left subclavian artery during endovascular repair of traumatic descending thoracic aortic transection. *J Vasc Surg* 2013; **57**: 684–90.e1.

39. Cooper DG, Walsh SR, Sadat U, *et al.* Neurological complications after left subclavian artery coverage during thoracic endovascular aortic repair: a systematic review and meta-analysis. *J Vasc Surg* 2009; **49**: 1594–601.

40. Acher CW, Wynn M. A modern theory of paraplegia in the treatment of aneurysms of the thoracoabdominal aorta: an analysis of the technique specific observed/expected ratios for paralysis. *J Vasc Surg* 2009; **49**: 1117–24.

Anesthesia considerations for cardiothoracic trauma

Mark A. Gerhardt and Glenn P. Gravlee

Objectives

(1) Understand the pathophysiology and treatment of cardiothoracic trauma.
(2) Discuss the anesthetic implications of trauma to the heart, great vessels, lungs, thoracic wall, and intrathoracic airways.

Introduction

Thoracic trauma, particularly to the heart or great vessels, accounts for 20–25% of trauma mortality. In out-of-hospital traumatic cardiopulmonary arrest, hypovolemia has been implicated as a primary factor in traumatic fatalities.[1] Most significant injuries to the cardiac or great vessel structures are immediately fatal. Cardiac tamponade and tension pneumothorax from blunt or penetrating truma can be rapidly fatal if not diagnosed and treated. It is imperative that anesthesiologists understand trauma of the heart and great vessels so that appropriate and expeditious care can be provided. Supplemental material can be accessed via the internet on the websites shown in Table 30.1 (see also Chapter 29).

The management of cardiothoracic trauma continues to evolve, with notable modification in clinical strategy, imaging, and surgical interventions. Advances in imaging technology,

Table 30.1 Trauma websites

www.aast.org
www.acls.net
www.americanheart.org
www.amtrauma.org
www.asahq.org
www.bt.cdc.gov
www.east.org
www.itaccs.com
www.sccm.org
www.trauma.org

specifically computed tomography (CT) (see Chapter 11), and the application of minimally invasive surgical techniques, predominantly endovascular stent repair (see Chapter 29), have refined patient management strategies. Historically, trauma anesthesiology has held fast to the "golden hour" dogma. It has been suggested, however, that the concept of the golden hour be discarded with realignment of trauma care to match recent clinical experience and evidence-based medicine.[2] Clinical practice is shifting to a deliberate approach, with acquisition of more detailed diagnostic data prior to emergent surgical exploration.[3,4] Additionally a "damage control" strategy, incorporated from the military experience, is leading to improved outcomes (see Chapters 18 and 38). Fluid management, including the use of massive transfusion protocols (MTPs) and hemostatic pharmacological adjuncts (tranexamic acid [TXA], factor concentrates), have been applied to trauma patients (see Chapter 6). Pain management for rib and/or sternal fractures has improved, and there are a number of effective techniques that provide excellent analgesia for thoracic trauma such as thoracic epidural anesthesia (TEA) and paravertebral nerve block (see Chapters 15 and 16).[5–7]

Cardiothoracic anatomy

The thorax contains vital organs and vasculature that are protected by the bony structures of the vertebral column, sternum, and ribs. Inferiorly the thorax is demarcated by the diaphragm, while the structures of the neck and lung apices are found superiorly. The primary organs within the thorax are the heart, lungs, great vessels, and esophagus. Significant injury to the heart, lungs, or great vessels can be rapidly fatal. Some structures have fibrous anchor points that limit the mobility of the mediastinal structures. These regions are clinically relevant, because shear forces during blunt trauma (especially deceleration injuries) are more likely to result in avulsions or disruption at the anchor points. The heart is immobile at the junction of the vena cava with the right atrium, the posterior left atrial wall where the four pulmonary veins enter, and the aortic valve annulus. The proximal descending thoracic aorta is fixed at the ligamentum arteriosum just distal to the subclavian artery, and this is the typical site of

Trauma Anesthesia, 2nd Edition, ed. Charles E. Smith. Published by Cambridge University Press. © Charles E. Smith, 2015.

injury in traumatic aortic transection. Additionally, the thoracic aorta is immobilized by the diaphragmatic hiatus as it exits the thorax and at the aortic valve annulus.

The great vessels consist of the aorta, pulmonary arteries, pulmonary veins, vena cava, and their major intrathoracic branches. The great vessels occupy a central mediastinal location and connect with the base of the heart. The apex of the heart lies in the left thoracic cavity. The heart is contained within the pericardium, a tough fibrous sac that limits cardiac motion. Rapid accumulation of fluid in the pericardial space, particularly following penetrating cardiac trauma or aortic transection, can result in cardiac tamponade and hypotension.

The surface anatomy of the heart has important relationships with respect to trauma. Trauma mechanisms that have an impact on the anterior chest create risk for anterior cardiac structures, particularly penetrating wounds. The right heart comprises the majority of the anterior presentation of the heart. The right atrium (RA) is superior and the right ventricle (RV) lies inferiorly. Together, the RA and RV form a crescent that wraps around the ellipsoidal left ventricle (LV). The RV free wall forms the vast majority of the anterior surface area of the heart and is thus the most likely structure to be injured from a stab wound to the anterior chest. The left anterior descending coronary artery (LAD) courses over the ventricular septum that separates the LV and RV. A portion of the LV inferiorly is at risk for trauma originating anteriorly. The entire heart is encased by the pericardial sac, with outlets at the base for the great vessels. The pericardium slides freely over the body and apex of the heart but is adherent at the base. Pericardial fluid can accumulate because there is no anatomic fluid outlet. Thus, bleeding into the pericardial space with subsequent compression of the heart is the only physical recourse, and this can lead to cardiac tamponade.

Initial assessment
Imaging (see also Chapter 11)

Helical CT is the standard imaging modality for the initial assessment of thoracic trauma (including cardiac trauma).[8–10] CT is rapid (minutes) and robust, giving detailed information about abnormal anatomy of all thoracic structures. The consequences of the traumatic wound, including simple/tension pneumothorax, pericardial effusion, hemorrhage, and violation of anatomic structural integrity, are all revealed by CT (Fig. 30.1). The versatility of CT imaging has resulted in wide dissemination of this diagnostic modality. Most trauma centers have CT capabilities in the emergency department, allowing detailed imaging of the entire body within minutes of admission. Helical CT and focused assessment with sonography for trauma (FAST) scans are the preferred diagnostic modalities to evaluate blunt or penetrating trauma to the thoracic organs (see Chapters 10 and 11). Transesophageal echocardiography (TEE) remains invaluable for the assessment

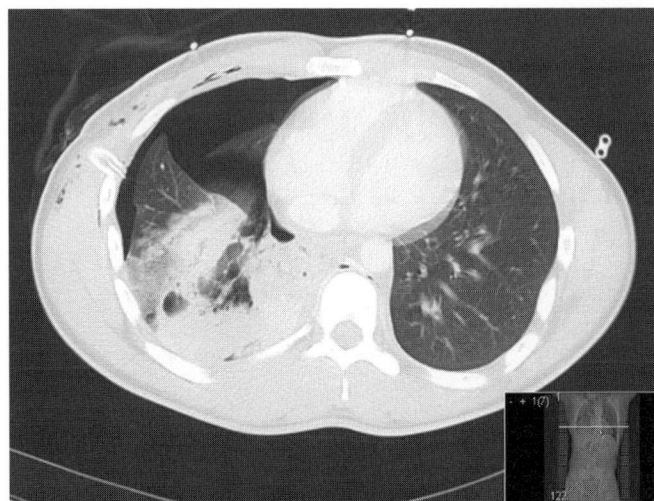

Figure 30.1 Helical CT identifying simple pneumothorax on the right. In addition to the lung collapse, right posterior hemothorax can be seen, along with a bullet path traversing the right chest wall. (Image acquired from trauma.org on 9 March 2013.)

of valvular function and cardiac structure and function during the intraoperative period (see Chapter 10).

Abbreviated Injury Scale (AIS)

The American Association for the Surgery of Trauma (AAST) created the Abbreviated Injury Scale (AIS) as an assessment tool for categorizing the impact of specific organ injuries on patient survival.[11] The AIS score is associated with predicted survival outcome (Table 30.2). An AIS score of 6 (= grade VI) is fatal. The severity of injury is nonlinear between AIS scores, in that the difference between AIS-1 and AIS-2 is less than that between AIS-4 and AIS-5. The AIS scores can be combined with those from other injury sites (e.g., abdomen, head) to calculate the clinical condition.

Damage control resuscitation (DCR)

Damage control resuscitation (DCR) was conceptualized and refined by the military.[12–14] Three essential elements govern the DCR strategy: (1) abbreviated initial surgical intervention, with the goal of gaining rapid control of immediate, life-threatening injuries without definitive correction; (2) ICU stabilization of clinical abnormalities such as acidosis, unstable hemodynamic status, and inadequate end-organ oxygen delivery; (3) return to the operating room (OR) for staged repair (see Chapter 18). The success of this military strategy has resulted in its adoption by civilian trauma medicine. It should be noted that, with the exception of pneumothorax and chest tube thoracostomy, the majority of cases had abdominal, orthopedic, or blast/burn trauma rather than cardiac or great vessel wounds.[12–14] Over the last decade, thoracic trauma was identified in 2049 of 23,797 military casualties (8.6%) with a mean AIS score of 2.9 ± 0.9.[15] Penetrating trauma occurred in 61.5%, with explosive device fragmentation as the mechanism

Table 30.2 Cardiac organ injury scaling

AIS grade/ severity	Injury description
I. Minor	Blunt cardiac injury with minor ECG abnormality Nonspecific ST or T wave changes, PAC, PVC, persistent sinus tachycardia Blunt or penetrating pericardial wound without cardiac injury, cardiac tamponade or cardiac herniation
II. Moderate	Blunt cardiac trauma with heart block or ischemic changes without heart failure Penetrating tangential wound not extending through endocardium, without tamponade
III. Serious	Blunt cardiac injury with sustained or multifocal PVC Blunt or penetrating cardiac injury with septal rupture, PI, TR, papillary muscle dysfunction or distal coronary artery occlusion without HF Blunt pericardial laceration with cardiac herniation Blunt cardiac injury with HF Penetrating tangential myocardial wound not extending through endocardium, with tamponade
IV. Severe	Blunt or penetrating cardiac injury with septal rupture, PI, TR, papillary muscle dysfunction or distal coronary artery occlusion with resultant HF Blunt or penetrating cardiac injury with AV or MV incompetence Blunt or penetrating cardiac injury of the RV, RA, or LA
V. Critical	Blunt or penetrating cardiac injury with proximal coronary artery occlusion Blunt or penetrating LV perforation Stellate injuries < 50% tissue loss of RV, RA, or LA
VI. Not survivable	Blunt avulsion of the heart Penetrating wound producing > 50% loss of a cardiac chamber

NOTE: Advance one grade for multiple penetrating wounds to a single chamber or injury of multiple chambers.
Modified from trauma.org (accessed March 5, 2013).
AIS, Abbreviated Injury Scale; AV, aortic valve; ECG, electrocardiograph; HF, heart failure; LA, left atrium; MV, mitral valve; PAC, premature atrial contractions; PI, pulmonic insufficiency; PVC, premature ventricular contractions; RA, right atrium; RV, right ventricle; TR, tricuspid regurgitation.

for the vast majority. Pneumothorax (51.8%) and pulmonary contusion (50.2%) were the most common injuries. Chest tube thoracostomy was the sole surgical intervention in 47%. Risk factors associated with a poor outcome were acute respiratory distress syndrome (ARDS) and inhalational injuries.[15]

Management of fluid resuscitation in trauma patients is undergoing rigorous evaluation.[2] Traditionally trauma resuscitation has emphasized rapid reversal of hypotension with crystalloid fluid therapy augmented by colloid fluids and/or blood products, especially packed red blood cells (pRBC). An alternative DCR strategy is directed towards preservation/ restoration of hemostatic pathways as the primary goal. Recently the use of "hypotensive resuscitation" and administration of blood products (fresh frozen plasma [FFP] in a 1:1 ratio of FFP:pRBC) rather than crystalloid fluids has yielded improved outcomes.[2] Military DCR has had success with an empiric FFP:pRBC:platelet ratio of 1:1:1 in trauma patients.[13] Massive transfusion therapy is presented in detail in Chapter 6.

Pharmacological therapy to augment hemostasis is now widely employed. The CRASH-2 clinical trial results concluded that the antifibrinolytic drug tranexamic acid (TXA) administered within 3 hours of injury improved survival and other outcomes.[16] Trauma patients are now commonly treated with TXA in the field even prior to hospital admission. It is unknown if patients with blunt/penetrating cardiac or great vessel injury derive similar benefit. Empiric factor VIIa administration to trauma patients with refractory bleeding has been reported.[17] Military patients received transfusion therapy for trauma. Propensity-score matched groups ($n = 266$/group) were compared in patients who were treated with factor VIIa with patients who did not receive factor VIIa. Massive transfusion was utilized in 50% of each group. There was no difference between groups in complications (21%) or mortality (control 14%; treated 20%).[17] A meta-analysis reached a similar conclusion, that factor VIIa did not improve survival in trauma patients.[18] A case report of a patient with a gunshot wound to the chest with refractory bleeding that responded to factor VIIa therapy is representative of the evidence favoring factor VIIa administration.[19] Factor VIIa is best reserved for patients with refractive coagulopathy. With the likely exception of prophylactic TXA, hemorrhage from the heart or major vascular conduits is a surgical problem that is unlikely to respond to empiric pharmacological therapy. Consequently, factor VIIa should not be administered empirically to patients with uncontrolled hemorrhage from blunt or penetrating thoracic trauma.

Anesthetic considerations

Cardiothoracic procedures create unique anesthetic issues that require excellent communication between the surgeon(s) and anesthesiologist(s) prior to OR entry. Pneumothorax (Fig. 30.2) is common, and chest tube(s) placement should be completed prior to anesthetic induction to prevent the development of tension pneumothorax after the institution of positive-pressure ventilation. Cardiac trauma (Table 30.2) can result in injury to a variety of anatomic structures. Surgical approach dictates patient position and need for lung isolation. Possible surgical approaches include: sternotomy, right and/or (lateral) left thoracotomy, clam-shell and thoracoabdominal incisions (see Chapter 29). Lateral thoracotomy is most often facilitated by one-lung ventilation (see Chapter 33), assuming that complicating factors such as ARDS or bilateral pulmonary

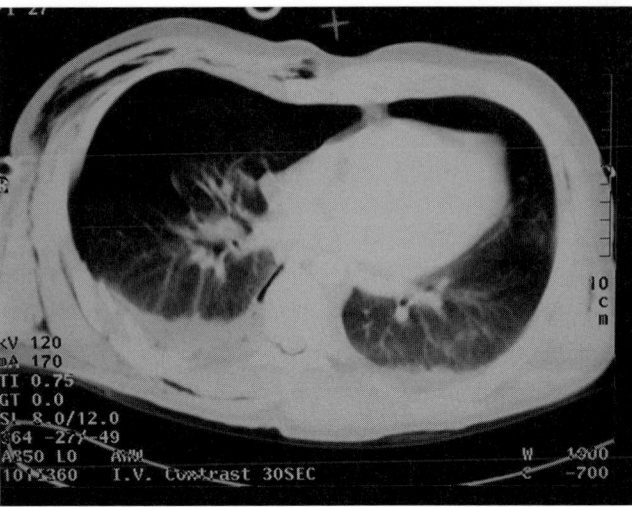

Figure 30.2 Helical CT demonstrating a tension pneumothorax. Note the right lung atelectasis and shift of the heart and mediastinum to the left secondary to the tension pneumothorax. Note also the prominent subcutaneous emphysema. Air trapping has resulted in an enlarged right chest. (Image acquired from trauma.org on 9 March 2013.)

Table 30.3 Associated injuries in blunt chest trauma patients with and without cardiac injury: autopsy results.

Associated injury	With cardiac trauma, $n = 96$	Without cardiac trauma, $n = 208$	p-value
Thoracic aorta	47%	27%	0.001
Hemothorax	81%	59%	< 0.001
Rib fractures	91%	71%	< 0.001
Sternum fracture	32%	13%	< 0.001
Intraabdominal	77%	48%	< 0.001

Modified from Teixeira et al. 2009.[21]

contusions do not preclude its safe use. The lung isolation technique must balance the intraoperative and postoperative advantages and limitations of the double-lumen tube, bronchial blocker, or intentional advancement of a single-lumen endotracheal tube into a main bronchus (see Chapter 33). Surgical techniques include open, minimally invasive, video-assisted thoracoscopic surgery (VATS), and robotic-assisted thoracotomy. The use of cardiopulmonary bypass (CPB) should include discussion of planned cannulation sites, whether left heart bypass with a centrifugal pump or full CPB is anticipated, and finally whether hypothermic (< 20 °C) circulatory arrest will be used.

Cardiac trauma

Trauma, including to the heart and great vessels, can be divided into blunt and penetrating mechanisms. Blunt trauma is produced by three mechanisms: deceleration, direct energy transfer, and compression.[20] Rapid deceleration results in shear forces on the heart and great vessels. Depending on the force vector and body positioning during deceleration, various injuries result such as blunt cardiac and aortic injuries. In blunt trauma with a fatal outcome, patients with a cardiac injury also had a higher incidence of associated injuries (Table 30.3).[21] In this chapter we explicitly use the term aortic transection, which results from blunt trauma. Aortic transection at the attachment of the ligamentum arteriosum is the most common deceleration injury. Direct energy transfer occurs during impact of the thorax. The classic example is the steering wheel impacting the anterior chest during a motor vehicle collision (MVC). Resultant injuries depend on the force of impact. The majority of blunt cardiac trauma results in myocardial contusion (part of the "spectrum" of blunt cardiac trauma). Compression is a trauma mechanism unique to the thorax which can occur when an external force traps and crushes the heart (and/or other organs) between the sternum and thoracic spine. This mechanism may be concomitant with direct energy transfer, and both may be responsible for injury, particularly organ rupture. Chest compressions during cardio-pulmonary resuscitation (CPR) are an iatrogenic cause of blunt cardiac trauma that may produce injury.

Penetrating cardiac trauma further may be subdivided into low- and high-velocity injuries. Stab wounds constitute the prototypical low-velocity wound, whereas most gunshot wounds (GSWs) are high-velocity. High-velocity wounds transfer significant energy to surrounding tissue (Fig. 30.1), often resulting in more tissue destruction than that produced by the projectile's specific pathway. Risk factors for death following chest wall blunt trauma include age > 65 years, ≥ 3 rib fractures, preexisting cardiac/pulmonary disease, and pneumonia.[22]

The experience and innovation of military medicine has been invaluable in improving management of blunt and penetrating thoracic trauma (see Chapter 38). The incidence of death from penetrating chest trauma was 63% during the American Civil War and was markedly reduced in World War II (10%) and the Korean War (2%).[15] Mortality rates increased during the Vietnam War (3%) and the Iraq/Afghanistan operations (8.3%).[15] Superficial examination of these increased death rates probably fail to correct for improved initial treatment and rapid casualty transportation, which has allowed AIS-4/AIS-5 patients to arrive at medical facilities while still alive. In the past, these patients would have expired in the field.

Blunt cardiac trauma

Cardiac rupture

Cardiac rupture secondary to blunt chest trauma is a common mechanism of death. An excellent forensic study of blunt cardiac trauma noted that cardiac injury is a risk factor for death at the accident scene (Table 30.3).[21] Trauma fatalities with a full autopsy ($n = 304$) were separated into two groups (with or without cardiac injury). The study population had an average age of 43 years, was predominantly male (71%), and 39% were intoxicated. MVCs accounted for 50% of the cases,

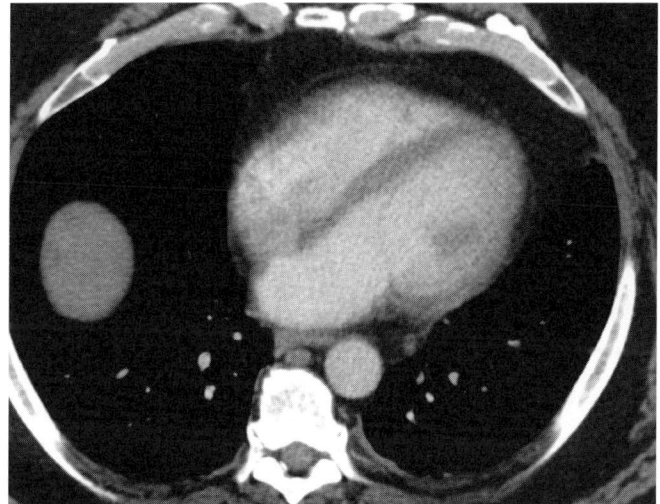

Figure 30.3 Helical CT of thorax. There are no notable abnormalities. (Used with permission from Co *et al.* 2011.[8])

Table 30.4 Clinical manifestations of myocardial contusion

Dysrhythmias, bundle branch block
Decreased cardiac function, wall motion abnormalities
Elevated myocardial enzymes
Right heart failure

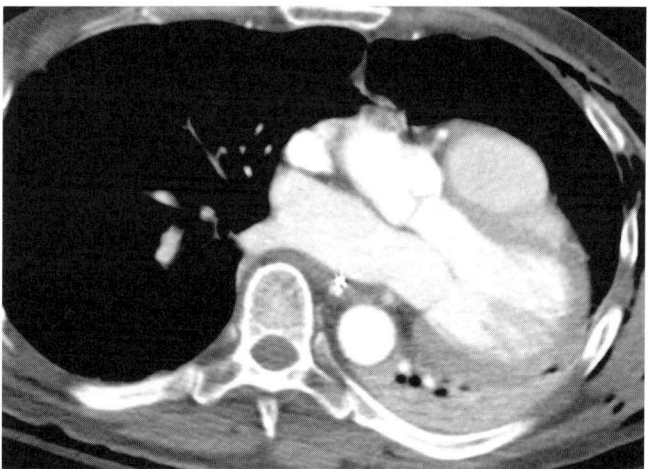

Figure 30.4 Cardiac luxation. Compare this CT scan with the normal CT scan in Figure 30.3. Note the posterior position of the heart in the left hemithorax. The apex is visible, as are the tricuspid and aortic valves. (Used with permission from Co *et al.* 2011.[8])

followed by vehicle versus pedestrian collisions (37%). The incidence of cardiac injury was 32%. The right heart possessed the most injuries with the RA and RV injured in 30% and 27% respectively. Transmural rupture was found in 64%. In this subpopulation multiple chambers (26%) demonstrated injury along with transmural injury to the RA (25%) and RV (20%). Death was pronounced at the scene in 78%, with expiration occurring during transport for the remaining 22%. Data regarding patients with cardiac trauma with rupture who presented alive were not reported. Pericardial rupture is noteworthy in that cardiac luxation (cardiac herniation)[23] can result (compare Fig. 30.3 with 30.4), presenting clinically with signs/symptoms identical to cardiac tamponade.

Myocardial contusion

Myocardial contusion (also called cardiac contusion) is common in blunt chest trauma patients. Controversy exists about the diagnostic criteria and clinical significance of myocardial contusion (Table 30.4). A diagnosis of blunt cardiac trauma consistent with myocardial contusion is typically made from a history of chest trauma along with abnormalities in the electrocardiogram (ECG), cardiac enzymes, and/or echocardiography. However, the possibility of myocardial contusion is not ruled out even with normal results from these cardiac evaluations. Furthermore, the majority of patients diagnosed with cardiac contusions have unremarkable recovery from a cardiac standpoint. Although some authors have called for abolishing myocardial contusion as a clinical entity, it seems reasonable to recognize that histopathologic changes,[24] as well as alteration in clinical risk factors and patient management, result from cardiac contusion.

At the cellular level, blunt cardiac trauma can result in myocardial hemorrhage, edema, inflammation, and cell necrosis. During histopathologic examination, cellular disruption is noted and correlates linearly with the force of blunt trauma.[24]

Damage at the tissue and cellular level is heterogeneously distributed, with patchy areas of trauma interspersed with normal-appearing myocardium. This results in abnormal electrical conduction and contractility of the damaged myocardium. Cardiac contractile dysfunction resulting from myocardial contusion typically improves over time.[25]

Clinically, the RV is at greatest risk for blunt cardiac trauma, as this is the most anterior chamber of the heart.[26] RV contusion can result in RV contractile dysfunction, which in turn leads to systemic hypotension from decreased LV filling. RV contusion is frequently associated with pulmonary contusion, which can synergistically contribute to right heart failure. Pulmonary contusion results in increased interstitial pulmonary edema and hemorrhage, diffusion abnormalities, and hypoxia, which all contribute to increased pulmonary vascular resistance and hence pulmonary arterial pressures. The contribution made by positive-pressure ventilation further augments pulmonary arterial pressures. Mechanical ventilation, decreased pulmonary compliance (with increased peak and plateau airway pressures), and utilization of positive end-expiratory pressure (PEEP) all serve to increase mean airway pressure, which translates into increased pulmonary arterial pressure. Concomitant pneumothorax and hemothorax can add to the increased intrathoracic pressure. Pulmonary contusion can cause acute pulmonary hypertension, which can manifest as right heart failure, especially when combined with abnormal RV systolic function.

ECG abnormalities are noted in essentially all patients. Cardiac arrhythmia is a typical sign of myocardial contusion. Sinus tachycardia is the most common abnormality, but can only be attributed to myocardial contusion when other causes of tachycardia have been ruled out, notably hypovolemia and pain. All dysrhythmias have been associated with myocardial contusion, including supraventricular arrhythmias, conduction delays, and ventricular dysrhythmias. Fatal ventricular arrhythmias can result from a reentry mechanism in myocardial contusion,[27] although this is rare. ECG changes consistent with ischemia or myocardial infarction should prompt investigation, as blunt trauma can cause coronary artery dissection.[28]

Definitive diagnosis of myocardial contusion is difficult. A clinical history of chest trauma, even a minor low-speed impact, is the only constant feature of the diagnosis. Physical examination may reveal signs suggestive of trauma. Fractures of the ribs, sternum, or clavicle are particularly correlated with myocardial contusion. Chest radiographs showing sternal or rib fractures, pulmonary contusion, pneumothorax, hemothorax, or widened mediastinum should raise suspicion of myocardial contusion. The primary diagnostic modalities for myocardial contusion are ECG, troponin I, and transthoracic echocardiography (TTE), although TEE may have superior diagnostic capabilities (see Chapter 10).[29]

Patients with myocardial contusion are at increased risk for hypotension and arrhythmias.[20] Risk factors associated with perioperative mortality in myocardial contusion patients include atrial fibrillation, aortic rupture, and advanced age.[20] Patients who display any arrhythmia during a procedure or have hypotensive episodes attributed to myocardial contusion should have increased postoperative observation and monitoring.

Cardiac luxation (cardiac herniation)

Cardiac luxation is classically associated with postoperative ICU care of patients following a right pneumonectomy. Post-surgical luxation occurs on the surgical side and is more commonly noted to the right. Blunt cardiac trauma can disrupt the pericardium. If the rent in the pericardial sac is sufficient in size the heart can herniate through the defect. The constriction and torsion created after luxation mechanically hinders cardiac function (Figs. 30.3, Fig. 30.4). Traumatic cardiac luxation has only been reported into the left hemithorax.[23] It is extremely important to note that the clinical presentation of cardiac luxation is virtually identical to cardiac tamponade. Both cardiac tamponade and cardiac luxation are potentially treatable mechanisms causing hypotension and death after blunt cardiac trauma. CT and FAST scan can narrow the differential diagnosis. Cardiac luxation is distinguished on CT by displacement of the heart apex into the left posterior chest and pneumopericardium in association with pneumothorax.[23]

Penetrating cardiac trauma

Penetrating cardiac trauma (Fig. 30.5) is produced by low- and high-velocity mechanisms. Cardiac tamponade and

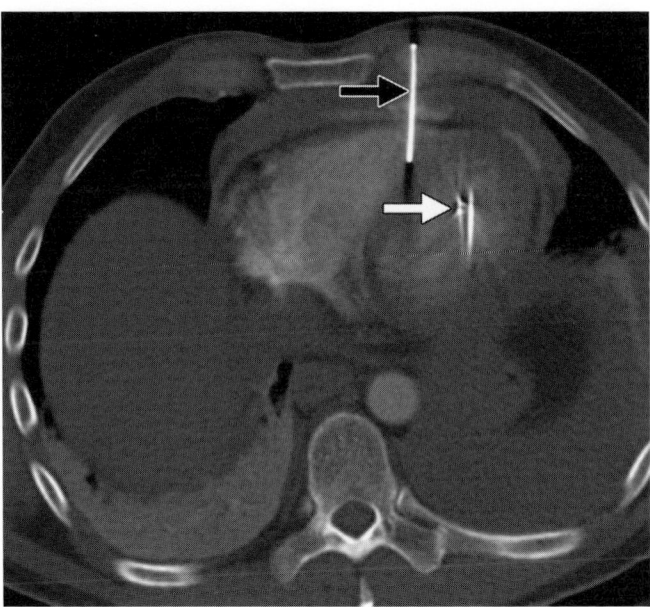

Figure 30.5 Penetrating cardiac trauma from two nail-gun foreign bodies, which are both visible. The tip of one nail (black arrow) is in the intraventricular septum. Note also the pericardial fluid accumulating anteriorly. Hemothorax is visible in the right posterior chest. (Used with permission from Co *et al.* 2011.[8])

exsanguination are immediately life-threatening complications of penetrating cardiac trauma. Prompt recognition and treatment is required to avoid poor outcomes. In a study of 711 penetrating cardiac trauma patients, there was a 47% mortality rate (stab wounds 54%, GSW 42%).[30] Right heart wounds were noted in 64% of penetrating cardiac trauma victims (24% RA, 40% RV), while LV injury was noted in 40%. Approximately 5% of patients suffered injury to a coronary artery, predominantly the LAD. Additional defects reported were the creation of a ventricular septal defect (VSD) and damage to the mitral valve. Occasionally, penetrating cardiac trauma can occur from a blunt injury. If sufficient blunt force to the thorax results in fracture of the rib or sternum, the sharp bone fragments can be displaced into the heart with a resultant penetrating wound.

Mortality from penetrating heart trauma is high. In a study of 117 patients, mortality from stab wounds was 15%, whereas GSWs resulted in an 81% mortality.[31] Cardiac tamponade was noted in 53% of the patients with stab wounds, but mortality was only 8% in this subpopulation. The authors concluded that cardiac tamponade was associated with improved survival in patients with stab wounds of the heart. Exsanguination was an important contributing factor in the fatalities.

Anesthetic considerations

Anesthetic management of penetrating cardiac trauma should be directed toward recognizing and treating life-threatening injuries such as cardiac tamponade, tension pneumothorax, and exsanguination. A history of chest trauma, physical examination findings of Beck's triad (distended neck veins, hypotension, and muffled heart tones), or pulsus paradoxus supports the diagnosis of cardiac tamponade. The neck veins may not be distended when tamponade is accompanied by severe hypovolemia. ECG may show electrical alternans. Rapid diagnosis of cardiac tamponade can be obtained with ultrasonography.

FAST is routine for the initial assessment of trauma patients and can easily detect pericardial fluid (see Chapters 2 and 10). Emergent thoracotomy may have a role in improving outcomes in penetrating, but not blunt, thoracic trauma.[32] Alternatively, a pericardial window can be performed under local anesthesia to drain pericardial fluid and stabilize the patient while preparations are made for transport to the OR for definitive care. The anesthesiologist should insure large-bore venous access to allow for rapid fluid administration as required (see Chapter 5). Chest tube placement should be strongly considered prior to or coincident with anesthetic induction because of the risk of pneumothorax. Note that positive-pressure ventilation, including mask ventilation, can convert a simple pneumothorax to a tension pneumothorax, accelerate a developing tension pneumothorax, or create a tension pneumothorax. In addition, positive-pressure ventilation can reduce venous return to the heart, and exacerbate the effects of cardiac tamponade.

The choice of induction agents is less important than the selection of an appropriate dose. Hemodynamic stability during induction and tracheal intubation in cardiac surgical patients with LV dysfunction was best achieved with midazolam (0.15 mg/kg) compared to etomidate (0.2 mg/kg), thiopental (5 mg/kg), and propofol (1.5 mg/kg).[33] The midazolam group had no change in heart rate or mean arterial pressure (MAP) from baseline to post-intubation. Etomidate was least effective at maintaining baseline hemodynamics (increased heart rate and blood pressure), although it should be noted that the dose administered was relatively low whereas the upper limit of the usual dose range was used for the other agents. In patients with cardiac tamponade, ketamine (with preservation of spontaneous respiration) has historically been the drug of choice if the patient is deemed hemodynamically safe for induction. Alternatively a pericardial window under local anesthesia should be used to relieve tamponade and allow appropriate anesthetic intervention. Video-assisted thoracoscopic surgery (VATS) is acceptable for chronic stable patients requiring a pericardial window but is contraindicated in acute, unstable trauma patients. Stab wounds of the heart can usually be repaired without the use of CPB. Temporary asystole can be induced with adenosine, which allows the surgeon time to accurately place the required number of sutures in a semi-bloodless and motionless field to adequately control hemorrhage.[34] A rapid bolus of adenosine, 6–12 mg IV, results in acute inhibition of the sinus node and some or all of the following: sinus bradycardia, transient atrioventricular block, and asystole. During the period of asystole, the heart is rendered completely flaccid and more amenable to manipulation, especially when dealing with the lateral wall.[34] Owing to

adenosine's ultra-short half-life, asystole lasts for approximately 15–20 seconds, with prompt restoration of sinus rhythm afterward. ECG monitoring, pacing backup, corrective measures for untoward hemodynamic effects (e.g., ephedrine, low-dose epinephrine, phenylephrine), and defibrillation capabilities are required. Hypotension and bronchospasm can occur after adenosine. Certain injuries will require CPB, such as pulmonary artery lacerations and VSD repair.

GSWs of the heart have several unique considerations for anesthetic management. The potential exists for transmediastinal injury, including the great vessels and the esophagus. Traumatic esophageal perforation may be worsened with TEE, so that placement of a TEE probe may be contraindicated. Missile embolus can occur with GSWs of the heart. This occurs when the bullet or shrapnel fragment penetrates a vascular structure and then is carried by blood flow until it lodges in the arterial tree at a remote site where it can produce end-organ ischemia. The trauma team can be distracted by the penetrating cardiac trauma and neglect to search for missile embolus preoperatively. Appropriate evaluation for missile embolus should occur prior to leaving the OR, to avoid prompt return for embolectomy.

Trauma of the great vessels

Endovascular stenting of most arterial vascular defects, except the pulmonary artery (PA), has been clinically demonstrated and is now considered the best surgical option for many vascular injuries, with improved survival and decreased paraplegia (see Chapter 29).[35] The AAST has published a multicenter trial which forms the foundation for the dramatic changes in trauma vascular surgery.[36–38] Paradigm shifts in the clinical diagnosis of major vascular trauma mirror those discussed earlier for cardiac trauma. Helical CT has become the imaging modality of choice for the diagnosis of vascular trauma (see Chapter 11).[37] Clinical presentation varies depending on the location and extent of the injury (Table 30.5). Operative repair strongly favors minimally invasive endovascular stent techniques rather than open surgical techniques.[36] Delayed repair of thoracic aortic trauma has shown improved survival outcomes.[38] While the surgical management of great vessel trauma has been simplified, decisions about anesthetic management remain challenging. The confounding issue for the anesthesiologist is which primary or potential procedures should the anesthetic plan accommodate? If the surgical plan is an endovascular repair via percutaneous femoral access, adequate anesthesia can be achieved with local or regional anesthesia and/or sedation.[39] In contradistinction, if the surgeon has to convert to an open procedure, the complexity of anesthetic care shifts to the other end of the spectrum, becoming perhaps the most challenging case in the field of anesthesiology. Possible anesthetic techniques involve use of lung isolation and/or partial left heart bypass or full CPB with deep hypothermic circulatory arrest. Because the rate of emergently converting to an open procedure is small, each case

Table 30.5 Factors associated with traumatic aortic injury

Trauma mechanism
High-speed, head-on motor vehicle collision (MVC)
Motor vehicle collision with passenger death
Fall > 30 feet

Site of anatomic immobilization
Junction of vena cava with right atrium
Posterior left atrium at confluence with 4 pulmonary veins
Aortic valve annulus
Proximal descending thoracic aorta at ligamentum arteriosum
Aorta at diaphragmatic hiatus

Table 30.6 Thoracic vasculature organ injury scaling

AIS grade/ severity	Injury description
I. Mild	Intercostal artery/vein Internal mammary artery/vein Bronchial artery/vein Esophageal artery/vein Hemiazygous vein Unnamed artery/vein
II. Moderate	Azygous vein Internal jugular vein Subclavian vein Innominate vein
III. Serious	Carotid artery Innominate artery Subclavian artery
IV. Severe	Thoracic aorta, descending Inferior vena cava (intrathoracic) Pulmonary artery, primary intraparenchymal branch Pulmonary vein, primary intraparenchymal branch
V. Critical	Thoracic aorta, ascending and/or arch Superior vena cava Pulmonary artery, main trunk Pulmonary vein, main trunk
VI. Not survivable	Uncontained total transection of thoracic aorta Uncontained total transection of pulmonary hilum

Note: Advance one grade for multiple grade III/IV if > 50% of circumference. Decrease one grade for IV/V if < 25% circumference.
Modified from trauma.org (accessed March 5, 2013).
AIS, Abbreviated Injury Scale.

should be considered individually, accounting for surgeon experience and relevant patient factors. Endovascular stents have also been used in pediatric patients to repair traumatic aortic rupture.[40]

Blunt injury to the great vessels

Thoracic aortic transection

Blunt trauma can result in rupture or avulsion of the great vessels within the thoracic cavity. Table 30.6 shows a continuum of thoracic vascular injuries rated by severity. The thoracic aorta is particularly prone to damage when rapid deceleration is the mechanism of injury, resulting in thoracic aortic partial or complete transection. Falls and MVCs are prototypical scenarios that can produce aortic transection (Table 30.6). The thoracic aorta is anchored at the aortic annulus, the ligamentum arteriosum, and the diaphragmatic hiatus. These points of attachment immobilize small sections of the thoracic aorta, which is otherwise freely mobile within the chest. Traumatic aortic transection is distinguished from thoracic aortic aneurysmal (TAA) disease in that aortic transection is an *acute* life-threatening event involving disruption of all layers of the aortic wall, whereas TAA is a weakening and expansion of some of the layers of the aortic wall without immediate rupture. The majority, up to 90%, of TAA patients with frank rupture of the aorta die prior to hospital arrival.[41] Patients who survive to hospital admission have a contained rupture that requires prompt diagnosis and treatment. The classic dogma has maintained that these patients are "time bombs" that could deteriorate at any moment, and therefore should be rushed to the OR for open repair. Evidence-based medicine suggests that patients with acute aortic transection who survive to reach the hospital may have a better acute prognosis than previously believed.[25,38] Therefore, an immediately life-threatening injury, such as exsanguination from rupture of the spleen, should take precedence over the potentially life-threatening aortic transection. The aortic injury should then be promptly treated. If the patient is hemodynamically stable, an aortic disruption can be managed medically (see below) and watched carefully for signs of further deterioration necessitating urgent or emergent surgery. The natural long-

term result of this lesion would be an aortic pseudoaneurysm that would necessitate elective surgical repair because of the eventual likelihood of fatal rupture.

Patients with aortic transection can have variable clinical presentations. The vital signs may reflect an increased sympathetic state (hypertension and tachycardia) caused by pain, anxiety, and inadequate oxygen delivery to vital organs. A contained rupture in the proximal descending thoracic aorta may induce downstream ischemia as a result of interrupted distal aortic flow from the aortic disruption itself or from hematoma compressing the distal thoracic aorta. Spinal cord ischemia and paraplegia can result. A partial or complete aortic transection may also have a dissection component, which involves separation of layers within the wall of the aorta. Extension of such a dissection into major arterial vessels may produce additional symptoms associated with the ischemic organ. Classically, the patient may complain of sharp, tearing chest pain with radiation to the back between the scapulae. Retrograde dissection can affect the coronary arteries, producing myocardial ischemia or infarction, pericardial tamponade, or acute aortic insufficiency. Dissection of the cranial vessels may produce mental status changes, neurologic deficits, or stroke. Dissection of the splanchnic vasculature can result in mesenteric ischemia, with pain out of proportion to the physical examination. Acute kidney injury and oliguria can result when there is renal arterial involvement or hypotension from a prerenal mechanism. Extension of the dissection distally into the iliac and femoral arterial tree can present with lower-extremity ischemia. Any combination of these symptoms can be present, depending on the specific organ perfusion state after dissection. Symptoms can worsen over time, which usually reflects extension of the dissection.

There are two systems to classify aortic dissection (Fig. 30.6). The Stanford classification system has greater clinically utility.[42] Aortic dissection that involves the ascending thoracic aorta is classified as type A and requires surgery for definitive management. Aortic dissection that involves the descending thoracic aorta is classified as type B and can be treated with an initial trial of medical management (aggressive control of blood pressure and heart rate). Patients who continue to display symptoms or whose symptoms worsen during medical management are considered to have failed therapy and require emergent surgery. The DeBakey classification system classifies aortic dissection based on anatomical location and extent of the dissection. DeBakey types I and II require surgical management, whereas types IIIA and IIIB can undergo a trial of medical management. Typical proximal descending aortic traumatic transection is most similar to a DeBakey type IIIa dissection, even though the actual injury most often is not a dissection.

Historically a widened mediastinum (Fig. 30.7) on chest x-ray and a history of blunt trauma triggered evaluation via aortography or TEE. CT has now replaced aortography and TEE as the gold-standard diagnostic modality for acute aortic transection.[8,9,37] Intraoperatively, TEE may be used to guide the management of open aortic cases under general anesthesia (Table 30.7).[43] Although TEE is not the initial imaging modality for traumatic injury of the heart (and great vessels), it does retain a primary role in evaluating cardiac valve and contractile function.

In 2008 the results of the AAST 2 review were published, supplanting the 1997 AAST 1 review on clinical management of aortic injury resulting from blunt trauma.[37] In the AAST 2 study, aortic injury (Figs. 30.8, 30.9) was diagnosed by CT in 93.3% of patients. This is radically different than AAST 1, where CT was used to make the diagnosis in 34.8% of patients. For the diagnosis of aortic injury, in AAST 1 compared to AAST 2, use of TEE and angiography changed from 87% to 1.0%, and from 11.9% to 8.3%, respectively. The time from aortic injury to repair increased from 16.5 hours to 54.6 hours. In the AAST 1 study, all patients had open repair, whereas only 35.2% were open repairs in AAST 2. The AAST 2 study showed improved outcomes, with mortality decreased from 22.0% to 13.0% ($p = 0.02$), and paraplegia decreased from

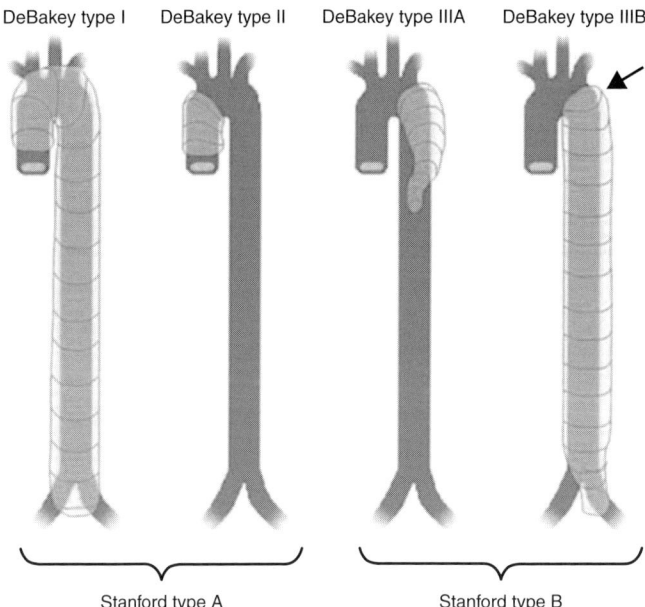

Figure 30.6 Schematic diagram of the Stanford and DeBakey classification schemes for aortic dissection. (Adapted from Miller R, ed., *Atlas of Anesthesia*, Vol. 8.; Reves J, ed., *Cardiothoracic Anesthesia*. London: Churchill Livingstone, 1999, p 6.10.)

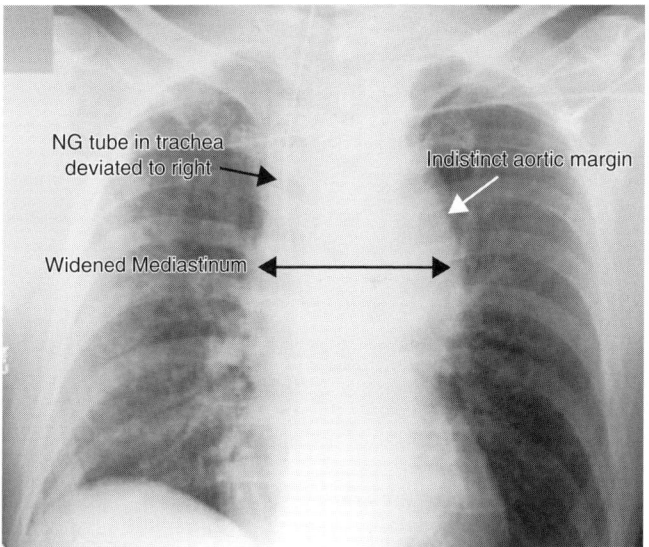

Figure 30.7 Chest x-ray in a trauma victim portraying a widened mediastinum suspicious for traumatic disruption of the proximal descending thoracic aorta.

8.7% to 1.6% ($p = 0.01$). Graft-related complications increased from 0.5% in AAST 1 to 18.4% in AAST 2. When comparing the AAST 2 endovascular stent group with the open repair group, the stent group had decreased mortality and blood transfusion.[36] In a separate analysis of the AAST 2 data, comparing early (< 24 hours; $n = 109$) and late (> 24 hours; $n = 69$) repair via endovascular stent, the delayed repair group had decreased mortality.[38] Importantly, the delayed group demonstrated improved survival with or without concomitant major associated trauma injuries.[38]

Table 30.7 Advantages and disadvantages of transesophageal echocardiography (TEE) in cardiothoracic trauma (see also Chapter 10)

Advantages	Disadvantages
Portability	Requires experienced specialist (operator dependent)
Ease of performance	Contraindicated in esophageal pathology
Ease of follow-up examinations	Potential to exacerbate unstable cervical spine injuries
No perceptible delay in primary or secondary survey	Potential airway problems if not tracheally intubated
Excellent imaging of aortic valve, proximal ascending aorta, distal aortic arch, descending thoracic aorta, cardiac function, and intracardiac lesions	Unable to visualize portions of the ascending aorta, proximal aortic arch, and brachiocephalic branches due to tracheal and bronchial air Decreased diagnostic ability if pneumomediastinum

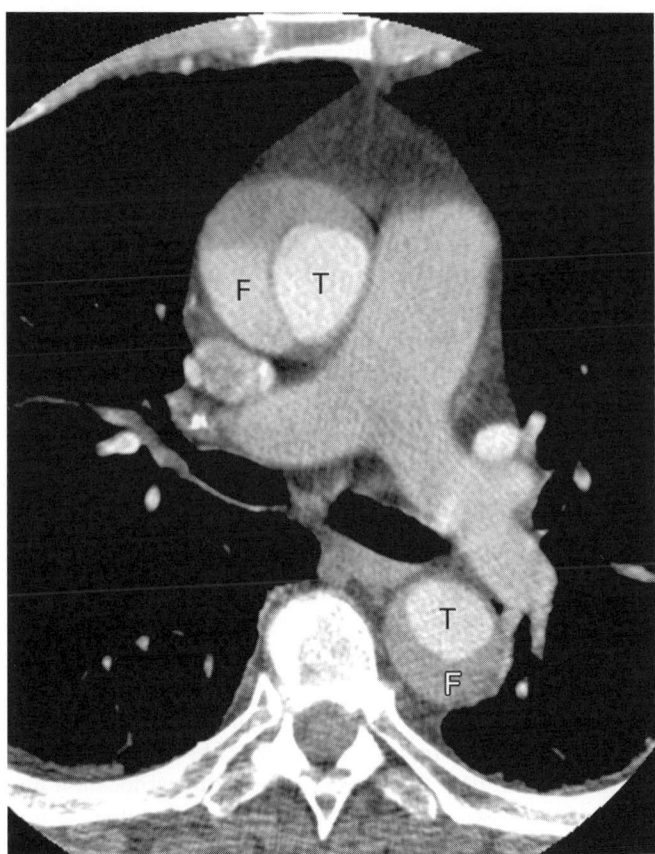

Figure 30.9 Thoracic CT of aortic dissection with intimal flaps. True (T) and false (F) lumen are noted in both the ascending and descending thoracic aorta at the level of the pulmonary artery bifurcation. (Used with permission from Hayter et al. 2006.[58])

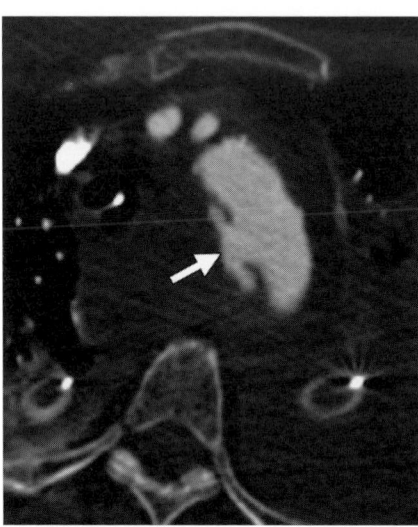

Figure 30.8 Thoracic CT demonstrating aortic leak of contrast material. The patient died immediately after the study. (Used with permission from Co et al. 2011.[8])

Open surgical repair is required in thoracic injury of the aortic root, ascending aorta, and/or arch, and in penetrating trauma of the great vessels. The surgical approach will depend on the type of transection (proximal descending aorta versus aortic root versus at the diaphragm), patient condition, and technical expertise and experience of the surgeon. These decisions dictate critical aspects of anesthetic management. Aortic rupture at the aortic root (aortic valve and sinuses of Valsalva) requires open surgical repair employing full CPB via median sternotomy. Repair or inspection of the endovascular intima of the aortic arch may require deep hypothermic circulatory arrest. The more common proximal descending aortic transection may or may not require CPB and is approached via left lateral thoracotomy. Endovascular stent repair of traumatic aortic transection does not require CPB. Endovascular stents have also been used in pediatric patients to repair traumatic aortic rupture.

Anesthetic considerations

Aggressive and precise control of the preoperative and intraoperative blood pressure is required to avoid extension of the transection or frank rupture and death. In addition to arterial blood pressure control, there is a concern that the shear forces generated from blood flow may worsen the transection. Pharmacological therapy to reduce heart rate and contractility is indicated. Traditionally, this has been achieved by utilizing continuous infusion of a rapidly acting vasodilator in combination with a β-adrenergic receptor antagonist (β-blocker). The most common regimen is probably infusions of esmolol and sodium nitroprusside (SNP), although other therapies have been effectively utilized and are acceptable (Table 30.8). Although nitroglycerin (NTG) has been employed as an antihypertensive agent, it would seem prudent to select agents that preferentially act on arterial rather than venous smooth muscle; thus we do not recommend NTG for blood pressure control in this setting. Pain may contribute to the hypertensive response. Rib fractures, especially if ≥ 3 ribs, can be treated with paravertebral nerve blockade.[5]

Table 30.8 Recommended pharmacological therapy options for preoperative blood pressure control in patients with aortic transection

Drug	Usual dose range	Loading dose	Add β-blocker	Notes
Esmolol	50–500 μg/kg/min	1–1.5 mg/kg	n/a	Rapid-acting β$_1$-AR antagonist
SNP	0.1–8.0 μg/kg/min	None	Yes	Cyanide toxicity a concern when used in high doses and/or renal dysfunction
Labetalol	0.5–3 mg/min	5–20 mg every 5 min to total of 300 mg	No	Antagonist at α$_1$-AR, β$_1$-AR, and β$_2$-AR
Nicardipine	2.5–15 mg/h	0.25–0.5 mg	Yes	CCB; improves coronary artery blood flow
Phentolamine	1–20 μg/kg/min	1–5 mg	Yes	Antagonist at α$_1$-AR and α$_2$-AR
Fenoldopam	0.03–3 μg/kg/min	None	Yes	↑ renal and mesenteric perfusion
Dexmedetomidine	0.2–0.7 μg/kg/h	≤ 1 μg/kg over 10–15 min	No	Sedative/sympatholytic via agonist action at central α$_2$-AR. If loading dose too rapidly given will initially ↑ BP followed by ↓ BP and ↓ HR.
Clevidipine	4–6 mg/h	0.5–1 mg	Yes	CCB with faster onset and offset than nicardipine

AR, adrenergic receptor; CCB, Ca^{2+} channel blocker; SNP, sodium nitroprusside; n/a, not applicable.

Cardiac β-adrenergic blockade should be instituted as quickly as possible to decrease the force of blood ejection from the heart. Esmolol is a β$_1$-adrenergic receptor antagonist with rapid onset and elimination. The goal of esmolol therapy is to decrease the heart rate and left ventricular contractile force, which in turn will attenuate the shear stress of blood flow at the transection site. A heart rate of ≤ 80 beats per minute would be a reasonable goal. Although esmolol is an excellent choice for heart rate control, additional agents will be required for control of arterial blood pressure if the patient is hypertensive. Labetalol is a nonspecific β-adrenergic receptor antagonist that also possesses α$_1$-adrenergic antagonist properties. Therefore, it can be utilized as a single agent to control both blood pressure and heart rate. Although prevention of tachycardia and attenuation of myocardial contractility are important to the management of thoracic aortic injury, the presence of other injuries and associated hemorrhage may at times counterbalance this concern and complicate decision making about β-adrenergic blockade.

Several other approaches to blood pressure control have been successfully employed in aortic dissection patients. Desirable features would include rapid onset, ease of dose adjustment, and availability to administer as a continuous infusion. SNP has a long and successful history in the treatment of hypertensive emergencies. SNP has several desirable characteristics, but it also causes reflex tachycardia that increases endovascular shear forces and requires concomitant β-blockade therapy. Moreover, SNP is metabolized to cyanide ion, and high-dose SNP therapy increases the risk of cyanide toxicity, especially in patients with renal dysfunction. This is relevant to aortic dissection in that tissue oxygen delivery may be compromised from impaired perfusion and ischemia, including to the kidneys. Nicardipine is a calcium-channel

blocking (CCB) drug that can be parenterally administered to produce systemic and coronary arterial vasodilatation. In patients with myocardial ischemia this may improve myocardial oxygen delivery. The pharmacologic effects of nicardipine do not dissipate as rapidly as SNP. Clevidipine is a CCB with shorter half-life than nicardipine.[44] Phentolamine is a nonspecific α-adrenergic antagonist that results in arterial vasodilatation. Although phentolamine is commonly associated with the management of pheochromocytoma, it is an effective short-acting medication that can be applied to the patient with aortic transection. In recent years, its clinical availability has been inconsistent.

Fenoldopam is a D$_1$-dopamine receptor agonist utilized clinically for the treatment of hypertension.[45] Impaired perfusion and ischemia of the renal and abdominal organs cause concern during aortic dissection. Fenoldopam enhances perfusion of the renal and mesenteric vasculature and thus may have a unique role in treating the hypertension associated with aortic dissection. In patients undergoing elective repair of aortic aneurysm, fenoldopam controlled crossclamp hypertension. Additionally, fenoldopam achieved better preservation of renal function than sodium nitroprusside and dopamine,[46–48] although this benefit has not been observed in other reports.[49] During TAA repair fenoldopam was associated with a decrease in mortality.[48,50] Fenoldopam is administered parenterally by continuous infusion. Although low-dose fenoldopam (0.03–0.05 μg/kg/min) augments renal and mesenteric perfusion, the antihypertensive actions are achieved in the 0.1–3 μg/kg/min dose range. Fenoldopam is devoid of effects on the adrenergic receptors, and thus concomitant β-adrenergic receptor antagonism with esmolol by continuous infusion (or metoprolol) is probably required to control heart rate and decrease endovascular shear forces.

Dexmedetomidine is considered by some to be the sedative of choice in trauma patients [51] and may have a role in the preoperative therapy of thoracic aortic transection, especially if sedation is required. Dexmedetomidine is a potent α_2-adrenergic agonist that produces sedation without respiratory depression.[51] In trauma patients additional effects of dexmedetomidine include analgesia, neuroprotection against traumatic brain injury, attenuation of withdrawal syndromes, and sympatholysis.[51,52] In experimental rat models, dexmedetomidine attenuates lung injury from pulmonary contusion, positive-pressure ventilation barotrauma, ischemia reperfusion injury to vital organs, and sepsis.[53–57] The sympatholysis is produced via a centrally mediated mechanism which reduces catecholamine levels. Although no studies have examined dexmedetomidine use in the aortic transection patient population, there are distinct clinical and theoretical advantages that may be imparted in contained aortic rupture patients. Inhibition of catecholamine secretion results in smoothing of hemodynamic variability, lowering of the arterial blood pressure and heart rate, and reduction of the shear forces on the arterial wall. The mechanism of sedation is distinct from the γ-aminobutyric acid$_A$ (GABA$_A$) agonists (e.g., midazolam) in that the dexmedetomidine effects are mediated by the endogenous adrenergic sleep pathways of the locus ceruleus. Thus, patients appear to be sleeping but are easily aroused and can be cooperative with physical examination without adjustment of the dexmedetomidine infusion. Dexmedetomidine is available for continuous intravenous infusion (0.2–0.7 µg/kg/h) following a loading dose of ≤ 1 µg/kg administered for 10–15 minutes. Rapid administration of the dexmedetomidine loading dose should be avoided because it may initially cause hypertension via stimulation of peripheral vascular α_2-adrenergic receptors (vasoconstriction) followed by bradycardia and hypotension. Contraindications to the use of dexmedetomidine include hypovolemia, hypotension, heart block, and congestive heart failure prior to administration.

Invasive pressure monitoring is indicated (see also Chapters 5 and 9). The preferred site of arterial catheter placement will depend on the type of aortic transection and potential surgical considerations. A *right* radial arterial catheter is preferred in proximal descending thoracic transection because the surgeon may need to place the aortic crossclamp proximal to the left subclavian artery. A left-sided arterial catheter would then be excluded from arterial blood flow, and thus the ability to continuously monitor the blood pressure would be lost. Likewise a *left* radial arterial catheter is indicated for a proximal ascending aortic disruption or transection to avoid problems with innominate artery crossclamping. Cannulation of the ipsilateral brachial or axillary artery should be considered if a catheter cannot be placed into the desired radial artery. Aortic arch repair requires profound hypothermic circulatory arrest. Because there is no blood pressure to measure during circulatory arrest, the arterial catheter site can be on either the right or left side. If partial cardiac bypass will be used to repair a proximal descending aortic transection, placement

of a second arterial catheter to measure lower-extremity blood pressure is advocated by many anesthesiologists. Femoral arterial catheter placement may be complicated by a false lumen. CT can identify a false lumen and the distal extension. Figure 30.9 shows a dissection flap in the ascending aorta at the level of the pulmonary artery bifurcation.[58] Extension of the true and false lumens into the descending thoracic aorta is noted. The use of a pulmonary artery catheter (PAC) is typically indicated.[59]

Many anesthesiologists feel that an oximetric and/or continuous cardiac output PAC provides valuable real-time information in the management of critically ill trauma patients.[60] A fall in mixed venous oxygen saturation derives from increased oxygen consumption or decreased oxygen delivery (see Chapter 9). Oxygen delivery is governed by cardiac output, hemoglobin concentration, and arterial oxygen saturation.

TEE can play a pivotal role in the management of patients during aortic surgery.[61] TEE provides rapid, accurate diagnosis of aortic transection or dissection, evaluates cardiac structural integrity and function, and can identify associated life-threatening conditions such as cardiac tamponade (see Table 30.7 and Chapter 10).[61]

Surgical repair of aortic transection has an impact on airway management. Ascending aortic transection can be managed with a single-lumen endotracheal tube similar to most cardiac anesthetic cases. Descending aortic transections (open repair) generally require the utilization of lung isolation techniques to facilitate surgical exposure and repair (see Chapter 33).[62–64] Although a double-lumen tube can adequately accomplish this goal, we prefer the placement of a bronchial blocker (e.g., Arndt or Cohen) through a single-lumen tracheal tube, which offers several advantages in this patient population. The aortic hematoma can displace and distort the intrathoracic airway, particularly below the carina. Placement of the endobronchial portion of the double-lumen tube can cause trauma to the distorted airway and erode into the aortic hematoma. These patients have significant postoperative pulmonary challenges that are ideally managed with a single-lumen endotracheal tube. Additionally, frequently significant intraoperative hemorrhage requires large-volume resuscitation, which can cause marked edema of the upper airway and preclude safe exchange of a double-lumen to a single-lumen endotracheal tube at the conclusion of the procedure. Blunt chest trauma is associated with pulmonary contusion and hypoxia, which require expert adjustment of mechanical ventilation. Removal of pulmonary secretions is limited in double-lumen tubes, as is bronchoscopic examination of the airway. The use of a bronchial blocker for lung isolation attenuates or obviates these difficulties in the postoperative period (see also Chapter 33).

The anesthesiologist should anticipate significant blood loss and the possibility of coagulopathy. Adequate intravenous access should be obtained and should include a minimum of two large-bore peripheral intravenous catheters or their equivalent in the central venous circulation (see Chapter 5). Packed red blood cells, fresh frozen plasma, and platelets should be immediately available during the operative course. Thermal conservation measures should be employed early in the operative course to limit the adverse effect of hypothermia on hemostasis (see Chapter 14).[65] Obtaining a coagulation profile via thromboelastography or thromboelastometry will guide rational blood component therapy administration.[66]

Treatment of postoperative pain will be required after thoracotomy (see Chapters 15 and 16). Parenteral opioid therapy can be supplemented with a regional anesthetic technique after consideration of the risk–benefit ratio. Thoracic epidural analgesia (TEA) has significant risks, complicating TEA placement in the immediate postoperative period: abnormal coagulation status and the risk of neurologic deficit from the procedure. If TEA is selected, catheter placement should be deferred until these issues have resolved. Placement of a paravertebral nerve block catheter might have less risk of neuraxial hematoma and, when appropriately inserted, appears to offer equivalent analgesia to TEA.[67,68] Multiple intercostal nerve blocks with local anesthetic can provide effective pain relief for thoracotomy incisions but will require repeat placement every 6–8 hours.

Blunt injury of arterial vessels

Injuries to major arterial branches of the thoracic aorta are less common than traumatic aortic transection. The specific vessel injured depends on the force vector and patient position at time of impact (Table 30.5). The mechanism of injury could include either deceleration or traction. Disruption of the cranial vessels should be suspected when hematoma of the neck, bruits, mental status changes, or focal neurologic deficits are found. Avulsion of the left subclavian artery is associated with brachial plexus injury.

Diagnosis is more difficult than in aortic rupture. Although TEE is excellent for the rapid diagnosis of proximal ascending aorta and descending aortic abnormalities, it has little value in detecting injuries of aortic branch vessels. Penetrating trauma can masquerade as blunt trauma in the presence of rib, sternal, or clavicular fractures. Displacement of these fractures can avulse or puncture the vascular structures of the thorax. A large, left hemothorax on chest x-ray may provide a clue to the correct diagnosis.

Penetrating injury to the great vessels

Similar to penetrating cardiac trauma, the clinical presentation varies greatly depending on the site and extent of the wound. Attenuation of active hemorrhage and restoration of end-organ perfusion is the primary goal. Unlike blunt trauma, there may be a role for emergency room thoracotomy to gain proximal control of the thoracic aorta for hemostasis. Rapid hemorrhage and hypotension are the primary concerns in penetrating trauma. Penetrating trauma of the proximal pulmonary arteries, terminal pulmonary veins, or vena cava has a very high mortality rate (~75%). Surgical repair is challenging and may require CPB. Fractures of the sternum or rib(s) can avulse the internal mammary or intercostal arteries, respectively. Chest x-ray may reveal a hemothorax. It is important to recognize that these vessels are frequently lacerated iatrogenically. The entry site for needle decompression of a tension pneumothorax is the midclavicular line in the second intercostal space. If the entry site is too medial, the internal mammary artery can be injured. Chest tube placement can be complicated by laceration of an intercostal artery.

Blast injury

Although traditionally associated with military casualties, trauma secondary to explosion is a growing concern because of the global spread of terrorist activity (see Chapter 38). Bomb detonation seems most likely to occur in settings designed to produce the greatest number of injuries. Anesthesiologists are likely to have a critical role in the management of blast injury,[69] given that triage and resuscitation of multiple trauma victims will be required simultaneously. Among the many possible injuries, injury to the lungs most often requires immediate treatment, and chest trauma has been reported in 40% of casualties (Table 30.9).[70] The differential diagnosis includes air embolism, penetrating thoracic trauma, and blunt thoracic trauma. Air emboli in the pulmonary and systemic circulation are the primary mechanisms of death.[69]

Explosions create direct and indirect trauma. The sudden increase in atmospheric pressure, termed blast overpressure, is a primary trauma mechanism responsible for direct trauma. Parameters governing blast overpressure include the amount and type of explosive utilized and the distance from the blast. The inverse square of the distance correlates with blast force. Blast overpressure of 35 psi will result in significant pulmonary injury, whereas 65 psi has a 99% resultant mortality. Indirect injuries can occur from projectiles generated from the explosive force (shrapnel), collapse of a building following the explosion, fire created by the explosion, and victims being thrown forcibly into other objects.

Triage of patients is the first priority in disaster management.[69] Patients are initially assigned to one of four groups: minor injury, delayed treatment, immediate life-saving treatment, and expectant (death is unavoidable). It is important to recognize that delayed presentation of additional blast injuries is common. Thus, patients need to be reassessed frequently. The number of victims that present to the emergency department in the first hour following an explosion has been used for resource utilization planning, as this often represents about half of the total number of expected patients.[69]

Organs exposed to atmospheric pressure or with air–fluid interfaces are the most susceptible to blast overpressure trauma. Tympanic membrane rupture is the most common injury following explosion,[71] followed by blast lung injury. Victims can present with the blast lung injury triad of apnea, bradycardia, and hypotension. The Centers for Disease

Table 30.9: Clinical Manifestations of Blast Injury

Head

    Brain injury

    Laryngeal injury

    Tympanic membrane rupture

    Skull fracture

Thoracic

    Cardiac

        Cardiac contusion

        Dysrhythmia

        Hypotension

        Myocardial ischemia

        Penetrating cardiac trauma

    Pulmonary

        Air embolism

        Apnea

        Bronchopleural fistula

        Dyspnea

        Hypoxia

        Pneumothorax

        Pulmonary contusion

Abdominal

    Hemorrhage

    Organ rupture

    Penetrating trauma

    Perforation

        Peripheral

        Traumatic limb amputation

    Secondary trauma

        Crush injury

        Thermal injury

Control and Prevention (CDC) recommends prophylactic bilateral thoracostomy tube placement in all suspected blast lung injury patients because of the risk of life-threatening pneumothorax.

Laryngeal and pulmonary injuries complicate airway management. Laryngeal fracture, dislocation of cartilaginous structures, hemorrhage, and penetrating injury of airway structures can make tracheal intubation difficult (see Chapter 3). Inspiratory stridor requires immediate evaluation and may signal impending loss of airway. Alveolar rupture from blast overpressure is common, and initiation of positive-pressure ventilation may hasten the development of a tension pneumothorax. Bronchopleural fistula or hemoptysis may require institution of lung isolation techniques.

Cardiac injury can occur in blast injury patients. Cardiac dysrhythmia is a common manifestation of blast injury. Arrhythmogenic mechanisms include myocardial contusion, neurally mediated reflexes, and coronary artery embolism (especially air embolism).[69] Tachycardia, bradycardia, ventricular fibrillation, and asystole have been noted following blast injury. Patients should be monitored for ECG abnormalities, and Advanced Cardiac Life Support (ACLS) protocols should be employed to treat unstable electrical disturbances. Coronary artery air embolism deserves special consideration because it is believed to be a major cause of death following blast injury.[69] Myocardial ischemia and myocardial infarction may be found. Penetrating cardiac trauma from shrapnel can cause cardiac tamponade that requires prompt treatment for survival.[72] Distinguishing these diagnostic possibilities can be difficult.

Anesthetic considerations

Appropriate preparation to care for multiple patients with reversible, immediately life-threatening injuries is the first priority. The institutional disaster plan should be activated to recruit sufficient personnel for acute care. Establishing a chain of command and deployment of an anesthesiologist to the emergency department as an integral component of the initial assessment and management of patients has been shown to improve outcomes.[73] All elective procedures should be canceled to allow immediate access to operative suites. Patients require triage upon presentation to identify those most likely to benefit from immediate care. The goal of initial therapy is to stabilize the patient; definitive procedures should be delayed, and medical resources (personnel and operating rooms) redirected to additional patients as quickly as possible.

Preoperative assessment should be balanced with the clinical scenario; it may not be feasible to obtain a complete history and laboratory evaluation prior to anesthetic care. Minimal preoperative evaluation should probably include a chest radiograph and determination of hematocrit. Securing adequate large-bore intravenous access is routine (see Chapter 5). Arterial catheter placement is probably indicated for most blast injury patients to monitor blood pressure and the severity of pulmonary injury (using arterial blood gases). Placement of central venous catheters or a pulmonary artery catheter should be guided by the patient's condition. When deciding to use TEE intraoperatively, the possibility of esophageal injury from the blast overpressure must be considered. Prophylactic chest tubes should be placed bilaterally prior to anesthetic induction in any patient with suspected pulmonary injury. Broad-spectrum antibiotic prophylaxis should be administered.[74]

Considerations for anesthetic induction in blast injury patients are similar to those for all trauma victims: patients should be considered to be at risk for aspiration (full stomach), to be underresuscitated, and to have undiagnosed injuries. Administration of a fluid bolus prior to induction may improve hemodynamic stability during induction. There are no contraindications to succinylcholine per se as a result of the acute injury. Once intubated, ventilator settings should be selected to minimize airway pressures and allow permissive hypercapnia.[69]

Lung injury resulting in systemic air embolism is frequently seen in blast injury victims.[75] Anesthetic maintenance should *avoid the use of nitrous oxide*, which diffuses rapidly into closed air-filled spaces within the body. The resultant expansion of the air embolism will worsen the patient's condition. Fluid management can be complex. The blast injury patient requires sufficient fluid administration to provide acceptable organ perfusion. Provision of a systolic blood pressure $> 100\,\text{mmHg}$ and heart rate ≤ 120 beats per minute has been suggested as acceptable.[71] Concomitant morbidities (e.g., coronary vascular disease) or ongoing blood loss may alter the management goals. Heat conservation measures are routine (e.g., warm room, warmed IV fluids, convective and gelpad warming) because hypothermia contributes to worsening coagulopathy and increased oxygen utilization (see Chapter 14).

Surgical considerations

Preoperative evaluation and diagnosis of traumatic blast lesions will guide the choice of surgical approach. This has anesthetic implications regarding positioning the patient, appropriate placement of monitors, and provision for airway management (e.g., lung isolation). Indications for surgery are shown in Table 30.10. Patients with suspected cardiac trauma can undergo surgical exploration by subxiphoid pericardial window, open surgical exposure, or video-assisted thoracoscopic surgery (VATS). The choice is guided by the clinical scenario and suspicion of injury along with surgeon preference and experience. If minimally invasive methods (VATS, pericardial window) are selected for initial evaluation, the anesthesiologist must be prepared for immediate conversion to an open procedure. Pericardial window has the advantage that it can be performed under local anesthesia if required, and it is both diagnostic and therapeutic for cardiac tamponade, a common cause of hypotension following thoracic trauma. If active hemorrhage is discovered during tamponade the incision will be extended and the chest is entered via median sternotomy (see also Chapter 29).

VATS procedures have gained wide popularity and have the advantage that the chest tube sites can be utilized to introduce the videoscope. Patients undergoing VATS experience less pain and less impairment in pulmonary function when compared to thoracotomy. The use of VATS is therefore expanding in stable trauma patients for the diagnosis and treatment of continued chest tube bleeding, retained hemothorax, posttraumatic empyema, suspected

Table 30.10 Indications for surgery after cardiothoracic trauma

Acute indications
Cardiac tamponade
Acute deterioration or cardiac arrest in the trauma center
Penetrating truncal trauma
Vascular injury at the thoracic outlet
Loss of chest wall substance
Massive air leak from chest tube
Tracheobronchial tear
Great vessel laceration
Mediastinal traverse of a penetrating object
Missile embolism to the heart or pulmonary artery
Placement of inferior vena caval shunt for hepatic vascular injury

Subacute indications
Traumatic diaphragmatic hernia
Cardiac septal or valvular lesion
Nonevacuated clotted hemothorax
Chronic thoracic aortic pseudoaneurysm
Posttraumatic empyema
Lung abscess
Tracheoesophageal fistula
Missed tracheal or bronchial tear
Innominate artery/tracheal fistula
Traumatic arterial venous fistula

Modified from Wall MJ, Storey JH, Mattox KL. Indications for thoracotomy. In Mattox KL, Feliciano DV, Moore EE, eds., *Trauma*, 4th edition. New York, NY: McGraw-Hill, 2000, pp. 473–82.

diaphragmatic injuries, persistent air leaks, and mediastinal injuries. Contraindications to VATS include hemodynamic instability, injuries to the heart and great vessels, inability to tolerate one-lung ventilation, prior thoracotomy, coagulopathy, and indications for emergent thoracotomy or sternotomy. Because the VATS procedure requires lung isolation, this creates unique challenges to the anesthesiologist in the trauma setting. Many blunt trauma patients will have associated injuries that markedly alter the standard management of lung isolation, including facial/airway trauma, unstable cervical spine, and requirements for continued hemodynamic resuscitation. Furthermore, patients might not tolerate one-lung ventilation secondary to hypoxia, particularly, if there is an associated pulmonary contusion or pulmonary embolism (originating from long-bone fractures), which impairs alveolar oxygen diffusion. Positive findings on VATS exploration may result in conversion to an open procedure. In several small case series, conversion to thoracotomy was necessary in 10 of 99 patients.

The surgical approach to great vessel injury is more complex and relates to the specific injury but can be broadly divided into median sternotomy and thoracotomy approaches. Extension of the median sternotomy into the neck allows access to the cranial vessels. If required, a thoracotomy incision can be extended via transverse sternotomy and contralateral thoracotomy ("clamshell") to gain access to both thoracic cavities.

Noncardiac thoracic trauma
General principles and initial management

Blunt or penetrating thoracic trauma may involve the heart or great vessels as noted earlier, but may also induce injury specific to the larynx, tracheobronchial tree, lungs, or chest wall (Table 30.11).[76] Table 30.12 shows the AIS for blunt and penetrating lung injuries. There is a high incidence of extrathoracic injuries associated with major blunt thoracic trauma, such as head trauma and musculoskeletal injuries (Table 30.13). Initial physical examination should involve

Table 30.11 Incidence of injuries in patients with blunt thoracic trauma presenting to the operating room for emergency surgery

Type of injury	Incidence (%)
Rib fractures	67
Pulmonary contusion	65
Pneumothorax	30
Hemothorax	26
Flail chest	23
Diaphragmatic injury	9
Myocardial contusion	5.7
Aortic tear	4.8
Tracheobronchial injury	0.8
Laryngeal injury	0.3

Modified from Devitt JH, McLean RF, Koch JP. Anaesthetic management of acute blunt thoracic trauma. *Can J Anaesth* 1991; **38**: 506–10.

Table 30.12 Lung organ injury scaling

AIS grade/ severity	Injury description
I. Mild	Contusion: unilateral, < 1 lobe
II. Moderate	Contusion: unilateral, single lobe Laceration: simple pneumothorax
III. Serious	Contusion: unilateral, > 1 lobe Laceration: persistent (> 72 hours) air leak from distal airway Hematoma: nonexpanding intraparenchymal
IV. Severe	Laceration: major airway leak (segmental or lobar) Hematoma: expanding intraparenchymal Vascular: primary branch intrapulmonary vessel disruption
V. Critical	Vascular: hilar vessel disruption
VI. Not survivable	Uncontained total transection of pulmonary hilum

Note: Advance one grade for bilateral injuries.
Modified from trauma.org (accessed March 5, 2013).
AIS, Abbreviated Injury Scale.

inspection and auscultation of the thorax to assess for obvious injuries and to determine whether breath sounds are present bilaterally. Laryngeal injury should be suspected in any patient with hoarseness, subcutaneous emphysema in the neck, and/or hemoptysis. Tracheal and bronchial compromise by compression or direct injury should be suspected if there is upper airway obstruction, stridor, obvious trauma at the base of the neck, or significant sternal fracture with a palpable defect in the region of the sternoclavicular joint. If breath sounds are unequal, then either a pneumothorax or hemothorax is likely. If the patient is stable, then a chest x-ray should be done to confirm the diagnosis. If the patient is not stable, or if an x-ray is not immediately available, then a tube thoracostomy should be performed. This will serve to relieve a pneumothorax resulting from blunt bronchial tears or to reexpand the lung in the event of hemothorax resulting from trauma to pulmonary veins or arteries. In many trauma centers, bilateral chest tube placement is considered routine if there is evidence of thoracic trauma.

If the initial tube thoracostomy reveals a continuing air leak, then a bronchial tear probably is causing a bronchopleural fistula, which may compromise gas exchange (even after chest tube placement) sufficiently to warrant immediate bronchoscopy, temporizing lung isolation with a bronchial blocker or a double-lumen endobronchial tube (see Chapter 33), or surgical repair. In general, the air leak will be minimized by continuation of spontaneous ventilation, but if the leak is massive, effective ventilation may not be possible without immediate surgical repair or lung isolation. As with blast injury, a bronchial tear may also result in life-threatening air embolus through gas entrainment into disrupted pulmonary veins that lie in close proximity to the airway injury. Classic findings are hemoptysis, sudden cardiac or cerebral dysfunction after initiating positive-pressure ventilation (e.g., after rapid sequence intubation), air in retinal vessels, and air in arterial blood gas.[75] Treatment is supportive and may include avoidance of high peak airway pressures during

Table 30.13 Extrathoracic injuries associated with thoracic trauma

Injury	Incidence (%)
Skull fracture	10
Cerebral concussion	38
Cerebral contusion	13
Facial fractures	8
Vertebral column	11
Upper limbs	20
Lower limbs	26
Pelvic fractures	14
Abdomen	32

Modified from Besson A, Saegesser F. *Color Atlas of Chest Trauma and Associated Injuries*. Oradell, NJ: Medical Economics Books, 1983, pp. 12–14.

mechanical ventilation, avoidance of positive-pressure ventilation to the affected side (mandating one-lung ventilation), and adequate volume resuscitation. Hyperbaric oxygen therapy may be of value in cases of cerebral air embolism.[5,75]

If the initial tube thoracostomy reveals a large amount of blood and the patient is hemodynamically unstable despite adequate fluid resuscitation, urgent thoracotomy is indicated with or without lung isolation as time and circumstances permit (Table 30.10). Pulmonary vascular injury is often self-limited, however, so simple drainage of the hemothorax via a tube thoracostomy may suffice as treatment. If hemodynamic instability coexists with a massive hemothorax that does not remit after chest tube insertion, this suggests aortic or proximal pulmonary arterial disruption, either of which will require immediate thoracotomy for patient survival. Most thoracic trauma can be managed with chest tubes and observation if it does not involve the heart or great vessels.

In penetrating thoracic injury, the wound(s) itself typically guides initial therapy. A knife wound into the pulmonary region typically induces a pneumothorax, hemothorax, or both. The wound should be covered with a nonpermeable dressing to isolate the hemithorax from atmospheric pressure; then reexpansion of the ipsilateral lung may be achieved by placement of a chest tube. A bullet wound requires assessment of entry and exit points, which will dictate appropriate management based on the principles articulated above.

Anesthetic considerations for specific noncardiac thoracic injuries

Laryngeal injury

Direct blows to the neck can produce a "clothesline" type injury that crushes the cervical trachea against the vertebral bodies, transecting tracheal rings or the cricoid cartilage. Shear forces on the trachea create damage at its relatively fixed points – the cricoid cartilage and the carina. Major injuries affecting the airway should be recognized and addressed during the primary survey. The method of choice for securing the airway in patients with laryngeal trauma and airway compromise with stridor is awake fiberoptic bronchoscopic-assisted intubation while maintaining spontaneous ventilation (see Chapter 3). Blind intubation techniques are contraindicated in the setting of airway injury. Oversedation and neuromuscular relaxants are also best avoided, as these may result in loss of the airway. Emergency cricothyroidotomy may be required. Associated injuries include skull base or intracranial damage, open neck wounds, cervical spine, and esophageal or pharyngeal injury.

Tracheobronchial injury

Intrathoracic rupture of the trachea or major bronchi results from blunt chest trauma generating great force with shearing of the more mobile distal bronchi from relatively fixed proximal structures during rapid deceleration.[77–79] Furthermore, the cervical trachea is protected by the mandible and sternum anteriorly and by vertebrae posteriorly. More than 80% of ruptures of bronchi are within 2.5 cm of the carina. Diagnostic findings include hemoptysis, dyspnea, subcutaneous and mediastinal emphysema, and hypoxia. A large pneumothorax is present if there is free communication between the rupture of the tracheobronchial tree and the pleural cavity (bronchopleural fistula). In this situation, the tube thoracostomy shows continuous bubbling of air in the water seal, and suction may fail to reexpand the lung. The chest x-ray demonstrates pneumothorax, pleural effusion, pneumomediastinum, or subcutaneous air (Fig. 30.10). Overall, 90% of these patients will have extraanatomic air seen on the admission chest x-ray. Helical CT scan may be helpful in establishing the diagnosis. Fiberoptic bronchoscopy should be carried out promptly whenever tracheobronchial rupture is suspected, because it is the most reliable means of establishing the diagnosis (Fig. 30.11). Airway management of patients with bronchial injuries may require placement of a double-lumen tube or bronchial blocker (see Chapter 33). Extreme caution should be exercised during airway instrumentation, particularly double lumen tube placement, to avoid extension of the injury. Fiberoptic bronchoscopy should be used for all facets of airway management. Tracheobronchial injuries should be repaired surgically with thoracotomy as soon as possible to diminish the risk of repeated pulmonary infections, severe bronchial

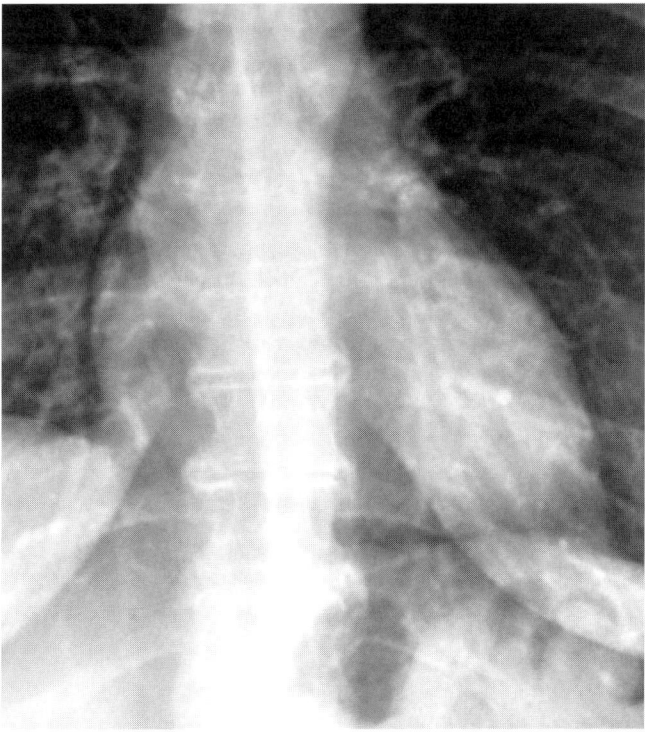

Figure 30.10 Chest x-ray remarkable for pneumopericardium. The diagnosis of pneumopericardium should prompt investigation to determine the location and extent of the injury. Anesthetic considerations include direct visualization (bronchoscopically) of the airway including distally into at least the right and left main bronchial branches. (Used with permission from Co et al. 2011.[8])

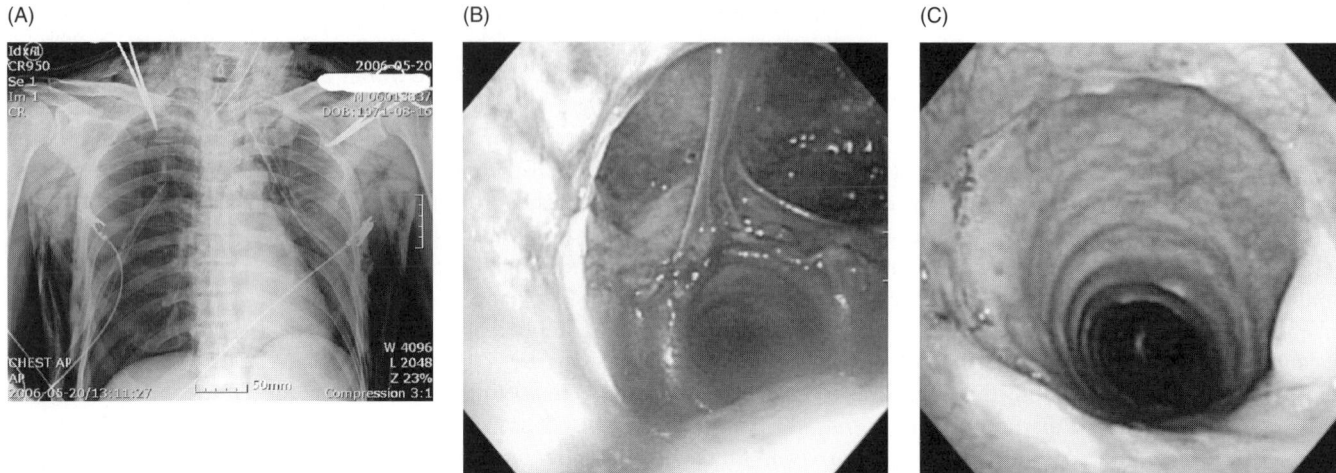

(A)　(B)　(C)

Figure 30.11 Tracheal transection secondary to blunt chest trauma. (**A**) Markedly abnormal endotracheal tube position and subcutaneous emphysema noted on chest x-ray. (**B**) Fiberoptic bronchoscopy through endotracheal tube reveals complete tracheal avulsion. (**C**) Trachea following surgical repair. (Used with permission from Shim et al. 2008.[77]) *A black and white version of this figure will appear in some formats. For the color version, please refer to the plate section.*

stenosis, or mediastinitis (Fig. 30.11). Resuscitation and anesthetic care are directed toward airway control, maintenance of adequate pulmonary ventilation, and management of blood loss.

Tension pneumothorax

A tension pneumothorax (Fig. 30.2) develops when air enters the pleural space from the lung or through the chest wall via a "one-way-valve"-like opening, which allows entry of air but no exit. The progressively increasing intrathoracic pressure in the affected hemithorax leads to complete collapse of the affected lung, shifting the mediastinum toward the contralateral side and severely impairing central venous return. In addition to ipsilateral lung collapse, compression of the contralateral lung by the displaced mediastinum occurs, further impairing ventilatory capacity, resulting in hypoventilation and hypoxemia. Decreased venous return by elevated intrathoracic pressure leads to profound hypotension and cardiac arrest if untreated.

Clinically, tension pneumothorax is characterized by chest pain, dyspnea, tachycardia, hypotension, contralateral tracheal deviation, and ipsilateral lung hyperresonance with the absence of breath sounds. A chest x-ray or CT reveals widening of the intercostal spaces and downward displacement of the diaphragm on the ipsilateral side of the tension pneumothorax, while the trachea and mediastinum are deviated away toward the contralateral side. Treatment should not be delayed waiting for radiologic confirmation. Increasingly this diagnosis is made at the bedside using ultrasound. The classic diagnostic sign is loss of pleural movement during breathing. Treatment consists of immediate decompression with a needle or tube thoracostomy. Needle thoracostomy is a temporizing maneuver converting the injury to a less severe simple pneumothorax. It is performed by placing a needle in the second intercostal space in the midclavicular line. Medial, parasternal placement should be avoided because injury of the internal mammary artery can occur. For definitive

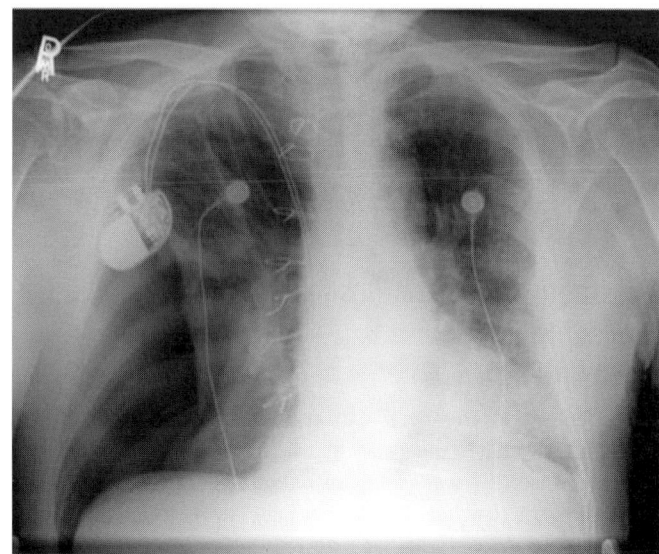

Figure 30.12 Chest x-ray showing right pneumothorax. A simple pneumothorax can transform into a tension pneumothorax, especially under general anesthesia, because of positive-pressure ventilation and/or administration of N_2O.

treatment, tube thoracostomy should be performed in the fifth intercostal space just anterior to the midaxillary line on the affected side. If the lung does not fully reexpand after tube thoracostomy and there is a large ongoing air leak, the airways should be evaluated bronchoscopically to exclude airway injury. However, in most cases, no further treatment will be required after chest tube insertion.

A simple pneumothorax (Fig. 30.12; see also Fig. 30.1) caused by any disruption of pleural space (e.g., subclavian or internal jugular venous catheter insertion) can transform into a tension pneumothorax, especially under general anesthesia, because of application of positive-pressure ventilation and/or the administration of nitrous oxide. Furthermore, diagnosis of the pneumothorax during general anesthesia is difficult, but it should be suspected when various combinations of hypotension, hypoxia, elevated airway pressures, absent breath sounds on either side with hyperresonance to percussion, distended neck veins, and a deviated trachea are present. PEEP should be avoided, and nitrous oxide is contraindicated. Chest tube placement should occur prior to, or in experienced hands concurrent with, induction or any positive-pressure ventilation (including mask ventilation) in any patient with pneumothorax.

Open pneumothorax ("sucking chest wound")

Open pneumothorax results from a large defect of the chest wall usually caused by a wound that creates a communication between the pleural space and the external environment. As the size of this chest wall defect approaches two-thirds the diameter of the trachea, air passes preferentially through the lower-resistance injury tract with each respiratory effort rather than through the normal airways. In an open or "sucking" wound of the chest wall, the lung on the affected side is exposed to atmospheric pressure, and equilibration between intrathoracic pressure and atmospheric pressure is immediate, resulting in the lung's collapse and a shift of the mediastinum to the unaffected side. The severe venoarterial shunting that occurs in both lungs produces profound ventilation/perfusion mismatch. The patient's effective oxygenation and ventilation is thereby severely compromised, leading to hypoxia and hypercarbia. This is an immediately life-threatening condition.

In the spontaneously ventilating patient, open pneumothorax is initially treated by application of a sterile occlusive dressing with Vaseline gauze, which must be large enough to cover the entire wound, and which is taped securely on three sides. This will then act as a one-way valve so that air can escape the pleural space but not reenter. Taping all edges of the dressing before a chest tube is placed is contraindicated because accumulation of air in the affected thoracic cavity will lead to the development of tension pneumothorax.

Tube thoracostomy should be performed as soon as possible at a remote site away from the wound. If the chest wall defect is relatively small, the pleura may soon seal and no further intervention is necessary. In patients with airway or breathing difficulty, early intubation and initiation of positive-pressure ventilation should be considered. For large, open chest wall defects, surgical debridement of dead and devitalized tissue and closure of the wound (with or without prosthetic patch) are often required under general anesthesia.

Massive hemothorax

Massive hemothorax is defined as a rapid accumulation of more than 1500 mL of blood in the pleural space. Such a massive hemorrhage usually indicates great vessel or major branch injury, especially on the left side. Large pulmonary lacerations or intercostal vessel injury can result in left or right hemothorax. One hemithorax can accommodate as much as 50–60% of the entire blood volume. Tension hemothorax may

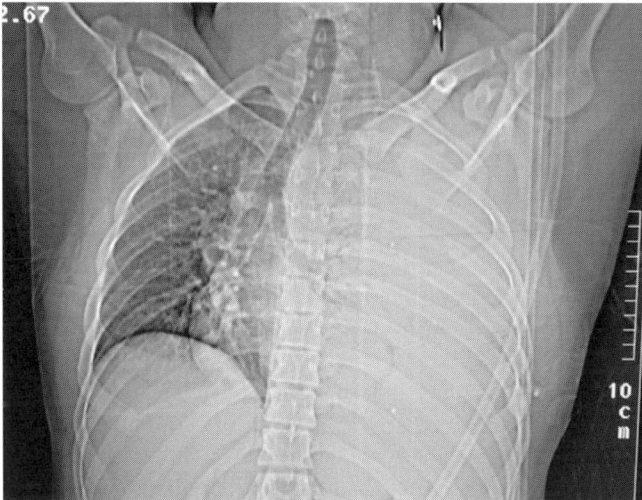

Figure 30.13 Chest x-ray of left tension hemothorax with marked shift of trachea to the right. (Image acquired from trauma.org on 9 March 2013.)

induce hemodynamic instability by loss of intravascular volume and by decreased central venous return with increasing intrathoracic pressure and mediastinal shift (Fig. 30.13). Tension hemothorax is a medical emergency and should be treated similarly to tension pneumothorax, with the expectation that the patient might be hypovolemic as well. Diagnosis is easily made by chest x-ray or ultrasound. Hemothorax also causes respiratory compromise by lung compression secondary to blood accumulation. A trauma patient in shock, associated with the absence of breath sounds and/or dullness on one side of the chest, should be treated for massive hemothorax until proven otherwise. The initial management includes simultaneous resuscitation and decompression of the chest cavity with a large (36–40 Fr) chest tube. Autotransfusion of the blood from massive hemothorax is highly desired whenever possible. A moderate hemothorax (< 1500 mL) that stops bleeding after tube thoracostomy can generally be treated by closed drainage alone. Most cases of hemothorax can be adequately treated by a tube thoracostomy and restoration of circulating blood volume. Bleeding from the lung generally stops within a few minutes after lung expansion, although initially it may be profuse. An urgent thoracotomy should be strongly considered for an initial chest tube output of greater than 1500 mL or with continued bleeding of more than 250 mL per hour for more than three consecutive hours, or requiring persistent blood transfusion.

Pulmonary contusion

Similar to the heart, the lungs can be injured by deceleration forces even in the absence of bony fractures of the chest wall. The frequency and extent of lung contusions are proportional to the severity of thoracic injuries. Alveolar hemorrhage and parenchymal destruction are maximal during the first 24 hours after injury and usually resolve within 7 days.[80] Pulmonary contusion decreases pulmonary compliance and increases intrapulmonary shunt fraction. Symptoms and signs of pulmonary contusion are dyspnea, hypoxemia, cyanosis, tachycardia, and decreased or absent breath sounds. Hemorrhage, edema, and microatelectasis are the morphologic consequences of pulmonary contusion. Chest x-ray changes tend to lag behind the patient's condition and laboratory values, and the extent of lung injury is usually greater than suspected radiologically. Pulmonary contusion is more readily diagnosed on helical CT (Fig. 30.14). Often these injuries are self-limiting and require only supplemental oxygen and time for healing. Occasionally, one or both lungs may be severely injured by contusion, resulting in compromised alveolar gas exchange and the need for mechanical ventilation.

Antibiotic therapy may be indicated to treat pneumonia and other infections. Early application of continuous positive airway pressure (CPAP) improves ventilation/perfusion mismatch, functional residual capacity, and lung compliance, and enhances efficiency of gas exchange and spontaneous ventilation.[5] Spontaneous breathing and biphasic intermittent positive airway pressure (BiPAP) results in more efficient oxygenation and ventilation than with controlled mechanical ventilation. Limiting peak and plateau pressures and tidal volume and avoiding overdistension during mechanical ventilation are important management strategies in patients with lung injury, including pulmonary contusion (see Chapter 19). Pressure-controlled ventilation minimizes peak and plateau airway pressures and may help prevent barotrauma. Lung contusions usually begin to resolve in 2–5 days if other pulmonary complications are not superimposed. Although PEEP and increased FiO_2 are initially required, a strategy of limiting peak and plateau pressure and of using small tidal volumes to avoid overdistension during mechanical ventilation is applied to the degree possible. This strategy has been associated with improved survival at 28 days, a higher rate of weaning from mechanical ventilation, and a lower rate of barotrauma in nontrauma patients with early ARDS. The degree of metabolic acidosis at the time of admission identifies patients with the highest probability of developing acute lung injury after trauma.[81]

Pulmonary parenchymal repair or resection, including tractotomy and repair, wedge resection, lobectomy, or pneumonectomy, is required in less than 2% of blunt thoracic trauma and 6% of penetrating thoracic trauma victims.[82]

Pulmonary contusion should always be considered when there is an unexpectedly high alveolar-to-arterial PO_2 difference in the course of resuscitation from or surgical repair of any thoracic injury. Rib fractures are often associated with pulmonary contusion in the area adjacent to the fractures. Pneumonia and ARDS may occur with subsequent long-term disability.

Flail chest

When rib fractures occur at multiple sites in more than three ribs on the same side, the chest wall in the injured area moves paradoxically, that is, it moves inward during inspiration and outward during expiration. This manifests as inefficient ventilation, and this commonly coexists with pulmonary contusion, pneumothorax, or hemothorax. Flail chest injury usually results from a direct impact such as lateral compression of the chest wall following a "T-bone" MVC, or anterior chest compression of the driver against the steering wheel. Flail chest causes pain with respiratory movement, decreased vital capacity, decreased functional residual capacity, and pulmonary contusion. The underlying pulmonary injury can cause shunt and ventilation/perfusion mismatch. Even in the absence of other thoracic injury, a patient with a flail thoracic segment may require mechanical ventilation to reduce the work of breathing (Table 30.14). Elective surgical stabilization may be required in some cases. Adjunct techniques such as epidural

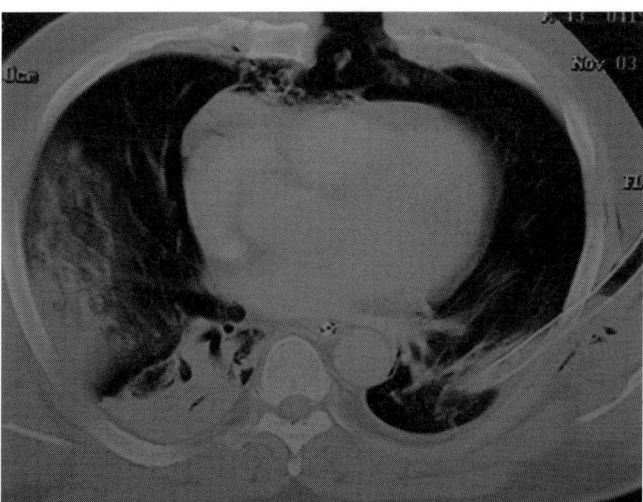

Figure 30.14 Helical CT of the thorax notable for a right lung pulmonary contusion. Also visible are the right hemothorax, sternal fracture, and left chest tube. (Image acquired from trauma.org on 9 March 2013.)

Table 30.14 Flail chest: indications for tracheal intubation and mechanical ventilation

Pulmonary function criteria/dose	Indication
PaO_2	≤ 70 mmHg with rebreathing mask
$PaCO_2$	> 50 mmHg
Respiratory rate	> 35/min or ≤8/min
Vital capacity	≤ 15 mL/kg
Negative inspiratory force	≤ 20 cm H_2O
PaO_2/FiO_2 ratio	≤ 200
Dead-space tidal volume ratio	> 0.6
FEV_1	≤ 10 mL/kg
Shunt fraction (Qs/Qt)	> 0.2

Modified from Cogbill TH, Landercasper J. Injury to the chest wall. In Mattox KL, Feliciano DV, Moore EE, ed. *Trauma*, 4th edition. New York, NY: McGraw-Hill, 2000, pp. 483–505.

analgesia or continuous thoracic paravertebral block may allow the patient to breathe more comfortably and either avoid or minimize the duration of mechanical ventilatory support.

Traumatic asphyxia

Traumatic asphyxia is a rare syndrome resulting from a severe crush injury to the thoracic wall by a very heavy object. The crush injury produces a marked elevation in thoracic and superior vena caval pressure. Concurrent closure of the glottis further promotes a significant increase in venous pressure, resulting in the reversal of venous flow in the valveless veins and capillary rupture of the head and neck. The craniocervical cyanosis, facial edema, petechiae, and subconjunctival hemorrhage mark the strikingly moribund appearance of this syndrome. Loss of consciousness, seizures, confusion, temporary or permanent blindness, hematuria, hemotympanum, epistaxis, and cerebral edema may also be present. Associated chest wall and intrathoracic injuries are common. Treatment includes supportive care in ICU with airway and ventilation maintenance, oxygen supplementation, and 30-degree elevation of the head of the bed. Operative treatment may be required for associated injuries.

Esophageal rupture

Esophageal trauma, if unrecognized, leads to mediastinitis and bacterial necrosis due to contamination of the mediastinal space by esophageal contents. Symptoms consist of excruciating pain in the epigastrium, which radiates to the chest and/or back. Dyspnea, cyanosis, and shock may follow. Emphysema and pneumothorax or hydropneumothorax develop, especially in the left chest, and become visible radiographically. Rupture of the esophagus is rare after blunt trauma but may occur after penetrating trauma or after instrumentation of the esophagus (e.g., gastric tube, intubating laryngeal mask airway, tracheoesophageal Combitube, TEE probe). Failure to release cricoid pressure in the presence of active vomiting during rapid sequence intubation may also lead to esophageal tears. Esophagoscopic visualization of localized blood in the esophagus or an actual laceration is diagnostic. The principles in the management of major esophageal injuries are those of early operation, one-lung ventilation, surgical debridement and repair when possible, and wide drainage. Extensive tissue destruction or associated major mediastinal contamination, such as occurs when repair is delayed by more than 12–16 hours, are indications that esophagectomy with delayed reconstruction or esophageal exclusion and diversion should be considered.

Rib, sternum, and scapular fractures

Rib fractures contribute significantly to the morbidity and mortality associated with chest injuries (Table 30.15). Fracture of three or more ribs is an independent risk factor for morbidity. The elderly and patients with poor respiratory reserve are particularly vulnerable. Fractured ribs cause severe pain, which can be more debilitating and harmful than the injury itself.

Table 30.15 Chest wall organ injury scaling

AIS grade/severity	Injury description
I. Mild	Contusion: any size Laceration: skin and subcutaneous Fracture: < 3 ribs (closed) or nondisplaced clavicle (closed)
II. Moderate	Laceration: skin, subcutaneous and muscle Fracture: ≥ 3 adjacent ribs (closed), open or displaced clavicle, nondisplaced sternum, closed scapular body
III. Serious	Laceration: full thickness including pleura Fracture: open, displaced or flail sternum; unilateral flail segment < 3 ribs
IV. Severe	Laceration: avulsion of chest wall tissues and underlying rib fractures Fracture: unilateral flail chest ≥ 3 ribs
V. Critical	Fracture: bilateral flail chest

Note: Advance one grade for bilateral injuries.
Modified from trauma.org (accessed March 5, 2013).
AIS, Abbreviated Injury Scale.

Because pain characteristically occurs with inspiration, the patient tends to splint the chest wall and therefore hypoventilates. Pain limits the patient's ability to cough and breathe deeply, resulting in sputum retention, atelectasis, and a reduction in functional residual capacity. These factors, in turn, result in decreased lung compliance, ventilation/perfusion mismatch, and hypoxemia. There may be paradoxical respiration, as occurs with flail chest. There may be associated hemopneumothoraces and pulmonary contusions. Crushing injuries produce multiple fractures, the sites being dependent on the direction of the compressing forces. Lower rib fractures are associated with injuries to the spleen and liver (see Chapters 31 and 32). Impacting the anterior chest on a steering wheel during an MVC often fractures the sternum and several ribs anteriorly on both sides. Costovertebral dislocation may occur at any level. Fractures may be transverse or oblique and the fragments can override. Occasionally a pointed fragment can be pushed inward, tearing the pleura and underlying lung and causing a pneumothorax. In the elderly patient with atrophic, decalcified ribs, fractures can result from low-energy trauma events including minor falls or even aggressive coughing. Failure to control pain, compounded by the presence of pulmonary contusion, flail segment, and other insults, can result in respiratory complications, including respiratory failure and subsequent pneumonias.[5]

Acute pain control utilizing regional anesthesia is particularly important for analgesia in traumatic rib fracture(s) (see Chapters 15 and 16).[5,83] Appropriate regional techniques for rib fractures include peripheral nerve block of intercostal nerves, paravertebral block, and epidural anesthesia (see Chapter 16). Paravertebral block and TEA are particularly amenable to catheter placement and continuous infusion. We frequently place "single shot" paravertebral block urgently/emergently for severe thoracic pain. This promptly relieves the pain and quiets the labored respiration that may be accentuating paradoxical motion of the chest. Furthermore, this strategy facilitates acquisition of any diagnostic studies and provides a comfortable, cooperative patient for definitive acute pain catheter placement. TEA and paravertebral block provide superior analgesia and appear to be equally effective.[7,84] We prefer to place a paravertebral catheter for unilateral rib fractures. In the absence of mitigating factors, we are equivocal in our choice of bilateral paravertebral catheters or TEA for bilateral rib fractures. After initial dosing, we administer a local anesthetic with opioid (0.2% ropivacaine with 4 µg/mL fentanyl) continuous infusion at 4–10 mL/hour initial rate for either a paravertebral or epidural catheter. Further details of regional analgesia techniques are presented in Chapter 16.

Acute pain management with regional anesthesia improves patient outcomes in trauma patients.[5,83] Increased bronchial secretions must be removed if patients are to avoid an obstructive type of pneumonia that is particularly dangerous in the elderly. Elderly patients with multiple rib fractures and cardiopulmonary disease are at increased risk for complications that lead to prolonged length of hospitalization and readmission to the hospital.[85] Epidural analgesia provides excellent pain relief for patients with multiple rib fractures and helps facilitate an effective cough. Benefits of epidural analgesia include improved vital capacity, functional residual capacity, airway resistance, and dynamic lung compliance. Patients receiving continuous epidural analgesia have been shown to have decreased ventilator days, shorter ICU stays, shorter hospitalizations, and decreased incidence of tracheostomy when compared with control-matched groups with similar injury severity indices.[86–89] Intercostal nerve blocks have been utilized for many years to alleviate rib fracture pain. The chief limitation is that the relief of pain is temporary, lasting 6–12 hours or less. There is also a risk of pneumothorax. Rapid vascular absorption of local anesthetics can occur, with a risk of toxicity. Continuous intercostal nerve blockade has also been described.[5] An interpleural catheter placed for thoracic pain allows for continuous infusions or intermittent injections to provide prolonged pain relief. The major concerns with interpleural catheter placement are that the peak plasma levels of local anesthetics are relatively high and pain relief is not achieved consistently. In addition, in patients with thoracostomy tubes, there is a risk of suctioning the injected local anesthetics. This risk is minimized by placing the catheter distant from the thoracostomy tube or delaying the suction of the thoracostomy tube for 15–30 minutes after injection of the local anesthetic through the interpleural catheter. The use of interpleural catheters is patient-position dependent. The tip of the catheter can migrate in certain patients, leading to inadequate analgesia.

If coughing is inadequate, tracheal aspiration by catheter or by bronchoscopy and occasionally via tracheal intubation may be necessary. The ribs usually become fairly stable within 10 days to 2 weeks. Firm healing with callus formation is seen after about 6 weeks.

Postoperative considerations following cardiothoracic trauma

After cardiothoracic trauma, patients often require support of the respiratory and cardiovascular systems and optimization of ventilation, hemodynamics, and oxygen delivery in the ICU. Care is directed toward management of general problems such as fluids, pain control, nausea and vomiting, head injuries, agitation, temperature maintenance, and complications of unsuspected drug abuse. Serial chest x-rays, assessment of chest tube drainage, and monitoring for complications related to the initial trauma such as pulmonary contusion, blunt cardiac injuries, retained hemothorax, empyema, pulmonary cavitary lesions, and noncardiothoracic injuries (e.g., head, spinal cord, abdominal, retroperitoneal, orthopedic, and vascular injuries) may be necessary. Specific postcardiothoracic trauma complications include ARDS, multiple organ system failure, and sepsis, the last two being the major late causes of death in trauma.

In patients with traumatic lung injury, the incidence of ARDS, empyema, recurrent pneumothorax, pneumonia, bleeding/hemothorax requiring reoperation, and mortality has been found to be higher with blunt injuries (versus penetrating), low blood pressure at thoracotomy, and increasing amount of lung resection.[82]

Postoperative complications after cardiac trauma include intracardiac shunts, valvular lesions, ventricular aneurysms, wall motion abnormalities, arrhythmias, and conduction blocks. Retained foreign body and aortocaval and aortopulmonary fistula may also occur in survivors of penetrating cardiac trauma.

Summary

- With severe blunt trauma, the heart and great vessels are most often disrupted at one of four "anchor points": the aortic root, the posterior left atrium, the cavo-right atrial junction, and the proximal descending thoracic aorta.
- Blunt trauma can cause myocardial contusion, most often to the right ventricle, which can present as hypotension and/or arrhythmia. Diagnostic findings that tend to confirm this diagnosis include cardiac isoenzyme elevations, ECG changes, and TEE changes, but there is no "gold standard" for diagnosis of this entity.
- Penetrating wounds to the heart most often injure the right ventricle and carry a high mortality, especially with gunshots. The cause of death is either exsanguination or cardiac tamponade.
- Aortic disruptions typically occur at the attachment site of the ligamentum arteriosum in the proximal descending aorta. These often cause immediate exsanguination, but life

can be spared if the aortic adventitia or parietal pleura contains the rupture, in which case downstream ischemia to abdominal organs and to the spinal cord can result from decreased aortic blood flow before or during surgical repair.

- Surgical and anesthetic management of descending thoracic aortic traumatic disruptions has changed dramatically in the past few years. Endovascular stenting is now the surgical technique of choice. Outcomes are improved compared to open procedures.

- Blast injury can cause several different types of trauma, but the most common thoracic injury is barotrauma leading to pneumothorax, so early chest tube insertion is often critical for those who acutely survive the blast. Air embolus is the most frequent cause of death.

- Compression of the sternum against the vertebral column is a mechanism of injury unique to the thorax, and it can result in rupture of any thoracic organ or heart chamber.

- The acute management of suspected pneumothorax or hemothorax involves emergency placement of a chest tube. Most hemothoraces do not require thoracotomy, and if they do, often video-assisted thoracotomy suffices.

- Aside from the usual diagnostic and therapeutic considerations, nonvertebral fractures in the thoracic cage often require regional analgesic techniques such as thoracic epidural or paravertebral catheters to improve breathing and either avoid or reduce the duration of endotracheal intubation.

Questions

(1) Which of the following cardiothoracic anatomic locations is *not* an anchor point subject to avulsion from deceleration forces during an automobile accident?
   a. Junction between venae cavae and right atrium
   b. Posterior left atrium
   c. Proximal descending aorta
   d. Aorta at diaphragmatic hiatus
   e. Mitral valve annulus

(2) A 21-year-old unrestrained driver experiences a deceleration injury with his chest against a steering wheel in an automobile that lacks an airbag. ST segments are abnormal in leads V_1 and V_2 and plasma troponin I levels are increased. A chest x-ray shows a fluffy "butterfly" central infiltrate pattern, sternal fracture, and prominent pulmonary vascular markings. The mediastinum and cardiac silhouette appear normal. Which of the following pathologic combinations is most likely?
   a. Pulmonary contusion and right ventricular dysfunction
   b. Thoracic aortic transection and pulmonary edema
   c. Left anterior descending coronary rupture and left ventricular failure

   d. Aortic root (proximal ascending aorta) rupture and pericardial effusion
   e. Pulmonary arterial injury and left ventricular contusion

(3) A 42-year-old man who was in a domestic dispute has a butcher knife sticking out of his chest. The knife is going straight into the parasternal portion of the left fifth intercostal space. Which of the following cardiac structures is most likely to be injured?
   a. Interventricular septum
   b. Lateral wall of right atrium
   c. Anterior wall of right ventricle
   d. Left anterior descending coronary artery
   e. Apex of left ventricle

(4) An unidentified and unconscious young man presents to the operating room with a bullet entry wound in the right anterior fourth intercostal space and an exit wound in the left posterior paraspinous muscles at approximately T8. Blood pressure 70/50 mmHg, heart rate 110 bpm, respirations 28 per minute, SpO_2 92% on face mask O_2. After obtaining a chest x-ray and placing bilateral chest tubes and intubation, the next action should be:
   a. Perform a transesophageal echocardiogram
   b. Perform a transthoracic echocardiogram
   c. Obtain a thoracic CT scan
   d. Place a radial arterial catheter
   e. Change to a double-lumen endobronchial tube

(5) In a blunt deceleration-type injury, the most common site for aortic disruption is:
   a. Aortic valve
   b. Junction of ascending aorta and innominate artery
   c. Junction of subclavian artery and descending thoracic aorta
   d. Diaphragmatic hiatus
   e. Bifurcation of abdominal aorta

(6) The most common outcome of a traumatic aortic rupture is:
   a. Long-term survival with medical management
   b. Long-term survival with immediate surgical repair
   c. Long-term survival with elective surgical repair
   d. Delayed death from pseudoaneurysm rupture
   e. Immediate death

(7) Which of the following diagnostic modalities is *least* specific for diagnosing a suspected acute traumatic rupture of the descending thoracic aorta?
   a. Magnetic resonance imaging
   b. Spiral CT scan
   c. Transesophageal echocardiography
   d. Chest x-ray
   e. Aortography

(8) A 32-year-old man will soon undergo anesthesia for repair of a traumatic transection of the proximal descending aorta. He has received morphine sulfate 14 mg intravenously, which has reduced his back pain

from a score of 10 of 10 to 4 of 10, and he is now sleepy unless stimulated. His blood pressure is 174/102 mmHg, heart rate is 105 bpm, and respirations are 12 per minute. Which of the following interventions is most appropriate at this time?

a. Initiate a nitroglycerin infusion IV
b. Place a thoracic aortic catheter and administer epidural ropivacaine
c. Administer additional morphine IV
d. Administer a dexmedetomidine loading dose IV push
e. Initiate esmolol and nitroprusside IV infusions

(9) A 22-year-old woman was near an outdoor explosion and was thrown against a wall. She never lost consciousness. Physical examination reveals impaired hearing, bruises on her back, and no other obvious injuries. She is conscious, dyspneic, and apprehensive. Blood pressure 90/60 mmHg, heart rate 110 bpm, respirations 32 per minute, room air SpO$_2$ 86% without splinting or an obvious flail chest. Breath sounds are present but somewhat diminished bilaterally. After administering oxygen by face mask, your next action should be:

a. Intubate and initiate positive-pressure ventilation
b. Perform a transthoracic echocardiogram
c. Insert bilateral chest tubes
d. Perform a tracheostomy
e. Order a chest x-ray

(10) A 25-year-old man experienced blunt trauma from a blast injury 1 hour ago. A transthoracic echocardiogram reveals a large pericardial effusion with diastolic invagination of the right ventricle. Other diagnostic studies have ruled out pleural effusion and intraabdominal blood. A subxiphoid pericardial window is planned. Blood pressure 75–80/50 mmHg with 15 mmHg pulsus paradoxus, pulse 120 bpm, respirations 28 per minute. Which of the following anesthetic options is most appropriate?

a. Rapid sequence induction with propofol 2 mg/kg and intubation followed by positive-pressure ventilation
b. Administration of nitrous oxide analgesia (60% N$_2$O, 40% O$_2$) by face mask
c. Local anesthesia for the surgical field accompanied by intravenous sedation using midazolam
d. Placement of a laryngeal mask airway under propofol anesthesia with attempts to preserve spontaneous ventilation
e. Thoracic epidural anesthesia

(11) Three days after experiencing blunt thoracic trauma that caused a mild pulmonary contusion and dissection of his proximal left subclavian artery, a 35-year-old man is having endovascular stent repair with vascular access to be acquired percutaneously in the right groin. BP 120/62 mmHg, pulse 74 bpm, respirations 16 per minute;, SpO$_2$ 95% on 2 liters per minute nasal cannula O$_2$. Which of the following regional anesthetic techniques is *not* appropriate?

a. Subarachnoid block with hyperbaric bupivacaine
b. Placement of a right femoral peripheral nerve block
c. Local anesthesia for the surgical field accompanied by intravenous sedation using midazolam
d. Placement of right T10–L2 paravertebral nerve blocks with 0.75% ropivacaine
e. Lumbar epidural anesthesia

(12) A 22-year-old woman experienced blunt trauma from a motor vehicle crash. She has femur fracture and bilateral single rib fractures from the steering wheel impact. Her past medical history is significant for a one pack/day tobacco abuse since age 14 and mild asthma. Her only medication is an oral contraceptive. An open reduction and internal fixation of the femur is planned. Immediately prior to induction she complains of dyspnea. You administer oxygen via face mask with manual CPAP. Over the next minute the blood pressure decreases to 70/50 mmHg (from 125/75 mmHg), and pulse increases from 90 bpm to 120 bpm. She is increasingly agitated. Which of the following options is most appropriate?

a. Rapid sequence induction and intubation followed by positive-pressure ventilation
b. Administration of nitrous oxide analgesia (60% N$_2$O, 40% O$_2$) by face mask
c. Intercostal nerve blocks accompanied by intravenous sedation using midazolam
d. Placement of a laryngeal mask airway under propofol anesthesia with attempts to preserve spontaneous ventilation
e. Bilateral needle thoracostomy

(13) Which statement about imaging modalities is *incorrect*?

a. Helical CT can diagnose pneumothorax but not tension pneumothorax
b. TEE is the modality of choice for cardiac valve function
c. Chest x-ray is sufficient for diagnosis of tension hemothorax
d. FAST scanning includes evaluation for pericardial fluid
e. Helical CT can distinguish between cardiac tamponade and cardiac luxation

(14) A 21-year-old man presents following a motor vehicle crash. He is dyspneic and has massive subcutaneous emphysema of his anterior chest and neck. The most appropriate next step is:

a. Rapid sequence induction and intubation followed by positive-pressure ventilation
b. Awake blind nasal intubation
c. Awake fiberoptic intubation
d. Tracheostomy
e. CPAP mask

(15) Pharmacological effects of dexmedetomidine include all of the following, *except*:
  a. Analgesia
  b. Sedation
  c. Attenuation of withdrawal syndromes
  d. Amnesia
  e. Neuroprotection

Answers

(1) e
(2) a
(3) c
(4) b
(5) c
(6) e
(7) d
(8) e
(9) e
(10) c
(11) b
(12) e
(13) a
(14) c
(15) d

References

1. Lockey D, Crewdson K, Davies G. Traumatic cardiac arrest: who are the survivors? *Ann Emerg Med* 2006; **48**: 240–4.

2. Tobin JM, Varon AJ. Review article: update in trauma anesthesiology: perioperative resuscitation management. *Anesth Analg* 2012; **115**: 1326–33.

3. Cook CC, Gleason TG. Great vessel and cardiac trauma. *Surg Clin North Am* 2009; **89**: 797–820, viii.

4. Navid F, Gleason TG. Great vessel and cardiac trauma: diagnostic and management strategies. *Semin Thorac Cardiovasc Surg* 2008; **20**: 31–8.

5. Ho AM, Karmakar MK, Critchley LA. Acute pain management of patients with multiple fractured ribs: a focus on regional techniques. *Curr Opin Crit Care* 2011; **17**: 323–7.

6. De Cosmo G, Aceto P, Gualtieri E, Congedo E. Analgesia in thoracic surgery: review. *Minerva Anestesiol* 2009; **75**: 393–400.

7. Chelly JE. Paravertebral blocks. *Anesthesiol Clin* 2012; **30**: 75–90.

8. Co SJ, Yong-Hing CJ, Galea-Soler S, et al. Role of imaging in penetrating and blunt traumatic injury to the heart. *Radiographics* 2011; **31**: E101–15.

9. Singh KE, Baum VC. The anesthetic management of cardiovascular trauma. *Curr Opin Anaesthesiol* 2011; **24**: 98–103.

10. Restrepo CS, Gutierrez FR, Marmol-Velez JA, Ocazionez D, Martinez-Jimenez S. Imaging patients with cardiac trauma. *Radiographics* 2012; **32**: 633–49.

11. Moore EE, Malangoni MA, Cogbill TH, et al. Organ injury scaling. IV: Thoracic vascular, lung, cardiac, and diaphragm. *J Trauma* 1994; **36**: 299–300.

12. Blackbourne LH, Baer DG, Eastridge BJ, et al. Military medical revolution: military trauma system. *J Trauma Acute Care Surg* 2012; **73**: S388–94.

13. Blackbourne LH, Baer DG, Eastridge BJ, et al. Military medical revolution: prehospital combat casualty care. *J Trauma Acute Care Surg* 2012; **73**: S372–7.

14. Blackbourne LH, Baer DG, Eastridge BJ, et al. Military medical revolution: deployed hospital and en route care. *J Trauma Acute Care Surg* 2012; **73**: S378–87.

15. Ivey KM, White CE, Wallum TE, et al. Thoracic injuries in US combat casualties: a 10-year review of Operation Enduring Freedom and Iraqi Freedom. *J Trauma Acute Care Surg* 2012; **73**: S514–19.

16. Roberts I, Shakur H, Coats T, et al. The CRASH-2 trial: a randomised controlled trial and economic evaluation of the effects of tranexamic acid on death, vascular occlusive events and transfusion requirement in bleeding trauma patients. *Health Technol Assess* 2013; **17**: 1–79.

17. Wade CE, Eastridge BJ, Jones JA, et al. Use of recombinant factor VIIa in US military casualties for a five-year period. *J Trauma* 2010; **69**: 353–9.

18. Nishijima DK, Zehtabchi S. Evidence-based emergency medicine/critically appraised topic. The efficacy of recombinant activated factor VII in severe trauma. *Ann Emerg Med* 2009; **54**: 737–44.e1.

19. Smith JE, Fawcett R, Randalls B. The use of recombinant activated factor VII in a patient with penetrating chest trauma and ongoing pulmonary hemorrhage. *Mil Med* 2012; **177**: 614–16.

20. Orliaguet G, Ferjani M, Riou B. The heart in blunt trauma. *Anesthesiology* 2001; **95**: 544–8.

21. Teixeira PG, Georgiou C, Inaba K, et al. Blunt cardiac trauma: lessons learned from the medical examiner. *J Trauma* 2009; **67**: 1259–64.

22. Battle CE, Hutchings H., Evans PA. Risk factors that predict mortality in patients with blunt chest wall trauma: a systematic review and meta-analysis. *Injury* 2012; **43**: 8–17.

23. Leibecke T, Stoeckelhuber BM, Gellissen J, et al. Posttraumatic and postoperative cardiac luxation: computed tomography findings in nine patients. *J Trauma* 2008; **64**: 721–6.

24. Bertinchant JP, Robert E, Polge A, et al. Release kinetics of cardiac troponin I and cardiac troponin T in effluents from isolated perfused rabbit hearts after graded experimental myocardial contusion. *J Trauma* 1999; **47**: 474–80.

25. Pretre R, Chilcott M. Blunt trauma to the heart and great vessels. *N Engl J Med* 1997; **336**: 626–32.

26. Sutherland GR, Calvin JE, Driedger AA, Holliday RL, Sibbald WJ. Anatomic and cardiopulmonary responses to trauma with associated blunt chest injury. *J Trauma* 1981; **21**: 1–12.

27. Robert E, de La Coussaye JE, Aya AG, et al. Mechanisms of ventricular arrhythmias induced by myocardial contusion: a high-resolution mapping study in left ventricular rabbit heart. *Anesthesiology* 2000; **92**: 1132–43.

28. Sato Y, Matsumoto N, Komatsu S, et al. Coronary artery dissection after blunt

chest trauma: depiction at multidetector-row computed tomography. *Int J Cardiol* 2007; **118**: 108–10.

29. Chirillo F, Totis O, Cavarzerani A, *et al.* Usefulness of transthoracic and transoesophageal echocardiography in recognition and management of cardiovascular injuries after blunt chest trauma. *Heart* 1996; **75**: 301–6.

30. Wall MJ, Mattox KL, Chen CD, Baldwin JC. Acute management of complex cardiac injuries. *J Trauma* 1997; **42**: 905–12.

31. Degiannis E, Loogna P, Doll D, *et al.* Penetrating cardiac injuries: recent experience in South Africa. *World J Surg* 2006; **30**: 1258–64.

32. Hunt PA, Greaves I, Owens WA. Emergency thoracotomy in thoracic trauma-a review. *Injury* 2006; **37**: 1–19.

33. Singh R, Choudhury M, Kapoor PM, Kiran U. A randomized trial of anesthetic induction agents in patients with coronary artery disease and left ventricular dysfunction. *Ann Card Anaesth* 2010; **13**: 217–23.

34. Lim R, Gill IS, Temes RT, Smith CE. The use of adenosine for repair of penetrating cardiac injuries: a novel method. *Ann Thorac Surg* 2001; **71**: 1714–15.

35. Hoffer EK, Forauer AR, Silas AM, Gemery JM. Endovascular stent-graft or open surgical repair for blunt thoracic aortic trauma: systematic review. *J Vasc Interv Radiol* 2008; **19**: 1153–64.

36. Demetriades D, Velmahos GC, Scalea TM, *et al.* Operative repair or endovascular stent graft in blunt traumatic thoracic aortic injuries: results of an American Association for the Surgery of Trauma Multicenter Study. *J Trauma* 2008; **64**: 561–70.

37. Demetriades D, Velmahos GC, Scalea TM, *et al.* Diagnosis and treatment of blunt thoracic aortic injuries: changing perspectives. *J Trauma* 2008; **64**: 1415–19.

38. Demetriades D, Velmahos GC, Scalea TM, *et al.* Blunt traumatic thoracic aortic injuries: early or delayed repair– results of an American Association for the Surgery of Trauma prospective study. *J Trauma* 2009; **66**: 967–73.

39. Lachat ML, Pfammatter T, Witzke HJ, *et al.* Endovascular repair with bifurcated stent-grafts under local anaesthesia to improve outcome of ruptured aortoiliac aneurysms. *Eur J Vasc Endovasc Surg* 2002; **23**: 528–36.

40. Karmy-Jones R, Hoffer E, Meissner M, Bloch RD. Management of traumatic rupture of the thoracic aorta in pediatric patients. *Ann Thorac Surg* 2003; **75**: 1513–17.

41. Williams JS, Graff JA, Uku JM, Steinig JP. Aortic injury in vehicular trauma. *Ann Thorac Surg* 1994; **57**: 726–30.

42. Fann JI, Miller DC. Aortic dissection. *Ann Vasc Surg* 1995; **9**: 311–23.

43. Burns JM, Sing RF, Mostafa G, *et al.* The role of transesophageal echocardiography in optimizing resuscitation in acutely injured patients. *J Trauma* 2005; **59**: 36–40.

44. Lord MS, Augoustides JG. Perioperative management of pheochromocytoma: focus on magnesium, clevidipine, and vasopressin. *J Cardiothorac Vasc Anesth* 2012; **26**: 526–31.

45. Murphy MB, Murray C, Shorten GD. Fenoldopam: a selective peripheral dopamine-receptor agonist for the treatment of severe hypertension. *N Engl J Med* 2001; **345**: 1548–57.

46. Gilbert TB, Hasnain JU, Flinn WR, Lilly MP, Benjamin ME. Fenoldopam infusion associated with preserving renal function after aortic cross-clamping for aneurysm repair. *J Cardiovasc Pharmacol Ther* 2001; **6**: 31–6.

47. Halpenny M, Rushe C, Breen P, *et al.* The effects of fenoldopam on renal function in patients undergoing elective aortic surgery. *Eur J Anaesthesiol* 2002; **19**: 32–9.

48. Papia G, Klein D, Lindsay TF. Intensive care of the patient following open abdominal aortic surgery. *Curr Opin Crit Care* 2006; **12**: 340–5.

49. Oliver WC, Nuttall GA, Cherry KJ, *et al.* A comparison of fenoldopam with dopamine and sodium nitroprusside in patients undergoing cross-clamping of the abdominal aorta. *Anesth Analg* 2006; **103**: 833–40.

50. Sheinbaum R, Ignacio C, Safi HJ, Estrera A. Contemporary strategies to preserve renal function during cardiac and vascular surgery. *Rev Cardiovasc Med* 2003; **4** (Suppl 1): S21–8.

51. Tobias JD. Dexmedetomidine in trauma anesthesiology and critical care. *Trauma Care* 2007; **17**: 6–18.

52. Gerlach AT, Dasta JF. Dexmedetomidine: an updated review. *Ann Pharmacother* 2007; **41**: 245–52.

53. Koca U, Olguner CG, Ergur BU, *et al.* The effects of dexmedetomidine on secondary acute lung and kidney injuries in the rat model of intra-abdominal sepsis. *ScientificWorldJournal* 2013; **2013**: 292687.

54. Wu X, Song X, Li N, *et al.* Protective effects of dexmedetomidine on blunt chest trauma-induced pulmonary contusion in rats. *J Trauma Acute Care Surg* 2013; **74**: 524–30.

55. Geze S, Cekic B, Imamoglu M, *et al.* Use of dexmedetomidine to prevent pulmonary injury after pneumoperitoneum in ventilated rats. *Surg Laparosc Endosc Percutan Tech* 2012; **22**: 447–53.

56. Schoeler M, Loetscher PD, Rossaint R, *et al.* Dexmedetomidine is neuroprotective in an in vitro model for traumatic brain injury. *BMC Neurol* 2012; **12**: 20.

57. Zhang XY, Liu ZM, Wen SH, *et al.* Dexmedetomidine administration before, but not after, ischemia attenuates intestinal injury induced by intestinal ischemia-reperfusion in rats. *Anesthesiology* 2012; **116**: 1035–46.

58. Hayter RG, Rhea JT, Small A, Tafazoli FS, Novelline RA. Suspected aortic dissection and other aortic disorders: multi-detector row CT in 373 cases in the emergency setting. *Radiology* 2006; **238**: 841–52.

59. Kirton OC, Civetta JM. Do pulmonary artery catheters alter outcome in trauma patients? *New Horiz* 1997; **5**: 222–7.

60. Shoemaker WC, Wo CC, Chien LC, *et al.* Evaluation of invasive and noninvasive hemodynamic monitoring in trauma patients. *J Trauma* 2006; **61**: 844–53.

61. Karski JM. Transesophageal echocardiography in the intensive care unit. *Semin Cardiothorac Vasc Anesth* 2006; **10**: 162–6.

62. Campos JH. Lung isolation techniques. *Anesthesiol Clin North America* 2001; **19**: 455–74.

63. Campos JH. Current techniques for perioperative lung isolation in adults. *Anesthesiology* 2002; **97**: 1295–301.

64. Campos JH. Which device should be considered the best for lung isolation: double-lumen endotracheal tube versus bronchial blockers. *Curr Opin Anaesthesiol* 2007; **20**: 27–31.

65. Sessler DI. Temperature monitoring and perioperative thermoregulation. *Anesthesiology* 2008; **109**: 318–38.

66. Shore-Lesserson, L. Evidence based coagulation monitors: heparin monitoring, thromboelastography, and platelet function. *Semin Cardiothorac Vasc Anesth* 2005; **9**: 41–52.

67. Casati A, Alessandrini P, Nuzzi M, *et al.* A prospective, randomized, blinded comparison between continuous thoracic paravertebral and epidural infusion of 0.2% ropivacaine after lung resection surgery. *Eur J Anaesthesiol,* 2006; 1–6.

68. Davies RG, Myles PS, Graham JM. A comparison of the analgesic efficacy and side-effects of paravertebral vs epidural blockade for thoracotomy–a systematic review and meta-analysis of randomized trials. *Br J Anaesth* 2006; **96**: 418–26.

69. Leissner KB, Ortega R, Beattie WS. Anesthesia implications of blast injury. *J Cardiothorac Vasc Anesth* 2006; **20**: 872–80.

70. Gutierrez de Ceballos JP, Turegano Fuentes F, Perez Diaz D, *et al.* Casualties treated at the closest hospital in the Madrid, March 11, terrorist bombings. *Crit Care Med* 2005; **33**: S107–12.

71. DePalma RG, Burris DG, Champion HR, Hodgson MJ. Blast injuries. *N Engl J Med* 2005; **352**: 1335–42.

72. Biocina B, Sutlic Z, Husedzinovic I, *et al.* Penetrating cardiothoracic war wounds. *Eur J Cardiothorac Surg* 1997; **11**: 399–405.

73. Shamir MY, Weiss YG, Willner D, *et al.* Multiple casualty terror events: the anesthesiologist's perspective. *Anesth Analg* 2004; **98**: 1746–52.

74. Wolf YG, Rivkind A. Vascular trauma in high-velocity gunshot wounds and shrapnel-blast injuries in Israel. *Surg Clin North Am* 2002; **82**: 237–44.

75. Ho AM, Ling E. Systemic air embolism after lung trauma. *Anesthesiology* 1999; **90**: 564–75.

76. O'Connor JV, Adamski, J. The diagnosis and treatment of non-cardiac thoracic trauma. *J R Army Med Corps* 2010; **156**: 5–14.

77. Shim HS, Noe MH, Kim IK, Shin NK, Lee SH. Anesthetic management of a patient with complete trachial transection by blunt trauma: a case report. *Korean J Anesthesiol* 2008; **54**: 454–8.

78. Chow E, Farrar DJ. Right heart function during prosthetic left ventricular assistance in a porcine model of congestive heart failure. *J Thorac Cardiovasc Surg* 1992; **104**: 569–78.

79. Nakagiri T, Inoue M, Nakagawa J, Okumura M. Blunt tracheal transection repair requiring open abdominal management. *Ann Thorac Surg* 2011; **92**: 2248–50.

80. Cohn SM. Pulmonary contusion: review of the clinical entity. *J Trauma* 1997; **42**: 973–9.

81. Eberhard LW, Morabito DJ, Matthay MA, *et al.* Initial severity of metabolic acidosis predicts the development of acute lung injury in severely traumatized patients. *Crit Care Med* 2000; **28**: 125–31.

82. Karmy-Jones R, Jurkovich GJ. Blunt chest trauma. *Curr Probl Surg* 2004; **41**: 211–380.

83. Keene DD, Rea WE, Aldington D. Acute pain management in trauma. *Trauma* 2011; **13**: 167–79.

84. Simon B, Ebert J, Bokhari F, *et al.* Management of pulmonary contusion and flail chest: an Eastern Association for the Surgery of Trauma practice management guideline. *J Trauma Acute Care Surg* 2012; **73**: S351–61.

85. Alexander JQ, Gutierrez CJ, Mariano MC, *et al.* Blunt chest trauma in the elderly patient: how cardiopulmonary disease affects outcome. *Am Surg* 2000; **66**: 855–7.

86. Ullman DA, Fortune JB, Greenhouse BB, Wimpy RE, Kennedy TM. The treatment of patients with multiple rib fractures with continuous thoracic epidural narcotic infusion. *Reg Anesth* 1989; **14**: 43–7.

87. Wisner DH. A stepwise logistic regression analysis of factors affecting morbidity and mortality after thoracic trauma: effect of epidural analgesia. *J Trauma* 1990; **30**: 799–804.

88. Mackersie RC, Karagianes TG, Hoyt DB, Davis JW. Prospective evaluation of epidural and intravenous administration of fentanyl for pain control and restoration of ventilatory function following multiple rib fractures. *J Trauma* 1991; **31**: 443–9.

89. Bulger EM, Edwards T, Klotz P, Jurkovich GJ. Epidural analgesia improves outcome after multiple rib fractures. *Surgery* 2004; **136**: 426–30.

Chapter

31

Abdominal trauma: surgical considerations

Jeffrey A. Claridge and Jana Hambley

Objectives

(1) Provide a brief overview of the priority of surgical interventions for trauma.
(2) Provide an overview of the operative interventions for specific injuries resulting from abdominal trauma.

Introduction

"The abdomen rules" in trauma is a common phrase that may be overstated, but it is a useful philosophy when caring for traumatically injured patients. When dealing with traumatically injured patients it is important to remember this simple and very important concept. Although the abdomen may not be the most commonly injured area of the body or the area most commonly associated with fatal outcomes, the priority of abdominal trauma for both the surgical and the anesthesia teams is paramount. Identifying and addressing surgical issues of the abdomen promptly will allow the greatest opportunity for better outcomes. Because of the many different abdominal structures, the methods of treatment and approaches for surgical intervention vary. In most cases of abdominal injury, no operative intervention will be required This chapter will give a brief overview of surgical interventions for trauma, then it will focus on the operative interventions that may be required for abdominal injury involving different abdominal structures.

Laparotomy

While most abdominal trauma is managed nonoperatively, in general, the trauma laparotomy remains the mainstay of trauma operative intervention.

Basic surgical approach

The patient is prepared with a sterile cleansing solution, with an emphasis on a large area in the event that unforeseen interventions are needed. As a general rule, the operative team should be prepared to prep the patient from chin to knees. A midline abdominal incision is the most effective method to gain exposure in trauma. An incision is made from the

xyphoid to the pubis over the midline. Upon entering the abdomen in blunt trauma, the patient is eviscerated and the abdomen is explored systematically by quadrant. Packing may be used to control bleeding, with laparotomy pads placed superior to the liver and spleen, and within the paracolic gutters. With penetrating injury, the bowels are eviscerated and exploration is focused on the injured region.[1] Further interventions will be based on the findings of this initial exploration.

In a stable trauma patient, the initial trip to the operating room is often the only one needed. During this operation, the patient's injuries are assessed. Definitive procedures are then performed to repair the traumatic injuries. For example, this approach would be used in performing a small bowel resection for an isolated gunshot wound.

Damage control laparotomy

When a patient presents with unstable vital signs and multiple traumatic injuries, it is often not possible to repair those injuries definitively on the first trip to the operating room. Instead, the practice of "damage control" has emerged to address this (see Chapter 18). The goal of damage control is to quickly identify injuries and stabilize the patient. The key goals of the initial operation are to stop bleeding and control gastrointestinal spillage. There are three main stages to damage control procedures:

(1) abbreviated resuscitative surgery with a focus on controlling hemorrhage and abdominal contamination
(2) intensive care resuscitation with rewarming and correction of coagulopathy
(3) definitive surgical intervention with repair of injuries and abdominal closure[2]

Laparoscopy

Laparoscopy is occasionally used in trauma and can be effective in specific situations, particularly to explore the left upper quadrant when there is concern for diaphragmatic injury following penetrating trauma.[3] Likewise, laparoscopy has a role in diagnosing intraperitoneal injuries after trauma.

Trauma Anesthesia, 2nd Edition, ed. Charles E. Smith. Published by Cambridge University Press. © Charles E. Smith, 2015.

Laparoscopy is less invasive than a laparotomy and causes less blood loss. With laparoscopy, however, there are concerns for missed injuries and the difficulty it poses for fully examining the bowel, especially if blood is present in the abdomen. A special concern to the anesthesiologist is the possibility of exacerbating a pneumothorax in a patient with a diaphragmatic injury due to insufflation of gas.

Bedside laparotomy

Bedside laparotomy is an intervention that can be performed in very unstable patients located in a surgical intensive care unit. This method can be especially challenging if it is not frequently used, as organizing staff, controlling an airway, and providing sedation will need to be carefully arranged. It is typically only done in the situation of reopening a recent laparotomy or concern for abdominal compartment syndrome.

Liver and biliary injuries

The liver is the most frequently injured organ in blunt trauma. Interventions for hepatic injury range from nonoperative management to complex surgical repairs and resections. Injuries to the liver are graded on a scale from I to VI based on injury severity (Table 31.1).[4] This grading scheme is more often used to compare outcomes than necessarily guide treatment.

Table 31.1 Liver injury scale

I	Hematoma	Subcapsular, < 10 cm surface area
	Laceration	Capsular tear, nonbleeding, < 1 cm deep
II	Hematoma	Subcapsular, nonexpanding, 10–50% surface area, or intraparenchymal < 10 cm deep
	Laceration	Capsular tear, active bleeding, 1–3 cm deep, < 10 cm in length
III	Hematoma	Subcapsular, > 50% surface area or expanding in size, ruptured subcapsular hematoma with active bleeding, intraparenchymal > 10 cm diameter or expanding in size
	Laceration	> 3 cm deep
IV	Hematoma	Ruptured intraparenchymal hematoma with active bleeding
	Laceration	Parenchymal disruption of 25–75% of hepatic lobe
V	Laceration	Parenchymal disruption of > 75% of hepatic lobe
	Vascular	Juxtahepatic venous injury (retrohepatic vena cava or major central hepatic veins)
VI	Hepatic avulsion	

Modified from http://www.trauma.org/archive/scores/ois-liver.html (accessed April 2014).

Blunt liver injury

The management of blunt liver injury is an area in which surgical care has evolved. While previously operative intervention was standard, the paradigm has changed so that most patients are now managed nonoperatively. Most patients with blunt hepatic injury are hemodynamically stable on presentation.[5] The traumatic impact in these injuries traverses the segments of the liver, and injures primarily the hepatic veins, which allows for hemostasis to occur without operative interventions. Instead, these patients have been found to have improved outcomes without surgical intervention.[6] The Eastern Association for the Surgery of Trauma (EAST) has recently changed its practice management guidelines to state that "nonoperative management of blunt hepatic injuries currently is the treatment modality of choice in hemodynamically stable patients irrespective of the grade of injury or patient age."[7]

Operative management of hepatic injuries

Injuries to the liver frequently cause large amounts of bleeding. The patient therefore may be hemodynamically unstable on arrival to the operating room, making communication and planning for adequate resuscitation between all caregivers extremely important. The patient may already have symptoms of hypothermia or a developing coagulopathy. The anesthesia team should be prepared to transfuse the patient as needed, and in many institutions a massive transfusion protocol (MTP) may be activated (see Chapter 6). The first step of an operation for hepatic trauma is to identify and attempt to stop hemorrhage. Upon opening the abdomen, a large amount of blood may be immediately evacuated. The anesthesia and surgical teams should be ready to address this through resuscitative efforts. Communication is key to catch up with the fluid and blood losses already present prior to arrival in the operating room.

Perihepatic packing is an effective and frequently used treatment for hepatic injury and is used to quickly gain control of hemorrhage. For this maneuver, the wound is compressed with a surgical sponge between the chest wall, diaphragm, and retroperitoneum. Earlier use of perihepatic packing has been associated with better survival rates.[8]

For more extensive hepatic injuries, other methods to achieve hemostasis are employed. Occasionally large sutures may be placed to approximate a bleeding wound. "Finger fracture" is a method by which large bleeding hepatic veins may be isolated. For this method, the surgeon carefully uses his or her finger to extend the hepatic wound until bleeding vessels can be clearly identified and ligated or repaired. If this method is employed, it is important to be aware that the process may at first cause increased bleeding before the repair is achieved.[4] For penetrating injuries, tamponade with a balloon or surgical packing may be used. In cases of severe injury to part of the liver, an emergent segmental resection may be performed. This method is employed when there is massive bleeding related to hepatic venous injury, massive parenchymal tissue destruction, or a major bile leak. It is most successful when undertaken by an experienced trauma or hepatobiliary surgeon.[9]

Shunting procedures are used in the repair of retrohepatic caval injury, and include an atrial–caval shunt, balloon shunt, or venovenous bypass. All share the same clinical goal of bypassing the injured retrohepatic vena cava and replacing blood into venous circulation. When there is a possibility of severe hepatic injury or retrohepatic caval injury, these procedures must be planned for early on. They often involve additional steps before the first incision is even made, such as preparing for thoracoabdominal exposure in the case of atrial–caval shunting, or assembling all necessary equipment for venovenous bypass.[10,11] Patients in need of these interventions will frequently already have experienced large amounts of hemorrhage and may already exhibit coagulopathy.

Extrahepatic injuries to the structures of the portal triad are extremely rare, accounting for just 0.07–0.2% of all traumas. However, these injuries carry a very high mortality rate, with only about 50% of patients surviving. Patients usually present in shock and should be treated by emergent laparotomy with hematoma evacuation and packing. Resuscitation and correction of coagulopathy play a large role in achieving hemostasis in these cases.[12]

There may be times when a patient's liver bleeding cannot be effectively controlled in the operating room. It may be very effective to quickly temporarily close the patient and transfer him or her to the angiography suite. The anesthesiologist may need to be prepared to assist with care and transfer of this patient in an expeditious manner.

Splenic trauma

The spleen is the second most frequently injured organ in abdominal trauma. As with hepatic injuries, a grading scale has been developed for injuries to the spleen (Table 31.2).[13]

Nonoperative management of splenic injury

Frequently splenic injuries are managed nonoperatively. This practice started in pediatric populations, who were commonly found to be hemodynamically stable following traumatic injury to the spleen. These populations had better clinical outcomes without any operative interventions. Nonoperative management has been found to be preferable to operative intervention in many adults as well. Guidelines from EAST state that "Nonoperative management of blunt splenic injuries is now the treatment modality of choice in hemodynamically stable patients, irrespective of the grade of injury, patient age, or the presence of associated injuries."[14] Hemodynamically stable patients typically have less severe injury in the case of splenic trauma.

In some instances, a patient who is initially hemodynamically stable may fail nonoperative management. This can occur in a patient who is hemodynamically stable upon presentation, but then becomes unstable. Other failed attempts at nonoperative management may occur in patients older than 55, who

Table 31.2 Splenic organ injury scaling system

I	Hematoma	Subcapsular, < 10% surface area
	Laceration	Capsular tear, < 1 cm deep
II	Hematoma	Subcapsular, 10–50% surface area, < 5 cm diameter
	Laceration	1–3 cm deep (not involving a trabecular vessel)
III	Hematoma	Subcapsular, > 50% surface area or expanding, ruptured subcapsular or parenchymal hematoma. Intraparecnchymal hematoma > 5 cm or expanding
	Laceration	> 3 cm deep or involving trabecular vessels
IV	Laceration	Involving segmental or hilar vessels producing major devascularization (> 25% of spleen)
V	Laceration	Completely shattered spleen
	Vascular	Hilar vascular injury that devascularizes spleen

Modified from http://www.trauma.org/archive/scores/ois-spleen.html (accessed April 2014).

require more than 4 units of blood transfusion, who have persistent leukocytosis, who exhibit peritonitis, who have worsening radiographic evidence of injury, or who have intraabdominal compartment syndrome.[15]

Operative management of splenic injury

Patients who exhibit hemodynamic instability following splenic trauma must undergo operative exploration. Some centers will pursue operative exploration in patients who have multisystem trauma, severe brain damage, another injury that is associated with the splenic lesion and may require operative repair, age greater than 55 years, or a previously diseased spleen. Some studies have demonstrated that up to 45% of patients with splenic trauma will require emergency surgery.[16] When preparing for operative intervention, it is important to be aware of the possibility of injury to structures surrounding the spleen. Most frequently, the diaphragm, stomach, small bowel, or pancreas may be concurrently injured. A nasogastric tube placed in preparation for surgery can be helpful in assessing for gastric injury. This also allows for better surgical exposure of the splenic anatomy and access to the short gastric vessels.

Primary repair of the spleen, or splenorrhaphy, while it rarely occurs, can be undertaken by several different methods. The spleen may be repaired by suturing closed a lacerated area. Often, electrocautery or argon beam cautery is used to stop bleeding from the injured parenchyma. Fibrin coagulation products may also be used for hemostasis. These methods are used for less severe splenic injuries, grades I–III. Splenectomy is performed in the hemodynamically unstable patient with a high-grade splenic injury, grade IV or V. The operative procedure begins by mobilizing the spleen and packing the retrosplenic area. When a splenectomy will be performed, control of the vasculature is achieved through ligation at the hilum. Occasionally, due to the segmental nature of splenic blood supply, a partial splenectomy may be performed, preserving some of the spleen's function. However, in this day and age the spleen is generally removed very quickly, and if this is the only source of bleeding the operation can be finished within an hour.

Hollow viscus injury: stomach and small bowel

Hollow viscus organs include the stomach and small bowel. These structures are commonly injured in penetrating traumas, with 80% of gunshot and 30% of stab wound victims presenting with injuries to the stomach or small intestine. According to EAST, 1.25% of all trauma admissions present with a hollow viscus injury.[17] Hollow viscus injuries occur less frequently with blunt trauma; however, they still make up one-third of all blunt abdominal trauma injuries that require operation. When a patient presents with a solid organ injury, the likelihood of a concurrent injury to the stomach or small intestine also rises. In general, suspicion or recognition of a hollow viscus injury necessitates operative exploration. In a hemodynamically stable patient, this operation will likely provide definitive injury repair. However, as discussed previously, a hemodynamically unstable patient may undergo a damage control procedure with future return to the operative suite for definitive injury repair.

Stomach

Injuries to the stomach occur with high-force mechanisms; therefore gastric injuries are frequently associated with additional severe intraabdominal injuries. These additional injuries are often the cause of an increased mortality seen with gastric injury.[18] Patients with gastric injury frequently exhibit signs of peritonitis on physical exam due to peritoneal irritation secondary to acidic gastric secretions. Blood in the gastric tube may be noted. A grading scale for stomach injuries is shown in Table 31.3.[19]

Table 31.3 Stomach injury scale

I	Contusion/hematoma Partial thickness laceration
II	Laceration in gastroesophageal junction or pylorus < 2 cm Laceration in proximal 1/3 stomach < 5 cm Laceration in distal 2/3 stomach < 10 cm
III	Laceration in gastroesophageal junction or pylorus > 2 cm Laceration in proximal 1/3 stomach ≥ 5 cm Laceration in distal 2/3 stomach ≥ 10 cm
IV	Tissue loss/devascularization < 2/3 stomach
V	Tissue loss/devascularization > 2/3 stomach

Modified from http://www.aast.org/library/traumatools/injuryscoringscales.aspx (accessed April 2014).

Operative intervention for gastric injury

There are several general considerations when beginning to operate for traumatic gastric injury. First, to improve operative exposure a nasogastric tube should be carefully placed. If return from the nasogastric tube contains sanguineous fluid, the operative team should have high suspicion for gastric injury. Second, when positioning the patient, a reverse Trendelenburg position can improve gastric exposure and exposure of the surrounding area to better assess injuries. Finally, if a diaphragmatic injury is identified there is a risk of gastric content contamination of the pleural space, which will require evacuation. The team may need to prepare for a thoracotomy to wash out the pleural space, or alternatively may place a thoracostomy tube to allow the gastric fluids to drain. Less frequently, the diaphragmatic injury may need to be extended to allow better irrigation and cleaning of the contaminated area.[20]

Gastric injuries are treated according to their severity. Grade I and II injuries are repaired primarily with evacuation of a hematoma if present and primary closure of the laceration. Grade III injuries are also closed primarily; however, due to the size of these injuries they may be stapled rather than hand-sewn. Grade IV injures may require a partial gastrectomy. In the case of severe grade V injuries, a total gastrectomy with Roux-en-Y esophagojejunostomy may be required.[19] As a general principle, whenever an anterior gastric wound is present, the surgeon must carefully examine the stomach to ascertain the presence of a posterior wound. The anesthesiologist may help with this by providing insufflation through the nasogastric tube.

Small bowel

While the small bowel is the organ most commonly injured after penetrating abdominal trauma, blunt injuries to the small intestine are uncommon, with only 0.3% of all blunt trauma admissions having small bowel perforation.[21] Injuries to the small bowel can prove difficult to diagnose with current imaging modalities. The likelihood of small bowel injury increases with the presence of other intraabdominal injuries to solid organs, with a higher incidence found with concurrent liver or colon injury.[22] Intraluminal contents of the small bowel vary with anatomic location, with proximal small bowel fluid relatively sterile and with similar bacterial species to those found within gastric secretions. The bacterial content of small bowel contents increases and its speciation changes with distance from the pylorus. In the ileum and jejunum the bacterial content increases to 10^5–10^8 CFU/mL of Gram-negative and Gram-positive species. This should be considered when making perioperative antibiotic decisions. A grading scale for small bowel injuries is shown in Table 31.4.[19]

Operative intervention for small bowel injury

The type of surgical intervention will be based upon the degree of small bowel injury. In a stable patient definitive repair is performed at the time of presentation with the necessary

Table 31.4 Small bowel injury scale

I	Hematoma	Contusion/hematoma without devascularization
	Laceration	Partial wall thickness, no perforation
II	Laceration	Less than 50% of circumference
III	Laceration	Greater than 50% of circumference
IV	Laceration	Transection of small bowel
V	Laceration	Transection of small bowel with segmental tissue loss
	Vascular	Devascularized segment of small bowel

Modified from http://www.aast.org/library/traumatools/injuryscoringscales.aspx (accessed April 2014).

Table 31.5 Duodenal injury scale

I	Hematoma involving single portion of duodenum Partial thickness laceration without perforation
II	Hematoma involving more than one portion Laceration with disruption < 50% of circumference
III	Laceration with 50–75% disruption circumference of D2 Laceration with 50–100% disruption circumference of D1, D3, D4
IV	Laceration with > 75% disruption circumference of D2 Involving ampulla or distal common bile duct
V	Massive disruption/laceration of duodenopancreatic complex Devascularization of duodenum

Modified from http://www.aast.org/library/traumatools/injuryscoringscales.aspx (accessed April 2014).

complete surgical interventions. However, some patients present hemodynamically unstable, acidotic, or coagulopathic; in these cases the entire surgical team must be prepared to set up quickly and expeditiously complete the procedure. In all cases of small bowel injury it is helpful to decompress the small bowel through the placement of a nasogastric tube. After opening the abdomen, the entire length of small bowel is carefully examined for injury. Any mesenteric injuries are also noted, and bleeding vessels may be clamped.[23]

Grade I injuries are repaired primarily by suture repair of serosal tears or inversion of small hematomas. Grade II lesions, laceration of less than 50% of the small bowel circumference, are debrided and closed primarily. Resection is usually not recommended, even in cases with multiple small bowel perforations, unless it would be a more expeditious procedure than primary repair.[19] Grade III and IV injuries, when the small intestine is transected by more the 50% of its circumference or completely transected, are repaired through surgical resection and anastomosis. In some cases, the mesentery must also be resected and repaired. With grade V injury, causing devascularization to a segment of small bowel, the entire segment must be resected to viable tissue along with mesentery, and the bowel and mesentery surgically anastomosed.

In unstable patients with severe injury, damage control principles are employed to control bleeding and provide simple, temporizing repairs. These patients are left with an open abdominal wound to complete resuscitative efforts in an intensive care setting. They are then returned to the operating room in 24–48 hours for further intervention.

Retroperitoneal structures: duodenum and pancreas

Traumatic injury to the retroperitoneal structures of the duodenum and pancreas is a rare occurrence, as these organs are located in a protected area behind the peritoneum and abdominal structures. Injury is observed most frequently in penetrating trauma or with a direct and forceful insult to the region, such as a crush injury seen in a motor vehicle collision (MVC).[24] The pancreas and duodenum are rarely injured in

isolation: because of their anatomic proximity these organs are frequently both injured at one time. Furthermore, the incidence of injury to these organs increases with other intraabdominal injuries, and worse outcomes are observed when other organs are damaged. Concomitant splenic injury in particular contributes to worse morbidity and mortality outcomes.[25] An additional difficulty in assessing retroperitoneal injuries is their location which may "wall off" damage or the spillage of fluid, causing delayed development of peritoneal and systemic signs and potentially a delay in diagnosis. Obesity can further complicate the case making exposure even more difficult.

Operative management of duodenal injury

Table 31.5 shows a grading scale for duodenal injury.[26] The extent of operative intervention required for duodenal injury will depend on the nature of the injury. Nasogastric decompression should be performed at the beginning of the operation.

After abdominal entry, the duodenum will be exposed through a Kocher maneuver, which involves medial reflection of the hepatic flexure of the colon from its lateral attachments toward the midline, followed by mobilization of the C-loop of the duodenum from the retroperitoneum. The entire duodenum should then be visually inspected.

A grade I hematoma is managed nonoperatively with nasogastric decompression and bowel rest. This injury does not require operative intervention unless nonoperative management fails. A grade I or II laceration must be repaired operatively, with simple suture approximation and repair. Grade III injury, greater than 50% circumferential disruption, can usually be managed with primary duodenorrhaphy. However, if the second part of the duodenum distal to the ampulla is injured, a more extensive repair will be required, usually a Roux-en-Y duodenojejunostomy or an end-to-end duodenojejunostomy.[26]

Grade IV and V duodenal injuries are complicated and often involve complex intraoperative decision making. Grade

Table 31.6 Pancreatic injury scale

I	Major contusion/hematoma without duct injury or tissue loss Major laceration without duct injury or tissue loss
II	Hematoma involving more than one portion Disruption/laceration < 50% of circumference
III	Distal transection of parenchymal injury with duct injury
IV	Proximal (to right of superior mesenteric vein) transection or parenchymal injury
V	Massive disruption of pancreatic head

Modified from http://www.aast.org/library/traumatools/injuryscoringscales.aspx (accessed April 2014).

IV injuries, which involve the ampulla or common bile duct, have several operative repair options: (1) pancreatoduodenectomy, (2) reimplantation of the ampulla or distal common bile duct into a Roux-en-Y limb of jejunum, (3) reimplantation of the common bile duct into the duodenum or primary anastomosis of the common bile duct. A final and frequently required approach to severe grade IV injury is delayed reconstruction. This approach is also used as the first step in management of grade V injuries, or devascularization of the duodenum or severe disruption of the duodenal–pancreatic complex, when the injury is often best managed through an abbreviated damage control procedure with planned take-back for further reconstruction in 24–48 hours.[27]

Operative management of pancreatic injury

Traumatic injury to the pancreas provides a particular challenge to the surgeon. The management of these injuries is evolving, particularly in low-grade, blunt injuries. A grading scale for pancreatic injuries is shown in Table 31.6.[26] Recent studies have found that it may be safe to manage grade I or II injuries nonoperatively.[28] In these cases it is important to ensure that there is no disruption to the main pancreatic duct, and therefore endoscopic retrograde cholangio-pancreatogram (ERCP) or magnetic retrograde cholangio-pancreatogram (MRCP) may be performed to investigate ductal involvement. When a grade I or II pancreatic injury is discovered intraoperatively, surgical hemostasis with drain placement is usually sufficient treatment.

Grade III injuries, distal injuries with ductal disruption, are managed based on the amount of pancreatic tissue involved. With a distal injury involving the duct, a distal pancreatectomy can be performed if 50% of the pancreas will remain to preserve organ function. A grade IV injury with more proximal involvement of the duct is often managed in a similar fashion with resection of damaged tissue and oversewing of the duct and damaged tissue. Rarely, a Roux-en-Y pancreaticojejunostomy will be performed to preserve distal pancreatic tissue function if otherwise less than 20% of pancreatic tissue would remain.

Grade V injuries, which involve massive disruption of the pancreatic head, are especially challenging. In centers with staff who are trained in the procedure and with a patient whose clinical status will support an extended operative time, it has been shown that a pancreaticoduodenectomy, or Whipple procedure, can be performed at the time of trauma with outcomes similar to elective procedures.[29] However, because high-grade pancreatic injuries are frequently accompanied by other severe traumatic injuries, these patients are frequently unstable. It has been shown that in such patients a damage control approach may be safest, with definitive operation performed after the patient is adequately resuscitated.[30]

Injury to both duodenum and pancreas

Because of their anatomic proximity, the duodenum and pancreas are frequently both injured by the same traumatic event. The degree of injury to each organ will determine what interventions are performed. Low-grade injuries to both organs can be managed with operative debridement, hemostasis, and drainage. When there is an intermediate degree of injury to the duodenum with concurrent injury to the pancreas, the pyloric exclusion procedure is usually performed to protect the healing duodenum.[27] However, some recent studies have begun to question this practice, and surgical recommendations may be changing. High-grade injuries, as discussed above, may require more extensive operative intervention or damage control procedures. It should be noted that concurrent pancreas and duodenal injury significantly increases the complication and mortality rates for these patients.[26]

Colon and rectum injury

Most colon and rectal trauma occurs secondary to penetrating injury, with gunshot wounds being the most frequent cause. Such injuries are observed rarely in blunt trauma, and are usually secondary to high-impact blunt trauma when they do occur. One of the most important considerations in both colon and rectal trauma is antibiotic coverage, due to the heavy organismal load of these structures. Coverage of both aerobes and anaerobes should be accounted for, especially *E. coli* and *B. fragilis*. It has been shown that inadequate antibiotic coverage is an independent risk factor for intraabdominal sepsis in these cases. Current recommendations are that monotherapy can provide adequate coverage, and that it should be continued for no more than 24 hours, in the absence of established peritonitis.[31]

Patient positioning is also an important perioperative consideration. In cases of suspected rectal injury, preoperative preparation for lithotomy position or conversion to supine position may be necessary for improved surgical access. These maneuvers will require the assistance of all operative suite team members.

Table 31.7 Colon injury scale

I	(a) Contusion or hematoma without devascularization
	(b) Partial-thickness laceration
II	Laceration < 50% of circumference
III	Laceration > 50% of circumference
IV	Transection of the colon
V	Transection of the colon with segmental tissue loss

Modified from http://www.aast.org/library/traumatools/injuryscoringscales. aspx (accessed April 2014).

Colon injury

While grading scales for colonic injury have been developed, as for many other organs, in practice colonic injury is divided into two categories that direct surgical management: (1) non-destructive injury, involving less than 50% of the bowel wall without devascularization, and (2) destructive injury, involving greater than 50% of colon circumference, complete transection of colon, significant tissue loss, or devascularization of a segment of colon.[32] These clinical classifications correspond with the American Association for the Surgery of Trauma (AAST) scale, with grades I and II corresponding to nondestructive injury, and grades III–V comprising destructive injury (Table 31.7).[33]

Operative intervention for colon injury

Patients with nondestructive colon injuries should undergo primary repair of the injury without need for diversion. Patients with destructive colon injury will require colon resection and anastomosis unless they are in shock. The anatomic boundaries of resection and anastomosis will depend on the injury location. In patients with significant comorbid disease or a high transfusion requirement, anastomosis with diversion has been shown to be beneficial in preventing complications of suture line failure and intraabdominal abscess.[32] Prior to abdominal closure all patients should undergo abdominal washout.

Operative management of rectal trauma

Most distinctions in the operative management of rectal injuries are based on anatomic location. Intraperitoneal rectal injuries, involving the anterior and lateral upper two-thirds of the rectum, are generally managed in the same manner as colon injuries, due to their similarity to the left colon. These injuries frequently can be repaired primarily. Extraperitoneal injuries can occasionally be repaired. However, many of these injuries are inaccessible for this type of repair, and in these cases proximal diversion provides appropriate management and allows for the injury to heal without fecal contamination. In the past, presacral drainage and rectal washout was commonly performed intraoperatively. These practices, however, have

been called into question in some recent studies, and should be used selectively.[32,34] The surgical team must also be aware that many rectal injuries are accompanied by regional vascular injury, especially of the iliac vessels, or by bladder injury.

Abdominal vascular trauma

Patients suffering from trauma to the abdominal vasculature present frequently, with the most common sites of major abdominal hemorrhage coming from the viscera, mesentery, and the great vessels. In nearly 25% of gunshot wounds to the abdomen, a major vessel will be injured.[35] The incidence is approximately half as frequent in blunt abdominal trauma and stab injuries. In blunt injuries, vessels may be damaged by deceleration or crush injuries. These injuries present with vessel avulsion, complete vessel disruption, or intimal tearing with possible luminal thrombosis. Penetrating injuries can cause complete transection of the vessel, resulting in hemorrhage or vessel thrombosis. Less frequently a hematoma or arteriovenous fistula may form. When the penetrating injury results from a gunshot, an intimal flap may form within the vessel, resulting in thrombosis.[36] Vascular injuries are classified by anatomic zone, with specific operative interventions and considerations for each zone.

General operative considerations

Patients presenting with abdominal vascular trauma are frequently unstable and may have already lost large amounts of blood from the intravascular space prior to arrival in the operating room. Therefore, one of the most important determinants of outcome is the time from presentation to operation. It is of utmost importance that the surgical, anesthesia, and other teams work together to minimize this time.[37] There are many other perioperative considerations when caring for a patient with intraabdominal vascular injury. The patient will be "prepped" in a sterile fashion from chin to knees to allow for many potential operative interventions. It is also important to be sure that necessary blood products are readily available, and an MTP should be activated (see Chapter 6), or an auto-transfusion device prepared for intraoperative use. Because of the risk of hypothermia-induced coagulopathy, warming considerations are mandatory (see Chapter 14). The operating room should be warmed ($\geq$ 29 °C), and convective warming applied. All fluids and blood products should be warmed. A nasogastric tube, thoracostomy tubes, and body cavities may be irrigated with warm saline to increase body temperature. Some centers practice a low threshold for thoracotomy and aortic crossclamping. This procedure may be initiated in a patient with systolic blood pressure less than 70 mmHg, in an effort to maintain cerebral and coronary perfusion. However, in patients whose shock is not responsive to this maneuver, further operative intervention is considered futile.[38]

After opening the abdomen through a large midline incision, a rapid visual inspection is performed. Free blood and clots are evacuated, and any obvious bleeding is controlled with the packing of solid organs, or temporary clamping of bleeding vessels. Repair is deferred until all injuries are identified.

Zone 1 injury

Zone 1 includes the great vessels found in the anatomic midline. It is subdivided into two regions: the supramesocolic zone 1 and inframesocolic zone 1.

Zone 1: supramesocolic region

The supramesocolic zone 1 includes the suprarenal aorta, celiac axis, superior mesenteric artery, proximal renal arteries, and superior mesenteric vein. When operating in this zone, the surgeon will begin by gaining proximal control of the aorta at the diaphragmatic hiatus. Access to the aorta is obtained by reflecting all left-sided viscera. However, the operative team should be aware of a possible hyperfibrinolytic state that may occur when the aorta is crossclamped. It is thought that this occurs secondary to hepatic hypoperfusion, and it should be carefully monitored.

Patients with aortic injury have predictably low survival outcomes, between 21% and 50% in various studies.[35] Puncture wounds to the aorta may be primarily repaired by suture. However, more severe injuries may require resection of the injured vessel with grafting. If this is required, aortic bypass will need to be performed. The anesthesia team should be aware of the risk of lower-extremity compartment syndrome, which can occur with crossclamping of the aorta and subsequent reperfusion of the lower extremities after unclamping. Lower-extremity compartment pressures may need to be monitored in these cases.

Injuries to the celiac axis and superior mesenteric artery and vein are rare and mortality is high. When the celiac axis is damaged, primary repair should be performed. If simple repair is not possible, the artery should be ligated. Any damaged branches should likewise be ligated.[39] Depending on the nature of the injury to the superior mesenteric artery, this vessel may be repaired primarily or a graft may be used. For damage control a shunt may be left in place. When the superior mesenteric vein is injured, it can frequently be sutured for primary repair. However, it can also successfully be ligated.[35]

Zone 1: inframesocolic region

The vessels in the inframesocolic region of zone 1 include the infrarenal abdominal aorta and the inferior vena cava. Exposure of vessels in this region requires reflection of left-sided viscera and evisceration of the small bowel with opening of the retroperitoneum. The inferior vena cava can usually be repaired primarily after exposure of the injury. If the vena cava is clamped for control, the operative teams should be aware of the potential development of right heart strain. In younger patients with uncontrollable vena cava injury, the vessel can be ligated. When the vena cava is ligated, the patient should be monitored for the development of lower-extremity compartment syndrome. Generally, operative teams are able to achieve survival rates close to 70% for patients with vena cava injury. Injury to the infrarenal aorta is managed with techniques similar to those used for the suprarenal aorta.

Zone 2 injury

The vessels encountered in zone 2 include the renal arteries and veins. Renal artery injury is repaired primarily if possible. However, if there are multiple injuries to the artery, concurrent severe kidney injury, or long kidney ischemic time, a nephrectomy may be performed. Occasionally, the kidney may be salvaged through autotransplantation, but this is seldom indicated. Endovascular repair is also becoming a more commonly used intervention for renal artery repair. The renal vein can be a source of significant hemorrhage with a penetrating injury. However, with blunt trauma it is not uncommon for bleeding from a renal vein injury to tamponade within the retroperitoneum. Venorrhaphy should be performed if possible. If the surgeon is unable to achieve repair, a nephrectomy is a viable option.[35]

Zone 3 injury

Zone 3 contains the common, external, and internal iliac arteries and veins within the pelvic retroperitoneum. These vessels are most commonly injured with penetrating trauma or severe pelvic fracture. Common or external iliac artery injuries should be repaired or shunted if possible, as ligation will lead to ipsilateral lower-extremity ischemia. The iliac veins should be repaired by suturing if possible; however, ligation of these vessels is generally well tolerated if required. Fecal contamination is a common problem when repairing the iliac vessels, occasionally requiring that the vessel be shunted or ligated until fecal contamination is cleared and the vessel can be repaired by synthetic graft placement.

Porta hepatis injury

The structures found within the porta hepatis include the portal vein, hepatic artery, and common bile duct. When a hematoma is found in this region, the Pringle maneuver is performed by controlling the proximal hepatoduodenal ligament with a tape or clamp prior to exploring the injured area. Hepatic artery injuries are extremely rare; however, when the hepatic artery is injured, ligation is generally well tolerated to control the injury. Injuries to the portal vein are more difficult to control because of its posterior location, fragile vessel wall, and high blood volume. Venorrhaphy is the preferred repair technique. Other methods that can be used when primary anastomosis is not possible include grafting, transposition of the splenic vein, portacaval shunt creation, or venovenous shunt creation with the superior mesenteric vein. In a damage control procedure, it is possible to ligate the portal vein with patient survival.

Endovascular repair

Endovascular techniques have recently begun to be applied in traumatic injury to abdominal vasculature. This is an area of growing interest, and will likely have a greater role in the future.

Summary

The abdomen is frequently injured in trauma, making it an important area for surgical intervention. While nonoperative approaches have been found to be superior in some types of solid organ injury, the trauma laparotomy remains a mainstay of operative care.

The liver is the most frequently injured abdominal organ, and treatment of traumatic hepatic injuries ranges from non-operative management to resection or venous shunting procedures. Likewise, many splenic injuries may be managed nonoperatively in stable patients; however, splenectomy for injury to the organ is commonly performed. Hollow viscus, stomach, or intestinal injuries are repaired based on degree of injury. This may range from primary repair to resection. The retroperitoneal duodenum and pancreas provide a particular operative challenge, and can require complex surgical repairs.

Abdominal vascular injuries are identified by anatomic region. Repair focuses on injury identification and hemorrhage control. Vascular injuries frequently have a high mortality rate.

In all cases of abdominal trauma, it is important to maintain good communication between anesthetic and surgical teams, as the patient may have a sudden change in status or newly discovered injury. In these cases, all people working in the operative suite will have important roles in resuscitation and injury management.

Questions

(1) The stages of damage control laparotomy for trauma include:
   a. Abbreviated resuscitative surgery to control hemorrhage and abdominal contamination; intensive care resuscitation; definitive surgical intervention at a later time
   b. Abbreviated resuscitative surgery to control hemorrhage and abdominal contamination; observation on a regular nursing floor; repeat surgical exploration
   c. Expeditious abdominal wound exploration with definitive repair of all damaged structures
   d. Resuscitation in intensive care unit until patient is stable to undergo complete operative repair of all injuries
   e. Using smaller incision techniques for trauma laparotomy to minimize further tissue damage

(2) A 24-year-old man presents to the emergency department after a motor vehicle collision. He is found to have a 2 cm liver laceration in the left hepatic lobe. On presentation, vital signs are HR 88, BP 110/76, RR 16, O_2 saturation 98%. A repeat set of vitals after 1 hour is HR 89, BP 112/83, RR 15, O_2 saturation 99%. Which of the following is the best course of management for this patient's injuries?
   a. Exploratory laparotomy and segmental hepatic resection
   b. Laparoscopy with suture repair of laceration for hemostatsis
   c. Admit to intensive care unit for hemodynamic monitoring; an operation may be required if the patient develops hemodynamic instability
   d. Discharge the patient home with follow-up in gastroenterology clinic the following day
   e. Transfuse fresh frozen plasma to prevent hepatic hemorrhage from developing

(3) A pediatric patient who is hemodynamically stable and has a low-grade splenic injury should:
   a. Promptly receive vaccination for pneumococcus and meningococcus
   b. Be managed nonoperatively, unless the patient becomes hemodynamically unstable
   c. Have scheduled serial abdominal imaging to ensure that the splenic injury does not worsen
   d. Be evaluated by hematology consultant given concern for new onset of immunodeficiency
   e. Be evaluated for possible partial spleen autotransplantation

(4) A patient who presents following traumatic injury and is found to have a solid organ injury:
   a. Has a higher likelihood of also having a hollow viscus injury
   b. Requires immediate operative repair
   c. Should be given red blood cell transfusion immediately on presentation as the patient likely lost a large amount of blood
   d. Is unlikely to require inpatient care if he/she is stable on presentation
   e. Should undergo serial FAST exams to assess for intraabdominal hemorrhage

(5) When preparing a patient with abdominal gunshot wounds and suspected gastric injury for operation, it is important to place a nasogastric tube for which of the following reasons?
   a. Because return of bloody fluid provides further evidence of gastric injury, providing information to the operative team and allowing for better operative planning
   b. A nasogastric tube can be used to help identify the anatomy of the stomach and surrounding area
   c. Insufflation of the nasogastric tube provides a means of identifying gastric injury
   d. Both (a) and (c)
   e. All are correct

(6) In the instance of traumatic injury to the small bowel:
  a. It is unlikely that any other intraabdominal structures will be injured
  b. Serosal tears or small hematomas should be repaired primarily by suturing
  c. Mesenteric injuries can be observed due to the extensive small intestine collateral blood supply
  d. All injuries to the small intestine should be definitively repaired on the first trip to the operating room, even in an unstable patient, because of the risk of bacterial contamination
  e. The small intestine is relatively sterile, so perioperative antibiotics are rarely needed

(7) When managing a traumatic injury to the pancreas, the surgeon should:
  a. Proceed to perform a Whipple procedure for definitive repair of any injury
  b. Ensure that there is no injury to the pancreatic duct by either ERCP or MRCP prior to choosing a nonoperative treatment strategy
  c. Perform a distal pancreatectomy
  d. Not consider any concomitant duodenal injuries in his/her operative plan, as these structures have little effect on one another
  e. Plan for nonoperative management in nearly all cases

(8) A patient presents to the emergency department following a gunshot wound involving her rectum. When considering perioperative antibiotics you will be certain to provide broad-spectrum coverage, including coverage for these two most commonly found organisms:
  a. *E. coli* and *B. fragilis*
  b. *E. coli* and *C. dificile*
  c. *E. coli* and *S. aureus*
  d. *S. aureus* and *S. pneumoniae*
  e. *C. perfringens* and anaerobes

(9) When caring for a patient with hemorrhage secondary to abdominal vascular trauma, one should:
  a. Keep the patient's body temperature slightly hypothermic to prevent neurologic sequela
  b. Not use a nasogastric tube, as no hollow viscus has been injured
  c. Only prep the injured area, as a wide sterile prep will waste valuable time
  d. Avoid using warming devices
  e. Notify the blood bank, or follow other pertinent hospital procedures, to obtain large amount of blood products rapidly

(10) Which of the following is true regarding injury to abdominal vasculature?
  a. The zone 2 vessels include the aorta and inferior vena cava
  b. The Pringle maneuver involves compressing the gastric pylorus to prevent gastric content spillage
  c. Endovascular techniques should never be used in trauma
  d. In a young, healthy, patient the iliac vein may be ligated to achieve control of bleeding, and this is generally well tolerated
  e. When the vena cava is clamped for control of hemorrhage, one must be cautious of the development of left heart strain

Answers

(1) a
(2) c
(3) b
(4) a
(5) e
(6) b
(7) b
(8) a
(9) e
(10) d

References

1. Hershberg A. Chapter 27. Trauma laparotomy: principles and techniques. In Mattox KL, Moore EE, Feliciano DV, eds., *Trauma*, 7th edition. New York, NY: McGraw-Hill, 2013.

2. Shapiro M, Jenkins D, Schwab CW, *et al.* Damage control: collective review. *J Trauma* 2000; **49**: 969–78.

3. Villavicencio R, Aucar J. Analysis of laparoscopy in trauma. *J Am Coll Surg* 1999; **189**: 11–20.

4. Fabian TC, Bee TK. Chapter 29. Liver and biliary tract. In Mattox KL, Moore EE, Feliciano DV, eds., *Trauma*, 7th edition. New York, NY: McGraw-Hill, 2013.

5. Malhotra AK, Fabian TC, Croce MA, *et al.* Blunt hepatic injury: a paradigm shift from operative to nonoperative management in the 1990s. *Ann Surg* 2000; **231**: 804–13.

6. Croce MA, Fabian TC, Menke PG, *et al.* Nonoperative management of blunt hepatic trauma is the treatment of choice for hemodynamically stable patients. *Ann Surg* 1995; **221**: 744–55.

7. Stassen NA, Bhullar I, Cheng JD, *et al.* Non-operative management of blunt hepatic injury: an Eastern Association for the Surgery of Trauma practice management guideline. *J Trauma* 2012; **73**: S288–93.

8. Caruso DM, Battistella FD, Owings JT, *et al.* Perihepatic packing of major liver injuries. *Arch Surg* 1999; **134**: 958–63.

9. Palanco P, Leon S, Pineda J, *et al.* Hepatic resection in the management of complex injury to the liver. *J Trauma* 2008; **65**: 1264–9.

10. Richardson JD, Franklin GA, Lukan JK, *et al.* Evolution in the management of hepatic trauma: a 25-year perspective. *Ann Surgery*. 2000; **232**: 324–30.

11. Schrock T, Blaisdell W, Mathewson C, *et al.* Management of blunt trauma to

the liver and hepatic veins. *Arch Surg* 1968; **96**: 698–704.

12. Jurkovich GJ, Hoyt DB, Moore FA, *et al.* Portal triad injuries. *J Trauma* 1995; **39**: 426–34.

13. Wisner DH. Chapter 30. Injury to the spleen. In Mattox KL, Moore EE, Feliciano DV, eds., *Trauma*, 7th edition. New York, NY: McGraw-Hill, 2013.

14. Stassen NA, Bhullar I, Cheng JD, *et al.* Selective nonoperative management of blunt splenic injury: an Eastern Association for the Surgery of Trauma practice management guideline. *J Trauma* 2012; **73**: S294–300.

15. Beuran M, Gheju I, Venter MD, *et al.* Non-operative management of splenic trauma. *J Medicine and Life*. 2012; **1**: 47–58.

16. Harbrecht BG, Peitzman AB, Rivera L, *et al.* Contribution of age and gender to outcome of blunt splenic injury in adults: multicenter study of the Eastern Association for the Surgery of Trauma. *J Trauma* 2001; **51**: 887–95.

17. Watts DD, Fakhry SM. Incidence of hollow viscus injury in blunt trauma: an analysis from 257,557 trauma admissions from the East multi-institutional trial. *J Trauma* 2003; **54**: 289–94.

18. Bruscagin V, Coimbra R, Rasslan S, *et al.* Blunt gastric injury. A multicentre experience. *Injury*. 2001; **32**: 761–4.

19. Diebel LN. Chapter 31. Stomach and small bowel. In Mattox KL, Moore EE, Feliciano DV, eds., *Trauma*, 7th edition. New York, NY: McGraw-Hill, 2013.

20. Coimbra R, Pinto MCC, Aguiar JR, Rasslan S. Factors related to the occurance of postoperative complications following penetrating gastric injuries. *Injury*. 1995; **26**: 463–6.

21. Fakhry SM, Watts DD, Luchette FA, *et al.* Current diagnostic approaches lack sensitivity in the diagnosis of perforated blunt small bowel injury: analysis from 275,557 trauma from the EAST multi-institutional HVI trial. *J Trauma* 2003; **54**: 295–306.

22. Hackam DJ, Ali J, Jastaniah S, *et al.* Effects of other intra-abdominal injuries on the diagnosis, management, and outcome of small bowel trauma. *J Trauma* 2000; **49**: 606–10.

23. Guarino J, Hassett JM, Luchette FA. Small bowel injuries: mechanisms, patterns, and outcome. *J Trauma* 1995; **39**: 1076–80.

24. Degiannis E, Boffard K. Duodenal injuries. *Br J Surg* 2000; **87**: 1473–9.

25. Blocksom JM, Tyburski JG, Sohn RL, *et al.* Prognostic determinants in duodenal injuries. *Am Surg* 2004; **70**: 248–55.

26. Biffl WL. Chapter 32. Duodenum and pancreas. In Mattox KL, Moore EE, Feliciano DV, eds., *Trauma*, 7th edition. New York, NY: McGraw-Hill, 2013.

27. Carillo EH, Richardson JD, Miller FB. Evolution in the management of duodenal injuries. *J Trauma* 1996; **40**: 1037–46.

28. Duchesne JC, Schmieg R, Islam S, *et al.* Selective nonoperative management of low-grade blunt pancreatic injury: are we there yet? *J Trauma* 2008; **65**: 49–53.

29. Asensio JA, Petrone P, Roldan G, *et al.* Pancreaticoduodenectomy: a rare procedure for the management of complex pancreaticoduodenal injuries. *Am Coll Surg* 2003; **197**: 937–42.

30. Seamon MJ, Kim PK, Stawicki SP, *et al.* Pancreatic injury in damage control laparotomies: is pancreatic resection safe during the initial laparotomy? *Injury* 2009; **40**: 61–5.

31. Demetriades D, Murray J, Chan L, *et al.* Penetrating colon injuries requiring resection: diversion or primary anastomosis? An AAST prospective multicenter study. *J Trauma* 2001; **50**: 765–75

32. Sharpe JP, Magnotti LJ, Weinberg JA, *et al.* Adherence to a simplified management algorithm reduces morbidity and mortality after penetrating colon injuries: a 15-year experience. *J Am Coll Surg* 2012; **214**: 591–7.

33. Demetriades D, Inaba K. Chapter 33. Colon and rectal trauma. In Mattox KL, Moore EE, Feliciano DV, eds., *Trauma*, 7th edition. New York, NY: McGraw-Hill, 2013.

34. McGrath V, Fabian TC, Croce MA, *et al.* Rectal trauma: management based on anatomic distinctions. *Am Surg* 1998; **64**: 1136–41.

35. Asensio JA, Chahwan S, Hanpeter D, *et al.* Operative management and outcome of 302 abdominal vascular injuries. *Am J Surg* 2001; **180**: 528–33.

36. Feliciano DV, Dente CJ. Chapter 34. Abdominal vascular injury. In Mattox KL, Moore EE, Feliciano DV, eds., *Trauma*, 7th edition. New York, NY: McGraw-Hill, 2013.

37. Cushman JG, Feliciano DV, Renz BM, *et al.* Iliac vessel injury: operative physiology related to outcome. *J Trauma* 1997; **42**: 1033–40.

38. Wiencek RG, Wilson RF. Injuries to the abdominal vascular system: how much does aggressive resuscitation and prelaparotomy thoracotomy really help? *Surgery* 1987; **102**: 731–6.

39. Asensio JA, Petrone P, Kimbrell B, *et al.* Lessons learned in the management of thirteen celiac axis injuries. *South Med J* 2005; **98**: 462–6.

Chapter

32

Anesthetic considerations for abdominal trauma

Henry G. Chou and William C. Wilson

Objectives

(1) Review the anesthetic management of abdominal trauma, including considerations for resuscitation, preoperative preparation, intraoperative management, and acute postoperative care.
(2) Discuss the anesthetic and surgical implications of specific abdominal organ injuries.
(3) Describe the principles of nonoperative management of abdominal trauma.

Introduction

The abdomen is frequently injured following trauma, is a major site for posttraumatic bleeding, and is difficult to evaluate and monitor clinically. Furthermore, uncontrolled hemorrhage is the major acute cause of death immediately following abdominal trauma.[1] Therefore, patients often present to the operating room for exploratory laparotomy following acute abdominal trauma.

The abdomen is aptly named, having been derived from the Latin terms *abdere*, "to hide," and *omen*, which may be a contraction of omentum or omen in the sense of presage (insight was said to be gained by the ancients during inspection of the abdominal contents). The term first appeared in the English literature in 1541 in a translation of Galen's *Terapeutyke*, as l'abdomen.[2]

This chapter describes the anesthetic management of abdominal trauma, including the resuscitation considerations, preoperative preparation, intraoperative management, and acute postoperative care.

Anatomic considerations

The mechanism of injury and wound location assists the clinician in predicting the organs injured, magnitude of blood loss, and expected scope of surgery (see Chapter 31). The abdomen can be divided into four anatomic compartments (Table 32.1); thoracic, peritoneal (true abdomen), retroperitoneal, and pelvic spaces. Clinical evaluation of these spaces is difficult by physical examination alone, especially in the acute trauma patient.

The intrathoracic abdomen lies beneath the rib cage and includes the diaphragm, liver, spleen, and stomach. Surface anatomical landmarks demarcating the intrathoracic abdomen include the region between the inframammary crease and the costal margin. During exhalation (with both spontaneous breathing and positive-pressure ventilation), the diaphragm often ascends to the third thoracic vertebra. Thus, a high association of intraabdominal injury occurs in patients with concomitant blunt or penetrating thoracic trauma.

The hollow viscera (stomach, small and large bowel) are almost completely contained within the true abdomen, as is the omentum, gravid uterus, and the dome of the bladder (when full of urine). At the end of inhalation (during both spontaneous and positive-pressure ventilation), the liver and spleen are pushed inferiorly by the diaphragm into the true abdomen.

The pelvic abdomen is surrounded by the bony pelvis. Fractures and other trauma to the pelvis can injure these contents (Table 32.1). The bony surroundings of the pelvis make diagnosis of injuries difficult without additional procedures. Pelvic fractures often result in significant retroperitoneal hemorrhage (see Chapters 27 and 28).

The retroperitoneal abdomen contains the great vessels, kidneys, ureters, pancreas, the second and third portions of the duodenum, and some segments of the colon. Ongoing hemorrhage (e.g., injury to great vessels, kidneys, etc.) or contamination from a missed injury to a hollow viscus represent the greatest concern following injury to the retroperitoneal structures. Aortic and caval injuries typically present with hemorrhagic shock, whereas renal, pancreatic, and duodenal injuries can manifest several days following the trauma as subsequent renal insufficiency, pancreatitis, or infection.

Classification of injuries

Accurate categorization of abdominal injury expedites workup and improves intraoperative management. Categorization into blunt versus penetrating trauma has traditionally been used for predicting likelihood of structures injured, for determining the most appropriate diagnostic modality, and for predicting morbidity and mortality.

Table 32.1 Anatomic compartments of the abdomen, organs contained, recommended order of diagnostic studies, and perioperative considerations

Abdominal compartment	Organs contained	Diagnostic exam	Perioperative considerations
Intrathoracic abdomen	Diaphragm	CXR, CT	Possible thoracic injury
	Liver	CT, US, DPL	Bleeding, coagulopathy
	Spleen	CT, US, DPL	Bleeding, sepsis
	Stomach, first part of duodenum	CXR (free air), CT	Peritoneal soiling
Pelvic abdomen	Urethra	RUG	No Foley until after RUG
	Bladder	Cystogram	Urine output may be misleading
	Rectum	Rectosigmoidoscopy	Peritoneal soiling
	Small intestine	CT (with oral contrast)	Increased fluid loss
	Uterus, tubes, ovaries	CT (shield if gravid), US	Bleeding, fetal demise, infertility (late complication)
Retroperitoneal abdomen	Great vessels	Arteriogram, CT, US, Venogram	Hypotension, massive bleeding, compartment syndromes
	Kidneys and ureters	CT, IVP, US	Urine output may be misleading
	Pancreas	CT	Missed injury, pancreatitis
	Duodenum – second and third parts	CT (with oral contrast)	Postop gastric outlet obstruction
True abdomen	Small intestine	CT (with oral contrast)	Fluid losses, missed injury
	Large intestine	CT (with oral contrast)	Peritoneal soiling
	Gravid uterus	US (radiation concern)	Fetal monitoring issues, cesarean delivery

CT, computed tomography; CXR, chest x-ray; IVP, intravenous pyelogram; RUG, retrograde urethrogram; US, ultrasound.

Blunt abdominal trauma

Two types of forces are involved in blunt abdominal trauma: compression and deceleration. Compression of the abdominal cavity against a fixed object such as a safety belt or steering wheel results in a rapid increase in intraluminal pressure, which can then cause bowel rupture and tears or hematomas of solid organs. Deceleration forces cause shearing and stretching of elements located between fixed and mobile structures. These forces typically result in injury to the mesentery, large vessels, and solid organ capsule, such as a liver tear at the ligamentum teres. Solid organs, especially spleen and liver, are most commonly injured following blunt abdominal trauma (Table 32.2).

An increased probability of intraabdominal injury occurs when signs of seatbelt trauma are present, such as seatbelt abrasion or hematoma of the abdominal wall, or fracture of the lumbar spine.[3] Seatbelts became widely used in the 1960s and led to a decrease in mortality due to ejection from the vehicle. However, the "seatbelt sign" has become an indicator that significant deceleration has occurred, with the interface of deceleration forces occurring at the locations where the belt contacts the patient. Ecchymosis and abrasions on the neck and upper chest (secondary to the use of a shoulder harness) have been associated with increased likelihood of aortic tears and cervical vascular injuries.[4]

The incidence of major intraabdominal injury approaches 90% if the diaphragm is ruptured.[5] Major pelvic fractures are also associated with an increased risk of intraabdominal organ injury (including bladder rupture). The incidence of intraabdominal organ injury increases incrementally with pelvic,

Table 32.2 Frequency of organ injury following blunt and penetrating abdominal trauma

Organ injured	Blunt trauma (%)	Penetrating trauma (%)
Liver	15	37
Spleen	25	7
Small bowel	< 1	26
Stomach	< 1	19
Colon	< 1	17
Vascular	2	13
Retroperitoneal hematoma	13	10
Kidney	7	4
Urinary bladder	6	< 1
Mesentery and omentum	5	10
Pancreas	3	4
Diaphragm	2	5
Urethra	2	< 1
Duodenum	< 1	2
Biliary system	< 1	1

chest, and head injuries, ranging from 40% with single-site trauma to 75% with trauma to all three locations.[6]

Patients with severe blunt trauma must have their abdomens evaluated for injury by using an objective study rather than physical exam alone. This is particularly true in patients with a significant mechanism of injury (e.g., high-speed deceleration), competing pain, and/or altered mental status. The most common objective techniques for evaluating the abdomen include computed tomography (CT) scans (see Chapter 11), focused assessment with sonography for trauma (FAST) (see Chapter 10), and diagnostic peritoneal lavage (DPL). In hemodynamically stable patients, the diagnostic study of choice is a CT scan.[7] When the patient is hemodynamically unstable, but no obvious indication for immediate surgery exists, the abdomen can be initially evaluated by FAST or (less commonly) DPL.

Penetrating abdominal trauma

The size of the object impaling the abdomen, as well as the location and force transmitted to the organs, determines the severity of intraabdominal injury. Significant injury to intraabdominal structures occurs 80–90% of the time following a gunshot wound and 25–35% of the time following stab wounds. The magnitude of injury resulting from a projectile is directly related to its kinetic energy and its composition, which affects its tendency to fragment or yaw (see Chapter 1). The incidence of organ injury with penetrating trauma is directly related to the volume occupied by the organ. Bowel, liver, and major vascular injuries predominate following penetrating abdominal trauma (Table 32.2). Given the location of the diaphragm during exhalation, penetrating injuries should be assumed to have entered the abdomen when thoracic wound sites are at or below nipple level.

Prehospital care (see also Chapter 2)

The airway is assessed for patency, and oxygen is administered immediately upon arrival of the emergency medical services (EMS) team. The airway must be considered first during initial evaluation, as loss of the airway for longer than 3–4 minutes can result in brain injury or death. If the patient has respiratory failure, the trachea should be intubated. Maintenance of adequate gas exchange is the fundamental responsibility of prehospital personnel. Airway concerns and complications are summarized in Table 32.3 (see Chapter 3 for a complete review of airway considerations for trauma).

Placement of two large-bore upper-extremity intravenous (IV) catheters should occur immediately after securing the airway. However, excessive time should not be wasted at the scene attempting to establish IV access in the patient (see Chapter 5). Administration of IV fluid in the form of crystalloid prior to arrival in the operating room (OR) should only proceed as necessary to maintain a systolic blood pressure of 90–100 mmHg, which ensures adequate perfusion of the major organs. Additional crystalloid used to achieve pressures above this range is probably not warranted prior to hemorrhage control in most previously healthy trauma patients. Indeed, Bickell *et al.* reported that patients with penetrating torso injuries receiving IV crystalloid resuscitation prior to the OR

Table 32.3 Airway complications to avoid in abdominal trauma

Complication	Treatment and comments
Hypoxia	Supplemental O_2 via face mask should be immediately instituted; failure to administer O_2 can promote hypoxemia and worsen prognosis.
Failure to intubate/ventilate	Evaluate airway – if predictably difficult, consider awake intubation (see Chapter 3).
Esophageal intubation	Problem of recognition, not commission. Any ETT placed in the field must be verified by the trauma team.
Aspiration	Aspiration risk is increased following abdominal trauma, compelling use of RSI. However, if the patient is both cooperative and hemodynamically stable, but thought to have a difficult airway, awake intubation should be considered.
Hypotension	Always start an IV and have fluids and vasopressors ready prior to intubating the trachea.
Conversion of partial into a complete airway obstruction	Maintain spontaneous ventilation in the stridorous patient. Have surgical airway supplies and TTJV available prior to intubation.
Exacerbation of cervical spine injury	With blunt abdominal trauma and penetrating trauma with C-spine proximity, the C-spine is immobilized using in-line stabilization.

C-spine, cervical spine; ETT, endotracheal tube; IV, intravenous; RSI, rapid sequence intubation; TTJV, transtracheal jet ventilation.

had a lower survival than those receiving no fluid, or "delayed resuscitation" (62% vs. 70%).[8] Other studies assessing the utility of hypertonic saline and colloid solutions have not demonstrated a clear benefit. See Chapter 8 for a complete review of this topic.

After addressing the trauma patient's airway, breathing, and circulation (ABC), the prehospital effort is focused on minimizing the transport time. Abdominal wound care should include placement of sterile dressings over injuries and applying direct pressure to active bleeding sites. In the event of bowel evisceration, saline-soaked dressings should be used to cover the organs to minimize evaporative losses and tissue desiccation. Imbedded foreign bodies are not to be removed. The use of military antishock trousers (MAST) for abdominal trauma was curtailed during the last decade.

Hospital resuscitation and diagnosis

Once the patient arrives at the hospital, the "primary survey" is initiated to identify and treat life-threatening injuries (ABCDEs as outlined by Advanced Trauma Life Support [ATLS]). The next focus in the abdominal trauma patient, after ensuring that life-threatening hemorrhage is not ongoing uncontrolled within the abdomen, becomes identification of other abdominal injuries and decision making regarding the need for emergent operation or urgent radiographic evaluation.

History and physical examination

Historical information is accepted from the paramedics, police, or bystanders transporting the patient, as well as from the patient (if conscious and lucid). Important information includes the circumstances and mechanism of injury. Patients with abdominal scars should be queried regarding type of prior surgery. Patients with altered mental status should have rapid blood glucose checked for hypoglycemia, and a trial of naloxone should be considered for those patients with putative signs of opioid overdose in the setting of hypotension.

The abdominal exam proceeds in an orderly fashion, with the recognition that abdominal findings may range from subtle signs to overt peritoneal irritability resulting from gastric, small intestinal, or colonic perforation. Associated injuries can mimic peritoneal signs, such as lower rib fractures and abdominal wall contusions, or distract the patient from abdominal complaints, such as extremity and pelvic fractures. The abdominal exam is difficult under ideal circumstances, and notoriously unreliable in the presence of head injury, shock, hypoxia, spinal cord injury, metabolic derangements, or intoxication.

Rectal and bimanual vaginal examination is important to identify possible injury and bleeding and to assess neurogenic tone. The Cullen sign, or periumbilical ecchymosis, and Grey–Turner sign, or flank ecchymosis, can indicate retroperitoneal injury, but usually take several hours to develop. Direct abdominal wall contusions and abrasions are also important and often indicate underlying abdominal organ injuries.

Hemodynamic instability, such as persistent hypotension despite at least 2 L of crystalloid administration, during the initial workup of abdominal trauma should trigger strong consideration for immediate blood transfusion and transfer to the OR for further evaluation, or exploratory laparotomy. Hypotension and shock following trauma in a patient with a normal chest radiograph, and without a large scalp laceration or major extremity injury, is due to intraabdominal or retroperitoneal bleeding until proved otherwise. An initial crossmatch for 6 units of packed red blood cells (pRBCs) and 6 units of fresh frozen plasma (FFP) should be ordered at this time, and type O Rh-positive or negative (for girls and women of childbearing age) or type-specific blood should be utilized in the meantime if needed. Early use of plasma is advocated, using a relatively high ratio of FFP to pRBCs (e.g., 1:1, see Chapter 6).

Laboratory studies

Extensive initial laboratory evaluation is unnecessary, and lab studies should be limited to a few tests. These include hematocrit, serum chemistry, and coagulation studies. With evidence of midabdominal trauma, where pancreatic injury is possible, lipase and amylase should be sent with initial studies. An arterial blood gas should be obtained for evaluation of oxygenation, ventilation, and tissue perfusion. If the patient is hypotensive during resuscitation or has an admission base deficit ≤ -6, blood type and screen is indicated, as transfusion is likely to be required. Occult rectal blood is assessed with a hemoccult test. Urinalysis for detection of hematuria is also obtained. When indicated, blood or urine ethanol and toxicology screens should be performed for correlation with mental status.

Diagnostic studies

Diagnostic modalities are selected on the basis of clinical information and guidelines, including mechanism of injury, history and physical examination, and the hemodynamic state of the patient (see also Chapter 11). A comparison of the various diagnostic studies along with organs injured is summarized in Table 32.1.

Chest radiograph

The chest radiograph is usually the first study performed during a trauma resuscitation because it provides important information for both chest and abdominal injuries. Thoracic bowel gas, a displaced nasogastric tube, or disruption of normal diaphragmatic contour can indicate a ruptured diaphragm. Diaphragmatic rupture is associated with other major abdominal injuries approximately 90% of the time. The presence of free air under the diaphragm following blunt trauma indicates bowel perforation. Splenic injury should be suspected in patients with left lower rib fractures, whereas patients with right lower rib fractures are likely to have an associated liver injury.[9] The chest radiograph should be scrutinized for pneumothorax, hemothorax, pulmonary contusion, aspiration, widening of the mediastinum, and evidence of diaphragmatic rupture.

Pelvis radiograph

A radiograph of the pelvis is used in blunt abdominal trauma to rule out a pelvic fracture. These injuries are important to detect, as posterior element fractures are associated with retroperitoneal hemorrhage, whereas anterior element fractures are associated with genitourinary injuries (see Chapter 27). An abdominal radiograph can help in patients with penetrating trauma, because it can delineate the trajectory and final location of the missiles, facilitated by the placement of radiopaque markers on the wound entrance and exit sites.

Focused assessment with sonography for trauma (FAST)

Ultrasound is rapid, noninvasive, and sensitive for visualizing free intraperitoneal fluid and pericardial fluid.[10] In the context of traumatic injury, free fluid is usually due to hemorrhage. Ultrasound can also detect certain solid organ injuries and is the initial imaging modality of choice for pregnant trauma patients.[11] Ultrasound facilitates rapid, noninvasive, serial examinations, is cost-effective, and can be performed during the resuscitation (see Chapter 10).

Although widely used for trauma in Europe in the 1970s and 1980s, ultrasound was formally introduced in the United States in the early 1990s as a quick and noninvasive method to screen for intraabdominal injury after blunt trauma.[11–14] Seven years after the first reports in the United States on ultrasound in trauma, 79% of surveyed Level I trauma centers had incorporated FAST examination into their trauma resuscitation, and 63% of the remaining centers were developing protocols to use FAST examination in the evaluation of blunt abdominal trauma.[12] The current reliance on FAST has resulted in rare use of DPL and a decreased incidence of subsequent exploratory laparoscopy/laparotomy.[13,14] Most centers now use FAST as a screening tool to decrease the use of CT scanning as well.[15,16] ATLS endorses the use of FAST in the evaluation of blunt trauma in adults and children.[17]

FAST surveys four anatomic areas for free fluid: (1) perihepatic, (2) perisplenic, (3) pelvis, and (4) pericardium. Despite the widespread acceptance of FAST, some have questioned its utility in the evaluation of blunt abdominal trauma because of missed injuries.[18]

Drawbacks of FAST include poor visualization of hollow structures such as bowel, and organs behind air-density interfaces. Intraabdominal injuries in which there is no free fluid, such as contained solid organ hematomas and lacerations, may be missed. Important retroperitoneal bleeding may also be difficult to detect with the FAST exam. Finally, ultrasound does not differentiate free intraperitoneal blood from ascites, which may result in false positives in cirrhotics. Thus, understanding the limitations guides decision making regarding additional testing (e.g., CT scanning) or exploratory laparotomy. Echocardiography (transthoracic and transesophageal) can be particularly helpful in diagnosing cardiac and great vessel injuries following abdominal–thoracic trauma (see Chapter 10).[19]

Diagnostic peritoneal lavage (DPL)

DPL was introduced in 1965 and is highly sensitive for intraabdominal injury.[20] The procedure has largely been replaced by ultrasound because DPL is invasive and time-consuming.[21] Furthermore, many believe DPL is overly sensitive, thus leading to a higher percentage of nontherapeutic laparotomies with subsequent morbidity.[22] Table 32.4 summarizes indications, contraindications, and criteria for a positive DPL. Of note, the indications for DPL are relatively limited when FAST is available. If the aspirate returns 5–10 mL of blood, the study

Table 32.4 Indications, contraindications, and positive values for diagnostic peritoneal lavage (when FAST is not available)

Indications	Comments
Altered mental status	Due to any source of CNS dysfunction, including head trauma, intoxication, hypothermia, metabolic derangement
High-energy transfer, but equivocal exam	High-speed MVC, fall from a height, MCC, bicycle collision, auto vs. pedestrian
Multiple injuries with unexplained shock	In the absence of head laceration, obvious extremity deformity, or bleeding, and the presence of a normal CXR, bleeding is in the abdomen until proven otherwise
Noncontiguous or thoracoabdominal injuries	Abdominal hemorrhage must be controlled prior to orthopedic fixation, and concomitantly with repair of head or chest injuries
Spinal cord injury	Physical examination is altered with denervation
Scheduled for prolonged general anesthesia for repair of other injuries	Inability to serially examine the abdomen, and possibility of confounding blood loss issues
Contraindications	**(Relative)**
Prior abdominal surgery	These patients should undergo
Pregnancy	CT or immediate operation
Morbid obesity	
Obvious need for surgery	
Positive DPL	**Comments**
RBC > 100,000/mm^3	> 1000/mm^3 positive (penetrating)
WBC > 500/mm^3	Bloody or pink lavage also positive
Amylase > 200 U/L	Bile, GI contents also positive

CNS, central nervous system; CT, computed tomography; CXR, chest x-ray; DPL, diagnostic peritoneal lavage; GI, gastrointestinal; MCC, motorcycle collision; MVC, motor vehicle collision; RBC, red blood cell count; WBC, white blood cell count.

is positive. If not, 1 L of warm normal saline is infused into the peritoneal cavity. Once in the abdomen, the bag is lowered to the floor, allowing the intraperitoneal fluid to siphon back into the bag. Injuries missed by DPL include diaphragmatic, retroperitoneal, bladder, and bowel wounds. False-positive results from a DPL are generally related to technical errors such as iatrogenic bleeding into the peritoneum from the DPL incision.

Computed tomography (CT)

CT has been used to evaluate the abdomen of hemodynamically stable trauma patients since 1981 and is particularly useful in identification of hemoperitoneum, solid organ, and retroperitoneal injury (see Chapter 10).[23] A complete abdominal CT scan traditionally utilizes both enteral and parenteral contrast. However, several studies reported that omission of oral contrast did not jeopardize making the essential diagnoses and significantly shortened the time to scan.[24] CT is particularly good for the detection and grading of discrete injuries to liver, spleen, and retroperitoneal structures (see Chapter 31). It is also the best technique for evaluating the abdomen in patients with concomitant injuries to the chest or pelvis.[25]

Drawbacks of abdominal CT include the requirement for patient transport to the scanner, exposure to IV contrast and radiation, relative expense, and time. Abdominal CT is not suitable for unstable trauma patients. In addition, contrast is contraindicated in those with renal insufficiency or contrast allergy. Abdominal CT can occasionally miss injuries to the diaphragm, bowel, and mesentery. However, the newer 64- and 128-multidetector helical CT scanners allow rapid scan times and higher resolution. Many trauma centers have dedicated CT scanners within, or adjacent to, the emergency department or trauma resuscitation suite.

Diagnostic laparoscopy

Laparoscopy provides direct visualization of active hemorrhage and solid organ and bowel injuries in a less invasive fashion than laparotomy, and initially reduced the frequency of negative trauma laparotomies.[26] However, laparoscopy is cumbersome for running the small bowel and does not visualize the dome of the liver or retroperitoneal structures. Complications of laparoscopy include trocar misplacement with damage to bowel, bladder, solid organ, or vascular structures.[27] Insufflation of carbon dioxide can create a tension pneumothorax in the presence of diaphragmatic tear, subcutaneous emphysema (with preperitoneal insufflation of gas), or intravenous gas embolism with solid organ or venous injury. Unstable patients may not tolerate the pneumoperitoneum, which results in decreased venous return and cardiac output. Furthermore, the increased airway pressure may confound the diagnosis of pneumothorax. However, minimally invasive laparoscopy techniques involving a single 5 mm port and minimal abdominal insufflation at 8–10 mmHg may cause less physiologic perturbation during general anesthesia.[28] The role of laparoscopy in trauma continues to evolve as both a diagnostic and a therapeutic modality.

Exploratory laparotomy

Exploratory laparotomy is the ultimate diagnostic modality, and its indications for abdominal trauma are listed in Table 32.5. Additional indications include significant bleeding via the nasogastric tube or rectum, ongoing bleeding from an unknown source, and stab wounds with known vascular,

Table 32.5 Indications for exploratory laparotomy in abdominal trauma

Unexplained hypotension or shock
Uncontrolled hemorrhage
Signs of peritonitis
Gunshot wound to abdomen
Ruptured diaphragm
Pneumoperitoneum on admission chest radiograph
Evisceration of bowel or omentum

biliary, or bowel injury. Surgical priorities during laparotomy are as follows:

(1) locate and control hemorrhage
(2) locate bowel injuries and control fecal contamination
(3) identify injuries to other abdominal organs and structures
(4) determine whether temporizing measures are most appropriate (i.e., damage control), or if definitive repair of injury should occur (see Chapter 18)

Emergency thoracotomy

An emergency resuscitative thoracotomy should be considered for penetrating abdominal trauma patients who lose their vital signs shortly before or after arrival to the emergency department, or in those who present with uncontrollable hemorrhage from the wound.[29,30] A left anterolateral approach is used to facilitate proximal aortic control, and open cardiac massage. Because of dismal survival rates, emergency thoracotomy is rarely indicated for blunt trauma patients except in the case of pericardial tamponade detected with ultrasound (see Chapters 29 and 30).

Other diagnostic procedures

Proctosigmoidoscopy should be performed for suspected rectal or sigmoid colon injury and can be done rapidly with minimal or no sedation. Because this is an unprepared examination, visualization may be limited. Full-thickness tears, hematomas, or sites of active arterial bleeding are indications for prompt surgical exploration. Retrograde urethrogram should be considered for patients with pelvic fracture, symphysis pubis diastasis, blood at the urethral meatus, or prostate displacement.

Anesthetic and surgical implications of specific organ injury
Solid organ injuries

The liver is the most commonly injured solid organ following penetrating trauma and the second most commonly injured organ following blunt trauma. Early death from abdominal trauma most commonly results from uncontrolled hemorrhage, and late death is most commonly attributable to sepsis.[31] Clinical findings suggestive of liver injury following blunt trauma include fractures of the right lower ribs, elevated right hemidiaphragm, right pleural effusion, pneumothorax, and right upper quadrant tenderness. Nonoperative management is now the initial treatment of choice for hemodynamically stable patients with isolated blunt liver trauma, with success rates approaching 95%.[31]

The spleen is the most commonly injured abdominal organ following blunt trauma, and is also frequently injured following penetrating trauma to the left thorax or abdomen. Hypotension from hemorrhage is the most common initial finding. Splenic injury should be suspected in patients with left lower rib fractures, left upper quadrant tenderness, or left shoulder pain. With splenic injury, there exists a significant incidence of additional intraabdominal damage following blunt or penetrating trauma.[32]

Nonoperative management is practiced for solitary splenic injuries in hemodynamically stable patients. Splenic preservation is practiced when able for both adult and pediatric trauma, but debate exists regarding the minimal amount of residual spleen required to confer immunity against encapsulated organisms. Overwhelming postsplenectomy sepsis can occur due to loss of immune responses, and subsequent pneumococcal infections carry an associated 80% mortality. Therefore, polyvalent pneumococcal vaccine must be given postoperatively following emergency splenectomy.[33]

Blunt pancreatic injury is usually due to an anteroposterior compression mechanism that crushes the pancreas against the vertebral column. Physical findings include burning epigastric and back pain, tenderness, or ileus. Laboratory findings include elevated amylase and lipase. CT is the gold standard for evaluation of pancreatic injury.

The kidney is commonly injured following deceleration injuries and can bleed extensively into the retroperitoneal space. Renal injury is suspected with hematuria, fractures of lower posterolateral ribs, or flank pain and tenderness. Diagnosis may require ultrasound, CT, intravenous pyelogram, and angiogram if renal vascular injury is suspected.

Hollow organ injuries

Injury to the stomach is commonly caused by penetrating trauma. The most common initial finding suggestive of gastric injury is blood via the mouth or nasogastric tube. Symptoms include rapid onset of epigastric pain and peritonitis due to release of gastric contents into the peritoneum. Radiographic findings include free air under the diaphragm on abdominal or chest films, displaced nasogastric tube, or extravasation of oral contrast medium.

The small bowel is the most frequently injured hollow organ in penetrating trauma, because of its relative volume, followed by stomach, then colon. Making the diagnosis of blunt injury to the small bowel, without exploratory laparotomy, is difficult. Elevated amylase and alkaline phosphatase in

the DPL fluid is highly suggestive of small bowel trauma.[34] CT findings suggestive of small bowel injury include bowel wall thickening, free intraperitoneal air, free fluid without evidence of solid organ injury, and mesenteric hematoma. Small bowel trauma can present with only vague generalized pain, with peritonitis after many hours. Duodenal injury may present with referred pain to the back.

Colon injuries are common after gunshot wounds, and less so following blunt trauma. Symptoms of bowel injury are usually caused by spillage of intestinal contents, rather than from blood loss. Peritonitis occurs more frequently with colon injuries than from small bowel injuries because of the increased bacterial contamination. Colonic injuries are associated with increased risk of abdominal abscess. Unrecognized colonic injuries often have devastating complications.

Abdominal vascular injuries

Patients with abdominal vascular injury usually present with profound hemorrhagic shock. Venous access is preferably located in the upper extremities to avoid fluid loss to the abdomen (see Chapter 5). On rare occasions, the surgical incision may need to be extended to a median sternotomy, whereafter vascular control can be obtained at the intrapericardial inferior vena cava. Saphenous vein cutdown lines or femoral venous catheters must not be relied on in the setting of significant intraabdominal trauma, because of the possibility of inferior vena cava (IVC) injury, and/or the need for temporary IVC clamping. This results in a 60% decrease in venous return and subsequent hemodynamic deterioration. Concurrent clamping of the abdominal aorta can be employed as a temporizing measure to maintain perfusion pressure to the brain and heart during periods of IVC disruption. In addition, the utilization of high-capacity fluid warming devices for the rapid administration of blood products into tributaries of the superior vena cava can be life-saving.

Retroperitoneal injuries

The retroperitoneum is a hidden area of the abdomen, not readily evaluated by physical exam, FAST, or DPL. Major retroperitoneal structures include the great vessels, pancreas, kidneys and ureters, and the second and third portions of the duodenum. When trauma to this area is likely, CT should be used for evaluation if the patient is stable (see Chapter 11). Ultrasound can provide some information about renal injury but does not stage injuries to the same degree of reliability as CT. Retroperitoneal hematoma formation from active pelvic bleeding may require external fixation or angiography to evaluate and treat with embolization (see Chapter 27).[24]

Rupture of the diaphragm

Diaphragmatic rupture is seen in 2–3% of patients with blunt abdominal trauma. Left hemidiaphragm rupture occurs in 70–75% of injuries, presumably due to the protective effect of the underlying liver on the right. The diagnosis of diaphragmatic rupture can be made on radiographs by finding a displaced nasogastric tube, interruption of the normal diaphragmatic contours, and intrathoracic displacement of (normally) intraabdominal contents. When the chest radiograph is taken during mechanical ventilation, the abdominal contents may revert to near-normal position, thus masking the injury. Peritoneal lavage is unreliable for diagnosis, although drainage of peritoneal lavage fluid via thoracostomy tube is definitive. A delay in diagnosis of diaphragmatic tear increases morbidity and mortality, and gastric herniation places the patient at increased risk of aspiration.

Pregnancy

Trauma is the leading cause of nonobstetric death in women between the ages of 14 and 44 years (see Chapter 37). Fetal injury and death following blunt and penetrating abdominal trauma are common, as the gravid uterus displaces viscera and acts as a shield. Aggressive maternal resuscitation remains the best strategy for promoting fetal survival. Indeed, the major cause of fetal death is maternal shock. Fetal mortality approaches 80% in cases of maternal shock.[35,36] When the mother survives, the major cause of fetal death is complete (6–66% of cases) or incomplete (30–80% of cases) placental separation.[37] Other common causes of fetal demise and peripartum hemorrhage include uterine rupture, direct trauma to the fetus, amniotic fluid embolus, and disseminated intravascular coagulation (DIC).

Ultrasound should be performed as soon as possible to detect trauma to the uteroplacental unit, which may lead to fetal–maternal hemorrhage and alloimmunization of an Rh-negative mother against an Rh-positive fetus. A Kleihauer–Betke test should be performed if this type of injury is suspected, and Rh immune globulin should be administered.

Amniotic fluid embolus can lead to cardiopulmonary arrest, inflammation, and overwhelming DIC. Under these circumstances, cesarean delivery should be performed as soon as possible (see Chapter 37). Limited data are available to support postmortem cesarean delivery in pregnant trauma patients suffering a cardiac arrest for hypovolemic shock.[38] Postmortem cesarean delivery has been occasionally successful if performed within 5–10 minutes of maternal death for causes other than hypovolemic traumatic shock.[39]

If cardiac arrest occurs in the first half of gestation, the purpose of cardiopulmonary resuscitation (CPR) is to resuscitate the mother; delivery of the fetus in this period of gestation may not improve the mother's chances of survival. However, after 24 weeks of pregnancy there are data to suggest that delivery can improve maternal survival.[40–42]

An extensive literature review by Katz suggests that a patient beyond 24 weeks gestation in cardiopulmonary arrest cannot be resuscitated without delivery.[43] He suggested that the delivery be called perimortem cesarean delivery and emphasized its urgency. The data in this article support the "four minute rule." Cesarean delivery should be started within 4 minutes of cardiopulmonary arrest and the baby delivered by the fifth minute (see Chapter 37).

Combined injuries
Abdomen and head injuries

Initial abdominal evaluation in patients with severe head injury and hemodynamic instability is best accomplished by FAST exam or DPL.[44] The decision to proceed with immediate laparotomy in the hemodynamically unstable patient with head injury can be based on these results.[45] If free intraperitoneal blood is detected, intraabdominal injury is assumed. After laparotomy, the stabilized patient can then undergo head CT. However, immediate head CT and concomitant abdomen and chest CT should precede laparotomy for patients demonstrating signs of herniation who respond to initial resuscitation.[46] The 64- or 128-slice helical CT allows a combined head, chest, and abdomen scan to be obtained in about 5 minutes. If both the head and abdomen CT demonstrates an operable lesion, then cranial and abdominal operations can be done concomitantly.

Abdomen and chest injuries

Life-threatening hemorrhage is common in major thoracoabdominal trauma. Resistant hypoxemia from rib fractures, or from chest wall and pulmonary contusions, can necessitate tracheal intubation and mechanical ventilation. The unreliability of physical examination, thoracostomy output, and prediction of bullet trajectory must be emphasized. Intraoperative clues of ongoing hemorrhage, such as occult intercostal artery laceration, retroperitoneal hemorrhage, and other causes outside of the operative field must be sought when patients experience unexplained deterioration.

Abdomen and pelvic fracture or extremity injuries

Important considerations in concomitant pelvic, extremity, and abdominal injuries include persistent retroperitoneal hemorrhage and increased risk of deep venous thrombosis.[47,48] The presence of abdominal pain or tenderness is associated with a higher incidence of intraabdominal injury. The lack of these findings, however, does not preclude injury in the presence of concomitant extraabdominal injury with competing pain.[49] Thus, definitive investigation with abdominal CT, DPL, or laparotomy is necessary to rule out intraabdominal injury in these patients. Hypotension in the patient with pelvic fractures should trigger consideration for retroperitoneal hemorrhage, suggesting the need for pelvic stabilization, and the possible need for angiographic evaluation and treatment. Furthermore, blood loss in these patients can be significant and, despite initially normal hematocrits, frequently requires early transfusion.

Preparation for anesthesia and surgery

Much of the preparation for surgery should already be completed during the initial hospital resuscitation and workup of the abdominal trauma patient. However, the anesthesiologist may enter the resuscitation or evaluation at any stage in the process, and must verify that all of the important work performed up to that point has been done correctly. Preparation for anesthesia and surgery begins with a survey of ABCs, IV access, laboratory data, cardiopulmonary monitoring, and positioning considerations.

Establishing or confirming presence of definitive airway

Establishing or confirming a definitive airway is the first priority. Rapid sequence induction and intubation is generally indicated. However, as noted in Table 32.3, patients with anatomic, pathologic, or historical indicators of difficult intubation should be considered for awake intubation, preferably utilizing a fiberoptic bronchoscope. The fiberoptic bronchoscope can be safely used for intubation even in patients with full stomachs following trauma. Indeed, Ovassapian *et al.* described 108 consecutive patients at high risk for aspiration who were intubated using an awake fiberoptic technique without a single case of aspiration.[50]

Intravenous access

Two large-bore peripheral IV catheters should be established and secured (see Chapter 5). Catheters are preferably located in venous systems that drain into the superior vena cava. Femoral or saphenous venous catheters should be avoided in patients with significant abdominal trauma. The utility of catheters draining into the IVC may be compromised should the IVC be clamped or packed during the surgical procedure. However, in extremis, access is established wherever possible.

Placement of a large-bore cordis introducer in the internal jugular vein is helpful for both volume administration and central venous pressure monitoring (see Chapter 5).

Evaluation of preoperative volume status

A quick evaluation of the patient's volume status can be made by measuring the blood pressure and heart rate, palpating the peripheral pulse, and assessing skin color and turgor and the quality of mucous membranes.

Systolic pressure variation is a technique for gauging intravascular volume status that anesthesiologists have employed for decades.[51] Arterial blood pressure has long been known to decrease with positive-pressure ventilation. The systolic pressure variability method of quantifying these changes directly correlates with intravascular depletion and fluid responsiveness in both animal experiments and clinical studies (see Chapter 9).[51] Variations of this technology are widely used,

and are often referred to as "dynamic measure of fluid responsiveness."

Review of available lab and radiographic data

All current laboratory data must be evaluated. Electrolyte imbalances, such as hypo- or hyperkalemia and acidosis, must be corrected and/or rechecked if lab error is suspected. The chest and cervical spine radiographs should be reviewed by the anesthesiologist prior to induction. The presence of rib fractures, hemopneumothorax, and spine fractures should all be considered in the determination of anesthetic technique, monitoring, and postoperative plans for the traumatized patient.

Monitoring for major abdominal injury

Intraoperative monitoring for major abdominal injury includes standard American Society of Anesthesiologists (ASA) guidelines, as well as arterial and central venous access. Ability to monitor exhaled gas CO_2 and nitrogen concentration is necessary for screening of air emboli. Monitoring considerations for trauma resuscitation are more fully covered in Chapter 9.

Positioning for abdominal trauma surgery

The supine position with arms out is optimal for venous and arterial access, as well as application of a convective warming blanket. However, if all the lines are already in place, the arms can be tucked, thereby improving surgical access for upper abdomen exploration. The spatial needs of special retractors should be considered. Padding of dependent body parts is required to minimize hypoperfusion and pressure-induced tissue ischemia. These issues should be negotiated between the surgical, anesthetic, and nursing teams prior to the patient's OR arrival to minimize conflict, misunderstanding, and surgical delay.

Induction and maintenance of anesthesia

The goals for anesthetic management of the abdominal trauma patient are summarized in Table 32.6. Besides physiologic stability, analgesia and amnesia should be provided once the patient's hemodynamic status becomes stable enough to tolerate anesthetic drugs.

General anesthesia for abdominal trauma

Hypotension at induction of anesthesia for trauma is a common and important complication to avoid. Peri-induction hypotension can be triggered by numerous processes directly attributable to anesthesia, including (1) suppression of endogenous catecholamines that serve to elevate systemic blood pressure despite significant hypovolemia, (2) direct myocardial depressant effects and/or vasodilator effects of certain induction drugs, and (3) initiation of positive-pressure

Table 32.6 Goals of general anesthesia for abdominal trauma

1. Reestablish and maintain normal hemodynamics

a. For hypotension, fluids first, then vasopressors.
b. Frequent evaluation of base deficit, hematocrit, urinary output
c. Titration of additional anesthetics if robust blood pressure

2. Maximize surgical exposure and minimize bowel edema

a. Limit fluids according to needs
b. Limit blood loss by allowing anesthetic catch-up
c. Muscle relaxation should be optimized
d. Nasogastric or orogastric tube to decompress bowel
e. Avoid N_2O

3. Limit hypothermia

a. Monitor core temperature
b. Warm intravenous fluids and blood
c. Keep patient covered and room warm ($> 28\,°C$)
d. Apply convective warming blanket

4. Help limit blood loss and coagulopathy

a. Encourage surgeon to stop and pack if blood loss excessive
b. Frequently monitor hematocrit, ionized Ca, coagulation studies
c. Provide calcium for large citrated product administration
d. Administer plasma, platelets, cryoprecipitate, and factor VIIa or prothrombin complex concentrate (PCC), as clinically indicated.

5. Limit complications to other systems

a. Monitor intracranial pressure, maintain cerebral perfusion pressure > 70 mmHg
b. Monitor peak airway pressures and tidal volumes. Be vigilant for pneumothorax
c. Measure urine output
d. Monitor peripheral pulses

ventilation that drives down $PaCO_2$ and decreases venous return.

Immediately following induction, the abdominal incision itself can cause hypotension by release of tamponaded abdominal bleeding; this occasionally results in a torrent of abdominal hemorrhage. Thus, the patient's abdomen should be prepped from the sternal notch to below the knees, and draped prior to induction, and the surgeons should be gowned and ready with scalpel in hand during induction of anesthesia in an actively hemorrhaging patient.

Induction principles

It is frequently stated that "more soldiers were killed in World War II by thiopental than by bullets." Indeed, Halford wrote a compelling negative critique of thiopental to that effect following the Japanese attack of Pearl Harbor.[52] However, in the same issue of *Anesthesiology*, Adams and Gray presented a case, with an accompanying editorial, clarifying that it is not necessarily the drug, but rather the dose, that leads to lethality in the traumatized patient.[53] On balance, massively traumatized patients should not receive propofol, thiopental, or other

drugs with negative inotropic or vasodilator properties for induction (see Chapter 7).

Comatose patients, those in severe shock, and especially those in complete cardiopulmonary arrest on admission, require nothing more than oxygen and possibly a neuromuscular blocking drug until the patient's blood pressure and heart rate rebound enough to allow anesthetic drugs to be added. Awake traumatized patients demonstrating signs of hypovolemia are generally best induced with etomidate, 0.1–0.2 mg/kg, because thiopental and propofol may cause profound hypotension in hypovolemic patients.[54] Ketamine is also a suitable induction drug.

Maintenance

Sedative and amnesic drugs should be titrated as blood pressure allows, because the provision of oxygen and neuromuscular relaxants alone can result in recall.[55] Anesthesia can be maintained with inhalational agents or with intravenous drugs such as propofol, with opioid supplementation as necessary.

All of the induction drugs mentioned above could be used as IV maintenance. However, repeated doses or prolonged infusions of etomidate will cause adrenal suppression. Trauma patients with hemorrhagic shock too severe to tolerate anesthetic drugs (other than neuromuscular blockade) should receive scopolamine as an amnesic. Later, benzodiazepines or propofol can be titrated in for amnesia.[56] However, there is no particular requirement for total IV anesthesia for abdominal trauma, and inhaled drugs are typically less expensive and possess equally satisfactory anesthetic results (as long as nitrous oxide is avoided).

All volatile anesthetics produce dose-dependent depression of myocardial contractility. Desflurane, isoflurane, and sevoflurane maintain cardiac output better than older agents such as enflurane or halothane, mainly through a peripheral vasodilatory effect. Whereas halothane (no longer available in USA) maintains blood pressure better at the same minimal alveolar concentration (MAC) level than isoflurane,[57] there are no absolute contraindications of any volatile drug for abdominal trauma. Yet halothane and sevoflurane have been occasionally avoided because of a theoretical potential for liver and renal injury, respectively. Nitrous oxide (N_2O) should be avoided to limit bowel and closed-space gas accumulation.

Halothane has very infrequently been associated with the development of fulminant hepatitis. The National Halothane Study conducted in the 1960s found that halothane was not associated with hepatic injury more frequently than other anesthetics.[58] However, abdominal trauma patients with pre-existing liver disease or hepatic injury constitute a special group. Halothane is associated with carboxylesterase antibodies that may be injurious to the liver.[59] Also, halothane is known to decrease hepatic blood flow to a far greater degree than any other inhaled drug. Conversely, isoflurane increases hepatic artery blood flow at both 1 and 2 MAC and is the authors' maintenance drug of choice for trauma patients with liver dysfunction. Halothane is no longer available in the USA.

It is best to avoid halothane in abdominal trauma in countries still using it, because hepatic blood flow may already be compromised by hypotension, ischemia, and direct hepatic injury.

Sevoflurane reacts with carbon dioxide absorbents to produce "compound A." Because of concern about the potential nephrotoxicity of compound A, sevoflurane was not released in the United States until 1995, 4 years after release in Japan, with a package insert warning to use fresh gas flow rates ≥ 2 L/minute. Despite this concern, sevoflurane has been used safely since 1991 in Japan without significant nephrotoxicity. Although nephrotoxicity was demonstrated in rats, investigators have been unable to demonstrate significant renal injury following low-flow sevoflurane in humans.[60] More sensitive tests of renal injury have demonstrated renal injury associated with compound A. One study demonstrated that 1.25 MAC sevoflurane plus compound A produced dose-related injury to glomeruli and tubules.[61] Given the possibility of renal toxicity resulting from sevoflurane and the high risk of hypotension and toxin exposure (e.g., aminoglycosides, IV contrast, rhabdomyolysis) with abdominal trauma, sevoflurane is probably best reserved for brief periods of administration in the multiply injured trauma patient. Because recovery from anesthesia has been shown to proceed slightly faster with desflurane than with sevoflurane,[62] the former agent may be preferred when rapid wakeup is considered beneficial.

The routine use of N_2O is discouraged in abdominal trauma, because N_2O will preferentially fill gas-containing structures, such as pneumothorax, pneumocephalus, and obstructed bowel, causing these structures to expand. Gas-containing structures expand because the blood: gas partition coefficient of N_2O is 34 times greater than that of nitrogen. Thus, the capacity of the blood to bring N_2O to gas-containing structures is greater than its capacity to remove nitrogen. Nitrous oxide can support combustion and should be avoided if electrocautery is used near any distended segment of bowel containing gas. In patients with solitary abdominal or extremity injuries, N_2O can be used during the last 15–30 minutes to promote rapid awakening and resumption of protective reflexes. However, in severely injured patients requiring postoperative mechanical ventilation, there is no benefit to the use of N_2O. Furthermore, when there is a risk of pneumocephalus or pneumothorax, N_2O should be avoided altogether.

Neuraxial regional anesthesia and abdominal trauma

Spinal and epidural anesthesia are contraindicated in the unstable abdominal trauma patient because it is impractical (the patient may not be able to assume the lateral or sitting position for drug placement), takes time to set up, and can result in several deleterious side effects, such as sympathectomy-mediated hypotension, local anesthetic-induced seizures, total spinal anesthesia, or cardiac arrest. During World War I, neuraxial blockade was frequently employed, causing Admiral Sir Gordon Taylor to proclaim

spinal anesthesia to be "the best form of euthanasia" he knew for war injuries. Regional anesthesia and analgesia are most useful in hemodynamically stable trauma patients with painful injuries, as discussed in Chapters 16 and 28.

Adjunctive management and complications

Administration of shed abdominal blood

The use of salvaged blood from abdominal trauma was previously considered to be contraindicated, because of the possibility of bacterial or fecal contamination. However, several studies have demonstrated the safety and efficacy of transfusing intraabdominally salvaged blood, under certain circumstances.[63,64] For noncontaminated intraabdominal blood involving liver, spleen, or retroperitoneal injury from stab wounds, cell-saver devices are used at many trauma centers.

Massive transfusion

A massive transfusion protocol (MTP) may be activated to insure rapid and timely administration of blood products, including coagulation factors (see Chapter 6). Adverse consequences of massive transfusion include coagulopathy, hypothermia, hypocalcemia, hyperkalemia, and hemolysis.[65,66] Nonsurvivors of penetrating trauma who received massive volume replacement are more likely to be hypothermic, acidotic, and coagulopathic than survivors.[67] Indeed, massive transfusion is the most important predictor of coagulopathy following abdominal trauma. The likelihood of coagulopathy (prothrombin time [PT] or partial thromboplastin time [PTT] equal to or greater than twice normal) following massive transfusion in seriously injured patients is predicted by persistent hypothermia, acidosis, hypotension, and Injury Severity Score (ISS). With all four risk factors (pH ≤ 7.10, temperature $\leq 34\,°C$, systolic blood pressure ≥ 70 mmHg, ISS ≥ 25), 98% of patients will develop a life-threatening coagulopathy.[68] There is an increasing reliance on point-of-care coagulation testing (e.g., thromboelastography, thromboelastometry) in the abdominal trauma patient.[69]

Thermal management

Hypothermia is a major comorbidity of trauma, as discussed in Chapter 14. Besides impaired thermoregulation, loss of heat from radiation (exposure), conduction (unwarmed IV infusions), evaporation, and convection (exposed abdominal surfaces), and redistribution of warm core blood to the periphery in the setting of drug use and spinal cord injury contribute. Furthermore, pharmacologic paralysis prevents normal heat production mechanisms (e.g., shivering), and vasodilating anesthetic agents impair heat conservation mechanisms (e.g., vasoconstriction).

Hypothermia affects the platelet coagulation process, promotes platelet sequestration, reduces drug metabolism, and induces vasoconstriction. Combined hypothermia and acidosis reflect a decrease in cardiac output and tissue perfusion. The hypothermic myocardium is susceptible to ectopy, especially ventricular dysrhythmias. Many studies have identified hypothermia as a factor associated with increased morbidity and mortality in severely injured patients.[70] Moderate hypothermia (35.5–34.5 °C), however, is neuroprotective and may be tolerated in certain conditions, especially when clinical manifestations of bleeding are absent.[71]

Neuromuscular blockade

Muscle relaxation facilitates exposure during exploratory laparotomy for trauma. Accordingly, neuromuscular relaxants should be routinely used in these patients (see Chapter 13). Reversal of neuromuscular blockade is generally not required in patients expected to be mechanically ventilated for several hours or days following abdominal trauma surgery. Rocuronium is often used in trauma patients because of its rapid onset, and vecuronium is often used because of its minimal effects upon the hemodynamic system. No particular neuromuscular blockade drugs are contraindicated in abdominal trauma, unless hepatic or renal insufficiency is present (see Chapter 13), in which case cisatracurium is favored because of its nonhepatic and nonrenal elimination properties. Owing to potential histamine release, atracurium, mivacurium, curare, and metocurine are generally avoided in hypotensive patients.[72]

Acid–base management

Acid–base status is measured via arterial blood gas, and the derived base deficit is useful in guiding resuscitative efforts. Acidosis impairs myocardial contractility in response to both endogenous and exogenous catecholamines. However, the oxyhemoglobin dissociation curve is shifted rightward by acidosis, thereby improving oxygen delivery to tissues. Lactic acidosis should be treated by improving oxygen delivery (including fluid replacement). Although controversial, some physicians would treat pH ≤ 7.10 with sodium bicarbonate and temporary hyperventilation.

Antibiotics

Preoperative (empiric/prophylactic) antibiotic therapy in patients with intraabdominal injury begins with broad-spectrum coverage of both Gram-positive and Gram-negative bacteria, especially anaerobes and enterobacteriacea. A third- or fourth-generation cephalosporin in combination with metronidazole is recommended by the American College of Surgeons. A single preoperative dose of an appropriate antibiotic is adequate prophylaxis for penetrating and blunt abdominal injuries. Postoperative antibiotics should be reserved for late (> 12 hours post injury) operations and for enteric perforations.

If the patient has sustained gross spillage of gut contents, or has received a massive transfusion, antibiotics should be repeated more frequently. The optimal duration of treatment under these circumstances is not well established.[73] Data suggest that, in high-risk penetrating colonic trauma, 24 hours of broad-spectrum antibiotics is as efficacious as 5 days of therapy.[74] Fever and leukocytosis are imprecise indicators of the need for continued postoperative antibiotic administration in the severely traumatized patient.

Polyvalent pneumococcal vaccine given early after splenectomy substantially reduces the incidence of overwhelming sepsis.[75] Some advocate waiting 2 weeks following the trauma prior to its administration, because postoperative elevated stress hormones may attenuate the immunologic response. Administration of additional vaccines against *Neisseria meningitidis* and *Haemophilus influenzae* should be considered, as these organisms, like *Streptococcus pneumoniae*, are encapsulated and difficult to combat in the asplenic patient. Others administer the polyvalent pneumococcal vaccine early to decrease the risk of the patient being inadvertently discharged prior to having been vaccinated at all. Tetanus prophylaxis must be considered in every trauma patient, but especially in those with contaminated wounds or perforated bowel injuries.[76]

Other intraoperative complications

The anesthesiologist must maintain increased vigilance for the delayed presentation of occult complications such as intrathoracic, retroperitoneal, and extremity bleeding, as well as for diaphragmatic rupture, tension pneumothorax, pericardial tamponade, or intracranial bleeding (manifested as increasing intracranial pressure or pupil dilation). Additional considerations in patients with significant abdominal trauma include the possible development of venous air embolism, most often resulting from pulmonary vascular or hepatobiliary injury. Minimizing the risk of this potentially lethal complication requires maintenance of adequate intravascular volume and vigilance for the early signs of venous air embolism such as hypotension, sudden decreased end-tidal CO_2 concentration on the capnograph, or increased end-tidal nitrogen concentration.

Considerations related to the surgical approach

Standard approach to exploratory laparotomy

The anesthesiologist should understand the standard surgical approach to anticipate problems and monitor progress of the case. The standard exploratory abdominal incision is midline, extending from the xiphoid process to the pubic symphysis. Following entry into the peritoneal cavity, the small bowel is evacuated, and the abdomen is divided into four quadrants and packed with lap pads. The first priorities are to stop hemorrhage and control contamination; each quadrant is then explored sequentially. The next priority is to temporarily close any major contaminating visceral tears. Having accomplished these primary aims, a more thorough evaluation of each organ is undertaken, and specific injuries are sought and repaired. If the patient becomes hemodynamically unstable or has hemorrhage that is difficult to control, the area is packed again, and anesthetic "catch-up" is allowed, with infusion of blood products and/or pressors if necessary (see Chapter 6).

In certain very unstable patients, "damage control" can be achieved at the initial operation, with later return to the OR for staged repair, as discussed below and more completely reviewed in Chapter 18.

Pringle maneuver

Complex hepatic injuries (grades III–V) generally require temporary portal triad occlusion (Pringle maneuver) to gain operative visibility and vascular control. The Pringle maneuver involves isolation and control of the hepatic inflow vessels, including occlusion of the hepatic artery, portal vein, and common bile duct. The Pringle maneuver is used to stem the rapid loss of blood, allowing the surgeon to then expose and ligate lacerated vessels and bile ducts. Hemodynamic changes associated with the Pringle maneuver reflect decreased right heart venous return. If abdominal bleeding is not controlled with packing and the Pringle maneuver, this usually reflects damage to the retrohepatic vena cava or hepatic vein, which will require isolation and control of both the supra- and infrahepatic vena cava.

Atrial–caval shunt placement

In certain situations, such as massive retrohepatic injury, a shunt may be placed between the infrahepatic vena cava and the right atrium in an effort to bypass the injury. To place an atrial–caval shunt, a right thoracotomy or median sternotomy is required. Typically, the abdominal incision is extended to a median sternotomy. The shunt is placed through the right atrial appendage into the inferior vena cava distal to the hepatic region, but superior to the renal veins.[77] The danger of venous air embolism always exists with hepatic trauma and repair. Most bleeding hepatic injuries, including blunt retrohepatic caval injuries, can be managed with precise surgical packing.

Damage control, anesthetic "catch-up," and planned reoperation

"Damage control" is the term applied to abbreviated operations in unstable, severely injured patients with metabolic derangements (coagulopathy, hypothermia, and acidosis) in whom prolonged initial operations would be dangerous (see Chapter 18).[69] The initial surgery is abbreviated to allow aggressive correction of metabolic derangements before definitive reconstruction of bowel injuries. Shorter operative times have been associated with increased survival and decreased morbidity, despite deferment of definitive organ repairs.[78,79] The damage control concept is not new. Indeed, many surgeons and anesthesiologists have advocated abbreviated

procedures for years, especially following hepatic injuries.[80] However, it is now being more rigorously employed. Hirshberg and Mattox have organized the concept of damage control surgery into three phases: initial control, stabilization, and delayed reconstruction.[81]

The initial damage control period involves rapid temporary cessation of bleeding and hollow visceral spillage. Occasionally, this period will alternate between brief epochs of abbreviated operative therapy and periods of anesthetic catch-up, where temporary packing occurs while the patient's intravascular volume is restored, allowing subsequent emergency control procedures to be performed. Following initial control of vascular bleeding and bowel spillage, temporary abdominal closure occurs. Some patients have so much bowel edema from resuscitation that the fascia cannot be approximated without the interposition of a sterile plastic or silastic closure (which is removed at later reoperation).[82]

The stabilization period is typically carried out in the intensive care unit (ICU). After transport to the ICU, the focus is on continued fluid resuscitation, aggressive warming measures, control of coagulopathic bleeding (thrombocytopenia, decreased factor levels, hypothermia), and normalization of acidosis. Reoperation generally occurs in 24–72 hours. Provisional abdominal packing is associated with increased morbidity and mortality when the duration of packing exceeds 72 hours.[83] Complications include abscess formation and sepsis due to residual foreign body fragments, necrotic tissue, blood, and/or bile. Other complications include acute respiratory distress syndrome (ARDS), jaundice, hepatorenal syndrome, DIC, bile peritonitis, and postoperative hemorrhage. During the delayed reconstruction, primary repair of bowel injuries, definitive survey of additional injuries, and copious abdominal irrigation occurs.

Nonoperative management

The trend of nonoperative management of liver injuries stems from the experience that bleeding often stops by the time of laparotomy in many patients with solitary liver injuries (with arterial extravasation) due to the natural hemostatic qualities of liver parenchyma. Providing that patients are hemodynamically stable and without other intraabdominal injuries requiring laparotomy, nonoperative management is usually successful. One study reported that 70 of 72 (97%) of liver injuries following blunt abdominal trauma were successfully managed nonoperatively.[84] When CT demonstrates extravasation of contrast, angiographic embolization of bleeding vessels can supplement nonoperative management.

Nonoperative management of the spleen occurs for similar reasons. Additionally, overwhelming postsplenectomy sepsis and increased risk of Gram-positive infections place increased emphasis on splenic conservation. The benefits derived from nonoperative management of splenic trauma must be balanced against the potential risk of transfusion-related bacterial and viral diseases. Laparoscopic blood salvage for transfusion may further shift the balance toward splenic salvage.[85] Laparoscopy not only enables examination of the spleen, but also salvage of intraperitoneal blood for transfusion. Interestingly, nonoperative management is now being advocated for rupture of the diseased spleen, as the combination of splenectomy and immunosuppression renders these patients particularly susceptible to sepsis.[86]

Bowel injury is more than twice as common with two solid organ injuries, and 6.7 times more likely with three solid organ injuries, compared with a solitary solid organ injury.[87] However, indications for surgery remain the same (e.g., peritonitis, free air).

Postoperative ICU considerations

Postoperative ICU considerations include monitoring for and prevention of ongoing bleeding and shock, coagulopathy, hypothermia, abdominal compartment syndrome, acute lung injury, deep venous thrombosis and pulmonary emboli, and sepsis. In addition, nutrition in the form of early enteral feeding should be initiated.

Abdominal compartment syndrome

Abdominal compartment syndrome is a condition of increased intraabdominal pressure usually due to bowel and interstitial tissue edema following trauma in patients with shock and massive fluid resuscitation.[88] The increased intraabdominal pressure results in impairment of circulation, decreased tissue perfusion, and organ dysfunction (cardiovascular, renal, gut, pulmonary).[89] The tense abdomen leads to increased peak airway pressures, hypercarbia, and oliguria. Decreased thoracic venous return, with decreased cardiac output and decreased renal function due to hypoperfusion, are components of the syndrome. In addition, increased intraabdominal pressure causes decreased tidal volume, increased ventilatory pressures, and increased atelectasis. Increased intraabdominal pressure can also cause venous hypertension and elevate intracranial pressure.

Abdominal compartment pressures may be monitored by attaching an indwelling Foley catheter to a pressure transducer, leveled to the symphysis pubis, inserting 100 mL of sterile saline, and measuring the subsequent pressure.[90] Pressures greater than 20–25 mmHg accompanied with organ failure require decompression.[91] Normal postoperative abdominal pressure is 0–5 mmHg. At pressures greater than 10 mmHg, hepatic arterial blood flow decreases, at 15 mmHg cardiovascular changes occur, and at 15–25 mmHg oliguria occurs, with anuria occurring at pressures between 30 and 40 mmHg.[89] These patients require emergency decompressive laparotomy to relieve the symptoms. However, opening the abdomen results in a rapid decrease in intraabdominal pressure with a resultant reperfusion syndrome that can lead to hypotension and asystole unless proper preparations are made.[92]

Preparation for decompression of abdominal compartment syndrome involves maneuvers similar to those taken immediately prior to clamp removal during an open thoracic aortic aneurysm repair: (1) intravascular volume is increased, (2) dopamine or other vasopressors are prepared and ready to go, (3) acidosis is treated with sodium bicarbonate, and (4) preparation is completed to increase minute ventilation and transiently decrease peak end-expiratory pressure (PEEP) and driving pressure. The increased minute ventilation is necessary to eliminate CO_2 from released lactate from the gut and from administered bicarbonate. Calcium chloride is administered to protect against increased potassium washed out from the gut. Calcium is also useful to bolster the transient hypocalcemia following sodium bicarbonate administration. Morris et al. recommend 2 L of normal saline, with 50 g mannitol and 50 mEq sodium bicarbonate per liter IV prior to abdominal wall release.[92]

Deep venous thrombosis: screening, prophylaxis, and therapy

The prevalence of deep venous thrombosis in trauma patients was determined in a prospective study in which serial impedance plethysmography and lower-extremity contrast venography was used; lower-extremity deep venous thrombosis was found in 201 of 349 (58%) patients, and 18% were proximal.[93] Despite routine prophylaxis, trauma patients remain at increased risk for venous thromboembolism. A 5-year retrospective review of pulmonary embolism by Rogers et al. identified four high-risk groups on the basis of injury.[94] Head injuries, spinal cord injuries, complex pelvic fractures, and hip fractures accounted for 92% of pulmonary emboli in patients on the trauma service. Prophylactic vena cava filters were found to be efficacious in decreasing the likelihood of pulmonary embolism in high-risk trauma patients. In addition, subcutaneous heparin, early mobilization, venous compression stockings, and sequential compression devices should all be considered to reduce risk of deep venous thrombosis.

Sepsis

Postoperative sepsis can occur from peritoneal soiling, prolonged tracheal intubation, intravascular lines, and pre-injury pneumonia. Bacteremia can be classified as early onset, occurring within 96 hours after trauma, and late onset, appearing after 96 hours following trauma.[95] Gram-positive cocci are isolated more frequently in early-onset bacteremia. In addition, the risk of early-onset bacteremia is increased by the presence of pulmonary contusion or aspiration pneumonia, and with high magnitude of abdominal injuries. Intravascular catheters and endotracheal tubes do not appear to represent risk factors for early-onset bacteremia, but did increase the risk of late-onset bacteremia, especially when mechanical ventilation was required for more than seven days.

Late complications

Complications following surgical procedures for abdominal trauma carry high mortality and morbidity rates. Risk factors include missed injuries, anastomotic breakdown with peritonitis, wound infection or dehiscence, bowel ischemia or obstruction, and abscess or fistula formation. Missed injuries are associated with serious morbidity following abdominal trauma.[96] One study reviewed missed injuries following trauma to the torso.[97] The most common presentation was delayed hemorrhage, with the colon, thoracic vasculature, chest wall arteries, and diaphragm the most frequently involved sites. Half of the injuries were overlooked during the diagnostic workup, and half were missed during surgery.

Stress ulceration may occur as a result of decreased gastric blood flow and subsequent loss of protective mucous, and has been shown to occur in up to 20% of ICU patients. Acid damage to exposed submucosal structures can lead to gastritis, ulceration, and frank hemorrhage. Proton-pump inhibition, histamine-2 receptor antagonism, and topical agents that bind to exposed mucosa should be considered to avoid this complication.

Pulmonary complications, such as pneumonia, aspiration pneumonitis, and ARDS, are common postoperatively in the critically injured patient, as is sepsis. Additional considerations with abdominal trauma include bacterial translocation due to splanchnic hypoperfusion and ischemia, and liver damage resulting in decreased metabolic efficacy and decreased clotting factor production.

Summary

The management of patients with abdominal trauma has become more complex, but also safer, with the improved imaging capabilities available to the clinician. In patients with abdominal trauma accompanied by significant intraabdominal hemorrhage and hypotension, an awake preparation should be considered, with surgeons gowned, gloved, and ready to incise prior to rapid sequence induction. The most hemodynamically stable anesthetic agents available should be used to manage these patients. Prior to surgery the presence and patency of two large-bore intravenous catheters, which drain into the superior vena cava, should be ensured. For combined thoracic and abdominal trauma one catheter above the diaphragm and one below may be prudent.

A cell-saver autotransfusion device should be used with significant hemoperitoneum in the absence of fecal contamination. Early consideration should be given to damage control and planned, staged, reoperation when extended periods of hemorrhagic shock accompany surgery.

The abdominal compartment syndrome requires careful hemodynamic monitoring and emergent decompression. Post-decompression release of lactate and subsequent hemodynamic compromise should be anticipated. Subsequent staged closure of the abdomen can occur after the patient's bowel edema resolves.

Questions

(1) The number one cause of early death following abdominal trauma is:
  a. Missed hollow viscus injury
  b. Uncontrolled hemorrhage
  c. Abdominal sepsis
  d. Missed solid organ injury

(2) There is increased risk of intraabdominal injury when each of the following is present, *except*:
  a. Seatbelt abrasion/hematoma
  b. Fracture of lumbar spine
  c. Gastric bubble in left chest on chest radiograph
  d. Open extremity fractures

(3) Of the following options, the least objective examination of the abdomen is:
  a. Computed tomography of the abdomen
  b. Serial physical examinations of the abdomen
  c. Diagnostic peritoneal lavage (DPL)
  d. Focused assessment with sonography for trauma (FAST)

(4) Compared with FAST, DPL is:
  a. More sensitive
  b. Less able to differentiate ascites from blood
  c. Less invasive
  d. More operator-dependent

(5) Patients with abdominal trauma are at increased risk of aspiration. Accordingly, which of the following statements is correct?
  a. Rapid sequence induction and intubation (RSI) is always indicated following abdominal trauma.
  b. Hemodynamically stable and cooperative patients with anatomic, pathologic, or historical indications of difficult intubation are candidates for an awake intubation technique.
  c. Fiberoptic intubation techniques are contraindicated in abdominal trauma patients because of the excessively high aspiration rate.

(6) Initial intravenous access following abdominal trauma is most satisfactorily achieved by placing:
  a. Two large-bore IVs in the lower extremities
  b. One large-bore IV in an upper extremity and one in a lower extremity
  c. Two large-bore IVs in the upper extremities

(7) Hypotension following induction of anesthesia in the abdominal trauma patient can occur due to:
  a. Suppression of endogenous catecholamines by the induction drug
  b. Direct myocardial depression of vasodilatation of the induction drug
  c. Initiation of positive-pressure ventilation
  d. Abdominal incision with release of the tamponade effect of abdominal hemorrhage
  e. All of the above

(8) Which of the following statements is true regarding the appropriateness of volatile anesthetic drugs for abdominal trauma?

   a. Although halothane is not associated with increased hepatic injury compared with the others, it should be avoided in patients with known liver injury or preexisting liver dysfunction

   b. Sevoflurane can cause nephrotoxicity in rats and has been shown to commonly impair renal function in trauma patients

   c. The routine use of N_2O in trauma patients is acceptable, as long as a nasogastric tube is in place

(9) Which of the following statements best illustrates the use of a cell saver in anesthetized patients following abdominal trauma?

   a. Always contraindicated

   b. Safe and effective except in the case of biliary system injury

   c. Safe and effective in the absence of injury to the urinary tract

   d. Safe and effective except in the setting of microbial contamination following injury to hollow visceral structures (e.g., stomach or colon perforation)

(10) Venous air embolism can occur following trauma to the following structure(s):

   a. Lungs

   b. Liver

   c. Vena cava

   d. Other large vessels

   e. All of the above

Answers

(1) b
(2) d
(3) b
(4) a
(5) b
(6) c
(7) e
(8) a
(9) d
(10) e

References

1. Demetriades D, Murray J, Charalambides K, *et al.* Trauma fatalities: time and location of hospital deaths. *J Am Coll Surg* 2004; **198**: 20–6.

2. Skinner HA. *The Origin of Medical Terms.* Baltimore, MD: Williams & Wilkins, 1949.

3. Appleby JP, Nagy AG. Abdominal inquiries associated with the use of seatbelts. *Am J Surg* 1989; **157**: 457–8.

4. Berne JD, Norwood SH, McAuley CE, Villareal DH. Helical computed tomographic angiography: an excellent screening test for blunt cerebrovascular injury. *J Trauma* 2004; **57**: 11–17.

5. Rodriguez-Morales G, Rodriguez A, Shatney CH. Acute rupture of the diaphragm in blunt trauma: Analysis of 60 patients. *J Trauma* 1986; **26**: 438–44.

6. Burgess AR, Eastridge BJ, Young JW, *et al.* Pelvic ring disruptions: effective classification system and treatment protocols. *J Trauma* 1990; **30**: 848–56.

7. Hoff WS, Holevar M, Nagy KK, *et al.* Practice management guidelines for the evaluation of blunt abdominal trauma: EAST Practice Management Guidelines Work Group. *J Trauma* 2002; **53**: 602–15.

8. Bickell WH, Wall MJ, Pepe PE, *et al.* Immediate versus delayed fluid resuscitation for hypotensive patients with penetrating torso injuries. *N Engl J Med* 1994; **331**: 1105–9.

9. Shweiki E, Klena J, Wood GC, Indeck M. Assessing the true risk of abdominal solid organ injury in hospitalized rib fracture patients. *J Trauma* 2001; **50**: 684–8.

10. Healy MA, Simons RK, Winchell RJ, *et al.* A prospective evaluation of abdominal ultrasound in blunt trauma: is it useful? *J Trauma* 1996; **40**: 875–85.

11. Richards JR, Schleper NH, Woo BD, Bohnen PA, McGahan JP. Sonographic assessment of blunt abdominal trauma: A 4-year prospective study. *J Clin Ultrasound* 2002; **30**: 59–67.

12. Boulanger BR, Kearney PA, Brenneman FD, *et al.* Utilization of FAST (Focused Assessment with Sonography for Trauma) in 1999: results of a survey of North American trauma centers. *Am Surg* 2000; **66**: 1049–55.

13. Liu M, Lee CH, P'eng FK. Prospective comparison of diagnostic peritoneal lavage, computed tomographic scanning, and ultrasonography for the diagnosis of blunt abdominal injury. *J Trauma* 1993; **35**: 267–70.

14. Rozycki GS. Surgeon performed ultrasound: its use in clinical practice. *Ann Surg* 1998; **228**: 16–28.

15. Boulanger Rose JS, Levitt MA, Porter J, *et al.* Does the presence of ultrasound really affect computed tomographic scan use? A prospective randomized trial of ultrasound in trauma. *J Trauma* 2001; **51**: 545–50.

16. McKenney MG, McKenney KL, Hong JJ, *et al.* Evaluating blunt abdominal trauma with sonography: a cost analysis. *Am Surg* 2001; **67**: 930–4.

17. American College of Surgeons, Committee on Trauma. *ATLS: Advanced Trauma Life Support for Doctors (Student Course Manual)*, 9th edition. Chicago, IL: ACS, 2012.

18. Miller MT, Pasquale MD, Bromberg WJ. Not so fast. *J Trauma-Injury Infection & Critical Care* 2003; **54**: 52–60.

19. Kennedy NJ, Ireland MA, McConaghy PM. Transoesophageal echocardiographic examination of a patient with venacaval and pericardial tears after blunt chest trauma. *Br J Anaesth* 1995; **75**: 495–7.

20. Root HD, Hauser CW, McKinley CR, *et al.* Diagnostic peritoneal lavage. *Surgery* 1965; **57**: 633–7.

21. Davis JR, Morrison AL, Perkins SE, Davis FE, Ochsner MG. Ultrasound: impact on diagnostic peritoneal lavage, abdominal computed tomography, and

resident training. *Am Surg* 1999; **65**: 555–9.

22. Drost TF, Rosemurgy AS, Kearney RE, Roberts P. Diagnostic peritoneal lavage: limited indications due to evolving concepts in trauma care. *Am Surg* 1991; **57**: 126–8.

23. Stuhlfaut JW, Anderson SW, Soto JA. Blunt abdominal trauma: current imaging techniques and ct findings in patients with solid organ, bowel, and mesenteric injury. *Semin Ultrasound CT MR* 2007; **28**: 115–29.

24. Tsang BD, Panacek EA, Brant WE, Wisner DH. Effect of oral contrast administration for abdominal computed tomography in the evaluation of acute blunt trauma. *Ann Emerg Med* 1997; **30**: 7–13.

25. Mckersie RC. Intra-abdominal injury following blunt trauma: identifying the high risk patient using objective risk factors. *Arch Surg* 1989; **124**: 809–13.

26. Smith RS, Fry WR, Morabito DJ, Koehler RH, Organ CH. Therapeutic laparoscopy in trauma. *Am J Surg* 1995; **170**: 632–6.

27. Ivatury RR, Simon RJ, Stahl WM. A critical evaluation of laparoscopy in penetrating abdominal trauma. *J Trauma* 1993; **34**: 822–8.

28. Carey JE, Koo R, Miller R, Stein M. Laparoscopy and thoracoscopy in evaluation of abdominal trauma. *Am Surg* 1995; **61**: 92–5.

29. Grove CA, Lemmon G, Anderson G, McCarthy M. Emergency thoracotomy: appropriate use in the resuscitation of trauma patients. *Am Surg* 2002; **68**: 313–16.

30. Rhee PM, Acosta J, Bridgeman A, *et al.* Survival after emergency department thoracotomy: review of published data from the past 25 years. *J Am Coll Surg* 2000; **190**: 288–98.

31. Ahmed N, Vernick JJ. Management of liver trauma in adults. *J Emerg Trauma Shock* 2011; **4** (1): 114–19.

32. Traub AC, Perry JF. Injuries associated with splenic trauma. *J Trauma* 1981; **21**: 840.

33. Green JB, Shackford SR, Sise MJ, *et al.* Late septic complications in adults following splenectomy for trauma: a prospective analysis in 144 patients. *J Trauma* 1986; **26**: 999–1004.

34. McAnena OJ. Peritoneal lavage enzyme determinations following blunt and penetrating abdominal trauma. *J Trauma* 1991; **31**: 1161–4.

35. Pearlman MD, Tintinalli JE, Lorenz RP. Blunt trauma during pregnancy. *N Engl J Med* 1990; **323**: 1609–13.

36. Rothenberger D, Quattlebaum FW, Perry JF, Zabel J, Fischer RP. Blunt trauma: a review of 103 cases. *J Trauma* 1978; **18**: 173–9.

37. Doan-Wiggins L. Trauma in pregnancy. In Benrubi GI, ed., *Obstetric and Gynecologic Emergencies*. Philadelphia, PA: Lippincott, 1996, pp. 57–76.

38. Brown HL. Trauma in pregnancy. *Obstet Gynecol* 2009; **114**: 147–60.

39. Hauswald M, Kerr NL. Perimortem cesarean section. *Acad Emerg Med* 2000; **7**: 726.

40. De Pace NL, Betesh JS, Kotler MN. Postmortem cesarean section with recovery of both mother and offspring. *JAMA* 1982; **248**: 971–3.

41. Parker J, Balis N, Chester S, Adey D. Cardiopulmonary arrest in pregnancy, successful resuscitation of mother and infant after immediate cesarean section in labor ward. *Aust N Z J Obstet Gynaecol* 1996; **36**: 207–10.

42. McCartney CJ, Dark A. Cesarean delivery during cardiac arrest in late pregnancy. *Anesthesia* 1998; **53**: 310–11.

43. Katz VL, Dotters DJ, Droegemueller W. Perimortem cesarean delivery. *Obstet Gynecol* 1986; **68**: 571–6.

44. Blow O, Bassam D, Butler K, *et al.* Speed and efficiency in the resuscitation of blunt trauma patients with multiple injuries: the advantage of diagnostic peritoneal lavage over abdominal computerized tomography. *J Trauma* 1998; **44**: 287–90.

45. Wisner DH, Victor NS, Holcroft JW. Priorities in the management of multiple trauma: intracranial versus intra-abdominal injury. *J Trauma* 1993; **35**: 271–6.

46. Winchell RJ, Hoyt DB, Simons RK. Use of computed tomography of the head in the hypotensive blunt-trauma patient. *Ann Emerg Med* 1995; **25**: 737–42.

47. Biffl WL, Smith WR, Moore EE, *et al.* Evolution of a multidisciplinary clinical pathway for the management of unstable patients with pelvic fractures. *Ann Surg* 2001; **233**: 843–50.

48. Cullinane DC, Schiller HJ, Zielinski MD, *et al.* Eastern Association for the Surgery of Trauma practice management guidelines for hemorrhage in pelvic fracture: update and systematic review. *J Trauma* 2011; **71**: 1850–68.

49. Ferrera PC, Verdile VP, Bartfield JM, Snyder HS, Salluzzo RF. Injuries distracting from intraabdominal injuries after blunt trauma. *Am J Emerg Med* 1998; **16**: 145–9.

50. Ovassapian A, Krejcie TC, Yelich SJ, *et al.* Awake intubation in the patient at high risk of aspiration. *Br J Anaesth* 1989; **62**: 13–16.

51. Pizov R, Segal E, Kaplan L, *et al.* The use of systolic pressure variation in hemodynamic monitoring during deliberate hypotension in spine surgery. *J Clin Anesth* 1990; **2**: 96–100.

52. Halford F. A critique of intravenous anesthesia in war surgery. *Anesthesiology* 1943; **4**: 67–9.

53. Adams RC, Gray HK. Intravenous anesthesia with pentothal sodium in the case of gunshot wound associated with accompanying severe traumatic shock and loss of blood: report of a case. *Anesthesiology* 1943; **4**: 70–3.

54. Weiskopf RB, Bogetz MS, Roizen MF, Reid IA. Cardiovascular and metabolic sequelae of including anesthesia with ketamine or thiopental in hypovolemic swine. *Anesthesiology* 1984; **60**: 214–19.

55. Bogetz MS, Katz JA. Recall of surgery for major trauma. *Anesthesiology* 1984; **61**: 6–9.

56. Sanchez-Izquierdo-Riera JA, Caballero-Cubedo RE, Perez-Vela JL, *et al.* Propofol versus midazolam: safety and efficacy for sedating the severe trauma patient. *Anesth Analg* 1998; **86**: 1219–24.

57. Scheller MS. New volatile anesthetics: desflurane and sevoflurane. *Semin Anesth* 1992; **11**: 114–22.

58. Bunker JP, Forrest WH, Mosteller F, ed. *The National Halothane Study: a Study of the Possible Association Between Halothane Anesthesia and Postoperative Hepatic Necrosis*. Washington, DC: US Government Printing Office, 1969.

59. Smith GC, Kenna JG, Harrison DJ, *et al.* Autoantibodies to hepatic microsomal carboxylesterase in halothane hepatitis. *Lancet* 1993; **342**: 963–4.

60. Kharasch ED, Frink EJ Jr, Zager R, *et al.* Assessment of low-flow sevoflurane and

isoflurane effects on renal function using sensitive markers of tubular toxicity. *Anesthesiology* 1997; **86**: 1238–53.

61. Eger EI, Gong D, Koblin DD, *et al.* Dose-related biochemical markers of renal injury after sevoflurane versus desflurane anesthesia in volunteers. *Anesth Analg* 1997; **85**: 1154–63.

62. Eger EI, Bowland T, Ionescu P, *et al.* Recovery and kinetic characteristics of desflurane and sevoflurane in volunteers after 8-h exposure, including kinetics of degradation products. *Anesthesiology* 1997; **87**: 517–26.

63. Smith LA, Barker DE, Burns RP. Autotransfusion utilization in abdominal trauma. *Am Surg* 1997; **63**: 47–9.

64. Brown CVR, Foulkrod KH, Sadler HT, *et al.* Autologous blood transfusion during emergency trauma operations. *Arch Surg* 2010; **145** (7): 690–4.

65. Crosson JT. Complications associated with massive transfusions. *Clin Lab Med* 1996; **16**: 873–82.

66. Sihler KC. Napolitano LM: Complications of massive transfusion. *Chest* 2010; **137** (1): 209–20.

67. Mitchell KJ, Moncure KE, Onyeije C, Rao MS, Siram S. Evaluation of massive volume replacement in the penetrating trauma patient. *J Natl Med Assoc* 1994; **86**: 926–9.

68. Cosgriff N, Moore EE, Sauaia A, *et al.* Predicting life-threatening coagulopathy in the massively transfused trauma patient: hypothermia and acidosis revisited. *J Trauma* 1997; **42**: 857–61.

69. Kashuk JL, Moore EE. The emerging role of rapid thromboelastography in trauma care. *J Trauma* 2009; **67**: 417–18.

70. Gentilello LM, Jurkovich GJ, Stark MS, Hassantash SA, O'Keefe GE. Is hypothermia in the victim of major trauma protective or harmful? A randomized, prospective study. *Ann Surg* 1997; **226**: 439–47.

71. Koshimizu T, Saitoh K, Mitsuhata H, *et al.* Massive bleeding from the ruptured liver and the inferior vena cava controlled with autotransfusion and cerebral ischemia treated with mild hypothermia. *Masui* 1997; **46**: 978–82.

72. Wilson WC. Anesthesia for colorectal surgery. In Block GE, Moosa AR, eds., *Operative Colorectal Surgery.* Philadelphia, PA: Saunders, 1994, pp. 107–26.

73. Hirshberg A, Mattox K. Duration of antibiotic treatment in surgical infections of the abdomen. Penetrating abdominal trauma. *Eur J Surg Suppl* 1996; (576): 6–7.

74. Kirton OC, O'Neill PA, Kestner M, Tortella BJ. Perioperative antibiotic use in high-risk penetrating hollow viscus injury: a prospective randomized, double-blind, placebo-control trial of 24 hours versus 5 days. *J Trauma* 2000; **49**: 822–32.

75. Reihner E, Brismar B. Management of splenic trauma-changing concepts. *Eur J Emerg Med* 1995; **2**: 47–51.

76. Rhee P, Nunley MK, Demetriades D, Velmahos G, Doucet JJ. Tetanus and trauma: a review and recommendations. *J Trauma* 2005; **58**: 1082–8.

77. Kudsk KA, Sheldon GF, Lim RC. Atrial-caval shunting after trauma. *J Trauma* 1982; **22**: 81–5.

78. Bender JS, Bailey CE, Saxe JM, Ledgerwood AM, Lucas CE. The technique of visceral packing: recommended management of difficult fascial closure in trauma patients. *J Trauma* 1994; **36**: 182–5.

79. Brenneman FD, Rizoli SB, Boulanger BR. Abbreviated laparotomy for damage control: a case report. *Can J Surg* 1994; **37**: 237–9.

80. Carmona RH, Peck DZ, Lim RC. The role of packing and planned reoperation in severe hepatic trauma. *J Trauma* 1984; **24**: 779–84.

81. Hirshberg A, Mattox KL. Planned reoperation for severe trauma. *Ann Surg* 1995; **222**: 3–8.

82. Howdieshell TR, Yeh KA, Hawkins ML, Cue JI. Temporary abdominal wall closure in trauma patients: indications, technique, and results. *World J Surg* 1995; **19**: 154–8.

83. Abikhaled JA, Granchi TS, Wall MJ, Hirshberg A, Mattox KL. Prolonged abdominal packing for trauma is associated with increased morbidity and mortality. *Am Surg* 1997; **63**: 1109–12.

84. Meredith JW, Young JS, Bowling J, Roboussin D. Nonoperative management of blunt hepatic trauma: the exception or the rule? *J Trauma* 1994; **36**: 529–34.

85. Collin GR, Bianchi JD. Laparoscopic examination of the traumatized spleen with blood salvage for autotransfusion. *Am Surg* 1997; **63**: 478–80.

86. Guth AA, Pachter HL, Jacobowitz GR. Rupture of the pathologic spleen: is there a role for nonoperative therapy? *J Trauma* 1996; **41**: 214–18.

87. Nance ML, Peden GW, Shapiro MB, *et al.* Solid viscus injury predicts major hollow viscus injury in blunt abdominal trauma. *J Trauma* 1997; **43**: 618–22.

88. Malbrain ML, Cheatham ML, Kirkpatrick A, *et al.* Results from the International Conference of Experts on Intra-abdominal Hypertension and Abdominal Compartment Syndrome. I. Definitions. *Intensive Care Med* 2006; **32** (11): 1722–32.

89. Schein M, Wittmann DH, Aprahamian CC, Condon RE. The abdominal compartment syndrome: the physiological and clinical consequences of elevated intra-abdominal pressure. *J Am Coll Surg* 1995; **180**: 745–53.

90. Iberti TJ, Kelly KM, Gentili DR, Hirsch S, Benjamin E. A simple technique to accurately determine intra-abdominal pressure. *Crit Care Med* 1987; **15**: 1140–2.

91. Kron IL, Harman PK, Nolan SP. The measurement of intra abdominal pressure as a criteria for abdominal re-exploration. *Ann Surg* 1984; **199**: 28–30.

92. Morris JA, Eddy VA, Blinman TA, *et al.* The staged celiotomy for trauma. Issues in unpacking and reconstruction. *Ann Surg* 1993; **217**: 576–86.

93. Geerts WH, Code KI, Jay RM, Chen E, Szalai JP. A prospective study of venous thromboembolism after major trauma. *N Engl J Med* 1994; **331**: 1601–6.

94. Rogers FB, Shackford SR, Ricci MA, Wilson JT, Parsons S. Routine prophylactic vena cava filter insertion in severely injured trauma patients decreases the incidence of pulmonary embolism. *J Am Coll Surg* 1995; **180**: 641–7.

95. Antonelli M, Moro ML, D'Errico RR, *et al.* Early and late onset bacteremia have different risk factors in trauma patients. *Intensive Care Med* 1996; **22**: 735–41.

96. Sung CK, Kim KH. Missed injuries in abdominal trauma. *J Trauma* 1996; **41**: 276–82.

97. Hirshberg A, Wall MJ, Allen MK, Mattox KL. Causes and patterns of missed injuries in trauma. *Am J Surg* 1994; **168**: 299–303.

Intraoperative one-lung ventilation for trauma anesthesia

George W. Kanellakos and Peter Slinger

Objectives

(1) Review the indications for one-lung ventilation in trauma.
(2) Describe the physiologic effects of one-lung ventilation in trauma.
(3) Review the modern management of one-lung ventilation, including treatment for intraoperative hypoxemia.
(4) Discuss lung isolation techniques and relevant bronchial anatomy.
(5) Discuss the advantages and disadvantages of equipment options for achieving lung isolation.

Introduction

Trauma patients who have one or more of the "deadly dozen" thoracic injuries[1,2] are difficult to manage and require expert clinical management.[3–6] These are airway obstruction, tracheobronchial disruption, tension pneumothorax, open pneumothorax, flail chest, pulmonary contusion, massive hemothorax, cardiac tamponade, myocardial contusion, aortic disruption, traumatic diaphragmatic tear, and esophageal disruption. Treatment is made more difficult by the presence of occult injuries, requiring constant clinical reassessment. The traditional classification of blunt versus penetrating thoracic trauma is important, and both mechanisms lead to significant respiratory injury, at any level within the tracheobronchial tree. All trauma algorithms place the utmost emphasis on early diagnosis. This can result in an emergency room thoracotomy (with 7% survival rate) or delayed surgery in the operating room.[4] All cases require a secure airway, with the potential for lung isolation and one-lung ventilation (OLV).

Indications for lung isolation in trauma patients

Traditionally, the approach to lung isolation is divided into absolute and relative indications (Table 33.1).[7] There are two guiding principles:

(1) Lung protection: prevent contralateral lung soiling from blood or secretions (pus), or to prevent further lung injury secondary to positive-pressure ventilation, as in the case of a bronchopleural fistula or severe pulmonary contusion.
(2) Surgical procedures: to facilitate surgical management, essential in video-assisted thoracoscopic surgery (VATS).

The decision to establish OLV should be made on a case-by-case basis. A discussion with members of the healthcare team, particularly surgical colleagues, can be helpful in establishing an agreed-upon treatment plan. This is because OLV can be established by a number of techniques, which can vary significantly from patient to patient depending on the type of injury, clinical stability, planned surgical procedure, or surgeon or anesthesiologist preference. One technique is not always the best, with anesthesiologists often differing in their approaches, being influenced by personal experience and comfort level.[8]

Advanced Trauma Life Support (ATLS) primary and secondary surveys can help guide treatment, including airway management (see Chapter 3). Rapid sequence induction (RSI) with direct laryngoscopy and in-line cervical stabilization is often performed to secure the airway.[9] The patient's normal anatomy must be assessed to determine whether intubation would be difficult without the presenting injuries. Difficult intubations can be unexpected in nontrauma patients, and

Table 33.1 Indications for lung isolation

Absolute	Relative
Infection	Surgical exposure
Hemorrhage	High: thoracic aneurysm, dissection, or rupture
Bronchial disruption or fistula	High: pneumonectomy
Unilateral bullous disease	High: upper lobectomy
Lung lavage	Low: esophagectomy
Video-assisted thoracoscopic surgery (VATS)	Low: middle, lower lobectomy
Differential ventilation	Low: thoracoscopy

Adapted from Brodsky & Lemmens 2003.[7]

Trauma Anesthesia, 2nd Edition, ed. Charles E. Smith. Published by Cambridge University Press. © Charles E. Smith, 2015.

normal airways become significantly more difficult in trauma situations. Secondary and tertiary plans are necessary, with a thorough knowledge of the difficult airway algorithm (see Chapter 3).

There are multiple signs and symptoms that may be present to help guide airway management as well as the urgency for intervention.[3,5,10,11] The presence of hoarseness, stridor, hemoptysis, subcutaneous emphysema, mediastinal emphysema on chest x-ray, or a persistent air leak through a chest tube are all important signs to be recognized. These can indicate the presence of airway disruption, and they are usually caused when high intrathoracic pressure is exerted against a closed glottis. Management is complicated because the location of the injury is often unknown. This makes intubation more difficult, but also emphasizes the necessity of airway visualization to avoid further injury. Studies indicate that up to 80% of injuries occur within 2.5 cm of the carina, which helps provide an area of focus for the clinician.[12,13] Bronchoscopy is necessary for confirmation, and to safely secure the airway in these patients it is recommended that spontaneous respiration be maintained. However the airway is secured, treatment with a chest tube should be expected, as positive-pressure ventilation might reveal an undetected injury leading to tension pneumothorax.[14] When there is a high probability of lung injury it is prudent that chest drainage tubes be placed prophylactically prior to the initiation of positive-pressure ventilation.

In high tracheal injuries, establishing OLV is usually not necessary to stabilize the patient, but it may be necessary for the surgical repair. Management usually involves passing an endotracheal tube (ETT) past the lesion under direct vision and then ventilating normally. When a bronchial or carinal injury is present, the management becomes far more complicated. Blind insertion of any tube should be avoided, making the availability of fiberoptic bronchoscopy essential. Even though the presence of blood or secretions may make this difficult, bronchoscopy should always be attempted, as instituting OLV in these patients can be critical for stabilizing the patient and avoiding further injury.

In addition to tracheal or bronchial injuries, OLV is also necessary for other thoracic injuries. Vascular injuries vary significantly in their management, and surgical repair is often necessary. When bleeding occurs within the airway, lung isolation for contralateral lung protection is indicated. Stabilization of the patient often occurs only when OLV is established, but occasionally it is not tolerated and oxygenation is compromised. When OLV cannot be tolerated, many techniques can be instituted to manage hypoxemia, and these are described later in this chapter. Occasionally, hypoxemia can only be corrected with intermittent two-lung ventilation. Care must be taken to minimize airway pressures, because initiating ventilation to the injured lung can produce further injury, including more bleeding, pneumothorax, and air embolism.[15,16] Another approach includes differential lung ventilation, with the injured lung exposed to much lower airway pressures.

Aside from lung parenchymal vascular injuries, open surgical repair of descending thoracic transection can be facilitated by OLV. However, these patients most often undergo endovascular repair without the need for OLV (see Chapters 29 and 30).

Esophageal injuries account for the last main category of thoracic trauma that requires lung isolation. Esophageal injury is uncommon because of the protected location of the esophagus, but it can still occur with penetrating trauma or ingestible agents. Surprisingly, the most common cause of esophageal injury is iatrogenic, accounting for 43% of all injuries of the esophagus.[17] Iatrogenic injuries include surgical trauma, nasogastric tube placement, traumatic intubations, and transesophageal echocardiography. Surgical repair of midesophageal injuries often requires a thoracotomy approach, where once again OLV is advantageous but not critical to the repair.

Another select group of trauma patients who provide challenges to the anesthesiologist are patients with cervical spine injury that require lung isolation for thoracic surgical procedures. Often the standard approach of using a double-lumen tube (DLT) in these patients is not feasible, secondary to greater difficulty of insertion relative to normal ETTs. Common approaches to establish lung isolation include the use of a bronchial blocker placed through a more easily placed ETT or the placement of a DLT via a tube exchange technique.

One-lung ventilation
Physiologic effects

Ventilation and oxygenation during OLV are complex topics that are well described elsewhere.[18] To summarize, when compared with normal ventilation, two-lung ventilation in the lateral decubitus position with the chest open results in ventilation/perfusion (V/Q) mismatch. This is mostly due to compression of the dependent lung by gravitational, mediastinal, and abdominal forces resulting in relatively greater ventilation to the nondependent lung. Combined with decreased perfusion to the nondependent lung due to gravity, the physiologic state leads to a reduction in PaO_2 and an increased P_AO_2–PaO_2 gradient. When OLV is superimposed, oxygenation is further impaired because of the increased shunt that is created. By not ventilating one lung, one would expect a 50% cardiac shunt, but this is not what is observed clinically. The measured PaO_2 decreases far less than predicted, and the observed shunt measures only 20–30% of the cardiac output. The most significant mechanism that accounts for this observation is hypoxic pulmonary vasoconstriction (HPV).[19] Factors affecting HPV are numerous and beyond the scope of this chapter. In general, the lung responds to atelectasis or a reduction in PaO_2 by increasing pulmonary vascular resistance, leading to a reduction of blood flow through the nonventilated or "hypoxic" lung. Clinically, this results in most patients easily tolerating the V/Q mismatch introduced by OLV. In addition, there are numerous interventions that can be applied to help reduce the

Table 33.2 Management of one-lung ventilation

Step 1: Two-lung ventilation until chest opening
Step 2: Assess proper tube placement and patency
Step 3: FiO_2 at 100%[19,20]
Step 4: Tidal volume 6 mL/kg
Step 5: Respiratory rate • Conventional: maintain $PCO_2 = 40$ mmHg • Current: "permissive hypercapnia" when extreme parameters reached[21,22]
Step 6: CPAP of 5–10 cm H_2O to nondependent lung[23,24] • May interfere significantly in VATS procedures
Step 7: PEEP of 5–10 cm H_2O to dependent lung[25,26] • Harmful if preexisting intrinsic PEEP or auto-PEEP is high[29]
Step 8: Increase CPAP to nondependent lung to 10–15 cm H_2O
Step 9: Equalize PEEP to dependent lung and CPAP to nondependent lung
Step 10: Intermittent ventilation of nondependent lung
Step 11: HFV to nondependent lung[30] • Although superior to CPAP, not practical due to complexity
Step 12: Inhaled nitric oxide • Benefit limited to patients with pulmonary hypertension[31]
Step 13: Pulmonary artery compression

CPAP, continuous positive air pressure; HFV, high frequency ventilation; PCO_2, partial pressure of carbon dioxide; PEEP, peak end-expiratory pressure; VATS, video-assisted thoracoscopic surgery.
Adapted from Benumof 1995 and Triantafillou et al. 2003.[30,31]

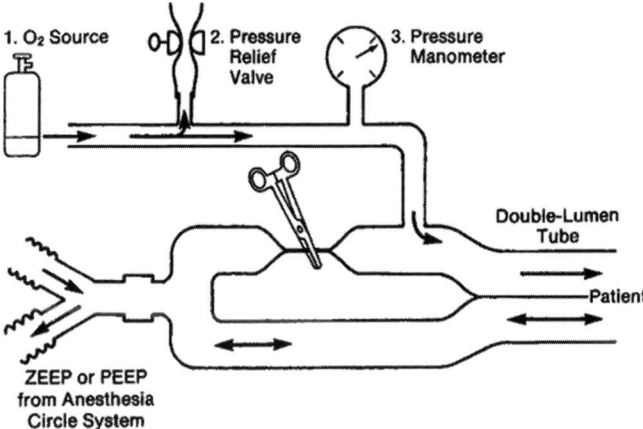

Figure 33.1 Components of CPAP systems. Three components of continuous positive airway pressure systems: (1) oxygen source, (2) pressure regulator (relief valve), and (3) pressure manometer. (Reproduced from Benumof 1995,[20] with permission from Elsevier.)

degree of hypoxemia (see next section). It should be noted that most problems regarding OLV revolve around hypoxemia, while the $PaCO_2$ is significantly less affected as a result of oxygen–hemoglobin dissociation characteristics.

Management of one-lung ventilation and hypoxemia

Classic management of one-lung ventilation has been described by Benumof.[20,21] There have been updates to this approach, and Table 33.2 is a summary of conventional and current management techniques. Of the interventions listed for correcting hypoxemia, the most important or successful intervention after ensuring an FiO_2 of 100% is the application of continuous positive airway pressure (CPAP) to the nondependent lung. It is extremely rare for severe hypoxemia (PaO_2 < 50 mmHg) not to be corrected when CPAP is applied.[27,32] In the operative setting, it is recommended to discuss starting CPAP with surgical colleagues, because it often produces minor expansion of the surgical lung. Many CPAP equipment systems have been described in the literature. Figure 33.1 shows an example of the three components that are common to all of these systems. These include an oxygen source, a

pressure regulator, and a manometer to measure the resulting pressure.

Volume control versus pressure control

Although there have been numerous advances in equipment, one of the most important advances in OLV strategies lies in ventilatory management. It has become evident that traditional OLV strategies, particularly ventilatory tidal volumes of 10 mL/kg with respiratory rates of 8–12 breaths per minute, contribute to lung injury (see Chapter 19).[33,34] This is true in healthy patients, and it becomes more important in thoracic trauma where the lung has already been injured.[35–38] Patients who are relatively healthy and require OLV are easily managed by using traditional volume-control settings, but this no longer qualifies as standard care for thoracic anesthesia. The concept of "volutrauma" to a healthy lung can no longer be ignored, and many studies have shown that healthy lungs ventilated in this manner release the inflammatory mediators that are commonly seen in patients with acute respiratory distress syndrome (ARDS).[39–43] The debate concerns whether this is clinically significant.[44,45] Many authors advocate that lung-protective strategies currently used to treat ARDS patients should be applied to patients undergoing OLV. Clinically, this translates to tidal volumes of 6 mL/kg or lower, with respiratory rates adjusted to maintain normocapnia. In difficult ventilatory cases, an increase in PCO_2 or "permissive hypercapnia" has become an acceptable approach to help limit the degree of lung injury secondary to volutrauma.[24]

In addition to the suggested decreased tidal volumes and airway pressures, it should be noted that there are significant differences in the ventilation pattern between volume-controlled ventilation (VCV) and pressure-controlled ventilation (PCV) settings. For any given tidal volume in VCV, the same volume can be achieved in PCV with significantly lower airway pressures.[46] This is due to the mechanical delivery characteristics of each mode of ventilation and the interaction with lung compliance. In healthy patients not undergoing OLV, this is usually not significant, because airway pressure seldom becomes elevated. However, in thoracic surgical patients undergoing thoracotomies in the lateral position, airway pressures using VCV can rise significantly. Peak airway pressures of 30 cmH$_2$O and plateau pressures of 20 cmH$_2$O are relatively common occurrences. These pressures should trigger the anesthesiologist to make adjustments, primarily by converting to PCV.

Lung isolation techniques

Innovation in lung isolation has benefited the modern-day anesthesiologist with a surplus of options for establishing lung isolation. What once was a major undertaking is now routine and should be part of the skills of all anesthesiology trainees. The options more commonly available are summarized in Table 33.3. It is up to the anesthesiologist to be familiar with

these choices, and this is particularly important in the trauma patient. Their availability varies according to institution preference and budget. Although double-lumen tubes might be standard in most institutions, more specialized equipment might not be available, or might be used so infrequently that clinicians are uncomfortable with its use. Most clinicians would agree that the gold standard for establishing OLV is with a DLT, as compared with the main alternative, bronchial blockers (BBs). This is based primarily on the assumption that the quality of OLV is best when a DLT is used. In the past this would have been considered true, but both types of technology have undergone major improvement in their design, making the quality of lung isolation between the two indistinguishable in many cases.[47] In trauma patients, DLTs become less ideal for lung isolation, because of their size and the difficulty of placement, particularly when airways are compromised. In these patients, BBs are more easily placed and suitable despite their limitations. These limitations must be considered,

Table 33.3 Common options for lung isolation

Options	Advantages	Disadvantages
Double-lumen tubes (DLT) 1. Direct laryngoscopy 2. Via tube exchanger 3. Fiberoptically	Quickest to place successfully Repositioning rarely required Bronchoscopy to isolated lung Suction to isolated lung CPAP easily added Can alternate OLV to either lung easily Placement still possible if bronchoscopy not available	Size selection more difficult Difficult to place in patients with difficult airways or abnormal tracheas Nonoptimal postoperative two-lung ventilation Laryngeal trauma Bronchial trauma
Bronchial blockers (BB) 1. Arndt 2. Cohen 3. Fuji 4. EZ Blocker 5. Fogarty catheter	Size selection rarely an issue Easily added to regular ETT Allows ventilation during placement Easier placement in patients with difficult airways and in children • Bilateral blocker balloons • Allows for sequential lung isolation without repositioning Postoperative two-lung ventilation easily accomplished by withdrawing blocker Selective lobar lung isolation possible CPAP to isolated lung possible	More time needed for positioning Repositioning needed more often Bronchoscope essential for positioning Nonoptimal right lung isolation due to RUL anatomy Bronchoscopy to isolated lung impossible Minimal suction to isolated lung Difficult to alternate OLV to either lung
Univent	Same as bronchial blockers Less repositioning than BBs	Same as bronchial blockers Higher air flow resistance than regular ETT Larger diameter than regular ETT
Endobronchial tubes	Like regular ETTs, easier placement in patients with difficult airways Longer than regular ETT Short cuff designed for lung isolation Tube is reinforced	Bronchoscopy necessary for placement Does not allow for bronchoscopy, suctioning, or CPAP to isolated lung Difficult right lung OLV
Endotracheal tube advanced into bronchus	Easier placement in patients with difficult airways	Does not allow for bronchoscopy, suctioning, or CPAP to isolated lung Cuff not designed for lung isolation Difficult right lung OLV

CPAP, continuous positive air pressure; ETT, endotracheal tube; OLV, one-lung ventilation.

however, because the placement of a bronchial blocker might be simple and provide excellent lung collapse, but it quickly becomes impractical if suctioning the isolated lung is essential. The pros and cons of each device must be considered in relation to the patient's anatomy and injuries.

Provided that institutions are equipped appropriately, it has been suggested that the major barrier to establishing and maintaining lung isolation today is not the choice of equipment, but rather the operator's limited knowledge of bronchial anatomy.[48] Without proper knowledge of bronchial anatomy, bronchoscopic placement of any endobronchial tube or device is set up for failure. Despite user preference and bias, most equipment choices for lung isolation work very well – but they fail when used inappropriately or in the wrong clinical setting. For example, successful DLT placement may be impossible when the anesthesiologist fails to recognize anatomic variations in bronchial segments, such as a carinal right upper lobe take-off. The failure to recognize anatomic features and their interaction with lung isolation equipment is a major barrier to successful lung isolation. This particularly applies to the thoracic trauma patient, where injuries can interact with tube placement to a greater extent.

Bronchial anatomy

Knowledge of bronchial anatomy is critical if lung isolation is to be successful. It is a subject that is not emphasized in medical education and is even neglected to some degree in anesthesiology residency training. Applying or correlating that knowledge during hands-on bronchoscopy is difficult and requires practice. A thorough working knowledge of bronchial anatomy makes the troubleshooting of any problems that may arise with OLV far more efficient and safe.

There are a number of anatomic structures that must be familiar to the bronchoscopist. Table 33.4 summarizes these structures, with a few clinical pointers that can be used to help identify them.

Fiberoptic bronchoscopy

Fiberoptic bronchoscopy has become the gold standard in providing anesthetic care to thoracic surgery patients. Although proper functioning of endobronchial devices can be verified clinically, their proper placement and/or evaluation during procedures can only be accomplished with bronchoscopy.[49] The placement of some devices (for example, the Arndt endobronchial blocker) is totally dependent on the use of a fiberoptic bronchoscope. For these reasons, every surgical procedure that requires lung isolation must have a bronchoscope readily available. When a difficult clinical scenario is encountered, the clinician must be familiar with normal anatomy and tube placement. This is especially true when anatomic variations arise. It is recommended that all clinicians take every opportunity to practice bronchoscopy and identify anatomy whenever possible.

Table 33.4 Bronchial anatomy (supine patient)

Anatomical structure	
Trachea and carina 1. flat membranous trachea posteriorly (semicircular-shaped lumen) 2. bifurcation is sharp 3. first-generation bronchi are large and have no bifurcations in sight	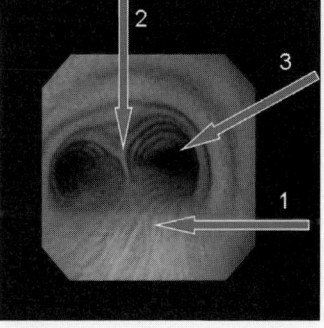
Left mainstem bronchus (LMB) 1. long, average length 5 cm 2. bifurcation of left upper and lower lobes not visible	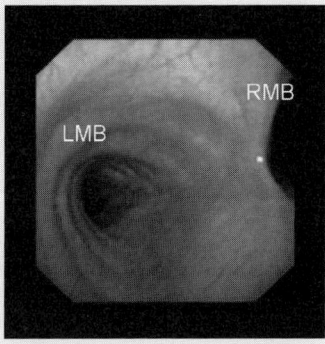
Left upper lobe (LUL) and left lower lobe (LLL) bronchi 1. longitudinal bundles usually more prominent into lower lobe (dashed lines) 2. LLL-LUL carina angled horizontally (~ 8–2 o'clock position)	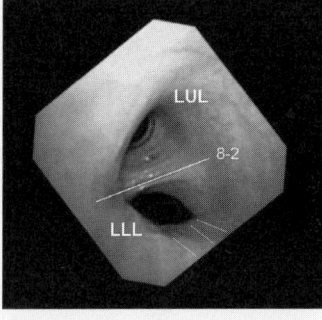
Right mainstem bronchus (RMB) 1. short, average length 2.5 cm (dashed line) 2. followed by longer right bronchus intermedius (RBI) 3. right upper lobe (RUL) bifurcation visible	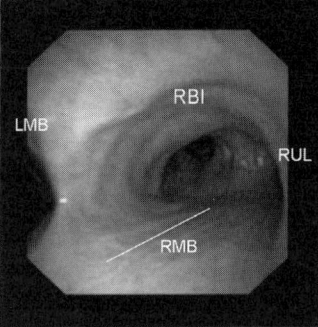

Table 33.4 *(cont.)*

Anatomical structure

Right upper lobe bronchus (RUL)
1. characteristic bronchial trifurcation

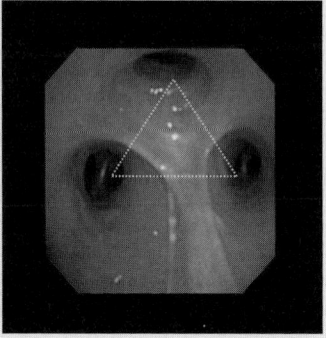

Right bronchus intermedius (RBI)
1. longitudinal bundles usually more prominent into right lower lobe (dashed lines in proximal view)
2. linear alignment of bronchi (dashed line in distal view)
3. right lower lobe (RLL) with segmental bronchi immediately visible
4. right middle lobe (RML) with segmental bronchi not visible
5. angle of RML-RLL carina, if followed proximally, would line up with right upper lobe take-off (not visible in figure)

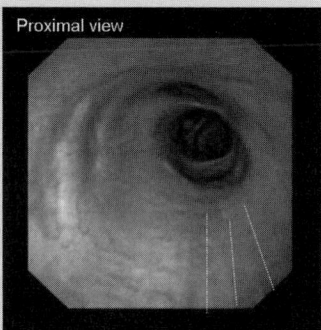

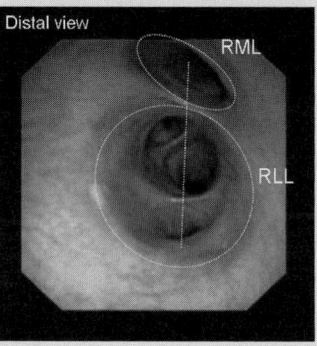

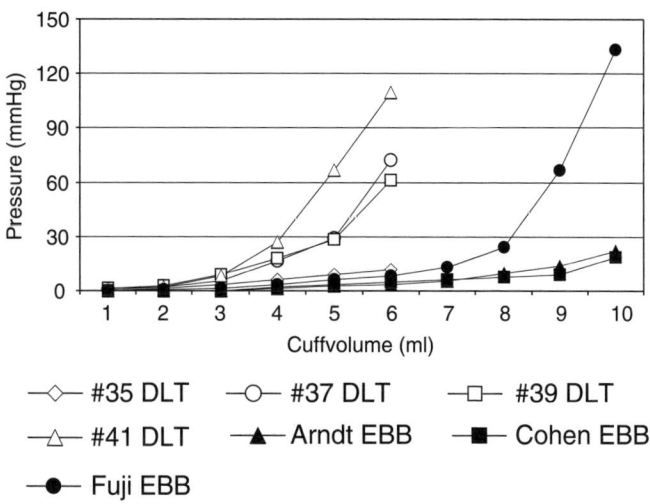

Figure 33.2 The mean pressures exerted by endobronchial devices on the model bronchus, under static conditions. DLT, double-lumen tube; EBB, endobronchial blocker.

Bronchoscopy does not only mean becoming familiar with tracheobronchial anatomy; in addition, the operator must anticipate practical problems that arise with everyday use. Other reasons for technique failure are inexperience and insufficient planning. For example, during the placement of a bronchial blocker, the operator must anticipate that an adult bronchoscope will not be useful if the patient has a 7.0 mm endotracheal tube in place. The blocker and the adult bronchoscope will not fit simultaneously in this tube. Alternatively, an adult bronchoscope provides exceptional suctioning but will not fit within a 35 Fr DLT. In thoracic trauma, where time is limited, proper preparation can make the difference in achieving successful outcomes.

Equipment

Table 33.3 is a comparison chart that summarizes the advantages and disadvantages of the common technology available for lung isolation. One of the main concerns of past DLTs and present BBs is the pressure they exert against the bronchus, potentially leading to bronchial injury. A study comparing the pressures exerted by the cuffs of modern endobronchial devices shows that in all devices, when appropriately inflated, the cuffs fail to exert a bronchial wall pressure that exceeds 30 mmHg (Fig. 33.2).[50]

Double-lumen tubes (DLTs)

Bjork and Carlens first described DLTs in 1950. Today there are many manufacturers of DLTs, and since 1950 there have been many changes made in their design. The most notable change has been the introduction of a highly visible, low-pressure cuff.[51] DLTs are used routinely for lung isolation and are considered the gold standard. Proper sizing is important, because tubes that are too small have been associated with iatrogenic injury due to being placed too deep in the airway or by causing bronchial injury secondary to hyperinflated cuffs.[52] Tubes that are too large simply do not fit into the bronchus or cause excessive swelling of the airway due to trauma. A guide to selecting the appropriate size of DLT is presented in Table 33.5.

Placing a DLT can be challenging at times, but it can become significantly more difficult in trauma patients. First, laryngoscopy can be more difficult due to cervical spine considerations and because patients often are uncooperative. Second, the airway itself can be compromised, and as DLTs are very large they have a greater probability of causing injury than regular ETTs. The recommended depth of insertion is 29 cm for a patient 170 cm tall.[53] When placed with a blind

Table 33.5 Recommendations for DLT size

Males	Height < 170 cm: 39 Fr	Height > 170 cm: 41 Fr
Females	Height < 160 cm: 35 Fr	Height > 160 cm: 37 Fr

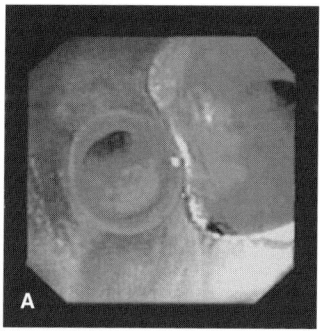 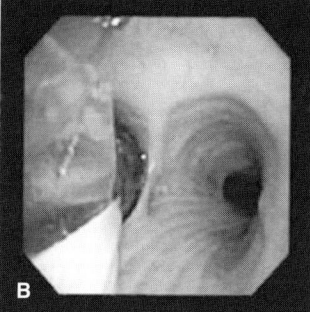

Figure 33.3 Correct positioning of right and left double-lumen tubes. (**A**) Right DLT. Within the bronchial lumen, the center channel should reveal the opening of right bronchus intermedius. The side port should show patent right upper lobe bronchus. The bronchial cuff position should then be checked through the tracheal lumen. (**B**) Left DLT. Within the tracheal lumen, the blue bronchial cuff should be slightly visible.

technique, DLT malposition can occur in approximately 30% of patients. Whenever ventilation is impaired, the anesthesiologist must check the position of the tube and deflate the bronchial cuff until the problem has been corrected. This requires fiberoptic bronchoscopy, which, as discussed, has become standard care. Figure 33.3 shows the correct placement of right and left DLTs.

In the situation where the left mainstem bronchus is injured or is the planned location of surgery, it is advantageous to use a right-sided DLT. Placement of right DLTs is never straightforward, as positioning requires greater precision to avoid obstruction of the right upper lobe (RUL). A quick method to correctly place a right-sided DLT involves taking note of the RUL location with fiberoptic bronchoscopy, advancing the DLT past the opening, then slowly retracting the tube while rotating in the direction of the RUL orifice. Correct placement is confirmed when the orifice to the RUL is visible through the side opening of the DLT (Fig. 33.3) and when the bronchial cuff is successfully inflated so that the left mainstem bronchus is unobstructed. Anomalous RUL anatomy, estimated in 1 in 250 people, is one reason why right DLTs fail in providing adequate lung isolation. Change in tube position due to patient positioning or surgical movement, however, is the most common reason for failure of right DLTs to provide adequate lung isolation.

It should be noted that video laryngoscopes (i.e., Glide-Scope, C-MAC) have quickly made their way into the practice of many anesthesiologists. They have the ability to convert a difficult intubation into one that is easy to manage, a benefit that can also be applied to thoracic trauma. Because DLTs are more difficult to insert, and trauma patients present with unique airway challenges, it should be remembered that DLT placement can be facilitated with the use of such a scope.

The main difficulty encountered clinically is limited space in mouth opening. In these situations, the problem can be overcome by placing the DLT into the oral cavity prior to inserting the fiberoptic laryngoscope. This decreases the potential for cuff rupture, and when the DLT is shaped with the same curvature as the laryngoscope blade, the probability of successful intubation is increased. Prior to advancing the DLT past the glottic opening, fiberoptic bronchoscopy is again recommended.

The main technique that is used to place DLTs in patients with difficult airways involves the use of an airway exchange catheter. These catheters are discussed in more detail below (see *Postoperative ventilation*).

One patient group in thoracic trauma requires special consideration. These are patients with a tracheostomy, who occasionally require lung isolation. There are multiple techniques for establishing OLV in these patients. Options include the placement of a regular ETT through the tracheostomy site with advancement into the appropriate bronchus. An alternative to the regular ETT, and a better choice, is the endobronchial tube (see Table 33.3). It has a flexible design and a short, distal cuff that is better suited to lung isolation. The use of a DLT or BB through the tracheostomy is an acceptable option, but it must be noted that the bulk of the equipment lies outside the patient and may become cumbersome to manage. If the anatomy permits, lung isolation can also be achieved by removing the tracheostomy tube just before advancing an ETT or DLT through the glottic opening. It should be noted that DLTs are available in a short design specifically tailored to the tracheostomy patient (Fig. 33.4).

Bronchial blockers (BBs)

Bronchial blockers consist of a very thin, relatively stiff "catheter" equipped with an inflatable distal cuff. They are designed to be placed within an endotracheal tube and directed into either lung, depending on the clinical situation. The blocker can be placed external to the ETT, but this makes successful lung isolation more difficult. A benefit of BB technology is the ability to provide lobar lung isolation, which is impossible to do with other equipment. Figure 33.2 shows how BBs, when used appropriately with 7 mL of cuff volume or less, exert a mean pressure less than 30 mmHg against the bronchus wall.[50] All models available today have this configuration, with some form of modification engineered to help direct the distal tip or balloon. Blockers have many advantages over other choices in achieving lung isolation, which have recently only become significant due to their technological advances.

There is a belief that BBs provide less satisfactory surgical conditions than DLTs. Many believe this to be true and, in fact, there is probably enough evidence in the literature to support such a claim, but only in certain clinical scenarios. The success rate of adequate lung deflation with a BB is dependent on the operative side, for reasons related to anatomy. It has been shown that the quality of lung deflation during video-assisted

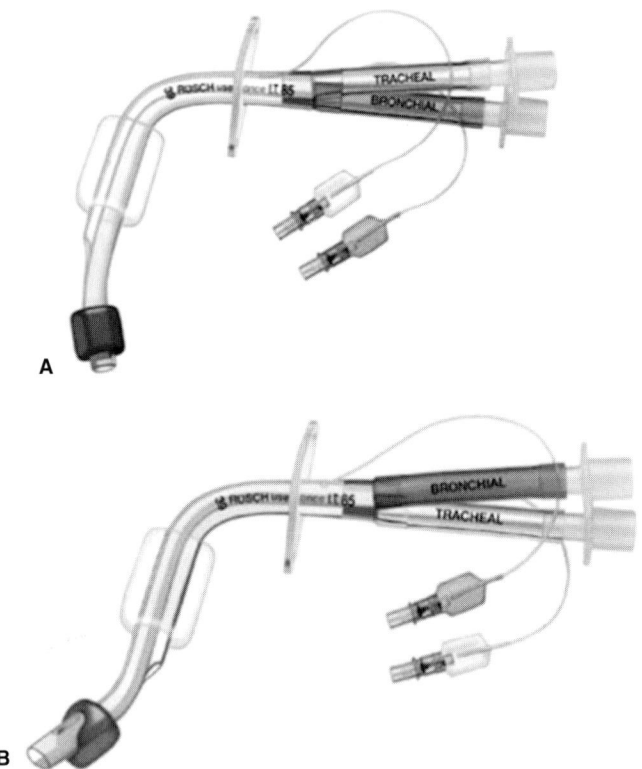

Figure 33.4 Double-lumen tube ("tracheopart") for patients with tracheostomy. (**A**) Left DLT. (**B**) Right DLT. (Adapted from www.rusch.com.)

thoracoscopic surgery (VATS), which requires excellent lung deflation conditions, is equal between left DLTs and left BBs when left-sided surgery is undertaken. With respect to right-sided surgery, left DLTs provided surgical conditions that were described as "excellent or fair" for all patients. In contrast, 44% of patients who had right-sided surgery and received a right BB had "poor" conditions.[54] This suggests that BBs placed in the left mainstem bronchus and left DLTs are equally effective for left-sided thoracoscopic surgery, and presumably for other left-sided thoracic surgical procedures. It should be noted, however, that left BBs took nearly twice as long to place correctly compared with left DLTs and were associated with a significantly greater number of malpositions. From this study, it was clear that right DLTs were superior to BBs for right-sided lung isolation.

The increased time to position BBs is due to a number of factors including time spent assembling the multiple parts and time required to direct the tip of the blocker (not always straightforward). Placement is difficult unless a trained assistant is present. This is offset by the ability to continue ventilating the patient. When directing the blocker into the desired bronchus is difficult, one way to increase the likelihood of success is to start with the endotracheal tube extremely high in the trachea. Blocker shafts are relatively stiff, and directing the tip is difficult. An ETT close to the carina would require a sharp turn with the stiff blocker, something that is difficult to do with the bronchoscope. By placing the tip of the ETT high in the trachea, a small deflection there translates to an

Table 33.6 Comparison of common bronchial blockers

Arndt
- center channel for CPAP or suctioning
- tip is directed with wire loop tightly wrapped around bronchoscope
- wire loop removed through center channel
- wire loop can be reinserted if repositioning required
- spherical balloon shape

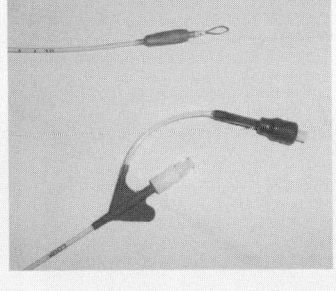

Fuji Uniblocker
- center channel for CPAP or suctioning
- tip is directed by torquing the blocker, taking advantage of preformed angle proximal to balloon
- spherical balloon shape
- same blocker technology from Univent tube

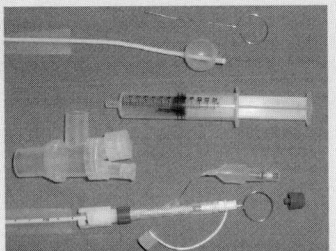

Cohen
- center channel for CPAP or suctioning
- tip is directed by turning wheel 90°
- tip deflects in the direction of the arrow
- spherical balloon shape
- caution: turning wheel excessively can stress the mechanism, causing it to malfunction

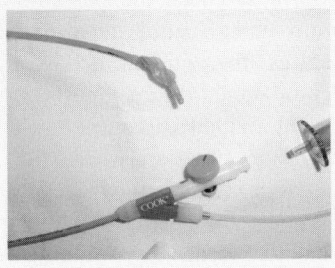

EZ Blocker
- two blocker balloons
- each balloon sits in a mainstem bronchus
- color coded, bronchus to be blocked corresponds to color of pilot balloon
- high-pressure balloons

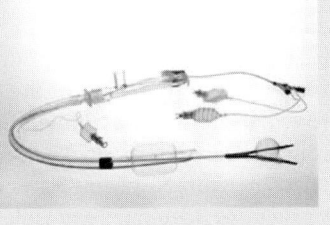

improved ability to direct the distal tip left or right. Table 33.6 is a summary of the pros and cons of a few of the bronchial blockers more commonly available.

Endobronchial tubes

Endobronchial tubes are long single-lumen tubes that are wire-reinforced. They are highly flexible and come equipped with a guiding stylet for stiffness. They differ significantly from regular ETTs, the main differences being in length and cuff design.

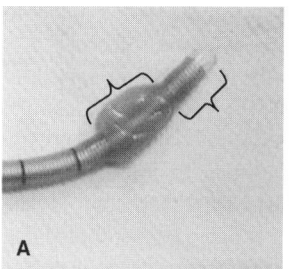
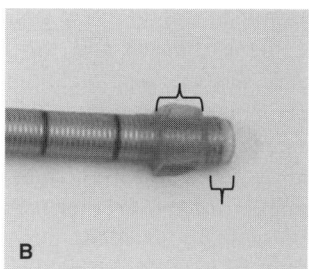

Figure 33.5 (**A**) Old versus (**B, C**) new endobronchial tubes.

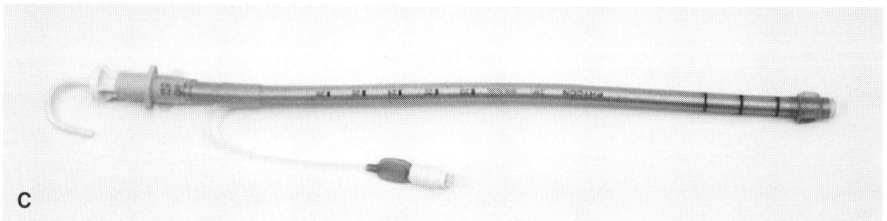

Figure 33.5A shows an older version of an endobronchial tube with a cuff similar to that found on regular endotracheal tubes. Newer versions of the tube (Fig. 33.5B, C) have cuffs very similar to those found on DLTs, making them far more ideal for lung isolation. Similar to DLTs, when an endobronchial tube is advanced past the glottic opening, the stylet should be removed and replaced with a fiberoptic bronchoscope. The tube is then advanced to its final location under direct visual guidance. In this case the bronchoscope is essential in helping direct the tube to the appropriate bronchus, because of the highly flexible nature of the tube.

Univent tubes

The Univent tube, despite having a BB, deserves to be discussed separately because of its unique structure. As described in Table 33.6, the Univent's blocker has been removed by the manufacturer and is now available as a separate unit (Fuji Uniblocker). Nevertheless, the original unit is still available, and is used in many institutions. It has a channel along the main ETT that holds the blocker, and when the tube is placed in the trachea, the blocker is advanced. It is then directed into the appropriate bronchus under fiberoptic guidance. To help facilitate tip direction, the blocker shaft is rotated or "torqued" while advancing the blocker into the bronchus. Further facilitation can be achieved by turning the ETT or the patient's head to one side. Once in position, this blocker may require less repositioning than the other blockers, possibly due to a relatively more "fixed" position at the tip of its ETT.

As with BBs, the main advantage of the Univent tube is that the blocker can be removed, allowing for easy conversion to postoperative ventilation, if necessary. It must be remembered, however, that for any given size of Univent tube, the outer diameter is significantly greater than for normal ETTs. This requires the selection of a Univent tube to be smaller, thereby reducing the internal diameter even further and increasing airway resistance. With the emergence of modern BBs, there no longer is a place for the Univent tube in clinical settings.

Postoperative ventilation

The clinical management of difficult thoracic surgery cases requires careful perioperative planning and technical execution. Patient disposition can be equally challenging, especially the decision to extubate the trachea or to change the DLT to a standard ETT. The anesthesiologist can be faced with difficult management decisions regularly, especially with trauma patients, patients with difficult airways, or patients who have had prolonged surgery and now have airways that are compromised. The decision to extubate the trachea is not always clear, and it becomes more difficult in the presence of a DLT. Even if extubation is not planned, postoperative care in an intensive care unit (ICU) can be complicated by the fact that many of the caregivers are not familiar with the ventilatory management of a patient with a DLT. For example, a DLT that is slightly malpositioned not only causes ventilatory problems, but in some cases it can be life-threatening or jeopardize the surgical repair.

When OLV is to be continued for a prolonged period, maintaining a DLT may be necessary, even in the ICU setting. The ability to suction and perform regular bronchoscopy through a DLT is critical. However, when OLV is no longer necessary, many patients still require short-term postoperative two-lung ventilation. Not surprisingly, anesthesiologists are reluctant to do this in the presence of a DLT. In addition to the expertise needed to manage a DLT, there is also a widespread belief that DLTs have increased airway resistance versus regular ETTs, making spontaneous respiration even more difficult. One study comparing the airflow resistance between multiple tubes, including DLTs, revealed that flow resistance in smaller DLTs is in fact lower than that in corresponding single-lumen ETTs (Fig. 33.6).[55] This study concluded that changing DLTs to single-lumen ETTs on the basis of increased airway resistance is not necessary. It is also interesting to note that the resistance within Univent tubes was found to be higher than in regular single-lumen tubes, leading to the recommendation that Univent tubes should be replaced at the end of a

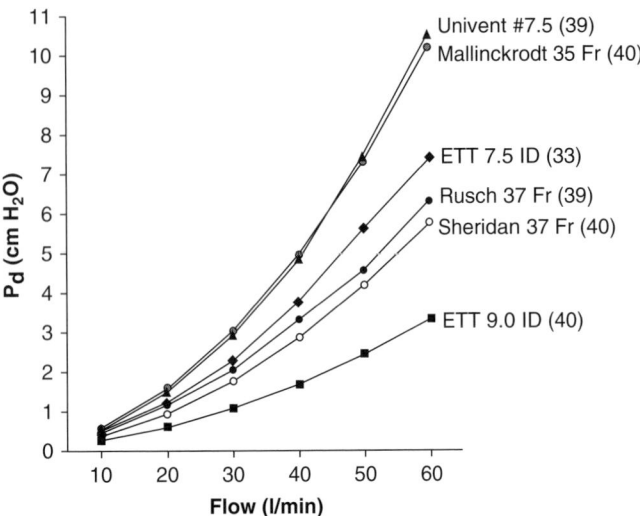

Figure 33.6 Flow resistances of single-lumen, double-lumen, and Univent tubes. Pressure differential (Pd), an indicator of flow resistance, versus airflow in a subset of the tubes studied. The double-lumen tubes and the Univent tube all have approximately equivalent external circumferences in millimeters, shown in parentheses. These tubes could be used clinically for a small adult patient. Two sizes of single-lumen ETTs are shown for comparison. (Reproduced from Slinger & Lesiuk 1998,[51] with permission from Elsevier.)

case as well. These findings should be emphasized, especially in patients where reintubation is expected to be difficult and losing the airway is a concern.

In these clinical scenarios BB technology becomes advantageous. BBs can be removed at the termination of a case, leaving a regular ETT to provide normal postoperative ventilation. The risk of losing the airway is therefore diminished, and there is a benefit of having a tube that does not irritate the carina, as is the case with DLTs. The benefit of BBs in trauma cases is therefore obvious. The disadvantage of no suctioning can be overcome by temporarily deflating the cuff, suspending ventilation, and quickly suctioning prior to cuff reinflation. However, BBs are still used infrequently and DLTs remain standard for OLV. Many anesthesiologists therefore elect to remove a DLT at the end of a case and replace it with a regular ETT. If this approach is taken, safety with airway tube exchangers must be emphasized.

Tube exchangers

Airway tube exchange is a maneuver burdened with risk. This cannot be overemphasized, as even attempting a tube exchange is usually based on a known or expected difficult airway. This scenario is common in thoracic surgery, especially in thoracic trauma patients. Preplanning is the key principle that is critical to a successful tube exchange. Table 33.7 presents a suggested approach to airway tube exchanges, using the Cook Airway Exchange Catheter, a commonly available tube exchanger designed for DLTs.

There are a few clinical "pearls" that can be employed to increase the success rate of tube exchanges. First, it is always

important to apply a very generous amount of lubricant to both the exchanger and the internal lumen of the ETT. Second, the use of a rigid fiberoptic laryngoscope (Glide-Scope, WuScope, C-MAC) for assisting in a tube exchange offers many advantages. The view of the larynx is greatly enhanced, and when there is resistance at the larynx to passing a tube over the exchanger, this view allows the anesthesiologist to adjust the tube appropriately, increasing the efficiency and safety. Third, the tube exchanger size should be chosen carefully. The largest exchanger that fits into the smallest ETT should always be used, if possible. This allows for a smaller gap between the exchanger and the edge of the ETT, which is the main source of resistance when passing the ETT through the larynx. If resistance is encountered, it is almost always caused by a laryngeal structure (i.e., arytenoids, vocal cords, epiglottis) becoming lodged within this gap. Excess pressure applied at this point only makes the tube more difficult to pass and increases the probability of laryngeal injury significantly. Success is better achieved by applying *continuous mild to moderate pressure* at the site of resistance while slightly rotating and advancing the tube. This allows for the bevel of the ETT to pass over the structure that is lodged within its lumen, resulting in a loss of resistance and tube advancement.

Summary

Lung isolation for thoracic trauma is a difficult procedure that inherently carries a high degree of risk. Meticulous planning and equipment checking is necessary for a positive outcome. Indications for lung isolation should always be reviewed and a plan discussed with the surgical team. Thorough knowledge of lung isolation techniques and bronchial anatomy is essential, since patient characteristics often dictate the best technique of choice. The interaction of the tube with patient anatomy and injury should be considered when choosing a lung isolation method. When lung isolation is established and positive-pressure ventilation is instituted, care should be taken to prevent and treat potential complications. Modern ARDS lung ventilation strategies will reduce the risk of lung injury. Intraoperative hypoxemia should always be expected and treated promptly. Finally, the anesthesiologist must consider multiple factors when planning postoperative management, including method of ventilation, choice of ETT, patient location, and expected duration of intubation.

Questions

(1) **A bronchopleural fistula in the left mainstem bronchus is best managed with:**
   a. Univent tube
   b. Bronchial blocker
   c. Left double-lumen tube

Table 33.7 Approach to airway tube exchange

Steps	Comments
A. Is tube exchange indicated?	• The risk of losing the airway should never be minimized; therefore, indications for tube exchange should always be reviewed.
B. Assemble equipment	• Laryngoscope (or GlideScope, WuScope, C-MAC) • Endotracheal tubes (at least two sizes) • Airway exchange catheter • Lubricant • Dry gauze or sponge (to provide traction when rotating tube in step I below) • Fiberoptic bronchoscope • Oxygen insufflation source • Suction • Assistance for handling equipment
C. Test equipment	• Add lubricant liberally to catheter, internal lumen of ETT, and bronchoscope. • Test exchanger and bronchoscope in DLT and ETT to confirm easy passage. • Remove ETT and exchange catheter connectors for easier passage. • Attempt to insufflate oxygen through exchange catheter. • Ensure suction is working. • Confirm bronchoscope is connected.
D. Ventilate with 100% FiO$_2$	• All airway maneuvers should begin with preoxygenation.
E. Ensure adequate muscle paralysis	• A patient that begins coughing during airway manipulation significantly reduces tube exchange success.
F. Insert laryngoscope	• Provides a better "chin lift," displaces the tongue, and provides a more direct path for the tube exchange. • Establish a view of the larynx. • Apply suction, if necessary.
G. Insert exchange catheter into patient's DLT (or ETT)	• Usually requires an assistant. • Take into consideration depth of insertion by observing markings on exchange catheter (premeasure with an external tube, if necessary). • An exchange catheter advanced too deep can cause severe injuries, especially as they are very stiff. Consider using the newest model by Cook that is equipped with a soft, flexible tip. • An exchange catheter not advanced deep enough risks losing the airway during the exchange.
H. Remove patient tube	• Care must be taken to keep exchange catheter from moving out with tube.
I. Insert new tube over exchange catheter and advance into airway (most difficult step)	• It is important to keep exchange catheter depth constant in order to avoid injury. • Care must be taken not to damage the cuff along the patient's teeth. • When the tube touches the larynx, resistance will be felt. Excessive pressure only makes advancement more difficult and causes injury. *Moderate to low* pressure should be applied while slowly rotating the tube. This allows the bevel of the ETT to "unhook" itself from an obstruction and then advance. If the advancing pressure is too strong, the distal tip of the ETT will not rotate well and cause tissue trauma. Use gauze to help grip tube, if necessary. • The obstruction is usually visible with laryngoscopy, helping to direct tube rotation. • Complete 360° rotation may be necessary to overcome obstruction.
J. Remove tube exchanger	• Immediately check correct tube placement with bronchoscope, P$_{ET}$CO$_2$, and auscultation.

DLT, double-lumen tube; ETT, endotracheal tube; P$_{ET}$CO$_2$, end-tidal CO$_2$

d. Right double-lumen tube

e. Endobronchial tube

(2) A 25-year-old patient undergoing video-assisted thoracoscopic bullectomy develops mild hypoxemia during one-lung ventilation. All of the following are appropriate initial interventions, *except*:

a. Checking tube position with fiberoptic bronchoscopy

b. Adding 5 cmH$_2$O of PEEP to the ventilated lung

c. Increasing FiO$_2$ to 100%

d. Adding CPAP to the nonventilated lung

e. Adding 10 cmH$_2$O of PEEP to the ventilated lung

(3) Which of the following is *not* an absolute indication for lung isolation?

a. Hemorrhage

b. Thoracoscopy

c. Bronchopleural fistula

d. Lung lavage

e. Video-assisted thoracoscopic surgery

(4) In this endoscopic image of the airway, which bronchus is the arrow pointing to?

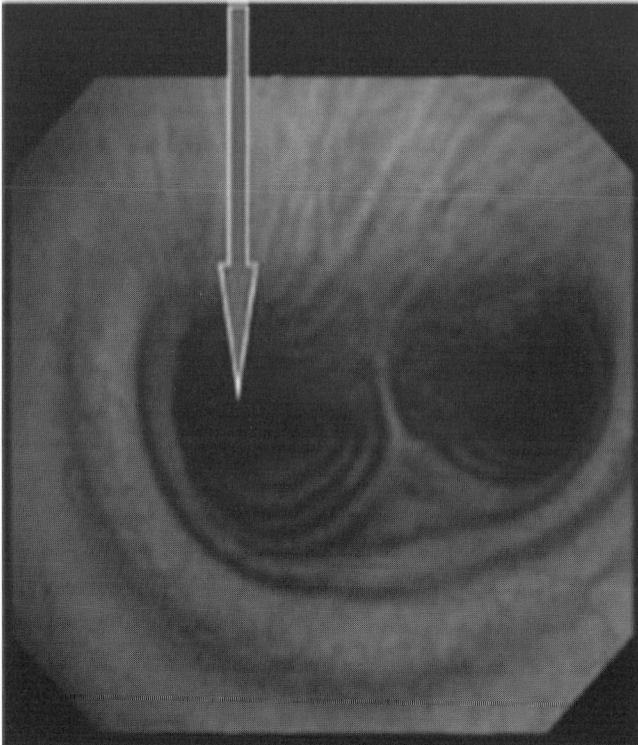

Figure 33.Q4

a. Right bronchus intermedius

b. Right lower lobe bronchus

c. Left lower lobe bronchus

d. Left mainstem bronchus

e. Right mainstem bronchus

(5) The white circle shows the opening of which bronchus?

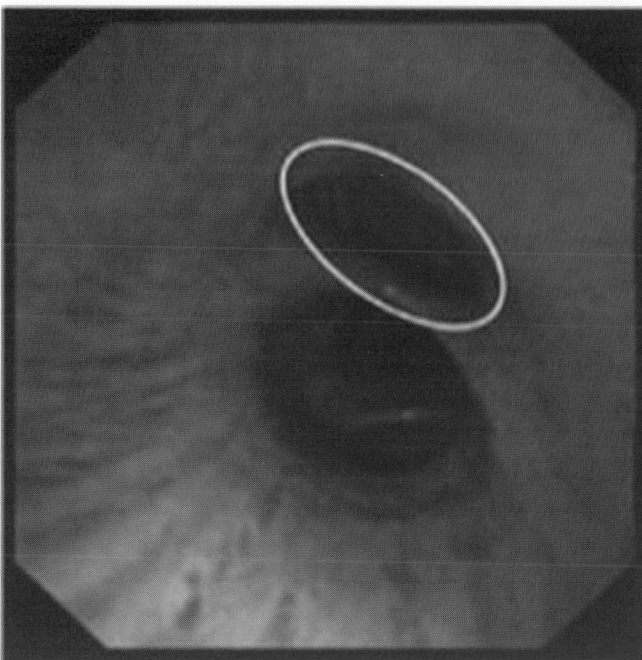

Figure 33.Q5

a. Right upper lobe bronchus

b. Right middle lobe bronchus

c. Right lower lobe bronchus

d. Left upper lobe bronchus

e. Left lower lobe bronchus

(6) The arrow is pointing to which bronchus?

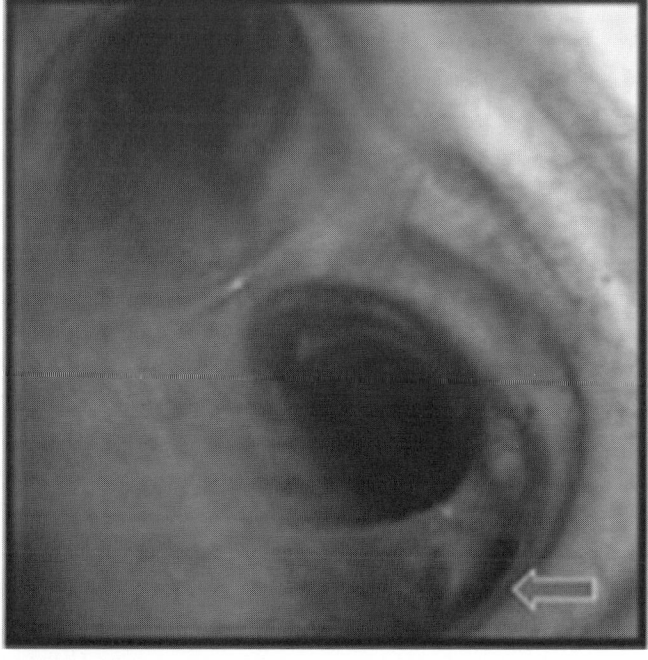

Figure 33.Q6

a. Left mainstem bronchus
b. Right mainstem bronchus
c. Right bronchus intermedius
d. Right lower lobe bronchus
e. Right upper lobe bronchus

(7) The following statements are all true with respect to double-lumen tubes and bronchial blockers, *except*:
a. Double-lumen tubes are more difficult to insert in difficult airways
b. Both double-lumen tubes and bronchial blockers allow for CPAP to be applied to the nonventilated lung
c. Both double-lumen tubes and bronchial blockers allow for bronchoscopy of the nonventilated lung
d. Bronchial blockers can be used for selective lobar isolation
e. Bronchial blockers provide a simple method for postoperative ventilation

(8) The cuff of a bronchial blocker typically requires how many milliliters of air to provide lung isolation?
a. 1
b. 3
c. 5
d. 7
e. 9

(9) A spontaneously breathing patient with a severe right-sided pulmonary contusion and hemothorax is in the emergency room. Severe hypotension occurs immediately following intubation with positive-pressure ventilation. The patient has received 3 L of normal saline and a chest tube that drained only 200 mL of blood. Besides tension pneumothorax, the most likely cause for the hypotension is?
a. Cardiac tamponade
b. Endobronchial intubation
c. Air embolism
d. Severe hypovolemia
e. Myocardial infarction

(10) Management of one-lung ventilation includes all of the following, *except*:
a. Respiratory rate of 8–12 breaths per minute
b. Tidal volume 8–12 mL/kg
c. PEEP to the dependent lung
d. CPAP to the nondependent lung
e. FiO_2 of 100%

Answers

(1) d
(2) d
(3) b
(4) e
(5) b
(6) e
(7) c
(8) d
(9) c
(10) b

References

1. Cipolle M, Rhodes M, Tinkoff G. Deadly dozen: dealing with the 12 types of thoracic injuries. *JEMS* 2012; 37 (9): 60–5.

2. Yamamoto L, Schroeder C, Morley D, Beliveau C. Thoracic trauma: the deadly dozen. *Crit Care Nursing Q* 2005; 28 (1): 22–40.

3. Kingsley CP. Perioperative anesthetic management of thoracic trauma. *Anesthesiol Clin N Am* 1999; 17: 183–95.

4. Meredith JW, Hoth JJ. Thoracic trauma: when and how to intervene. *Surg Clin North Am* 2007; 87: 95–118, vii.

5. Moloney JT, Fowler SJ, Chang W. Anesthetic management of thoracic trauma. *Curr Opin Anesthesiol* 2008; 21: 41–6.

6. Thierbach AR, Lipp MDW. Airway management in trauma patients. *Anesthesiol Clin N Am* 1999; 17: 63–81.

7. Brodsky JB, Lemmens HJ. Left double-lumen tubes: clinical experience with 1,170 patients. *J Cardiothorac Vasc Anesth* 2003; 17: 289–98.

8. Fouche Y, Tarantino DP. Anesthetic considerations in chest trauma. *Chest Surg Clin N Am* 1997; 7: 227–38.

9. American Society of Anesthesiologists. Practice guidelines for management of the difficult airway: an updated report by the American Society of Anesthesiologists Task Force on Management of the Difficult Airway. *Anesthesiology* 2003; 98: 1269–77.

10. Kummer C, Netto FS, Rizoli S, Yee D. A review of traumatic airway injuries: potential implications for airway assessment and management. *Injury* 2007; 38: 27–33.

11. Simon B, Ebert J, Bokhari F, *et al.* Management of pulmonary contusion and flail chest: an Eastern Association for the Surgery of Trauma practice management guideline. *J Trauma Acute Care Surg* 2012; 73 (5 Suppl 4): S351–61.

12. Symbas PN, Justicz AG, Ricketts RR. Rupture of the airways from blunt trauma: treatment of complex injuries. *Ann Thorac Surg* 1992; 54: 177–83.

13. Velly JF, Martigne C, Moreau JM, *et al.* Post traumatic tracheobronchial lesions. A follow-up study of 47 cases. *Eur J Cardiothoracic Surg* 1991; 5: 352–5.

14. Kshettry VR, Bolman RM, 3rd. Chest trauma. Assessment, diagnosis, and management. *Clin Chest Med* 1994; 15: 137–46.

15. Brownlow HA, Edibam C. Systemic air embolism after intercostal chest drain insertion and positive pressure ventilation in chest trauma. *Anaesth Intensive Care* 2002; 30: 660–4.

16. Ho AM, Ling E. Systemic air embolism after lung trauma. *Anesthesiology* 1999; 90: 564–75.

17. English GM, Hsu SF, Edgar R, Gibson-Eccles M. Oesophageal trauma in patients with spinal cord injury. *Paraplegia* 1992; 30: 903–12.

18. Slinger P. *Principles and Practice of Anesthesia for Thoracic Surgery.* New York, NY: Springer, 2011.

19. Scanlon TS, Benumof JL, Wahrenbrock EA, Nelson WL. Hypoxic pulmonary vasoconstriction and the ratio of hypoxic lung to perfused normoxic lung. *Anesthesiology* 1978; 49: 177–81.

20. Benumof JL. Conventional and differential lung management of one-lung ventilation. In Benumof JL, ed., *Anesthesia for Thoracic Surgery*. Philadelphia, PA: Saunders, 1995, pp. 406–31.

21. Triantafillou AN, Benumof JL, Lecamwasam HS. *Physiology of the Lateral Decubitus Position, the Open Chest, and One-Lung Ventilation*. Philadelphia, PA: Elsevier, 2003.

22. Winter PM, Smith G. The toxicity of oxygen. *Anesthesiology* 1972; **37**: 210–41.

23. Ni Chonghaile M, Higgins B, Laffey JG. Permissive hypercapnia: role in protective lung ventilatory strategies. *Curr Opin Crit Care* 2005; **11**: 56–62.

24. O'Croinin D, Ni Chonghaile M, Higgins B, Laffey JG. Bench-to-bedside review: Permissive hypercapnia. *Crit Care* 2005; **9**: 51–9.

25. Capan LM, Turndorf H, Patel C, *et al.* Optimization of arterial oxygenation during one-lung anesthesia. *Anesth Analg* 1980; **59**: 847–51.

26. Cohen E, Eisenkraft JB, Thys DM, Kirschner PA, Kaplan JA. Oxygenation and hemodynamic changes during one-lung ventilation: effects of CPAP10, PEEP10, and CPAP10/PEEP10. *J Cardiothorac Anesth* 1988; **2**: 34–40.

27. Hogue CW. Effectiveness of low levels of nonventilated lung continuous positive airway pressure in improving arterial oxygenation during one-lung ventilation. *Anesth Analg* 1994; **79**: 364–7.

28. Michelet P, Roch A, Brousse D, *et al.* Effects of PEEP on oxygenation and respiratory mechanics during one-lung ventilation. *Br J Anaesth* 2005; **95**: 267–73.

29. Slinger PD, Kruger M, McRae K, Winton T. Relation of the static compliance curve and positive end-expiratory pressure to oxygenation during one-lung ventilation. *Anesthesiology* 2001; **95**: 1096–102.

30. Godet G, Bertrand M, Rouby JJ, *et al.* High-frequency jet ventilation vs continuous positive airway pressure for differential lung ventilation in patients undergoing resection of thoracoabdominal aortic aneurysm. *Acta Anaesthesiol Scand* 1994; **38**: 562–8.

31. Rocca GD, Passariello M, Coccia C, *et al.* Inhaled nitric oxide administration during one-lung ventilation in patients undergoing thoracic surgery. *J Cardiothorac Vasc Anesth* 2001; **15**: 218–23.

32. Fujiwara M, Abe K, Mashimo T. The effect of positive end-expiratory pressure and continuous positive airway pressure on the oxygenation and shunt fraction during one-lung ventilation with propofol anesthesia. *J Clin Anesth* 2001; **13**: 473–7.

33. Baudouin SV. Lung injury after thoracotomy. *Br J Anaesth* 2003; **91**: 132–42.

34. Gama de Abreu M, Heintz M, Heller A, *et al.* One-lung ventilation with high tidal volumes and zero positive end-expiratory pressure is injurious in the isolated rabbit lung model. *Anesth Analg* 2003; **96**: 220–8.

35. Slutsky AS, Ranieri VM. Ventilator-induced lung injury. *N Engl J Med* 2013; **369**: 2126–36.

36. Serpa Neto A, Cardoso SO, Manetta JA, *et al.* Association between use of lung-protective ventilation with lower tidal volumes and clinical outcomes among patients without acute respiratory distress syndrome: a meta-analysis. *JAMA* 2012; **308**: 1651–9.

37. Severgnini P, Selmo G, Lanza C, *et al.* Protective mechanical ventilation during general anesthesia for open abdominal surgery improves postoperative pulmonary function. *Anesthesiology* 2013; **118**: 1307–21.

38. Futier E, Constantin JM, Paugam-Burtz C, *et al.* A trial of intraoperative low-tidal-volume ventilation in abdominal surgery. *N Engl J Med* 2013; **369**: 428–37.

39. Crimi E, Slutsky AS. Inflammation and the acute respiratory distress syndrome. *Best Pract Res Clin Anaesthesiol* 2004; **18**: 477–92.

40. Grichnik KP, D'Amico TA. Acute lung injury and acute respiratory distress syndrome after pulmonary resection. *Semin Cardiothorac Vasc Anesth* 2004; **8**: 317–34.

41. Licker M, de Perrot M, Spiliopoulos A, *et al.* Risk factors for acute lung injury after thoracic surgery for lung cancer. *Anesth Analg* 2003; **97**: 1558–65.

42. Slinger PD. Acute lung injury after pulmonary resection: more pieces of the puzzle. *Anesth Analg* 2003; **97**: 1555–7.

43. Acute Respiratory Distress Syndrome Network. Ventilation with lower tidal volumes as compared with traditional tidal volumes for acute lung injury and the acute respiratory distress syndrome. *N Engl J Med* 2000; **342**: 1301–8.

44. Gal TJ. Con: low tidal volumes are indicated during one-lung ventilation. *Anesth Analg* 2006; **103**: 271–3.

45. Slinger P. Pro: low tidal volume is indicated during one-lung ventilation. *Anesth Analg* 2006; **103**: 268–70.

46. Senturk NM, Dilek A, Camci E, *et al.* Effects of positive end-expiratory pressure on ventilatory and oxygenation parameters during pressure-controlled one-lung ventilation. *J Cardiothorac Vasc Anesth* 2005; **19**: 71–5.

47. Campos JH, Kernstine KH. A comparison of a left-sided Broncho-Cath with the torque control blocker univent and the wire-guided blocker. *Anesth Analg* 2003; **96**: 283–9.

48. Campos JH, Hallam EA, Van Natta T, Kernstine KH. Devices for lung isolation used by anesthesiologists with limited thoracic experience: comparison of double-lumen endotracheal tube, Univent torque control blocker, and Arndt wire-guided endobronchial blocker. *Anesthesiology* 2006; **104**: 261–6.

49. Slinger PD. Fiberoptic bronchoscopic positioning of double-lumen tubes. *J Cardiothorac Anesth* 1989; **3**: 486–96.

50. Roscoe A, Kanellakos GW, McRae K, Slinger P. Pressures exerted by endobronchial devices. *Anesth Analg* 2007; **104**: 655–8.

51. Benumof JL. Improving the design and function of double-lumen tubes. *J Cardiothorac Anesth* 1988; **2**: 729–33.

52. Mirzabeigi E, Johnson C, Ternian A. One-lung anesthesia update. *Semin Cardiothorac Vasc Anesth* 2005; **9**: 213–26.

53. Brodsky JB, Benumof JL, Ehrenwerth J, Ozaki GT. Depth of placement of left double-lumen endobronchial tubes. *Anesth Analg* 1991; **73**: 570–2.

54. Bauer C, Winter C, Hentz JG, *et al.* Bronchial blocker compared to double-lumen tube for one-lung ventilation during thoracoscopy. *Acta Anaesthesiol Scand* 2001; **45**: 250–4.

55. Slinger PD, Lesiuk L. Flow resistances of disposable double-lumen, single-lumen, and Univent tubes. *J Cardiothorac Vasc Anesth* 1998; **12**: 142–4.

Pediatric trauma and anesthesia

M. Jocelyn Loy

Objectives

(1) Describe the differences between pediatric and adult trauma.

(2) Explain the initial evaluation and management priorities in an injured pediatric patient.

(3) Describe the developing physiologic and anatomic characteristics of infants and children.

(4) Identify anatomic characteristics of the pediatric airway and describe the associated implications for airway management after trauma with potential cervical spine injury.

(5) Describe fluid options and blood product resuscitation for a bleeding pediatric patient.

(6) Explain the anesthetic considerations applicable to the care of an injured child, and how trauma influences the choice of medications and other elements of the anesthetic plan.

(7) Describe the physiology and pharmacology of drugs used in the management of injured infants and children.

(8) Describe the alternatives available for the management of pediatric acute postoperative pain.

Introduction

Trauma remains the leading cause of mortality and serious long-term morbidity in the pediatric population. In the US, a significant majority of pediatric trauma occurs in motor vehicle collisions (MVCs). Injuries related to falls and sports comprise the second largest group. Other causes include drowning, child abuse, and burns. Falls from heights are most common in toddlers, while older children sustain more traumatic injuries from motor vehicle and bicycle-related accidents.[1] Homicide is the leading cause of traumatic death in infants, 50% occurring in the first 4 months after birth.[2] Pediatric injuries vary from minor and isolated to severe, multiple, and potentially fatal, involving several organ systems. Evaluation and assessment of the pediatric trauma patient requires an efficient, organized, and systematic approach to properly identify, prioritize, and treat the most life-threatening injuries and to achieve a favorable outcome, with minimal to no long-term functional limitations.

Management principles of pediatric trauma patients are similar to those of adults, but modified according to the age group of the child. Children are not just small adults. Their unique, developing psychologic, anatomic, and physiologic characteristics pose special challenges to anesthesiologists and the entire trauma care team. Optimal management of the pediatric trauma patient depends on adequate knowledge and understanding of these unique characteristics.

Initial assessment and management

Primary survey

The main goal of the primary survey is to rapidly find all potentially life-threatening injuries to prioritize management for efficient resuscitation and achieve hemodynamic stability (see Chapter 2). This requires immediate assessment of the "ABCDEs" of the Advanced Trauma Life Support (ATLS) protocol and constant reevaluation of the adequacy of resuscitation strategies.

Airway with C-spine control

Evaluation of the airway in an injured child can be complex. Injury to the airway or nearby structures may distort normal anatomy and render mask ventilation and tracheal intubation difficult. Preexisting conditions that may complicate emergency airway management include congenital abnormalities, such as micrognathia (mandibular hypoplasia), macroglossia, and cleft palate, and the presence of obstructive sleep apnea with or without obesity.

Assessment of the airway for signs of airway compromise or obstruction takes priority (see Chapter 3). Inability to establish, maintain, and secure a patent airway for oxygenation and ventilation can lead to hypoxia, hypercarbia, bradycardia, and cardiac arrest. Inspection of the airway includes the face, mouth, mandible, nose, and neck. It is important to look for edema, foreign bodies, secretions, blood, loose or missing teeth, and fractures of the mandible, and cervical spine (C-spine). Any trauma victim, especially one with a closed

Trauma Anesthesia, 2nd Edition, ed. Charles E. Smith. Published by Cambridge University Press. © Charles E. Smith, 2015.

head injury, is presumed, until proved otherwise, to have C-spine injury and a "full stomach." C-spine precautions should be maintained, and techniques that minimize the risk of pulmonary aspiration should be used at all times. The anesthesiologist may be called on to help with airway management in the emergency room, or may first encounter the child in the operating room; hence, knowledge and appreciation of the peculiarities of the pediatric airway is mandatory.

Healthy neonates and young infants have large heads, including prominent occiputs relative to body size, so that, in the supine position, the neck is naturally flexed on the chest and the head may be flexed on the neck (Fig. 34.1).[3,4] This has several important implications. The natural head and neck flexion of the obtunded or sedated young infant often results in significant airway obstruction, which may be relieved by gently lifting the chin up and forward (anteriorly) to slightly extend the head on the neck. Otherwise, an oral airway can be inserted with relatively no movement of head and neck. In suspected C-spine injury, a more neutral, straight head and neck position should be achieved by placing a blanket or pad under the supine infant or young child's torso (Fig. 34.2).[4,5] Direct laryngoscopy may be facilitated by some of this natural supine flexion of neck on chest, as only slight additional extension of head on neck may be needed to achieve a good

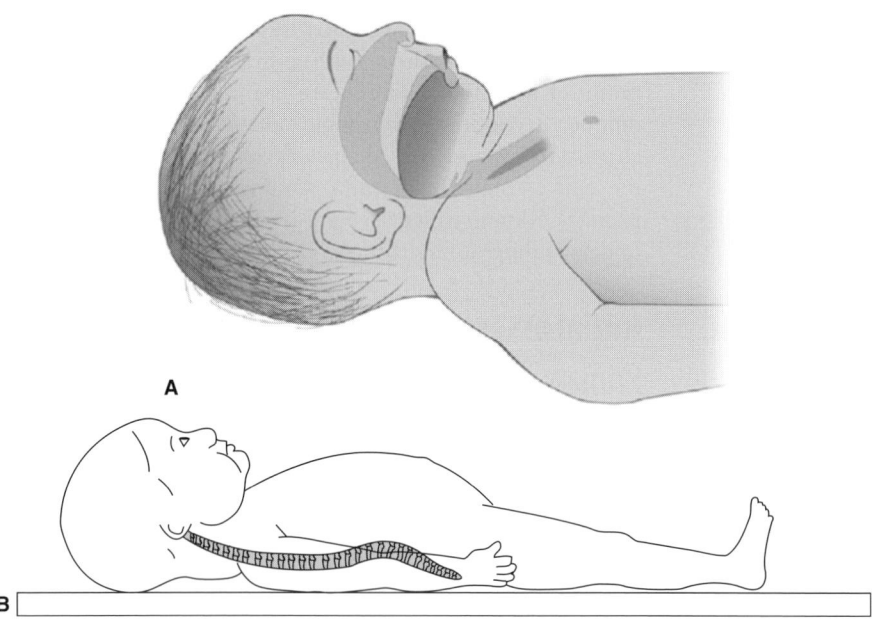

Figure 34.1 In the supine position, because of the relatively large occiput, the neck of an infant or a young child is naturally flexed on the chest, while the head may be additionally flexed on the neck. This may result in partial or significant airway obstruction in a sedated or obtunded infant or young child. (Courtesy of medical illustrator at MetroHealth Medical Center.)

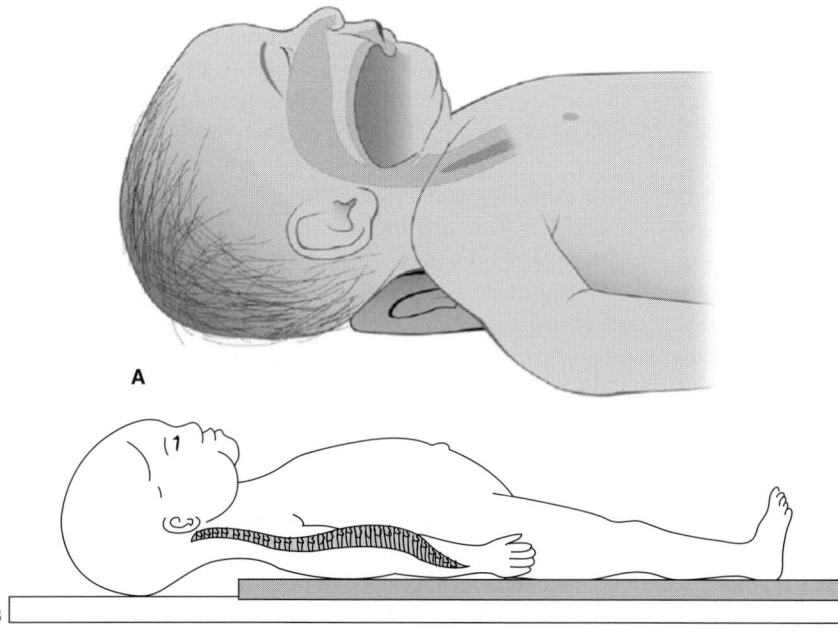

Figure 34.2 A blanket or pad placed under the torso of a supine infant or young child will achieve a neutral, straight head and neck position. (Courtesy of medical illustrator at MetroHealth Medical Center.)

"sniffing position" for optimal laryngeal visualization. In general, in infants and young children, the pad belongs under the body, not under the head.

Neonates and young infants are obligate nose breathers until 3–5 months of age, so any secretions or blood in their relatively narrow nasal passages can lead to airway obstruction. Furthermore, the supine, obtunded, or sedated young infant's relatively large tongue tends to fall against the soft palate, epiglottis, and posterior pharyngeal wall, resulting in upper airway obstruction and difficulty with mask ventilation and direct laryngoscopy for intubation. Insertion of an oral airway, with the aid of a tongue depressor if needed, helps relieve the obstruction. The most appropriate size oral airway for the child is one that is approximately as long as the distance from the child's lips to the angle of the mandible. A good face-mask seal should be achieved by holding the face mask with the fingers pressing on the mandible only, avoiding pressure on the soft tissues in the submandibular area. Pressure on the submandibular soft tissue may actually push the tongue onto the palate and pharyngeal wall, leading to further airway obstruction in proportion to the amount of pressure applied. In infants, pressure should be applied to the bone, not the soft tissue.

The larynx in infants and children is more cephalad, approximately at the level of the C3–C4 vertebrae in infants, compared with the C5–C6 level in adults.[6] This may give the impression that the infant larynx is more anterior during direct laryngoscopy. The floppy, narrow, and more omega-shaped infant epiglottis is also angled more posteriorly than the adult epiglottis, and this, combined with the shallower vallecula, may make it more difficult to lift the epiglottis during direct laryngoscopy. Application of external inferior laryngeal pressure and/or use of a straight laryngoscope blade to pick up the epiglottis may aid in visualization of the glottis. The more anterocaudal attachment of the vocal cords in infants occasionally results in the tip of the endotracheal tube (ETT) getting hung up on the shelf of tissue anterior to the anterior commissure during intubation. Navigating the ETT tip past this natural obstruction is facilitated by maintaining gentle forward pressure on the ETT while rotating or turning it longitudinally. More than 90 degrees of rotation may be needed. The tube should be gently twisted into the trachea.

The length of the trachea is only 4–5 cm in infants and approximately 7 cm by 18 months of age, so right mainstem intubation or ETT dislodgement can occur with correspondingly small movements of the infant's head. Constant vigilance and frequent reassessment are recommended. Flexion of the head may lead to mainstem intubation, whereas head extension may result in extubation. When choosing the appropriately sized ETT, keep in mind that in children less than 5 years old, the narrowest part of the upper airway is at the level of the cricoid cartilage, not at the glottis as in adults (Fig. 34.3).[7] The size of the ETT appropriate for the patient's age may be estimated by comparing the tube size with that of the infant's or child's fifth finger, or by using the formula: ETT tube size

Table 34.1 Pediatric endotracheal tube sizes

Age	Internal diameter (mm)	
	Uncuffed ETT	Cuffed ETT
Premature infant (< 1 kg)	2.5–3.0	—
Term newborn	3.0–3.5	3.0
< 6 mo	3.5	3.5
6–12 mo	4.0	3.5
1–2 yr	4.5	4.0
3–4 yr	5.0	4.5
5–6 yr	5.5	5.0
7–8 yr	6.0	5.5
8–10 yr	6.5	6.0
>10 yr	7.0–7.5	6.5–7.0

Uncuffed ETT size = 4 + (¼) age in years. Use 0.5 mm size smaller for cuffed ETTs greater than size 3.0.

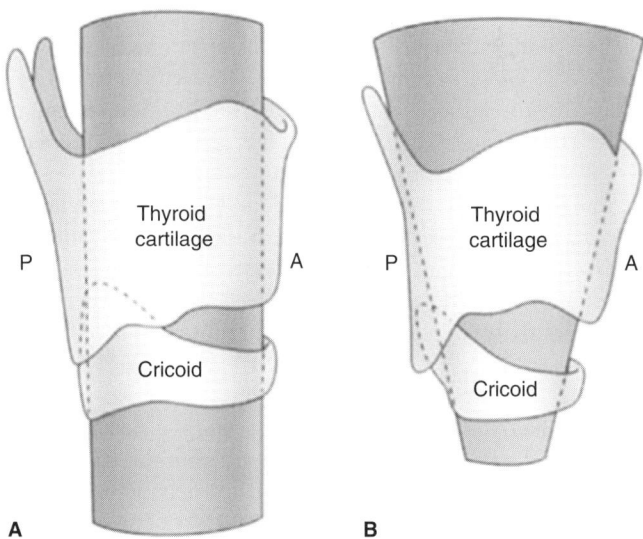

Figure 34.3 The narrowest portion of the cylindrical-shaped larynx of an adult (**A**) occurs at the glottic opening, whereas the narrowest part of the funnel-shaped larynx of an infant (**B**) occurs in the subglottic area at the level of the cricoid cartilage. A, anterior; P, posterior. (Courtesy of medical illustrator at MetroHealth Medical Center; redrawn from Cote CJ, Todres ID. The pediatric airway. In Cote CJ, Ryan JF, Todres ID, *et al.*, eds., *A Practice of Anesthesia for Infants and Children*. Philadelphia, PA: Saunders, 1992.)

(diameter in mm) = 4 + (1/4)age (Tables 34.1 and 34.2). An air leak around the ETT at 15–20 cmH$_2$O pressure and easy passage of the tube into the trachea clinically suggests that the ETT size is appropriate.

Whether cuffed or uncuffed tubes should be used to intubate the trachea of infants and young children remains somewhat controversial, though most recent evidence suggests that, at least for tubes sized 3.5 and larger, cuffed ETTs are the better choice. Traditional teaching that only uncuffed ETTs should be used in children less than 8 or 10 years old[8,9] is based

Table 34.2 Guidelines for endotracheal tube size (millimeters)

Newborns	3.0–3.5
Newborns to 1 year	3.5–4.0
1 year	4.0–4.5
2 years and older	4 + (1/4)age

Use 0.5 size smaller for cuffed ETTs greater than size 3.0.

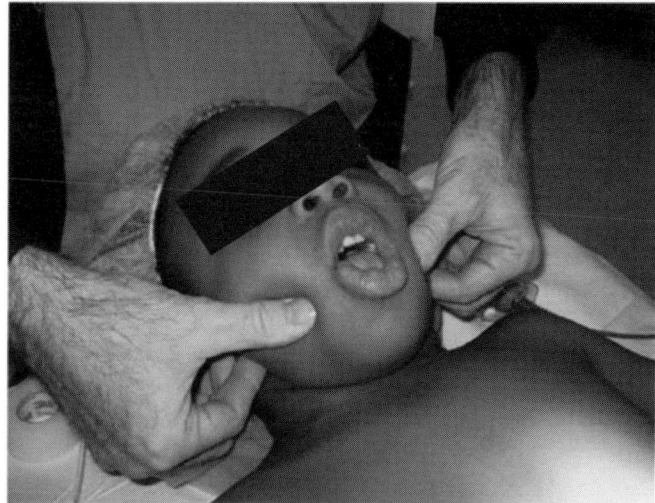

Figure 34.4 Jaw thrust with mouth-opening maneuver. Lifting the angles of the mandible upward and outward opens the airway by moving the jaw and tongue forward, relieving the obstruction.

on reports from the early 1960s describing the development of mucosal ischemia and subglottic stenosis associated with prolonged use of oversized uncuffed ETTs. It has also been pointed out that an uncuffed ETT has a larger diameter and thus offers less airway resistance and reduced work for spontaneous breathing. It was claimed that the uncuffed tubes might avoid the subglottic trauma described after use of high-pressure, low-volume cuffed ETTs. Subsequent studies showed that the risk of subglottic stenosis is significantly related to the duration of intubation,[10] ETT size,[11,12] and use of overinflated cuffed ETTs;[13,14] and this risk is not related to whether or not the ETT is cuffed.[15,16] Newer low-pressure, high-volume cuffed tubes that are appropriately sized, positioned, and inflated offer many advantages over uncuffed ETTs.[17,18] These advantages include more efficient and less traumatic intubation with less need for multiple attempts, better control of tidal volume with less air leak during mechanical ventilation and application of positive end-expiratory pressure (PEEP), better controlled and more cost-effective inhalational anesthesia with lower fresh gas flows and less environmental pollution, and decreased risk of aspiration[19] and infection. Because cuffed ETTs have slightly larger outer diameters than uncuffed tubes, the appropriate cuffed ETT is one half-size smaller than calculated by the formula above (Table 34.1). For example, for a healthy 4-year-old, a cuffed ETT one half-size smaller than 4 + 4/4, that is a size 4.5 cuffed tube, would be appropriate. The air leak around a cuffed tube at peak inflation pressure of 20–25 cmH$_2$O may be adjusted by inflating the cuff to approximately 20 cmH$_2$O (16 mmHg) to help avoid mucosal ischemia. The use of a slightly smaller cuffed tube eliminates the time and trauma associated with the need to replace an uncuffed ETT with excessive air leak or an oversized uncuffed tube that was used in an effort to minimize air leak.[16] The development of new ultra-thin-walled ETTs that have larger internal diameters might further help end the ETT cuff controversy.

The following formula may be used as a guide to determine the appropriate depth of the ETT placement (in centimeters from lips to tip of ETT) for children older than 2 years: 13 + (1/2) age; for under 1 year old: 8 + weight in kilograms.[20] The appropriate depth of ETT insertion may also be approximated by multiplying the internal diameter of the ETT (in millimeters) by 3. For example, the appropriate depth of a 5 mm ETT is usually 15 cm. Besides auscultation, other maneuvers that will help confirm the appropriate depth of the ETT clinically include palpating the inflated cuff externally between the

level of the cricoid cartilage and the sternal notch,[21] or deliberate right mainstem bronchial intubation followed by withdrawal of the ETT until equal and bilateral breath sounds are heard.[22] Besides direct visualization of the ETT passing between the vocal cords into the trachea, further confirmation of ETT placement and position can be obtained by chest x-ray or fiberoptic endoscopy.

During the initial evaluation, all trauma patients should receive supplemental oxygen, and oxygen saturation should be monitored by pulse oximetry. Supplemental oxygen delivered through nasal cannula or face mask may be satisfactory for a conscious injured child without respiratory distress. Certain maneuvers, such as chin lift or jaw thrust, will help improve or establish patency of an obstructed or partially obstructed upper airway. Chin lift involves using the fingers of one hand to gently lift the mandible upward, to move the chin anteriorly. Care should be taken not to hyperextend the neck during the performance of this maneuver. Jaw thrust with mouth opening is a two-handed airway maneuver done by grasping the angles of the jaw to displace the mandible forward and upward by using one hand on each side (Fig. 34.4). Jaw thrust has been shown to be more effective than the chin-lift maneuver in establishing a patent airway in children when tonsils and adenoids are prominent or hypertrophied.[23,24] Applying incremental pressure on the mandible during the jaw-thrust maneuver can also help assess the level of consciousness of an unconscious child.[25] Placing an oral airway in a conscious patient is not recommended as this can induce gagging and vomiting, with the risk of pulmonary aspiration. If desaturation occurs with a face mask and a patent airway, then a 100% oxygen nonrebreather system and tracheal intubation should be considered. Before attempting intubation, a properly working suction system, an adequate source of oxygen, varied sizes of airway devices, and a table or list of calculated drug dosages should be readily available. If direct laryngoscopy is

Table 34.3 Indications for endotracheal intubation

a. Loss of consciousness or altered level of consciousness with inability to protect the airway
b. Inability to maintain patency of airway or clear secretions
c. Provide positive-pressure ventilation and adequate oxygenation
d. Significant burn with airway injury

initially unsuccessful, then insertion of a laryngeal mask airway (LMA) can be a temporary life-saving measure until endotracheal intubation is accomplished by an alternative method. Endotracheal intubation is the definitive airway normally used to provide or maximize oxygenation, control or support ventilation, and help protect the patient from pulmonary aspiration (Table 34.3).

Nasotracheal intubation or passage of a nasogastric tube is relatively contraindicated in the presence of a basilar skull fracture, because of the potential for the ETT to penetrate the thin cribriform plate and injure the brain.

Emergency tracheostomy is not commonly done in children. A preferred alternative is needle cricothyroidotomy using a 12, 14, or 16 gauge angiocatheter. This provides satisfactory oxygenation but most likely will not provide adequate ventilation. Surgical cricothyroidotomy is rarely indicated in infants and small children, but can be performed in children older than 12 years whose cricothyroid membrane is more easily palpable. It should be noted that the exact age at which a surgical cricothyroidotomy can be safely performed is controversial and has not been well defined. Different sources list lower age limits ranging from 5 to 12, and Pediatric Advanced Life Support (PALS) defines the pediatric airway as age 1–8 years. A conservative approach is to use 12 years as the cutoff age.

Cervical spine (C-spine) injury

C-spine fractures are less likely in children than in adults, because of the greater mobility of the spine and relative laxity of the ligaments present in children. Pediatric C-spine injuries are different from adult injuries (until the age of 8–10 years), resulting mainly from anatomical differences. Children have relatively underdeveloped neck muscles and large heads in proportion to their bodies. Children's vertebral bodies are wedged anteriorly and tend to slide forward with flexion. Younger children have horizontally angled or flat articulating facets, cartilaginous endplates, and elastic, lax interspinous ligaments. These characteristics predispose children to upper cervical injuries, spinal cord injury without radiographic evidence of abnormality (SCIWORA), and severe ligamentous injuries. Age-related differences in behavior and risk exposure also lead to variation in the type of cervical injury. Falls and MVCs are common among children less than 10 years of age, while sports-related injuries and MVCs are predominant in children over 10 years of age.[26] C-spine injuries in children less than 8 years old are more commonly at the C1–C3 level because of the more horizontal facets. Adolescents are more

prone to lower cervical injuries. SCIWORA, occurring in up to 50% of pediatric spinal cord injuries,[27] makes spinal cord injury in children more difficult to diagnose and potentially catastrophic if unrecognized. Because up to two-thirds of children with spinal cord injury have normal spine x-rays, careful history and neurologic exam are essential in its diagnosis. Pseudosubluxation of cervical vertebrae (C2–C3) and incomplete ossification are normal findings that may contribute to the difficulty in diagnosing spinal cord injuries in children. Risk of C-spine injury is increased in children with Down's syndrome, Klippel–Fiel syndrome, Chiari malformation, and other pathologic conditions that may be associated with C-spine instability. Anteroposterior and lateral cervical spine radiographs are basic imaging studies for spine clearance. Computed tomography (CT) is useful, providing more definition of bony abnormalities. Magnetic resonance imaging (MRI) has been used to detect ligamentous and soft tissue injuries, the extent of spinal cord injuries, the presence of hematoma formation, and herniated disks not visualized by other imaging modalities. Prognosis after C-spine injury is related to the severity of the initial neurologic insult. Children generally have a more favorable outcome than adults, especially those with incomplete injuries.

To minimize secondary injury after an initial insult, the C-spine should be protected until C-spine injury has been ruled out. Patients should be maintained supine on a rigid backboard, with head blocks or sandbags on each side of the head strapped securely onto the backboard, and a rigid cervical collar in place to minimize neck flexion and extension. If the need for tracheal intubation arises, the patient should be preoxygenated with 100% oxygen, and manual in-line stabilization of the head and neck without traction should be maintained by one trained person while another trained provider performs a rapid sequence intubation. Traction on the possibly injured neck is not recommended and may be harmful. The goal of cervical stabilization is immobility, not traction. The neck should remain stabilized after intubation and during transport of the injured child.

Breathing and ventilation

To evaluate breathing and assess ventilation, abnormalities in respiratory rate and pattern, presence of stridor, grunting, nasal flaring, sternal, intercostal or subcostal retractions, head bobbing, and use of accessory muscles of respiration should be noted. The chest should be observed for symmetry of expansion and paradoxical or "rocking boat" pattern of breathing that suggests airway obstruction, and bilateral and equal breath sounds in the axillary areas should be ascertained. End-tidal carbon dioxide ($ETCO_2$) monitoring is a valuable tool for providing information about carbon dioxide retention and adequacy of ventilation. Positive-pressure ventilation via manual bag and mask must be monitored carefully in pediatric patients to avoid barotrauma and gastric distention that could compromise ventilation and increase the risk for pulmonary aspiration. Suctioning through an orogastric tube decompresses the stomach but must be done with care to avoid traumatizing fragile mucous membranes. Flail chest may present with asymmetry of the chest. The differential diagnosis of unilateral decreased or absent breath sounds includes endobronchial intubation, pneumothorax, or hemothorax, any of which require prompt intervention to ensure adequate oxygenation and ventilation.

Circulation and hemorrhage control

Hemorrhagic shock is not an uncommon presentation in children who have sustained multiple injuries. Recognition of shock and identification of the probable cause may be critically important. Treatment goals are prompt control of hemorrhage and restoration of organ perfusion and tissue oxygenation. Initial assessment includes blood pressure, pulse rate and rhythm, and peripheral pulses and perfusion. Delayed capillary refill (longer than 2 seconds), cool extremities, cyanosis, and skin mottling are signs suggestive of poor perfusion. Absolute reliance on the blood pressure can be misleading, resulting in a delay in recognition and management with potentially fatal consequences. Blood pressure is a poor indicator of hypovolemia in children, because they are often able to maintain a normal blood pressure despite significant hypovolemia by compensatory vasoconstriction and tachycardia. Blood pressure change may not be manifested until 30–40% of the child's circulating blood volume has been lost.[28] Marked tachycardia is one of the early signs of hypovolemic shock in pediatric patients. Persistent tachycardia with absent or narrow pulse pressure implies impending cardiovascular collapse.

Immediate restoration of circulating blood volume to maintain adequate blood pressure, cardiac output, and perfusion of vital organs is crucial. Initial resuscitation includes the administration of warmed isotonic crystalloid solution, preferably lactated Ringer's as a 20 mL/kg bolus, which may be repeated once or twice. If the child remains hemodynamically unstable despite aggressive crystalloid fluid resuscitation, administration of colloids and blood products should be strongly considered. Type-specific, crossmatched packed red blood cells (pRBCs), in 10–20 mL/kg increments, are preferable, but if fully crossmatched blood is not immediately available, type-specific, partially crossmatched pRBCs or type-specific unmatched blood can be given. Otherwise, type O Rh-negative pRBCs can be given until type-specific blood is available. If the patient remains hemodynamically compromised, vasopressors may be indicated. Vasopressin maintains its efficacy in hypoxia and severe acidosis (see Chapter 6) and can be used in critically ill children as a rescue therapy in refractory shock and cardiac arrest, although there are few data to support its use in injured children. In case of failure to restore organ perfusion despite these aggressive supportive measures, thorough and continuing reevaluation for other causes of bleeding should be performed. Acidosis, myocardial contusion, pericardial tamponade, tension pneumothorax, or unrecognized internal bleeding may require early and immediate surgical intervention to achieve hemostasis.

Favorable signs suggestive of adequate response to volume resuscitation include return of normal blood pressure, pulse pressure greater than 20 mmHg, pulse rate and skin color approaching normal, improvement in level of consciousness and acid–base status, and adequate urine output. Placement of a urinary catheter allows accurate monitoring of urine output and facilitates assessment of the response to volume resuscitation. Adequate urine output is generally considered to be 2 mL/kg/h in infants (< 1 year old), 1 mL/kg/h in children, and 0.5 mL/kg/h in adolescents and adults (Table 34.4).

Vascular access

Obtaining intravenous (IV) access in pediatric patients, especially those less than 18 months of age, may be challenging.[29] In pediatric trauma patients with hypovolemia or shock, obtaining peripheral IV access can be a nightmare, even in the most experienced hands. The hypovolemic child needs at least two relatively large-bore peripheral IV lines: 22 gauge for newborns and infants up to 3 years old, 20 gauge for children 4–8 years old, 20 or 18 gauge for those older than 8 years. Vascular access may be obtained peripherally or centrally, percutaneously or by cutdown, or through an intraosseous (IO) route (Table 34.5). The saphenous vein can be peripherally accessed medial to the medial malleolus. Extravasation of some drugs, such as IV sodium bicarbonate and calcium, can cause tissue necrosis and sloughing. Therefore, peripheral IV access should be free-flowing and not infiltrated before injecting medications.

Central line (internal jugular or subclavian vein) cannulation is not recommended for primary IV access, because of the risks of pneumothorax and hemothorax and because the head and neck should not be manipulated if C-spine injury has not been ruled out. If there is a high suspicion of injury to the

Table 34.4 Normal hemodynamic parameters[5]

Age (years)	Weight (kg)	Heart rate (bpm)	Blood pressure (mmHg)	Respiratory rate (per min)	Urine output (mL/kg/h)
Infant–1	0–10	< 160	> 60	< 60	2
1–3	10–14	< 150	> 70	< 40	1.5
3–5	14–18	< 140	> 75	< 35	1.0
6–12	18–36	< 120	> 80	< 30	1.0
> 12	36–70	< 100	> 90	< 30	0.5

Table 34.5 Preferred sites for venous access in children[5]

1. Percutaneous peripheral
2. Intraosseous (IO)
3. Percutaneous femoral
4. Venous cutdown: saphenous vein
5. Percutaneous external jugular vein

inferior vena cava from abdominal and pelvic trauma, accessing the femoral vein should be avoided (see Chapter 5).

If percutaneous venous access, the preferred route, is not established in three attempts or in 90 seconds, placement of an IO needle should be considered.[5] The IO route is a simple, reliable, and effective alternative when peripheral intravascular access is difficult to obtain, especially in children less than 6 years old. To obtain IO vascular access, insert a bone marrow needle or a Cook IO infusion needle into the proximal tibia approximately 1–3 cm below and medial to the tibial tuberosity.[3,30] Direct the needle caudally to avoid the epiphyseal plate. Drugs given via the IO route should be flushed with at least 5 mL of saline to ensure delivery to the central circulation. Crystalloids, as well as blood products and medications, can be infused at rates up to 40 mL/min using up to 300 mmHg pressure.[31] IO needle placement is contraindicated in patients with osteogenesis imperfecta, ipsilateral fractured extremity, or infection at the planned cannulation site. Complications are uncommon but may be severe; therefore, the IO route is only a temporary measure until more definitive intravenous access has been obtained. Complications include compartment syndrome, fat embolism, tibial fracture, growth plate injuries, cellulitis, and osteomyelitis.

Disability/neurologic evaluation

Disability refers to the initial neurologic evaluation that will serve as the basis for comparison with subsequent assessments. The mnemonic AVPU refers to awareness (A), response to verbal (V) stimuli and pain (P), and unresponsive to stimuli (U).

The classic Glasgow Coma Scale (GCS: see Chapter 35, Table 35.1) used in adults for initial assessment of neurologic status and prognosis is not very reliable in children of all ages. It has been shown that in the absence of ischemic–hypoxic injury, children with severe traumatic brain injury and unfavorable GCS score (GCS 3–5) can recover independent function.[32] To be applicable to infants and young children, the GCS verbal scoring has been modified (Table 34.6). A more general Pediatric Trauma Score (PTS) may be used for triage purposes (Table 34.7).

Exposure/environmental control

Traumatized children should be completely undressed to facilitate thorough examination. Infants and children lose body heat quickly because they have large surface areas relative to body weight, thinner skin with less subcutaneous fat, and higher metabolic rates. Temperature must be closely monitored, and measures should be taken to keep pediatric trauma patients warm. Ambient room temperature should be adjusted to more than 24 °C, even before the child's arrival. Warm blankets may be used to cover all exposed areas after the initial assessment. Forced-air convective heating blankets have been shown to be effective in preventing hypothermia.[33] All fluids and blood products should be infused through fluid warmers

Table 34.6 Glasgow Coma Scale (GCS)

Response	Score
Eye opening	
Spontaneous	4
To shout/speech	3
To pain	2
No response	1
Motor response	
Spontaneous/obeys commands	6
Localizes pain	5
Flexion withdrawal	4
Decorticate posturing	3
Decerebrate posturing	2
No response	1
Verbal response, modified for children	
Appropriate words, social smile, fixes and follows	5
Cries, consolable/inappropriate words	4
Persistently irritable/incomprehensible words	3
Restless, agitated, moans	2
No response	1

GCS: ≤ 8, severe injuries; 9–12, moderate injuries; 13–15, minor injuries.

Table 34.7 Pediatric Trauma Score (PTS)

Variable	+2	+1	−1
Weight (kg)	> 20	10–20	< 10
Airway patency	normal	maintained	unable to maintain
Systolic blood pressure (mmHg)	> 90	50–90	< 50
Neurologic status	awake	obtunded	comatose
Open wound	none	minor	major/penetrating/burns
Skeletal trauma	none	closed	open/multiple

Pediatric TS: 9–12, minor trauma; 6–8, potentially life-threatening; 0–5, life-threatening; <0, usually fatal.

(see also Chapter 14). Transfusing cold blood rapidly through a central line may lead to arrhythmias.

Secondary survey

The secondary survey includes a thorough evaluation of each organ system, a head-to-toe examination of the injured patient, and reevaluation of hemodynamic parameters. The following information can be obtained by using the mnemonic

AMPLE: allergies (A), medications (M), past medical and surgical histories (P), last meal (L), and events (E) related to the injury. Additional indicated diagnostic procedures should be performed according to clinical need and ATLS approach. Consultation with other services is done as necessary.

Anesthetic considerations

Preoperative evaluation

The trauma anesthesia team should be involved early in the care of the pediatric trauma patient to maximize efficiency and optimize adequate operating room (OR) preparation and availability. Preoperative evaluation starts with the history and physical exam. However, obtaining information in pediatric trauma patients may be limited because of the severity of the injury, unavailability of family or relatives, and, occasionally, the need to move an unstable patient to the OR for immediate surgical intervention. Family members, if available, can provide information about the child's drug allergies, medical conditions, prior surgeries and anesthetic experience, and any family history of anesthetic complications. Otherwise, preliminary information can be obtained from the transport team or emergency room physician. It is also important to note the course of events and treatment given at the scene of the accident and in the emergency department, the type and amount of fluids and blood products given, available ancillary laboratory data, electrocardiogram (ECG), and results of radiologic studies. Physical examination should include vital signs, neurologic status, and a quick, organized organ system evaluation. The presence of adequate free-flowing intravenous lines, orogastric or nasogastric tubes, chest tubes, urinary catheters, and an intracranial pressure (ICP) monitoring device should also be noted.

Understanding the physiologic, anatomic, and pharmacologic characteristics of pediatric patients, and how certain aspects of pediatric trauma differ from adult trauma, contributes to safe conduct of anesthesia and may improve outcome. Specific modification of anesthetic techniques and equipment may be required. Major anesthetic considerations in the management of urgent surgery in the pediatric trauma patient include the presence of gastric contents ("full stomach"), airway management, monitoring, anesthetic agents, and fluid and blood resuscitation.

Intraoperative management

Adequate preparation and availability of an operating room (OR) for trauma is vital in the care of severely injured children. The anesthesia machine should be checked and properly functioning. All appropriate monitors, equipment, heating devices and rapid infusion systems, defibrillator, and resuscitation "crash" cart should be readily available, along with airway equipment of various sizes and a "difficult airway cart" including equipment for establishing an airway using fiberoptic

endoscopy or another alternative technique with which the anesthesiologist is comfortable.

It is logical to use an individualized approach in the conduct of anesthesia for the pediatric trauma patient. The decision making should be influenced by the type and severity of injury, preoperative airway management, anticipated airway difficulty, hemodynamic stability, and neurologic status of the patient.

Monitors

No monitor can satisfactorily substitute for the vigilant pediatric trauma anesthesiologist, but monitors provide useful information that can aid in the timely application of necessary therapeutic interventions (see Chapter 9). Standard monitors include noninvasive BP, ECG, pulse oximeter, expiratory capnogram, precordial or esophageal stethoscope, temperature probe, and FiO_2 monitor. The pulse oximeter measures arterial oxygen saturation and evaluates adequacy of oxygenation and peripheral tissue perfusion. In the presence of vasoconstriction due to hypovolemia, hypothermia, or shock, pulse oximetry becomes unreliable. Exhaled CO_2 monitoring (capnography) is used to confirm endotracheal intubation, follow the adequacy of ventilation and effectiveness of cardiopulmonary resuscitation (CPR) (closely related to pulmonary blood flow and cardiac output), and estimate arterial partial pressure of carbon dioxide ($PaCO_2$). The concentration of expired CO_2 is normally within 2–3 mmHg of that in the arterial blood.[7] In the mechanically ventilated neonate or young infant, the dead-space volume between the breathing circuit and the ETT may be relatively more significant than in an adult, resulting in higher dead space to tidal volume ratio and less accurate, lower, $ETCO_2$ values. High oxygen flows, hypovolemia, or low cardiac output, increased alveolar–arterial gradient, and high respiratory rates are other factors that may cause a decrease in the $ETCO_2$ value. Monitoring the trend as much as the actual $ETCO_2$ value is, therefore, especially important in infants and young children. Laboratory blood gas analysis may be used to determine the relationship between $ETCO_2$ and actual arterial $PaCO_2$. Continuous temperature monitoring is a requisite in the care of an injured child, to help avoid the adverse effects of hypothermia (Table 34.8).

Table 34.8 Effects of hypothermia

Increased oxygen consumption
Left shift of oxyhemoglobin dissociation curve
Coagulopathy with prolonged bleeding
Metabolic and lactic acidosis, hypoglycemia
Apnea
Depressed myocardial contractility, arrhythmias
Impaired drug metabolism, delayed emergence from anesthesia
Increased mortality[34]

Invasive monitors to consider include an arterial line, a central venous catheter, a urinary catheter, and/or an ICP monitoring device. Invasive arterial blood pressure measurement is useful, but urgent surgery should not be delayed if attempts to place an arterial line are unsuccessful. An arterial line allows accurate, continuous beat-to-beat blood pressure measurement, especially useful when intraoperative major changes in blood pressure are expected, and it also provides access to obtain blood samples for analysis. Aside from urine output and central venous pressure (CVP) monitoring, respiratory cycle variations in the contour of the arterial waveform during mechanical ventilation may predict a favorable response to fluid resuscitation (arterial pulse contour analysis: see Chapter 9).[35]

Induction of anesthesia

Pediatric trauma patients are brought urgently to the OR most commonly because of hemodynamic instability, often due to penetrating chest injury or acute head bleed. Transport of the unstable trauma patient to the OR can be challenging and potentially dangerous because lines, airways, and even vital signs may be lost en route. Efficient airway and breathing assessment and inventory of lines should be performed immediately upon arrival of the child in the OR. When transferring the child to the OR table, C-spine precautions should be maintained. Resuscitation should be continued during placement of invasive monitors (arterial line, urinary catheter) and establishment of additional IV access.

The primary responsibility of the anesthesiologist is focused first on airway, breathing, and circulation. If the trachea is already intubated, correct placement and position of the ETT should be confirmed by symmetry of chest expansion, presence of bilateral, equal breath sounds, and a normal $ETCO_2$ waveform on the capnogram or a color change when using a portable $ETCO_2$ detector before beginning mechanical ventilation to ensure adequate oxygenation and ventilation.

Infants and children may come to the OR conscious or semiconscious on supplemental oxygen through a nasal cannula or face mask. They will most often require endotracheal intubation for the surgical procedure, so a reasonable and safe plan to secure the airway must be formulated. Alternative means of establishing an airway should be immediately available at hand in case direct laryngoscopy proves to be difficult. This underscores the need to be familiar and knowledgeable with the American Society of Anesthesiologists (ASA) difficult airway algorithm (see Chapter 3).

All emergency trauma patients are presumed to have full stomachs, and many are at risk for C-spine injuries. Rapid sequence induction and intubation (RSI) with manual in-line C-spine stabilization is generally indicated. An assistant maintains the head and neck in anatomic alignment with the body by holding the child's head on both sides just under the child's mastoid processes,[31] so that extreme flexion and extension of the head during intubation is prevented. RSI minimizes the time between loss of airway reflexes and protection of the airway with an ETT. It begins with preoxygenation using 100% oxygen for 3–5 minutes or four maximal breaths, followed by intravenous injection of an anesthetic induction agent and a muscle relaxant while a trained assistant applies cricoid pressure as the child loses consciousness. Direct laryngoscopy is performed as soon as the muscle relaxant has taken effect. In-line C-spine stabilization is maintained throughout. Once the induction agent and muscle relaxant are given, manual ventilation by facemask is generally avoided unless there is concern for hypoxia and hypercarbia. ETT placement is confirmed by continuous presence of a normal $ETCO_2$ capnogram, auscultating bilateral equal breath sounds in the axillary areas, and absence of gastric sounds in the stomach. Cricoid pressure is maintained until ETT tube placement has been confirmed and the ETT cuff inflated. If the child is combative and uncooperative with preoxygenation, a "modified" RSI is an option. The term "modified" refers to bag-mask ventilation prior to intubation. Gentle positive-pressure ventilation by bag and mask is performed after the muscle relaxant is given. Inflation pressures should ideally be limited to less than 15–20 cmH$_2$O to minimize gastric distention. Alternatively, inhalation induction can be used in a combative child with cricoid pressure applied as the child loses consciousness. The risks and benefits of each induction technique need to be carefully considered, especially regarding aspiration and exacerbation of injuries due to excessive movement. Compared with adults, younger pediatric patients desaturate more quickly even with short periods of apnea, such as may occur during induction and intubation, because they have higher oxygen consumption due to increased metabolic rate, and lower oxygen reserve due to decreased functional residual capacity. This emphasizes the importance of adequate preoxygenation. A properly working suction system should be readily available prior to direct laryngoscopy in the event of passive regurgitation or vomiting. Oxygen should also be provided after any failed intubation attempt.

The rigid C-collar, C-spine stabilization, and application of cricoid pressure potentially can all serve to make direct laryngoscopy and intubation technically more difficult. The anterior part of the rigid collar is usually removed before induction while an assistant stabilizes the child's head in the neutral position. C-spine stabilization occasionally interferes with visualization of the vocal cords, converting a grade 2 laryngeal view of the vocal cords into a grade 3 view (Fig. 34.5).[36] The use of a gum elastic bougie can be a life-saving tool in this scenario, where the bougie is inserted first and acts as a stylet to guide the passage of the ETT into the trachea. The smallest cuffed ETT that will fit over a pediatric gum elastic bougie is 3.5 mm internal diameter (ID), whereas the adult size gum elastic bougie will fit into a cuffed ETT 6.5 mm ID and larger.

Cricoid pressure, the Sellick maneuver, is used routinely in patients with a full stomach to theoretically protect against gastric distention, passive regurgitation, and pulmonary aspiration. However, optimal application of cricoid pressure is difficult to achieve and its application is operator-dependent. Even though cricoid pressure remains widely practiced during RSI,[37,38] concerns about its safety and efficacy have been raised.[39,40] The benefit of cricoid pressure has been questioned because there has been no proof that its introduction into clinical practice has improved patient outcome.[41] Cricoid pressure may be ineffective even when applied by experienced personnel,[42] and it may actually increase the risk for failed intubation and regurgitation.[41] Cricoid pressure is applied by placing the thumb and middle finger on either side of the cricoid cartilage and the index finger above, preventing lateral movement of the cricoid.[43] Another method is to place the palm of the hand on the sternum and apply pressure to the cricoid cartilage using only the index and middle fingers,[44] with the assistant personnel applying the maneuver standing on the left side of the patient. Cricoid pressure is relatively contraindicated in patients with known or suspected laryngeal injury or hypertrophied lingual thyroid tissue. Cricoid pressure in these instances may lead to complete airway obstruction.

If a difficult airway, especially with difficult direct laryngoscopy, is anticipated, spontaneous ventilation may be maintained while an inhalational agent is used to deepen the level of anesthesia in preparation for a fiberoptic-assisted intubation. In this case, adequate bag-mask ventilation should be confirmed prior to administering a muscle relaxant. Fiberoptic intubation allows visualization of the glottis without any neck movement, but the presence of blood and debris in the airway may make visualization difficult (see Chapter 3). If a difficult intubation was unexpected, an LMA can usually be easily and quickly inserted to reestablish or maintain oxygenation and ventilation until a more definitive airway can be established. An LMA may also be used as a conduit to facilitate fiberoptic tracheal intubation.

A hypovolemic child is sensitive to the vasodilating and negative inotropic effects of volatile anesthetic agents, propofol, barbiturates, and other drugs associated with histamine release, such as morphine, meperidine, and atracurium. The key to safe anesthetic management of the hemodynamically unstable pediatric trauma patient is the administration of relatively small incremental doses of any selected agents. Anesthetic induction agents are effective in reduced doses because the hypovolemic child has a decreased volume of distribution while blood flow to the brain and heart are maintained close to normal, and because concentrations of drug-binding serum proteins are reduced by the dilutional effects of fluid resuscitation. Any of the major intravenous induction agents can be used as long as the chosen agent is titrated carefully to minimize deleterious effects.

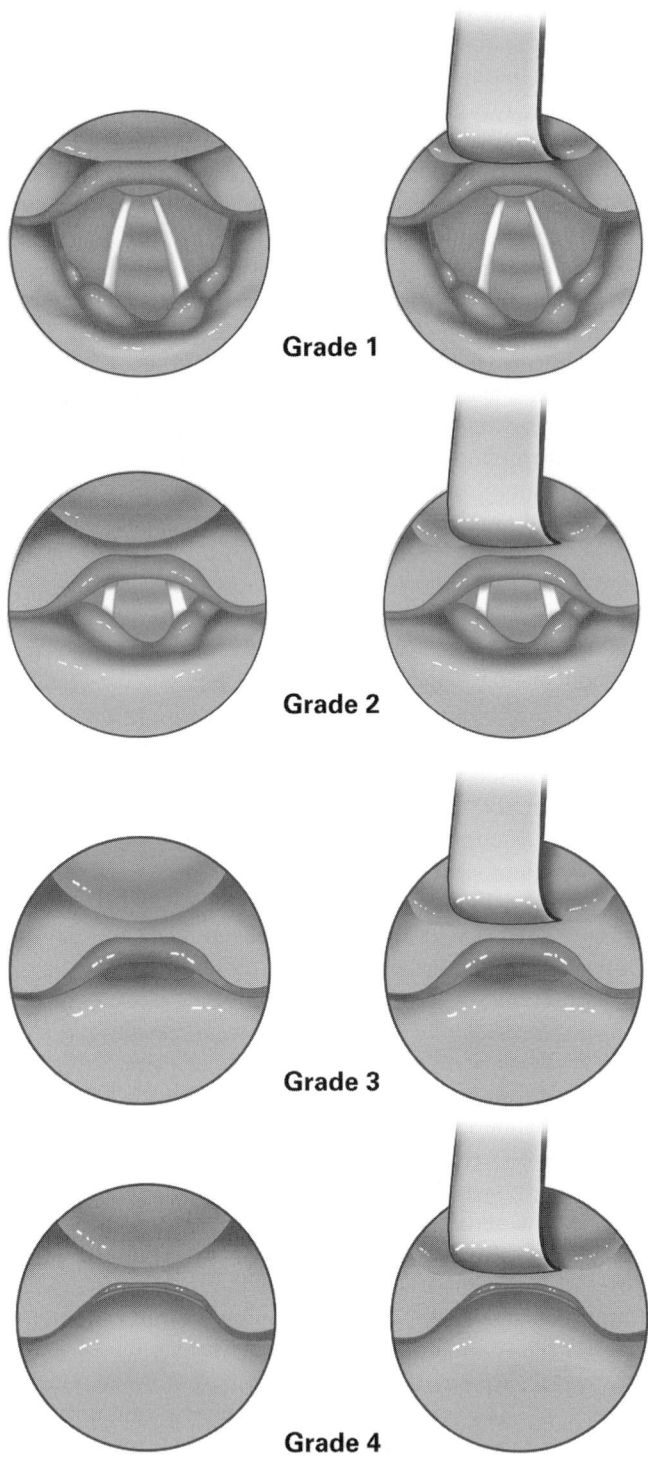

Cormack and Lehane Laryngeal Grades

Figure 34.5 Cormack and Lehane classification. Grading based on the degree of visualization of the glottic opening during direct laryngoscopy. Grade 1, entire glottis visible; grade 2, posterior portion of glottis visible; grade 3, only tip of epiglottis is visible; grade 4, only soft palate is visible. (Courtesy of medical illustrator at MetroHealth Medical Center; redrawn from Cormack and Lehane 1984.[36]) *A black and white version of this figure will appear in some formats. For the color version, please refer to the plate section.*

Sodium thiopental (3–6 mg/kg IV) causes myocardial depression and venodilatation; therefore, cautious and slow intravenous titration is necessary to minimize significant decreases in blood pressure in the hypovolemic patient. Thiopental is rapid-acting, lowers intraocular pressure (IOP), and does not cause pain on injection. It is a good choice in children with head injury and ICP, because it causes dose-dependent decreases in cerebral oxygen consumption, cerebral blood flow, and ICP and reduces epileptiform activity. Induction doses of propofol (2–3 mg/kg IV) may also be expected to decrease BP due to a decrease in systemic vascular resistance, cardiac contractility, and preload. Propofol has more pronounced hypotensive effects than thiopental, especially in inadequately hydrated patients (see also Chapter 7). A major clinical disadvantage with propofol is pain on injection, especially when it is given into the small veins of infants and children. Propofol may, therefore, not be the best choice for RSI. Crying can lead to air swallowing and gastric distention, increasing the risk of aspiration. The use of lidocaine, 0.5–1 mg/kg IV, prior to propofol injection may help attenuate the pain. Propofol decreases cerebral blood flow and intracranial pressure. It also has antiemetic, anticonvulsant, and antipruritic properties.

Ketamine may be the ideal anesthetic induction agent for the hypotensive, hypovolemic, severely injured child who needs urgent or emergent surgery to control hemorrhage. An induction dose of ketamine, followed by a continuous maintenance infusion, may actually elevate and help maintain blood pressure while providing complete anesthesia including analgesia and amnesia. Ketamine (1–3 mg/kg IV) is an N-methyl-D-aspartate (NMDA) receptor antagonist that has indirect cardiovascular effects through central stimulation of the sympathetic nervous system and inhibition of norepinephrine reuptake, leading to increased systemic blood pressure, heart rate, and cardiac output, which is often beneficial to patients in acute hypovolemic shock. Rarely, the direct myocardial-depressant, hypotensive effect of ketamine may be unmasked in patients whose catecholamine stores are maximally depleted. Induction doses of ketamine minimally affect the ventilatory drive and do not depress upper airway reflexes. Ketamine causes some increase in salivation that may be attenuated by an anticholinergic premedication, such as atropine (0.01–0.02 mg/kg IV) or glycopyrrolate (0.01 mg/kg IV). Ketamine has been reported to increase IOP.[45] Ketamine has also been shown to increase ICP,[46] cerebral oxygen consumption, and cerebral blood flow, and thus is usually avoided in patients with space-occupying intracranial lesions.

Etomidate (0.2–0.3 mg/kg IV) is a short-acting, nonbarbiturate sedative hypnotic without analgesic properties that provides hemodynamic stability because of its minimal effects on the cardiovascular system. It is associated with myoclonus, and, like propofol, it causes pain on injection due to its propylene glycol additive. Etomidate possesses both anticonvulsant and proconvulsant properties. Like thiopental, etomidate decreases cerebral metabolic rate, cerebral blood flow, and

ICP. Its major drawback is adrenocortical suppression, especially after prolonged continuous infusions.[47,48]

Succinylcholine (1.5–2 mg/kg IV) is a depolarizing muscle relaxant and may be the drug of choice for RSI because of its rapid onset (30–60 seconds) and brief duration of action (5–10 minutes). In the event that tracheal intubation is unexpectedly difficult and bag-mask ventilation becomes inadequate, quick recovery from succinylcholine neuromuscular blockade allows return of spontaneous respiratory efforts. Due to their relatively large volume of distribution, infants require larger doses of succinylcholine (2–3 mg/kg IV) than do adults. Succinylcholine, especially when given repeatedly, may produce transient bradycardia,[49,50] junctional rhythm, and sinus arrest in children.[51] Pretreatment with a vagolytic agent such as atropine (0.01–0.02 mg/kg IV) is indicated before a repeat dose of succinylcholine is given. Routine administration of prophylactic atropine (or glycopyrolate) before an initial dose of succinylcholine in children to maintain cardiovascular stability and prevent bradycardia remains controversial,[52,53] and this practice varies widely.[52] Atropine produces a bimodal sinoatrial node response such that small doses slow and larger doses accelerate nodal activity.[54] The administration of atropine 10 μg/kg may reduce the incidence of, but not prevent, arrhythmias following the first dose of succinylcholine.[52,55] Infants under 6 months of age appear to have parasympathetic dominance.[56,57] This incomplete maturation of the sympathetic nervous system may account for the clinically observed marked vagal responses of neonates to a variety of stimuli,[58] such as direct laryngoscopy and intubation. Desire to minimize the occurrence of this reflex-induced bradycardia may partly explain the continued use of "prophylactic" atropine in infants and neonates. Though the debate goes on, the majority of practitioners use prophylactic atropine before repeated doses of succinylcholine.[50,59] The mechanism of the cardiovascular effects of succinylcholine remains unexplained.[60,61] Succinylcholine transiently increases IOP, intragastric and lower esophageal sphincter pressures, and ICP. Hyperkalemic cardiac arrest has occurred after succinylcholine administration to children with undiagnosed myopathy. Succinylcholine is contraindicated in patients with muscular dystrophies, major denervation injury, burns more than 24 hours old, a history of malignant hyperthermia, disuse atrophy, neuromuscular disorders, prolonged immobility with disease, or hyperkalemia (see also Chapter 13).

Rocuronium is a nondepolarizing muscle relaxant frequently used as an alternative to succinylcholine. Larger doses of rocuronium (0.9–1.2 mg/kg IV) are required to facilitate rapid onset of neuromuscular blockade for intubation. These doses of rocuronium may prolong its duration of action to as much as 90 minutes. Rocuronium does not cause histamine release. After injecting thiopental, the intravenous line should be flushed before administering rocuronium, which precipitates with thiopental.

Vecuronium is another nondepolarizing muscle relaxant that does not cause histamine release or adverse cardiovascular effects. Its onset of action is slower than that of rocuronium. Vecuronium, 0.25 mg/kg IV, provides good intubating conditions in 60–90 seconds. It is an acidic compound that can be deactivated in alkaline solution such as commercial preparations of thiopental. Therefore, thiopental should be flushed from the intravenous line before administering vecuronium.

Maintenance of anesthesia

The overall clinical status of the injured child, associated injuries, nature of the surgical procedure, and postoperative ventilatory needs dictate choice of technique and selection of agents used in the maintenance of anesthesia. A balanced general anesthetic using volatile agents, opioids, and muscle relaxants may be used for maintenance in hemodynamically stable patients. A narcotic-based anesthetic technique, using fentanyl or remifentanil with muscle relaxant, and an amnesic agent, would be more appropriate for unstable patients who cannot tolerate volatile agents. Sevoflurane, isoflurane, and nitrous oxide are inhalational anesthetic agents widely used in pediatric anesthesia. All inhalational agents cause a dose-dependent myocardial depression, peripheral vasodilatation, and systemic hypotension. The less commonly used halothane and enflurane decrease cardiac output with minimal effect on systemic vascular resistance, while isoflurane and desflurane can profoundly decrease systemic vascular resistance but have minimal effect on the cardiac output, both because of tachycardia. Sevoflurane is associated with no or minimal change in systemic blood pressure and increase in heart rate. In the injured child, perfusion to the heart and brain may be maintained despite poor perfusion to other organs, so inhalational anesthetic requirements are reduced. Isoflurane is the preferred agent for neurosurgical pediatric patients because it has less cerebral effects at 1 MAC (minimum alveolar concentration) values.

Nitrous oxide is 34 times more soluble than nitrogen and tends to rapidly diffuse into and expand any air-containing cavities. Therefore, the use of nitrous oxide should be avoided in children with suspected or known pneumothorax, air embolism, or pneumocephalus.

Hypotensive pediatric trauma patients may not tolerate even reduced concentrations and doses of anesthetic agents. Amnesic agents such as benzodiazepines or scopolamine may be administered to help prevent recall or intraoperative awareness. An opioid-based anesthetic technique, supplemented with carefully titrated volatile agents, may be well tolerated. Fentanyl provides good analgesia and maintains hemodynamic stability. Fentanyl can be given IV as a bolus of 2–20 µg/kg, depending on the procedure, or infused at a rate of 0.02–0.03 µg/kg/min. An alternative to fentanyl is remifentanil, a narcotic with a short half-life and lack of drug accumulation even with prolonged infusion. It can be titrated at a rate of 0.01–1.0 µg/kg/min. It is recommended that the IV tubing containing the remifentanil be connected to an intravenous line close to the patient to avoid opioid-induced bradycardia and chest wall rigidity associated with bolus doses of remifentanil that would otherwise be given whenever the IV line is flushed. Because of its rapid offset, adequate postoperative analgesia should be established before stopping the remifentanil infusion.

Rapid changes in the ventilatory and hemodynamic status can occur intraoperatively, so constant vigilance is imperative. Positive-pressure ventilation may expand a small undiagnosed pneumothorax leading to compromised circulation, oxygenation, and ventilation. Lung contusion may lead to progressive hypoxemia and hypercarbia. Occult bleeding can result in unexplained hypotension and shock.

Large amounts of IV fluids may be required to replace body fluid deficits and blood loss during surgery. Isotonic crystalloid solution is the IV fluid of choice for initial replacement of fluid losses associated with hemorrhagic shock, major surgery, and trauma to rapidly restore circulating blood volume and vital organ perfusion. Intraoperative fluid management includes replacement of preoperative deficits, provision of maintenance fluids, and replacement of ongoing losses.

An accurate estimate of preoperative blood loss in pediatric trauma patients is difficult, if not impossible. To estimate the intraoperative maintenance for pediatric patients, the "4–2–1 rule" formula (Table 34.9) is commonly used. With this formula, the required maintenance fluid for a 23 kg child will be 4 mL/kg/h for the first 10 kg, plus an additional 2 mL/kg/h for the next 10 kg, plus another 1 mL/kg/h for weight greater than 20 kg, for a total of 63 mL/h (40 + 20 + 3). Glucose-containing solutions should be avoided, unless necessary in cases of hypoglycemia or in patients at risk for hypoglycemia, for example, neonates. Glucose-containing solutions contribute to hyperosmolality, intraoperative hyperglycemia, and osmotic diuresis, and have been shown to worsen neurologic outcome after cerebral ischemia.[62,63]

A relatively small amount of blood loss may be detrimental to an infant or child, whose normal pre-injury circulating blood volume is small relative to that of an adult. Replacement fluids include crystalloids, colloids, and blood products. Preoperative and intraoperative fluid losses are mostly isotonic and are appropriately replaced by lactated Ringer's or 0.9% normal saline solutions. Lactated Ringer's solution is slightly hypotonic (273 mOsm/L; sodium, 130 mEq/L; chloride, 108 mEq/L) and contains electrolytes. It appears to be the most physiologic solution, especially when given in large volumes. In contrast, normal saline (308 mOsm/L; sodium, 154 mEq/L; chloride, 154 mEq/L) leads to hyperchloremic metabolic acidosis when large volumes are infused. Colloids such as 5% albumin have been used in pediatric patients,[64] with limited

Table 34.9 "4–2–1 rule" for hourly maintenance fluid requirement

Weight (kg)	Fluid (mL/kg/h)
0–10	4 for each kg
10–20	40 + 2 for each kg between 10 and 20
> 20	60 + 1 for each kg over 20

data to show their advantage over crystalloids.[65,66] Hetastarch, a colloid solution, has limited usefulness because it is associated with platelet dysfunction and clinical coagulopathy when more than 15–20 mL/kg are infused.[67] Primarily based on studies in adults, Hextend, a solution of 6% hetastarch in lactated Ringer's solution, is less likely to result in clinical coagulopathy even when infused in relatively large volumes, when compared with Hespan, a solution of 6% hetastarch in normal saline.[68–71] Limited data support the use of hetastarch in children.[72] One study suggests that 6% hetastarch is safe and as effective a volume expander as 5% albumin in children older than 1 year.[73] Debate continues over the best choice of fluid for volume resuscitation. Balanced salt solutions, crystalloids, distribute to the extracellular space with only 20–30% of the infused volume remaining in the intravascular space after 2 hours; thus, 3–4 times the volume of blood lost must be infused to maintain normovolemia. Proponents of colloids argue that the need for larger volumes of crystalloid to restore adequate circulating blood volume promotes more tissue edema and reduction in oxygen delivery to the tissues after the acute phase of resuscitation.

Third-space fluid losses depend on the severity of the injury and the extent of the surgery. The composition of this third-space fluid is similar to that of extracellular fluid, so balanced salt solution is again the preferred fluid for replacement. An accurate estimate of actual fluid loss is impossible, so fluid replacement should be guided by cardiovascular response and urine output. A guideline commonly used is presented in Table 34.10.

Initially, each 1 mL of blood loss should be replaced with 3 mL of crystalloids, combined with colloids (1 mL per 1 mL of blood loss) to maintain normovolemia. The hematocrit should be monitored whenever blood loss is moderate or greater. When a predetermined lower limit of hematocrit has been reached, blood products are indicated. Red blood cell transfusion is initiated to increase, maintain, or optimize the oxygen-carrying capacity of the intravascular volume. The use of other blood products, such as fresh frozen plasma (FFP), platelets, and cryoprecipitate or other factors, should be guided by coagulation studies and clinical signs of coagulopathy or disseminated intravascular coagulopathy (DIC), except in the situation of severe blood loss, where a massive transfusion protocol (MTP) may be necessary (see Chapter 6).

Indications for blood transfusion are similar to those in adults. The decision to transfuse will be influenced by preoperative hematocrit, estimated blood volume (EBV), the presence and nature of coexisting illnesses, rate of bleeding, and the clinical response of the patient to volume resuscitation. Knowledge of the estimated blood volume (Table 34.11) and the acceptable hematocrit in the pediatric patient (Table 34.12) will aid the anesthesiologist in determining the maximum blood loss that can be safely tolerated, beyond which blood transfusion becomes an important consideration. Maximum allowable blood loss (MABL) may be calculated as:

$$MABL = \frac{(\text{initial hematocrit} - \text{target hematocrit})}{\text{Initial hematocrit}} \times EBV$$

To estimate the amount of pRBCs needed to reach the targeted hematocrit value, the following formula may be used:

$$\text{Volume of PRBCs(mL)} = \frac{\text{desired hematocrit} - \text{present hematocrit}}{\text{hematocrit of PRBC (approximately 60\%)}} \times EBV$$

The hematocrit of pRBCs is approximately 60–70%, so 100 mL of pRBC will provide 60–70 mL of red blood cells. pRBCs (10 mL/kg) will increase the hematocrit by 5–10% and hemoglobin by approximately 3 g/dL. Platelets and FFP should be given when blood loss exceeds 1–2 blood volumes or when results of coagulation profile studies are abnormal. Platelets (10 mL/kg) will raise the platelet count to about 50,000/μL. FFP (10–15 mL/kg) is indicated to treat coagulopathy. It is important to remember that FFP has a high citrate concentration and that citrate chelates calcium, so rapid infusion of large volumes of FFP can lead to severe hypocalcemia and hypotension,[7] if unrecognized or not treated. Infusion of blood products in the same tubing as calcium-containing solutions, such as lactated Ringer's, should be avoided because the anticoagulant citrate present in the blood products may bind to

Table 34.10 Replacement of third-space and evaporative surgical fluid losses

Surgical trauma	Fluid replacement (mL/kg/h)
Minimal	1–2
Moderate	4–6
Severe	6–10

Table 34.11 Estimated blood volume in relation to age

Age	Blood volume (mL/kg)
Premature infant	90–100
Newborn	80–90
3 months to 1 year	70–80
> 1 year	70

Table 34.12 Normal and acceptable hematocrits in pediatric patients[74]

	Normal hematocrit	Acceptable hematocrit
Premature	40–45	35–40
Newborn	45–65	35–40
3 months	30–42	25
1 year	34–42	20–25
6 years	35–43	20–25

calcium and become inactivated, resulting in clot formation. The pediatric dose of cryoprecipitate is 1 unit/10 kg weight.

Recombinant activated coagulation factor VIIa (rFVIIa) is approved for treatment of bleeding in hemophilia or von Willebrand disease with inhibitor antibodies. Even with limited pediatric data and clinical experience, its off-label use has been effective in controlling life-threatening traumatic and intraoperative bleeding unresponsive to conventional supportive intervention (pRBC, FFP, platelets).[75–80]

Massive blood loss is defined as the loss of one or more circulating blood volumes (see also Chapter 6). Massive blood transfusion may lead to coagulopathy as a result of dilutional thrombocytopenia and reduction in clotting factors (Table 34.13). With the first blood volume lost, approximately 40% of the starting platelet count is lost. Losing the second blood volume will lead to loss of another 20% of the starting platelets, with yet another 10% of the starting platelet count lost when the third blood volume is lost.[81] Obtaining laboratory studies such as prothrombin time (PT), partial prothrombin time (PTT), and platelet count will help evaluate the presence and severity of coagulopathy. Other tests, such as platelet function analyzer, thromboelastography (TEG), and thromboelastometry (ROTEM), may also be helpful if available. The presence of increased fibrinogen split products and low fibrinogen level is suggestive of trauma-induced coagulopathy or DIC requiring transfusion of FFP, platelets, and cryoprecipitate. A pediatric trauma MTP is feasible and allows for rapid provision of plasma, pRBCs, and platelets to injured children with hemorrhagic shock and coagulopathy.[82]

Damage control resuscitation includes rapid control of surgical bleeding and hemostatic resuscitation. Hemostatic resuscitation refers to early administration of packed red blood cells (pRBC) with FFP and platelets in a 1:1:1 unit ratio. This strategy minimizes crystalloid and colloid hemodilution that exacerbates coagulopathy and the vicious cycle of coagulopathy, acidosis, and hypothermia (the lethal triad). However, larger studies are warranted to determine if such a strategy will improve outcome in pediatric trauma patients.

Pediatric patients are prone to hypothermia, especially when exposed to a cold operating room, cold irrigation fluids, cold IV fluids and blood products, and the effects of anesthesia on thermoregulation. The presence of large open wounds and exposure of body cavities during surgery aggravate evaporative heat loss. All possible measures should be taken to restore

Table 34.13 Complications of massive transfusion

Citrate toxicity and hypocalcemia
Hyperkalemia
Metabolic acidosis
Hypothermia
Coagulopathy or DIC
Shift of oxyhemoglobin dissociation curve to the left

normothermia and avoid its adverse effects (Table 34.8). Techniques to prevent hypothermia include warming all IV fluids, transfused blood products, surgical preparation, and irrigation fluids, using convective warming systems and overhead radiant warmers, and increasing the ambient temperature of the operating room to $\geq 28\,^\circ C$. Wrapping the head and uninvolved exposed extremities is also effective, because children, especially infants, lose heat significantly from their heads. Humidifying and warming the breathing gas is also indicated.

Emergence and postoperative considerations

The severity and type of initial injury, intraoperative surgical course, and the need for postoperative ventilatory support influence the decision to extubate the child's trachea at the conclusion of surgery. Children with minor injuries can be extubated at the end of the procedure if the following criteria are met: child is awake and alert, vital signs are stable without any inotropic support, and the child is euthermic and maintaining adequate oxygenation and ventilation with spontaneous respirations and reversal of neuromuscular blockade. If the decision has been made to keep the child intubated, then transport to the intensive care unit must be carefully planned. Transport monitors, full oxygen tank and bag-mask, emergency airway equipment, fluids, and resuscitation drugs should be readily available. Spine precautions should be maintained throughout if the spine has not been cleared, and reassessment of the adequacy of oxygenation and ventilation should be confirmed every time the patient is moved.

Head trauma

More than half of pediatric trauma patients sustain serious head injuries, the major cause of morbidity and mortality in children.[27,83] The child's relatively large head helps explain the higher incidence of closed head injury associated with MVCs and falls in infants and young children (see also Chapters 21 and 35).

Child abuse is the leading cause of head injury in infants less than 1 year old, and accidental head injury is the most common cause of mortality in children older than 1 year of age.[84] The relatively rapid brain growth with increasing brain water content during the first 2 years of life, combined with relatively lower cerebrospinal fluid and cerebral blood volumes, makes the young brain more vulnerable to traumatic injury and ischemia. Compared with adults, blunt head trauma in children is less likely to cause focal mass lesions or intracranial hematomas, but more likely to lead to diffuse brain swelling with elevated ICP.[85]

Head trauma varies from scalp injury to skull fracture, hematoma formation, cerebral concussion, and intracranial bleed. Because the scalp is highly vascular, blood loss from scalp injury in a child can be significant, even leading to hemodynamic instability in an infant. Most pediatric skull fractures are linear and do not require surgery unless the underlying brain and vasculature is damaged. Child abuse should be suspected in the presence of multiple fractures inconsistent with the child's reported history. A scalp hematoma in a child is suggestive of an underlying skull fracture and is a sensitive predictor of intracranial injury.[86] Epidural hematomas are less common in pediatric than adult trauma. Sixty to eighty percent of pediatric cranial epidural hematomas are associated with skull fracture.[27] Epidural hematomas are most commonly due to bleeding from middle meningeal artery injury, whereas subdural hematomas are due to tears in the cortical bridging veins. In contrast to adults, children with subdural hematomas may have no associated skull fractures.[1] Expansion of a hematoma may lead to neurologic deterioration requiring emergent surgical evacuation to decrease morbidity. Intracerebral bleeding, usually requiring great force, is less common in children, but its presence portends a poor prognosis.[84]

Children older than 3 years of age with severe head injury have better outcomes than adults with similar injury.[5] Hypotension from isolated head injury is unusual, but can occur in infants with open cranial sutures and fontanelles. A gradual increase in ICP is compensated by expansion of the cranium; however, rapid increase in intracranial volume is poorly tolerated. Normal ICP varies with age (Table 34.14),[87] and increases more rapidly in children than in adults. The level of consciousness in a child with head injury can deteriorate quickly, so frequent reassessment is recommended. As isolated trauma to the brain does not usually lead to hypotension; if the brain-injured child is hypotensive, other injuries should be sought.

Goals of the anesthesiologist caring for the child with head injury perioperatively are to provide adequate anesthesia and analgesia, optimize surgical conditions, support vital functions, ensure adequate oxygenation and ventilation, minimize cerebral edema, and prevent further brain injury from increased ICP, or from hypoxemia, hypercarbia, acidosis, hypo/hyperglycemia, and hypotension. Special care must also be given to prevent further damage from potentially coexistent C-spine injury. Adequate intravascular volume and cerebral perfusion pressure (CPP) should be maintained. CPP depends primarily on mean arterial pressure (MAP):

$$CPP = MAP - (CVP \text{ or } ICP)$$

MAP should be at least 50 mmHg in infants and at least 60–70 mmHg in children to maintain adequate cerebral perfusion.[88] Hypotension has been shown to significantly increase morbidity and mortality in children with head injury.[89] Even a single episode of hypotension perioperatively can affect outcome in adults and pediatric patients.[83] Adult patients with intraoperative hypotension (< 90 mmHg) have a threefold

increase in mortality compared to normotensive patients.[90] Judicious use of intravascular fluid replacement is necessary to avoid overhydration with the potential to promote cerebral edema. Normovolemia is the goal. For initial fluid resuscitation, maintenance, and replacement, normal saline (154 mEq/L of sodium) may be preferable to lactated Ringer's (130 mEq/L of sodium). Hypercapnia results in cerebral vasodilatation with subsequent increase in ICP and impairment of cerebral oxygen transport, and so should be avoided. Maintenance of normocapnia, $PaCO_2$ 35–40 mmHg, is recommended to ensure adequate oxygenation (PaO_2 100 mmHg at FiO_2 of 40%).[91] Mild or prophylactic hyperventilation ($PaO_2 < 35$ mmHg) is not necessary in the absence of increased ICP. In fact, the vasoconstrictive effects of hyperventilation decrease cerebral blood flow and may exacerbate secondary brain injury.[92] Hyperventilation may actually be detrimental if the $PaCO_2$ is kept below 30 mmHg.[1,93] However, hyperventilation during the first 24 hours after severe traumatic brain injury may be a necessary option briefly during acute neurologic deterioration such as impending brain herniation or for longer periods of refractory increased ICP.[94] The use of positive end-expiratory pressure (PEEP) to provide or improve oxygenation may increase ICP and affect CPP, and therefore should be avoided.

Mannitol (0.25–1.0 g/kg) given intermittently has been used effectively to help decrease brain swelling in the euvolemic brain-injured patient. Serum osmolarity should be maintained below 320 mOsm/L to minimize the occurrence of acute tubular necrosis and renal failure.[95] Mannitol reduces blood viscosity, resulting in reflex vasoconstriction in the presence of intact cerebral blood flow (CBF) autoregulation. It rapidly reduces ICP but the effect is transient, lasting less than approximately 75 minutes.[95] Mannitol has a slow osmotic effect lasting up to 6 hours, and its safe use depends on an intact blood–brain barrier to prevent cerebral edema.[95] Mannitol use has not been shown to improve neurological outcome.[96] There are reports on the efficacy of hypertonic saline (3% saline) to control ICP after severe pediatric traumatic brain injury, but clinical experience is limited (see Chapter 21).[95] Hypertonic saline may be considered in patients who are refractory to mannitol.

Anticonvulsants, such as phenytoin, may be administered prophylactically to reduce the incidence of early (first week) posttraumatic seizures with concomitant increase in ICP and $CMRO_2$ in young pediatric patients and infants.[97] The increased excitability of the developing brain increases the risk of posttraumatic seizures in infants and small children compared with adults.[96,98] Phenytoin decreases the incidence of early seizures but has no effect on late-occurring seizures (more than 7 days after injury) or overall outcome.[99] Corticosteroids have not proved to be generally beneficial in pediatric head trauma, so routine steroid use in not currently indicated.

A child with increased ICP or brain swelling may need an ICP monitor or a ventriculostomy catheter device that also allows therapeutic drainage of cerebrospinal fluid. Other strategies to maintain normal ICP include cerebrospinal fluid

Table 34.14 Normal intracranial pressure (ICP, mmHg)[87]

Infants	0–6
Toddlers	6–11
Adolescents	13–15

drainage and use of sedatives and barbiturates to decrease cerebral metabolic requirements. For refractory intracranial hypertension, barbiturate coma and decompressive craniectomy might be necessary. Patients with head injury may develop hyperglycemia from increased gluconeogenesis and glycogenolysis in response to release of cathecholamines and cortisol, and glucose intolerance that may lead to secondary brain injury. Data in children and adults have shown that hyperglycemia after traumatic brain injury is associated with poor neurologic outcome.[100,101] There are currently insufficient data to support the hypothesis that treatment of hyperglycemia will improve outcome.[63,102]

Additional anesthetic concerns include (1) full stomach with the risk of regurgitation and aspiration, (2) potential cervical injury requiring C-spine precautions that make endotracheal intubation more difficult, and (3) elevated ICP. One of the main goals during induction is to minimize or prevent severe increases in ICP that may result in secondary brain injury from cerebral ischemia. Preoperative sedation may be minimized or avoided to lower the risk for respiratory depression, hypoxia, and hypercarbia. Standard monitors include BP (noninvasive or arterial catheter), ECG, pulse oximeter, stethoscope (precordial or esophageal), capnogram, temperature, and a nerve stimulator (see Chapter 9). If the child's head is above the heart intraoperatively, then the arterial line transducer should be zeroed at the level of the external auditory meatus to assess the cerebral perfusion pressure more accurately. Adequate IV access and blood products should always be available in anticipation of possible sudden and severe hemodynamic changes.

Induction should include a smooth, modified RSI. Drugs that provide hemodynamic stability should be chosen for induction and muscle relaxation. Most commonly used induction agents, except ketamine, lower ICP by decreasing CBF and cerebral metabolism. There are conflicting reports on the effects of ketamine on cerebral hemodynamics (Table 34.15). It has been shown to increase, decrease, or not change ICP.[103] Thiopental (4–6 mg/kg IV) may be the induction agent of choice, with the advantages of painless injection and anticonvulsant properties. Thiopental causes dose-dependent decrease in CBF, cerebral metabolic requirement for oxygen (CMRO$_2$), and ICP. It has a direct myocardial depressant effect resulting in decrease in cardiac contractility and BP leading to reduction in CPP. In hypovolemic patients, these effects may be detrimental. Propofol decreases systemic vascular resistance and preload, causing a significant decrease in MAP. Therefore, thiopental and propofol should be used with caution in hemodynamically unstable trauma patients. Etomidate is a good alternative agent that provides cardiovascular stability with less direct myocardial depressant effect. It may be the induction agent of choice for hemodynamically unstable patients because of its minimal effect on blood pressure with maintenance of MAP and CPP.

Other maneuvers that may help decrease ICP include elevating the head at 30 degrees and keeping the head in the

Table 34.15 Effects of anesthetic drugs on the brain

	CMRO$_2$	CBF	ICP
Thiopental	↓↓	↓↓	↓↓
Propofol	↓↓	↓↓	↓↓
Etomidate	↓	↓	↓
Ketamine	↔	↑	↑↑ (?)
Opioids	↓ or ↔	↔	↔
Benzodiazepines	↓↓	↓	↓
Halothane	↓	↑↑	↑
Isoflurane	↓↓	↑	↑
Sevoflurane	↓↓	↑	↑
Desflurane	↓↓	↑	↑
N$_2$O	↑	↑ or ↔	↑

CMRO$_2$, cerebral metabolic oxygen requirements; CBF, cerebral blood flow; ICP, intracranial pressure.
↑, increased ↓, decreased, ↔, unchanged.

midline position to optimize cerebral venous drainage while maintaining CPP. Lidocaine, 1.5–2.0 mg/kg, IV, 90 seconds before intubation, and fentanyl (1–3 µg/kg IV) may help blunt the hemodynamic response associated with direct laryngoscopy and therefore minimize increases in ICP. There is, however, no evidence that lidocaine pretreatment for RSI improves neurological outcome after head trauma.[104] Hypoxia, hypercarbia, and acidosis may exacerbate intracranial hypertension, so induction and endotracheal intubation should be performed smoothly and efficiently. Succinylcholine (1.5–2 mg/kg IV) is the preferred muscle relaxant for RSI (see Chapter 13). Relatively large doses of rocuronium (1.2 mg/kg IV) will provide good intubating conditions with onset time approaching that of succinylcholine. Use of muscle relaxants helps minimize coughing, straining, and physical movements that may increase ICP.

Anesthesia may be maintained with inhalational anesthetic agents, supplemented with narcotics, such as fentanyl. Regional CMRO$_2$ is tightly coupled with CBF such that CBF increases with increased CMRO$_2$. All inhalational anesthetics are cerebral vasodilators and produce a dose-dependent increase in CBF and ICP. However, these inhalational agents decrease CMRO$_2$. Isoflurane produces small increases in CBF that can be prevented by passive hyperventilation,[105] and reduces CMRO$_2$ to a greater degree than halothane because of its direct effect that decreases cortical electrical activity.[106] Thus, it has been suggested that isoflurane is relatively more neuroprotective while maintaining and providing cardiovascular stability. Nitrous oxide increases both CBF and CMRO$_2$ and is best avoided.

IV anesthetic agents generally reduce or do not change CBF and ICP. Fentanyl, by boluses or continuous infusion, is the opioid most commonly used to supplement general anesthesia. It has the advantage of providing hemodynamic stability with minimal or no effect on ICP. Slow IV administration is recommended to minimize the occurrence of bradycardia, especially in neonates, whose cardiac output is relatively more heart-rate-dependent than is that of older infants and children. There appears to be no significant difference in neurologic outcomes between patients anesthetized with IV agents and those receiving inhalational agents.[96,107] Maintaining the $PaCO_2$ at normal to slightly low levels will prevent hypercarbia. Judicious use of IV fluids and blood products is mandatory to minimize cerebral edema, which might compromise cerebral perfusion. Glucose-containing solutions are best avoided unless serum glucose is ≤ 70 mg/dL (3.9 mmol/L).[96,108] Infants and children are susceptible to heat loss, so fluids and blood products should be warmed to help avoid the adverse effects of hypothermia. Because hyperthermia ($> 38\,°C$) also increases metabolic demand, CBF, and ICP, which can worsen secondary brain injuries, the goal should be to maintain normothermia. The use of therapeutic hypothermia in children with traumatic brain injury remains controversial (see Chapter 35).[109]

Abdominal trauma

Most pediatric abdominal injuries are due to blunt trauma and commonly involve more than one organ. The presence of multiple organ system injuries can make abdominal physical examination difficult and unreliable. Abdominal injuries can be potentially life-threatening if initially unrecognized, with mortality rates as high as 8.5%.[110]

Children are at greater risk for sustaining intraabdominal organ injuries after blunt trauma because of their body habitus and immature musculoskeletal systems.[111] Compared with adults, children's intraabdominal organs are proportionally larger and are relatively closer together. Their abdominal wall has thinner musculature, cushioned by less fat and connective tissue, and their more compliant rib cage offers less protection to the underlying organ structures from a traumatic impact. With a given impact, a small child experiences more force per body surface area unit than does an adult. Therefore, the child is more likely to suffer significant multiple organ injury. The spleen is the most frequently injured abdominal organ, followed by the liver, intestine, and pancreas (Table 34.16).[110,111] Intraabdominal hemorrhage is therefore most likely due to splenic injury. Diagnosis of solid organ injuries can be supported by contrast-enhanced CT in addition to frequent reevaluation and repeated examination. Surgical repair of hepatic and splenic injuries can be challenging.

Surgical hemostasis may prove difficult, and massive blood loss and intraoperative hemodynamic instability are possible. Unless the child is hemodynamically unstable, a more conservative, nonoperative approach may be preferable in an attempt to preserve organ function. Because the spleen of a child provides an important immunologic function against some infections, and the relative risk of sepsis is increased in

Table 34.16 Frequency of abdominal organ injuries in children[110,111]

	Blunt (%)	Penetrating (%)
Liver	15	22
Spleen	27	9
Pancreas	2	6
Kidney	27	9
Stomach	1	10
Duodenum	3	4
Small bowel	6	18
Colon	2	16
Others	17	6

postsplenectomy patients, splenectomy is rarely indicated in a child. Children are less likely than adults to require surgical intervention after splenic injury.[112] Obtaining serial hematocrit and aggressive fluid and blood resuscitation play a crucial part in the selective and conservative nonoperative management of these injuries.

Improvements in noninvasive diagnostic modalities have led to the selective nonsurgical approach to pediatric abdominal trauma. Focused abdominal sonography for trauma (FAST) is a cost-effective method of detecting intraperitoneal fluid in hemodynamically unstable children.[113] However, it requires a skilled and properly trained operator. Many injured children present with intraabdominal injuries with no more than minimal free fluid,[111] so the diagnosis might be missed. Compared with CT, FAST is superior for identifying blood in the peritoneum, but, for stable patients, CT is superior for identifying intraabdominal injuries and for providing comprehensive anatomic information on the nature and extent of injuries.[111,114] Diagnostic peritoneal lavage (DPL) is an invasive procedure that may detect the presence of hemoperitoneum, but it does not help in identifying the source of abdominal bleeding and is unable to detect a retroperitoneal bleed, if the child is hemodynamically stable and is under close supervision and monitoring.

Most blunt injuries involving the spleen and liver can be managed nonoperatively. Conservative, nonoperative management demands careful observation, frequent repeated examination, and close monitoring of vital signs in a pediatric intensive care setting by pediatric trauma surgeons for at least 24 hours. Immediate access to the OR for possible urgent surgical exploration is a prerequisite in the event of deteriorating clinical status, hemodynamic instability, developing peritonitis, or transfusion requirements of more than 30–40 mL/kg. Adequate IV access should be maintained at all times. Hemodynamic instability with distended abdomen is a main indication for emergent exploratory laparotomy. Thus, the clinical status of the injured child dictates the need for diagnostic imaging studies. Modern, high-quality noninvasive diagnostic imaging may be used to provide comprehensive anatomic information on the nature and extent of internal injuries.

Posttraumatic paralytic ileus in children may be more likely than in adults to compromise ventilation as the diaphragm is pushed superiorly by distended abdominal viscera. This complication may be alleviated by nasogastric decompression.

Retroperitoneal injuries are more difficult to evaluate and can be misleading. Diagnosis may be delayed without overt signs of peritoneal irritation. Penetrating abdominal wounds with obvious abdominal pain, tenderness, and blood loss necessitate surgical exploration.

A child with blunt abdominal trauma is more likely than an adult to sustain renal injury. Surgical intervention may be indicated for ongoing bleeding, or for extravasation of urine or contrast medium on CT scan.

Pancreatic and bowel injuries may occur with blunt or penetrating abdominal trauma from seatbelts or bicycle handle bars. Frequent physical examination accompanied by radiologic imaging will aid in diagnosis and decision making regarding surgical exploration. Injuries of the pancreas and intestine frequently require surgical intervention.[99,111]

Anesthetic considerations for an injured child with abdominal trauma include gastric decompression to decrease the potential risk of pulmonary aspiration.

Thoracic trauma

A child is more likely to sustain blunt chest trauma than penetrating injury. Falls and MVCs are frequent causes of trauma to the chest in young children, while penetrating injuries from stab wounds and gunshot wounds are more commonly seen in adolescents older than 13 years.[115] A child with penetrating injury to the chest is more likely to require surgical exploration than is an adult (50% vs. 15%).[116]

Anatomic differences between children and adults lead to differences in chest injury profiles. The more compliant chest wall, with its cartilaginous and incompletely ossified ribs, makes a child more vulnerable to intrathoracic injuries without evidence of rib or sternal fractures. It takes a greater force to fracture the ribs of a child than those of an adult. The presence of rib fractures in a child signifies massive impact transmitted to the thorax and should alert caregivers to the increased likelihood of severe injuries to the lungs, heart, and mediastinum. The lung is the most frequently injured thoracic organ in a child,[117] and it is not unusual to find lung contusion without rib fracture. Fracture of the first rib in a child should suggest the possible presence of major vascular injury that may require surgery. Frequent monitoring of arterial blood gases will help detect early signs of pulmonary contusion, manifested by worsening hypoxemia and hypercarbia, even before clinical signs and radiologic changes are evident. Minimal pulmonary contusion may resolve within a few days. Severe lung contusion can cause respiratory compromise and acute respiratory distress that may require endotracheal intubation for mechanical ventilatory support with PEEP. Lung contusion may first manifest intraoperatively with decreased pulmonary compliance contributing to hypoxemia and respiratory acidosis.

Pneumothorax should be suspected when there is unilateral decreased or absent breath sounds and hyperresonance, tachypnea, hypotension, and contralateral tracheal and mediastinal shift. Migration of an ETT into the right mainstem bronchus may also present with absent breath sounds over the left chest. Therefore, appropriate ETT depth should be reconfirmed to avoid confusion. A small pneumothorax, which may not be seen in the initial chest x-ray, may become clinically apparent after initiation of mechanical ventilation in the OR and in association with the use of nitrous oxide. Because a child has more mobile mediastinal structures than an adult, unrecognized tension pneumothorax may be more likely to result in life-threatening respiratory compromise and circulatory collapse. Therefore, clinically significant pneumothorax should be emergently decompressed by inserting a needle in the second intercostal space in the midclavicular line until an indwelling chest tube is placed. Hemothorax is most frequently a result of penetrating chest injury. It produces dullness and unilateral decreased or absent breath sounds. A large accumulation of blood within the pleural cavity may compromise respiratory function and calls for prompt chest tube placement for drainage of blood and lung reexpansion. Surgical intervention is indicated when thoracic bleeding exceeds 30 mL/kg in 8 hours or if the child is in hemorrhagic shock. The pediatric trauma anesthesiologist should be aware that blood lost in the thoracic cavity may be significant enough to cause hypovolemic shock in a child.

Cardiac contusion may present with dysrhythmias and unexplained hypotension (see Chapter 30). Monitoring includes continuous ECG and BP measurement. Echocardiography is indicated for symptomatic patients with cardiovascular instability (see Chapter 10). Management is mainly supportive. Cardiac tamponade is caused by penetrating injury to the heart with resultant accumulation of blood within the pericardium. It is characterized by unexplained tachycardia and hypotension, muffled or distant heart sounds, narrow pulse pressure, distended neck veins, and jugular venous distension due to increased central venous pressure. Emergency surgical drainage is the definitive treatment.

A child with thoracic injury may be taken to the OR for a thoracic procedure or for surgical intervention for other trauma-related organ injuries. It is important for the anesthesiologist to be aware of thoracic injuries that may be initially unrecognized preoperatively, and to be prepared to respond efficiently when these injuries suddenly manifest themselves during surgery by causing hemodynamic instability and respiratory compromise. Evaluating the severity of the injury and the presence of other organ system injuries will help determine anesthetic induction technique and airway management. Initiation of mechanical ventilation and use of nitrous oxide intraoperatively may unmask a previously undetected pneumothorax, or expand a small pneumothorax compromising oxygenation and ventilation. Chest tubes should be placed for clinically significant pneumothoraces before initiation of mechanical ventilation. The effects of pulmonary contusion may manifest during surgery with increasing oxygen requirement and peak inspiratory pressures needed to maintain adequate arterial oxygenation. Peak inspiratory pressure should also be monitored closely to help prevent breakdown of fresh surgical repairs.

In addition to standard routine monitors, arterial line placement for accurate continuous BP measurement and frequent blood gas analysis is helpful. Adequate oxygenation before and during induction of patients with chest injury is crucial. A young infant has 2–3 times more oxygen consumption per kilogram than an adult, and is more likely to desaturate quickly with relatively mild airway obstruction or during the short period of apnea that occurs during endotracheal intubation. Maintenance of anesthesia may require the use of up to 100% oxygen with volatile anesthetic agents carefully titrated as tolerated, supplemented with narcotics and a muscle relaxant. Postoperative mechanical ventilation in an intensive care environment may be necessary, depending on the nature and severity of injury and extent of surgical repair.

Bone injuries

Occult bleeding that continues for hours after injury will have greater consequences for a child than for an adult. Fractures of the pelvis or long bones may be associated with loss of more than 25% of a child's circulating blood volume, leading to hypotension and shock. A high index of suspicion is mandatory following routine evaluation. Diagnosis of occult bleeding can be difficult, especially in a young child or an infant who is not able to communicate verbally, and in the presence of other injuries that alter mental status. Adequate IV access that will allow aggressive fluid and blood resuscitation is important. All fluids and blood products should be warmed before administration, and the clinician must be prepared to diagnose and treat the adverse consequences of massive blood transfusion.

Acute postoperative pain management

Management of postoperative pain is a fundamental part of the anesthetic care of an injured child (see also Chapters 15 and 16). Inadequate treatment of pain may lead to detrimental physiologic and behavioral consequences.[118] Understanding how the developmental changes occurring during childhood affect the pharmacokinetics and pharmacodynamics of drugs is essential to provide adequate analgesia while avoiding potential medication overdose.

Assessment of pain and adequacy of treatment in a child are challenging and dependent on the child's age, ability to understand and communicate, and social development. A child less than 3 years old or a critically injured child may not be able to verbalize the presence or severity of pain. An older child may understand and be able to communicate pain but may deny or underreport pain because of fear. Different pain-rating scales have been used for verbal children 7 years and older, such as the visual analog scale (VAS), the verbal numeric rating scale (scale 0 for no pain to 10 for worst pain), and the graphic rating scales.[119] For a preverbal child, caregivers may use an objective rating system that includes monitoring of vital signs (increased sympathetic activity as a result of stress response to pain) and assessment of behavior.

Nonopioid analgesics are used primarily for mild and moderate pain (Table 34.17). Examples are acetaminophen and nonsteroidal anti-inflammatory drugs (NSAIDs). For both of these agents, increasing doses above a "ceiling effect" will not provide more analgesia, but is more likely to lead to undesirable effects. Hence, these analgesics are used in combination with an opioid (opioid-sparing effect). Acetaminophen is an antipyretic with minimal anti-inflammatory properties. It inhibits cyclooxygenase (COX) centrally,[120] in contrast to the NSAIDs that inhibit peripheral COX, preventing the formation of prostaglandins and thromboxane. Thus, acetaminophen is devoid of NSAID-related side effects, such as gastritis, alteration in renal function, bleeding, and bronchospasm. Hepatic necrosis with fulminant hepatic failure has been associated with acetaminophen overdose.[120] Advantages of NSAIDs include the absence of respiratory depression or sedation. Ketorolac is a parenteral NSAID available in the United States. It has been reported to interfere with bone healing[121] and platelet aggregation, and thus may be best avoided in patients at risk of bleeding.[122]

Opioids are commonly used to treat moderate to severe pain. If given at equipotent doses, most opioids have similar analgesic and side-effect profiles. The response to treatment of pain is characterized by patient-to-patient variability, which mandates careful titration to obtain the desired level of analgesia while avoiding opioid-related serious complications. Common side effects include bradycardia, nausea and vomiting, sedation, respiratory depression, pruritus, urinary

Table 34.17 Nonopioid analgesics

Drug	Dose (< 60 kg) (mg/kg)	Route and interval	Maximum daily dose
Acetaminophen	10–15	PO q 4 h	90 mg/kg/day children
	LD: 30–40	PR	75 mg/kg/day infants
	MD: 20–30	PR q 4–6 h or PR q 8 h	
Ibuprofen	6–10	PO q 4–6 h	40 mg/kg/day
Naproxen	5–10	PO q 12 h	20 mg/kg/day
Ketorolac	LD: 0.5–0.1	IV, IM	2 mg/kg/day or 120 mg/kg/day
	MD: 0.5	IM, IV q 6 h	5 days only

IV, intravenously; LD, loading dose; MD, maintenance dose; PO, orally; PR, rectally.

Table 34.18 Commonly used opioid analgesics

Drugs	Equianalgesic IV dose (mg/kg)	Interval and route
Codeine*	0.5–1.0	q 4–6 h PO
Hydrocodone	0.05–0.1	q 4 h PO
Oxycodone	0.15	q 4 h PO
Fentanyl	0.001	q 1–2 h IV
Hydromorphone	0.015–0.02	q 3 h IV
Meperidine	1	q 3–4 h IV
Morphine	0.1	q 2–3 h IV

IV, intravenously; PO, orally.
* Risk of fatal and life-threatening adverse events in children with genetic variation of liver enzyme that leads to ultrarapid metabolism of codeine to morphine (see http://www.medscape.com/viewarticle/779598, accessed April 2013).

Table 34.19 Patient (parent or nurse)-controlled analgesia (PCA)

Drugs	Bolus (µg/kg)	Rate (boluses/ hour)	Lock-out interval (min)	1-hour limit (µg/kg)
Morphine	20	5	6–10	100
Hydromorphone	4	5	6–10	20
Fentanyl	0.5	5	6–8	2.5

Low-dose continuous, background, or basal infusion of opioids is an option provided by the PCA pumps. However, its use remains controversial because of the potential risk of overdose.[123,124] Commonly used background infusion rates are: morphine, 20–30 µg/kg/h; hydromorphone, 3–4 µg/kg/h; fentanyl, 0.5 µg/kg/h.

Table 34.20 Continuous opioid infusion

Drugs	Infusion rate (µg/kg/h)
Morphine	25 for children 5–10 for infants 2–6 months old
Hydromorphone	3–5
Fentanyl	0.5

retention, ileus, and constipation. Commonly used opioids include codeine, oxycodone, hydrocodone, and morphine (Table 34.18). Careful monitoring is required when administering opioids to neonates and infants, who, because of pharmacokinetic differences, are generally at increased risk for hypoventilation and apnea. Life-threatening cases of respiratory depression, and death, have been reported after codeine use for pain relief. This is likely due to genetic variation in the liver enzyme cytochrome P450 isoezyme 2D6 (CYP2D6), which converts codeine into morphine. The genetic variation speeds up that metabolism, resulting in higher than normal levels of morphine in the blood after codeine treatment.

Ketamine is another analgesic used for short painful procedures in children. Ketamine, 0.25–0.5 mg/kg IV, can provide analgesia for 10–15 minutes; 1–2 mg/kg is for more painful procedures such as closed reduction of a fractured or dislocated bone or burn dressing changes.

Various strategies are available to manage pain postoperatively. As-needed (PRN) intermittent boluses of IV opioid analgesics may be ineffective to control pain, because of patient-to-patient variability in analgesic requirements. Methods available to manage breakthrough pain include the use of IV patient-controlled analgesia (PCA) (Table 34.19), continuous IV opioid infusion, and continuous patient or parent/nurse-controlled epidural analgesia. PCA has been used for children more than 6 years of age in treating moderate to severe pain. It has been shown to be safe and effective, with high satisfaction among patients, families, and nursing staff.[123] For children less than 6 years old, and for critically injured patients with physical or cognitive impairment, PCA by proxy (nurse- or parent-controlled) has been used. PCA computer-driven infusion pumps are programmed to deliver intermittent doses of opioid when needed (demand) with or without concurrent continuous infusion (basal or "background"). Appropriate pumps allow setting of drug dose, dosage interval

(lockout interval), and maximum number of doses per hour (1-hour limit). This method gives the child a sense of satisfaction as a participant in her/his care by allowing her/him some control in obtaining more pain relief while reducing the risk of overdose.

Patients who are unable to use PCA owing to young age or to physical or cognitive constraints may benefit from carefully monitored continuous IV opioid infusions (Table 34.20) with additional bolus doses for breakthrough pain.

Regional anesthesia decreases anesthetic requirement if used in combination with general anesthesia. It also may provide effective postoperative analgesia without the side effects associated with systemic opioids. Contraindications to regional blockade include parental refusal, coagulopathy, infection at the intended site of the block, sepsis, and allergy to local anesthetics. Proper patient selection, knowledge of the relevant anatomy, and proficiency in the required technical skills and knowledge of the local anesthetic pharmacology are important considerations for the performance of regional analgesia and anesthesia. Local infiltration of surgical site, caudal, lumbar, or thoracic epidural analgesia, and peripheral nerve blocks are useful adjuncts to postoperative analgesia. Caudal epidural block is relatively easy to perform in infants and young children and produces reliable analgesia, reduces intraoperative opioid requirements, and provides superior postoperative pain relief for surgeries involving the lower extremities and lower abdomen. A caudal epidural catheter can be inserted for the continuous infusion of local anesthetic.

The relative safety of performing regional blocks in anesthetized children has been the subject of debate and controversy. The consensus of pediatric anesthesiologists appears to be that performing regional blocks in an immobile, anesthetized child improves safety and success rate compared with attempting the same block in an uncooperative, moving, awake child. The long record of safety in performing these blocks in anesthetized children supports the continuing use of this practice.[125–127]

Summary

Trauma is the leading cause of long-term morbidity and death in children. Effective management of injured children requires coordinated, multidisciplinary expertise and a team approach to improve outcome and survival. Prompt and systematic evaluation for identification, prioritization, and timely management of fatal injuries is crucial. The primary survey focuses on airway management, obtaining vascular access, resuscitation, and prevention of secondary brain injury. The secondary survey includes a thorough head-to-toe evaluation, assessment for neurologic disability, and diagnostic imaging studies. Knowledge and understanding of the unique characteristics and needs of traumatized children will help optimize their care, management, and outcome.

Acknowledgments

The author would like to thank Gregory J. Gordon, MD, beloved guru and mentor of pediatric anesthesia, for his great support, helpful suggestions, and editorial assistance in preparing this chapter.

Questions

(1) The leading cause of mortality and serious long-term morbidity in the pediatric population is:
   a. Congenital anomalies
   b. Infectious diseases
   c. Trauma
   d. Malignancy
   e. Pulmonary diseases

(2) The leading cause of traumatic death in children aged 1–19 years is:
   a. Motor vehicle collision
   b. Fall from height
   c. Thermal injury
   d. Homicide
   e. Gunshot wound

(3) In suspected C-spine injury in an infant, a more neutral, straight head and neck position should be achieved in the supine infant by:
   a. Placing a blanket or pad under the torso
   b. Placing a blanket or pad under the neck
   c. Gently extending the head on the neck
   d. Gently flexing the head on the neck
   e. Placing a blanket or pad under the head

(4) During intubation of an infant, the endotracheal tube seems to hang up at the level of the glottis. The best method to use next to intubate this infant is to:
   a. Insert a stylet in the tube and apply firm forward pressure
   b. Withdraw the tube and try again
   c. Apply cricoid pressure
   d. Extend the head on the neck
   e. Rotate the tube longitudinally

(5) The most appropriate cuffed oral endotracheal tube for a normal 4-year-old child is size:
   a. 3.0
   b. 3.5
   c. 4.0
   d. 4.5
   e. 5.0

(6) The best maneuver to improve upper airway patency in an injured, semiconscious child is:
   a. Perform a chin lift
   b. Flex the head on the neck
   c. Perform a two-handed jaw thrust
   d. Insert an oral airway
   e. Insert a nasal airway

(7) A toddler presents to the ED after a fall. Physical exam reveals hemorrhagic shock. Peripheral IV access has failed despite several attempts over the last 2 minutes. The next route to be attempted should be:
   a. Intraosseous in an unfractured tibia
   b. Percutaneous in another peripheral site
   c. Saphenous vein cutdown on the uninjured leg
   d. Subclavian percutaneous
   e. Internal jugular vein percutaneous

(8) Hypothermia in an injured child is most effectively treated by using:
   a. Warm hospital "bath" blanket to cover all exposed areas
   b. Appropriately directed overhead heat lamps
   c. A pediatric warming mattress
   d. Warm intravenous fluids
   e. Forced-air convective warming system

(9) For the hypotensive, hypovolemic, severely injured child who needs urgent surgery to control hemorrhage, the best anesthetic induction agent is:
   a. Sevoflurane (inhalation induction)
   b. Ketamine
   c. Methohexital
   d. Propofol
   e. Thiopental

(10) The preferred fluid for initial volume replacement in the hypovolemic pediatric trauma patient is:
   a. Lactated Ringer's
   b. Hextend
   c. Hypertonic saline (3%)
   d. Normal saline (0.9%)
   e. Albumin (5%)

(11) According to the "4–2–1 rule," hourly maintenance fluid requirement of a 22 kg 5-year-old boy is:
   a. 40 mL

b. 52 mL

c. 60 mL

d. 62 mL

e. 82 mL

(12) Compared with an adult, an infant or young child injured in a motor vehicle collision is more likely to sustain injury to her/his:

    a. Head

    b. Extremities

    c. Chest

    d. Abdomen

    e. Pelvis

(13) Appropriate management of the child with head trauma includes all of the following, *except*:

    a. Maintenance of normal or higher mean arterial pressure

    b. Hyperventilation to keep $PaCO_2$ less than 30 mmHg for up to first 72 hours post injury

    c. Mannitol to decrease brain swelling

d. Phenytoin to prevent seizures with concomitant increase in intracranial pressure

e. Cerebrospinal fluid drainage if necessary to lower intracranial pressure

Answers

(1) c

(2) a

(3) a

(4) e

(5) d

(6) c

(7) a

(8) e

(9) b

(10) a

(11) d

(12) a

(13) b

References

1. Ross AK. Pediatric trauma: anesthetic management. *Anesthesiol Clin N Am* 2001; **19**: 309–37.

2. Christian C. Assessment and evaluation of the physically abused child. *Clin Fam Pract* 2003; **5** (1): 21–46.

3. American Academy of Pediatrics and American Heart Association. Basic life support for the PALS healthcare provider. In *PALS Provider Manual*. Dallas, TX: American Heart Association, 2002, pp. 43–80.

4. Herzenberg JE, Hensinger RN, Dedrick DK, *et al.* Emergency transport and positioning of young children who have an injury of the cervical spine. The backboard may be hazardous. *J Bone Joint Surg Am* 1989; **71-A**: 15–22.

5. American College of Surgeons. Extremes of age: pediatric trauma. In *Advanced Trauma Life Support (ATLS) for Doctors*, 7th edition. Student Course Manual. Chicago, IL: ACS, 2004, pp. 243–62.

6. Finucane BT. *Principles of Airway Management*. Philadelphia, PA: FA Davis, 1988.

7. Cote CJ. Pediatric anesthesia. In Miller RD, ed., *Miller's Anesthesia*, 6th edition. Philadelphia, PA: Churchill Livingstone, 2005, pp. 2367–407.

8. Motoyama EK. Endotracheal intubation. In Motoyama EK, Davis PJ, ed., *Smith's Anesthesia for Infants and Children*, 5th edition. St. Louis, MO: Mosby, 1990, pp. 269–75.

9. Fisher DM. Anesthesia equipment for pediatrics. In Gregory GA, ed., *Pediatric Anesthesia*, 3rd edition. New York, NY: Churchill Livingstone, 1994, pp. 197–225.

10. Joshi VV, Mandavia SG, Stern L, Wiglesworth FW. Acute lesions induced by endotracheal intubation. *Am J Dis Child* 1972; **124**: 646–9.

11. Stocks JG. Prolonged intubation and subglottic stenosis. *Br Med J* 1966; **2**: 1199–200.

12. Stamm D, Floret D, Stamm C *et al.* Subglottic stenosis following intubation in children. *Arch Fr Pediatr* 1993; **50**: 21–5.

13. Hawkins DB. Glottic and subglottic stenosis from endotracheal intubations. *Laryngoscope* 1977; **87**: 339–46.

14. Honig EG. Persistent tracheal dilatation: onset after brief mechanical ventilation with a "soft-cuff" endotracheal tube. *South Med J* 1979; **72**: 487–90.

15. Deakers TW, Reynolds G. Cuffed endotracheal tubes in pediatric intensive care. *J Pediatr* 1994; **125**: 57–62.

16. Khine HH, Corddry DH, Kettrick RG, *et al.* Comparison of cuffed and uncuffed endotracheal tubes in young children during general anesthesia. *Anesthesiology* 1997; **86**: 627–31.

17. Fine GF, Borland LM. The future of the cuffed endotracheal tube. *Pediatr Anesth* 2004; **14**: 38–42.

18. Weiss M, Gerber AC. Cuffed tracheal tubes in children: things have changed. *Pediatr Anesth* 2006; **16**: 1005–7.

19. Browning DH, Graves SA. Incidence of aspiration with endotracheal tubes in children. *J Pediatr* 1983; **102**: 583–4.

20. Lau N, Playfor SD, Rashid A, Dhanarass M. New formulae for predicting tracheal tube length. *Pediatr Anesth* 2006; **16**: 1238–43.

21. Okuyama M, Imai M, Sugawara K, Okuyama A, Kemmotsu O. Finding appropriate tube position by the cuff palpation method in children. *Masui* 1995; **44**: 845–8.

22. Bloch EC, Ossey K, Ginsberg B. Tracheal intubation in children: a new method for assuring correct depth of tube placement. *Anesth Analg* 1988; **67**: 590–2.

23. Roth B, Magnusson J, Johansson I, *et al.* Jaw lift: a simple and effective method to open the airway in children. *Resuscitation* 1998; **39**: 171–4.

24. Bruppacher H, Reber A, Keller JP, *et al.* The effects of common airway maneuvers on airway pressure and flow in children undergoing adenoidectomies. *Anesth Analg* 2003; **97**: 29–34.

25. European Resuscitation Council. Part 9: Pediatric Basic Life Support. *Resuscitation* 2000; **46**: 301–41.

26. Proctor MR. Spinal cord injury. *Crit Care Med* 2002; **30** (11 Suppl): S489–99.

27. Cantor RM, Leaming JM. Evaluation and management of pediatric major trauma. *Emerg Med Clin N Am* 1998; **16**: 229–56.

28. Schwaitzberg SD, Bergman KS, Harris BH. A pediatric trauma model of continuous hemorrhage. *J Pediatr Surg* 1988; **23**: 605–9.

29. Losek JD, Szewczuga D, Glaeser PW. Improved prehospital pediatric ALS care after an EMT-paramedic clinical training course. *Am J Emerg Med* 1994; **12**: 429–32.

30. Fiser DH. Intraosseous infusion. *N Engl J Med* 1990; **322**: 1579–81

31. Badgwell MJ. The traumatized child. *Anesthesiol Clin N Am* 1996; **14**: 151–71.

32. Lieh-Lai MW, Theodorou AA, Sarnaik AP, *et al.* Limitations of the Glasgow Coma Scale in predicting outcome in children with traumatic brain injury. *J Pediatr* 1992; **120**: 195–9.

33. Sessler DI, Moayeri A. Skin surface warming: heat flux and central temperature. *Anesthesiology* 1990; **73**: 218–24.

34. Jurkovich GJ, Greiser WB, Luterman A, Curreri PW. Hypothermia in trauma victims: an ominous predictor of survival. *J Trauma* 1987; **27**: 1019–24.

35. Michard F. Changes in arterial pressure during mechanical ventilation (Review). *Anesthesiology* 2005; **103**: 419–28.

36. Cormack RS, Lehane J. Difficult tracheal intubation in obstetrics. *Anaesthesia* 1984; **39**: 1105–11.

37. Rosen M. Anaesthesia for obstetrics (Editorial). *Anaesthesia* 1981; **36**: 145–6.

38. Standards and guidelines for cardiopulmonary resuscitation (CPR) and emergency cardiac care (ECC). *JAMA* 1986; **255**: 2905–89.

39. Schwartz DE, Cohen NH. Questionable effectiveness of cricoid pressure in preventing aspiration. *Anesthesiology* 1995; **83**: 432.

40. Kron SS. Questionable effectiveness of cricoid pressure in preventing aspiration. *Anesthesiology* 1995; **83**: 431.

41. Brimacrombe JR, Berry AM. Cricoid pressure. *Can J Anaesth* 1997; **44**: 414–25.

42. Howells TH, Chamney AR, Wraight WJ, Simons RS. The application of cricoid pressure: an assessment and a survey of its practice. *Anaesthesia* 1983; **38**; 457–60.

43. Sellick BA. Cricoid pressure to prevent regurgitation of stomach contents during induction of anaesthesia. *Lancet* 1961; **2**: 404–6.

44. Cowling J. Cricoid pressure: a more comfortable technique. *Anaesth Intensive Care* 1983; **10**: 93–4.

45. Yoshikawa K, Murai Y. The effect of ketamine on intraocular pressure in children. *Anesth Analg* 1971; **50**: 199–202.

46. Gardner AE, Olson BE, Lichtiger M. Cerebrospinal-fluid pressure during dissociative anesthesia with ketamine. *Anesthesiology* 1971; **35**: 226–8.

47. Wagner RL, White PF. Etomidate inhibits adrenocortical function in surgical patients. *Anesthesiology* 1984; **61**: 647–51.

48. Longnecker DE. Stress-free: to be or not to be? *Anesthesiology* 1984; **61**: 643–4.

49. Williams CH, Deutsch S, Linde HW, Bullough JW, Dripps RD. The effects of intravenously administered succinylcholine on cardiac rate, rhythm and arterial blood pressure in anesthetized man. *Anesthesiology* 1961; **22**: 947–54.

50. Green DW, Bristow AS, Fisher M. Comparison of i.v. glycopyrrolate and atropine in the prevention of bradycardia and arrhythmias following repeated doses of suxamethonium in children. *Br J Anaesth* 1984; **56**: 981–5.

51. Robinson AL, Jerwood DC, Stokes MA. Routine suxamethonium in children. A regional survey of current usage. *Anaesthesia* 1996; **51**: 874–8.

52. McAuliffe G, Bissonnette B, Boutin C. Should routine use of atropine before succinylcholine in children be reconsidered? *Can J Anaesth* 1995; **42**: 724–9.

53. Shorten GD, Bissonette B, Hartley E, Nelson W, Carr AS. It is not necessary to administer more than 10 micrograms.kg-1 of atropine to older children before succinylcholine. *Can J Anaesth* 1995; **42**: 8–11.

54. Das G, Talmers FN, Weissler AM. New observations on the effects of atropine on the sinoatrial node and atrioventricular nodes in man. *Am J Cardiol* 1975; **36**: 281–5.

55. Goudsouzian NG. Turbe del ritmo cardiaco durante intubazione tracheale nei bambini. *Acta Anaesthesiol Ital* 1981; **32**: 393–6.

56. Hirsch EF. *Innervation of the Vertebrate Heart.* Springfield, IL: Charles C Thomas, 1970, pp. 125–33.

57. McAuliffe G, Bissonnette B, Boutin C. Should atropine be routine in children? *Can J Anaesth* 1996; **43** (7): 754.

58. McGowan FX, Steven JM. Cardiac physiology and pharmacology. In Cote CJ, Todres ID, Goudsouzian NG, Ryan JF, eds., *A Practice of Anesthesia for Infants and Children*, 3rd edition. Philadelphia, PA: Saunders, 2001, pp. 353–90.

59. Parnis SJ, Van der Walt JH. A national survey of atropine by Australian anaesthetists. *Anaesth Intensive Care* 1994; **22**: 61–5.

60. Jonsson M, Dabrowski M, Gurley DA, *et al.* Activation and inhibition of human muscular and neuronal nicotinic acetylcholine receptors by succinylcholine. *Anesthesiology* 2006; **104**: 724–33.

61. Naguib M, Lien CA. Pharmacology of muscle relaxants and their antagonists. In Miller RD, ed., *Miller's Anesthesia*, 6th edition. Philadelphia, PA: Churchill Livingstone, 2005, pp. 481–572.

62. Seiber FE, Smith DS, Traystman RJ, Wollman H. Glucose: a reevaluation of its intraoperative use. *Anesthesiology* 1987; **67**: 72–81.

63. Lam AM, Winn HR, Cullen BF, *et al.* Hyperglycemia and neurological outcome in patients with head injury. *J Neurosurg* 1991; **75**: 545–51.

64. Soderlind M, Salvignol G, Izard P, Lonnqvist PA. Use of albumin, blood transfusion and intraoperative glucose by APA and ADARPEF members: a postal survey. *Pediatr Anesth* 2001; **11**: 685–9.

65. Robertson NR. Use of albumin in neonatal resuscitation. *Eur J Pediatr* 1997; **156**: 428–31.

66. Greenough A. Use and misuse of albumin infusions in neonatal care. *Eur J Pediatr* 1998; **157**: 699–702.

67. Treib J, Haass A, Pindur G. Coagulation disorders caused by hydroxyethyl starch. *Thromb Haemost* 1997; **78**: 974–83.

68. Gan TJ, Bennett-Guerrero E, Phillips-Bute B, *et al*. Hextend, a physiologically balanced plasma expander for large volume use in major surgery: a randomized phase III clinical trial. Hextend Study Group. *Anesth Analg* 1999; **88**: 992–8.

69. Martin G, Bennett-Guerrero E, Wakeling H, *et al*. A prospective, randomized comparison of thromboelastographic coagulation profile in patients receiving lactated Ringer's solution, 6% hetastarch in balanced-saline vehicle, or 6% hetastarch in saline during major surgery. *J Cardiothorac Vasc Anesth* 2002; **16**: 441–6.

70. Roche AM, James MF, Grocott MP, Mythen MG. Coagulation effects of in vitro serial haemodilution with a balanced electrolyte hetastarch solution compared with a saline-based hetastarch solution and lactated Ringer's solution. *Anaesthesia* 2002; **57**: 950–5.

71. Roche AM, James MF, Bennett-Guerrero E, Mythen MG. A head-to-head comparison of the *in vitro* coagulation effects of saline-based and balanced electrolyte crystalloid and colloid intravenous fluids. *Anesth Analg* 2006; **102**: 1274–9.

72. Paul M, Dueck M, Herrmann J, Holzki J. A randomized, controlled study of fluid management in infants and toddlers during surgery: hydroxyethyl starch 6% (HES 70/0.5) vs. lactated Ringer's solution. *Pediatr Anesth* 2003; **13**: 603–8.

73. Brutocao D, Bratton SL, Thomas JR, *et al*. Comparison of hetastarch with albumin for postoperative volume expansion in children after cardiopulmonary bypass. *J Cardiothorac Vasc Anesth* 1996; **10**: 348–51.

74. Berry FA. Practical aspects of fluid and electrolyte therapy. In Berry FA, ed., *Anesthetic Management of Difficult and Routine Pediatric Patients*, 2nd edition. New York, NY: Churchill Livingstone, 1990, pp. 89–120.

75. Morenski JD, Tobias JD, Jimenez DF. Recombinant activated factor VII for cerebral injury-induced coagulopathy in pediatric patients: report of three cases and review of literature. *J Neurosurg* 2003; **98**: 611–16.

76. Kulkarni R, Daneshmand A, Guertin S, *et al*. Successful use of activated recombinant factor VII in traumatic liver injuries in children. *J Trauma* 2004: **56**: 1348–52.

77. Heisel M, Nagib M, Madsen L, *et al*. Use of recombinant factor VIIa (rFVIIa) to control intraoperative bleeding in pediatric brain tumor patients. *Pediatr Blood Cancer* 2004; **43**: 703–5.

78. Tofil NM, Winkler MK, Watts RG, Noonan J. The use of recombinant factor VIIa in a patient with Noonan syndrome and life-threatening bleeding. *Pediatr Crit Care Med* 2005; **6**: 352–4.

79. Tobias JD. Synthetic factor VIIa to treat dilutional coagulopathy during posterior spinal fusion in two children. *Anesthesiology* 2002; **96**: 1522–5.

80. Tobias JD, Berkenbosch JW, Russo P. Recombinant factor VIIa to treat bleeding after cardiac surgery in an infant. *Pediatr Crit Care Med* 2003; **4**: 49–51.

81. Cote CJ, Liu LM, Szyfelbein SK, *et al*. Changes in serial platelet counts following massive blood transfusion in pediatric patients. *Anesthesiology* 1985; **62**: 197–201.

82. Hendrickson JE, Shaz BH, Pereira G *et al*. Implementation of a pediatric trauma massive transfusion protocol: one institution's experience. *Transfusion* 2012; **52**: 1228–36.

83. Tepas JJ III, DiScala DL, Ramenofsky ML, Barlow B. Mortality and head injury: the pediatric perspective. *J Pediatr Surg* 1990; **25**: 92–6.

84. Lam WH, Mackersie A. Paediatric head injury: incidence, aetiology and management. *Paediatr Anaesth* 1999; **9**: 377–85.

85. Bruce DA, Alavi A, Bilaniuk L, *et al*. Diffuse cerebral swelling following head injuries in children: the syndrome of "malignant brain edema". *J Neurosurg* 1981; **54**: 170–8.

86. Schutzman SA, Greenes DS. Pediatric minor head trauma. *Ann Emerg Med* 2001; **37**: 65–74.

87. Welch, K. The intracranial pressure in infants. *J Neurosurg* 1980; **52**: 693–9.

88. White JR, Dalton HJ. Pediatric trauma: post-injury care in the pediatric intensive care unit. *Crit Care Med* 2002; **30** (11 Suppl): S478–88.

89. Pigula FA, Wald SL, Shackford SR, Vane DW. The effect of hypotension and hypoxia on children with severe head injuries. *J Pediatr Surg* 1993; **28**: 310–14.

90. Pietropaoli JA, Rogers FB, Shackford SR *et al*. The deleterious effect of intraoperative hypotension on outcome in patients with severe head injuries. *J Trauma* 1992; **33**: 403–7.

91. Mazzola CA, Adelson PD. Critical care management of head trauma in children. *Crit Care Med* 2002; **30** (11 Supp)l: S393–401.

92. Muizelaar JP, Marmarou A, Ward JD, *et al*. Adverse effects of prolonged hyperventilation in patients with severe head injury. A randomized clinical trial. *J Neurosurg* 1991; **75**: 731–9.

93. Bullock R, Chestnut R, Clifton G, *et al*. Guidelines for management of severe traumatic brain injury. *J Neurotrauma* 2000; **17**: 451–553.

94. Kochanek, PM, Carney N, Adelson PD, *et al*. Guidelines for the acute medical management of severe traumatic brain injury in infants, children and adolescents, second edition. Chapter 13: Hyperventilation. *Pediatr Crit Care Med* 2012; **13** (1 Suppl): S58–60.

95. Kochanek, PM, Carney N, Adelson PD, *et al*. Guidelines for the acute medical management of severe traumatic brain injury in infants, children and adolescents, second edition. Chapter 8: Hyperosmolar therapy. *Pediatr Crit Care Med* 2012; **13** (1 Suppl): S36–41.

96. Tarun B, Dewhirst E, Sawardekar A, *et al*. Perioperative management of the pediatric patient with traumatic brain injury. Review article. *Pediatr Anesth* 2012; **22**: 627–40.

97. Kochanek, PM, Carney N, Adelson PD, *et al*. Guidelines for the acute medical management of severe traumatic brain injury in infants, children and adolescents, second edition. Chapter 17: Anti-seizure prophylaxis. *Pediatr Crit Care Med* 2012; **13** (1 Suppl): S72–5.

98. Leisemer K, Bratton SL, Zebrack CM *et al*. Early posttraumatic seizure in moderate to severe pediatric traumatic brain injury: rates, risk factors and clinical features. *J Neurotrauma* 2011; **28**: 755–62.

99. Khan A, Banerjee A. The role of prophylactic anticonvulsant in moderate to severe head injury. *Int J Emerg Med* 2010; **3**: 187–91.

100. Sharma D, Jelacic J, Chennuri R *et al*. Incidence and risk factors for

perioperative hyperglycemia in children with traumatic brain injury. *Anesth Analg* 2009; **108**: 81–9.

101. Rovlias A, Kotsou S. The influence of hyperglycemia on neurological outcome in patients with severe head injury. *Neurosurgery* 2000; **46**: 335–42.

102. Smith RL, Lin JC, Adelson PD *et al.* Relationship between hyperglycemia and outcome in children with severe traumatic brain injury. *Pediatr Crit Care Med* 2012; **13**: 85–91.

103. Albenese J, Arnaud S, Rey M, *et al.* Ketamine decreases intracranial pressure and electroencephalographic activity in traumatic brain injury patients during propofol sedation. *Anesthesiology* 1997; **87**: 1328–34.

104. Robinson N, Clancy M. In patients with head injury undergoing rapid sequence intubation, does pretreatment with intravenous lignocaine/lidocaine lead to an improved neurological outcome? A review of the literature. *Emerg Med J* 2001; **18**: 453–7.

105. Wade JG, Stevens WC. Isoflurane: an anesthetic for the eighties? *Anesth Analg* 1981; **60**: 666–83.

106. Newberg LA, Michenfelder JD. Cerebral protection by isoflurane during hypoxemia and ischemia. *Anesthesiology* 1983; **59**: 29–35.

107. Kochanek PM, Carney N, Adelson P *et al.* Guidelines for the acute medical management of severe traumatic brain injury in infants, children and adolescents, second edition. Chapter 15: Analgesics, sedatives and neuromuscular blockade. *Pediatr Crit Care Med* 2012; **13**: (1 Suppl): S64–7.

108. Kochanek PM, Carney N, Adelson P *et al.* Guidelines for the acute medical management of severe traumatic brain injury in infants, children and adolescents, second edition. Chapter 16: Glucose and nutrition. *Pediatr Crit Care Med* 2012; **13**: (1 Suppl): S68–71

109. Kochanek PM, Carney N, Adelson P *et al.* Guidelines for the acute medical management of severe traumatic brain injury in infants, children and adolescents, second edition. Chapter 9: Temperature control. *Pediatr Crit Care Med* 2012; **13**: (1 Suppl): S42–5.

110. Saxena AK, Nance ML, Lutz N, Stafford PW. Pediatric abdominal trauma. *MedScape* 2013. www.emedicine.com/ped/topic3045.htm (accessed September 2014).

111. Gaines BA, Ford HR. Abdominal and pelvic trauma in children. *Crit Care Med* 2002; **30**: (11 Suppl): S416–23.

112. Powell M, Courcoulas A, Gardner M, *et al.* Management of splenic trauma: significant differences between adults and children. *Surgery* 1997; **122**: 654–60.

113. Thourani VH, Pettitt BJ, Schmidt JA, *et al.* Validation of surgeon-performed emergency abdominal ultrasonography in pediatric trauma patients. *J Pediatr Surg* 1998; **33**: 322–8.

114. Furnival R. Controversies in pediatric thoracic and abdominal trauma. *Clin Pediatr Emerg Med* 2001; **2**: 48–62.

115. Othersen HB. Cardiothoracic injuries. In Touloukian JR, ed., *Pediatric Trauma*, 3rd edition. St. Louis, MO: Mosby, 1990, pp. 266–311.

116. Peterson RJ, Tiwary AD, Kissoon N, *et al.* Pediatric penetrating thoracic trauma: a five-year experience. *Pediatr Emerg Care* 1994; **10**: 129–31.

117. Peterson RJ, Tepas JJ, Edwards FH, *et al.* Pediatric and adult thoracic trauma: age-related impact on presentation and outcome. *Ann Thoracic Surg* 1994; **58**: 14–18.

118. Zwass MS, Polaner DM, Berde CB. Postoperative pain management. In Cote CJ, Todres ID, Goudsouzian NG, Ryan JF, eds., *Practice of Anesthesia for Infants and Children*, 3rd edition.

Philadelphia, PA: Saunders, 2001, pp. 675–97.

119. Wong DL. *Whaley and Wong's Essential of Pediatric Nursing*, 5th edition. St. Louis, MO: Mosby., 1997, pp. 1215–16.

120. Brislin RP, Rose JB. Pediatric acute pain management. *Anesthesiol Clin N Am* 2005; **23**: 789–814.

121. Gerstenfeld LC, Thiede M, Seibert K, *et al.* Differential inhibition of fracture healing by nonselective and cyclo-oxygenase-2 selective nonsteroidal anti-inflammatory drugs. *J Orthop Res* 2003; **21**: 670–5.

122. Gunter JB, Vaurghese AM, Harrington JF. Recovery and complications after tonsillectomy in children: a comparison of ketorolac and morphine. *Anesth Analg* 1995; **81**: 1136–41.

123. Berde CB, Lehn BM, Yee JD, *et al.* Patient-controlled analgesia in children and adolescents: a randomized, prospective comparison with intramuscular administration of morphine for postoperative analgesia. *J Pediatr* 1991; **118**: 460–6.

124. Monitto CL, Greenberg RS, Kost-Beyerly S, *et al.* The safety and efficacy of parent-nurse controlled analgesia in patients less than six years of age. *Anesth Analg* 2000; **91**: 573–9.

125. Rose JB. Acute pain management in children. In Litman RS, ed., *Pediatric Anesthesia: the Requisites in Anesthesiology*. Philadelphia, PA: Mosby, 2004, pp. 212–18.

126. Krane EJ, Dalens BJ, Murat I, *et al.* The safety of epidurals placed during general anesthesia. *Reg Anesth Pain Med* 1998; **23**: 433–8.

127. Giaufre E, Dalens B, Gombert A. Epidemiology and morbidity of regional anesthesia in children: a 1-year prospective survey of the French Language Society of Pediatric Anesthesiologists. *Anesth Analg* 1996; **83**: 904–12.

Intensive care unit management of pediatric brain injury

Maroun J. Mhanna, Elie Rizkala, and Dennis M. Super

Objectives

(1) Review the significance and incidence of traumatic brain injury in children, as well as the impact of preventive care.

(2) Recognize when a child with a closed head injury is developing intracranial hypertension.

(3) Describe the pathophysiology of primary brain injury as well as the process leading to the secondary injury.

(4) Evaluate first-tier and second-tier therapies for the management of severe traumatic brain injury in children.

Introduction

Severe traumatic brain injury (TBI) is a leading cause of mortality and morbidity in children. In 2011, the leading cause of death in children (age 1–19 years) in the United States was unintentional injuries ($n = 20{,}192$, 35.6%) followed by homicide (11.4%) and intentional self-harm (10.1%).[1] A significant percentage of these injuries involved the brain. For example, during an 18-month period in King County, Washington (Seattle area, comprising a population of 1.8 million), there were 1806 children under 18 years of age with TBI, of which 45 were moderate to severe injuries. This corresponds to incidence rates of 296 and 7.6 per 100,000 child years, respectively. Falls were the most common cause in preschool children, at 86%, whereas in the children over 10 years of age it was either being hit by an object or via a vehicular collision at 67%.[2] At 1 year post injury, 61% of children with moderate to severe TBI still required rehabilitative services.[3] At 2 years following the injury, there was improvement in function; however the quality of life in moderately to severely injured children was still reduced when compared to their pre-injury status. For example, in the severely injured group the Pediatric Quality of Life Score (which assesses physical, emotional, social, and school functioning of children 2 years and older) was 89.6 before the injury and 68.1 at 24 months following the injury, with each 5 point decrease being clinically significant.[4] Besides preventing these injuries, the hallmark of care depends on early recognition and treatment of children with TBI. In this chapter, we present the epidemiology, pathophysiology, and rationale for various treatment modalities. In addition, clinical guidelines are reported in an algorithm format to aid the clinician caring for these critically ill children.

Clinical presentation

The clinical presentation of children with TBI can initially range from a normal neurological presentation to that of minimal to no neurological function. The initial evaluation consists of a history, set of vital signs, and physical examination. The history should include the following: mechanism of injury (height of fall, speed of impact, extraction time); presence of headache, vomiting, altered mental status (Glasgow Coma Scale score [GCS] < 15, drowsiness, irritability, amnesia, visual disturbance, loss of consciousness, confusion); and the development of seizures. Vital signs consist of a blood pressure, heart rate, respiratory rate, and oxygen saturation (SpO_2). With elevated intracranial pressure (ICP), the patient may develop Cushing's triad, which is bradycardia, hypertension, and an abnormal respiratory pattern (Cheyne–Stokes, hyperpnea, apnea). The physical examination consists of a focused neurological examination composed of an assessment for spinal cord injury (step-off between vertebrae, paralysis of an extremity, loss of rectal tone), signs of intracranial hypertension (3rd nerve impairment – dilated pupil; 6th nerve damage – loss of lateral gaze; Parinaud's syndrome – loss of upward gaze), presence of basilar skull fracture (periorbital bruising, hemotypanum, mastoid bruising, spinal fluid otorrhea and rhinorrhea), other facial/skull injuries, and the GCS.[5]

The GCS consists of the patient's best motor, eye, and verbal response (Table 35.1). The Pediatric GCS is also a 15-point scale with more developmentally appropriate responses for children under 4 years of age (Table 35.1). The Pediatric GCS performs in the same manner as the GCS. Both of these scoring systems have been used to guide therapy (GCS ≤ 8 or a declining GCS prior to transport, proceed with intubation) as well as in grading the severity of the TBI (mild: GCS 13–15 with any neurological symptoms; moderate: GCS ≤ 12 but motor response > 3; and severe: motor response ≤ 3).[3,5]

Following the initial assessment, the patient then proceeds to the appropriate neuroimaging studies, which usually consist of a noncontrast computed axial tomography scan of the head

---

Trauma Anesthesia, 2nd Edition, ed. Charles E. Smith. Published by Cambridge University Press. © Charles E. Smith, 2015.

Table 35.1 Assessing neurological function: Glasgow Coma Scale (GCS) and Pediatric GCS

Glasgow Coma Scale	Score	Pediatric Glasgow Coma Scale (children < 4 years old)	Score
Best motor response		**Best motor response**	
Follows commands	6	Moves purposefully	6
Localizes pain	5	Withdraws from touch	5
Withdraws from pain	4	Withdraws from pain	4
Flexion response to pain	3	Flexion (decorticate) to pain	3
Extension to pain	2	Extension to pain	2
No motor response	1	No motor response	1
Best verbal response		**Best verbal response**	
Orientated	5	Smiles, interacts	5
Confused conversation	4	Cries, consolable	4
Inappropriate words	3	Intermittent consolable, moans	3
Incomprehensible	2	Inconsolable, agitated	2
No verbal response	1	No verbal response	1
Best eye opening		**Best eye opening**	
Spontaneous	4	Spontaneous	4
To verbal commands	3	To verbal commands	3
To pain	2	To pain	2
No eye opening	1	No eye opening	1
Summation of all three categories			
Range	3 to 15		3 to 15

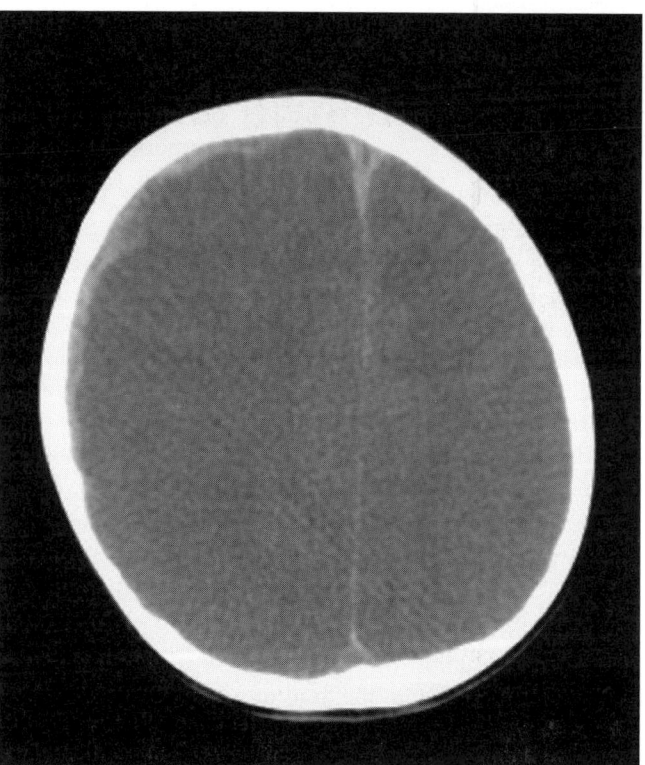

Figure 35.1 A head CT scan showing an acute right subdural hematoma and generalized cerebral edema in a 6-year-old child victim of a motor vehicle collision.

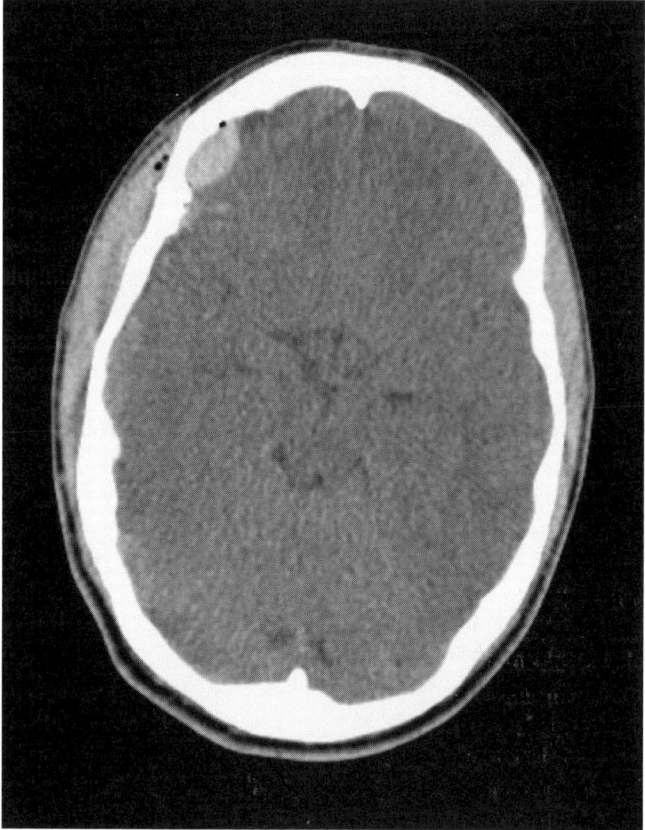

Figure 35.2 A head CT scan showing a right temporal–frontal epidural hematoma following a bike accident in an unhelmeted 14-year-old adolescent.

and possibly radiographs of the spine. The purpose of these scans is to assess the degree of cerebral edema (size of the ventricles, open cisterns), the presence of intracranial hemorrhages (cerebral contusions, subarachnoid hemorrhages, subdural hematomas, and epidural hematomas), and the magnitude of midline shifts, as well as to identify potential fractures (Figs. 35.1, 35.2).[5,6]

During the initial hours following the injury, cerebral hemorrhage and edema can increase in size, resulting in elevated ICP and worsening neurological function. To reduce potential morbidity from increased ICP, the clinician needs to follow these children closely and institute appropriate interventions to reduce the rising pressures. Through programs designed to prevent TBI (see Chapter 41) coupled with close monitoring and aggressive treatment of TBI, we hope to reduce this leading cause of morbidity and mortality that our children face.

Pathophysiology of TBI in children

The anatomy of a child's brain is different than an adult's, making it more susceptible to significant injury from rapid acceleration–deceleration as well as from rotational forces (see also Chapter 34). The damage from the initial injury may be focal or diffuse (primary injury), and it may be further compounded by a host of cellular responses leading to secondary injury (see also Chapters 20 and 21).[7–9]

Anatomical differences in a child's brain

By the age of 2 years, the intracranial volume of the toddler's brain is approximately 72% of that of an adult. Hence, a child's head comprises almost 10% of its body mass, in contrast to the adult's 2%.[2] In addition, the head of a child is supported by relatively weak neck muscles that are less able to protect the head from the rotational and deceleration forces from the initial injury. Also, in children, the periosteum of the inner table of the skull, the falx cerebri, the tentorium, and the falx cerebelli contain dural veins that are easily torn by rapid acceleration–deceleration forces. The dura in children is not affixed to the inner table of the skull, which with rapid changes in force can increase the child's risk for intracerebral hemorrhage.[2,5,10] Because of the relative lack of brain myelination in children, these axons are more susceptible to developing diffuse axonal injury, further compounding the morbidity from the initial insult.[11,12]

Primary injury

Primary injury occurs at the moment of impact. The primary injury may cause focal damage to brain tissue (i.e., hematomas, contusions, lacerations) or diffuse injury secondary to shear forces resulting in vascular injury and/or tearing of white matter fibers (i.e., axons). The primary injury is irreparable. Other than prevention, little can be done to treat the primary brain injury. Hence, the focus of treating TBIs in children is the prevention and treatment of secondary injuries (e.g., increased ICP).

Secondary injury

Secondary injury is usually delayed, peaking at 3–5 days post injury. A cascade of cytochemical reactions leads to ischemic brain injury and neuronal death (Fig. 35.3). This cascade involves increased ICP, disruption of the blood–brain barrier, cerebrovascular dysregulation, cerebral swelling, excitotoxicity, oxidative stress, inflammation, and apoptosis.

Intracranial hypertension is one of the most common causes of secondary brain injuries in children. ICP increases as the volume of the injured brain becomes larger in the confined space of rigid calvarium. The volume increase can come from the brain parenchyma (hemorrhage, cerebral volume), cerebrospinal fluid (hydrocephalus), or cerebral blood volume (vasodilatation). When intracranial hypertension compromises cerebral perfusion, there is further cellular damage resulting in worsening cerebral edema and eventual displacement and herniation of the brain. Normal ICP varies

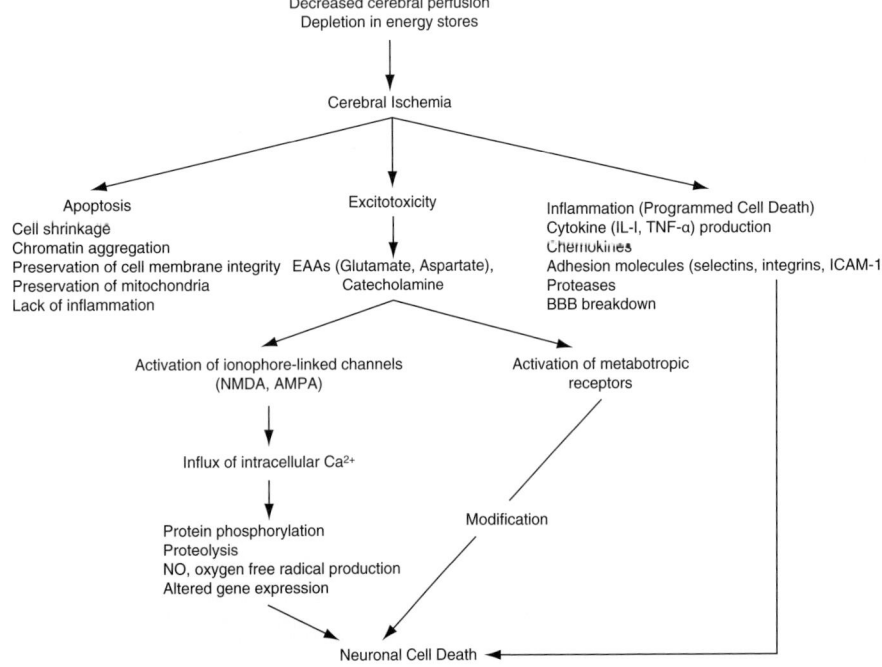

Figure 35.3 Proposed mechanisms involved in secondary damage after severe TBI in infants and children. (Reproduced from Bayir *et al.* 2003,[7] with permission.)

with age. In infants, a normal ICP is 8–10 mmHg, whereas less than 15 mmHg is considered normal for an older child. Intracranial hypertension is defined as having an ICP in excess of 20 mmHg for more than 5 minutes.[13]

Cerebral blood flow (CBF) in the uninjured brain is a highly regulated process involving a dynamic coupling of cerebral blood flow to neuronal activity.[14] In normal brain tissue, vascular tone is controlled by the release of vasodilators such as nitric oxide (NO), endothelium-derived hyperpolarization factor, and prostanoids. During injury, vasoconstriction develops secondary to decreased NO bioavailability and release of endothelin-1.[15,16] The resulting vasoconstriction may have a role in further injury of the brain by posttraumatic hypoperfusion. In children with TBI, impaired cerebral autoregulation is greatest following moderate (GCS 9–12) to severe (GCS ≤ 8) injury. The impaired cerebral autoregulation is also associated with a poorer outcome.[17]

Cerebral swelling or edema contributes to intracranial hypertension by increasing the volume of the brain parenchyma. This increased volume can then lead to secondary ischemia via compression of the vascular bed and may eventually lead to brain herniation. Cerebral swelling may be secondary to cellular swelling, blood–brain barrier injury, and/or osmolar swelling. In diffusion-weighted magnetic resonance imaging, the cerebral swelling in patients with TBI was predominantly cellular. A low apparent diffusion coefficient was noted in the brain tissue, indicating high water content.[18] Cellular swelling occurs predominantly in the astrocyte foot. Glutamate uptake, acidosis, and arachidonic acid can all lead to astrocyte swelling.[19] Disruption of the blood–brain barrier can also be a significant contributor to cerebral edema, with its disruption being maximal during the first hours following the injury.[19]

Excitotoxicity is the process in which a variety of excitatory neurotransmitters trigger a biochemical cascade leading to neuronal death (Fig. 35.4). Excitatory neurotransmitters (glutamate, aspartate, homocysteine) coupled with catecholamines (dopamine, norepinephrine) lead to the activation of ionophase-linked channels (*N*-methyl-D-aspartate or NMDA). The activation of the channels leads to the influx of sodium and calcium ions into the neurons.[20] The high intraneuronal calcium concentration activates calpains, caspases, calcineurin, NO systems, endonucleases, and phosphatases, which further injure the glia.[21] Excessive stimulation of these calcium-sensitive processes causes organelle failure and neuronal somatic cytoskeletal damage leading to neuronal death. The excitotoxicity process may be the cause of neuronal death observed in the cortical and hippocampal tissue, which, in turn, leads to the cognitive dysfunction frequently observed following closed head injuries. Further evidence supporting the role of the excitotoxicity pathway is seen in the high levels of glutamate in the spinal fluid of children with closed head injuries, with the highest values noted in abused children.[22]

Oxidative stress from mitochondrial damage can also lead to secondary neuronal injury. The mechanical stretching of neurons induces mitochondrial dysfunction with the overproduction of free radicals.[23] The reactive oxygen species and the reactive nitrogen species in isolation are insufficient to kill the neurons. When reactive oxygen species are combined with NO, the highly reactive species peroxynitrite is formed, which leads to cellular death. These data highlight the enhanced vulnerability of sublethally injured neurons to secondary excitotoxic insults. Despite the clinical and laboratory evidence demonstrating a role for oxidative stress in TBI, clinical trials with antioxidants (tirilazad, selfotel) have been unsuccessful.[24,25] Possible reasons for the failure of these studies to demonstrate an effect include the limited brain-penetrating ability of these drugs, a delay in administration, or an inability to monitor the treatment effect on oxidant stress.

The **inflammatory response** to TBI, especially in the immature brain, is a vigorous one. The release of inflammatory cytokines (interleukin 1, tumor necrosis factor alpha) by

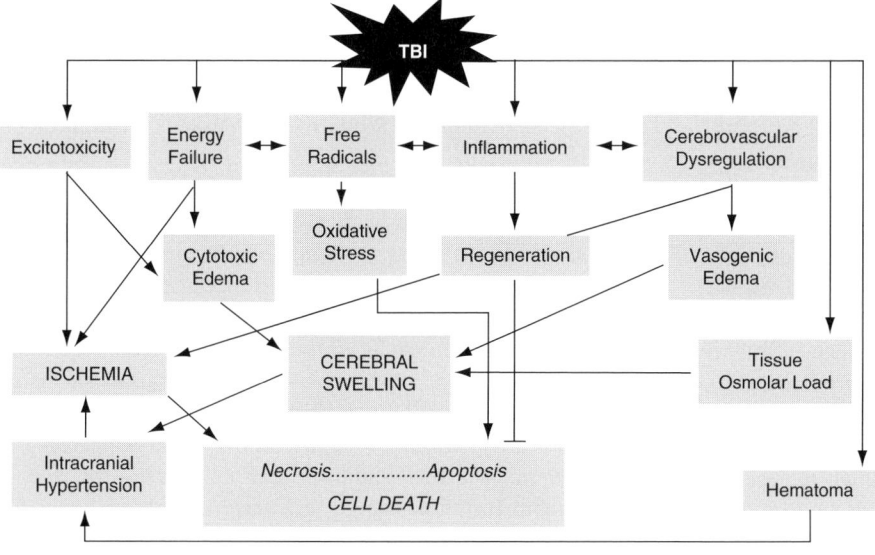

Figure 35.4 Schematic diagram representing events leading to ischemic brain injury. (Reproduced from Harukuni & Bhardwaj 2006,[8] with permission.)

ischemic neurons and by the supporting glial network leads to the generation of adhesion molecules (selectins, integrins, intracellular adhesion molecule 1). The release of the adhesion molecules results in the breakdown of the blood–brain barrier, culminating in edema formation.[26] Despite the laboratory evidence supporting the role of the inflammatory pathway in the development of cerebral edema secondary to TBI, clinical studies of anti-inflammatory agents have shown no therapeutic benefit.[27]

Apoptosis is programmed cell death. This process is an energy-dependent cascade that leads to cell shrinkage, nuclear condensation, DNA fragmentation, and formation of apoptotic bodies.[28] The two main pathways for apoptosis are the extrinsic pathway (receptor-dependent) and the intrinsic pathway (receptor-independent). Both pathways appear to play an active role in the body's response to TBI.[29]

Management of pediatric TBI

The basics of TBI treatment rely on ICP monitoring, control of ICP, and control of cerebral perfusion pressure (CPP). Unfortunately, few well-designed controlled studies have addressed the management of pediatric head trauma, but guidelines for the acute medical management of severe TBI in infants, children, and adolescents have been published.[30,31] These guidelines are based on consensus and expert opinions in the field. To maintain a low ICP and sustain an adequate CPP, several therapeutic modalities have been used including sedation, neuromuscular blockade, hyperosmolar therapy, corticosteroids, hyperventilation, hypothermia, cerebrospinal fluid (CSF) drainage, decompressive craniotomy, barbiturates, and seizure prophylaxis.

Intracranial pressure monitoring

Intracranial pressure (ICP) monitoring is appropriate in infants and children with severe TBI and GCS ≤ 8. The presence of open fontanelles and/or sutures in an infant with severe TBI does not preclude the development of intracranial hypertension or negate the utility of ICP monitoring.[32] *The goal is to maintain an ICP less than 20 mmHg*[33] *and CPP above 40–50 mmHg.*[31,34] There may be age-specific CPP thresholds, with 40 mmHg in infants, and 50 mmHg in adolescents.[31] A ventricular catheter, external strain gauge transducer, or catheter tip pressure transducer device can be used to monitor ICP. A ventriculostomy catheter device has the advantage of enabling therapeutic CSF drainage. A parenchymal catheter tip pressure transducer device can be used also to measure ICP and is advantageous when ventricular access is limited. These transducers have the potential for measurement differences and drift due to the inability to recalibrate.[35] By maintaining a low ICP coupled with an appropriate CPP, one assumes that there will be adequate oxygen delivery to the brain. Direct measurement of partial pressure of brain tissue oxygenation is feasible by brain tissue oxygen tension ($PbtO_2$) monitoring catheters. These catheters help determine the optimal CPP to maintain appropriate oxygen delivery to the brain and improve outcome, especially when it has been shown that reduced $PbtO_2$ is associated with poor outcome in pediatric severe TBI.[36] These catheters may be able to determine the optimal CPP for maintaining appropriate oxygen delivery to the brain and thus serve as a guide for supporting therapies.

The role of sedation and neuromuscular blockade

In experimental studies, pain and stress have been shown to increase cerebral metabolic rate, resulting in higher ICP.[37,38] Multiple studies have shown a direct relationship between noxious stimuli such as suctioning and increases in ICP.[39–41] Therefore, analgesia and sedation have an important role in the management of TBI. Sedatives and analgesics are also necessary to manage patients who are mechanically ventilated. Other benefits of sedatives include anticonvulsant and anti-emetic actions, prevention of shivering, and mitigation of the long-term psychological trauma of pain and stress.[42] The ideal sedative for patients with severe TBI is one that is rapid in onset and offset, is easily titrated to effect, has well-defined metabolism, neither accumulates nor has active metabolites, exhibits anticonvulsant actions, has no adverse cardiovascular or immune actions, and lacks drug–drug interactions, while preserving the neurologic examination.[43] Unfortunately, there is no ideal sedative or analgesic for patients with TBI. Agents used for sedation in TBI include lorazepam, midazolam, and thiopental, while analgesics include fentanyl and morphine. Premedication with lidocaine has been advocated before endotracheal tube suctioning to prevent a rise in ICP.

Few studies have addressed the role of analgesia and sedation in pediatric patients with severe TBI. In a case report, an increase in ICP was seen in an 11-year-old child with severe TBI following an infusion of 5 µg/kg of fentanyl.[44] In another study of 10 patients with severe TBI, including three adolescents, sufentanil (1 µg/kg over 6 minutes, followed by an infusion of 0.005 µg/kg/min) was associated with a significant increase in ICP (9 ± 7 mmHg) accompanied by a 24% decrease in mean arterial pressure and thus a 38% decrease in CPP. Therefore, caution should be exercised in the administration of a sufentanil bolus to patients with increased ICP.[45] However, pain can increase cerebral metabolic demands, arterial blood pressure, and CBF with subsequent increase in ICP in severe TBI. The use of analgesics remains essential in patients with multiple traumatic injuries.

The use of sedation is necessary to treat patients with severe TBI who are tracheally intubated and mechanically ventilated. In a study of eight patients (including one adolescent) with severe TBI, diazepam reduced the cerebral metabolic rate and CBF by approximately 25%, each without significant alteration of the blood pressure.[46] In another study of 12 patients (17–44 years old) the infusion of midazolam induced a decrease in mean arterial pressure and CPP and an increase in ICP in patients with ICP < 18 mmHg. However, in patients with ICP ≥ 18 mmHg, midazolam induced a slight decrease in ICP.[47]

Therefore, close monitoring of blood pressure, ICP, and CPP should be exercised when using these agents. Propofol has been used for sedation and control of ICP in head-injured patients.[48,49] However, deterioration in cerebrovascular pressure autoregulation with rapid propofol infusion rates may occur after head injury. Therefore, large propofol doses may increase the injured brain's vulnerability to secondary insults.[50] Several reports have also suggested that administration of propofol by continuous infusion is associated with an unexplained increased risk of mortality and severe metabolic acidosis in children.[51–55] Therefore, continuous infusion of propofol for either sedation or the management of refractory intracranial hypertension in infants and children with severe TBI is not recommended.[31] Etomidate at a single dose (0.3 mg/kg/dose) may be considered to control severe intracranial hypertension; however, the risk of adrenal suppression must be taken in consideration when using such medication.[31]

Neuromuscular blockade has been used to reduce ICP by reduction of intrathoracic pressures, thereby improving cerebral venous outflow. Neuromuscular blocking agents can also prevent shivering, posturing, and ventilator asynchrony.[56] In a prospective study of 20 patients (1–15 years old, six of whom had severe TBI) Vernon and Witte showed a small reduction of oxygen consumption and energy expenditure in critically ill children who were sedated and mechanically ventilated.[57] However, neuromuscular blockade is associated with multiple risks, including an increased risk of nosocomial pneumonia and myopathy. In addition, neuromuscular blockade has been associated with an increased intensive care unit (ICU) length of stay and will mask seizure activities.[56,58–60] *The use of neuromuscular blockade should be reserved to specific indications such as increased ICP with shivering, intracranial hypertension, and prevention of movement during patient transport.*[42] In the management of TBI, it is important to maintain adequate sedation and analgesia. Regardless of which agent is used, the patient must be monitored for drug-related side effects (Table 35.2).

The role of hyperosmolar therapy

Mannitol and hypertonic saline have been used as hyperosmolar agents to control intracranial hypertension. Mannitol reduces ICP by two different mechanisms. The first mechanism decreases blood viscosity, which in turn lowers cerebral vascular diameters. The reduced blood viscosity enhances blood flow through the cerebral vasculature. With an intact viscosity autoregulation reflex, as the viscosity decreases, the cerebral vasculature constricts, thus maintaining appropriate CBF while reducing cerebral blood volume. Viscosity autoregulation is a mechanism whereby a decrease in resistance to flow from the decreased blood viscosity is balanced by increased resistance from vasoconstriction, so that CBF remains the same. When autoregulation is impaired, CBF increases with a lower viscosity without the compensatory vasoconstriction.[62–65] The impairment of the viscosity autoregulation reflex seen in TBI has led some authorities to caution

Table 35.2 Dosage and side effects of commonly used sedatives and analgesics in traumatic brain injury. Information from Taketomo et al. 2003–04.[111]

	Dosage	Side effects
Sedatives		
Midazolam	Loading dose (0.01–0.05 mg/kg) Continuous infusion (0.02–0.1 mg/kg/h)	Cardiovascular depression
Lorazepam	0.05 mg/kg per dose (repeat every 4–6 h)	Cardiovascular depression Metabolic acidosis Liver function test abnormalities
Thiopental	1–5 mg/kg per dose (repeat as needed)	Cardiovascular depression
Analgesics		
Fentanyl	Loading dose (1–2 µg/kg) Continuous infusion (1–3 µg/kg/h)	Chest wall rigidity Dependence May increase intracranial pressure
Morphine	Intermittent dose (0.1–0.2 mg/kg per dose, may repeat every 2–4 h) Continuous infusion (0.01–0.04 mg/kg/h)	Cardiovascular depression

against the use of mannitol in TBI.[66,67] The effect of mannitol administration on blood viscosity is rapid but transient (< 75 minutes). The second mechanism for mannitol to reduce ICP is by an osmotic effect. The osmotic effect gradually shifts fluids from the interstitial space into the intravascular space. The osmotic effect of mannitol has a slower onset of action (15–30 minutes), lasts longer (6 hours), and requires an intact blood–brain barrier.[68,69] The effective bolus doses of mannitol to control increased ICP after TBI range from 0.25 to 1 g/kg of body weight. Euvolemia should be maintained by fluid replacement. A urinary catheter is recommended to avoid bladder distension and rupture. Serum osmolarity should be maintained below 320 mOsm/L.

Hypertonic saline is another hyperosmolar agent that has been used to decrease ICP. Hypertonic saline has an osmotic effect on the brain because of its high tonicity and ability to effectively remain outside the blood–brain barrier. In animal models the maximum benefit is observed with focal injury associated with vasogenic edema. The ICP reduction is seen for 2 hours or less and may be maintained for longer periods by using a continuous infusion of hypertonic saline. ICP reduction is thought to be caused by a reduction in water content in areas of the brain with an intact blood–brain barrier, such as the noninjured hemisphere and cerebellum. Other systemic effects seen with hypertonic saline include transient volume expansion, natriuresis, hemodilution, immunomodulation, and improved pulmonary gas exchange. Potential adverse effects with hypertonic saline include electrolyte abnormalities, cardiac failure, bleeding diathesis, phlebitis, central pontine myelinolysis, and rebound intracranial hypertension with uncontrolled administration.[70] A continuous infusion of 3% saline (ranging between 0.1 and 1.0 mL/kg/h) administered on a sliding scale (minimum dose needed to maintain ICP < 20 mmHg) is effective in controlling increased ICP. A serum osmolarity of 360 mOsm/L appears to be tolerated with hypertonic saline, even when used in combination with mannitol.[71,72] Khanna et al. showed a significant decrease in ICP and an increase in CPP with a continuous infusion of 3% saline in 10 children who failed conventional therapy to control their intracranial hypertension.[71] The 3% saline was administered via a sliding scale to achieve a target serum sodium level that would maintain an ICP at less than 20 mmHg. In their study, the mean duration of 3% saline infusion was 7.6 days (range 4–18 days). The highest serum sodium, serum osmolarity, and serum creatinine for their patients were 170 mEq/L (range 157–187 mEq/L), 364 mosm/L (range 330–431 mosm/L), and 1.3 mg/dL (range 0.4–5.0 mg/dL), respectively. In a double-blind crossover study in 18 children with TBI, Fisher et al. have shown that 3% saline at 6.5–10 mL/kg/dose significantly reduces ICP in comparison to normal saline.[73]

The role of corticosteroids

Steroids have been used in adults and children in an attempt to reduce edema in TBI. However, in a multicenter randomized controlled trial involving 10,008 adult patients (the CRASH trial), the use of steroids was associated with a higher risk of death within 2 weeks following enrollment (1052 [21.1%] vs. 893 [17.9%] deaths; relative risk 1.18, 95% CI 1.09–1.27, p < 0.0001).[74] At 6 months following enrollment, there was a higher risk of death or severe disability in the corticosteroid group than in the placebo group (death 1248 [25.7%] vs. 1075 [22.3%], relative risk 1.15, 95% CI 1.07–1.24, p < 0.0001; death or severe disability 1828 [38.1%] vs. 1728 [36.3%], relative risk 1.05, 95% CI 0.99–1.10, p = 0.079).[75] Therefore, steroids are not recommended in TBI.

The role of hyperventilation

Hyperventilation is a well-known cause of cerebral vasoconstriction causing a reduction in CBF and a decrease in ICP in the healthy brain. There is an approximately 3% reduction in global CBF for every 1 mmHg decrease in the $PaCO_2$. However, following severe TBI, global CBF is reduced by approximately 50% early after the injury, resulting in global and regional CBF levels that are near the ischemic threshold in adults.[76] Therefore, excessive hyperventilation in the face of critically low baseline CBF could cause cerebral ischemia or worsen preexisting cerebral ischemia.[77] In a study of 12 patients with head trauma (including three children, 1 month to 8 years old), Stringer et al. showed that hyperventilation-induced ischemia affects CBF in both injured and apparently intact brain tissues.[78] Skippen et al. also

showed that hypocapnia ($PaCO_2$ < 25 mmHg) was associated with more cerebral ischemic regions than normocapnia in a prospective study of 23 children with severe TBI who underwent CBF measurements at different $PaCO_2$.[79] In a retrospective cohort study, Curry et al. showed that severe hypocarbia independently predicted mortality in children with severe TBI.[80] Therefore, excessive hyperventilation should not be used routinely in children with TBI. As well, mild or prophylactic hyperventilation ($PaCO_2$ < 35 mmHg) should be avoided for the acute management of severe TBI in infants, children, and adolescents.[81] Mild hyperventilation ($PaCO_2$ 30–35 mmHg), however, may be considered for refractory intracranial hypertension. In these situations, monitoring CBF, jugular venous oxygen saturation, or brain tissue oxygen may be helpful in identifying cerebral ischemia when hyperventilation is considered.

The role of hypothermia

In ischemic stroke and TBI, hyperthermia (temperature > 38.5 °C) can be deleterious to the injured and noninjured brain. It has been shown in experimental models that hyperthermia enhances the release of neurotransmitters, exaggerates oxygen radical production, enhances blood–brain barrier breakdown, impairs recovery of energy metabolism, increases inhibition of protein kinases, and worsens cytoskeletal proteolysis.[82] However, hypothermia preserves the blood–brain barrier and reduces cerebral ischemia, edema, and tissue injury.[83–87] In a randomized controlled trial comparing the effect of moderate hypothermia (patients cooled to 33 °C at a mean of 10 hours after injury, and kept at 32–33 °C for 24 hours) and normothermia in 82 adult patients with severe closed head injuries, hypothermia did not improve the outcomes in patients with a GCS of 3 or 4 on admission. However, among patients with GCS of 5–7, hypothermia was associated with significantly improved GCS at 3 and 6 months but not at 12 months following the TBI.[88] In another randomized controlled multicenter trial of 392 patients (16–65 years of age with acute brain injury), hypothermia (temperature reaching 33 °C within 8 hours after injury and maintained for 48 hours) was not effective in improving outcomes 6 months following brain injury. However, fewer patients in the hypothermia group had high ICP than in the normothermia group.[89]

Hypothermia has not been extensively studied in children with TBI. In a study of 21 children, 48 hours of moderate hypothermia (32–34 °C) initiated within 6 hours of acute TBI was found to decrease the severity of intracranial hypertension and was safely tolerated.[90] In another randomized controlled trial, Adelson et al. studied the effect of moderate hypothermia (32–33 °C within 6 hours of injury and maintained for 48 hours) compared with normothermia (36.5–37.5 °C) in severe TBI in children younger than 13 years.[91] Forty-eight children were randomized, and an additional 27 patients were entered into a parallel single-institution trial of excluded patients. Moderate hypothermia was found to be safe in children of all ages and in children with delay of initiation of treatment up to

24 hours. Although hypothermia was associated with decreased mortality and lower ICP during the first 72 hours of injury, it was associated with an increased potential for arrhythmias and rebound ICP elevations (for up to 10–12 hours) after rewarming.[91] In another multicenter randomized controlled study, early hypothermia (32.5 ± 0.5 °C), initiated within 8 hours following TBI and continued for 24 hours, was associated with a trend toward an increase in mortality in 225 children with severe TBI.[92] Overall, there was 21% (23/108) death in the hypothermic group versus 12% (14/117) death in the normothermic group (*p* = 0.06). There was more hemodynamic instability, including hypotension and use of vasoactive agents, in the hypothermic group during the rewarming period than in the normothermic group. *Therefore, moderate hypothermia may be considered in refractory intracranial hypertension, but special attention should be given to the possibility of hemodynamic instability during rewarming, cardiac arrhythmias, and rebound intracranial hypertension after rewarming.*

The role of cerebrospinal fluid (CSF) drainage and decompressive craniectomy

Intraventricular catheter placement, or ventriculostomy, can be beneficial in children with severe TBI. A ventriculostomy allows diagnostic measurement of ICP and therapeutic drainage of CSF. The drainage of CSF reduces intracranial fluid volume and therefore lowers ICP.

Decompressive craniectomy (Fig. 35.5) has been shown to improve cerebral oxygenation[93] and cerebral blood flow velocity[94] in adult patients with cerebral edema. Few studies have been reported on the benefits of surgical decompression versus medical management in children with severe TBI. A case–control study of 35 pediatric and adult patients with malignant posttraumatic cerebral edema showed that bifrontal decompressive craniectomy had an advantage over medical management.[95] The advantage of the surgical decompression was mainly seen in young patients, in patients who underwent surgical decompression within 48 hours following their injury,

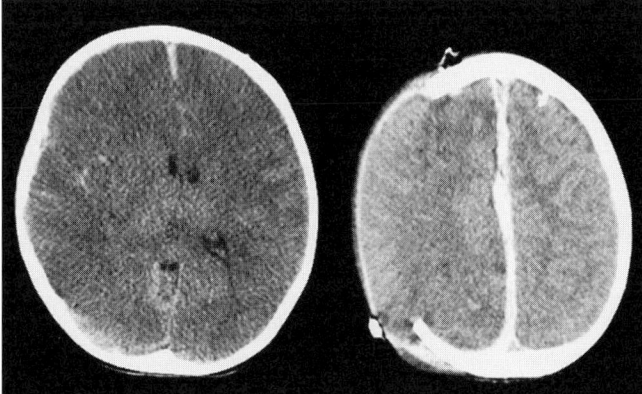

Figure 35.5 Head CT scans of a 6-year-old child victim of a car accident with a cerebral edema and midline shift (*left*) and post hemicraniectomy (*right*). Notice the herniation of the brain through the right hemicraniectomy and the development of an interhemispheric subdural hematoma.

and in patients who did not exhibit a sustained ICP greater than 40 mmHg. In another study of 27 children with TBI, 54% of children who had a bitemporal decompressive craniectomy within 24 hours of their injury were normal or had a mild disability 6 months following their injury, compared with only 14% of children in the control group.[96] A study of 23 children younger than 2 years of age with acute shaken-impact baby syndrome showed that decompressive craniectomy reduced mortality and hearing impairment in surgically treated children.[97] Patients with ICP less than 30 mmHg benefited most from the surgery. In a study of 18 children with TBI, decompressive craniectomy for diffuse brain edema was shown to improve ICP and brain oxygenation without increasing disability in survivors.[98] In another study of 23 children, decompressive craniectomy was effective in reducing ICP and was associated with good outcomes in surviving patients.[99] In a long-term follow-up study, decompressive craniectomy in 14 children with severe TBI resulted in a comparable outcome to 39 children with less severe TBI who did not have a craniectomy as part of their management.[100] Decompressive craniectomy may be indicated in patients with TBI who have early signs of neurologic deterioration or herniation or who have increased ICP refractory to medical management.[31] *Decompressive craniectomy is not indicated in children with irreversible brain damage.*

The role of barbiturate-induced coma

Barbiturates reduce ICP by suppressing cerebral metabolism and metabolic demands, leading to a decrease in cerebral blood volume and ICP. However, barbiturates also reduce blood pressure and therefore may adversely decrease CPP.[101] Eisenberg *et al.* showed that high-dose pentobarbital controlled ICP better than conventional therapy in 73 patients (15–59 years old) with severe head injury and intractable intracranial hypertension.[102] Hypotension was the major cardiovascular complication seen with barbiturate use in the study. A retrospective review of 25 children with severe TBI showed that high-dose barbiturates were associated with hypotension, cardiovascular depression, and arrhythmias.[103] In a study of 67 adult patients with severe head injury and refractory intracranial hypertension, Cormio *et al.* showed that, following a loading dose of pentobarbital, there was an ICP decrease of 12 mmHg and a mean arterial pressure decrease of 9 mmHg.[104] CPP, however, was unchanged. CBF, cerebral oxygen consumption, and arteriovenous oxygen difference also decreased following the loading dose of pentobarbital, by 20%, 31%, and 11%, respectively. In their study 45% of their patients had a good response (with a reduction in ICP from 34 ± 9 to 15 ± 5 mmHg) and 40% had a partial response (with a decrease in ICP that remained > 20 mmHg) after the initial loading dose of pentobarbital. Responders to pentobarbital had a better outcome than nonresponders. In comparison with nonresponders, responders to pentobarbital had cerebral oxygen consumption and arteriovenous oxygen differences that were greater prior to the barbiturate therapy and decreased more following the loading dose. *Therefore, barbiturate coma can be a useful treatment to reduce ICP in selected patients who do not have an overwhelmingly severe TBI with markedly reduced cerebral oxygen consumption.* The recommended dosage of pentobarbital is 10–15 mg/kg over 1–2 hours as a loading dose followed by a continuous infusion of 1 mg/kg/h, which may be increased to 5 mg/kg/h as a maintenance dose.[102] Dosage should be titrated to reach a burst suppression pattern on the electroencephalogram. In addition, patients should be hemodynamically monitored to maintain adequate systemic blood pressure and CPP.

The role of seizure prophylaxis

Seizure activity in the early posttraumatic period following head injury may cause secondary brain damage as a result of increased metabolic demands, raised ICP, and excess neurotransmitter release.[105] In an observational study of 477 children with head trauma, of whom 128 had severe TBI, the use of seizure medications was associated with a reduced mortality risk (odds ratio = 0.17, 95% CI = 0.04–0.70, p = 0.014).[106] However, in another prospective randomized trial of 102 children with moderate to severe head injury, phenytoin prophylaxis did not substantially reduce early posttraumatic seizures

(within 48 hours after injury) or survival and neurologic outcome 30 days after injury.[107] In a review of multiple studies, prophylactic antiseizure therapy was shown to reduce early seizures without reducing the occurrence of late seizures or having any effect on death or neurological disability;[105] and since young children (< 7 years of age) are more prone to early seizure,[108] *prophylactic antiseizure therapy might have a role in reducing the incidence of early posttraumatic seizures in children with severe TBI.* A note of caution with IV phenytoin must be made. If given too rapidly, IV phenytoin has been associated with severe hypotension and cardiac arrest. The drug should be administered at a rate not exceeding 1–3 mg/kg/minute, or 50 mg/minute, whichever is slower.

The role of head positioning

An improvement of ICP has been documented with head elevation at 30 degrees in patients with severe head injury. In a study of 38 patients with severe closed head injury, Ng *et al.* showed a significant decrease in ICP without a significant change in mean arterial pressure, CPP, global venous cerebral oxygenation, or regional cerebral oxygenation.[109] Hence, head elevation within 24 hours following TBI reduces ICP without concomitant alteration in cerebral oxygenation. In another

Table 35.3 Suggested guidelines for ICU management of patients with TBI

Central nervous system	1. Serial neurologic exams (in the absence of ICP monitoring and GCS > 8) 2. Head elevated at 30 degrees and in midline position 3. Sedation and pain control. Neuromuscular blockade if shivering and increased ICP 4. Maintain ICP < 20 and CPP 40–65 mmHg 5. Mannitol and saline 3% therapies
Respiratory system	1. Ventilator support (tidal volume, 6–8 mL/kg) 2. Titrate ventilator setting to maintain adequate oxygenation (pulse oximetry > 94%) and ventilation (PaCO$_2$ 35–40) 3. Serial arterial blood gazes (arterial line)
Cardiovascular system	1. Invasive hemodynamic monitoring (arterial line) 2. Central venous pressure (CVP) monitoring (central line) 3. Fluid resuscitation to maintain adequate CVP (5–10) 4. Pressors (such as phenylephrine) to sustain an adequate mean arterial blood pressure to support a CPP between 40 and 60 mmHg. 5. Inotropic support (such as Dopamine or epinephrine if signs of myocardial depression)
Gastrointestinal system/fluids and electrolytes	1. On admission keep patient NPO on isotonic solution (normal saline or Ringer's lactate) 2. Monitor patient's electrolytes and serum osmolarity (goal 300–320 mOsm/L) 3. Stress ulcer prophylaxis (H$_2$ blockers or proton pump inhibitors). 4. Resume feeds within 48 hours of the injury and advance as tolerated. 5. Serum glucose monitoring (goal of euglycemia. Consider continuous insulin infusion if hyperglycemia)
Renal system	1. Close monitoring of the urinary output (Foley catheter in place). 2. Monitor urine electrolytes and osmolarity if suspicious of diabetes insipidus, syndrome of inappropriate antidiuretic hormone secretion, or cerebral salt-wasting syndrome.
Hematology system	1. Monitoring of patient's hematocrit and coagulation 2. Correct coagulopathy (fresh frozen plasma, platelets, vitamin K, and factor VII)
Infectious disease	1. Temperature monitoring. Cooling blanket to maintain moderate hypothermia – normothermia (at 35–37 °C) 2. Daily surveillance cultures if patient on cooling blanket

CPP, cerebral perfusion pressure; GCS, Glasgow Coma Scale; ICP, intracranial pressure; ICU, intensive care unit; TBI, traumatic brain injury.

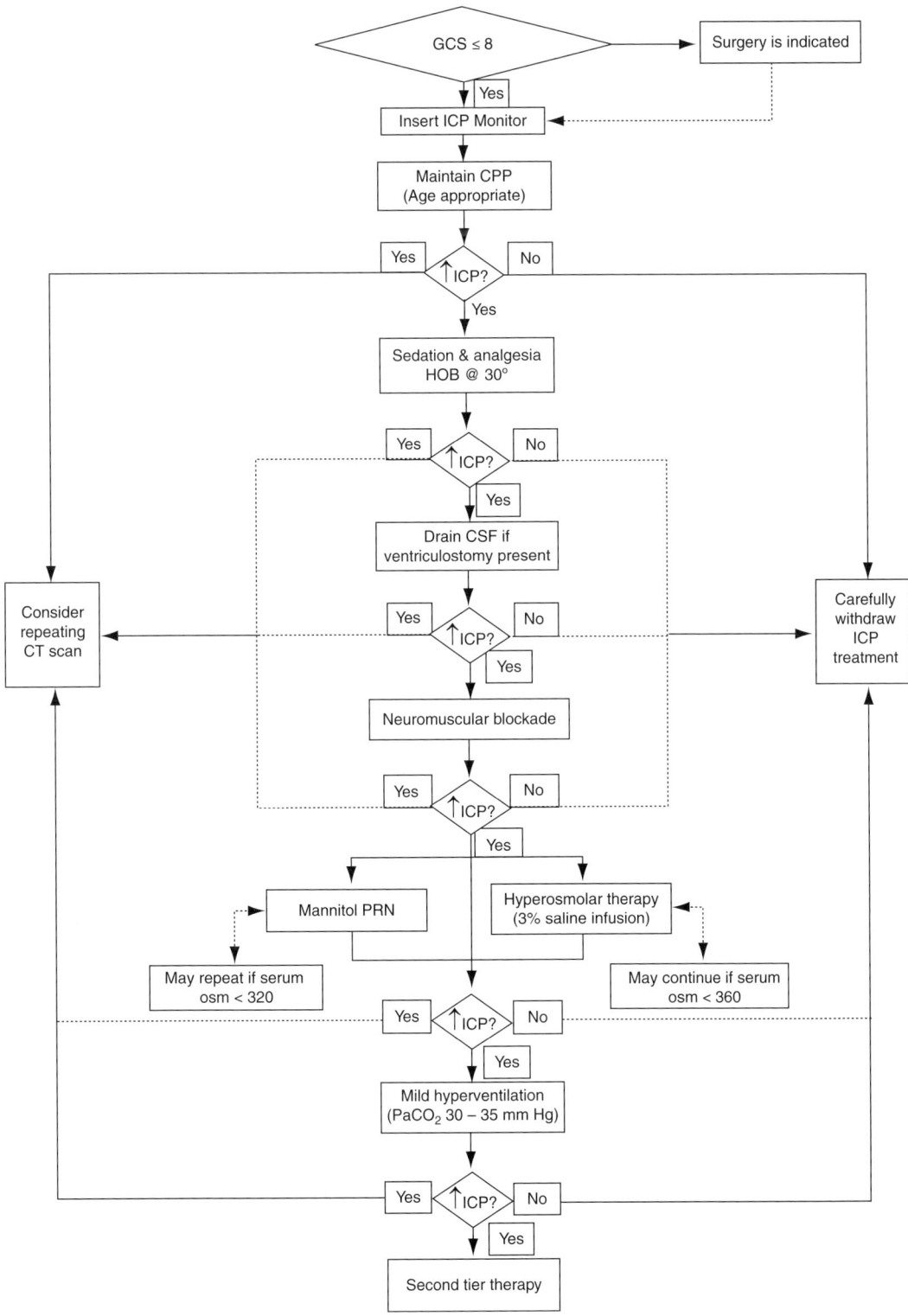

Figure 35.6 First-tier therapy of traumatic brain injury in children. CPP, cerebral perfusion pressure; CSF, cerebrospinal fluid; CT, computed tomography; GCS, Glasgow Coma Scale; HOB, head of bed; ICP, intracranial pressure; PRN, as needed. (Reproduced from Adelson 2003,[111] with permission.)

study of 22 patients with severe head injury, 30 degrees versus 0 degrees head elevation also significantly reduced ICP without reducing CPP, CBF, cerebral metabolic rate of oxygen, arteriovenous difference of lactate, or cerebrovascular resistance.[110] Therefore, elevation of the head of the bed to 30 degrees will improve ICP without compromising cerebral oxygenation. In addition, the head should be maintained in the midline position to avoid jugular compression, which may impair cerebral vascular drainage. Spinal precautions should be maintained until the cervical, thoracic, and lumbar spines can be cleared.

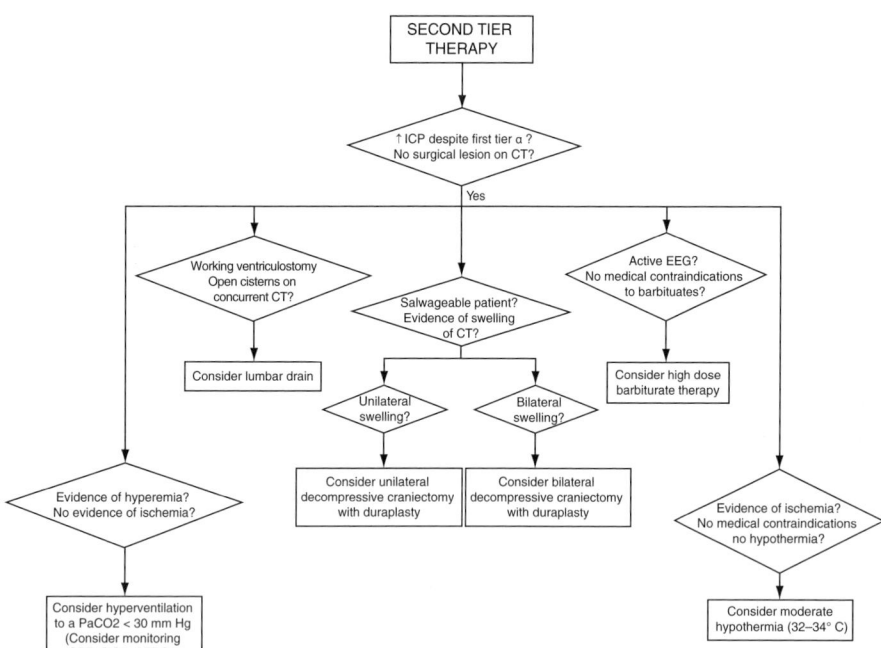

Figure 35.7 Second-tier therapy of traumatic brain injury in children. AJDO₂, arterial-jugular venous difference in oxygen content; CBF, cerebral blood flow; CT, computed tomography; EEG, electroencephalogram; ICP, intracranial pressure; SjO₂, jugular venous oxygen saturation. (Reproduced from Adelson 2003,[111] with permission.)

The role of other therapeutic modalities

Stress ulcer prophylaxis, adequate nutrition, and control of hyperglycemia are essential components of the management of high-risk, critically ill patients with severe TBI (Table 35.3).

A treatment algorithm for established intracranial hypertension in pediatric TBI, developed by an expert panel, might be used as a guideline to direct clinicians caring for children with severe TBI (Figs. 35.6, 35.7).[111]

Summary

Severe TBI is a leading cause of mortality and morbidity in children. The GCS is the landmark scoring system that is used to assess the severity of injury and to guide therapy. The anatomy of a child's brain is different than an adult's, making it more susceptible to injuries related to rapid acceleration–deceleration mechanisms. The brain damage could be primary, from the initial injury, or secondary, following a host of cellular responses and inflammation. The treatment of TBI relies on ICP monitoring, control of ICP, and control of CPP. Several therapeutic modalities have been used to lower the ICP and sustain an adequate CPP, including sedation, neuromuscular blockade, barbiturates and seizure prophylaxis, hyperosmolar therapy, hypothermia, CSF drainage, and decompressive craniotomy. Unfortunately, few well-designed controlled studies have addressed the management of pediatric TBI, and most of the current therapeutic modalities rely on consensus and expert opinion.

Questions

(1) A child presents to the emergency room unresponsive. With noxious stimulation his only response is decerebrate posturing. His Glasgow Coma Scale (GCS) score is:
   a. 3
   b. 4
   c. 6
   d. 8

(2) An indication to intubate a child's trachea (to protect his airways) who presents with a traumatic brain injury is:
   a. GCS ≤ 14
   b. GCS ≤ 12
   c. GCS ≤ 10
   d. GCS ≤ 8

(3) Secondary brain injury seen in children with traumatic brain injury is associated with all of the following, *except*:
   a. Disruption of the blood–brain barrier
   b. Cerebrovascular dysregulation
   c. It peaks at 24 hours post injury
   d. Oxidative stress, inflammation, and apoptosis

(4) Intracranial pressure monitoring is indicated in a child with:
   a. GCS ≤ 14
   b. GCS ≤ 12
   c. GCS ≤ 10
   d. GCS ≤ 8

(5) In traumatic brain injury in children the goal is to maintain the intracranial pressure (ICP) and cerebral perfusion pressure (CPP) at:
   a. ICP < 30 and CPP > 60
   b. ICP < 20 and CPP > 40
   c. ICP < 15 and CPP > 60
   d. ICP < 20 and CPP > 80

(6) How does mannitol reduce intracranial hypertension?

    a. By reducing the intravascular volume secondary to its diuretic effect

    b. By increasing blood viscosity and increasing serum osmolality

    c. By reducing blood viscosity and shifting fluid from the interstitial space into the intravascular space

    d. By reducing blood viscosity and shifting fluid from the intravascular space into the interstitial space

(7) In traumatic brain injury:

    a. Steroids significantly decrease cerebral edema

    b. Saline 3% solution increases cerebral edema

    c. Saline 3% solution decreases cerebral edema

    d. Steroids are indicated in adults but not in children with traumatic brain injury

(8) Hyperventilation:

    a. Decreases cerebral perfusion

    b. Increases cerebral perfusion

    c. Has no effect on cerebral blood flow in children with traumatic brain injury

    d. Increases cerebral blood volume

(9) In children with severe traumatic brain injury, which of the following is contraindicated as a continuous infusion for long-term sedation?

    a. Midazolam

    b. Phenobarbital

    c. Propofol

    d. Lorazepam

(10) The use of a continuous infusion of propofol for sedation in TBI may be associated with all of the following, *except*:

    a. Hyperlipidemia

    b. Metabolic acidosis

    c. Hyperglycemia

    d. Discoloration of urine

Answers

(1) b
(2) d
(3) c
(4) d
(5) b
(6) c
(7) c
(8) a
(9) c
(10) c

References

1. Hamilton BE, Hoyert DL, Martin JA, Strobino DM, Guyer B. Annual summary of vital statistics: 2010–2011. *Pediatrics* 2013; **131**: 548–58.

2. Koespell TD, Rivara FP, Vavilala MS, *et al.* Incidence and descriptive of epidemiologic features of traumatic brain injury in King County, Washington. *Pediatrics* 2011; **128**: 946–54.

3. Rivara FP, Koepsell TD, Wang J, *et al.* Incidence of disability among children 12 months after traumatic brain injury. *Am J Public Health*. 2012; **102**: 2074–9.

4. Rivara FP, Koepsell TD, Wang J, *et al.* Disability 3, 12, and 24 months after traumatic brain injury among children and adolescents. *Pediatrics* 2011; **128**: e1129–38.

5. Thiessen ML, Woolridge DP. Pediatric minor closed head injury. *Pediatr Clin N Am* 2006; **53**: 1–26.

6. Stocchetti N, Conte V, Ghisoni L, Canavesi K, Zanaboni C. Traumatic brain injury in pediatric patients. *Minerva Anestesiol.* 2010; **76**: 1052–9.

7. Bayir H, Kochanek PM, Clark RS. Traumatic brain injury in infants and children: mechanisms of secondary damage and treatment in the intensive care unit (Review). *Crit Care Clin* 2003; **19**: 529–49.

8. Harukuni I, Bhardwaj A. Mechanisms of brain injury after global cerebral ischemia (Review). *Neurol Clin* 2006; **24**: 1–21.

9. Okonkwo DO, Stone JR. Basic science of closed head injuries and spinal cord injuries (Review). *Clin Sports Med.* 2003; **22**: 467–81.

10. Schutzman SA, Barnes P, Duhaime AC, *et al.* Evaluation and management of children young than two years old with apparently minor head trauma: Proposed guidelines (Review). *Pediatrics* 2001; **107**: 983–93.

11. Bruce DA, Schut L, Bruno LA, Wood JH, Sutton LN. Outcome following severe head injuries in children. *J Neurosurg* 1978; **48**: 679–88.

12. Strich SJ. Lesions in the cerebral hemispheres after blunt head injury. *J Clin Pathol Suppl (R Coll Pathol)* 1970; **4**: 166–71.

13. James HE. Pediatric head injury: What is unique and different? *Acta Neurchir (Wien)* 1999; **739**: 85–8.

14. Koehler RC, Gebremedhin D, Harder DR. Regulation of the cerebral circulation: Role of astrocyles in cerebrovascular regulation. *J Appl Physiol* 2006; **100**: 307–17.

15. Andresen J, Shafi NI, Bryan RM. Endothelial influences on cerebrovascular tone. *J Appl Physiol* 2006; **100**: 318–27.

16. Armstead WM. Role of nitric oxide, cyclic nucleotides, and the activation of ATP-sensitive K+ channels in the contribution of adenosine to hypoxia-induced pial artery dilation. *J Cereb Blood Flow Metab* 1997; **17**: 100–8.

17. Vavilala MS, Lee LA, Boddu K, *et al.* Cerebral autoregulation in pediatric traumatic brain injury. *Pediatr Crit Care Med* 2004; **5**: 257–63.

18. Marmarou A, Signoretti S, Fatouros PP, *et al.* Predominance of cellular edema in traumatic brain swelling in patients with severe head injuries. *J Neurosurg* 2006; **104**: 720–30.

19. Kimelberg HK. Astrocytic swelling in cerebral ischemia as a possible cause of injury and target for therapy (Review). *Glia* 2005; **50**: 389–97.

20. Faden AI, Demediuk P, Panter SS, Vink R. The role of excitatory amino acids and NMDA receptors in traumatic brain injury. *Science* 1989; **244**: 798–800.

21. Tymianski M, Tator CH. Normal and abnormal calcium homeostatis in neurons: a basis for the pathophysiology of traumatic and ischemic central nervous system injury (Review). *Neurosurgery* 1996; **38**: 1176–95.

22. Ruppel RA, Kochanek PM, Adelson PD, *et al.* Excitatory amino acid concentrations in ventricular cerebrospinal fluid after severe traumatic brain injury in infants and children: the role of child abuse. *J Pediatr* 2001; **138**: 18–25.

23. Arundine M, Aarts M, Lau A, Tymianski M. Vulnerability of central neurons to secondary insults after in vitro mechanical stretch. *J Neurosci* 2004; **24**: 8106–23.

24. Marshall LF, Maas AI, Marshall SB, *et al.* Multicenter trial on the efficacy of using tirilazad mesylate in cases of head injury. *J Neurosurg* 1998; **89**: 519–25.

25. Morris GF, Juul N, Marshall SB, Benedict B, Marshall LF. Neurological deterioration as a potential alternative endpoint in human clinical trials of experimental pharmacological agents for treatment of severe traumatic brain injuries. Executive Committee of the International Selfotel Trial. *Neurosurgery* 1998; **43**: 1369–72.

26. Danton GH, Dietrich WD. Inflammatory mechanisms after ischemia and stroke (Review). *J Neuropathol Exp Neurol* 2003; **62**: 127–36.

27. Marklund N, Bakshi A, Castelbuono DJ, Conte V, McIntosh TK. Evaluation of pharmacological treatment strategies in traumatic brain injury (review). *Curr Pharm Des* 2006; **12**: 1645–80.

28. Kerr JF. History of the events leading to the formulation of the apoptosis concept (review). *Toxicology* 2002; **181–82**: 471–4.

29. Serbest G, Horwitz J, Jost M, Barbee K. Cell death and neuro-protection by poloxamer 188 after mechanical trauma. *FASEB J* 2006; **20**: 308–10.

30. Adelson PD. Guidelines for the acute medical management of severe traumatic brain injury in infants, children, and adolescents. *Crit Care Med* 2003; **31** (6 Suppl): S417–91.

31. Kochanek PM, Carney N, Adelson PD, *et al.* Guidelines for the acute medical management of severe traumatic brain injury in infants, children, and adolescents-second edition. *Pediatr Crit Care Med.* 2012; **13** (Suppl 1): S1–82.

32. Adelson PD. Guidelines for the acute medical management of severe traumatic brain injury in infants, children, and adolescents. Chapter 5. Indications for intracranial pressure monitoring in pediatric patients with severe traumatic brain injury. *Pediatr Crit Care Med* 2003; **4** (3 Suppl): S19–24.

33. Adelson PD Guidelines for the acute medical management of severe traumatic brain injury in infants, children, and adolescents. Chapter 6. Threshold for treatment of intracranial hypertension. *Pediatr Crit Care Med* 2003; **4** (3 Suppl): S25–7.

34. Adelson PD. Guidelines for the acute medical management of severe traumatic brain injury in infants, children, and adolescents. Chapter 8. Cerebral perfusion pressure. *Pediatr Crit Care Med* 2003; **4** (3 Suppl): S31–3.

35. Adelson PD. Guidelines for the acute medical management of severe traumatic brain injury in infants, children, and adolescents. Chapter 7. Intracranial pressure monitoring technology. *Pediatr Crit Care Med* 2003; **4** (3 Suppl): S28–30.

36. Figaji AA, Zwane E, Thompson C, *et al.* Brain tissue oxygen tension monitoring in pediatric severe traumatic brain injury. Part 1: Relationship with outcome. *Childs Nerv Syst* 2009; **25**: 1325–33.

37. Nilsson B, Rehncrona S, Siesjo BK. Coupling of cerebral metabolism and blood flow in epileptic seizures, hypoxia and hypoglycemia. In Purves M, ed., *Cerebral Vascular Smooth Muscle and Its Control.* Amsterdam: Excerpta Medica, Elsevier, 1978, pp. 199–218.

38. Rehncrona S, Siesjo BK. Metabolic and physiologic changes in acute brain failure. In Grenvik A, Safar P, eds., *Brain Failure and Resuscitation.* New York, NY: Churchill Livingstone, 1981, pp. 11–33.

39. White PF, Schlobohm RM, Pitts LH, *et al.* A randomized study of drugs for preventing increases in intracranial pressure during endotracheal suctioning. *Anesthesiology* 1982; **57**: 242–4.

40. Raju TNK, Vidyasagar D, Torres C, *et al.* Intracranial pressure during intubation and anesthesia in infants. *J Pediatr* 1980; **96**: 860–2.

41. Kerr ME, Weber BB, Sereika SM, *et al.* Effect of endotracheal suctioning on cerebral oxygenation in traumatic brain-injured patients. *Crit Care Med* 1999; **27**: 2776–81.

42. Adelson PD. Guidelines for the acute medical management of severe traumatic brain injury in infants, children, and adolescents. Chapter 9. Use of sedation and neuromuscular blockade in the treatment of severe pediatric traumatic brain injury. *Pediatr Crit Care Med* 2003; **4** (3 Suppl): S34–7.

43. Prielipp RC, Coursin DB. Sedative and neuromuscular blocking drug use in critically ill patients with head injuries. *New Horiz* 1995; **3**: 456–68.

44. Tobias JD. Increased intracranial pressure after fentanyl administration in a child with closed head trauma. *Pediatr Emerg Care* 1994; **10**: 89–90.

45. Albanese J, Durbec O, Viviand X, *et al.* Sufentanil increases intracranial pressure in patients with head trauma. *Anesthesiology* 1993; **79**: 493–7.

46. Cotev S, Shalit MN. Effects of diazepam on cerebral blood flow and oxygen uptake after head injury. *Anesthesiology* 1975; **43**: 117–22.

47. Papazian L, Albanese J, Thirion X, *et al.* Effect of bolus doses of midazolam on intracranial pressure and cerebral perfusion pressure in patients with severe head injury. *Br J Anaesth.* 1993; **71**: 267–71.

48. Spitzfaden AC, Jimenez DF, Tobias JD. Propofol for sedation and control of intracranial pressure in children. *Pediatr Neurosurg* 1999; **31**: 194–200.

49. Farling PA, Johnston JR, Coppel DL. Propofol infusion for sedation of patients with head injury in intensive care. *Anaesthesia* 1989; **44**: 222–6.

50. Steiner LA, Johnston AJ, Chatfield DA, *et al.* The effects of large-dose propofol on cerebrovascular pressure autoregulation in head-injured patients. *Anesth Analg* 2003; **97**: 572–6.

51. Bray RJ. Propofol infusion syndrome in children. *Paediatr Anaesth* 1998; **8**: 491–9.

52. Hanna JP, Ramundo ML. Rhabdomyolysis and hypoxia associated with prolonged propofol infusion in children. *Neurology* 1998; **50**: 301–3.

53. Cray SH, Robinson BH, Cox PN. Lactic acidemia and bradyarrhythmia in a

child sedated with propofol. *Crit Care Med* 1998; **26**: 2087–92.

54. Parke TJ, Stevens JE, Rice AS, *et al*. Metabolic acidosis and fatal myocardial failure after propofol infusion in children: five case reports. *BMJ* 1992; **305**: 613–16.

55. Canivet JL, Gustad K, Leclercq P, *et al*. Massive ketonuria during sedation with propofol in a 12 year old girl with severe head trauma. *Acta Anaesthesiol Belg* 1994; **45**: 19–22.

56. Hsiang JK, Chesnut RM, Crisp CB, *et al*. Early, routine paralysis for intracranial pressure control in severe head injury: Is it necessary? *Crit Care Med* 1994; **22**: 1471–6.

57. Vernon DD, Witte MK. Effect of neuromuscular blockade on oxygen consumption and energy expenditure in sedated, mechanically ventilated children. *Crit Care Med* 2000; **28**: 1569–71.

58. Durbin CG. Neuromuscular blocking agents and sedative drugs. Clinical uses and toxic effects in the critical care unit. *Crit Care Clin* 1981; **7**: 480–506.

59. Martin LD, Bratton SL, Quint P, *et al*. Prospective documentation of sedative, analgesic, and neuromuscular blocking agent use in infants and children in the intensive care unit: a multicenter perspective. *Pediatr Crit Care Med* 2001; **2**: 205–10.

60. Douglass JA, Tuxen DV, Horne M, *et al*. Myopathy in severe asthma. *Am Rev Respir Dis* 1992; **146**: 517–19.

61. Taketomo CK, Hodding JH, Kraus DM. *Lexi-Comp's Pediatric Dosage Handbook*, 10th edition. Hudson, OH: Lexi-Comp, 2003–2004.

62. Levin AB, Duff TA, Javid MJ. Treatment of increased intracranial pressure: a comparison of different hyperosmotic agents and the use of thiopental. *Neurosurgery* 1979; **5**: 570–5.

63. Muizelaar JP, Lutz HA, Becker DP. Effect of mannitol on ICP and CBF and correlation with pressure autoregulation in severely head injured patients. *J Neurosurg* 1984; **61**: 700–6.

64. Muizelaar JP, Wei EP, Kontos HA, *et al*. Mannitol causes compensatory vasoconstriction and vasodilation in response to blood viscosity changes. *J Neurosurg* 1983; **59**: 822–8.

65. Muizelaar JP, Wei EP, Kontos HA, *et al*. Cerebral blood flow is regulated by changes in blood pressure and in blood viscosity alike. *Stroke* 1986; **17**: 44–8.

66. Raphaely RC, Swedlow DB, Downes JJ, *et al*. Management of severe pediatric head trauma. *Pediatr Clin N Am* 1980; **27**: 715–27.

67. Bruce DA, Alavi A, Bilaniuk L, *et al*. Diffuse cerebral swelling following head injuries in children: the syndrome of "malignant brain edema." *J Neurosurg* 1981; **54**: 170–8.

68. Bouma GJ, Muizelaar JP. Cerebral blood flow, cerebral blood volume, and cerebrovascular reactivity after severe head injury. *J Neurotrauma* 1992; **9**: S333–48.

69. James HE. Methodology for the control of intracranial pressure with hypertonic mannitol. *Acta Neurochir* 1980; **51**: 161–72.

70. Qureshi AI, Suarez JI. Use of hypertonic saline solutions in treatment of cerebral edema and intracranial hypertension. *Crit Care Med* 2000; **28**: 3301–13.

71. Khanna S, Davis D, Peterson B, *et al*. Use of hypertonic saline in the treatment of severe refractory posttraumatic intracranial hypertension in pediatric traumatic brain injury. *Crit Care Med*. 2000; **28**: 1144–51.

72. Adelson PD. Guidelines for the acute medical management of severe traumatic brain injury in infants, children, and adolescents. Chapter 11. Use of hyperosmolar therapy in the management of severe pediatric traumatic brain injury. *Pediatr Crit Care Med* 2003; **4** (3 Suppl): S40–4.

73. Fisher B, Thomas D, Peterson B: Hypertonic saline lowers raised intracranial pressure in children after head trauma. *J Neurosurg Anesthesiol* 1992; **4**: 4–10.

74. Roberts I, Yates D, Sandercock P, *et al*. Effect of intravenous corticosteroids on death within 14 days in 10008 adults with clinically significant head injury (MRC CRASH trial): randomised placebo-controlled trial. *Lancet* 2004; **364**: 1321–8.

75. Edwards P, Arango M, Balica L, *et al*. Final results of MRC CRASH, a randomised placebo-controlled trial of intravenous corticosteroid in adults with head injury-outcomes at 6 months. *Lancet* 2005; **365**: 1957–9.

76. Marion DW, Darby J, Yonas H. Acute regional cerebral blood flow changes caused by severe head injuries. *J Neurosurg* 1991; **74**: 407–14.

77. Marion DW. Does hyperventilation cause secondary brain injury? *Crit Care Med* 2006; **34**: 1284–5.

78. Stringer WA, Hasso AN, Thompson JR, *et al*. Hyperventilation-induced cerebral ischemia in patients with acute brain lesions: Demonstration by Xenon-enhanced CT. *Am J Neuroradiol* 1993; **14**: 475–84.

79. Skippen P, Seear M, Poskitt K, *et al*. Effect of hyperventilation on regional cerebral blood flow in head-injured children. *Crit Care Med* 1997; **25**: 1402–9.

80. Curry R, Hollingworth W, Ellenbogen RG, *et al*: Incidence of hypo- and hypercarbia in severe traumatic brain injury before and after 2003 pediatric guidelines. *Pediatr Crit Care Med* 2008; **9**: 141–6.

81. Adelson PD Guidelines for the acute medical management of severe traumatic brain injury in infants, children, and adolescents. Chapter 12. Use of hyperventilation in the acute management of severe pediatric traumatic brain injury. *Pediatr Crit Care Med* 2003; **4** (3 Suppl): S45–8.

82. Ginsberg MD, Busto R. Combating hyperthermia in acute stroke: a significant clinical concern. *Stroke* 1998; **29**: 529–34.

83. Busto R, Dietrich WD, Globus MYT, *et al*. Small differences in intraischemic brain temperature critically determine the extent of ischemic neuronal injury. *J Cereb Blood Flow Metab* 1987; **7**: 729–38.

84. Marion DW, White MJ. Treatment of experimental brain injury with moderate hypothermia and 21-aminosteroids. *J Neurotrauma* 1996; **13**: 139–47.

85. Pomeranz S, Safar P, Radovsky A, *et al*. The effect of resuscitative moderate hypothermia following epidural brain compression on cerebral damage in a canine outcome model. *J Neurosurg* 1993; **79**: 241–51.

86. Smith SL, Hall ED. Mild pre- and posttraumatic hypothermia attenuates blood-brain barrier damage following controlled cortical impact injury in the rat. *J Neurotrauma* 1996; **13**: 1–9.

87. Clasen RA, Pandolfi S, Russell J, Stuart D, Hass GM. Hypothermia and

hypotension in experimental cerebral edema. *Arch Neurol* 1968; **19**: 472–86.

88. Marion DW, Penrod LE, Kelsey SF, *et al.* Treatment of traumatic brain injury with moderate hypothermia. *N Engl J Med* 1997; **336**: 540–6.

89. Clifton GL, Miller ER, Choi SC, *et al.* Lack of effect of induction of hypothermia after acute brain injury. *N Engl J Med.* 2001; **344**: 556–63.

90. Biswas AK, Bruce DA, Sklar FH, Bokovoy JL, Sommerauer JF. Treatment of acute traumatic brain injury in children with moderate hypothermia improves intracranial hypertension. *Crit Care Med* 2002; **30**: 2742–51.

91. Adelson PD, Ragheb J, Kanev P, *et al.* Phase II clinical trial of moderate hypothermia after severe traumatic brain injury in children. *Neurosurgery* 2005; **56**: 740–54.

92. Hutchison JS, Ward RE, Lacroix J, *et al.* Hypothermia therapy after traumatic brain injury in children. *N Engl J Med* 2008; **358**: 2447–56

93. Stiefel MF, Heuer GG, Smith MJ, *et al.* Cerebral oxygenation following decompressive hemicraniectomy for the treatment of refractory intracranial hypertension. *J Neurosurg* 2004; **101**: 241–7.

94. Bor-Seng-Shu E, Hirsch R, Teixeira MJ, De Andrade AF, Marino R. Cerebral hemodynamic changes gauged by transcranial Doppler ultrasonography in patients with posttraumatic brain swelling treated by surgical decompression. *J Neurosurg* 2006; **104**: 93–100.

95. Polin RS, Shaffrey ME, Bogaev CA, *et al.* Decompressive bifrontal craniectomy in the treatment of severe refractory posttraumatic cerebral edema. *Neurosurgery* 1997; **41**: 84–92.

96. Taylor A, Butt W, Rosenfeld J, *et al.* A randomized trial of very early

decompressive craniectomy in children with traumatic brain injury and sustained intracranial hypertension. *Childs Nerv Syst* 2001; **17**: 154–62.

97. Cho DY, Wang YC, Chi CS. Decompressive craniotomy for acute shaken/impact baby syndrome. *Pediatr Neurosurg* 1995; **23**: 192–8.

98. Figaji AA, Fieggen AG, Argent AC, Le Roux PD, Peter JC. Intracranial pressure and cerebral oxygenation changes after decompressive craniectomy in children with severe traumatic brain injury. *Acta Neurochir Suppl* 2008; **102**: 77–80.

99. Jagannathan J, Okonkwo DO, Dumont AS, *et al.* Outcome following decompressive craniectomy in children with severe traumatic brain injury: a 10-year single-center experience with long-term follow up. *J NeuroSurg* 2007; **106** (4 Suppl): 268–75.

100. Thomale UW, Graetz D, Vajkoczy P, Sarrafzadeh AS. Severe traumatic brain injury in children: a single center experience regarding therapy and long-term outcome. *Childs Nerv Syst.* 2010; **26**: 1563–73.

101. Roberts I. Barbiturates for acute traumatic brain injury. *Cochrane Database Syst Rev* 2000; (2): CD000033.

102. Eisenberg HM, Frankowski RF, Contant CF, Marshall LF, Walker MD. High-dose barbiturate control of elevated intracranial pressure in patients with severe head injury. *J Neurosurg* 1988; **69**: 15–23.

103. Kasoff SS, Lansen TA, Holder D, *et al.* Aggressive physiologic monitoring of pediatric trauma patients with elevated intracranial pressure. *Pediatr Neurosci* 1988; **14**: 241–9.

104. Cormio M, Gopinath SP, Valadka A, Robertson CS. Cerebral hemodynamic effects of pentobarbital coma in head-

injured patients. *J Neurotrauma* 1999; **16**: 927–36.

105. Schierhout G, Roberts I. Anti-epileptic drugs for preventing seizures following acute traumatic brain injury. *Cochrane Database Syst Rev* 2001; (4): CD000173.

106. Tilford JM, Simpson PM, Yeh TS, *et al.* Variation in therapy and outcome for pediatric head trauma patients. *Crit Care Med* 2001; **29**: 1056–61.

107. Young KD, Okada PJ, Sokolove PE, *et al.* A randomized, double-blinded, placebo-controlled trial of phenytoin for the prevention of early posttraumatic seizures in children with moderate to severe blunt head injury. *Ann Emerg Med* 2004; **43**: 435–46.

108. Asikainen I, Kaste M, Sarna S. Early and late posttraumatic seizures in traumatic brain injury rehabilitation patients: brain injury factors causing late seizures and influence of seizures on long-term outcome. *Epilepsia.* 1999; **40**: 584–9.

109. Ng I, Lim J, Wong HB. Effects of head posture on cerebral hemodynamics: Its influences on intracranial pressure, cerebral perfusion pressure, and cerebral oxygenation. *Neurosurgery* 2004; **54**: 593–7.

110. Feldman Z, Kanter MJ, Robertson CS, *et al.* Effect of head elevation on intracranial pressure, cerebral perfusion pressure, and cerebral blood flow in head-injured patients. *J Neurosurg* 1992; **76**: 207–11.

111. Adelson PD. Guidelines for the acute medical management of severe traumatic brain injury in infants, children, and adolescents. Chapter 17. Critical pathway for the treatment of established intracranial hypertension in pediatric traumatic brain injury. *Pediatr Crit Care Med* 2003; **4** (3 Suppl): S65–7.

Trauma in the elderly

Jeffrey H. Silverstein

Objectives

(1) Understand the basic physiology of aging.
(2) Utilize current concepts of elderly trauma outcomes to support triage decisions.
(3) Apply knowledge of those aspects of aging required to design and execute an anesthetic plan for an elderly trauma victim.

Introduction

When an elderly patient enters the trauma room, what is your first thought? Do you rush to be more aggressive, because elderly patients are more fragile and need more immediate and intensive trauma care? Do you question whether the resources and effort necessary to treat such a patient are likely to provide benefit to the patient or society, because the functional outcome for such patients is so poor? This chapter seeks to summarize current knowledge regarding the best approach to elderly trauma victims.

Life expectancy in the United States continues to rise. Persons reaching age 65 have an average life expectancy of an additional 19.2 years (20.3 years for females and 17.6 years for males).[1] The retiring baby boomer population is more active than previous generations of elderly, many driving into their nineties and pursuing a variety of activities that increase their exposure to traumatic injury. Unintentional injury is the sixth leading cause of death among patients 65–74 years of age, and the eighth leading cause for those over 75. This and other information can be accessed from the Web-based Injury Statistics Query and Reporting System (WISQARS) supported by the Centers for Disease Control and Prevention (http://www.cdc.gov/injury/wisqars).

Growing old is an inevitable consequence of life that is associated with specific changes that can be defined as aging or senescence. Other nonspecific alterations that are more prevalent in the aged should be conceptualized as age-related disease. It is useful for the clinician to distinguish *normative aging*, which is a statistical approach to defining aging in the population as a whole, and *successful aging*, which describes those individuals who have survived to advanced age with relatively little impairment.[2,3] In general, this chapter approaches aging as a normative concept, seeking to clarify where aspects of aging alter or inform the approach to trauma management.

A key concept in the assessment and management of the elderly patient is that tremendous variability marks the aging process. Trauma patients are always subject to individual assessment. This approach should be informed by the observation that all 25-year-old patients are more similar than all 70-year-old patients. Chronologic age is a predictor of physical status in the population, but can be misleading. Ever more elderly patients are highly functional. The trauma team should avoid a subconscious tendency to triage elderly patients to less intense evaluation and care. To this end, one of the earliest clinical assessments that should be made is to determine the functional status prior to the trauma in an aged patient.

This chapter will develop an approach to the elderly trauma patient from two perspectives. The first views aging as a composite of key physiologic changes that are of interest to the practicing anesthesiologist. In this section we will discuss maintenance of perfusion, in which the interrelated alterations in autonomic function, cardiac and pulmonary physiology, and the response to fluid therapy interact to affect the responses one might expect to see in a trauma or operating room environment. We will briefly discuss some of the issues associated with central nervous system (CNS) aging and perioperative care, and finally review the anesthetic pharmacology of the aged. Although the information presented is rarely derived from studies of geriatric trauma patients, our general understanding of aging physiology is fairly sophisticated, providing a reasonable basis for the trauma clinician to extrapolate from the available information to the specific clinical problem at hand. In the subsequent section, the trauma-specific information that subtends our current understanding of triage decisions and specific management paradigms will be discussed. This section presents data on multisystem trauma in geriatric patients separately from data on the most common form of geriatric trauma, fracture of the hip.

Trauma Anesthesia, 2nd Edition, ed. Charles E. Smith. Published by Cambridge University Press. © Charles E. Smith, 2015.

The physiology of aging

One of the areas of senescent physiology with an extensive base of information is cardiac aging. The depth and breadth of available information is beyond the scope of this chapter. For the trauma clinician, the chapter provides a systematic review of those aspects of cardiovascular aging that affect the capacity of the body to maintain appropriate perfusion of vital organs.

Senescence of the autonomic nervous system

The autonomic nervous system is the principal system charged with the maintenance of general homeostasis, particularly arterial blood pressure and perfusion. Cardiac output, blood pressure, and the regional distribution of cardiac output are primarily controlled by postganglionic sympathetic neurons. The sympathetic nervous system also contributes to the regulation of temperature control and energy metabolism through epinephrine release from the adrenal medulla. Whole-body sympathetic activity increases with age (see reviews by Seals and Esler[4,5]). Circulating levels of norepinephrine slowly increase by about 10–15% per decade. The heart, skeletal muscle, and gastrointestinal tract manifest an increase in sympathetic activity, but the kidneys are not clearly affected. Postganglionic activity is increased; however, tonic levels of epinephrine are unchanged due to the combination of decreased excretion and decreased clearance. Although the baseline level of the autonomic nervous system appears elevated, the elderly are not clearly hyperresponsive to stress.[5] However, there is growing recognition that the duration of the stress response in the elderly may be prolonged, resulting in chronic stress.[6] The implication of the delayed return to homeostasis is not clear, but this has implications for neuroplasticity[7] and for the development of dementia.[8]

α_1-Adrenergic function appears to be preserved in aging, while α_2-mediated responses appear to be decreased.[9–11] Even though autonomic activity appears increased, the cardiovascular behavior of the elderly, with slightly lower resting heart rate and limited ability to increase cardiac output, is similar to that noted in patients receiving β-adrenergic antagonists.[12]

Cardiovascular aging and physiology

Relatively few prospective evaluations of the hemodynamic response of elderly patients to trauma or under anesthesia have been published. Therefore, much of the basis for a physiologic approach to the elderly trauma patient is extrapolated from the exercise literature. This may not be an unreasonable extrapolation. In the absence of significant disease, a healthy elderly patient manifests a slightly altered physiologic state of normal perfusion at rest, as outlined in Table 36.1. Average resting heart rate is stable or declines slightly. Systolic blood pressure increases but diastolic does not. On average, cardiac output is maintained, with perhaps a slight increase in stroke volume. It is important for the anesthesiologist to appreciate that the aerobic capacity of healthy adults decreases with age (Fig. 36.1)[13] This change is not constant, with acceleration

Table 36.1 Alterations in cardiac physiology in the elderly, as compared to young patients

Parameter	Elderly at rest	Exercising elderly
Heart rate	No change or slight decrease	Limited ability to increase
Systolic blood pressure	Increased	Significant increase
Diastolic blood pressure	No change or minor increase	Slightly greater increase
Cardiac output	No change	Slightly less increase
Ejection fraction	No change	Less increase
Stroke volume	No change or slight increase	Greater increase

noted in each decade, particularly in men, and without apparent influence by physical activity. Interestingly, Hollenberg *et al.* have suggested that this limitation is primarily associated with alterations in pulmonary capacity (FEV_1).[14] Observations of the elderly in the operating room do not contradict the idea that the capacity to increase cardiac output is limited in comparison with younger patients. This is generally associated with a reduced capacity to increase heart rate. This limitation should be rarely encountered in the operating room, as current management paradigms emphasize lower heart rates to avoid myocardial ischemia.

The interplay between cardiovascular senescence and cardiovascular disease is complicated. An extensive review was provided by Lakatta and colleagues.[15–17] Nonetheless, a relatively basic understanding of the structural alterations to the vessels and heart that accompany even successful aging can assist in the development of a clinical approach to an elderly trauma victim. Aging is associated with a decrease in connective tissue compliance and distensibility, primarily due to increasing crossbridging between collagen and elastin filaments. The arteries, most prominently the aorta, become increasingly stiff and noncompliant in response to years of expanding and contracting with each systolic ejection. Stiffening, widening, and elongation of the aorta is often noted in chest radiographs of the elderly. The hemodynamically important result is that stiffening of the vascular tree results in a higher peak systolic pressure in the left ventricle: that is, there is a considerable increase in afterload. In addition, each pulse wave travels through the stiffer vascular tree and is reflected back toward the heart earlier and more strongly than in a young patient. Pulse wave velocity increases two- to threefold with aging. In the elderly this component is appended to the end-systolic afterload, as opposed to young cardiovascular systems where the reflected pulse wave tends to arrive after systole and thus not contribute to afterload. Measurement of blood pressure in the arm, either by noninvasive

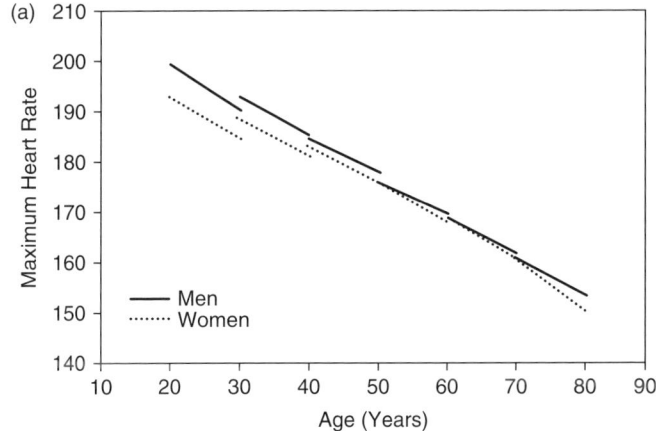

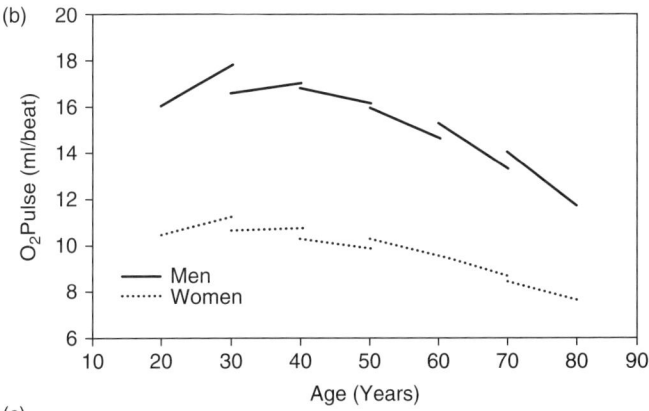

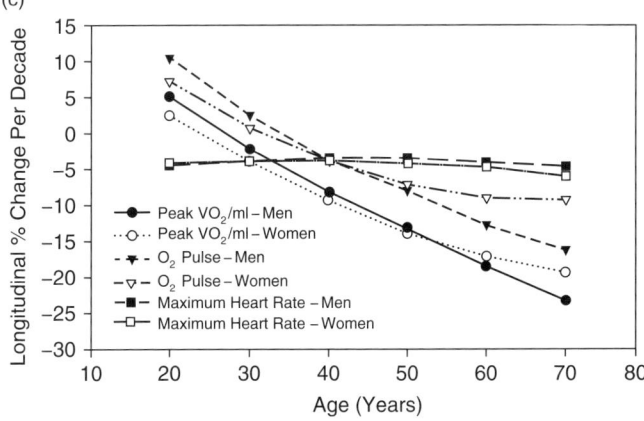

Figure 36.1 Longitudinal changes in maximal heart rate, oxygen (O_2) pulse and peak oxygen consumption (VO_2) by sex, predicted from the mixed-effects model. (A) Declines in heart rate are similar across age in men but steepen modestly with age in women. (B) O_2 pulse declines progressively more steeply with age, especially in men, leading to near convergence of O_2 pulse in elderly men and women. Note the similarity of these plots to those of peak VO_2 in (A). (C) The longitudinal percentage change per decade in maximal heart rate is only 4–5% per decade across the age span in both sexes. In contrast, longitudinal decline in O_2 pulse accelerates progressively with age, especially in men. Note the similarity in the shape and multitude of the decline in O_2 pulse to that of peak VO_2. (Reproduced from Fleg *et al.* 2005,[13] reproduced with permission.)

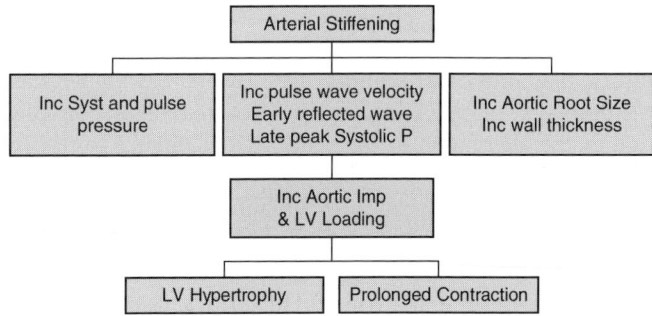

Figure 36.2 Cardiac adaptation to arterial stiffening in older men. Inc, increased; Imp, impedance; LV, left ventricle; P, pressure; syst, systolic.

The principal clinically relevant consequences of age-related alteration in aortic–arterial stiffness, *in the absence of disease states and severe deconditioning*, are concentric left ventricular hypertrophy and a substantial decline in diastolic compliance (Fig. 36.2). Unlike most other organs, the heart does not decrease in size with age. General cellular hypertrophy, as well as a marked increase in connective tissue, is the main cause of hypertrophy. By echocardiography, a 30% increase in left ventricular thickness has been described, primarily at the intraventricular septum.

Diastolic dysfunction is a state in which diastolic filling of the left ventricle is abnormal, whether left ventricular function (i.e., ejection fraction) is normal or the patient has symptoms. Heart failure with preserved systolic function, frequently called diastolic heart failure, is characterized by the presence of normal systolic function (left ventricular ejection fraction > 50%) and symptoms of heart failure with impaired diastolic function. These patients may become symptomatic from acute (as well as chronic) elevations in left ventricular end-diastolic pressure and/or left atrial pressure.[20,21] This pathology appears on top of a general 50% decline in early diastolic ventricular filling in the aged. The importance of atrial contraction to ventricular filling increases from 10% to 30% in elderly subjects. Diastolic dysfunction appears to be primarily related to systolic hypertension and is found more in elderly females than in elderly males. Altered diastolic relaxation results in increased left ventricular end-diastolic pressure, both at rest and during exercise. Exercise intolerance is present as commonly and as severely in diastolic as in systolic heart failure. Severe exercise intolerance is associated with an inability to increase stroke volume by way of the Frank–Starling mechanism despite severely increased left ventricular filling pressures. At any given stroke volume, higher pressures are generated. The Frank–Starling relationships are only relevant within the range of normal compliance. Factors that decrease ventricular preload, particularly a loss of effective atrial systole, can significantly alter cardiac output. These alterations can only be appreciated by echocardiography. All of the described potential alterations have to be considered with the understanding that cardiac output is essentially maintained in subjects who are carefully screened for occult disease.

cuff or by arterial catheter, underestimates the systolic pressure present in the aortic root. The reflected pulse wave is an important component of the chronic increase in afterload experienced by the elderly heart.[18,19]

Maximum aerobic capacity decreases with age. Individual conditioning and the presence of even occult coronary artery disease play important limiting roles. Lakatta has argued that the decline in oxygen consumption (VO_2 max) is not entirely due to the alterations in the central circulation. Age-related alterations in oxidation capacity per unit muscle, ability to shunt blood to exercising muscles, and/or muscle mass could also play a role. More recently, Hollenberg et al. have suggested that specific pulmonary limitations are involved.[14]

A number of major studies indicate a significant and increasing prevalence of coronary artery disease in elderly patients.[22] Thus, although pure age-related alterations in the cardiovascular system have been well described, the majority of elderly trauma patients in Western countries will have significant disease loads. Underlying disease combines with aging to increase risk from trauma.

Pulmonary aging and pathology

The elderly have a greater predisposition to pulmonary complications in the perioperative period, and this may be the primary cause of morbidity and mortality, rather than cardiac pathology.[23,24] The primary age-related alterations are: (1) decreased strength of the respiratory muscles, (2) progressive (20–30%) loss of alveolar surface area, (3) impaired nervous control of the ventilation, and (4) a reduction of the elastic recoil of lung tissue combined with stiffening of the chest wall.[25] The direct consequences of the reduced alveolar surface are a decreased oxygen-diffusing capacity and a slightly increased alveolar dead space. From youth to age 80, maximal diffusing capacity can decrease by up to 50%.

Old people must generate more power to attain necessary transpulmonary pressure for effective ventilation. The chest wall becomes stiffer and less compliant, while the lung parenchyma loses elastic recoil and becomes more compliant. The chest becomes more barrel-shaped with a flattened diaphragm. The new equilibrium of the opposing thoracic and pulmonary forces increases the interpleural pressure by 2–4 cmH$_2$O. The diaphragmatic efficacy is also impaired by a significant age-related loss of motor neurons. The work of breathing at rest is unchanged with age, but the work of breathing associated with vigorous exercise may exceed a 30% increase over a younger patient.[25]

A dangerous predisposition to hypoxemia exists in the perioperative period for elderly trauma patients. Carbon dioxide elimination is unchanged with age, but arterial oxygenation is progressively impaired.[26] Arterial oxygen tension falls approximately 5 mmHg per decade from 20 years of age. This is primarily due to an increased ventilation/perfusion maldistribution with shunt- and dead-space-like effects rather than decreased diffusing capacity. Alterations in hypocapnic bronchoconstriction and hypoxic pulmonary vasoconstriction may also contribute to the age-related ventilation/perfusion maldistribution. The magnitude of shunting can be markedly increased by atelectasis following induction of anesthesia, which occurs in more than 80% of elderly patients. Positive end-expiratory pressure has a limited impact on atelectasis, since the elastic recoil curves of atelectatic and nonatelectatic lung units can be quite different. Prolonged high-volume recruitment maneuvers followed by positive end-expiratory pressure may be effective. An increased tendency for upper airway collapse, decreased tonic activity of the upper airway muscles (pharyngeal collapse), and decreased ventilatory response to both hypercapnia and hypoxia are present in the elderly. Both hypercapnic and hypoxic respiratory drive are decreased to a greater degree in older people by both sedative drugs and pain medications. Finally, the elderly frequently manifest a decrease in upper airway protective reflexes, which increases the risk of aspiration.

In managing an elderly trauma victim, tracheal intubation should be undertaken early if considered. That is, if you are considering whether the trachea should be intubated, it probably should be – because, with limited respiratory reserve, such a patient will progress to respiratory arrest more rapidly than a younger patient. Denitrogenation (preoxygenation) takes longer in the elderly, but if time is available, full denitrogenation provides an important safety cushion. Tracheal intubation is usually no more difficult than in younger patients. Attention should be paid to maneuvers designed to decrease atelectasis during prolonged operations.

There are no specific recommendations for emergence and extubation of elderly trauma patients. Standard extubation parameters apply. Practitioners should evaluate the potential work of breathing and extubate the trachea as soon as the patient appears capable of maintaining such an effort.

Renal function

Renal function and, therefore, fluid and electrolyte balance are altered with aging; however, assessment of fluid status is not easy. The loss of elasticity and thinning of the dermis makes skin appear dehydrated in many patients, so skin turgor is difficult to interpret. A lack of thirst does not correlate with normal hydration status. As the possibility of inappropriately dilute urine exists in the elderly, even urine output must be evaluated with a degree of suspicion. Estimating equations for glomerular filtration rate allow the practitioner to develop an expectation of how quickly administered fluid and medications may be excreted. However, these equations are not often accurate for a given patient. Although an actual measurement of glomerular filtration rate is preferable, this is rarely applicable until the postoperative period.[27] Preferably, practitioners should use the Cockcroft–Gault formula.[28] Medications that require careful control of plasma levels should be managed with laboratory measurement of blood concentrations. In summary, the elderly response to disruption of fluid homeostasis and the current understanding of cardiovascular aging indicate that the therapeutic window for intravenous fluid is markedly narrowed.

CNS aging and dysfunction

The elderly brain does not significantly deteriorate in the absence of disease, although age-related CNS disease is common. Neurons represent a high-turnover cell type, with active new cell formation present in many areas of the brain. For patients with preexisting dementia or previous stroke, there is little in the way of coherent evidence to recommend a specific approach to trauma anesthesia. Maintaining cerebral perfusion is an important goal in both elective and trauma circumstances and, to date, does not require a unique plan for the geriatric patient.

There are CNS complications that are common in the perioperative period for elderly patients that can have an important influence on the long-term outcome of the trauma victim. A recent review of CNS dysfunction in the elderly discusses postoperative delirium and postoperative cognitive dysfunction.[29,30] Delirium is a disorder defined by specific behaviors, the primary features of which are (1) a change in mental status, characterized by a prominent disturbance of attention and reduced clarity of awareness of the environment, and (2) an acute onset, developing within hours to days and tending to fluctuate during the course of the day. Elderly patients should be screened for delirium both pre- and postoperatively. Delirium is clinically diagnosed by applying the Confusion Assessment Method (CAM).[31] The Confusion Assessment Method for use in the ICU (CAM-ICU) is available for patients who are tracheally intubated.[32] The development of delirium is associated with increased length of stay, increased hospital costs, increased morbidity and mortality, and perhaps with long-term cognitive problems.[29] Extensive work has been done on the prevention of delirium in patients with hip fracture (see below), but relatively little work has been done on elderly multisystem trauma patients.

Postoperative cognitive dysfunction occurs in a significant number of patients following elective surgery.[33] There are definitely individuals who have lost some level of function or had a personality change following surgery, particularly cardiac surgery. Making a determination for a specific patient requires a reliable baseline test from before surgery (or trauma). Therefore, in a practical sense, postoperative cognitive dysfunction is limited to findings from organized research studies. There is a great deal of controversy regarding exactly how much deterioration is clinically or epidemiologically significant, and which areas of cognitive function are most vulnerable. There are no studies that support any intervention to decrease the incidence of severity of postoperative cognitive dysfunction at the current time. Thus, the trauma clinician can do little more than be aware of this potential complication.

Pharmacologic alterations

With few exceptions, elderly patients require less anesthetic medications. However, sophisticated management of these patients requires a more detailed understanding of the physiologic alterations that underlie the altered requirements. Both pharmacodynamic and pharmacokinetic changes are involved in the altered impact of drugs on the elderly.[34] It is probably not reasonable to extrapolate from animal models, and the changes are unique for each drug, requiring individual studies to determine the impact of aging.[35–37] Lean body mass decreases with age, as does total body water, while total body fat tends to increase. Most drugs used by anesthesiologists are described by multicompartment pharmacokinetics models. The combination of decreased total body water and redistributed cardiac output tends to decrease the size of the central compartment, potentially increasing peak concentrations even though steady-state volume increases due to increased body fat.

The impact of hepatic aging varies from drug to drug. Both aging and anesthesia decrease liver blood flow, which probably impacts primarily the maintenance doses of anesthetic agent. Renal blood flow is inversely correlated with age, and there is a progressive decrease in the glomerular filtration rate with aging. Aging alters serum proteins differentially: albumin concentrations decrease with age, while α-1-acid glycoprotein increases with age. Depending on which protein primarily binds a drug, the active free fraction will either increase or decrease. Receptor sensitivity for specific drugs is highly variable with age.

In sum, a large number of highly variable changes impact the requirements for essentially all of the drugs used by anesthesiologists. Any individual patient may or may not demonstrate the changes that are experienced on average in this population.[34] Table 36.2 provides a limited overview of the alterations (or lack of alterations, for some drugs) seen in elderly patients. Various injuries and physical states associated with trauma may additionally alter the need for anesthetic drugs. There is, however, little direct pharmacokinetic or pharmacodynamic work that has been undertaken in elderly trauma victims.

Trauma care for the elderly

Fracture of the upper femur is a common injury that is relatively unique to the elderly population. Hip fractures are treated in almost all hospitals, even hospitals that would not generally accept trauma victims. Unlike multisystem trauma patients, in which the level of stress is frequently significant, hip fractures are frequently isolated injuries, so patients are treated with a reduction and fixation of the fracture with subsequent rapid transfer to geriatric and/or rehabilitation services. There is a fairly extensive literature on care of the hip fracture patient, and comparatively little on major trauma in the same patients. In this author's opinion, the hip fracture literature does not significantly illuminate the care of multisystem trauma victims. Therefore, the following discussion presents the approach to the hip fracture patient as a separate subset of geriatric trauma.

Table 36.2 Age-related pharmacologic changes of anesthetics and drugs in anesthesia practice

Anesthetic/drug	Pharmacodynamics	Pharmacokinetics	Anesthetic management
Inhalational anesthetics	↑ Sensitivity of the Brain (↓ cerebral metabolic rate)	Ventilation/perfusion mismatch with slow rise of alveolar/inspired ratio of inhaled gases; ↓ maximal cardiac output; ↓ volume of distribution	Minimum alveolar concentration (MAC) down 30%; slower induction and emergence; delayed but more profound onset of anesthesia
Hypnotics			
Thiopental	No change	↓ Central volume of distribution; ↓ intercompartmental clearance	Induction dose reduced by 15% (20-year-old patient: 2.5–5.0 mg/kg IV); 80-year-old patient: 2.1 mg/kg IV). Maintenance dose: same requirements 60 minutes after starting a continuation infusion. Emergence: slightly faster
Propofol	No change	↓ Central volume of distribution; ↓ intercompartmental clearance	Induction dose reduced by 20% (slower induction requires lower doses) (20-year-old: 2.0–3.0 mg/kg IV; 80-year-old: 1.7 mg/kg IV). Maintenance dose: same requirements 120 minutes after starting a continuous infusion. Emergence: slightly faster (?)
Midazolam	↑ Sensitivity of the Brain	↓ Clearance	Sedation/induction dose reduced by 50% (20-year-old: 0.07–0.15 mg/kg IV; 80-year-old: 0.02–0.03 mg/kg IV). Maintenance dose reduced by 25%. Recovery: delayed (hours)
Etomidate	No change	↓ Central clearance; ↓ volume of distribution	Induction dose reduced by 20% (20-year-old: 0.3 mg/kg IV; 80-year-old: 0.2 mg/kg IV). Emergence: slightly faster (?)
Ketamine	?	?	Use with caution: hallucinations, seizures, mental disturbance, release of catecholamines: avoid in combination with levodopa (tachycardia, arterial hypertension)
Opioids			
Fentanyl, alfentanil, sufentanil	↑ Sensitivity of the brain	No changes	Induction dose reduced by 50%. Maintenance doses reduced by 30–50%. Emergence: may be delayed
Remifentanil	↑ Sensitivity of the brain	↓ Central volume of distribution; ↓ intercompartmental clearance	Induction dose reduced by 50%. Maintenance dose reduced by 70%. Emergence: may be delayed
Muscle relaxants			
Succinylcholine	No change	↓ Plasma cholinesterase; ↓ muscle blood flow; ↓ cardiac output; ↓ intercompartmental clearance	Delayed onset time
Pancuronium, doxacuronium, pipecuronium, vecuronium, rocuronium	No change	↓ Muscle blood flow; ↓ cardiac output; ↓ intercompartmental clearance; ↓ clearance; ↓ volume of distribution	Delayed onset time. ↓ Maintenance dose requirements. ↑ Duration of action. Recommended dose reduced by 20%.
Atracurium Cisatracurium	No change	No change	No change
Reversal agents			
Neostigmine, pyridostigmine	No changes	↓ Clearance	↑ Duration of action; because muscle relaxants have a markedly prolonged duration of action, larger doses of reversal agents are needed in elderly patients

Table 36.2 (cont.)

Anesthetic/drug	Pharmacodynamics	Pharmacokinetics	Anesthetic management
Edrophonium	No change	No change	No change
Local anesthetics	↑ Sensitivity of the nervous tissue (?)	↓ Hepatic microsomal metabolism of amide local anesthetics (lidocaine (lignocaine), bupivacaine); ↓ plasma protein binding; ↑ cephalad spread	↓ Epidural (and spinal) dose requirements. Duration of spinal and epidural anesthesia seems clinically independent of age, ↑ toxicity (percent free drug)

Modified from Silverstein JH, Zaugg M. Chapter 69, Geriatrics. In Hemmings HC, Hopkins PM, eds., *Foundations of Anesthesia*, 2nd edition. St. Louis, MO: Mosby, 2005.

Hip fracture patients

Hip fractures are an important cause of mortality and functional dependence in the United States. Approximately 350,000 hip fractures occur annually in this country and this number is expected to increase to more than 650,000 by the year 2040.[38,39] For adults over age 65, the annual incidence of hip fracture is 818 per 100,000 persons, and women are two to three times more likely to experience a fracture than men. The mechanism of injury is almost always a fall. Extensive effort has been exerted to design effective fall prevention strategies.[40]

Patients presenting with a hip fracture should be assessed with the knowledge of the potential changes associated with physiologic senility, as described in the first section of this chapter, as well as with an understanding of the patient's comorbid conditions. Most elderly people take multiple drugs. Acquiring this history can be challenging, but it is important. The timing of operations remains a topic of discussion, with some studies reporting relatively little consequence to delayed repair, while others argue for urgent or emergent operation to minimize adverse effects.[41,42] In general, the literature does not support the need to operate within 24 hours to prevent major morbidity and mortality, but early surgery is associated with reduced pain and length of stay. There is a tendency toward fewer major complications among patients medically stable at admission operated on within 48 hours. Patients for whom surgery is delayed to manage multiple comorbidities are at increased risk.

Preoperative traction (skin or skeletal) to decrease pain and assist in reduction of the fracture does not appear to be effective.[43] Pain control remains, in general, suboptimal for hip fracture patients. In a small trial in Israel, hip fracture patients randomized to full epidural analgesia in the emergency department had improved pain control and a significant reduction in cardiac events compared with patients receiving standard parenteral opioids.[44] Early exploration of the use of regional nerve blocks (femoral nerve, 3-in-1, fascia iliaca) has provided encouraging evidence that pain control is improved and, in some cases, is associated with improved outcomes and decreased postoperative delirium.[45–48] Use of regional analgesia and anesthesia in the emergency setting represents an important clinical advance and is worthy of further study.[49] Pressure sores are a frequent and debilitating complication for the hip fracture patient and are worthy of preventive efforts.[50]

The choice of anesthesia for hip fracture, regional versus general, has been a raging controversy for about 100 years. The anesthesia literature has been nicely reviewed and summarized recently by Gulur and colleagues.[51] A meta-analysis for the *Cochrane Database* concluded that mortality at 1 month but not at 3 months following anesthesia was decreased in patients who had regional anesthesia.[52] However, even in this meta-analysis, when the authors excluded the oldest trial, in which the general anesthesia patients had a very high mortality, 1-month mortality was no longer different. There are reports that indicate that blood loss and deep venous thrombosis are decreased with regional anesthesia, but not of sufficient magnitude to influence patient outcomes. Multiple investigators have hypothesized that regional anesthesia would be associated with a decreased incidence of delirium, but the results have been mixed. The current state of the art appears to be that either general or regional anesthesia may be safely employed for the patient with a fractured hip.[53] Gulur *et al.* specifically mention current regimens for prophylaxis against thromboembolism and the use of perioperative β-blockade as potential reasons that the difference between anesthetic techniques has become less compelling as a determinant of outcomes.[51]

Modest hypovolemia is difficult to recognize in elderly patients. Skin turgor, expression of thirst, and urine output may all be misleading. Both diuretic use and reduced fluid intake predispose older patients to chronic volume depletion, which is exacerbated by hemorrhage, immobility, and starvation in preparation for surgery. Unrecognized hypovolemia may lead to poor tissue perfusion, and thus to covert suboptimal organ function or overt organ failure. Fluid overload can be just as detrimental as hypovolemia. The combination of a senescent heart, in addition to a high prevalence of chronic heart failure, chronic renal failure, and vascular disease in patents with hip fractures suggests enhanced sensitivity to the effects of suboptimal intravascular volume. If these patients are much more sensitive to too much and too little intravenous volume, what guidance is available to make an appropriate decision? Unfortunately, fluid administration for hip fracture patients is subject to the same controversies as those associated with fluid administration in both elective surgery and multi-system trauma. In the past few years, a steady stream of literature has been arguing, in general, for less fluid administration than had been standard practice.[54] This argument, noting that fluid loading for neuraxial blockade is ineffective, that limited quantities of fluid accumulate in traumatized tissue, and that there is a lack of evidence for a nonanatomical third space, is that "standard fluid regimens" produce fluid overload and that limited fluid administration should not be considered restricted, but rather appropriate therapy, avoiding excess fluid.

There are no recent studies of patients with hip fractures that specifically consider the role of colloid versus crystalloid, so the practitioner is forced to extrapolate from a large but inconclusive experience with primarily elective surgery that, for the most part, fails to show any advantage for colloid solutions.[55] The data to direct transfusion practices suggests that there are few advantages to liberal transfusion. The largest and most comprehensive study to date found that a liberal transfusion strategy (transfuse at $< 10\,g/dL$), compared with a restrictive strategy (transfuse at $< 8\,g/dL$), did not reduce rates of death or in-hospital morbidity in elderly patients at high cardiovascular risk, nor did it impact on the ability to walk independently on 60-day follow-up.[56]

Esophageal Doppler and central venous pressure monitoring have been evaluated in small studies of patients undergoing general anesthesia.[57] Additional monitoring tended to result in additional fluid administration and may convey some short-term benefit in terms of length of hospital stay. There are no current data suggesting improved functional outcomes for patients who have a specific monitoring technique employed to manage fluid balance following hip fractures. The potential for these techniques to induce iatrogenic injury must be considered. A major limitation for the clinician is the absence of any trials evaluating such strategies in patients receiving regional anesthesia, which is favored by many clinicians. Based on the current available data, it is not possible to recommend routine use of invasive (central venous pressure) or specific noninvasive (esophageal Doppler or transesophageal echo) monitoring in patients undergoing surgery for an uncomplicated hip fracture. An ongoing study of a noninvasive cardiac monitor may provide at new direction.[58]

Most clinicians would agree that postoperative care should include high-quality analgesia. In one randomized study of epidural analgesia for hip fracture patients, documented superior analgesia with improved patient satisfaction scores did result in improved rehabilitation.[59] Multimodal approaches have also been successfully employed, including the use of ketamine.[60] As described above, there is an evolving appreciation for the use of nerve blocks in analgesia programs.[45-48] There is an extensive literature on the value of organized care programs that include input from orthopedic surgeons, anesthesiologists, geriatricians, nurses, and rehabilitation specialists.[61-63] These programs have generally provided excellent

care, but the documented improvements have not generated sufficient interest to change standards of care. Payment schedules do not favor these approaches a,nd multiple barriers to implementation persist.[64]

In caring for postoperative hip fracture patients, attention should be paid to the prevention of decubitus ulceration. Certain decubitus wound protection strategies, such as foam and alternating pressure mattresses, appear to be effective and should be considered as part of the overall care plan.[63] The development of delirium has been independently associated with poor functional outcomes in hip fracture patients. A program designed by Edward Marcantonio that included a proactive geriatric consultation has been effective in decreasing the incidence of delirium by about one-third in hip fracture patients when compared with usual care.[61] The administration of preoperative antibiotics and postoperative prophylaxis for deep venous thrombosis are both strongly supported by randomized controlled trials.[43,65]

Multisystem trauma patients

In 2012, the Eastern Association for the Surgery of Trauma (EAST) published an updated practice management guideline regarding the evaluation and management of the geriatric trauma patient.[66] The group reviewed citations published between the years 2000 and 2008 with the intention of providing evidence-based guidelines for trauma management of the elderly. The current report concludes that effective evidence-based care of aging patients necessitates aggressive triage, correction of coagulopathy, and limitation of care when clinical evidence points toward an overwhelming likelihood of poor long-term prognosis. This publication represents the most extensive effort to provide a common approach to geriatric trauma patients to date and a substantial improvement over the original publication from 2001. It should be reviewed by all clinicians caring for elderly trauma victims. Its suggested algorithm is worthy of review (Fig. 36.3).

Given the physiology of aging, one might suspect that the impact of trauma on the elderly is greater than on young trauma victims. The Trauma Audit and Research Network (TARN), a United-Kingdom-based database, found that mortality begins to rise sharply after 45 years of age, doubling at age 75.[67] Unfortunately, this represents essentially no change in over two decades.[68] In the early reports, this effect was noted for all mechanisms of injury and all injury severity scores, and this has been supported in subsequent reports (Figs. 36.4, 36.5).[67-69] However, the EAST workgroup cautions that, although age has some impact on mortality projections for a population of geriatric trauma patients, it is not possible to support a specific age above which geriatric trauma in-hospital mortality can be predicted.[66] Perhaps of greater interest, the literature supports the concept that, for those who do survive trauma, the long-term outcomes in terms of function are reasonably good. A recent report indicated that 65% of the patients survive hospitalization and as many as 85% of

Care of the Injured Elder: An evidence-based flow diagram

Figure 36.3 Algorithm for geriatric trauma. (From Eastern Association for the Surgery of Trauma practice management guideline, 2012,[66] reproduced with permission from Wolters Kluwer Health.)

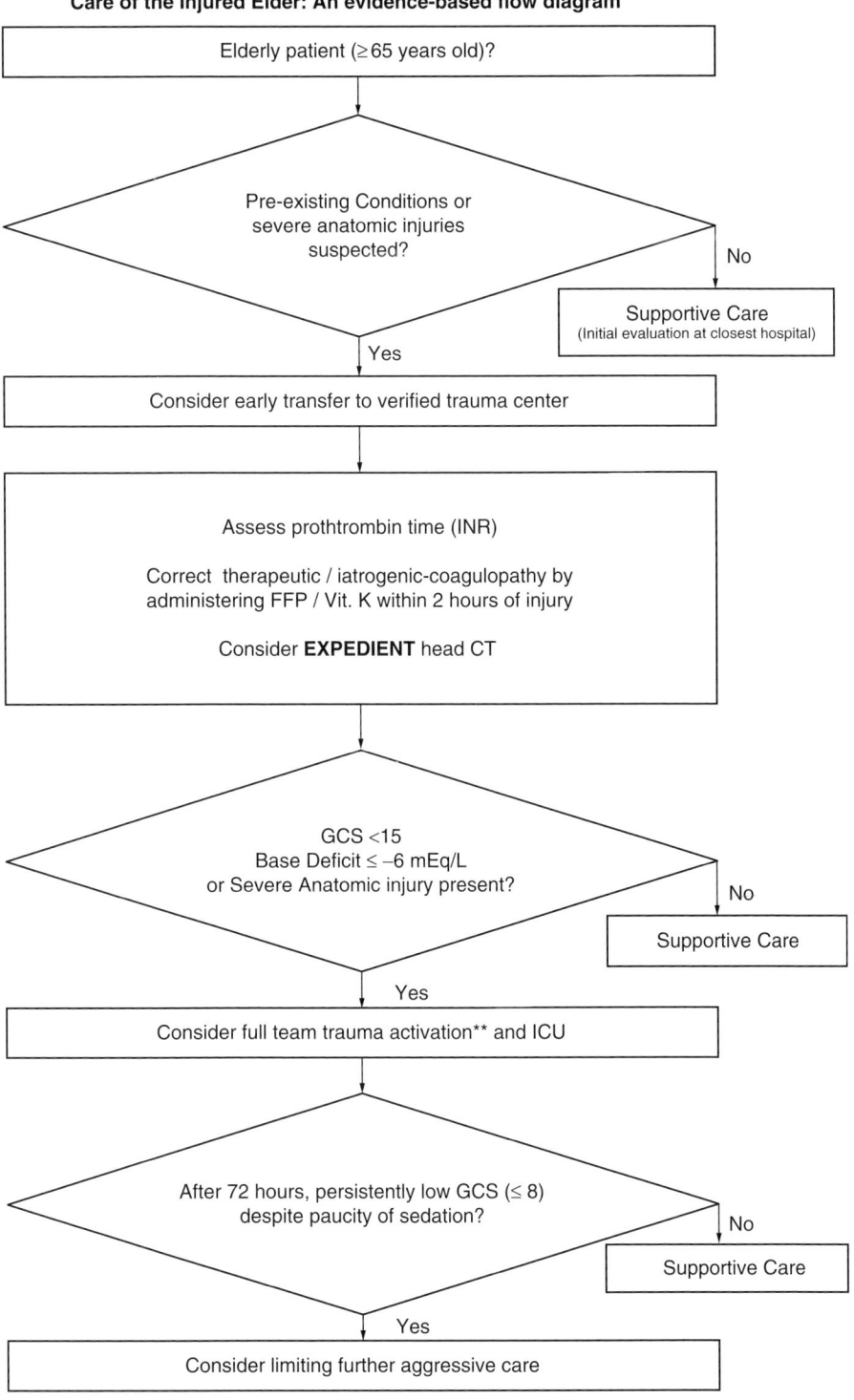

Elderly patient (≥65 years old)?

Pre-existing Conditions or severe anatomic injuries suspected?

No → Supportive Care (Initial evaluation at closest hospital)

Yes → Consider early transfer to verified trauma center

Assess prothrombin time (INR)

Correct therapeutic / iatrogenic-coagulopathy by administering FFP / Vit. K within 2 hours of injury

Consider **EXPEDIENT** head CT

GCS <15
Base Deficit ≤ –6 mEq/L
or Severe Anatomic injury present?

No → Supportive Care

Yes → Consider full team trauma activation** and ICU

After 72 hours, persistently low GCS (≤ 8) despite paucity of sedation?

No → Supportive Care

Yes → Consider limiting further aggressive care

**Evidence for benefit from full team activation derived from study of patients > 70 y.o.

survivors have been found to be functioning independently at home at follow-up intervals as long as 6 years post injury.[70,71] Based on this inability of age to predict early mortality and reasonable long-term functional outcomes for geriatric trauma patients surviving hospitalization, the EAST workgroup concluded that age "should not be used as the sole criterion for denying or limiting care."[66] Interestingly, the impact of pre-existing conditions on the outcome of trauma remains inconclusive.[72]

There are a number of indicators that have been associated with adverse outcomes which are useful to the clinician attempting to maximize the use of limited resources. It is

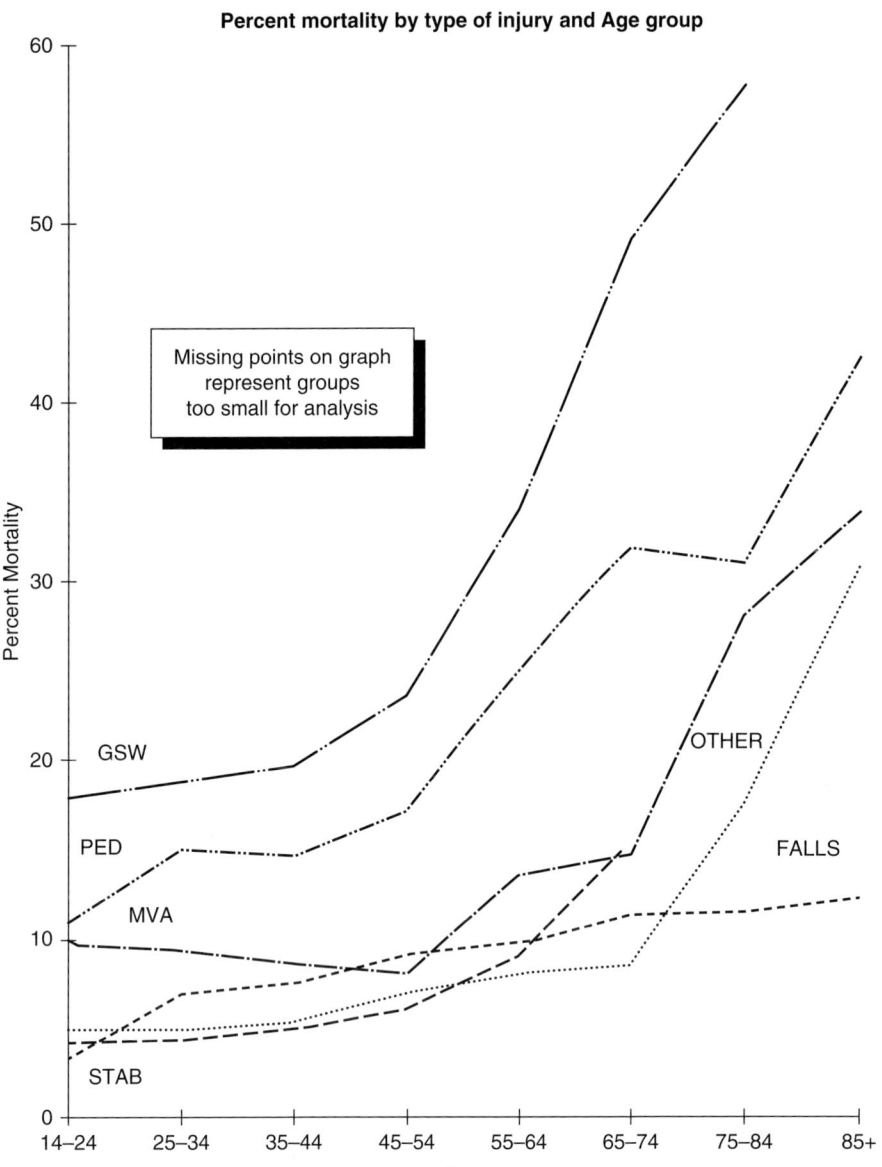

Percent mortality by type of injury and Age group

Figure 36.4 Percent mortality by type of injury. For all types of injury, mortality increases significantly with age. GSW, gunshot wound; MVA, motor vehicle accident (victim in the vehicle); STAB, stab wounds; PED, pedestrian accidents (victim outside of vehicle). (From Finelli FC, Jonsson J, Champion HR, *et al.* A case control study for major trauma in geriatric patients. *J Trauma* **29**: 1989; 541–8, reproduced with permission.)

important to realize that, for each finding, there is some level of controversy and most data come from retrospectively analyzed datasets. Nonetheless, these reports do provide some guidance to the clinician in his or her thinking about specific patients. Soles and Tornetta recommend that recognition of hypotension and hypoperfusion, despite normal or near normal vital signs on presentation, and early intensive monitoring and resuscitation improve survival.[73] Geriatric trauma patients are more likely to present in shock than similarly injured younger patients. The current guidelines no longer support indiscriminate use of pulmonary artery catheters and supranormal physiologic resuscitation, specifically noting the absence of level 1 or 2 evidence. The EAST group indicated that there is at best level 3 evidence to suggest that there is a benefit to optimization of cardiac index and the use of base deficit to determine resuscitation status.[66] Apart from the controversy described earlier regarding the tendency to administer less fluid to elderly surgical patients, there is little in the literature to guide the trauma practitioner. On the other side of the physiologic spectrum, elderly trauma patients who present with high systolic blood pressures appear to do better than younger patients, in whom elevated systolic blood pressure is found to predict mortality.[74]

When an elderly patient is involved in a traumatic event, age should not lower the threshold to triage victims directly to trauma centers. Nonetheless, even in the presence of a specific triage algorithm, Davis *et al.* found that patients over 55 were routinely not triaged correctly. The reasons for this were not clear, but it remains a concern given apparently improved outcomes in trauma centers.[75] On the basis of level 3 evidence,

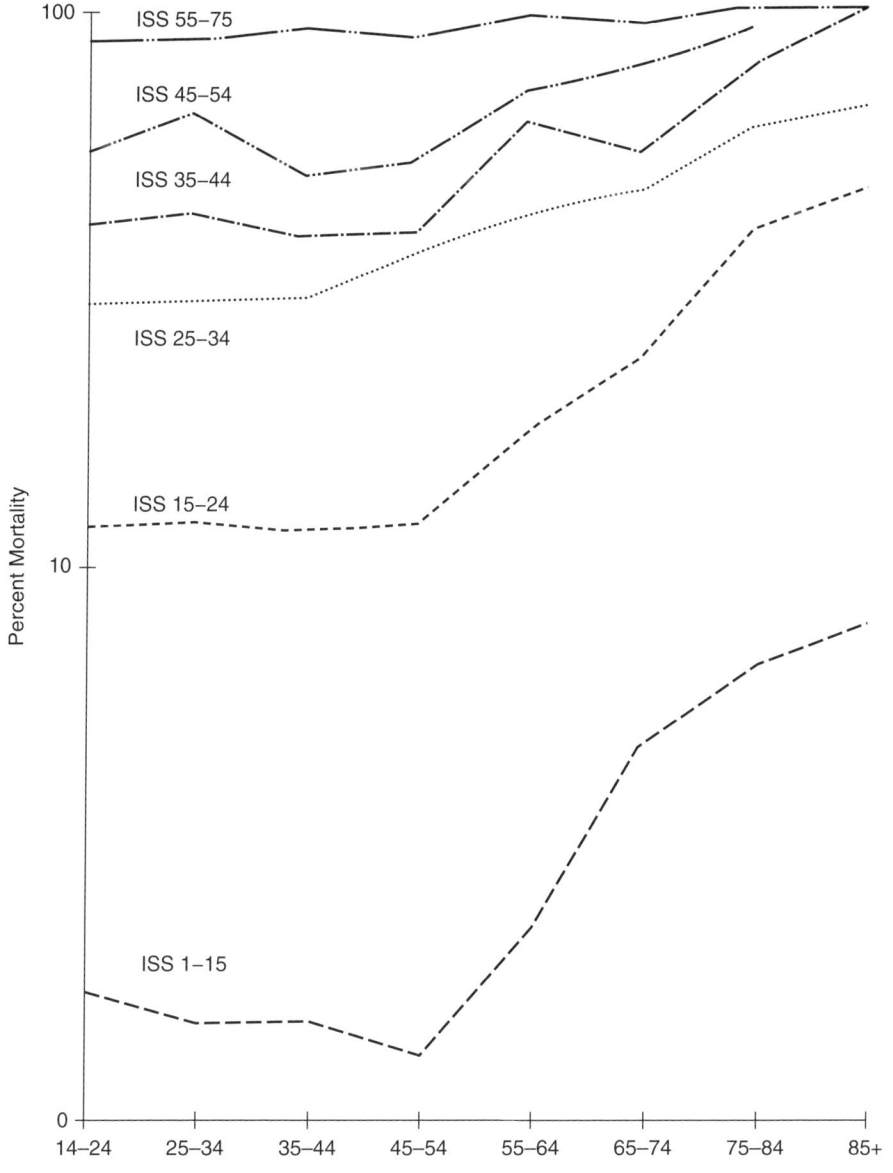

Percent Mortality by Injury Severity Score and Age Group

ISS 55–75

ISS 45–54

ISS 35–44

ISS 25–34

ISS 15–24

ISS 1–15

Percent Mortality

100

10

0

Age

14–24   25–34   35–44   45–54   55–64   65–74   75–84   85+

Figure 36.5 Percent mortality by Injury Severity Score (ISS). Even for ISS of 1–15, mortality increases after 54 years of age. (From Finelli FC, Jonsson J, Champion HR, *et al.* A case control study for major trauma in geriatric patients. *J Trauma* **29**: 1989; 541–8, reproduced with permission.)

the current guidelines recommend that elderly patients with one or more anatomic injuries should be treated at designated trauma centers, and preferably in an intensive care unit.[66]

Outcomes following traumatic brain injury in the elderly appear to be significantly worse than for younger patients, although the data supporting specific triage recommendations are lacking. The Glasgow Coma Scale (GCS) has been studied extensively, but experts are loath to suggest making triage decisions based solely on an admission GCS level. Nonetheless, patients with a GCS on admission of 7 or 8 have exceptionally bad outcomes.[66] The management of anticoagulation for elderly head trauma victims does appear crucial. Ivascu *et al.* studied a protocol to ensure rapid head computed

tomography, initiation of INR-correcting therapy within 1.9 hours, and full correction of coagulopathy within 4 hours of admission for elderly head trauma patients.[76,77] This approach demonstrated a greater than 75% decrease in mortality related to posttraumatic intracranial hemorrhage in elderly patients with coumadin-related coagulopathy.

Conclusions

Extensive information regarding the general physiologic alterations associated with aging, extensive knowledge of disease processes, and an understanding of trauma and resuscitation are all brought to bear in the care of elderly trauma victims.

Trauma clinicians can refine their approach to these patients by utilizing the available information, in particular, current concepts of pharmacology for the elderly. As for directly useful information to impact trauma care, apart from hip fractures, there is relatively little information available. The algorithm produced by the EAST group may be helpful.[66] Hopefully, this chapter will assist trauma clinicians to both become more proficient at caring for the elderly and more observant in searching for the keys to better trauma care for the elderly.

Questions

(1) **Concerning elderly multisystem trauma victims:**
   a. Those with a trauma score of 9 should be admitted to an ICU immediately
   b. Chronologic age should not be a basis for triage
   c. They have outcomes similar to younger patients following traumatic brain injury
   d. Age should lower the threshold for triage to a trauma center

(2) **In elderly patients with hip facture:**
   a. Transfusion using a hemoglobin threshold of 7 g/dL is as safe as using a 10 g/dL threshold
   b. Traction can be used to decrease pain
   c. Regional anesthesia improves all significant outcomes relative to general anesthesia
   d. Operating within 24 hours improves outcomes

(3) **When providing anesthesia to an elderly patient:**
   a. Both pharmacokinetic and pharmacodynamic alterations influence drug requirements
   b. Aging alters serum proteins in different way, so which protein binds a drug becomes important
   c. Requirements for nondepolarizing neuromuscular blockers are not altered with age
   d. All of the above are true

(4) **Following major surgery, elderly patients:**
   a. Rarely get emergence delirium
   b. Commonly suffer from delirium at 24–48 hours
   c. Routinely require 1–2 months to regain full consciousness
   d. Can be diagnosed with cognitive dysfunction postoperatively even without preoperative testing

(5) **In evaluating an elderly patient for surgery:**
   a. Patients with Parkinson's disease should never receive regional anesthesia
   b. Patients with dementing illness require additional volatile anesthetic
   c. Atelectasis will develop in the majority of patients receiving general anesthesia
   d. Evaluation of the airway requires observation of the size of the epiglottis

(6) **In the absence of coronary artery disease, an otherwise healthy elderly patient will have:**
   a. A slightly increased heart rate
   b. A decreased stroke volume
   c. A lower pulse pressure
   d. Decreased left ventricular diastolic relaxation

(7) **In evaluating an elderly trauma patient:**
   a. Chronologic age provides a good indication of organ function
   b. Preexisting disease is irrelevant
   c. A pulmonary artery catheter should be inserted in all patients older than 65 years
   d. Elderly patients who recover from trauma frequently retain their independence

Answers

(1) b
(2) a
(3) d
(4) b
(5) c
(6) d
(7) d

References

1. National Center for Health Statistics. *Health, United States, 2011: with special feature on socioeconomic status and health.* Hyattsville, MD: US Government Printing Office, 2012.

2. Rowe JW, Kahn RL. Successful aging. *Gerontologist* 1997; **37**: 433–40.

3. Rowe JW, Kahn RL. Successful aging and disease prevention. *Adv Ren Replace Ther* 2000; 7: 70–7.

4. Seals DR, Esler MD. Human ageing and the sympathoadrenal system. *J Physiol* 2000; **528**: 407–17.

5. Esler M, Hastings J, Lambert G, *et al.* The influence of aging on the human sympathetic nervous system and brain norepinephrine turnover. *Am J Physiol Regul Integr Comp Physiol* 2002; **282**: R909–16.

6. Aschbacher K, O'Donovan A, Wolkowitz OM, *et al.* Good stress, bad stress and oxidative stress: insights from anticipatory cortisol reactivity. *Psychoneuroendocrinology* 2013; **38**: 1698–708.

7. Bloss EB, Janssen WG, McEwen BS, Morrison JH. Interactive effects of stress and aging on structural plasticity in the prefrontal cortex. *J Neurosci* 2010; **30**: 6726–31.

8. Arikanoglu A, Akil E, Varol S, *et al.* Relationship of cognitive performance with prolidase and oxidative stress in Alzheimer disease. *Neurol Sci* 2013; **34**: 2117–21.

9. Tsai H, Pottorf WJ, Buchholz JN, Duckles SP. Adrenergic nerve smooth endoplasmic reticulum calcium buffering declines with age. *Neurobiol Aging* 1998; **19**: 89–96.

10. Tsai H, Buchholz J, Duckles SP. Postjunctional alpha 2-adrenoceptors in blood vessels: Effect of age. *Eur J Pharmacol* 1993; **237**: 311–16.

11. Buchholz J, Tsai H, Friedman D, Duckles SP. Influence of age on control of norepinephrine release from the rat tail artery. *J Pharmacol Exp Ther* 1992; **260**: 722–7.

12. Simoes RP, Bonjorno JC, Beltrame T, *et al.* Slower heart rate and oxygen consumption kinetic responses in the on- and off-transient during a discontinuous incremental exercise: effects of aging. *Rev Braz J Phys Ther* 2013; **17**: 69–76.

13. Fleg JL, Morrell CH, Bos AG, *et al.* Accelerated longitudinal decline of aerobic capacity in healthy older adults. *Circulation* 2005; **112**: 674–82.

14. Hollenberg M, Yang J, Haight TJ, Tager IB. Longitudinal changes in aerobic capacity: implications for concepts of aging. *J Gerontol A Biol Sci Med Sci* 2006; **61**: 851–8.

15. Lakatta EG, Levy D. Arterial and cardiac aging: major shareholders in cardiovascular disease enterprises: Part I: Aging arteries: a "set up" for vascular disease. *Circulation* 2003; **107**: 139–46.

16. Lakatta EG, Levy D. Arterial and cardiac aging: major shareholders in cardiovascular disease enterprises: Part II: The aging heart in health: links to heart disease. *Circulation* 2003; **107**: 346–54.

17. Lakatta EG. Arterial and cardiac aging: major shareholders in cardiovascular disease enterprises: Part III: Cellular and molecular clues to heart and arterial aging. *Circulation* 2003; **107**: 490–7.

18. Willum-Hansen T, Staessen JA, Torp-Pedersen C, *et al.* Prognostic value of aortic pulse wave velocity as index of arterial stiffness in the general population. *Circulation* 2006; **113**: 664–70.

19. Dolan E, Thijs L, Li Y, *et al.* Ambulatory arterial stiffness index as a predictor of cardiovascular mortality in the Dublin outcome study. *Hypertension* 2006; **47**: 365–70.

20. Kitzman DW, Daniel KR. Diastolic heart failure in the elderly. *Clin Geriatr Med* 2007; **23**: 83–106.

21. Lanier GM, Vaishnava P, Kosmas CE, *et al.* An update on diastolic dysfunction. *Cardiol Rev* 2012; **20**: 230–6.

22. Tung P, Albert CM. Causes and prevention of sudden cardiac death in the elderly. *Nat Rev Cardiol* 2013; **10**: 135–42.

23. Lawrence VA, Hilsenbeck SG, Mulrow CD, *et al.* Incidence and hospital stay for cardiac and pulmonary complications after abdominal surgery. *J Gen Intern Med* 1995; **10**: 671–8.

24. Lawrence VA, Hilsenbeck SG, Noveck H, Poses RM, Carson JL. Medical complications and outcomes after hip fracture repair. *Arch Intern Med* 2002; **162**: 2053–7.

25. Zaugg M, Lucchinetti E. Respiratory function in the elderly. *Anesthesiol Clin North America* 2000; **18**: 47, 58, vi.

26. Raine JM, Bishop JM. A difference in O_2 tension and physiological dead space in normal man. *J Appl Physiol* 1963; **18**: 284–8.

27. Malmrose LC, Gray SL, Pieper CF, *et al.* Measured versus estimated creatinine clearance in a high-functioning elderly sample: MacArthur foundation study of successful aging. *J Am Geriatr Soc* 1993; **41**: 715–21.

28. Spruill WJ, Wade WE, Cobb HH. Comparison of estimated glomerular filtration rate with estimated creatinine clearance in the dosing of drugs requiring adjustments in elderly patients with declining renal function. *Am J Geriatr Pharmacother* 2008; **6**: 153–60.

29. Deiner S, Silverstein JH. Postoperative delirium and cognitive dysfunction. *Br J Anaesth* 2009; **103** (Suppl 1): i41–6.

30. Silverstein JH, Timberger M, Reich DL, Uysal S. Central nervous system dysfunction after noncardiac surgery and anesthesia in the elderly. *Anesthesiology* 2007; **106**: 622–8.

31. Inouye SK, van Dyck CH, Alessi CA, *et al.* Clarifying confusion: the confusion assessment method: a new method for detection of delirium. *Ann Intern Med* 1990; **113**: 941–8.

32. Ely EW, Margolin R, Francis J, *et al.* Evaluation of delirium in critically ill patients: validation of the confusion assessment method for the intensive care unit (CAM-ICU). *Crit Care Med* 2001; **29**: 1370–9.

33. Deiner S, Silverstein JH. Long-term outcomes in elderly surgical patients. *Mt Sinai J Med* 2012; **79**: 95–106.

34. Shafer SL. The pharmacology of anesthetic drugs in elderly patients. *Anesthesiol Clin North America* 2000; **18**: 1, 29, v.

35. Trifiro G, Spina E. Age-related changes in pharmacodynamics: focus on drugs acting on central nervous and cardiovascular systems. *Curr Drug Metab* 2011; **12**: 611–20.

36. Shi S, Klotz U. Age-related changes in pharmacokinetics. *Curr Drug Metab* 2011; **12**: 601–10.

37. McLachlan AJ, Pont LG. Drug metabolism in older people: a key consideration in achieving optimal outcomes with medicines. *J Gerontol A Biol Sci Med Sci* 2012; **67**: 175–80.

38. Barrett-Connor E. The economic and human costs of osteoporotic fracture. *Am J Med* 1995; **98** (2A): 3S–8S.

39. Haentjens P, Lamraski G, Boonen S. Costs and consequences of hip fracture occurrence in old age: an economic perspective. *Disabil Rehabil* 2005; **27**: 1129–41.

40. Currie LM. Fall and injury prevention. *Annu Rev Nurs Res* 2006; **24**: 39–74.

41. Shiga T, Wajima Z, Ohe Y. Is operative delay associated with increased mortality of hip fracture patients? Systematic review, meta-analysis, and meta-regression. *Can J Anaesth* 2008; **55**: 146–54.

42. Simunovic N, Devereaux PJ, Sprague S, *et al.* Effect of early surgery after hip fracture on mortality and complications: systematic review and meta-analysis. *CMAJ* 2010; **182**: 1609–16.

43. Handoll HH, Queally JM, Parker MJ. Pre-operative traction for hip fractures in adults. *Cochrane Database Syst Rev* 2011; (12): CD000168.

44. Matot I, Oppenheim-Eden A, Ratrot R, *et al.* Preoperative cardiac events in elderly patients with hip fracture randomized to epidural or conventional analgesia. *Anesthesiology* 2003; **98**: 156–63.

45. Hogh A, Dremstrup L, Jensen SS, Lindholt J. Fascia iliaca compartment block performed by junior registrars as a supplement to pre-operative analgesia for patients with hip fracture. *Strategies Trauma Limb Reconstr* 2008; **3**: 65–70.

46. Dulaney-Cripe E, Hadaway S, Bauman R, *et al.* A continuous infusion fascia iliaca compartment block in hip fracture patients: a pilot study. *J Clin Med Res* 2012; **4**: 45–8.

47. Kunisawa T, Ota M, Suzuki A, Takahata O, Iwasaki H. Combination of high-dose dexmedetomidine sedation and fascia iliaca compartment block for

hip fracture surgery. *J Clin Anesth* 2010; **22**: 196–200.

48. Mouzopoulos G, Vasiliadis G, Lasanianos N, *et al.* Fascia iliaca block prophylaxis for hip fracture patients at risk for delirium: a randomized placebo-controlled study. *J Orthop Traumatol* 2009; **10**: 127–33.

49. Godoy Monzon D, Iserson KV, Vazquez JA. Single fascia iliaca compartment block for post-hip fracture pain relief. *J Emerg Med* 2007; **32**: 257–62.

50. Arblaster GM. Reducing pressure sores after hip fractures. *Prof Nurse* 1998; **13**: 749–52.

51. Gulur P, Nishimori M, Ballantyne JC. Regional anaesthesia versus general anaesthesia, morbidity and mortality. *Best Pract Res Clin Anaesthesiol* 2006; **20**: 249–63.

52. Parker MJ, Handoll HH, Griffiths R. Anaesthesia for hip fracture surgery in adults. *Cochrane Database Syst Rev* 2004; (4): CD000521.

53. Luger TJ, Kammerlander C, Gosch M, *et al.* Neuroaxial versus general anaesthesia in geriatric patients for hip fracture surgery: does it matter? *Osteoporos Int* 2010; **21** (Suppl 4): S555–72.

54. Brandstrup B. Fluid therapy for the surgical patient. *Best Pract Res Clin Anaesthesiol* 2006; **20**: 265–83.

55. Perel P, Roberts I. Colloids versus crystalloids for fluid resuscitation in critically ill patients. *Cochrane Database Syst Rev.* 2012; **6**: CD000567.

56. Carson JL, Terrin ML, Noveck H, *et al.* Liberal or restrictive transfusion in high-risk patients after hip surgery. *N Engl J Med* 2011; **365**: 2453–62.

57. Price JD, Sear JW, Venn RM. Perioperative fluid volume optimization following proximal femoral fracture. *Cochrane Database Syst Rev.* 2004; (1): CD003004.

58. Wiles MD, Whiteley WJ, Moran CG, Moppett IK. The use of LiDCO based fluid management in patients undergoing hip fracture surgery under spinal anaesthesia: neck of femur optimisation therapy – targeted stroke volume (NOTTS). Study protocol for a randomized controlled trial. *Trials* 2011; **12**: 213.

59. Foss NB, Kristensen MT, Kristensen BB, Jensen PS, Kehlet H. Effect of postoperative epidural analgesia on rehabilitation and pain after hip fracture surgery: a randomized, double-blind, placebo-controlled trial. *Anesthesiology* 2005; **102**: 1197–204.

60. Remerand F, Le Tendre C, Baud A, *et al.* The early and delayed analgesic effects of ketamine after total hip arthroplasty: a prospective, randomized, controlled, double-blind study. *Anesth Analg* 2009; **109**: 1963–71.

61. Marcantonio ER, Flacker JM, Wright RJ, Resnick NM. Reducing delirium after hip fracture: a randomized trial. *J Am Geriatr Soc* 2001; **49**: 516–22.

62. Foss NB, Christensen DS, Krasheninnikoff M, Kristensen BB, Kehlet H. Post-operative rounds by anaesthesiologists after hip fracture surgery: a pilot study. *Acta Anaesthesiol Scand* 2006; **50**: 437–42.

63. Beaupre LA, Cinats JG, Senthilselvan A, *et al.* Reduced morbidity for elderly patients with a hip fracture after implementation of a perioperative evidence-based clinical pathway. *Qual Saf Health Care* 2006; **15**: 375–9.

64. Kates SL, O'Malley N, Friedman SM, Mendelson DA. Barriers to implementation of an organized geriatric fracture program. *Geriatr Orthop Surg Rehabil* 2012; **3**: 8–16.

65. Mak JC, Cameron ID, March LM, National Health and Medical Research Council. Evidence-based guidelines for the management of hip fractures in older persons: an update. *Med J Aust* 2010; **192**: 37–41.

66. Calland JF, Ingraham AM, Martin N, *et al.* Evaluation and management of geriatric trauma: an Eastern Association for the Surgery of Trauma practice management guideline. *J Trauma Acute Care Surg* 2012; **73** (5 Suppl 4): S345–50.

67. Giannoudis PV, Harwood PJ, Court-Brown C, Pape HC. Severe and multiple trauma in older patients: incidence and mortality. *Injury* 2009; **40**: 362–7.

68. Champion HR, Copes WS, Sacco WJ, *et al.* The major trauma outcome study: establishing national norms for trauma care. *J Trauma* 1990; **30**: 1356–65.

69. Richter M, Pape HC, Otte D, Krettek C. The current status of road user injuries among the elderly in Germany: a medical and technical accident analysis. *J Trauma* 2005; **58**: 591–5.

70. Zietlow SP, Capizzi PJ, Bannon MP, Farnell MB. Multisystem geriatric trauma. *J Trauma* 1994; **37**: 985–8.

71. Grossman MD, Ofurum U, Stehly CD, Stoltzfus J. Long-term survival after major trauma in geriatric trauma patients: the glass is half full. *J Trauma Acute Care Surg* 2012; **72**: 1181–5.

72. Labib N, Nouh T, Winocour S, *et al.* Severely injured geriatric population: morbidity, mortality, and risk factors. *J Trauma* 2011; **71**: 1908–14.

73. Soles GL, Tornetta P. Multiple trauma in the elderly: new management perspectives. *J Orthop Trauma* 2011; **25** (Suppl 2): S61–5.

74. Ley EJ, Singer MB, Gangi A, *et al.* Elevated systolic blood pressure after trauma: tolerated in the elderly. *J Surg Res* 2012; **177**: 326–9.

75. Davis JS, Allan BJ, Sobowale O, *et al.* Evaluation of a new elderly trauma triage algorithm. *South Med J* 2012; **105**: 447–51.

76. Ivascu FA, Janczyk RJ, Junn FS, *et al.* Treatment of trauma patients with intracranial hemorrhage on preinjury warfarin. *J Trauma* 2006; **61**: 318–21.

77. Ivascu FA, Howells GA, Junn FS, *et al.* Rapid warfarin reversal in anticoagulated patients with traumatic intracranial hemorrhage reduces hemorrhage progression and mortality. *J Trauma* 2005; **59**: 1131–7.

Trauma in pregnancy

John R. Fisgus, Kalpana Tyagaraj, and Vanetta Levesque

Objectives

(1) Review the etiology of trauma in pregnant patients.

(2) Discuss the physiologic changes of pregnancy and their impact on anesthetic management of a pregnant trauma patient.

(3) List the various causes of maternal and fetal morbidity and mortality associated with different types of trauma.

(4) Be able to triage a pregnant trauma patient and understand the impact of gestational age on resuscitation.

(5) Review the principles of cardiorespiratory resuscitation in a pregnant patient, including perimortem cesarean delivery.

Introduction

The pregnant trauma patient presents significant challenges to all healthcare providers. The pregnant trauma victim represents two (or more) patients that are at risk, each needing evaluation and potentially treatment. Unfortunately trauma in pregnancy is not uncommon, complicating approximately 7% of all pregnancies and responsible for 0.3–0.4% of maternal hospital admissions.[1] Trauma is the most common cause of maternal death in the United States.[2] Mechanisms of trauma during pregnancy include motor vehicle collisions (MVCs), domestic violence,[3] falls,[4] and penetrating injuries .[5] Unique injuries due to the expanding uterus and developing fetus must be taken into consideration in the pregnant trauma patient.

Many providers are involved in the care of the pregnant patient: at the trauma scene, in the emergency department, and in the operating room. The anesthesiologist can play a key role in the care and management of the pregnant trauma victim. All anesthesiologists have training in obstetric anesthesia during their residency and frequently cover obstetric units in hospitals where pregnant patients are cared for. On the other hand, most nonobstetric physicians have little obstetric exposure and may be uncomfortable caring for the pregnant patient because of unfamiliarity with the physiologic changes of pregnancy or the evaluation of fetal well-being. This is not only a source of stress for other trauma providers, but can put maternal well-being at risk. Nonobstetric physicians may hesitate to order necessary diagnostic and therapeutic interventions for fear of doing the "wrong thing," all because the patient is pregnant. A multidisciplinary approach to the pregnant trauma patient, involving trauma surgeons, obstetricians, anesthesiologists, emergency medicine physicians, and other providers, is critical to deliver optimal care and achieve the best outcome possible.

With pregnancy comes the challenge of caring for two patients at once – the mother and the fetus. In general, providing optimal maternal care is the best strategy to optimize fetal survival.[6,7] In early pregnancy, the only way to save the fetus is to save the mother. The physiologic changes of pregnancy and fetal physiologic requirement will have an impact on the decision-making process.[8]

The trauma team must include providers familiar with the complications related to maternal trauma. Placental abruption, for example, is a major concern in abdominal trauma.[9,10] The pregnant patient may not exhibit significant symptoms initially. The fetus meanwhile may suffer serious compromise or even death. If not quickly recognized, placental abruption can eventually lead to maternal hypovolemia, hypotension, hypoxemia, and death from exsanguination. Abruption is but one of a number of sequelae related to pregnancy that the trauma team must be prepared to deal with.[11]

Physiologic changes in pregnancy
What makes the pregnant patient different?

Pregnancy produces a wide range of physiologic alterations that will affect maternal care (Table 37.1). Knowing the physiologic changes of pregnancy is imperative to correctly evaluate and safely manage the pregnant trauma victim. Most major organ systems are affected by these physiologic changes. Also, these changes are a dynamic process over the course of normal pregnancy. Thus, the knowledge of fetal gestational age is important not only for fetal evaluations and concerns, but also to know what physiologic changes in the mother can be expected at any point in time. Maternal disease states such as toxemia of pregnancy can further alter the physiologic maternal state and complicate care.

Trauma Anesthesia, 2nd Edition, ed. Charles E. Smith. Published by Cambridge University Press. © Charles E. Smith, 2015.

Table 37.1 Physiologic changes of pregnancy and their anesthetic implications

Physiologic changes	Anesthetic implications
Cardiovascular	
↑ Blood volume	Masks signs of hypovolemia
↑ Cardiac output	Masks signs of hypovolemia
↓ Blood pressure	
ECG changes	Mimic myocardial ischemia or cardiac contusion
↓ Cardiac filling pressures	
Aortocaval compression	Mimics hemorrhagic shock
Pulmonary	
↑ Functional residual capacity	Rapid onset of hypoxemia
	Increased uptake of inhaled agents
↑ Oxygen consumption	Rapid onset of hypoxemia
Alveolar hyperventilation and respiratory alkalosis	↓ Buffering capacity
Gastrointestinal	
↓ Gastric emptying	↑ Incidence of reflux and aspiration
↓ Gastroesophageal sphincter tone	
Displacement of small intestine into the abdomen	↑ Risk of upper abdominal penetrating injuries
Renal and genitourinary	
↑ Renal blood flow and glomerular filtration rate	Natriuresis
↓ Blood urea and creatinine	Fluid challenge is needed to differentiate prerenal vs. renal oliguria
Endocrine	
Diabetogenic state	Monitor glucose and electrolyte abnormalities
Hematologic	
↓ Hematocrit	Anemia, internal bleeding
↑ White blood cells	Infection
↑ Coagulation factors	Thromboembolic disease

Cardiovascular changes

Blood volume changes significantly during pregnancy. Maternal blood volume increases approximately 25%, beginning in the second trimester, then peaks in the third trimester at approximately 40–50% above baseline levels. The increase in blood volume is the result of an increase in both red blood cell mass and plasma volume. Plasma volume increases up to 40–50% above baseline.[12] The red blood cell mass also increases, but to a lesser extent, about 30% above baseline levels, which accounts for what is called the *physiologic anemia of pregnancy*.[13] The "normal" hematocrit of approximately 40% will decrease in pregnancy to between 29% and 32% by the end of the 34th week of gestation. The rise in maternal blood volume is seen as a protective physiologic effect for the mother, because potentially significant blood loss can occur during delivery.

Clinically, then, the parturient may suffer significant blood loss that may not be appreciated.[10] Maternal blood pressure/heart rate may remain relatively normal even with blood loss of up to 2 L. Maternal vital signs are maintained at the expense of uteroplacental blood flow as well as perfusion of other organs. Thus, fetal distress may be an earlier indicator of significant intravascular blood loss. Once blood loss exceeds 1.5–2 L, signs of maternal hypovolemia will likely become apparent. The relatively low hematocrit of pregnancy may be mistaken as a sign of blood loss from hemorrhage and raise concern that the patient needs further evaluation.

Cardiac output increases 30–50% throughout pregnancy, with up to half of the increase by the eighth week of gestation and peaking in the third trimester.[14] Early rise in cardiac output is a function of the increase in blood volume. Heart rate increases a modest 15% during this time. Blood pressure in normal pregnancy decreases by 20% as a result of a progesterone-induced decrease in systemic vascular resistance (SVR).[15] Central venous pressure (CVP) and pulmonary artery (PA) pressures also decrease in pregnancy. Thus, pregnant patients have lower filling pressures. Clinically, the assessment of hypovolemia can be more difficult – as heart rate and blood pressure are lower than in the nonpregnant state.

Electrocardiographic (ECG) changes occur during normal pregnancy. The heart is rotated left in pregnancy, resulting in a left axis deviation up to 20%. Nonspecific ST changes can occur, with the appearance of Q waves in leads II, III, and aVF resulting from the elevation of the diaphragm due to the expanding uterus. The ECG changes can be misinterpreted for myocardial contusion after chest trauma.

Uterine enlargement during pregnancy can lead to decreased venous return after the 20th week of gestation if the patient is placed supine. This condition is known as *supine hypotensive syndrome*, and it is critical that healthcare providers be familiar with this phenomenon of hypotension, which can mimic shock. Decreases in venous return may cause hypotension that can be detrimental for both mother and fetus. Because the uteroplacental blood flow lacks autoregulation, decreased blood pressure can lead to insufficient oxygen delivery to the fetus. It is essential that the pregnant patient not be placed supine after the 20th week of gestation. If the patient is supine, the uterus needs to be shifted – preferably leftward approximately 20–30% to relieve uterine obstruction of the inferior vena cava (IVC).[16] Cardiac output has been shown to increase as much as 25% after relieving uterine obstruction of the IVC by left uterine displacement.[17]

Pulmonary changes

Though a myriad of pulmonary parameters change during pregnancy, it is important to focus on the changes that have the most clinical ramifications.

Functional residual capacity (FRC) decreases in pregnancy by approximately 20% as a result of both diaphragmatic embarrassment and weight gain in pregnancy.[18] This, combined with an increased tendency for small airway collapse and ventilation/perfusion (V/Q) mismatching, results in a decrease in oxygen reserve.[19] At the same time, oxygen consumption increases from both the fetal metabolic demands and the maternal physiologic changes. Oxygen consumption is increased 20% at term.[18] The combination of decreased FRC and increased O_2 demand predisposes the parturient to rapid oxygen desaturation should apnea occur (e.g., during rapid sequence induction and intubation [RSI]). Maternal oxygenation/ventilation must be rapidly reestablished, or maternal cardiac arrest will follow.

Maternal tidal volume and respiratory rate increase in pregnancy in response to progesterone stimulation of the medullary respiratory centers. This causes a decrease in maternal PCO_2 to about 32 mmHg, which results in a respiratory alkalosis.[20] The renal response is to excrete bicarbonate to produce a compensatory metabolic acidosis. The management of the critically ill pregnant patient must keep in mind the altered acid–base parameters of pregnancy when managing ventilatory support.

As pregnancy progresses, airway edema and weight gain occur, which can result in difficult tracheal intubation. Failed intubation occurs eight times more frequently in the pregnant than in the nonpregnant patient. Moreover, the tissue of the maternal airway is more friable, such that multiple laryngoscopic attempts and/or traumatic attempts can result in bleeding and swelling of the airway with subsequent inability to bag-mask ventilate the lungs. Caution must be employed to minimize the risk of tissue trauma and edema due to unsuccessful attempts with conventional laryngoscopy. The clinical point to know is that tracheal intubation of the pregnant patient must be approached with care. It is critical that smaller endotracheal tubes (size 6.0–7.0 ETT) should be available for maternal intubations. Alternative methods of controlling and securing the airway must also be immediately available, such as videolaryngoscopy, laryngeal mask airway (LMA), gum elastic bougie, flexible fiberoptic bronchoscope, and surgical airway equipment (see Chapter 3).

Gastrointestinal changes

Progesterone levels increase in pregnancy, resulting in reduced smooth muscle tone, including the smooth muscle of the esophagus and esophageal sphincter. There is also a mechanical effect on the gastroesophageal junction that is a result of pressure from the expanding uterus on the stomach itself. The net result is to compromise the gastroesophageal sphincter.[21] Pregnant patients in the second/third trimester are then at increased risk of gastroesophageal reflux and potentially life-threatening aspiration of gastric contents. When tracheal intubation is anticipated, suction must be immediately available. Techniques such as RSI and cricoid pressure are used to minimize the aspiration risk (see Chapters 3 and 13). In the event the patient has eaten recently, medications that increase gastric emptying, such as metoclopramide, may be of use. Medications such as ranitidine can help raise gastric pH as prophylaxis against low pH gastric fluid aspiration when given 45 minutes to an hour prior to surgery.

Hematologic changes

Clotting factors increase significantly during pregnancy, leading to a hypercoagulable state. Serum fibrinogen level can increase 100% above normal values, while factors VII, VIII, IX, and X all increase.[21] At the same time, prothrombin, activated partial partial thromboplastin time (aPTT), and international normalized ratio (INR) all remain normal. The hypercoagulable state puts the patient at risk for pulmonary embolism. If fibrinogen levels are "normal" late in pregnancy, this may indicate the presence of a significant coagulopathy developing. Trauma-induced placental injury such as abruption can lead to disseminated intravascular coagulation (DIC) and hypofibrinogenemia.

Renal/genitourinary tract alterations

Increased renal blood flow and glomerular filtration rate result in a natriuresis. Progesterone can affect the smooth muscle of the ureter, allowing reflux. Hydronephrosis and hydroureter can occur in pregnancy secondary to uterine compression. It may therefore be difficult to evaluate fluid status by using urinary output as the sole parameter. Response to fluid challenges can sometimes be helpful in evaluating prerenal vs. renal causes of oliguria. Urinary tract infections are common in pregnancy as a result of ureteral reflux and can be a common source of fever.

Incidence and etiology of trauma

In the United States, the incidence of trauma in pregnancy ranges from 6% to 8%.[22,23] Maternal death rates have been reported as high as 11% after trauma.[24] Trauma is the leading cause of death for all women of childbearing age. Pregnant trauma victims tend to be younger, less severely injured, and more likely of African-American or Hispanic descent compared with nonpregnant victims of trauma. Drugs and alcohol are a factor in about 20% of maternal trauma.

Likewise, in the United States, MVCs account for almost two-thirds of all maternal trauma-related deaths, while falls and domestic violence comprise a large percentage of the rest. With MVCs, the use of seatbelts in pregnancy is an important factor in limiting injury.[25] The unrestrained pregnant driver is at higher risk of both maternal and fetal death, premature delivery (i.e., within 48 hours of trauma), and low-birth-weight

Table 37.2 Maternal injuries associated with trauma

1. Placental abruption
2. Premature rupture of membranes
3. Premature labor/delivery
4. Uterine rupture
5. Direct uterine/fetal injury from penetrating trauma more likely in the second and third trimester
6. Splenic rupture
7. Retroperitoneal hemorrhage
8. Hepatic injury
9. Hematoma
10. Bowel injury – uncommon due to protection from gravid uterus
11. Amniotic fluid embolism

Table 37.3 Direct and indirect fetal injuries from trauma

1. **Direct**
   a. Organ rupture
   b. Spinal/cranial fractures
   c. Intracranial hemorrhage
   d. Umbilical cord rupture
2. **Indirect**
   a. Placental abruption
   b. Uterine rupture
   c. Fetomaternal hemorrhage
   d. Preterm labor
   e. Isoimmunization

infants.[26] Unrestrained pregnant drivers were at higher risk of fetal death and significantly more blood loss compared with restrained pregnant trauma victims.[27] The restrained pregnant patient had no greater risk of poor pregnancy outcomes when compared with pregnant nontraumatized females.[28]

Minor trauma is very common during pregnancy and accounts for 90% of third-trimester injuries. With what would otherwise be "minor trauma," pregnancy-related complications occur in up to 10% of these cases.[29] Severe trauma in the third trimester occurs in only about 1% of cases of all pregnancies.

As would be expected, maternal/fetal mortality depends on the severity of the patient's injuries. Factors that are predictive of fetal demise include an Injury Severity Score (ISS) of more than 15, and abbreviated injury scores of ≥ 3 of the head, abdomen, thoracic, and lower extremities.[30] A Glasgow Coma Scale (GCS) score of ≤ 8 (see Table 35.1, Chapter 35), elevated base deficit, and abnormal uterine activity have also been predictive of poor fetal outcome.

Pregnancy-related complications are highest after assault, most likely because of trauma directed at the fetus. Fetal/neonatal death does not necessarily correlate with severity of maternal injury. Fetal loss occurs in 1–3% of cases considered "minor trauma." When trauma is considered "severe," fetal loss occurs in 50% of cases.[31] Risk of fetal mortality does not appear to be related to other factors such as medications, surgical procedures, or anesthesia.

Risk factors for maternal trauma

Risk factors for maternal trauma include young age (< 25 years), African-American or Hispanic race, use of illicit drugs and alcohol, domestic violence, noncompliance with proper seatbelt use, and low socioeconomic status.[32] The influence of intoxicating substances is significant. The data from the American College of Surgeons National Trauma Bank revealed that 19.6% and 12.9% of pregnancy-related traumas were attributable to the use of illicit drugs and alcohol respectively. One study showed that 45% of the pregnant patients with MVCs showed intoxicant use. Drug and alcohol abuse is also associated with significantly lower use of restraints while

driving than among nonusers (22% versus 46% respectively). Education about the use of illicit drugs and alcohol and proper use of seatbelts clearly has a role in preventing maternal injuries (see Chapter 41).

Mechanisms of injury

The most frequent mechanisms of maternal and fetal injury are summarized in Tables 37.2 and 37.3.[33]

Blunt injury

Blunt trauma is more common than penetrating injuries, and is often due to MVCs. Abdominal injuries may result (e.g., injury to a solid viscus: see Chapters 31 and 32). The severity of the impact is proportional to the force of the impact and exacerbated by the resistance of the abdominal wall. Blunt abdominal trauma is associated with splenic rupture and retroperitoneal hemorrhage. Injury to hollow viscera occurs at points of relative fixation such as the cecum, duodenum, and hepatic and splenic flexures. Hollow viscera are less likely to be injured because of greater mobility and ability to collapse when empty. Injury to solid abdominal organs can be managed nonoperatively in a stable pregnant patient. Unstable patients and those with injury to the intestines will benefit from early exploratory laparotomy, as hypotension and sepsis can be lethal for the fetus as well as the mother.

More challenging is the management of pelvic fracture, leading to massive hemorrhage, shock, and significant maternal and fetal death.[34] The most common cause of fetal death is placental abruption, causing prematurity, exsanguination, and hypoxemia (Table 37.4). When placental abruption occurs, loss of placental surface area up to 25% may be well tolerated by the fetus. Placental abruption of 50% or greater has a high likelihood of fetal loss.[21]

Penetrating injuries

Penetrating trauma typically result from either gunshot wounds (GSW) or stab wounds.[35] The gravid uterus is the most likely organ to be injured along with the liver and the small intestines. The gravid uterus can act as a shield for other viscera with abdominal injury, and injury to the organs is

Table 37.4 Placental abruption: clinical manifestations, complications, and management

Etiology	Hypertension	
	Trauma	
	Advanced age	
	Parity	
	Tobacco use	
	Cocaine use	
	Premature rupture of membranes	
	History of abruption	
Clinical manifestations	Vaginal bleeding	
	Uterine tenderness	
	Increased uterine activity	
	Ultrasound: retroplacental hematoma	
Complications	**Maternal**	**Fetal/neonatal**
	Hemorrhagic shock	Fetal distress
	Acute kidney injury	Fetal demise
	Coagulopathy	Prematurity
		Perinatal mortality and morbidity
Obstetric management	**Supportive management**	**Definitive management**
	Close monitoring of FHR	Continue pregnancy
	Large-bore IV access	• Preterm fetus
		• Minimal abruption
	Assess hematocrit	• No signs of fetal distress
	Assess coagulation	
	Blood for cross match	Induction of labor
	Left uterine displacement	• No evidence of fetal distress
	Supplemental oxygen	• Favorable cervix
		Cesarean delivery
		• Maternal instability
		• Fetal distress
Anesthetic management	Induction of labor	Consider epidural analgesia if no coagulopathy or hypovolemia
	Cesarean section	General anesthesia is preferred if fetal distress or hemodynamic instability
	General anesthesia	RSI with ketamine or etomidate
		Aggressive volume resuscitation
		Replacement with pRBC and coagulation factors
		Pitocin and other uterotonic agents to treat uterine atony

FHR, fetal heart rate; IV, intravenous; pRBC, packed red blood cells; RSI, rapid sequence induction.

avoided. Prognosis depends on the agent used to cause the injury and the site of injury. Stab wounds occur less frequently (23%) and have a better prognosis, as they are of low energy and organs slide away from the advancing instrument. Stab wounds are, however, more detrimental to the fetus than the mother. GSWs are a more common (73%) cause of penetrating injury during pregnancy and are more serious because all viscera and major vessels in the path of the bullet can be damaged. When the injury is confined to the uterus, maternal mortality is low (2.5%) but fetal mortality is high (40–71%).[21] The thick uterine musculature absorbs the energy from low-velocity penetrating injuries well. If the bullet has penetrated the uterus and the fetus is viable, cesarean delivery is indicated. Injury to the umbilical cord is rare, as are cord lacerations.

In the first trimester, the uterus is protected from both blunt and penetrating trauma by its position in the bony pelvis and its ligamentous suspension. As the uterus becomes an abdominal organ, the risk of injury increases. The mobility and elasticity of the uterus diminish the force of blunt trauma to the fetus. The amniotic fluid surrounds the fetus and acts as a buffer, protecting the fetus by dissipating the impact. The part of the membrane above the internal os is a weak point and can rupture. Placental abruption is the most frequent cause of fetal death.

Burn injuries

Burns are uncommon in pregnancy but still have important considerations (see also Chapters 39 and 40). Pregnancy, in general, does not affect the management of burns.[20] Maternal and fetal outcome depends on the severity of burns and associated complications.[36] Third spacing of fluids and intravascular volume depletion can result in uteroplacental hypoperfusion, fetal hypoxia, and fetal distress. Premature labor and death can be the result.[37]

Initial management consists of supplemental oxygen, assessment of extent and severity of the burn, and aggressive fluid management (see Chapter 39). The Parkland formula (4 mL per kg per % burn) can be used to estimate the 24-hour fluid requirement, with half of the fluid replacement in the first eight hours. Urine output should be monitored as a guide to adequacy of volume resuscitation. Fetal mortality increases with increasing severity of burns, with an almost 100% mortality rate associated with burns greater than 50%.[38,39] Tocolytic therapy is an option in case of preterm labor but must be instituted with caution. Tocolytic agents can have deleterious effects on fluid distribution in burn patients, with the potential for pulmonary edema.[40]

Carbon monoxide (CO) poisoning should be considered early in managing pregnant burn patients. CO crosses the placenta rapidly, and fetal hemoglobin has more affinity for CO than maternal hemoglobin. Fetal carboxyhemoglobin levels are higher than maternal levels, with slower fetal elimination.[41,42] Even in mildly symptomatic mothers, the chances of anatomic malformations and death of the fetus are high.[43,44] Hyperbaric oxygen therapy should then be considered early in the care of the pregnant patients with any injury where CO inhalation has occurred.

Initial care of the pregnant trauma patient
Prehospital care

The possibility of pregnancy should always be considered with all females of childbearing age. The primary concerns are airway management, spine immobilization, control of bleeding, limb splinting, support of vital signs, and care of other immediately life-threatening conditions such as tension pneumothorax (see Chapter 2). These initial areas are managed essentially the same way in all females of all ages. The airway of pregnant females can be significantly more challenging, with increased risks of aspiration, as will be discussed later. A distended abdomen in a female trauma patient may indicate intraabdominal bleeding, gravid uterus, or both. If pregnancy is confirmed by history and the gestation is more than 20 weeks, or if it is suspected by abdominal distention/ examination, uterine displacement (preferably leftward but not essential) should be initiated to avoid IVC obstruction.[45] If there is suspected spinal injury, the patient may have the entire backboard/bed tilted to avoid aortocaval compression while avoiding further spinal injury that could result from placing a wedge under the patient's hip.[46]

Transport and care of the pregnant trauma victim should in most cases be to a regional trauma center. Tachycardia, chest pain, possible loss of consciousness, and third-trimester pregnancies are independent risk factors for need of trauma-center care, and transport to this type of facility is indicated, if available.

Hospital care

When the patient is identified as pregnant, the trauma center needs to be notified as soon as possible so that the appropriate caregivers can be assembled in the emergency room for the patient's arrival. By using the multidisciplinary approach to the pregnant patient, optimal care may best be achieved by having a designated "obstetric trauma team." Having a designated team enables each member to have a clearly defined role. The obstetric trauma team should consist of trauma surgeons, obstetricians, anesthesiologists, emergency medicine physicians, pediatricians, and emergency room/labor room nurses, together with radiology and laboratory personnel. Each member of the team can initiate the therapeutic and diagnostic studies deemed necessary, with the coordination of studies and interpretation of results overseen by the team leader. Evaluations of different areas of concern then can be done simultaneously, maximizing time saved and helping to prevent errors of omission.

The primary and secondary surveys of the pregnant trauma patient remain essentially the same as for the nonpregnant patient, but with added attention to details relating to pregnancy (Table 37.5). Estimation of gestational age should be

Table 37.5 Advanced Trauma Life Support principles of initial assessment and evaluation of the pregnant trauma patient

Multidisciplinary approach. The obstetric, emergency, and trauma providers need to work together in an organized, coordinated fashion, according to ATLS protocols.

Pregnancy-related changes interfere with interpretation of signs and symptoms and laboratory data but do not interfere with management of trauma-related injuries.

The anesthesiologist can be a crucial link in the care of the obstetric trauma victim.

Many trauma caregivers lack knowledge of maternal physiologic change that can have an impact on care as well as assessing fetal well-being in the event of trauma.

Obstetric care providers are not experienced trauma caregivers.

In almost all cases, prompt resuscitation of the mother will maximize fetal chances of survival.

To save the life of the mother, prompt initiation of treatment is essential, even if pregnancy is jeopardized.

If maternal cardiac arrest does not respond to initial interventions *and* the fetus is viable/greater than 23 weeks gestation, emergent cesarean delivery should be considered, with the fetus delivered within less than 5 minutes of arrest.

If maternal death is imminent (fatal injury has clearly occurred), antepartum cesarean delivery may be considered to save the fetus.

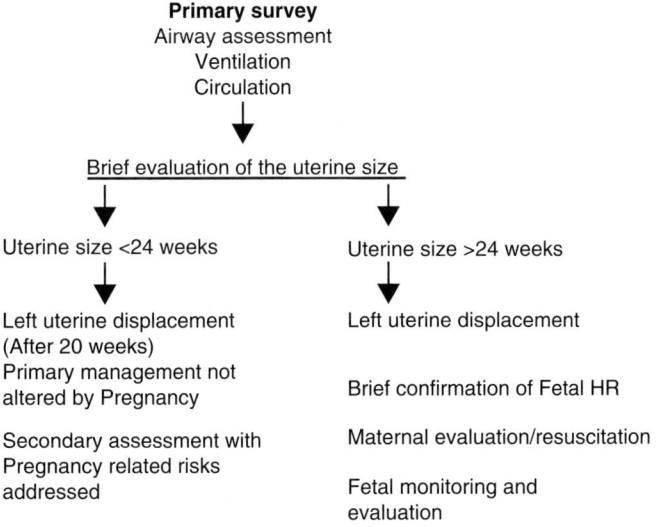

Primary survey
Airway assessment
Ventilation
Circulation

↓

Brief evaluation of the uterine size

Uterine size <24 weeks

Left uterine displacement
(After 20 weeks)
Primary management not altered by Pregnancy

Secondary assessment with Pregnancy related risks addressed

Uterine size >24 weeks

Left uterine displacement

Brief confirmation of Fetal HR

Maternal evaluation/resuscitation

Fetal monitoring and evaluation

Figure 37.1 Obstetric aspects of primary trauma management.

done as soon as possible, as uterine size, fetal age, and viability are critical factors affecting management and decision making in these patients (Fig. 37.1). If no clear history of gestational age is available, uterine size/gestational age can be estimated by physical exam or with the assistance of ultrasound. If it is determined that the pregnancy is viable ($\geq$ 24 weeks gestation),

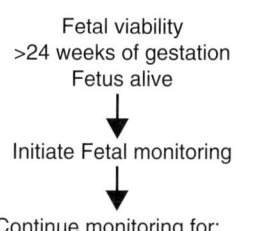

Fetal viability
>24 weeks of gestation
Fetus alive

Initiate Fetal monitoring

Continue monitoring for:
• Minimum of 4-6 hours (Minor trauma)
• Minimum of 24 hours (Severe trauma)
• Throughout period of maternal instability

Secondary evaluation of fetus by ultrasound
Rh immunoglobulin in Rh-negative patients

Figure 37.2 Fetal assessment in trauma.

Table 37.6 Difficulties of airway management in a pregnant trauma patient

Anatomic and physiologic changes of pregnancy
Mucosal edema
Increased oxygen requirements
Decreased functional residual capacity

Trauma-related injuries
Direct
• Facial fractures
• Cervical spine injuries

Indirect
• Airway obstruction
• Compromised protective laryngeal reflexes
• Decreased ability to clear secretions
• Inadequate ventilation
• Hypoxemia

fetal and uterine monitoring should be instituted during the secondary survey (Fig. 37.2).[20]

Initial care of all pregnant trauma patients should include the placement of supplemental oxygen. The airway is immediately examined to assess patency and the presence of protective reflexes, secretions, foreign bodies, and signs of injury. If any doubt about the airway exists, endotracheal intubation should be considered, because the mother can rapidly become hypoxic and fetal hypoxemia is a major cause of fetal distress. The maternal airway can be challenging owing to numerous factors (Table 37.6). Tissue edema, weight gain, and breast enlargement hinder visualization for intubation. Cervical spine injury may be a consideration, depending on the mechanism of trauma, further limiting allowable neck movement. After the first trimester of pregnancy, these patients are considered "full stomachs" that will require maneuvers such as cricoid pressure and RSI in an attempt to prevent passive regurgitation during intubation. Decreased FRC and increased oxygen consumption in pregnancy together cause the rapid development of hypoxemia in pregnant patients when apnea occurs.[19] With this in mind, should difficulty in intubation be encountered, alternative methods of airway control need to be immediately available. Mask ventilation with cricoid pressure, placement of a supraglottic device (e.g., LMA), or cricothyroidotomy may all be considered, depending on the circumstances (see Chapter 3). It must be kept in mind, however, that repeated attempts to intubate by using direct laryngoscopy can potentially cause tissue edema, bleeding, and possible loss of ability to ventilate by mask

Blood pressure, heart rate, and assessment of circulation must be done with the knowledge and understanding of how physiology of pregnancy differs from the nonpregnant state. Adequate mean arterial pressure must be established as soon as possible, because uterine perfusion of the placenta has no autoregulation and is blood-pressure dependent. Left uterine displacement should be instituted if the gestational age is greater than 20 weeks, either manually or by tilting the hip (if no injury contraindicates). Due to the significant increase in circulating blood volume in the second and third trimesters of pregnancy, significant hemorrhage may be initially

masked.[47,48] Fetal heart tones can be obtained with Doppler. If fetal bradycardia exists, all efforts need to be made to improve maternal oxygenation, circulation, and perfusion. This can include volume support with crystalloid, colloid, or blood products as indicated, as well as pressor support. Normal pregnancy decreases the response to drugs such as ephedrine/epinephrine, whereas the "toxemic" patient may be extremely sensitive to pressors. Maternal signs of adequate perfusion need to be assessed in parallel with the fetal assessment – patient mental status, pulse strength both central and peripheral, skin color, and capillary refill. Maternal heart rate is normally up to 15 bpm higher in pregnancy. If any circulatory compromise is suspected, two large-bore catheters for volume resuscitation with warm intravenous fluids need to be instituted.

Depending on gestational age, maternal medical condition, and fetal status, an emergency cesarean delivery may be necessary for both fetal and maternal management. These issues will be discussed later in the chapter.

If the patient is hemodynamically stable, the secondary survey should be instituted. Confirmatory evidence of fetal gestational age by pelvic exam should be done. Continuous fetal monitoring should be instituted as soon as possible. Gestational age of 24 weeks or greater is considered viable. Monitoring of uterine contractions may also be instituted at this time, though the presence of uterine contractions in the preterm period may not be indicative of labor. Uterine contractions can be secondary to uterine irritability, dehydration, and trauma, and often may subside with time. Vaginal speculum exam, looking for sources of bleeding or rupture of membranes, is an important part of the secondary assessment.[49] Pelvic and abdominal exam are done to evaluate the risk of peritoneal injury.

Laboratory testing includes complete blood count, type and crossmatch, blood gas analysis, and coagulation studies. Placental abruption may result in DIC and significant coagulopathy. Fibrinogen levels are elevated in normal pregnancy, so the presence of "normal" values can be a source of concern. A Kleihauer–Betke test can be used to assess whether fetal blood has entered the maternal circulation.[50,51] In Rh-negative mothers, this test can be done for the purpose of estimating the amount of fetal-to-maternal hemorrhage that has occurred. If the Rh-negative mother has a positive Kleihauer–Betke test, Rh immune globulin administration is indicated to decrease the risk of isoimmunization.[52] It is doubtful that this test has clinical value in the Rh-positive mother.

Imaging in pregnancy

Diagnostic evaluation of the pregnant patient should be geared toward the identification of maternal injuries and further assessment of the fetus.[32] In the diagnostic evaluation of a pregnant trauma patient, the safest and the most appropriate study that yields the best result must be used. Ultrasonography is a major tool in the initial evaluation of the pregnant trauma patient. There is no ionizing radiation used with ultrasonography, and all evidence indicates that it is safe for the fetus. Focused assessment with sonography for trauma (FAST) is an effective tool in assessing whether maternal intraabdominal injury has occurred (see Chapter 10). It can also be used to evaluate the fetus and placenta.[53–55] Diagnostic peritoneal lavage (DPL) is also used in the pregnant patient to identify peritoneal injury, especially if the results of FAST are equivocal.[56,57] The site of incision for open DPL is dictated by the size of the uterus (either above or below the umbilicus).[58] Whatever measures can be done to minimize exposure should be done. In general, little risk of radiation injury exists with basic radiographs after 20 weeks gestation. Earlier in pregnancy, especially in the first eight weeks, computed tomography (CT) scans of the abdomen expose the fetus to significantly more radiation than other types of x-rays.[59] The risks and benefits of such studies need to be evaluated in each individual case. CT scans of the head, neck, and chest allow the abdomen to be shielded, and therefore do not expose the fetus to the same radiation exposure as abdominal CTs (see Chapter 11). The benefit of timely and accurate diagnosis outweighs the typically low radiation risks to the fetus in the setting of trauma.

Ultrasound

Sonography is a well-established safe imaging technique in pregnancy without adverse effects on the fetus. It has a poor sensitivity for diagnosing placental abruption, with 50–80% of these conditions missed. Sonography is accurate to evaluate pelvic and intrauterine structures. The diagnostic yield does become increasingly limited by gestational age, with increasing body mass index and diminishing ability to evaluate visceral injuries, and is also dependent on operator experience. Advantages of ultrasound evaluation in pregnant trauma patients include the ability to carry out bedside evaluation, avoidance of exposure to ionizing radiation, and provision of diagnostic

information in patients too unstable for transport to the CT scanner. Fetal assessment with ultrasound can examine fetal heart rate, heart rate reactivity, amniotic fluid volume, respiratory effort, and gross body movements, as well as signs of placental abruption. Though not very sensitive for abruption, should there be signs of subchorionic hemorrhage or retroplacental hemorrhage during scanning, sonography may help in early diagnosis.

Magnetic resonance imaging

Although magnetic resonance imaging (MRI) is used to evaluate brain and spinal cord injury, it is rarely indicated in the emergency evaluation of the parturient (see Chapter 11).

Radiography

The dose of radiation absorbed with plain radiography is usually in the range 0.02–0.07 mrad, and this can be administered at any gestational age without harm to the fetus. An unshielded fetus will receive approximately 30% of the maternal absorbed dose. Still, care must be taken to avoid unnecessary imaging, and uterine shielding should be used when possible, especially if multiple films are necessary. All radiographs should be evaluated with the knowledge that physiologic changes of pregnancy affect their interpretation.

Angiography

Radiation exposure with fluoroscopy is influenced by the duration of the examination, the number of blood vessels evaluated, and the depth of the patient's tissues. Embolization is a useful tool to control hemorrhage from the pelvic vessels not involved in the circulation to the uterus. The typical exposure from fluoroscopy ranges from 2 to 10 rad/minute. Despite radiation reduction techniques, shielding, and limiting the time of the procedure where possible, the amount of radiation exposure varies considerably – but its use should not be denied as a life-saving intervention.

Computed tomography

To evaluate stable trauma patients, CT scans are the quickest and most sensitive noninvasive imaging studies available. Absorbed doses of ionizing radiation differ among various organs. Scanning the abdomen and pelvis exposes the fetus to larger radiation doses. Low-exposure techniques significantly attenuate the radiation exposure of the fetus. In 2008, the US Food and Drug Administration (FDA) issued a caution for radiologists to use the minimal amount of radiation, as there were reports that CT "sensitizing" of pacemakers and implantable cardioverter defibrillators (ICDs) could cause temporary misfiring of these devices. Now, five and a half years later, researchers who reviewed 10 years' worth of CT scans at their hospitals have found no signs of interference from CT imaging on implanted electronic cardiac devices.[60] Fortunately such devices are rarely found in pregnant patients.

Nuclear medicine

There is no indication for tagged isotope studies in pregnant patients except cerebral blood flow studies to confirm brain death. Technetium is one of the most commonly used isotopes, and typical exposures do not exceed 0.5 rad. The role of ventilation perfusion scanning in trauma is generally obsolete.

Surgical intervention and the role of anesthesia

One of the main decisions in managing the pregnant trauma patient is: does the patient need an exploratory laparotomy? If there is no evidence of peritoneal penetration or a ruptured intraabdominal organ, using physical exam, ultrasound/radiologic criteria, and/or DPL, then injury to the uterus or fetus is unlikely and surgical exploration is not indicated.

When surgical exploration is necessary to evaluate the type and severity of penetrating injuries, cesarean delivery may be required in the following situations:

(1) uterine size prohibits adequate abdominal exploration
(2) when necessary for the repair of an extrauterine injury
(3) for repair of a uterine injury in a woman with a viable fetus
(4) an injured and/or distressed viable fetus
(5) maternal cardiac arrest with a fetus of more than 23 weeks not responding to initial resuscitative efforts[61]

Anesthetic management

Anesthesia consultation should be sought early even if maternal injuries are considered minor and the patient is admitted to labor and delivery only for observation and fetal monitoring. Early evaluation of the patient for possible anesthesia risks is essential so that the anesthesia team can be prepared should surgical intervention be suddenly required.

Airway management of the pregnant trauma patient

With the pregnant trauma patient, the anesthesiologist utilizes the American Society of Anesthesiologists (ASA) algorithm for difficult airway management, with modifications related to the gestational effects of pregnancy (see Chapter 3). Difficult tracheal intubation occurs more frequently in the parturient (1 in 2500), and the incidence of failed intubation is 1 in 300, or eight times higher than in nonpregnant patients. Should trauma occur to the face, cervical spine, or neck, one would expect the level of difficulty to only increase.

If possible, airway management is ideally instituted in the operative setting where all tools for difficult airway management should be available. Supplemental O_2 is instituted with suction immediately available. Experienced personnel should be present to assist in airway management. If the patient is hypoxemic, has decreased ventilatory effort, is unable to clear secretions due to decreased level of consciousness or loss of protective airway reflexes, or has airway obstruction, then intubation should proceed rapidly. If significant difficulty in airway management is clearly anticipated, an alternative airway such as cricothyroidotomy or tracheostomy may be necessary, ideally performed by an experienced, skilled surgeon.

Should cervical spine injury be present or suspected, all precautions to prevent unnecessary movements of the neck are employed (see Chapter 3). Awake fiberoptic intubation can be done to minimize neck movement and decrease risk of aspiration. Topicalization with local anesthetics will facilitate airway manipulation. Benzocaine can be used for topicalization, but caution with dosing is needed as methemoglobinemia can occur with large doses. If indicated, small doses of midazolam can be safely used, with minimal depression of neonatal respiration. Nasotracheal fiberoptic intubation can be performed if no trauma to the face has occurred that would preclude this approach. But the nasal approach should be done with caution, because swelling of the nasal mucosa in pregnancy increases the likelihood of bleeding in this area, making visualization potentially much more difficult. Orotracheal fiberoptic intubation is the preferred approach. Should secretions and blood obstruct the view of the airway, retrograde oral intubation is another option.

Head trauma, shock, alcohol, and drug abuse can all contribute to an uncooperative patient, which may make awake fiberoptic intubation not only unrealistic but potentially dangerous. Patients who are combative can move during attempted intubation, with the potential of causing or worsening neurologic injury. RSI with cricoid pressure and in-line stabilization of the cervical spine is frequently and successfully utilized in the pregnant trauma patient (see Chapter 3). If time permits, and no contraindications are present, gastrointestinal prophylaxis should be considered prior to airway management, including the use of an H_2 receptor antagonist, metoclopramide, or a nonparticulate oral antacid such as sodium citrate. Preoxygenation prior to induction is mandatory, and alternative methods of airway management must be immediately available should intubation prove difficult.

Operative anesthetic management of pregnant trauma patients includes all the principles of anesthetic management of trauma patients as well as the principles of the pregnant patient undergoing nonobstetric surgery (Table 37.7). Patients

Table 37.7 Principles of anesthetic management of pregnant trauma patients

Optimization of gas exchange
Restoration of blood volume and tissue perfusion
Protection of brain and spinal cord
Maintenance of uteroplacental circulation and fetal oxygenation
Prevention of maternal awareness
Detection of unrecognized injuries
Correction of coagulopathy
Maintenance of normothermia
Avoidance of teratogenic drugs (during the first trimester)

may be fearful of anesthesia effects on the fetus and need reassurance that anesthesia itself is not in itself a cause of fetal loss or significant risk of fetal malformations even early in gestation. Preoperative pain medication and anxiolytics as indicated should be used, as elevated maternal circulating catecholamines from stress can potentially compromise uterine blood flow. All standard monitors should be used for surgery. Anesthetic goals include meticulous attention to details of airway management, ensuring adequate maternal cardiac output/blood pressure/perfusion and avoiding hypotension and hypoxemia. PCO_2 should be maintained in the normal range, as hyperventilation/hypocarbia/alkalosis may decrease uterine perfusion and fetal oxygenation. Fetal monitoring intraoperatively is done on a case-by-case basis once the fetus is considered viable.[62] Unfortunately, with abdominal procedures or in urgent situations, monitoring may not be practical. Fetal monitoring in itself has not been shown to improve fetal outcome.[63] Beat-to-beat variability, a highly sensitive indicator of fetal well-being, will be commonly lost under anesthesia, and this is a normal finding. Fetal bradycardia, however, is not expected, and once it occurs, maneuvers to improve maternal circulation/placental perfusion/fetal oxygenation should be instituted to try to resolve it. These measures can include ensuring adequate left uterine displacement, raising maternal blood pressure, increasing the inspired fraction of oxygen, and ensuring that surgical retraction/intervention is not a factor.[45] Tocolysis may be considered, but the other implications that this can have under anesthesia and its effects on maternal vital signs need to be taken into consideration (Table 37.8). Emergent cesarean delivery may be necessary if bradycardia does not resolve.

Medications

As a general rule, aggressive resuscitation of the pregnant trauma patient will be the best therapy for the fetus.[10,64] That is not to say that the medications used will not affect the fetus. After the first trimester of pregnancy, organogenesis is complete. Teratogenicity is usually not an issue at this stage of pregnancy. As it is, most medications used in the pregnant trauma patient are category B or C. Medications that affect uteroplacental blood flow, such as pressors, should be used as

Table 37.8 Anesthetic implications of tocolytic therapy

Tocolytic agents	Side effects		Anesthetic implications
	Maternal	**Fetal/neonatal**	
Beta-adrenergic agonists • Ritodrine • Terbutaline	Increased maternal heart rate Increased cardiac output Hypotension Arrhythmias Myocardial ischemia Pulmonary edema Hyperglycemia Hypokalemia Rebound hyperkalemia Fetal tachycardia	Neonatal hypoglycemia ? Neonatal IVH Transient decreased myocardial contractility	Avoid anesthesia until maternal tachycardia subsides (if possible) Delay GA for at least 10 minutes after discontinuation of β-agonists Avoid aggressive hydration Avoid agents like: atropine, glycopyrrolate, pancuronium, ketamine Avoid hyperventilation Avoid halothane Slow induction of epidural preferable to spinal anesthesia
Magnesium sulfate	Pulmonary edema Transient hypotension Chest pain and tightness Palpitations Blurred vision Sedation Toxic levels with abnormal renal function	? Increased perinatal mortality Neonatal hypotonia	↓ MAC for analgesics, sedatives Attenuation of hemodynamic response to endogenous and exogenous pressors Ephedrine is preferable to treat hypotension potentiation of depolarizing as well as nondepolarizing NMBA Possible modest ↑ in bleeding time
Prostaglandin synthetase inhibitors • Indomethacin	Nausea and heart burn Transient inhibition of platelet aggregation	Potential for premature closure of the ductus and persistent fetal circulation	No contraindication for regional anesthesia No coagulation studies indicated
Calcium-channel blocking agents • Nifedipine	Facial flushing Transient increase in heart rate Postpartum uterine atony	Does not affect uteroplacental or fetal circulation	Potentiation of volatile halogenated agents In combination with magnesium, may potentiate neuromuscular blockade

GA, general anesthesia; IVH, intraventricular hemorrhage; MAC, minimum alveolar concentration; NMBA, neuromuscular blocking agent.

needed for maternal care. Uteroplacental flow has no autoregulation, and thus adequate placental perfusion/fetal oxygen delivery is directly dependent on blood pressure. Drugs such as epinephrine can potentially decrease uterine flow by a direct effect, but the overall benefit of increasing uterine perfusion by raising maternal blood pressure usually predominates. Most β-blockers may be used in pregnancy, but esmolol readily crosses the placenta and has been associated with fetal acidosis.[65] The American College of Obstetricians and Gynecologists recommends giving the pregnant trauma patient tetanus toxoid as indicated.[23]

Anesthesia drugs are essentially safe in pregnancy. Any induction agent can be used to initiate anesthesia. Ketamine has the ability to increase uterine tone in the second trimester if doses greater than 2 mg/kg are used, which may decrease placental perfusion and fetal oxygen delivery.[66] Concern has been raised in the past regarding nitrous oxide (N_2O) and benzodiazepines. N_2O does have sympathomimetic properties and has the potential to vasoconstrict uterine vessels and decrease placental flow. If N_2O is used, a volatile anesthetic agent should also be used that would inhibit this effect. With benzodiazepines, early initial reports of an association with cleft palate have not been seen in follow-up studies.

Volatile anesthetic gases are best maintained below 2.0 MAC, as pregnant patients have decreased anesthetic requirement, and higher doses can decrease maternal blood pressure and cardiac output. If cesarean delivery occurs, volatile agents should be delivered at concentrations less than 1.0 MAC to avoid uterine relaxant effects that can increase maternal blood loss. Avoidance of isoflurane for long nonobstetric procedures may be advisable until questions regarding possible neurotoxic concerns raised by recent studies are further investigated.[67]

Tocolysis to prevent preterm labor has been done in the past by using magnesium and indomethacin. Indomethacin does not have an impact on anesthesia care. Magnesium can potentiate the effects of neuromuscular relaxants and cause hypotension, especially in volume-depleted patients.[68] The use of tocolytics has been questioned in trauma and probably should be avoided, because it may hinder the diagnosis and treatment of placental abruption. Tocolytics such as terbutaline and ritodrine can cause hypotension and tachycardia (Table 37.8). These effects are exacerbated by anesthesia if given within a short period of time (approximately 30 minutes of administration). Ventricular ectopy results, especially if ephedrine and/or atropine are given concomitantly. Excessive blood loss can result from residual uterine relaxation effects should emergency cesarean delivery become necessary.

CPR in pregnancy and perimortem cesarean delivery

Cardiac arrest occurs in approximately 1 in 30,000 pregnancies.[69] The incidence is higher among those with cardiovascular disease. In the setting of trauma, cardiac arrest can occur from multiple causes including hemorrhagic shock,

respiratory compromise, and tension pneumothorax (Table 37.9). Likelihood of survival is influenced by the timeliness and expertise of the resuscitation team. Obstetricians, anesthesiologists, neonatologists, and nursing staff must work efficiently and in an organized fashion to resuscitate these patients.[70] As these events happen unexpectedly, cooperation is essential to assemble needed equipment and perform resuscitation in the labor suite. When arrest occurs "in the field," the obstetric trauma team, with all necessary equipment, must be on standby in the emergency department for patient arrival in the event that emergency cesarean delivery be indicated to assist in maternal resuscitation.

The physiologic changes of pregnancy place the pregnant patient at significant risk of difficulty in resuscitation, should maternal arrest occur. The patient will rapidly become hypoxemic, and the uterus will obstruct some venous return during cardiopulmonary resuscitation (CPR), especially late in pregnancy, even if left uterine displacement is instituted. The uterus shunts anywhere from 20% to 30% of cardiac output (as opposed to the prepregnancy levels of 0.5–1.0%). Normal CPR, in the best of circumstances, can generate 25% of normal cardiac output. In pregnancy, cardiac output is increased by 30% or more, and with the uterus taking such a large percentage, this will potentially rob other maternal organs of adequate perfusion with CPR. In addition, the anatomic configuration of the patient, with gravid uterus and reduced chest wall compliance, may interfere with proper positioning and performance of effective CPR.

Basic life support and advanced life support protocols should be instituted (Table 37.11). In general, CPR in the pregnant patient follows the same resuscitation protocols. If spinal injury is present, manually displacing the uterus by hand may be one possible remedy. Shifting of the entire bed or backboard to one side may help relieve aortocaval compression, but may interfere with maintaining the proper positioning for chest compressions. Energy requirements for defibrillation appear to be similar to those in nonpregnant

Table 37.9 Causes of maternal cardiac arrest

1. Pulmonary embolism
2. Severe preeclampsia/eclampsia
3. Hemorrhage (obstetric or trauma-related)
4. Trauma
   a. Head trauma
   b. Penetrating/blunt thoracoabdominal trauma
5. Sepsis
6. Myocardial infarction
7. Congestive heart failure
8. Amniotic fluid embolism (see Table 37.10)
9. Iatrogenic causes
   a. Hypermagnesemia
   b. Failed airway management
   c. Complications of regional anesthesia
      i. High spinal
      ii. Local anesthetic toxicity

Table 37.10 Pathophysiology and management of amniotic fluid embolism

Definition
An anaphylactoid syndrome of acute peripartum hypoxia, hemodynamic collapse, and coagulopathy related to maternal exposure to fetal tissue during labor, vaginal delivery, or cesarean delivery. The exact etiology is unknown.

Pathophysiology: biphasic response

Early phase	Transient intense pulmonary vasospasm Acute right heart dysfunction and pulmonary hypertension Low cardiac output
Second phase	Ventilation/perfusion mismatch Hypoxemia and hypotension Left ventricular failure Pulmonary edema Consumptive coagulopathy

Clinical manifestations *
Hypotension 100%
Fetal distress 100%
Pulmonary edema or ARDS 93%
Cardiopulmonary arrest 87%
Cyanosis 83%
Coagulopathy 83%
Dyspnea 49%
Seizure 48%
Atony 23%
Bronchospasm 15%
Transient hypertension 11%
Cough 7%
Headache 7%
Chest pain 2%

Goals and methods of management
Maintenance of oxygenation
- Supplemental oxygen
- Intubation and ventilation
- Diuretics

Circulatory support
- CPR protocol
- Delivery of fetus
- Volume resuscitation
- Inotropes
- Afterload reduction

Correction of coagulopathy
- FFP, pRBCs, platelets, cryoprecipitate

Possible additional measures
- High-dose corticosteroids
- Epinephrine
- Cardiopulmonary bypass
- Nitric oxide
- Inhaled prostacyclin

* Clark SL, Hankins GD, Dudley DA, Dildy GA, Porter TF. Amniotic fluid embolism: analysis of the national registry. *Am J Obstet Gynecol* 1995; **172**: 1158–69.
CPR, cardiopulmonary resuscitation; FFP, fresh frozen plasma; pRBC, packed red blood cells.

Table 37.11 Principles of cardiopulmonary resuscitation (CPR) during pregnancy

1. Intubate the trachea soon after initiation of CPR, to facilitate oxygenation and ventilation and also to prevent aspiration.
2. Before 24 weeks, rescuer should be concerned mainly to save the mother.
3. After 24 weeks, goals of resuscitation should be to save both mother and the fetus.
4. Maintain left uterine displacement during CPR.
5. According to AHA guidelines, resuscitative measure should be followed including ventricular defibrillation algorithm and use of vasopressors such as epinephrine, norepinephrine, and dopamine.[71]
6. If initial efforts at resuscitation are unsuccessful, consider immediate delivery of the fetus. Optimal time from arrest to delivery is under 5 minutes.[72] Understand that cesarean delivery is to facilitate maternal resuscitation.
7. Cesarean delivery facilitates resuscitation by restoring venous return, decreasing metabolic demands, and allowing more effective chest compressions.[73–77]
8. If after delivery resuscitation is still ineffective, consider open-chest cardiac massage and cardiopulmonary bypass.[78–79]

AHA, American Heart Association.

Table 37.12 Maternal and fetal/neonatal complications of CPR

Maternal	Fetal/neonatal
Laceration of the liver	Cardiac arrhythmia
Uterine rupture	Asystole
Hemothorax	Neurological damage
Hemopericardium	Prematurity
	Hypoxia
	Acidosis

states.[71] The fetus is not harmed if the paddles are placed properly. If a fetal scalp monitor has been placed, the lead should be disconnected from the fetal heart rate monitor prior to defibrillation.

Use of sodium bicarbonate during resuscitation to reverse metabolic acidosis is controversial, because of evidence that it may worsen maternal intracellular acidosis in cardiac arrest. Sodium bicarbonate does not readily cross the placenta, and will likely not have a significant effect on the fetus. The most important consideration is restoration of placental perfusion and oxygen delivery to reverse fetal acidosis.

Maternal and fetal/neonatal complications of CPR during pregnancy

Maternal complications associated with CPR include laceration of the liver, uterine rupture, hemothorax, and hemopericardium (Table 37.12). Fetal complications related to maternal arrest include severe hypoxemia, neurologic damage, cardiac arrhythmias, and asystole. Possible mechanisms include uteroplacental vasoconstriction, maternal hypoxemia and acidosis, decreased maternal cardiac output, and central nervous system (CNS) complications from antiarrythmic drugs. The neonate in most cases will be hypoxic and acidotic, and depending on gestational age, may very well be preterm. Prompt resuscitation of the newborn by the neonatal team can significantly influence neonatal outcome.

Perimortem cesarean delivery

The decision to perform perimortem cesarean delivery should be based on the viability of the fetus, certainty of maternal death or unfavorable neurologic outcome, and duration of cardiac arrest. When cesarean delivery is being initiated, it is imperative that CPR be continued at optimal levels. Survival of the fetus after perimortem cesarean delivery is:

- 70% when delivered in less than 5 minutes
- 13% when delivered within 6–10 minutes
- 12% when delivered within 11–15 minutes

It is generally accepted, based on these data, that for most mothers who suffer cardiopulmonary arrest, cesarean delivery should be approached on the basis of what some have called the "4-minute" rule. That is, cesarean delivery should ideally be performed in under 5 minutes of maternal collapse and the neonate must be delivered by the fifth minute.[8,80] To achieve this goal is often difficult and requires tremendous preparation and coordination of the entire obstetric and trauma care team. Equipment for both fetal assessment and cesarean delivery may need to be permanently stocked in the emergency room. Obstetric and anesthesia staff must be immediately available to the emergency room for the anticipated arrival of the pregnant patient. Should arrest occur in labor and delivery or in the intensive care unit, it is imperative that the necessary equipment and personnel be readily available to both resuscitate and deliver the fetus. Pediatric/neonatal staff must also be available to manage the newborn.

Prevention of maternal mortality due to trauma

Prevention is the key to a decrease maternal mortality due to trauma (see Chapter 41). Potential preventive measures include education of the patients, education of the healthcare providers who routinely care for pregnant women, and education of the general public. The most common preventable causes are MVCs and domestic violence.

Education regarding proper use of seatbelts and airbags should be routinely done by the physicians. The lap belt portion should be placed under the pregnant woman's abdomen, over both anterior superior iliac spines and the pubic symphysis. The shoulder harness should be placed between the breasts. The lap and shoulder restraints should be applied tightly but comfortably. Placement of the lap belt over the dome of the uterus increases pressure transmission and is associated with fetal injury. Airbags should not be disconnected during pregnancy.

The frequency and nature of domestic violence seem to increase during pregnancy. It would be prudent to screen for domestic violence during the first prenatal visit, at least once in every trimester, and at the postpartum visit. Abuse may not be reported at the first visit or it may not start until later in pregnancy. Apart from asking the screening questions, the healthcare providers should be able to refer these patients to domestic violence services, mental health services, and legal services.

Summary

The pregnant trauma patient presents unique challenges to the trauma anesthesiologist. Pregnancy is associated with specific physiologic changes and unique injuries that must be considered along with concern for the developing fetus. A multidisciplinary approach to these patients using a designated obstetric trauma care team will offer both mother and fetus the greatest chance of successful outcomes. The anesthesiologist, with expertise in airway management, critical care, and the physiologic changes of pregnancy, can be a vital member of the team. Initial resuscitative efforts will be directed at the mother, with emphasis on maintaining uteroplacental perfusion and fetal oxygenation. The best maternal resuscitative efforts ensure better fetal outcome. In the event of cardiopulmonary arrest, if the pregnant patient does not respond within the first 4 minutes of CPR and the fetus is viable, emergency cesarean delivery should be considered to maximize both maternal and fetal chances of survival.

Key concepts

- A pregnant trauma patient poses unique challenges – caring for two lives, which involves an understanding of the potential injuries caused by the different types of traumatic injury and the impact of the physiologic changes of pregnancy on these injuries. The best strategy to optimize fetal well-being and care is to optimize maternal care.
- When the patient is identified as pregnant, the trauma center needs to be notified as soon as possible so that the appropriate caregivers can be assembled in the emergency room for the care of the pregnant trauma patient. Having a designated team enables each member to have a clearly defined role. The obstetric trauma team should consist of trauma surgeons, obstetricians, anesthesiologists, emergency medicine physicians, pediatricians, and emergency room/labor room nurses, together with radiology and laboratory personnel.
- All pregnant trauma patients should be considered "full stomach" after 12 weeks of gestational age.
- Left uterine displacement, especially after the 20 weeks of gestational age, is essential when caring for and resuscitating the pregnant trauma victim.

- Principles of CPR in a pregnant patient:
  - Intubate the trachea soon after initiation of CPR, to facilitate oxygenation and ventilation and also to prevent aspiration.
  - Before 24 weeks, the rescuer should be concerned mainly to save the mother.
  - After 24 weeks, the goals of resuscitation should be to save both mother and the fetus.
- Perimortem cesarean delivery. If initial efforts at resuscitation are unsuccessful, immediate delivery of the fetus should be considered. Optimal time from arrest to delivery is under 5 minutes.
- Understand that cesarean delivery is to facilitate maternal resuscitation. Cesarean delivery facilitates resuscitation by restoring venous return, decreasing metabolic demands, and allowing more effective chest compressions.
- If resuscitation is still ineffective after delivery, consider open-chest cardiac massage and cardiopulmonary bypass.
- A multidisciplinary approach to the pregnant trauma patient, involving trauma surgeons, obstetricians, anesthesiologists, emergency medicine physicians, and other providers, is critical to deliver optimal care and achieve the best outcomes possible.

Questions

(1) Which statement regarding physiologic changes of pregnancy is *false*?
   a. Cardiac output, systemic vascular resistance, and blood pressure are increased in normal pregnancy
   b. Intravascular volume increases as much as 40% in pregnancy
   c. Mechanical effects of the expanding uterus contribute to gastroesophageal reflux that is common in the later trimesters of pregnancy
   d. Renal blood flow and glomerular filtration rate are increased in normal pregnancy
   e. ECG changes that occur in normal pregnancy can be mistaken for myocardial infarction

(2) Factors that make the airway more difficult to manage in pregnancy include all of the following, *except*:
   a. Airway swelling and edema
   b. Maternal weight gain
   c. Easy friability of the mucosa
   d. Rapid desaturation when apnea occurs secondary to decreased functional residual capacity and increased oxygen consumption
   e. Decreased oral opening in pregnancy due to physiologic effects on the temporomandibular joint

(3) Which statement regarding the physiologic changes of pregnancy as related to trauma is *false*?
   a. The "low maternal hemoglobin" in pregnancy may be confused with blood loss from trauma
   b. Because of the changes in heart rate and blood pressure in normal pregnancy, the assessment of hypovolemia can be more difficult

   c. With autoregulation of uteroplacental blood flow, the mother is able to maintain adequate placental perfusion should hypotension occur
   d. Decreases in maternal PCO_2 are seen early in pregnancy as a response to the effects of progesterone on the medullary respiratory centers of the brain
   e. Clotting factors increase during pregnancy, placing the pregnant patient at increased risk for pulmonary embolism

(4) Which statement regarding trauma in pregnancy is *false*?
   a. Motor vehicle accidents account for almost two-thirds of all maternal trauma
   b. The use of seatbelts is a significant factor in maternal/fetal injury
   c. "Minor" third-trimester maternal injury results in almost 10% of pregnancy-related complications
   d. GCS ≤ 8, elevated base deficit, and abnormal uterine activity are predictive of poor fetal outcome
   e. The gravid uterus can shield other viscera from injury

(5) Initial management of the pregnant trauma patient should include all of the following, *except*:
   a. Airway evaluation and management
   b. Spine immobilization if indicated
   c. Left uterine displacement with a hip wedge if gestational age greater than 12 weeks
   d. Control of bleeding
   e. Limb splinting

(6) Regarding the initial hospital care of the pregnant trauma patient, identify the *incorrect* statement:
   a. The primary survey of the pregnant trauma patient is essentially unchanged compared with the nonpregnant patient
   b. Gestational age is unimportant to evaluate until the secondary survey is complete
   c. Supplemental oxygen should be instituted immediately
   d. Fetal heart tones should be evaluated as soon as possible during the secondary survey
   e. If maternal blood pressure is low, resuscitation with crystalloid/colloid and/or blood as needed should be promptly instituted

(7) Which statement regarding maternal diagnostic and radiologic evaluation is *false*?
   a. A Kleihauer–Betke test is vital to do in the Rh-positive pregnant trauma patient to assess the entrance of fetal blood in the maternal circulation
   b. FAST (focused abdominal ultrasound for trauma) is an effective tool in assessing whether maternal intraabdominal injury has occurred
   c. Diagnostic peritoneal lavage (DPL) can be used in the pregnant trauma patient to identify peritoneal injury, especially if FAST is equivocal

d. Uterine ultrasound is not sensitive for detecting placental abruption

e. CT scans of the abdomen expose the fetus to significantly more radiation than other types of x-rays

(8) **During surgery to explore the abdomen for possible injury, cesarean delivery would also be indicated in each of these situations,** *except***:**

a. Uterine size prohibits adequate abdominal exploration

b. For repair of a uterine injury in a woman with a viable fetus

c. When necessary for the repair of an extrauterine injury

d. Maternal cardiac arrest with a fetus less than 24 weeks and the mother is not responding to initial resuscitative efforts

e. When you have an injured and/or distressed viable fetus

(9) **All of the following statements are applicable to airway management of the pregnant trauma patient,** *except***:**

a. Patients who are unable to clear secretions adequately after trauma has occurred require tracheal intubation as soon as possible

b. Experienced assistants should help in the event that in-line stabilization of the cervical spine is necessary for tracheal intubation

c. Awake fiberoptic intubation is the method of choice in the combative pregnant trauma patient

d. Benzocaine local anesthetic use for topicalization of the airway has been complicated by methehemoglobinemia

e. Nasotracheal fiberoptic intubation may be contraindicated in a patient with facial fractures

(10) **Key features of anesthetic management for the pregnant trauma patient undergoing surgery include all of the following,** *except***:**

a. Maintenance of uteroplacental circulation and fetal oxygenation

b. Restoration of blood volume and tissue perfusion

c. Prevention of preterm labor

d. Maintenance of normothermia

e. Avoidance of teratogenic drugs during the third trimester

Answers

(1) a
(2) e
(3) c
(4) b
(5) c
(6) b
(7) a
(8) d
(9) c
(10) e

References

1. Colburn V. Trauma in pregnancy. *J Perinat Neonat Nurs* 1999; **13** (3): 21–32.

2. Lavin JP, Polsky SS. Abdominal trauma during pregnancy. *Clin Perinatol* 1983; **10**: 423–38.

3. Mighty H. Trauma in pregnancy. *Crit Care Clin* 1994; **10**: 623–34.

4. Petrone P, Asensio JA. Trauma in pregnancy: assessment and treatment. *Scand J Surg* 2006; **95**: 4–10.

5. Kaunitz AM, Hughes JM, Grimes DA. Causes of maternal mortality in the United States. *Obstet Gynecol* 1985; **65**: 605.

6. George ER, Vanderwaak T, Scholten DJ. Factors influencing pregnancy outcome after trauma. *Am Surg* 1992; **58**: 595–8.

7. Scorpio RJ, Esposito TJ, Smith LG, *et al.* Blunt trauma during pregnancy: factors affecting fetal outcome. *J Trauma* 1992; **32**: 213–6.

8. Moise KJ, Belfort MA. Damage control for the obstetric patient. *Surg Clin N Am* 1997; **77**: 835–52.

9. Hill DA, Lense JJ. Abdominal trauma in the pregnant patient. *Am Fam Physician* 1996; **53**: 1269–74.

10. Esposito TJ. Trauma during pregnancy. *Emerg Med Clin N Am* 1994; **12**: 167–99.

11. Shah KH, Simons RK, Holbrook T, *et al.* Trauma in pregnancy: maternal and fetal outcomes. *J Trauma* 1998; **45**: 83–6.

12. Capless EL, Clapp JF. Cardiovascular changes in early phase of pregnancy. *Am J Obstet Gynecol* 1988; **168**: 1449–53.

13. Clapp JF, Seawad BL, Sleamaker RH, Hiser J. Maternal physiological adaptations to early human pregnancy. *Am J Obstet Gynecol* 1988; **159**: 1456–60.

14. Ueland K, Hansen JM. Maternal cardiovascular hemodynamics. III. Labor and delivery under local and caudal analgesia. *Am J Obstet Gynecol* 1969; **103**: 8–17.

15. Ueland K, Akamatsu TJ, Eng M, *et al.* Maternal cardiovascular hemodynamics. VI. Cesarean section under epidural anesthesia without

epinephrine. *Am J Obstet Gynecol* 1972; **114**: 775–80.

16. Howard BK, Goodson JH, Mengert WF. Supine hypotension syndrome in late pregnancy. *Obstet Gynecol* 1953; **1**: 371–7.

17. Gamann WR, Ostheimer GW. Understanding the mother. In Ostheimer GW, ed., *Manual of Obstetric Anesthesia*. New York, NY: Churchill Livingstone, 1992, pp. 1–11.

18. Weinberger SE, Weiss ST, Cohen WR, *et al.* Pregnancy and the lung. *Am Rev Respir Dis* 1980; **121**: 559–81.

19. Campbell LA, Klocke RA. Implications for the pregnant patient. *Am J Respir Crit Care Med* 2001; **163**: 1051–4.

20. Shah AJ, Kilcline BA. Trauma in pregnancy. *Emerg Med Clin N Am* 2003; **21**: 615–29.

21. Maull KI. Maternal-fetal trauma. *Semin Pediatr Surg* 2001; **10**: 32–4.

22. Varela YB, Zietlow SP, Bannon MP, *et al.* Trauma in pregnancy. *Mayo Clin Proc* 2000; **75**: 1243–8.

23. Trauma during pregnancy. ACOG Technical Bulletin Number 161,

November 1991. *Int J Gynaecol Obstet* 1993; **40**: 165–70.

24. Weiss H, Songer T, Fabio A. Fetal deaths related to maternal injury. *JAMA* 2001; **286**: 1863–8.

25. Crosby WM, Costiloe JP. Safety of lap-belt restraint for pregnant victims of automobile collisions. *N Engl J Med* 1971; **284**: 632–6.

26. Wolf ME, Alexander BH, Rivera FP, *et al.* A retrospective cohort study of seatbelt use and pregnancy outcome after a motor vehicle crash. *J Trauma* 1993; **34**: 116–19.

27. Hyde LK, Cook LJ, Olson LM, Weiss HB, Dean JM. Effect of motor vehicle crashes on adverse fetal outcome. *Obstet Gynecol* 2003; **102**: 279–86.

28. Beck LF, Gilbert BC, Shults RA. Prevalence of seat belt use among reproductive-aged women and prenatal counseling to wear seat belts. *Am J Obstet Gynecol* 2005; **192**: 580–5.

29. Kettel LM, Branch DW, Scott JR. Occult placental abruption after maternal trauma. *Obstet Gynecol* 1988; **223**: 481–8.

30. Ikossi DG, Lazar AA, Morabito D, Fildes J, Knudson MM. Profile of mothers at risk: an analysis of injury and pregnancy loss in 1,195 trauma patients. *J Am Coll Surg* 2005; **200**: 49–56.

31. Pearlman MD, Tintinelli JE, Lorenz RP. A prospective controlled study of outcome after trauma during pregnancy. *Am J Obstet Gynecol* 1990; **162**: 1502–10.

32. Oxford CM, Ludmir J. Risk factors for maternal trauma: trauma in pregnancy. *Clin Obstet Gynecol* 2009; **52**: 611–29.

33. Romero VC, Pearlman M. Mechanisms of injury: maternal mortality due to trauma. *Semin Perinatol* 2011: **36**: 60–7.

34. Pearlman M. Management of trauma during pregnancy. *The Female Patient* 1996; **21**: 79–98.

35. Poole GV, Martin JN, Perry KG, *et al.* Trauma in pregnancy: role of interpersonal violence. *Am J Obstet Gynecol* 1996; **174**: 1873–5.

36. Amy B, McManus W, Goodwin C, *et al.* Thermal injury in the pregnant patient. *Surg Gynecol Obstet* 1985; **161**: 209–12.

37. Lavery J. Staten-McCormik M. Management of moderate to severe trauma in pregnancy. *Obstet Gynecol Clin N Am* 1995; **22**: 69–90.

38. Polko L, McMohan M. Burns in pregnancy. *Obstet Gynecol Surv* 1997; **53**: 50–6.

39. Schmitz J. pregnant patients with burns. *Am J Obstet Gynecol* 1971; **110**: 57.

40. Kuhlmann R, Cruikshank D. Maternal trauma during pregnancy. *Clin Obstet Gynecol* 1994; **37**: 274–93.

41. Longo LD, Hill EP. Carbon monoxide uptake and elimination in fetal and maternal sheep. *Am J Physiol* 1997; **232**: H324–30.

42. Longo LD. Carbon monoxide in the pregnant mother and fetus and its exchange across the placenta. *Ann N Y Acad Sci* 1970; **174**: 312.41.

43. Caravati EM, Adams CJ, Joyce SM, *et al.* Fetal toxicity associated with maternal carbon monoxide poisoning. *Ann Emerg Med* 1988; **17**: 714–17.

44. Cramer CR. Fetal death due to accidental carbon monoxide poisoning. *J Toxicol Clin Toxicol* 1982; **19**: 297–301.

45. Clark SL, Cotton DB, Privarnik JM, *et al.* Positional changes and central hemodynamic profile during normal third trimester pregnancy and post partum. *Am J Obstet Gynecol* 1991; **164**: 883–7.

46. Connoly AM, Katz VL, Bash KL, McMahon MJ, Hansen WF. Trauma in pregnancy. *Am J Perinatol* 1997; **14**: 331–6.

47. National Safety Council. *Accidents Facts.* Chicago, IL: National Safety Council, 1997.

48. Pak LL, Reece EA, Chen L. Is adverse pregnancy outcome predictable after blunt abdominal trauma? *Am J Obstet Gynecol* 1998; **179**: 1140–4.

49. Knudson MM, Rozycki GS, Pacquin, MM. Reproductive system trauma. In Moore EE, Feliciano DV, Mattox KL, eds., *Trauma*, 5th edition. New York, NY: McGraw-Hill, 2004, p. 851.

50. Davis BH, Olsen S, Bigelow NC, *et al.* detection of fetal red cells in fetomaternal hemorrhage using a fetal hemoglobin monoclonal antibody by flow cytometry. *Transfusion* 1998; **38**: 749–56.

51. Holland JG, Hume AS, Martin JN. Drug use and physical trauma: risk factors for preterm delivery. *J Miss State Med Assoc* 1997; **38**: 301–5.

52. Huzel PS, Remsburg-Bell EA. Fetal complication related to minor maternal trauma. *J Obstet Gynecol Neonatal Nurs* 1996; **25**: 121–4.

53. Goodwin H, Holmes J, Wisner D. Abdominal ultrasound examination in pregnant blunt trauma patients. *J Trauma* 2001; **50**: 689–94.

54. Ingeman J, Plewa M, Okasinski R, *et al.* Emergency physician use of ultrasonography in blunt abdominal trauma. *Acad Emerg Med* 1996; **3**: 931–7.

55. Ma O, Mateer J, DeBehnke D. Use of ultrasonography for the evaluation of pregnant trauma patients. *J Trauma* 1996; **40**: 665–8.

56. Rothenberger D, Quattlebaum F, Zabel J, *et al.* Diagnostic peritoneal lavage for blunt trauma in pregnant women. *Am J Obstet Gynecol* 1977; **129**: 479–81.

57. Ma O, Mateer J, Ogata M, *et al.* Prospective analysis of a rapid trauma ultrasound examination performed by emergency physicians. *J Trauma* 1995; **38**: 879–85.

58. Lazebnik N, Laebnik RS. The role of ultrasound in pregnancy related emergencies. *Radiol Clin N Am* 2004; **42**: 315–27.

59. Eliot G, Rao D. Pregnancy and radiographic examination. In Haycock CE, ed., *Trauma and Pregnancy*. Littleton, MA: PSG Publishing, 1985, p. 69.

60. Hussein AA, Abutaleb A, Jeudy J, *et al.* Safety of computed tomography imaging in patients with cardiac rhythm management devices: assessment of the FDA advisory in real-world practice. *J Am Coll Cardiol* 2014; **63**: 1769–75.

61. Selden BS, Burke TJ. Complete maternal and fetal recovery after prolonged cardiac arrest. *Ann Emerg Med* 1988; **17**: 346–9.

62. Runnebaum IB, Holeberg G, Katz M. Pregnancy outcome after repeated blunt abdominal trauma. *Eur J Obstet Gynecol Reprod Biol* 1998; **80**: 85–6.

63. Drost TF, Rosemurgy AS, Sherman HF, *et al.* Major trauma in pregnant women: maternal/fetal outcome. *J Trauma* 1990; **30**: 574–8.

64. Knupple RA, Drucker JE. *High Risk Pregnancy: a Team Approach*, 2nd edition. Philadelphia, PA: Saunders, 1993, p. 241.

65. Ducey JP, Knape KG. Maternal esmolol administration resulting in fetal distress and cesarean section in a term pregnancy. *Anesthesiology* 1992; **77**: 829–32.

66. Karsli B, Kaya T, Cetin A. Effects of intravenous anesthetic agents on pregnant myometrium. *Pol J Pharmacol* 1999; **51**: 505–10.

67. Carnini A, Eckenhoff MF, Eckenhoff RG. Interactions of volatile anesthetics with neurodegenerative-disease-associated proteins. *Anesth Clin N Am* 2006; **24**: 381–405.

68. Ostheimer GW. *Manual of Obstetric Anesthesia*. New York, NY: Churchill Livingstone, 1992.

69. Murphy N, Reed S. Maternal resuscitation and trauma. In Damos JR, Eisinger SH, eds., *Advanced Life Support in Obstetrics (ALSO) Provider Course Syllabus*. Leawood, KS: American Academy of Family Physicians, 2000, pp. 1–25.

70. Tweddale CJ. Trauma during pregnancy. *Crit Care Nurs Q* 2006; **29**: 53–67.

71. American Heart Association. Guidelines for cardiopulmonary resuscitation and emergency cardiac care. Emergency Cardiac Care Committee and Subcommittees, American Heart Association. Part III. Adult advanced cardiac life support. *JAMA* 1992; **268**: 2199–241.

72. Katz V, Dotters D, Droegemueller W. Perimortem cesarean delivery. *Obstet Gynecol* 1986; **68**: 571–6.

73. Selden BS, Burke TJ. Complete maternal and fetal recovery after prolonged cardiac arrest. *Ann Emerg Med* 1988; **17**: 346–9.

74. Oats S, Williams GL, Rees GA. Cardiopulmonary resuscitation in late pregnancy. *BMJ* 1988; **297**: 404–5.

75. Lindsay SL, Hanson GC. Cardiac arrest in near term pregnancy. *Anesthesia* 1987; **42**: 1074–7.

76. O'Connor RL, Sevarino FB. Cardiopulmonary arrest in the pregnant patient: a report of a successful resuscitation. *J Clin Anesth* 1994; **6**: 66–8.

77. DePase NL, Betesh JS, Kotler MN. Postmortem cesarean section with recovery of both mother and offspring. *JAMA* 1982; **248**: 971–3.

78. Lee R, Rodgers B, White L, Harvey R. Cardiopulmonary resuscitation of pregnant women. *Am J Med* 1986; **81**: 311–18.

79. Zakowski MI, Ramanathan S. CPR in pregnancy. *Curr Rev Clin Anesth* 1989; **10**: 106–11.

80. Mallampalli A, Powner DJ, Gardner MO. Cardiopulmonary resuscitation and somatic support of the pregnant patient. *Crit Care Clin* 2004; **20**: 747–61.

Field anesthesia and military injury

Nicholas T. Tarmey, Claire L. Park, Craig C. McFarland, and Peter F. Mahoney

Objectives

(1) Review the military environment and the constraints this imposes on resuscitation and anesthesia.
(2) Review the issues in resuscitation of the ballistic casualty.
(3) Discuss aspects of field anesthesia.

Introduction

Injuries from modern military munitions can be complex and devastating. Their management demands particular anesthetic and surgical skill sets including an understanding of time-critical injury.

In addition, casualty management in the deployed military setting is subject to a number of threats and constraints that influence how care can be delivered.

This chapter will consider the types of casualties that may present to the military provider, and how the care is influenced by situational constraints, and will suggest some anesthetic techniques that are appropriate for use in the field.

The military environment

The military environment presents a number of important constraints, all of which can challenge the safe and effective delivery of medical care. These include the threat of attacks on field medical units, the austerity of the environment, limited medical supplies, and the potential for large surges in casualty flow. Care delivered in this environment must be tailored to the circumstances of the conflict, and will often depend on working effectively with other nations' military and civilian medical systems.

Threat of attacks on field medical units

According to the Geneva conventions, medical units, personnel, and vehicles should expect protection from attack, provided they keep to their humanitarian role and do not engage directly in hostile actions.[1] Unfortunately this protection has proved of limited use in the recent conflicts in Iraq and Afghanistan, where there have been numerous instances of deliberate attacks on medical resources and personnel. The asymmetric nature of

modern warfare has also affected the nature of these risks, with the emerging threats of suicide attacks on military facilities and the infiltration of host-nation personnel by insurgent forces. Practically, this means that the medical response cannot be dissociated from the prevailing security situation, and casualty care has to be modified accordingly.

Current United Kingdom (UK) Battlefield Advanced Trauma Life Support (BATLS) teaching recognizes this situation and describes four levels of medical care: care under fire, tactical field care, field resuscitation, and advanced resuscitation.[2] Care for the casualty begins at the point of wounding and becomes increasingly advanced as the casualty is evacuated to a more permissive environment.

Care under fire

Care under fire emphasizes the primary need to win the fire fight (eliminate the immediate risk of further effective enemy gunfire) and deal with the threat. Medical intervention – if any – is limited to control of catastrophic hemorrhage with a tourniquet, rolling the casualty face down to minimize airway obstruction, and placing a chest seal over a penetrating chest wound. Care at this level will often be delivered by nonmedical military personnel, who must rely upon their own medical skills. At the time of writing (2013), all UK forces deploying to Afghanistan are trained to a high standard in battlefield first aid, including the immediate use of a Combat Application Tourniquet (CAT; Composite Resources, Inc. Rock Hill, SC) for massive external hemorrhage (Fig. 38.1).

The priority at this stage is to manage the threat and reach the next level of care. Summoning additional help or evacuation assets depends on an intact communication system and the state of the battle. The response to this request depends on what other military tasks are already in hand. For isolated units and individuals, help may take some time to arrive.

Tactical field care

Tactical field care is when the immediate threat has been dealt with but the environment is still not safe. Casualty assessment is done rapidly. Further interventions may include topical hemostatic dressings for control of catastrophic hemorrhage,

---

Trauma Anesthesia, 2nd Edition, ed. Charles E. Smith. Published by Cambridge University Press. © Charles E. Smith, 2015.

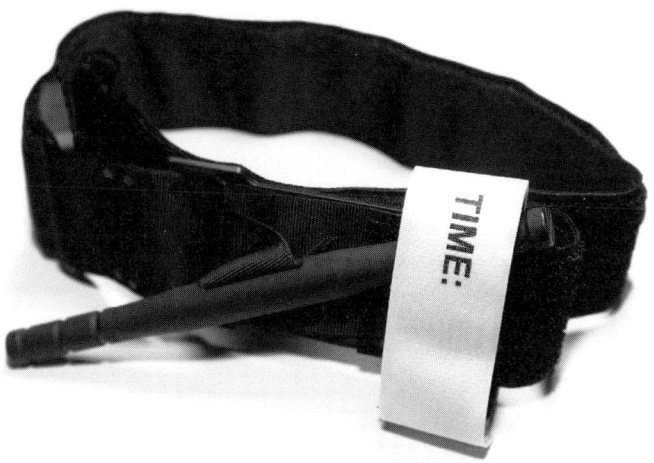

Figure 38.1 Combat Application Tourniquet. (Photo courtesy of N. Tarmey)

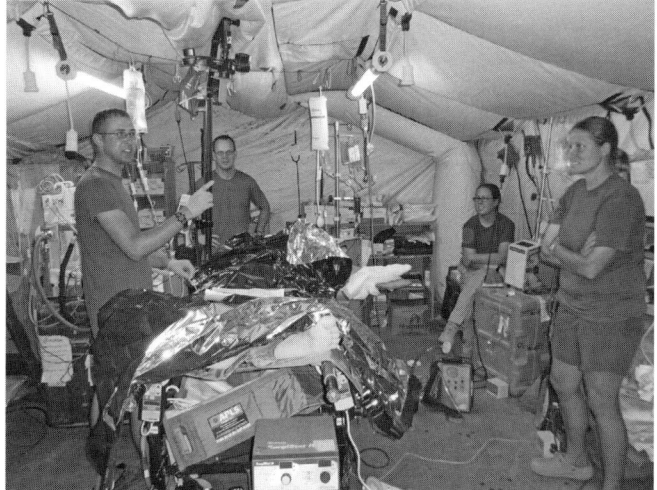

Figure 38.2 Role 2 field medical facility, Afghanistan, 2011. (Photo courtesy of C. Park.) *A black and white version of this figure will appear in some formats. For the color version, please refer to the plate section.*

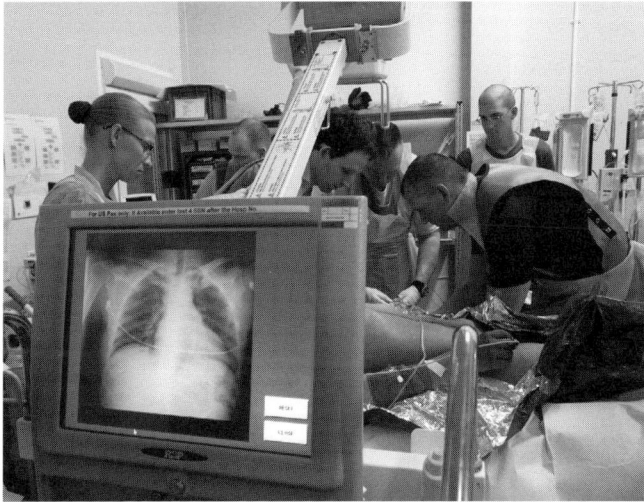

Figure 38.3 Casualty reception at the UK multinational Role 3 hospital, Afghanistan 2010. (Photo courtesy of N. Tarmey. Previously published inside the cover of *Journal of the Royal Army Medical Corps* 2010, Vol 156: reproduced with permission of the Editor.) *A black and white version of this figure will appear in some formats. For the color version, please refer to the plate section.*

basic airway maneuvers, needle decompression of tension pneumothorax, intravenous (IV) or intraosseous (IO) access, and limited fluid resuscitation.

Field resuscitation

Field resuscitation is conventionally delivered at the regimental aid post (RAP) or Role 1 facility, where a casualty will meet a medical officer for the first time. Here it is possible to conduct a more thorough examination and perform limited invasive procedures. As a small, mobile unit, the RAP is constrained by a lack of resources, and the priority remains to evacuate the casualty quickly to a higher level of care.

Advanced resuscitation

Advanced resuscitation is where the casualty will meet a full trauma team, which will usually include an emergency physician and an anesthesiologist. Depending on the type of facility, there will be diagnostic capability including x-ray and ultrasound.

Some facilities (Role 2 facilities) will also have the capability of performing surgery (Fig. 38.2). In a mature medical system, an established field hospital (a Role 3 facility) may evolve to include many of the resources found in a major civilian trauma center, including computed tomography (CT) and critical care capacity (Fig. 38.3). Nonetheless, a field hospital will still be constrained by the local security situation, the need to be mobile, and the limitations of the logistic chain. The concepts of advanced resuscitation are considered further in the next section.

Austerity of environment

Military personnel deployed on operations are likely to find themselves working in an environment where the local infrastructure has been damaged, if not destroyed (Fig. 38.4). The military system will need to provide its own infrastructure of shelter, water, sanitation, energy supply, and transport. The logistic support to the medical system will inevitably be limited by the state of battle and competition with other military priorities.

The degree of mobility required from a medical facility will also determine the standard of its infrastructure. A mobile medical facility has to move its personnel, shelter, food, water, and fuel, as well as medical supplies. All are competing for space and lift capacity. Mobile facilities are dependent on early evacuation of patients to avoid becoming fixed in place. In a more mature medical system, the field hospital may be located at an established military logistic base, where it can make use of a higher standard of in-theater infrastructure.

Limited supplies and equipment

Medical supplies have to compete in the military logistic system with other supplies and consumables. The longer and

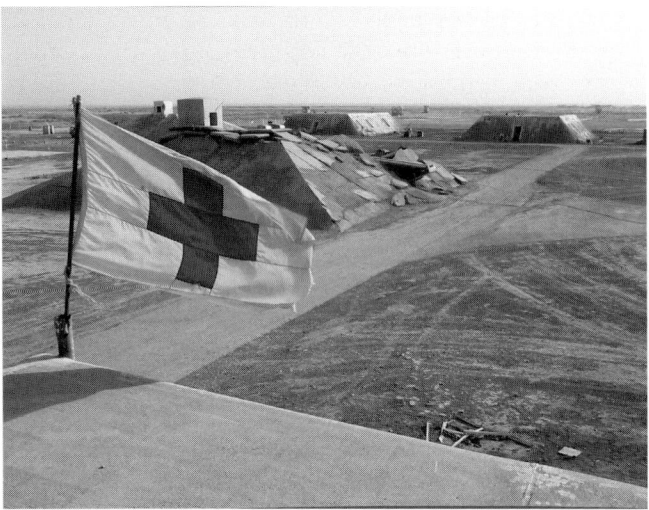

Figure 38.4 Medical facility located in battle-damaged infrastructure, Iraq, 2003. (Photo courtesy of N. Tarmey.)

more vulnerable the supply chain, the greater the need to make efficient use of consumables. The supply of blood and blood products is particularly problematic. These supplies have short shelf lives and depend upon an intact logistic chain of temperature-controlled transport to ensure they remain within a safe temperature range. When frequent resupply is not possible, in-theater blood donor panels can be used. These present problems of their own, including the potential for increased risks of infection and transfusion reactions.[3] It is anticipated that freeze-dried alternatives to fresh frozen plasma, factor concentrates (e.g., fibrinogen, prothrombin complex concentrates), and, possibly, synthetic oxygen carriers may provide alternative solutions to these problems.

Surge capacity

Military conflicts by their nature produce casualties at an unpredictable rate. The casualty load on a medical facility may increase steadily or a large number may arrive suddenly. When the number of casualties outstrips resources, triage is initiated. This situation may arise with few or many casualties depending on the facility and resources. The aim of triage is to "do the most for the most" by sorting casualties and prioritizing treatment to make the best use of limited resources.

Mobile surgical teams have traditionally been described by the number of casualties they can operate on prior to resupply. This description fails to account for multiply injured casualties, who may require a disproportionate amount of consumables. Instead, it may be better to describe resources by the number of body cavities and limbs that can be operated on prior to resupply.

In planning for surge capacity, it is also important to understand the rate of casualty flow that can be sustained by the medical facility. This will depend on the number of surgical cases that can be performed concurrently, the capacity for postoperative care, and the rate of onward evacuation. When

demand greatly outstrips capacity, a robust system of triage is essential to ensure that resources are used to the greatest effect.

Interaction with other medical systems

In recent conflicts, UK and US medical services have worked closely with other allied medical services to provide an integrated multinational medical capability. The Role 2 and Role 3 capabilities of each nation are fairly similar, whereas the approach to prehospital care varies more between nations. For example, the UK military helicopter-based prehospital team is led by an anesthesiologist or emergency medicine physician; in the US model this team is led by a specialist paramedic with advanced airway skills.

In a failed state, military medical services may initially be required to provide medical care for the civilian host-nation population. This does not provide a long-term solution, so it is essential to engage early with local facilities to plan and support the transfer of responsibility back to the host nation.

Engagement with nongovernmental organizations (NGOs) and local health leaders will help in this transition. This can be a sensitive area, especially where NGOs need to remain impartial in a conflict and cannot be seen to be working too closely with a military medical system. Local standards of health care will often fall short of established Western system standards, mostly because of disruption to structures and resources. The local system must continue to use local policies and standards that they are able to maintain when the military leaves.

When receiving casualties from civilian and allied military healthcare systems, they may arrive with poor documentation and incomplete treatment. The issue here is not to criticize the other system, as they may be working under immense difficulties and pressures, but to remind clinicians to take an objective look at each casualty transferred in and undertake a thorough examination and investigation.

Robust clinical governance is essential to ensure high-quality care in military medicine. Clinical governance systems are well established in the UK and US military, with continuous audit of performance indicators, systematic assessment of outcomes, detailed peer review of all deaths, and regular contemporaneous in-theater follow-up of repatriated casualties.[4]

Populations treated

Until the last part of the twentieth century war was mostly viewed as a face-to-face battle between two massed armies on a battlefield, otherwise described as symmetric warfare, where military casualties far exceeded civilian losses. More recently, warfare has changed, and this ratio is somewhat reversed. The asymmetric warfare of the twenty-first century is carried out in the midst of civilian populations, with terrorism targeting every continent.

The casualties treated in recent operations have included a significant number of civilians of all ages and medical conditions. Importantly, this includes a large number of children. One practical issue with children is estimating age and weight to allow calculation of drug and fluid doses. A solution is to use a system such as the Broselow tape (Armstrong Medical Industries Inc., Lincolnshire, Illinois) to estimate weight, drug doses, and equipment sizes. Host-nation children may be smaller than their Western counterparts, so calculations must be adjusted accordingly.

The number of civilians treated on an operation by the UK military depends on the nature and stage of the operation and is stated in the medical rules of engagement (MROE) for that particular theater of war. Life-, limb-, and eye-saving surgery will be provided for host-nation civilians and security forces, if the operational tempo allows the capacity to do so. During some operations, for example in disaster relief, the level of care provided to host nationals may be much greater than this. In addition, under the Geneva Conventions, coalition forces will provide emergency care and surgery for detainees and enemy forces injured in the conflict.[1]

In the case of civilian contractors, one must be aware of undeclared long-term medical and surgical histories. Recent UK and US experience includes patients with poorly managed cardiorespiratory disease, diabetes, immunological compromise, and malignant tumors. For the host nationals, disruption of the local healthcare service will often mean that acute and chronic health conditions have not been managed, and this will complicate resuscitation and anesthesia.

The military population at risk tends to be young and fit. Minimal medical problems and good reserve allow significant compensation in the early phases of severe injury. In addition, some prediction of likely injuries and casualty numbers can be made by using casualty templates from similar conflicts.

Resuscitation of the military casualty
Patterns of injury

Injuries on recent military operations have mostly been due to gunshot wounds (GSWs) and blast from improvised explosive devices (IEDs), with only a small proportion of casualties suffering blunt trauma.[5] This is in contrast to the UK civilian experience, where 56% of major trauma casualties are injured by blunt trauma.[6]

The ratio of GSWs to IEDs will vary according to the operational situation and enemy tactics employed. GSWs can affect any (and often multiple) body cavities.

In military trauma it is essential to maintain a high index of suspicion for serious injuries based on the mechanism of injury. In penetrating torso injuries the key surgical decision is often which cavity to open first. It is not uncommon for GSWs to the neck or abdomen to cross the spinal canal and cause significant spinal damage. High-velocity accurate GSWs to the head are usually nonsurvivable.[7] This contrasts with penetrating brain injuries from low-velocity fragments, which may result in a good neurological outcome.[8]

IED explosions can cause injury in three ways: by the primary blast shock wave, by secondary ballistic fragments,

and by the "tertiary injury" of the casualty or large objects being thrown by the blast. Injury patterns will vary depending on the design and placement of the IED, the proximity of the casualty to the device, and the degree of ballistic protection worn by the casualty.[5]

Blast injury tends to occur at the interface between tissues of different densities, notably in the form of perforated eardrums and blast lung (see also Chapter 30). When an IED is triggered by a soldier on foot, this blast may cause a very severe pattern of injury, with traumatic limb amputation and gross soft tissue damage complicated by secondary fragmentation. At the time of writing (2013), this has been the mechanism of injury for many of the most severely injured UK and US casualties in Afghanistan (Fig. 38.5).

Modern ballistic protection has done a great deal to protect personnel from fragmentation injuries. The use of ballistic eye protection has undoubtedly prevented sight loss, and the introduction of pelvic protection has been instrumental in decreasing pelvic injuries. Personnel injured by IEDs when travelling by armored vehicle tend to suffer a different pattern of trauma, with spinal injuries, lower limb fractures, and closed head injury. When blast occurs in an enclosed space, there is a significant risk of blast-related lung injury.[10]

Burns, disease, and nonbattle injury account for most of the remaining casualties in a military field hospital. A number of burn patients, both thermal and chemical, are seen in the deployed environment, and standard burns treatment applies (see Chapters 39 and 40). It is usually not appropriate for a field hospital to keep local patients to perform split skin grafts or flaps. Chemical, biological, radiological, and nuclear threats remain important in the military environment, and appropriate personal protective equipment is essential.

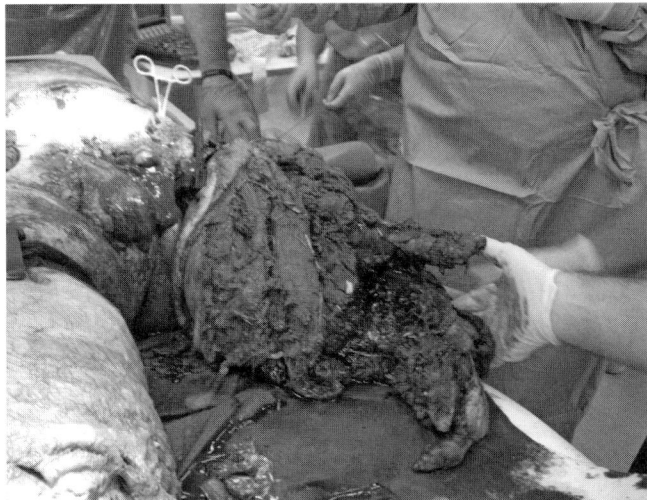

Figure 38.5 IED blast injury to the lower limbs, with proximal hemorrhage control from Combat Application Tourniquets and temporary surgical arterial ligation. (Reproduced from Parker 2011,[9] with permission of the Editor of the *Journal of the Royal Army Medical Corps.*) *A black and white version of this figure will appear in some formats. For the color version, please refer to the plate section.*

The <C>ABC paradigm

The UK military paradigm of <C>ABC places control of catastrophic hemorrhage, <C>, ahead of the traditional priorities of airway, breathing, and circulation. This recognizes the importance of immediate control of massive external hemorrhage to prevent early death on the battlefield.[11] This approach begins at the point of wounding, where immediate priorities include direct compression of bleeding wounds and the application of any limb tourniquets.

As the casualty is evacuated, compressive dressings and tourniquets are rechecked repeatedly. Bleeding may be reduced further with tightened or additional tourniquets or dressings, or with the use of pelvic and limb splinting and topical hemostatic agents. Throughout this process, the aim is to minimize blood loss while transporting immediately to a surgical facility. If there is ongoing major abdominal, pelvic, or thoracic hemorrhage, survival will depend upon rapid access to damage control surgery.

The military evacuation chain

In the symmetric warfare of the past, linear battlefields enabled casualties to be evacuated sequentially through echelons or "roles" of care. In current asymmetric warfare, helicopter-borne casualty evacuation (casevac) assets can retrieve a casualty from or near to the point of wounding, bypassing both Role 2 and often Role 1 facilities (Fig. 38.6). The UK physician-led medical emergency response team has the capability to begin Role 3 level resuscitation in flight and will take the casualty directly to the Role 3 trauma team. On arrival at the field hospital, a casualty in extremis may even bypass the emergency department and be transferred directly onto the operating table.[12]

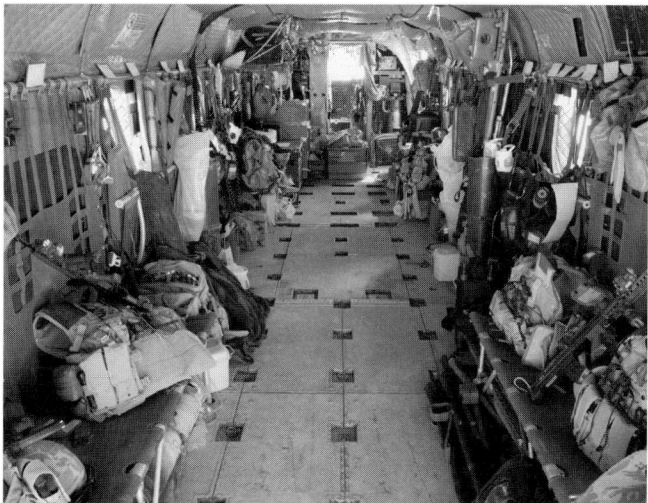

Figure 38.6 Chinook helicopter equipped for casualty evacuation by the UK Medical Emergency Response Team, Afghanistan, 2010. (Photo courtesy of N. Tarmey.) *A black and white version of this figure will appear in some formats. For the color version, please refer to the plate section.*

Casevac assets in theater are tasked by clinicians based in the patient evacuation control cell. Tasking is based primarily on mechanism and injuries sustained in addition to the casualty's location, available assets, and the operational situation. If a casualty has been transferred directly to a Role 2 facility for damage control resuscitation, an in-theater critical care air support team may be used for the onwards transfer to Role 3.

Triage of casualties, especially host-nation civilians, will depend on the threat situation and medical rules of engagement at the time. Medical rules of engagement are a set of agreed criteria stating who may be accepted for treatment, and under what circumstances. Treatment delivered will depend on the eventual destination, as many local civilian hospitals may be unable to manage ventilated patients. Critically ill military casualties are transported back to home (UK or US) Role 4 facilities by strategic critical care air support team. These teams are activated as soon as a soldier is admitted to the field hospital in a critical condition. In a well-established military medical system, casualties may reach the home Role 4 hospital within 24 hours of the initial injury.

Damage control resuscitation and surgery

From the point of wounding on the battlefield, through resuscitation and surgery to critical care, military casualties are managed according to the principles of damage control resuscitation and surgery. This incorporates the principles of permissive hypotension, hemostatic resuscitation, and damage control surgery (see Chapter 18).[13]

Permissive hypotension

Permissive hypotension is a strategy used in the initial management of traumatic bleeding, where moderate hypotension is tolerated to minimize blood loss before surgical control is achieved. This aims to balance the conflicting demands of maintaining organ perfusion and preventing hemodilution and early clot disruption.

The main clinical evidence for permissive hypotension comes from the prehospital environment, where withholding crystalloid resuscitation increased survival after civilian trauma.[14] These findings are applied on the battlefield with protocols that allow small (e.g., 250 mL) fluid challenges, titrated to the presence of a radial pulse or 90 mmHg systolic BP.

It is important to remember that this strategy compromises short-term organ perfusion and, if carried on for too long, will result in multiorgan failure. Emerging evidence from animal studies shows that limiting the period of permissive hypotension after blast injury to 60 minutes may be safer than prolonged hypotensive resuscitation.[15] Hypotensive resuscitation may be particularly harmful in brain trauma, where it is usually better to target a near-normal blood pressure (BP).[16] Patients will vary in their ability to tolerate hypotension, so the priority in all casualties is to reach a level of care where hemorrhage can be controlled and normal BP and perfusion restored as quickly as possible.[15]

Hemostatic resuscitation

Hemostatic resuscitation is a combination of strategies that aims to restore organ perfusion by replacing blood volume and targeting the effects of trauma-induced coagulopathy. It is widely accepted that coagulopathy after trauma can be caused by the "lethal triad" of hypothermia, acidosis, and dilution of clotting factors. More recently it has become clear that coagulopathy can also develop very early after severe trauma, apparently due to the release of multiple humoral factors in response to tissue hypoxia.[17] Hemostatic resuscitation aims to correct this coagulopathy through blood product transfusion, pharmacological adjuncts, and the restoration of tissue perfusion.

Blood product transfusion

An important part of the current military approach to hemorrhagic shock is the early use of blood and clotting products in ratios approximating whole blood (see Chapter 6). Early evidence for this approach came from a retrospective study from US field hospitals in Iraq, where transfusion of a higher ratio of plasma to packed red blood cells was associated with increased survival. Where resources permit, this is now applied

using military massive transfusion protocols (MTPs) that deliver plasma and blood in a 1:1 ratio until hemorrhage is controlled (Fig. 38.7).[18]

Although this approach is still not proven in a randomized trial, excellent outcomes have been achieved, with a UK study from Afghanistan in 2009 showing an 86% overall survival after massive transfusion.[19] In some settings, transfusion may even be projected forward of the field hospital, to allow an earlier move to hemostatic resuscitation. One example of this is the current (2013) physician-led UK medical emergency response team which carries blood and thawed plasma on a helicopter-based prehospital service in Afghanistan.

Military massive transfusion places high demands on the logistic cold chain to provide a ready supply of blood and clotting products. When resupply is delayed or prevented, it may be possible to activate an in-theater emergency blood donor panel. Although this overcomes the problems of transporting blood to the field hospital, considerable obstacles remain. Operating a donor panel places deployed laboratory staff under great pressure, especially if products are required immediately. Prescreening for blood-borne viruses may reduce the infection risk, but there remains the potential for serious transfusion reactions in nonleukodepleted blood.[3]

Transfused blood products can undoubtedly cause harm as well as benefit, so it is important to move to a more tailored transfusion as soon as the situation allows. In severe military

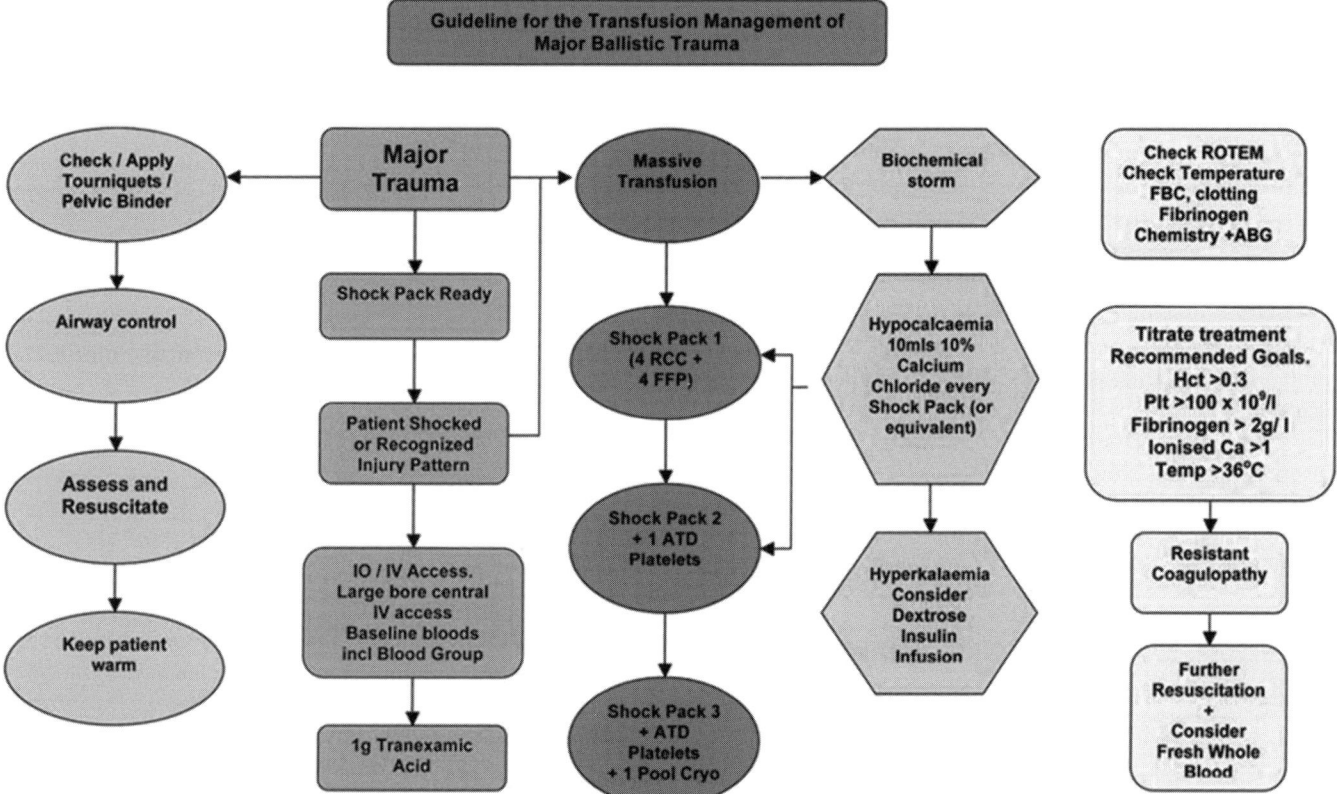

Figure 38.7 UK military massive transfusion protocol. (Reproduced from Doughty *et al.* 2011,[18] with permission of the Editor of the *Journal of the Royal Army Medical Corps.*) A black and white version of this figure will appear in some formats. For the color version, please refer to the plate section.

trauma this will not usually be possible until initial surgical control of hemorrhage is achieved. The emphasis should then switch towards individualized transfusion guided by the clinical findings and indices of coagulation.[20] The laboratory tests of prothrombin time and platelet count have traditionally been used, but recent UK military experience has shown that advanced coagulation monitoring using thromboelastometry is feasible in the deployed environment.[21] This type of monitoring may prove of greater value than in the civilian environment, given the even greater need to make the best possible use of limited blood supplies.

Pharmacological adjuncts

Although a number of drugs have been used to aid coagulation in military trauma, the mainstay of resuscitation remains the transfusion of blood and blood products. Recombinant activated human factor VIIa (rFVIIa) appeared useful in initial case series and observational studies, but a large randomized controlled trial in civilian trauma failed to show benefit.[22] This drug is now used rarely in military trauma and is typically reserved for cases where appropriate clotting product transfusion has proved impossible or ineffective. In contrast, tranexamic acid (TXA) has been shown to improve survival in both civilian and military trauma, and this is now given routinely as part of the UK military massive transfusion protocol.[23,24]

Damage control surgery

Damage control surgery is a strategy where the completeness of initial surgical repair is sacrificed in order to limit operating times and mitigate the combined physiological insults of trauma and surgery (see Chapters 18 and 31). As well as minimizing operating times, a key goal is to provide resuscitation seamlessly throughout surgery, so that patients may leave the operating room as physiologically restored as possible.[13]

Decision making on the extent of initial surgery should be a dynamic process, involving both anesthetic and surgical teams, with continuous reassessment of the patient's physiology. In some cases this team approach to damage control may allow more extensive initial surgery, permitting limb salvage where this would not otherwise be possible. In other cases the patient's condition or the tactical situation may dictate that only essential surgery for immediate control of hemorrhage can be performed.[25]

Crew resource management, communication, and human factors

Excellent communication and attention to the risks of human error are essential in the pressurized military medical environment. Clear, concise commands and communication are necessary for effective passage of information and team working.

It is worth considering how to optimize the effectiveness of the military complex trauma team. A team of similar competitive personalities does not always perform as well as one containing complementary personalities. Contrary to common belief, the best team is not always made up of the best individuals. Team size has consequences for its productivity, and more relevant than level of education or experience to team effectiveness is the level of "psychological safety" experienced within a team.

For an effective military trauma team to run well, there needs to be effective leadership and proficient followership, along with clear decision making. It is vital that the team leader maintains situational awareness and is able to anticipate and plan when physiological changes occur, and to provide the team with clear direction and early decision making.[26]

Nontechnical skills affect everyone in emergency situations. Rigorous training prior to deployment allows motor programs to be embedded so that routine actions are performed automatically, allowing more mental "bandwidth" to be available to take in everything else. This allows for an increased situational awareness and increased ability to anticipate and manage unforeseen problems. Awareness of one's own and others' ability to become task-focused, and of the possibility of fixation error, is vital. Training as a team allows all members to be aware of this and to compensate accordingly if not directly involved in the task. In addition to the injury pattern and evolving physiological response and interventions required, there is an added level of military situational awareness that is required, especially in the forward echelons of care and during forward casevac.

Interpreters are present at trauma calls to communicate with local nationals: whether civilians, security forces, or enemy combatants. Liaison officers are also needed for allied military casualties who do not speak English as their first language.

A standard handover format using the mnemonic AT-MIST is used by UK prehospital medical teams (Table 38.1). This ensures handover of all relevant information in a standardized format aiding reception of the information by the receiving clinician/team.

Field and military anesthesia
Timing and techniques of anesthesia

The military casualty's airway may require interventions at any stage of the evacuation chain. At Role 1 the skills and equipment for rapid sequence induction of anesthesia (RSI) do not exist – so the only option for a definitive airway is a surgical cricothyroidotomy under local anesthetic. For the medical emergency response team and Role 2 onwards, the anesthetic decisions and considerations are discussed below.

Anesthesia is just one part of the damage control resuscitation process, and the anesthetic must be given at the most appropriate stage in this process. The military anesthesiologist

Table 38.1 The AT-MIST handover format

A	Age
T	Time of injury
M	Mechanism
I	Injuries sustained
S	Signs and symptoms
T	Treatment given

Table 38.2 Indications for rapid sequence induction of anesthesia

1. Actual or impending loss of airway
2. Patients with a reduced conscious level who are unable to maintain their own airway
3. Head injured patients, especially if combative or with a low Glasgow Coma Scale (GCS: see Table 35.1 in Chapter 35).
4. Thoracic injuries or decreased level of consciousness causing ventilatory failure
5. Expected clinical course *
6. Humanitarian reasons (relief of distress and pain) *

* Numbers 5 and 6 are relative indications only, and will depend on a careful risk–benefit analysis, including the risks of rapid decompensation on induction of anesthesia and initiation of positive-pressure ventilation.

needs a full understanding of the casualty's cardiovascular status as well as the identified and potential injuries, necessitating a thorough understanding of the mechanism of injury.

BP and heart rate are unreliable indicators of a military casualty's cardiovascular status.[27] A young adult may lose up to 40% of his or her circulating volume yet compensate sufficiently to show little change in these vital signs. The presence of a radial pulse, along with serum lactate and base excess analysis where available, can be a more reliable way of assessing cardiovascular status prior to induction. The indication for RSI should be noted as an aid to decision making (Table 38.2).

An early priority in damage control resuscitation is to identify the main source(s) of bleeding. General anesthesia may be required to comfortably, safely, and rapidly perform the imaging required to achieve this. Source control of hemorrhage should not be delayed to pursue resuscitation; however, bolus administration of blood products at the time of anesthetic induction may help to prevent catastrophic vascular collapse. In the hemorrhaging patient this bolus therapy should be carefully monitored and balanced against the administration of anesthetic drugs to preserve a state of controlled hypotension.[28] In a few circumstances it may be more appropriate to anesthetize a bleeding patient on the operating table rather than in the emergency department.

Drugs for induction of anesthesia

There is no ideal induction agent. Any induction agent with familiarity can be used at an appropriate dose according to the hemodynamic status of the patient. Commonly used drugs in major trauma include ketamine, fentanyl, rocuronium, succinylcholine, and midazolam. Vasopressors are inappropriate in the management of hemorrhagic shock and should be avoided, because there is evidence of increased mortality in bleeding trauma patients.[29] Hypotension should be treated primarily using volume resuscitation with blood products where possible.

Ketamine is an agent with a number of useful properties for military and trauma anesthesia, including its tendency not to cause hypotension on induction of anesthesia. Two main concerns have prevented its widespread use in the UK and the US until recently. The first relates to its effects on intracranial pressure (ICP) in patients with traumatic brain injury (TBI) (see Chapter 21). The only patients in whom ketamine has previously been shown to cause an increase in ICP were self-ventilating patients with abnormal cerebral blood flow. A number of studies more recently have proven that ketamine does not increase ICP in ventilated patients with TBI, and confirms that the hemodynamic stability achieved improves cerebral perfusion pressure.[30,31]

The second concern relates to the sympathomimetic effects of ketamine in a normotensive bleeding patient. This effect can be counteracted by giving fentanyl as an adjunct to the ketamine at induction. A fentanyl dose of 1–3 µg/kg is appropriate for induction, which can be increased up to 15 µg/kg titrated to BP during ongoing resuscitation and surgery.

Fentanyl has been used for many years as part of a cardiostable anesthetic. Experience in major trauma suggests it can be used to reverse inappropriate vasoconstriction and improve microcirculatory perfusion. Titration of fentanyl will reveal evidence of ongoing hypovolemia through a fall in BP. This should then be addressed with the administration of blood products as appropriate.

High-dose rocuronium (1–1.2 mg/kg) can be used in place of succinylcholine (suxamethonium) for RSI. Major trauma patients who fulfill the criteria for requiring immediate intubation are unlikely to wake and breathe adequately. It negates the need for a second dose and, where available, there is the potential for immediate reversal of high-dose rocuronium with sugammadex, 16 mg/kg (see Chapter 13).[32]

Midazolam may be necessary to allow the safe induction of a combative head-injured patient, in order to allow adequate preoxygenation prior to induction. It is a more cardiostable alternative to a propofol infusion to maintain anesthesia in the initial stages of resuscitation.

Choice of airway technique

It is rare for casualties to arrive at the field hospital with injuries causing a difficult airway. When these injuries do occur they are often dramatic, with severe disruption to both soft tissue and bone. The proximity of the carotid vessels means that penetrating carotid injury may impact airway patency. From 2003 to 2008 there were 375 cases of face and/ or neck injury reported on the UK Joint Theatre Trauma

Registry.[33] Among these, there were only 28 penetrating neck injuries and 13 penetrating laryngotracheal injuries.

If tracheal compression from hemorrhage caused by penetrating neck trauma is suspected, the trachea should be intubated early under controlled conditions, rather than as an emergency when the airway is compromised, narrowed, or displaced (see Chapter 3). Partial severance of the trachea is a rare but potentially disastrous situation, and attempted endotracheal intubation may complete the disruption. Extreme care must be exercised with positioning of the head and neck.

There is a lack of robust evidence regarding the anesthetic management of penetrating neck injuries.[34] Current (2013) UK military consensus guidelines state that the approach for both anticipated and unanticipated difficult airways should be to use a Macintosh size 4 laryngoscope blade and a gum elastic bougie, and to have two suction devices ready to use. The cervical collar should be removed and manual in-line stabilization should be used during the RSI if cervical spine injury is suspected. Occasionally, the "plan A" for anticipated difficult intubation may instead be a surgical airway.

The requirement for cervical spine immobilization in ballistic injury is the subject of ongoing debate. The prevailing view is that for military-grade weapons producing high-energy-transfer wounds to the cervical spine, the vast majority of patients will die very rapidly after injury. If they survive to reach care and they have an unstable injury, this will be associated with neurological deficit. In the absence of neurological deficit, the bony cervical spine is likely to be stable.[35] In the ballistic casualty, the pragmatic approach for field care is that cervical spine immobilization should be maintained in the presence of blunt injury, or combined blunt and penetrating injury (IEDs), but not in isolated penetrating ballistic injury without neurologic deficit. In ballistic injury, cervical collars can conceal developing hematoma and tracheal deviation.

A "plan B" for securing the airway will depend on injury pattern, physiology, and the presence of anticipated difficult airway. The principles of standard civilian guidelines for the management of anticipated and unanticipated difficult intubation are appropriate (see Chapter 3).[36] Depending on circumstances, a surgical airway may be either plan A or plan B. The most appropriate person to perform this should be determined by the trauma team leader prior to the patient's arrival.

Human factors are crucial to the effective team management of a difficult airway. Early senior decision making is vital. It is important that all members of the team responsible for securing the airway realize that oxygenation of the patient is the most important aspect of the procedure, and that they do not become fixated on tracheal intubation in the event of difficulties. It should be noted that, despite traditional teaching, cricoid pressure may not always be effective and it can interfere with insertion of the laryngoscope and may impair the view of the larynx.[37] Although cricoid pressure remains standard practice, there should be a low threshold for relaxing or removing it in the event of difficulty.

Table 38.3 Head injury care bundle, adapted from 2013 United Kingdom Defence Medical Services (UK DMS consensus guidelines) [38]

1. PaCO$_2$ 4.5 to 5 kPa (34 to 38 mmHg).
2. PaO$_2$ > 8 kPa (> 60 mmHg) but < 26 kPa (< 195 mmHg)
3. ETT tie and C-spine collar not too tight
4. Head up 30 degrees (tilt whole trolley)
5. Adequate sedation and paralysis
6. Arterial line when possible. Aim MAP 80–90 mmHg
7. Aim CPP > 60 mmHg (assuming ICP of 20 mmHg if monitoring not available)
8. Hypertonic saline (e.g., 5%) if pupils become fixed and dilated
9. Central line. Vasopressors may be required *only* if isolated head injury and adequate fluid resuscitation

C-spine, cervical spine; CPP, cerebral perfusion pressure; ETT, endotracheal tube; ICP, intracranial pressure; MAP, mean arterial blood pressure; PaCO$_2$, partial pressure of carbon dioxide; PaO$_2$, partial pressure of oxygen.

Equipment, monitoring, and drugs are prepared by the anesthetic team, but the whole trauma team must be briefed on the plan for the RSI and the failed airway plan. Roles should be allocated to team members. The requirement for decompressive thoracostomy on commencing positive-pressure ventilation must be discussed, and a team member should be ready to perform this task, if necessary, immediately after intubation.

When head injury is suspected, an appropriate bundle of care should be followed in order to optimize cerebral perfusion and prevent secondary brain injury (Table 38.3).

Field anesthesia

In the field medical environment, medical gas supplies cannot be guaranteed, hence the use of drawover techniques, with air as the carrier gas and oxygen supplemented from concentrators or cylinders. The use of compressors and oxygen concentrators has simplified the provision of compressed gas supply. The UK military currently deploy with the Penlon Tri-Service Anaesthesic Apparatus (TSAA). Other systems have been designed for field use and are suitable for the military, for aid agencies, or in developing countries. The Penlon apparatus can be used as a simple drawover system with spontaneous ventilation (Fig. 38.8), as a manually controlled intermittent positive-pressure ventilation system, or with a mechanical ventilator (Fig. 38.9). Mechanical ventilation can be in drawover or pushover mode. The apparatus is compact and robust, and it has been used successfully in many operational environments.[39] The original description by Houghton included using two Oxford Miniature Vaporizers in series. The system can be further simplified to one vaporizer and resuscitation bag for forward use or in disaster settings. Disadvantages of the Oxford Miniature Vaporizer include lack of temperature compensation, the small volume of anesthetic agent it contains, and the potential risk of contaminating the circuit with liquid volatile agents should the vaporizer be tipped over, although this should not happen if the vaporizer is correctly secured.

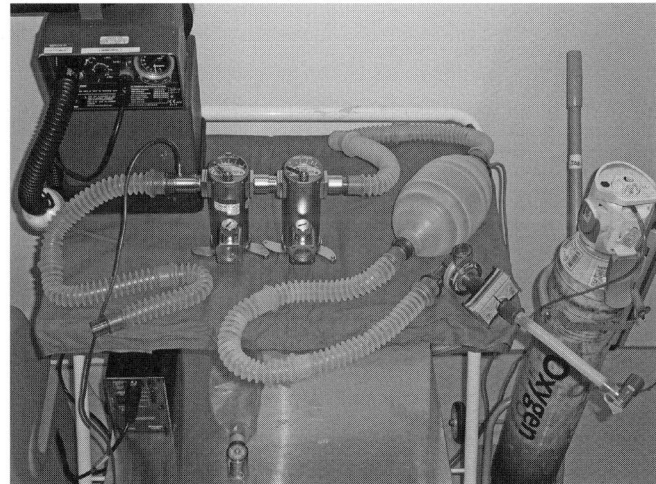

Figure 38.8 The Tri-Service Anesthetic Apparatus configured for spontaneous respiration. (Reproduced from Frazer and Birt 2010,[39] with permission of the Editor of the *Journal of the Royal Army Medical Corps*.)

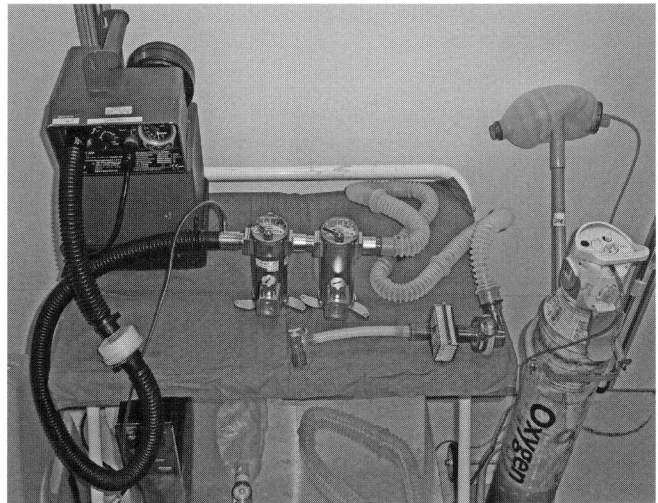

Figure 38.9 The Tri-Service Anesthetic Apparatus configured for mechanical ventilation. (Reproduced from Frazer and Birt 2010,[39] with permission of the Editor of the *Journal of the Royal Army Medical Corps*.)

The apparatus has been used successfully with enflurane, isoflurane, and halothane. Currently UK military practice usually involves air (supplemented with oxygen) as the carrier gas and isoflurane as the volatile agent. At the time of writing (2013) UK forces use the CompPAC ventilator.[40] If working with aid agencies, anesthetists can expect to have to use older, less expensive anesthetic agents. Where inhalational agents are neither available nor appropriate, intravenous anesthesia is an alternative.

Total intravenous anesthesia (TIVA)

The use of TIVA for war surgery has been documented since barbiturates were used during the Spanish Civil War (1936–39). The different techniques used have ranged from

Table 38.4 Example of anesthesia recipe

An infusion of 4 mg of propofol, 2.5 mg of ketamine, and 2.5 μg of fentanyl per mL of solution is easily administered. To mix the solution, add the following to 50 mL of saline:

- 40 mL of 1% propofol
- 250 μg (5 mL of 50 μg/mL) of fentanyl
- 250 mg (5 mL of 50 mg/mL) of ketamine

Use a standard 20 drops/mL drip set and, assuming an 80 kg patient, one drop per second equates to a propofol infusion rate of 150 μg/kg/min (or 9 mg/kg/h). One drop every three seconds equates to a propofol infusion rate of 50 μg/kg/min (or 3 mg/kg/h).

For most soldiers these rates provide good starting points for a range of anesthetics, and the infusion rates are easily titrated as needed, based on the patient's response to ongoing surgical stimuli. This infusion can be terminated at the end of the case or continued in the ICU at lower rates to provide sedation and analgesia.

ketamine increments to a mixture of agents given alone or in combination with a volatile anesthetic. Restall *et al.* described using a maintenance mixture of ketamine, midazolam, and vecuronium delivered by a syringe pump for tracheally intubated patients whose lungs were being ventilated with air.[41] This was felt to be an appropriate technique for the initial anesthetic for battle casualties. A later study found the ketamine/midazolam combination to be comparable to one based on propofol and alfentanil, and use of a propofol/alfentanil combination was first reported in the 1990–91 Gulf War.[42,43]

A subsequent technique for patients who could be allowed to breathe spontaneously (e.g., fasted casualties undergoing a delayed primary suture of a wound) involved a background infusion of ketamine, midazolam, and alfentanil supplementing the inhalation of isoflurane in oxygen-enriched air.[44] A propofol/remifentanil infusion is also suitable for field use with ventilated patients, allowing for a more rapid return to full arousal, although the time to first postoperative opioid requirement will also be reduced.

In the absence of intravenous infusion pumps or power supplies, intravenous anesthetics and anesthetic/analgesic mixtures can be injected into bags of compatible intravenous fluid and titrated to effect (Table 38.4).

Field regional anesthesia

A number of authors have described using regional anesthetic techniques in field conditions. These vary from simple infiltration of local anesthetics to nerve conduction blocks and spinal anesthesia. Military anesthetists have used central neuraxial blockade in the second world war, and peripheral nerve blocks in the Vietnam conflict and the Falklands War.[45] However, casualties injured by modern munitions containing preformed fragments have multiple penetrating injuries to different body areas and are often critically ill on admission, so regional anesthesia is rarely appropriate as a sole anesthetic.

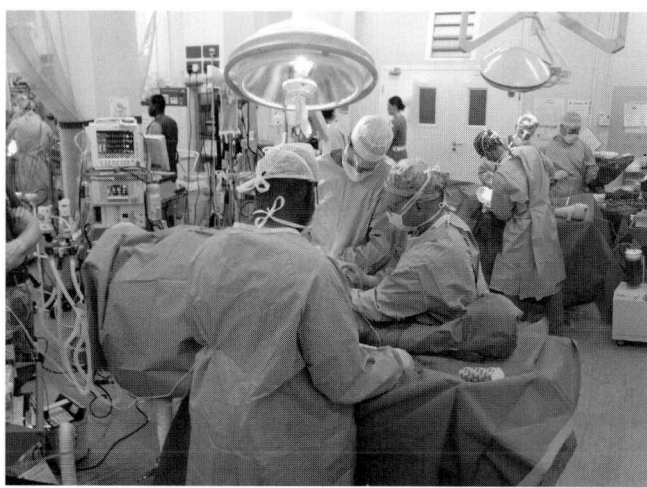

Figure 38.10 Three tables operating simultaneously at the UK Multinational Role 3 Hospital, Afghanistan, 2010. (Photo courtesy of N. Tarmey.) *A black and white version of this figure will appear in some formats. For the color version, please refer to the plate section.*

It is, however, used extensively to provide postoperative analgesia, as described below.

Anesthesia in an established field hospital

In contrast to the limitations of a forward surgical facility, an established field hospital may expand and develop during a prolonged conflict until it has facilities to rival many civilian trauma centers. Key improvements may include a greater range of specialist clinical personnel, ultrasound and CT diagnostic capability, a transfusion laboratory with regular resupply and emergency donor panel capability, and sufficient operating and critical care capacity to cope with a large surge in casualties (Fig. 38.10).

The military anesthetist's key roles in this environment remain unchanged from the forward surgical facility: supporting physiology through damage control resuscitation and providing anesthesia for damage control surgery. However, as part of a complex team with greater diagnostic and therapeutic capability, effective team working and communication become even more important. The military anesthetist's key priorities as the casualty progresses through the field hospital are summarized in Table 38.5.

Pain management

In contrast to the assertion that "severe wounds in soldiers are often associated with very little pain,"[46] 70% of injured UK soldiers surveyed in 2010 recalled moderate or severe pain on wounding.[47] Adequate pain relief has been very poorly managed by the military in the past. Failure to treat the pain of battlefield trauma may cause unnecessary suffering and psychological distress. Poor pain control may also impair healing and is associated with a higher incidence of chronic pain (see Chapter 17). Effective pain management is multimodal, and may require both pharmacological and nonpharmacological therapies (see Chapters 15 and 16). The treatment options vary based on the medical capability at each level of care. This section will focus on the acute and perioperative pain management strategies employed by anesthesiologists at the Role 3 field hospital.

Pain assessment is essential to enable effective pain management. The most effective scoring system has been found by the UK military to be the four-point scale (Table 38.6).[48] Pain scoring should occur with all nursing observations and be repeated following any intervention.

Acute pain management on admission

Nonpharmacological methods of analgesia include splinting fractured limbs prior to surgical fixation. Drugs used by the military for acute pain management include entonox (50% nitrous oxide in oxygen), fentanyl lozenges, parenteral opioids, and ketamine.

- **Inhaled entonox** is a rapid-onset analgesic that may be used by a cooperative patient. Offset is also rapid once administration is discontinued. The 50% oxygen in the mixture minimizes the risk of hypoxemia should there be any apneic periods.

- **Fentanyl lozenges** are fentanyl lollipops containing 400 or 800 μg of oral transmucosal fentanyl citrate. The lollipop has to be rubbed against the buccal mucosa, and it will take approximately 15 minutes to dissolve. Water may be needed if the patient has a dry mouth. 400 μg has a similar efficacy to 4–8 mg morphine IV. The time to peak effect is approximately 20 minutes, but there is a degree of effective analgesia after only about 5 minutes. It is particularly useful in multipatient scenarios where not all casualties have intravenous access.

- **Intramuscular morphine** is carried by every UK soldier in the form of a 10 mg autoinjector. IV or IO morphine may be given at any point in the evacuation chain. Its peak effect may not be seen for 10–20 minutes, so if immediate analgesia is essential to reduce a dislocation or fracture then IV fentanyl or IV ketamine is more appropriate.

- **Ketamine** has a rapid onset of analgesia (some effect after about 15 seconds when given IV, but 1–2 minutes for peak effect), and is particularly useful for procedural sedation. As it is a dissociative analgesic, patients appear "detached" and unresponsive but may moan or cry out, without any recollection when questioned later. A starting dose of 20–30 mg followed by 10–20 mg as needed is reasonable, but shocked patients may only need 20 mg in total. The analgesic offset may be rapid, and patients should be given IV morphine to ensure that analgesia continues after the effect of ketamine.

Postoperative analgesia

Standard postoperative regimes of simple oral analgesics supplemented by opioids as required form the basis of multimodal

Table 38.5 Priorities for trauma anesthesia in the field hospital

Aim	Priorities
Before casualty arrives	
Prepare the anesthetic team and equipment for the casualty's arrival.	Assess prehospital information, including: a. number and severity of casualties. b. AT-MIST report (see Table 38.1) c. airway at risk/already secured d. requirement for massive transfusion Prepare anesthetic team by: a. briefing anesthetic assistants b. checking availability of second anesthetist c. determining need to split anesthetic team between multiple casualties Check anesthetic equipment, including: a. airway equipment and ventilator b. anesthetic drugs c. large bore central access
Initial resuscitation in the emergency department	
Work as part of an effective trauma team to assess, resuscitate and prepare the casualty for surgery.	Remember team-working and 2-way communication with trauma team at every stage. Keep trauma team leader updated with casualty's physiological status. Catastrophic hemorrhage. Determine whether catastrophic hemorrhage has been controlled. If external control of ongoing catastrophic hemorrhage is not possible, all efforts should be directed towards gaining immediate surgical control of bleeding. This may involve induction of anesthesia in an unstable patient, with drug doses, fluid resuscitation and ventilation adjusted accordingly. Airway. Assess and treat, with RSI if indicated. Breathing. In severe hypovolemic shock, aim to minimize intrathoracic pressure during invasive ventilation by using low respiratory rate (e.g., 6/min) and zero PEEP. Circulation. Gain large bore central access if indicated.
Decision making on next stage of care	
Work with the trauma team leader to determine the next actions.	Provide guidance to team leader on physiology and anesthetic issues to decide: a. Immediate surgery or CT first? b. If surgery, which body cavity first? c. RSI prior to transfer to CT/ OR?
Transfer to and from CT	
Take primary responsibility for safe and timely transfer to and from CT	Check before transfer: a. tourniquets tight and effective b. airway secure c. working ventilator and sufficient oxygen supply d. venous access working and secure e. sufficient blood products available f. rapid infuser and ED transfusion team able to move with patient g. effective analgesia, sedation, and muscle relaxation h. protection from hypothermia Plan for next stage of care. When CT in progress, confirm readiness and plans for next destination (e.g., OR).
Operating room	

Provide seamless and effective damage control resuscitation throughout surgery.	Positioning on arrival:
	a. The default patient position is supine with both arms abducted on boards
	b. Apply forced-air warmer and commence warming as soon as possible
	c. Don't attempt arterial line placement until a strong radial pulse is palpable
	
	Handover from ED team leader:
	a. Handover does not begin until the patient is properly positioned and established on the anesthesia machine
	b. Information handed over should include:
	   i. list of injuries found
	   ii. treatment given so far
	   iii. transfusion running totals

Table 38.5 (*cont.*)

Aim	Priorities
	iv. outstanding issues
	v. provisional plan
	Maintenance of anesthesia:
	a. During hypovolemic shock, titrate fentanyl and volatile anesthetic carefully to physiology.
	b. When bleeding is controlled, carefully titrate in further analgesia (eg fentanyl *up to* 15 µg/kg) to improve analgesia, prevent excessive vasoconstriction and permit further volume resuscitation with blood and blood products.
	Hemostatic resuscitation:
	a. Before surgical control of hemorrhage:
	i. Keep ED transfusion team in OR.
	ii. Maintain circulating volume with empirical blood and products according to massive transfusion protocol.
	b. After effective surgical control of hemorrhage:
	i. Take handover of transfusion from ED team.
	ii. Beware overtransfusion and hypervolemia.
	iii. Move to tailored transfusion, guided by physiology and indices of coagulation.
	c. Remember:
	i. Don't treat hypovolemic shock with vasopressors.
	ii. Don't replace acute blood loss with crystalloid/colloid.
	iii. Warm aggressively to achieve normothermia.
	iv. Check and treat hyperkalemia/ hypocalcaemia.
	v. Use ROTEM to guide clotting product transfusion.
	Communication and team-working:
	a. Maintain effective 2-way communication with surgery, radiology, critical care and deployed medical director.
	b. Ensure surgeons aware of:
	i. current physiological status
	ii. coagulopathy on thromboelastometry/lab tests
	iii. plans for onward transfer, time constraints and resource limitations
	c. Ensure passage of information from surgeons, especially:
	i. tourniquets and vascular clamps being released or applied
	ii. difficult surgical control of hemorrhage
	iii. surgical evidence of coagulopathy
	d. Check CT report (verbal or written) for:
	i. radiological C-spine clearance
	ii. list of injuries found
	e. Remember Deployed Medical Director for:
	i. activation of emergency donor panel
	ii. referral for extra-hospital transfer
	iii. difficult futility decisions
	iv. resolution of areas of disagreement
	Preparation for postoperative care:
	a. Agree next destination (CT/critical care/aeromedical transfer).
	b. Ensure effective postoperative analgesia (systemic +/- regional).
	c. Handover to next team (in OR if possible).

CT, computed tomography; ED, emergency department; OR, operating room; PEEP, positive end-expiratory pressure; RSI, rapid sequence induction and intubation.

analgesia. If repeated doses of morphine are required, patient-controlled analgesia (PCA) can be delivered using an elastomeric pump. The current UK device is the Baxter Infusor PCA, which has the advantage of being entirely mechanical, with no electronic components, and safe for use during aeromedical transfer.[49]

PCA is not suitable for all patients. Effective use requires the patient to retain, understand, and apply the instructions for

Table 38.6 The four-point numerical pain rating scale[48]

0	No pain
1	Mild pain
2	Moderate pain
3	Severe pain

use, and where a patient does not meet the designated inclusion criteria a morphine infusion may be more appropriate, as is frequently the case with children or host-nation adults. Patients at risk of neural damage (e.g., those with amputations, crush injury, or spinal injury) are also started on 25–50 mg amitriptyline at night and 75 mg pregabalin twice a day.

Analgesia in the non-opioid-naive population of the local host nation may be a problem on some operations, and sufficient levels of opioid must be delivered, along with maximization of nonopioid techniques such as regional anesthesia. Neuropathic pain medications may help if pain is greater than expected, and clonidine can be useful for withdrawal symptoms as long as the patient is hemodynamically stable.

Regional anesthesia

Regional anesthesia can provide excellent opioid-sparing postoperative pain relief and is used regularly in the current field hospital setting in Afghanistan. Previously, there have been concerns with regards to difficulties in detection of compartment syndrome when the symptom of pain is removed. Current UK military consensus guidelines are that clinicians should be encouraged to use regional techniques.[49] In the military setting, casualties will often be repatriated within hours of injury, and they will be without access to surgical intervention for 12–24 hours during that period. Prophylactic fasciotomy is often performed early as part of the initial field hospital management if there are concerns with regards to potential compartment syndrome.

Ultrasound-guided peripheral nerve blocks and continuous peripheral nerve catheters are well suited to manage severe pain from these limb injuries (see Chapter 16). Single-shot blocks and catheters are currently inserted at the end of the damage control surgery with good effect. They often stay in situ for days to weeks during aeromedical evacuation and further dressing changes at the Role 4 hospital.[50] Common sites for catheter placement include interscalene or supraclavicular brachial plexus blocks for upper limb injuries, and femoral and popliteal sciatic nerve blocks as a combination for a below-knee amputation, with the femoral block alone for above-knee amputees.

Single-shot transversus abdominis plane (TAP) blocks are useful for relief of postoperative laparotomy pain, especially if an epidural may be difficult or contraindicated. If a catheter is inserted, the local anesthetic infusion may be given using an elastomeric infusion device. Where infusions are in use, facilities must be present for the management of life-threatening local anesthetic toxicity.

Epidural analgesia is highly effective in controlling acute pain after surgery or trauma to the chest, abdomen, pelvis, or lower limbs. The combination of excellent pain relief and minimal side effects provides high patient satisfaction compared with other methods of relieving pain. The UK military infuse either bupivacaine 0.125% or bupivacaine 0.1% and fentanyl 2 µg/mL at a rate of 7–15 mL/hr.

Concerns over the use of regional anesthesia include the risk of epidural hematoma in patients with trauma-induced coagulopathy, and the risk of epidural abscess or central nervous system infection in patients with systemic sepsis.

Trauma-induced coagulopathy affects a significant proportion of seriously injured military casualties, who may receive a massive transfusion before requiring peripheral or central regional analgesia. At the time of writing (2013) the current operational advice is adapted (with permission) from guidance produced by the Association of Anaesthetists of Great Britain and Ireland.[51] Following major trauma it is recommended that an assessment of potential coagulopathy is made before performing any regional anesthetic techniques. In assessing the degree of coagulopathy, it is recognized that coagulopathy in massive transfusion is a dynamic situation. Assessment should be made when hemorrhage is controlled and the patient has a stable cardiovascular system. An assessment of platelet function (e.g., by thromboelastometry) is desirable in patients who have received platelet transfusion.

Peripheral catheter techniques and single-shot techniques are considered on a patient-by-patient basis, weighing potential benefit against risk. Indwelling catheters present a higher infective risk than single-shot techniques, and invasive procedures must be conducted in an appropriately sterile environment. This may affect the ability to perform these techniques in forward surgical settings.

Central neuraxial blocks should not be performed (or catheters removed) within 12 hours of prophylactic low-molecular-weight heparin (LMWH), and further LMWH should not be administered within 4 hours of a procedure (block performed/catheter removed). Systemic sepsis remains a relative contraindication to central neuraxial anesthesia because of the presumed increased incidence of epidural abscess and meningitis.

All of the above techniques can also be used for children. Pediatric analgesic doses must be properly calculated, as these cannot always be extrapolated from adult doses. Assessment of pain may require a different tool, such as the Wong–Baker faces scale, which has been validated in smaller children and does not require translation.

Conclusion

Anesthesia for the multiply injured casualty is challenging. Anesthesia for the same casualty in a deployed environment is even more so. The practitioner working in this environment needs to understand the imposed constraints and be able to provide anesthesia by drawing on a variety of different techniques. This does not mean that the standard of care given to the casualty is reduced. Military practice is constantly looking at new technologies, new techniques, and new evidence to ensure that the best possible care can be delivered to casualties whatever the circumstances.

Questions

(1) Identify the correct statement regarding the care provided by UK and US military medical systems:
   a. All care is provided to UK and US military personnel
   b. Care for local national civilians will depend on the operational situation and the capacity of the system
   c. All care is provided for detainees
   d. All care is provided for enemy forces injured by UK or US military in the conflict
   e. All of the above

(2) True or false? Serious injuries to the head and chest are unlikely if a casualty is wearing correctly fitted and maintained body armor and helmet.

(3) Ketamine:
   a. Usually causes hypotension on induction of anesthesia
   b. Causes decreased salivary secretions
   c. Does not cause psychotropic effects
   d. Can be used safely in multiply injured patients with traumatic brain injury
   e. Does not have significant analgesic effects

(4) Identify the correct statement regarding the Triservice Anesthetic Apparatus:
   a. It uses a drawover system of anesthesia
   b. It can be used with spontaneous and manually controlled intermittent positive-pressure ventilation
   c. Oxford Miniature Vaporizers lack the ability to provide temperature compensation
   d. It can be used with or without supplemental oxygen from an oxygen concentrator
   e. All of the above are true

(5) Regarding postoperative pain management for military trauma, identify the correct statement:
   a. Pregabalin and amitriptyline should be started postoperatively in casualties who are at risk of neural damage
   b. Pain is rarely a problem in military casualties
   c. Elastomeric patient-controlled analgesia devices may interfere with the flight controls if used for patients who require aeromedical evacuation

   d. Peripheral nerve catheters must only remain in situ for 5 days
   e. Trauma induced coagulopathy prevents the use of epidurals in casualties who have undergone damage control resuscitation and massive transfusion

(6) True or false? In casualty care at the point of wounding, diagnosis and treatment of airway obstruction is the first priority.

(7) True or false? Hypotensive resuscitation (target systolic BP 80–90 mmHg) is suitable for all casualties.

(8) Identify the correct statement regarding damage control resuscitation and surgery:
   a. The aim is to achieve definitive repair of injuries at initial surgery
   b. Gaining rapid control of bleeding is a key priority
   c. The anesthetist should not be involved in decisions relating to surgery
   d. Blood product transfusion should be titrated according to PT and aPTT in early resuscitation
   e. Casualties should be allowed to cool naturally for neuroprotection

(9) True or false? Military medical practitioners can always expect protection under the Geneva Convention.

(10) Identify the correct statement regarding the military evacuation chain:
   a. Casualty care begins at the field hospital
   b. The traditional evacuation pathways of Role 1, through Role 2, to Role 3 must always be followed
   c. Analgesia is contraindicated before the casualty's physiology has been stabilized
   d. Casualty care begins at the point of wounding
   e. The number and rate of casualties presenting to a field hospital can be reliably predicted by mathematical models

Answers

(1) e
(2) False
(3) d
(4) e
(5) a
(6) False
(7) False
(8) b
(9) False
(10) d

References

1. Perrin P. Protecting the victims of armed conflicts. In Perrin P, editor. *Handbook on War and Public Health*. Geneva: International Committee of the Red Cross, 1996, pp. 377–403.

2. Ministry of Defence. *Battlefield Advanced Trauma Life Support*. Joint Service Publication 570. London: Defence Medical Services, 2008.

3. Gilstad C, Roschewski M, Wells J, *et al.* Fatal transfusion-associated graft-versus-host disease with concomitant immune hemolysis in a group A combat trauma patient resuscitated with group O fresh whole blood. *Transfusion* 2012; **52**: 930–5.

4. Willdridge DJ, Hodgetts TJ, Mahoney PF, Jarvis L. The Joint Theatre Clinical Case Conference (JTCCC): clinical governance in action. *J R Army Med Corps* 2010; **156**: 79–83.

5. Ramasamy A, Hill AM, Clasper JC. Improvised explosive devices: pathophysiology, injury profiles and current medical management. *J R Army Med Corps* 2009; **155**: 265–72.

6. Hodgetts TJ, Davies S, Russell R, McLeod J. Benchmarking the UK military deployed trauma system. *J R Army Med Corps* 2007; **153**: 237–8.

7. Surgical management of penetrating brain injury. *J Trauma* 2001; **51**: S16–25.

8. Coupland RM, Pesonen PE. Craniocerebral war wounds: non-specialist management. *Injury* 1992; **23**: 21–4.

9. Parker P, Consensus statement on decision making in junctional trauma care. *J R Army Med Corps* 2011; **157**: S293–6.

10. Leibovici D, Gofrit ON, Stein M, *et al.* Blast injuries: bus versus open-air bombings – a comparative study of injuries in survivors of open-air versus confined-space explosions. *J Trauma* 1996; **41**: 1030–5.

11. Hodgetts TJ, Mahoney PF, Russell MQ, Byers M. ABC to <C>ABC: redefining the military trauma paradigm. *EMJ* 2006; **23**: 745–6.

12. Tai NR, Russell R. Right turn resuscitation: frequently asked questions. *J R Army Med Corps* 2011; **157**: S310–4.

13. Midwinter MJ. Damage control surgery in the era of damage control resuscitation. *J R Army Med Corps* 2009; **155**: 323–6.

14. Bickell WH, Wall MJ, Pepe PE, *et al.* Immediate versus delayed fluid resuscitation for hypotensive patients with penetrating torso injuries. *N Engl J Med* 1994; **331**: 1105–9.

15. Doran CM, Doran CA, Woolley T, *et al.* Targeted resuscitation improves coagulation and outcome. *J Trauma Acute Care Surg* 2012; **72**: 835–43.

16. Harris T, Thomas GO, Brohi K. Early fluid resuscitation in severe trauma. *BMJ* 2012; **345**: e5752.

17. Brohi K, Singh J, Heron M, Coats T. Acute traumatic coagulopathy. *J Trauma Acute Care Surg* 2003; **54**: 1127–30.

18. Doughty HA, Woolley T, Thomas GO. Massive transfusion. *J R Army Med Corps* 2011; **157**: S277–83.

19. Allcock EC, Woolley T, Doughty H, *et al.* The clinical outcome of UK military personnel who received a massive transfusion in Afghanistan during 2009. *J R Army Med Corps* 2011; **157**: 365–9.

20. Tarmey NT, Woolley T, Jansen JO, *et al.* Evolution of coagulopathy monitoring in military damage control resuscitation. *J Trauma Acute Care Surg* 2012; **73 (Suppl 1)**: S417–22.

21. Doran CM, Woolley T, Midwinter MJ. Feasibility of using rotational thromboelastometry to assess coagulation status of combat casualties in a deployed setting. *J Trauma Acute Care Surg* 2010; **69 (Suppl 1)**: S40–8.

22. Hauser CJ, Boffard K, Dutton R, *et al.* Results of the CONTROL trial: efficacy and safety of recombinant activated Factor VII in the management of refractory traumatic hemorrhage. *J Trauma Acute Care Surg* 2010; **69**: 489–500.

23. Shakur H, Roberts I, Bautista R, *et al.* Effects of tranexamic acid on death, vascular occlusive events, and blood transfusion in trauma patients with significant haemorrhage (CRASH-2): a randomised, placebo-controlled trial. *Lancet* 2010; **376**: 23–32.

24. Morrison JJ, Dubose JJ, Rasmussen TE, Midwinter MJ. Military Application of Tranexamic Acid in Trauma Emergency Resuscitation (MATTERs) study. *Arch Surg* 2012; **147**: 113–19.

25. Mercer SJ, Tarmey NT, Woolley T, Wood PL, Mahoney PF. Haemorrhage and coagulopathy in the defence medical services. *Anaesthesia.* 2013; **68**: 49–60.

26. Midwinter MJ, Mercer S, Lambert AW, de Rond M. Making difficult decisions in major military trauma: a crew resource management perspective. *J R Army Med Corps* 2011; **157**: S299–304.

27. Victorino GP, Battistella FD, Wisner DH. Does tachycardia correlate with hypotension after trauma? *J Am Coll Surg* 2003; **196**: 679–84.

28. Pepe PE, Dutton RP, Fowler RL. Preoperative resuscitation of the trauma patient. *Curr Opin Anaesthesiol* 2008; **21**: 216–21.

29. Sperry JL, Minei JP, Frankel HL, *et al.* Early use of vasopressors after injury: caution before constriction. *J Trauma Acute Care Surg* 2008; **64**: 9–14.

30. Bourgoin A, Albanese J, Leone M, *et al.* Effects of sufentanil or ketamine administered in target-controlled infusion on the cerebral hemodynamics of severely brain-injured patients. *Crit Care Med* 2005; **33**: 1109–13.

31. Grathwohl KW, Black IH, Spinella PC, *et al.* Total intravenous anesthesia including ketamine versus volatile gas anesthesia for combat-related operative traumatic brain injury. *Anesthesiology* 2008; **109**: 44–53.

32. Jones RK, Caldwell JE, Brull SJ, Soto RG. Reversal of profound rocuronium-induced blockade with sugammadex: a randomized comparison with neostigmine. *Anesthesiology* 2008; **109**: 816–24.

33. Breeze J, Gibbons AJ, Shieff C, *et al.* Combat-related craniofacial and cervical injuries: a 5-year review from the British military. *J Trauma Acute Care Surg* 2011; **71**: 108–13.

34. Kummer C, Netto FS, Rizoli S, Yee D. A review of traumatic airway injuries: potential implications for airway assessment and management. *Injury* 2007; **38**: 27–33.

35. Bellamy RF. Combat trauma overview. In Zajtchuk R, Grande CM, eds., *Textbook of Military Medicine.* Falls Church VA: Office of the Surgeon General, US Army, 1995, pp. 1–42.

36. Henderson JJ, Popat MT, Latto IP, Pearce AC, Difficult Airway S. Difficult Airway Society guidelines for management of the unanticipated difficult intubation. *Anaesthesia* 2004; **59**: 675–94.

37. Jensen AG, Callesen T, Hagemo JS, *et al.* Scandinavian clinical practice guidelines on general anaesthesia for emergency situations. *Acta Anaesthesiol Scand* 2010; **54**: 922–50.

38. Ministry of Defence (UK). *Clinical Guidelines for Operations (CGOs).* Joint Service Publication 999. London: MoD, 2013. https://www.gov.uk/government/publications/jsp-999-clinical-guidelines-for-operations (accessed september 2014).

39. Frazer RS, Birt DJ. The Triservice Anaesthetic Apparatus: a review. *J R Army Med Corps* 2010; **156**: 380–4.

40. Roberts MJ, Bell GT, Wong LS. The CompPAC and PortaPAC portable ventilators bench tests and field experience. *J R Army Med Corps* 1999; **145**: 73–7.

41. Restall J, Tully AM, Ward PJ, Kidd AG. Total intravenous anaesthesia for military surgery: a technique using ketamine, midazolam and vecuronium. *Anaesthesia* 1988; **43**: 46–9.

42. Wilson RJ, Ridley SA. The use of propofol and alfentanil by infusion in military anaesthesia. *Anaesthesia* 1992; **47**: 231–3.

43. Bailie R, Craig G, Restall J. Total intravenous anaesthesia for laparoscopy. *Anaesthesia.* 1989; **44**: 60–3.

44. Restall J, Thompson MC, Johnston IG, Fenton TC. Anaesthesia in the field. Spontaneous ventilation–a new technique. *Anaesthesia* 1990; **45**: 965–8.

45. Jowitt MD, Knight RJ. Anaesthesia during the Falklands campaign. The land battles. *Anaesthesia.* 1983; **38**: 776–83.

46. Beecher HK. Pain in Men Wounded in Battle. *Ann Surg* 1946; **123**: 96–105.

47. Aldington DJ, McQuay HJ, Moore RA. End-to-end military pain management. *Philos Trans R Soc Lond B Biol Sci* 2011; **366**: 268–75.

48. Looker J, Aldington D. Pain scores: as easy as counting to three. *J R Army Med Corps* 2009; **155**: 42–3.

49. Clasper JC, Aldington DJ. Regional anaesthesia, ballistic limb trauma and acute compartment syndrome. *J R Army Med Corps* 2010; **156**: 77–8.

50. Devonport L, Edwards D, Edwards C, *et al.* Evolution of the Role 4 U.K. military pain service. *J R Army Med Corps* 2010; **156**: 398–401.

51. Association of Anaesthetists of Great Britain and Ireland. *Best Practice in the Management of Epidural Analgesia in the Hospital Setting.* London: Royal College of Anaesthetists, 2011. http://www.aagbi.org/sites/default/files/epidural_analgesia_2011.pdf (accessed September 2014).

Burn injuries: critical care in severe burn injury

Charles J. Yowler

Objectives

(1) Describe the classification system of burn depth.
(2) Outline the initial assessment of the severely burned patient.
(3) Determine burn size using the Lund–Browder diagram.
(4) Assess the airway and the need for intubation.
(5) Determine the fluid requirements for burn resuscitation.
(6) Determine the requirement for escharotomy.
(7) Describe the potential benefits and complications of early burn excision and grafting.

Introduction

Data from the United States in 2008 reveal that 450,000 patients were treated for burn injury, with 45,000 requiring hospitalization. Approximately 3500 people die from burn injury annually, with 75% of these deaths occurring at the scene of the fire. Many of the deaths are attributable to smoke inhalation and not the burn injury itself.[1]

While the leading cause of burn injury overall is a scald from hot liquids, many of these burns are minor and treated as outpatients. The etiologies of admissions to burn centers in the US are: 44% fire/flame, 33% scald, 9% contact, 4% electrical, 3% chemical, and 7% other. Overall, survival of burn patients treated at specialized burn centers exceeds 96%.[1] Thus, modern advances in surgery, anesthesia, and critical care have had a significant impact on the treatment of severe burn injuries.[2,3]

Cohorting burn victims in specialized care burn facilities resulted in clinical research studies that led to reductions in hypovolemic shock, respiratory and renal failure, sepsis, and malnutrition. As a result, the burn size that confers a 50% probability of death in patients aged 15–45 years has increased from 50% total body surface area (TBSA) in 1950 to 80% TBSA in 2000 (Table 39.1). Morbidity and mortality following a major burn injury are related to age of the patient, burn size, and the presence of an inhalation injury.[4–6] The greater the burn size the greater the fluid and heat loss to the environment, both of which contribute to organ hypoperfusion and shock. The inflammatory mediator response also increases

Table 39.1 Percent of total body surface area (TBSA) burn for an expected 50% mortality

Age (years)	Burn size (%)
0–5	70–80
5–20	80–90
30–50	70–80
50–60	50–60
60–70	30–40
> 70	20–30

with burn size, as does the degree of immunosuppression. Bacterial colonization increases with the size of the open wound and, in conjunction with the increase in immunosuppression, results in increased risk of life-threatening burn wound infection. Inhalation injury causes pulmonary dysfunction that is exacerbated by the large fluid resuscitation required following major burn injury. The resultant hypoxia and impaired oxygen delivery to tissue further impair organ function. Advanced age limits the ability of the burn patient to tolerate any organ dysfunction or subsequent infection.

Every organ is affected by the hypoperfusion and inflammatory mediator response of the initial injury,[7] and homeostasis does not return until definitive wound closure occurs, which may take weeks for a large burn. The significant metabolic changes that accompany a large burn persist for more than 9 months and impair return to normal function. Thus, the patient with severe burns poses unique challenges to the intensivist.[8]

Pathophysiology

Burn depth is classified as first, second, or third degree (Table 39.2). **First-degree burns** result from damage to the superficial layers of the epidermis. They are characterized by erythema and pain. No open wound is produced, and fluid loss and systemic response is minimal. First-degree burns are not considered significant, and they are not considered when burn size is calculated for fluid resuscitation. In fact, one of the

Trauma Anesthesia, 2nd Edition, ed. Charles E. Smith. Published by Cambridge University Press. © Charles E. Smith, 2015.

Table 39.2 Burn depth and treatment

Burn	Depth	Treatment
First-degree	Epithelium	Lotions, pain control
Superficial second-degree	Superficial dermis	Antibiotic ointments, pain control
Deep second-degree	Deep dermis	Antibiotic ointments, pain control, and may require excision and grafting
Third-degree	To subcutaneous tissue	Will usually require excision and grafting

Table 39.3 Indications for tracheal intubation

Inability to protect airway
Hypoxia
Stridor/hoarseness
Large third-degree facial burns
Carboxyhemoglobin > 20%

primary causes of overresuscitation and subsequent fluid overload in burn patients is inclusion of areas of first-degree burn in estimating burn size for resuscitation formulas. Areas of first-degree burn have to be appreciated but ignored in calculations of burn size for resuscitation.

Extension of thermal damage to the dermis results in **second-degree burns**. They may be further classified as **superficial** or **deep** second-degree burns. Superficial injury results in a very painful wound that is blistered or weeping. The wound is pink and blanches with light pressure. This wound typically heals within 10–20 days with minimal to no scarring if infection is avoided. Nevertheless, areas of superficial second-degree burn exceeding 20% TBSA may require fluid resuscitation and monitoring.

Deep second-degree burns extend to the deep dermis. The wounds are drier and are red rather than pink. Blanching is minimal and less pain is noted on compression of the wound. These burns will take more than 20 days to heal and can result in significant hypertrophic scarring. Depending on the burn location, size, and condition of the patient, skin grafting is usually recommended.

Coagulation of the entire dermis results in **third-degree burns**. These wounds may be charred or white to deep red. They are insensate to pain, although pressure may be noted with palpation. The skin is leathery in nature, and circumferential third-degree burns in extremities may compromise distal blood perfusion. Small third-degree burns will heal by the sloughing of skin followed by wound contracture and scarring, but burns of significant size will require excision and grafting.

Thermal injury causes release of inflammatory mediators that result in a systemic capillary leak syndrome and loss of fluid and plasma proteins into the interstitial tissue. The edema that follows this fluid leak further impairs tissue perfusion and viability. Hence the paradox of burn fluid resuscitation: too little fluid causes hypoperfusion of the wound and extension of cellular damage, whereas too much fluid causes excessive tissue edema, which impairs perfusion and also results in extension of injury.

The immediate hemodynamic response to a large burn is vasoconstriction and a fall in cardiac output.[9] The cardiac index typically falls by 50% within 30 minutes of burn injury

and is independent of plasma volume. In large burns, if the fluid loss is not immediately addressed, the combination of hypovolemia and impaired cardiac function will quickly lead to fatal burn shock. Patients with preexisting cardiac dysfunction typically cannot tolerate large burns and pose unique challenges to resuscitation. Thus, elderly patients tolerate large burns poorly. For example, while a burn size of 80% TBSA in a patient under 45 years old has an expected survival of approximately 50%, a burn of 30% TBSA is lethal to 50% of patients at age 70.

The capillary leak persists at significant rates for the initial 12–24 hours. Following adequate fluid resuscitation, cardiac function returns to normal by 48 hours after burn injury. By the end of the first burn week, the overall hemodynamic picture has reversed itself and the burn patient is vasodilated with supernormal cardiac output. By postburn day 10, the cardiac output typically plateaus at levels that approach 2.5 times predicted normal values. Cardiac output remains at significantly elevated levels until the wound is closed and the overall hypermetabolic response persists for 9–12 months.[9]

This hypermetabolic response is primarily due to the elevated catecholamine levels that follow burn injury, although elevated cortisol and inflammatory cytokines contribute to the response. The hypermetabolic response of high cardiac output, low systemic vascular resistance, low-grade fever, and elevated white blood cell count mimics the response to infection and makes sepsis difficult to recognize in these patients. It needs to be appreciated that an elderly patient who appears clinically to be doing poorly, but has a "normal" invasive hemodynamic profile following burn injury, may in fact be underresuscitated and require further fluids or inotropic agents.

Initial assessment and resuscitation

The initial assessment and resuscitation of patients with life-threatening burns are based on the principles outlined in the Advanced Trauma Life Support (ATLS) program of the American College of Surgeons (see Chapter 2). The airway and breathing are assessed and a decision made concerning the need for endotracheal intubation (Table 39.3). Inhalation injury is suspected in any patient exposed to smoke in an enclosed space. However, it should be noted that more than 90% of patients with exposure to smoke do not have a significant injury and do not require intubation. The signs of smoke exposure, such as soot in the nares or oropharynx, singed facial hair, and carbonaceous cough, are indications that smoke

Table 39.4 Carboxyhemoglobin levels and symptoms

Level (%)	Symptom
0–10	Minimal symptoms (frequently found in heavy smokers)
10–20	Nausea, headache
20–30	Drowsiness, weakness
30–40	Confusion, agitation
40–50	Coma, respiratory depression
> 50	Death

Table 39.5 Toxic compounds present in smoke

Gas	Source	Comments
Carbon monoxide	Organic material	Inhibits oxygen delivery and utilization
Carbon dioxide	Organic material	Decreased mental status
Nitrogen oxide	Paper, wood	Respiratory irritation, bronchospasm, pulmonary edema
Hydrogen chloride	Plastics	Severe respiratory irritation, bronchospasm, bronchorrhea
Hydrogen cyanide	Wool, plastics	Respiratory failure, inhibits oxygen utilization
Benzene	Plastics	Respiratory irritation, bronchospasm, bronchorrhea, coma
Aldehydes	Wood, cotton, paper	Severe respiratory mucosal damage
Ammonia	Nylon	Respiratory irritation, bronchospasm, bronchorrhea
Acrolein	Textiles, carpeting	Respiratory irritation, bronchospasm, bronchorrhea

exposure occurred; they are not signs that tracheal intubation is required. Symptoms that suggest a significant injury requiring tracheal intubation include hoarseness, stridor, dyspnea, and tachypnea. A decreased level of consciousness, hypoxia, and elevated blood levels of carbon monoxide are other findings that support the need for early tracheal intubation (see Chapter 40).

Laryngeal edema may occur secondary to heat or chemicals present in the smoke. Airway edema, if present, will increase for approximately 24 hours because of the chemical irritation and ongoing fluid resuscitation. Thus, early intubation is indicated if hoarseness or stridor is noted on exam. Early intubation is often not difficult, and a large endotracheal tube should be placed, if possible, since subsequent bronchoscopy is often required.[10]

Carbon monoxide is produced by the combustion of organic material, and carbon monoxide poisoning may accompany smoke exposure. Carbon monoxide binds to both hemoglobin and the mitochondrial cytochrome oxidase system, resulting in profound impairment of aerobic metabolism. Symptoms are directly related to carboxyhemoglobin (COHgb) concentrations (Table 39.4). Thus, all patients with exposure to smoke in an enclosed space should be placed on a 100% nonrebreather mask until an arterial blood gas with carbon monoxide level is obtained. Pulse oximetry is inaccurate in the presence of COHgb because it is interpreted as saturated hemoglobin. Since the brain and heart are most sensitive to decreases in oxygen delivery, decreased alertness and evidence of cardiac irritability or ischemia are the earliest signs of carbon monoxide poisoning. In the absence of these signs, COHgb levels of less than 20% may be treated with 100% mask ventilation with the expectation that concentrations will fall to nontoxic levels (< 10%) within 45 minutes. A COHgb level of greater than 20% implies an oxygen saturation of less than 80%, and endotracheal intubation with delivery of 100% oxygen should be considered. The inspired oxygen content should remain at 100% until COHgb levels fall to less than 10% and the cytochrome oxidase system returns to normal function. This is indicated by the reversal of the accompanying metabolic acidosis with a serum bicarbonate level greater than 20 mEq/L.

The use of hyperbaric oxygen remains controversial.[11–13] While carbon monoxide levels fall to normal more quickly with the use of hyperbaric oxygen, patients with large-surface-area burns are often in shock. One randomized trial of hyperbaric oxygen in burn patients with carbon monoxide poisoning had to be halted due to complications during the dives in these unstable patients. Thus, while hyperbaric oxygen may play a role in isolated carbon monoxide poisoning, its use is more problematic in hemodynamically unstable patients with large burns who are undergoing active resuscitation.

Cyanide is another asphyxiating agent that is released by the combustion of certain organic materials. Cyanide poisoning should be suspected in the presence of a closed-space smoke exposure if the patient has a profound metabolic acidosis not explained by the arterial carbon monoxide concentrations. A blood cyanide level of greater than 0.5 mg/L will confirm the diagnosis. Treatment consists of tracheal intubation with delivery of 100% oxygen and hemodynamic support. The use of sodium thiosulfate and intravenous (IV) hydroxocobalamin remains controversial for cyanide inhalation and is generally not recommended.

Other chemicals present in smoke (Table 39.5) can also directly irritate the respiratory epithelium. Impaired function of type II pneumocytes results in atelectasis, whereas decreased ciliary action results in pooling of secretions. The resulting chemical tracheobronchitis is frequently complicated by infection. Indeed, ventilator-associated pneumonia in patients with inhalation injury is the leading cause of death in patients who survive the initial burn resuscitation. Patients with acute respiratory distress syndrome (ARDS) secondary to inhalation injury should be treated with low tidal volumes (6–8 mL/kg), positive end-expiratory pressure (PEEP), and vigorous pulmonary toilet.[10] Pulmonary collapse due to inspissated secretions is common, and frequent bronchoscopy may be required. Steroids are not indicated and may increase the risk of pneumonia. The use of prophylactic antibiotics has not decreased the incidence of pneumonia, but has been associated with increased risk of antibiotic-resistant infection.

Some studies have indicated a possible role for high-frequency ventilation in patients with significant inhalation injury.[14] Volumetric diffusive respiration has been shown to decrease pulmonary injury and the incidence of ventilator-associated pneumonia in both adults and children with inhalation injuries. The volumetric diffusive respiration mode uses high-frequency percussive ventilation, which is also associated with increased clearing of secretions. Thus, this mode allows for delivery of oxygen at low volumes and pressures, while facilitating pulmonary toilet.

After the evaluation and treatment of disorders of the airway and breathing, the circulation must be assessed. Peripheral pulses may be weak or absent due to underresuscitation or proximal circumferential third-degree burns. Tachycardia is common and may be due to pain, not hypovolemic shock. Large peripheral IV access should be obtained, preferably in areas of unburned skin. In extensive burns, it may be necessary to place the IV through burned skin or to place central venous lines.

Intravenous fluid should consist of lactated Ringer's solution. Fluid resuscitation may require massive amounts of crystalloid solution, and the use of normal saline will result in a hyperchloremic acidosis. Although hypertonic solutions have been used for burn resuscitation, they have been associated with an increased incidence of renal failure.[15] Their administration should be confined to burn centers with extensive experience in the use of hypertonic solutions.

All of the various formulas used to estimate the amounts of fluid to be given to a burn patient are based on the TBSA burned. Figure 39.1 shows the Lund–Browder ("rule of nines") method to determine burn size. Surface area of various body

Complete the table to calculate the total area of burn involved.

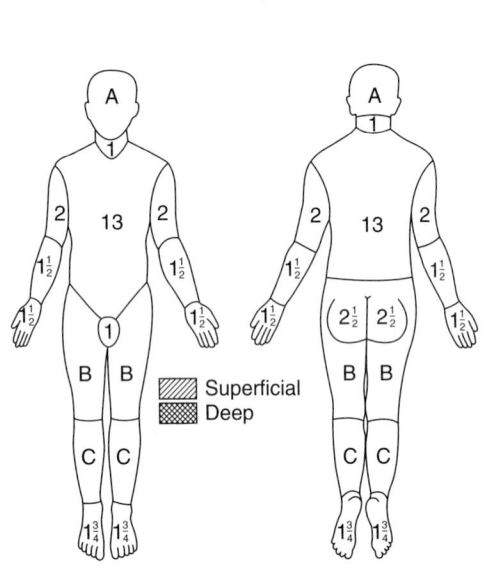

Figure 39.1 Lund–Browder ("rule of nines") burn diagram.

Region	%
Head	
Neck	
Ant. Trunk	
Post. Trunk	
Right arm	
Left arm	
Buttocks	
Genitalia	
Right leg	
Left leg	
Total burn	

Relative percentage of areas affected by growth

Age (years)	0	1	5	10	15	Adult
A - 1/2 of head	9 1/2	8 1/2	6 1/2	5 1/2	4 1/2	3 1/2
B - 1/2 of one thigh	2 3/4	3 1/4	4	4 1/4	4 1/2	4 3/4
C - 1/2 of one leg	2 1/2	2 1/2	2 3/4	3	3 1/4	3

parts changes with age, and this is also shown in this figure. Another useful method to determine the size of burns that are widely scattered is to use the patient's palm, including the palmar aspect of the fingers. This represents approximately 1% TBSA. By determining the size of the burn in relationship to the patient's hand an accurate estimate of burn size can be made. Once again, only second- and third-degree burns are used for the calculations.

The most widely used formula to estimate the initial fluid requirements for a burned patient is the Parkland formula. The 24-hour fluid requirement is estimated based on the formula: 4 mL per kg per % TBSA burned. Half of this amount of fluid is given in the first 8 hours following the burn, with the remainder given over the next 16 hours. For example, a 100 kg male receives burns covering 80% of his body. The formula $4(100)(80) = 32,000$. The 32 L of estimated fluid is divided such that 16 L is given over the initial 8 hours following burn injury. Thus the starting IV rate of lactated Ringer's solution is 2000 mL/hr. This example also emphasizes the complications that could occur if this volume of normal saline solution were to be administered.

Adjustments must be made for fluids received prior to arrival at the hospital. In the example above, if 6 L of crystalloid had been admitted in the initial 2 hours after burn injury, the remaining 10 L required for the initial 8-hour resuscitation would have to be delivered over 6 hours and the IV rate adjusted accordingly.

For children, the calculation of initial fluid requirement is more complex. A maintenance rate of D_5 lactated Ringer's solution should be administered continuously. In addition, 3 mL/kg/% burn of lactated Ringer's without glucose should be administered, half of this amount in the initial 8 hours and half over the subsequent 16 hours. Alternatively, the Galveston Pediatric Burn Resuscitation Formula may be utilized. Using this formula, the initial 24-hour fluid requirement is estimated as follows: 5000 mL/m^2 BSA burned + 2000 mL/m^2 BSA. The initial fluid rate is then changed as needed to maintain a urine output of 1 mL/kg.

Following this initial assessment of the patient, the secondary survey should be completed. Associated injuries are not uncommon following a significant burn injury.[16] Falls may occur in the attempt to leave a burning structure. It is unusual for burn patients to have alterations in mental status unless anoxic injury, carbon monoxide poisoning, or substance abuse has occurred. Thus, a patient "found down" at the site of the injury may have fallen and sustained a closed head injury. Elderly patients may have an acute coronary syndrome secondary to the stress/hypoxia associated with the injury. A thorough head-to-toe physical exam accompanied by appropriate imaging and laboratory studies will assist in the identification of these associated injuries and illnesses.

Preexisting chronic illnesses must be identified. Impaired cognition is an important contributor to burn injury, and a significant percentage of severely burned patients have a history of mental illness, dementia, or substance abuse.

Preexisting cardiac, respiratory, or renal disease will impact the success of resuscitation of the critically ill burned patient. Age, along with burn size and the presence of inhalation injury, is one of the determinants of burn survival. The elderly have thinner skin, which results in deeper burns requiring grafting, and have limited reserve to survive the initial injury plus the multiple complicated procedures required for burn reconstruction. Early discussions with the patient and family will facilitate the clinical decisions that have to be made concerning future treatment plans.

Finally, the adjuncts to the primary and secondary survey have to be performed. A Foley catheter is necessary to monitor urinary output during the resuscitation. Gastric ileus often accompanies large burn injury, and a nasogastric tube may be required. A gastric tube should certainly be placed in burns larger than 20% TBSA prior to transport to a tertiary burn center, to reduce the incidence of emesis with aspiration. All burn injuries are considered contaminated by the American College of Surgeons, and it is recommended that tetanus toxoid be administered in the absence of immunization in the 5 (not 10) years prior to burn injury.

The first 24 hours

Determination of ongoing fluid requirements is one of the most difficult tasks confronting the burns surgeon/intensivist. The administration of excess fluid to a patient with significant inhalation injury will result in further pulmonary edema, hypoxia, and mortality. However, underresuscitation will result in organ hypoperfusion and increase in pulmonary injury, hypoxia, and mortality. This is one of the many reasons that critically ill burn patients have improved outcomes when transferred to burn centers with experience in burn resuscitation.

Resuscitation of the burn patient is a continuous process that lasts 24–36 hours. As the capillary leak syndrome resolves at approximately 12 hours following burn injury, the fluid requirements of the patient will change. This is reflected in the fluid usage estimated by the Parkland formula. It must be emphasized, however, that the Parkland formula was derived from the mean fluid requirements of a large number of patients in a retrospective review. Any formula is merely an estimate; actual fluid administration must be based on the individual response of each patient to the resuscitation.

Urinary output is the most reliable guide to the adequacy of resuscitation. In the adult, the goal is 0.5 mL/hour; in children less than 30 kg, the goal is 1 mL/hour. Again, it must be emphasized that urinary outputs significantly greater than these recommendations reflect excess fluid administration that will negatively affect respiratory function. Urinary output may initially be unreliable in patients with alcohol intoxication or chronic diuretic use. Serial measurements of central venous pressure may offer additional information. However, central venous pressures of 4–6 mmHg may be adequate in healthy adults with acceptable urinary outputs.

As noted previously, cardiac output decreases immediately following large burns. This period of decreased cardiac function persists for approximately 48 hours, and the typical hypermetabolic response to burn injury is present at 5–7 days following burn injury. This period of cardiac dysfunction can become critical in the patient with preexisting compromise of cardiac function. A pulmonary artery catheter may be required to assess the adequacy of resuscitation in patients with preexisting heart or renal disease, age over 65 years, or severe inhalation injury. Fluid requirements greater than 6 mL/kg per percent TBSA are unusual, and placement of a pulmonary artery catheter may be needed to rule out unexpected cardiac dysfunction as an etiology for low urine outputs.

After the first 24 hours, increased fluid requirements are primarily due to evaporative loss from the open burn wound, and not from third-space loss. This evaporative fluid is primarily solute-free water, and intravenous fluids must replace this free water. Solutions such as half-normal saline are appropriate, with rates chosen to support the urine output goal. By this time, enteral nutrition has usually been started, and enteral volumes must be calculated into total fluid requirements.

Wound care

The burn wound consists of three zones. The **surrounding zone of hyperemia** consists of minimally injured skin, which becomes quickly hyperemic as angiogenesis occurs in attempts to heal the wound. The **central zone of coagulation** consists of necrotic tissue that will either be surgically excised or will slough with time. The **intervening zone of stasis** consists of injured cells that may either heal with time or proceed to die with further deeper conversion of the wound over the 24–48 hours following burn injury. The goal of fluid resuscitation and wound care is to maximize the viability of the zone of stasis.

Prolonged exposure of dermal and subdermal tissues will result in desiccation of these layers. Necrotic tissue in the wound serves as a nutrient layer for invading bacteria. Thus, the burn wound must remain moist and must be protected from bacterial overgrowth. Antibacterial ointments or emulsifications of antibiotics serve both to moisten and to protect the burn wound.

Small, superficial second-degree burns may be treated with any over-the-counter antibacterial ointment. However, burns large enough to require hospitalization have an increased risk of infection and require more effective agents. Silver sulfadiazine is commonly utilized. It is an effective antibiotic with minimal side effects. It commonly will cause neutropenia, but this usually resolves by the end of the first burn week and has not been associated with an increase of infections. It cannot be utilized in patients allergic to sulfa drugs, and *Pseudomonas* strains have been isolated that are resistant to its use. It inhibits epithelial cell replication and delays wound healing; thus it cannot be recommended for use in superficial second-degree burns that have a low risk of infection.

Mafenide acetate cream is another agent effective against a broad spectrum of bacteria. Its primary advantage is its absorption into tissue, making it an effective agent in areas of third-degree burns. However, it is painful if applied to areas of second-degree burns. It is a carbonic anhydrous inhibitor, and its use on large surface areas will result in a metabolic acidosis. It is available as a solution that causes minimal pain or acidosis. The cream is especially useful in areas of cartilage (ears, nose, etc.), where its absorption prevents invasive chondritis.

There are a number of products on the market based on the antibacterial properties of silver ion. Their advantage lies in the fact that the dressings are efficacious for a period of days following application, thus reducing the labor of burn care dressing changes. Silver ion is effective against all bacteria and fungi. However, it does not penetrate thick eschar or intact tissue, limiting its usefulness in established burn wound infections.

Escharotomy

Third-degree burns are hard and nonelastic. Circumferential third-degree burns of an extremity can act as a tourniquet and decrease blood flow to the distal limb. An escharotomy is an incision through the third-degree eschar to subcutaneous tissue that relieves the constriction. It is indicated in the presence of a circumferential third-degree burn with evidence of vascular compromise (diminished distal pulses, parathesias, abnormal capillary refill, etc.). It is essential that the incision be extended through the entire distance of the third-degree component of the burn, because even a 1 cm length may act as a tourniquet. A formal fasciotomy of the muscle is required only in the presence of a deep thermal burn involving the muscle or an electrical injury to the extremity.

In a similar manner, circumferential third-degree burns of the chest may compromise chest wall excursions, resulting in increased peak airway pressures, hypercapnia, and hypoxia. This effect will be exacerbated in the presence of significant inhalation injury. An escharotomy of the chest may be required to restore chest wall compliance.

Complications of resuscitation

There has been a trend toward more aggressive fluid resuscitation in the past decade. Whether this "fluid creep" is beneficial or detrimental is debatable.[17] One line of thought suggests that we have been historically underresuscitating many of the patients with severe burns. The countering opinion is that more fluids are being given in response to the increased usage of invasive hemodynamic monitoring devices despite the lack of evidence-based studies to support their use in the burn population. Whichever argument is correct, there is no question that there has been an increase in complications due to increased fluid use.

The increase in complications from overresuscitation has resulted in evaluation of the use of colloids in patients failing more traditional resuscitation formulae.[18–20] It is becoming more common to utilize colloid earlier in patients who have had their intravenous crystalloid rates increased to 6 mL/kg with persistent evidence of inadequate resuscitation.

Compartment syndromes may affect the muscle compartments of either the extremities or the abdomen.[21,22] Muscle compartment syndromes may occur in an extremity with deep burns in the presence of a large fluid resuscitation, and muscle compartment pressures should be obtained. If pressures are elevated above 30 mmHg, an escharotomy of the skin should be performed. Deeply burned extremities with associated fractures may require a fasciotomy (see also Chapter 28).

An increasing incidence of abdominal compartment syndrome has also been noted. Recent reports suggest that children, patients with circumferential abdominal burns, and patients with fluid requirements exceeding 6 mL/kg per percent TBSA burn are at risk for abdominal compartment syndrome and should have abdominal pressures monitored via Foley catheters. If these pressures are elevated above 30 mmHg (some utilize 20 mmHg) the abdominal pressure should be relieved. In the setting of burn resuscitation, this may be accomplished by placement of a peritoneal dialysis or diagnostic peritoneal lavage catheter and aspiration of abdominal fluid. If the pressures remain elevated after fluid aspiration, a decompressive laparotomy is required. The resultant open abdomen further complicates fluid management, and peritonitis can develop, especially if an adjacent abdominal burn wound becomes heavily colonized with *Pseudomonas*.

Early burn excision

Advances in resuscitation and topical antibiotics made it possible for patients with large surface area burns to survive 2–3 weeks following burn injury. However, a large number of patients eventually succumbed to invasive burn infections as surgeons waited for the burn wound to demarcate and slough prior to grafting. Advances in anesthesia and blood banking made it possible in the mid-1970s to attempt early excision and grafting of large surface area burns.

The advantages of early burn excision include decreased risk of infection, improved cosmetic result secondary to decreased hypertrophic scarring, decrease in hospital length of stay, and decreased mortality. However, performing a major excision in a recently resuscitated patient who remains 20 or more kilograms above his or her dry weight, with significant pulmonary compromise secondary to inhalation injury and an expected operative blood loss that will exceed one total blood volume, presents obvious challenges to the operative team.

Burn excisions may be either tangential or fascial. Tangential excision involves layer-by-layer excision until viable tissue is reached. This prolongs the time and blood loss of the excision. An excision directly to fascia limits operating time and blood loss but increases the cosmetic deformity. It is reserved for deep burns involving the subcutaneous tissues, or for elderly or massively burned patients where operative time and blood loss must be minimized.

Empiric use of systemic antibiotics does not reduce the incidence of burn wound infections. Blood supply is nonexistent to areas of third-degree burns, and therefore systemic antibiotics will not prevent infection in the eschar. While topical antibiotics are routinely employed, they cannot totally eliminate colonization of large burn wounds. Clinical studies have found a 20–40% incidence of bacteremia during burn excisions;[23] therefore, prophylactic preoperative antibiotics are routinely employed. The selection of the appropriate antibiotic depends on each hospital's biogram along with routine preoperative wound cultures. Gram-positive organisms predominate in the wound early after burn injury, with Gram-negative species (especially *Pseudomonas*) becoming more common during the second week following burn injury. Any empiric perioperative antibiotic use should be discontinued within 24 hours.

Burn excision often requires exposure of the entire patient, since areas that are not being grafted may be needed as donor sites. Maintenance of body temperature becomes a priority (see Chapters 14 and 40), since hypothermia exacerbates the coagulopathy that will occur due to the expected massive blood loss that invariably accompanies a large early excision. The operating room needs to be heated to near body temperature prior to the arrival of the patient, and external heating devices should be applied to areas not needed for the surgical procedure (see Chapter 14 and 40).

As noted previously, blood loss may be massive.[24] This may be underappreciated, since the blood does not enter suction canisters but instead lies on surgical sponges, drapes, and the floor. Close coordination between the surgeon and anesthesiologist is required to appropriately determine blood loss and appropriate transfusion requirements.

Conclusions

The burn unit, with its multidisciplinary approach to resuscitation, inhalation injury, infection, nutrition, burn excision, and reconstruction, has served as a model on which later specialty care units were organized. Research in the areas of "skin substitutes,"[25] novel methods of mechanical ventilation, and amelioration of the hypermetabolic response[26] will invariably result in further improvements in outcome.

Questions

(1) **All of the following increase mortality after burn injury, *except*:**
   a. Increasing age
   b. Increasing burn size
   c. Female gender
   d. Presence of inhalation injury

(2) **Larger burn size is associated with all of the following, *except*:**
   a. Increased heat loss
   b. Increased immune response
   c. Increased fluid loss
   d. Increased risk of burn infection

(3) **Which of the following statements is true?**
   a. First-degree burns are included in estimates of burn size for burn resuscitation
   b. All second-degree burns heal with minimal scarring
   c. Circumferential second-degree burns usually require escharotomy
   d. Third-degree burns will usually require excision and grafting

(4) **The hemodynamic response following burn injury is characterized by:**
   a. Immediate vasodilatation and increased cardiac output
   b. Immediate vasoconstriction and decreased cardiac output
   c. Late vasoconstriction and increased cardiac output
   d. Late vasoconstriction and decreased cardiac output

(5) **The hypermetabolic response following burn injury:**
   a. Begins immediately following burn injury
   b. May make it difficult to recognize sepsis
   c. Returns to normal within 4–6 weeks
   d. May be eliminated by adequate resuscitation

(6) **Which of the following statements concerning inhalation injury is *false*?**
   a. It should be suspected in patients exposed to closed-space fires
   b. It may be associated with elevated carbon monoxide levels
   c. It may increase the fluid requirement for resuscitation
   d. All patients with wheezing require intubation

(7) **Carbon monoxide poisoning is:**
   a. Present with COHgb levels > 5%
   b. Detected by pulse oximetry
   c. Suspected in patients with altered consciousness

   d. Treated by intubation and maintenance of oxygen saturations > 90%

(8) **The adequacy of burn resuscitation is best determined by:**
   a. Urine output
   b. Invasive hemodynamic parameters (cardiac output, pulmonary wedge pressures)
   c. Pulse
   d. The Parkland formula

(9) **Burn patients at increased risk for abdominal compartment syndrome include:**
   a. Elderly patients
   b. Abdominal burns
   c. Inhalation injury
   d. Fluid requirements greater than 6 mL/kg per percent burn

(10) **Systemic antibiotics:**
   a. Are given for the initial 10 days following burn injury
   b. Are given for the initial 10 days only if inhalation injury is present
   c. Are given preoperatively prior to burn excision
   d. Are given empirically for fevers > 38.5 °C

Answers

(1) c
(2) b
(3) d
(4) b
(5) b
(6) d
(7) c
(8) a
(9) d
(10) c

References

1. American Burn Association. *National Burn Repository: 2011 Report* Chicago, IL: ABA. http://www.ameriburn.org/2011NBRAnnualReport.pdf (accessed September 2014).

2. Pham TN, Gibran NS. Thermal and electrical injuries. *Surg Clin N Am* 2007; **87**: 185–206.

3. ABA Practice Guidelines Committee. Practice guidelines for burn care. *J Burn Care Rehabil* 2001; **22**: 1S–69S.

4. Ryan CM, Schoenfeld DA, Thorpe WP, *et al.* Objective estimates of the probability of death from burn injuries. *N Engl J Med* 1998; **338**: 362–6.

5. Spies M, Herndon DN, Rosenblatt JI, Sanford AP, Wolf SE. Prediction of

mortality from catastrophic burns in children. *Lancet* 2003; **361**: 989–94.

6. Sheridan RL, Remensnyder JP, Schnitzer JJ, *et al.* Current expectations for survival in pediatric burns. *Arch Pediatr Adolesc Med* 2000; **154**: 245–9.

7. Jeschke, MG, Chinkes DL, Finnerty CC, *et al.* Patholophysiologic response to severe burn injury. *Am Surg* 2008; **248**: 387–401.

8. Cancio LC, Lundy JB, Sheridan RL. Evolving changes in the management of burns and environmental injuries. *Surg Clin N Am* 2012; **92**: 959–86.

9. Williams FN, Herndon DN, Suman OE, *et al.* Changes in cardiac physiology after severe burn injury. *J Burn Care Res* 2011; **32**: 269–74.

10. Mosier MJ, Pham TN, Park DR, *et al.* Predictive value of bronchoscopy in

assessing the severity of inhalation injury. *J Burn Care Res* 2012; **33**: 65–73.

11. Wolf SJ, Lavonas EJ, Sloan EP, *et al.* Critical issues in the management of adult patients presenting to the emergency department with acute carbon monoxide poisoning. *Am Emerg Med* 2008; **51**: 138–52.

12. Annane D, Chadda K, Gajdos P, *et al.* Hyperbaric oxygen therapy for acute domestic carbon monoxide poisoning: two randomized controlled trials. *Intensive Care Med* 2011; **37**: 486–92.

13. Buckley NA, Juurlink DN, Isbister G, Bennett MH, Lavonas EJ. Hyperbaric oxygen for carbon monoxide poisoning. *Cochrane Database Syst Rev* 2011; (3): CD002041.

14. Cioffi WG, Rue LW, Graves TA, *et al.* Prophylactic use of high-frequency

percussive ventilation in patients with inhalation injury. *Am Surg* 1991; **213**: 575–80.

15. Huang PP, Stucky FS, Dimick AR. Hypertonic sodium resuscitation is associated with renal failure and death. *Ann Surg* 1995; **221**: 543–54.

16. Brandt CP, Yowler CJ, Fratianne RB. Burns with multiple trauma. *Am Surg* 2002; **68**: 240–3.

17. Cartotto RC, Innes M, Musgrave MA, Gomez M, Cooper AB. How well does the Parkland formula estimate actual fluid resuscitation volumes? *J Burn Care Rehabil* 2002; **23**: 258–65.

18. O'Mara MS, Slater H, Goldfarb IW, Caushaj PF. A prospective, randomized evaluation of intra-abdominal pressures with crystalloid and colloid resuscitation in burn patients. *J Trauma* 2005; **58**: 1011–18.

19. Lawrence A, Faraklas I, Watkins H, *et al.* Colloid administration normalizes resuscitation ratio and ameliorates "fluid creep." *J Burn Care Res* 2010; **31**: 40–7.

20. Faraklev I, Lam U, Cochran A, Stoddard G, Saffle J. Colloid normalizes resuscitation ratio in pediatric burns. *J Burn Care Res* 2011; **32**: 91–7.

21. Ivy ME, Atweh NA, Palmer J, *et al.* Intra-abdominal hypertension and abdominal compartment syndrome in burn patients. *J Trauma* 2000; **49**: 387–91.

22. Hobson KG, Young KM, Ciraulo A, Palmieri TL, Greenhalgh DG. Release of abdominal compartment syndrome improves survival in patients with burn injury. *J Trauma* 2002; **53**: 1129–33.

23. Mozingo DW, McManus AT, Kim SH, Pruitt BA. Incidence of bacteremia after burn wound manipulation in the early postburn period. *J Trauma* 1997; **42**: 1006–11.

24. Sheridan RL, Szyfelbein SK. Trends in blood conservation in burn care. *Burn* 2001; **27**: 272–6.

25. Brusselaers N, Pirayesh A, Hoeksema H, *et al.* Skin replacement in burn wounds. *J Trauma* 2010; **68**: 490–501.

26. Murphy KD, Lee JO, Herndon DN. Current pharmacotherapy for the treatment of severe burns. *Expert Opin Pharmacother* 2003; **4**: 369–84.

Objectives

(1) Understand the pathophysiology of a burn patient, including airway, respiratory, cardiac, hematologic, liver, and gastrointestinal functions, nutrition, metabolism, electrolyte abnormalities, thermoregulation, immune suppression, and renal function.

(2) Understand the preoperative requirements for surgery, including a thorough history and physical, proper laboratory tests, appropriate intravenous access, and preoperative medications.

(3) Understand the surgical process of wound care, excision and grafting, and alternative skin care.

(4) Safely administer intraoperative anesthetic management, including proper monitor selection, thermal regulation, ventilation, maintenance anesthesia, and calculation of the estimated blood loss during the excision.

(5) Give appropriate postoperative care, including the management of the airway and chronic pain control.

Introduction

Burn injury is regarded as one the most costly and challenging injuries in all of trauma care.[1] The skin is the largest organ of the human body, and it plays a very important role in physiology and the maintenance of body homeostasis. A large burn can alter the ability of almost all of the body's organs, and significantly increases the patient's risk for infection.[2] In 2013, the American Burn Association National Burn Repository reported 450,000 burn injuries that received medical treatment, 40,000 hospitalizations, and 3400 fire-related deaths.[3] About one-third of all burn admissions to the hospital are in children under age 15 years, and about 2000 of the burn-related deaths annually are in children.[2] Mortality is high with burn injuries, but there has been a significant improvement in survival secondary to the development of multidisciplinary burn teams, early and aggressive surgical treatments (see Chapter 39), advances in critical care, and improved understanding of burn pathophysiology.[4,5] This chapter reviews the pathophysiology of burns and the role of the anesthesiologist in the preoperative, surgical, intraoperative, and postoperative management of burns.

Pathophysiology of burns

Airway

Upper airway inhalation injury is usually due to a heat injury that leads to swelling and upper airway obstruction secondary to edema of the posterior pharynx and supraglottic regions.[2] Inhalation airway injury can occur after the inhalation of superheated air or steam and other toxic compounds found in smoke.[4] Chemical products of smoke include ammonia, nitrogen dioxide, sulfur dioxide, and chlorine. These chemicals dissolve in the airway to form acids that irritate the mucous membranes. Patients with significant burns to the face and neck are at increased risk of airway injury. Signs that are highly indicative of smoke exposure include facial burns, airway soot, carbonaceous sputum, and singed nasal hair.[1] Patients with increasing respiratory rate, increased secretions, stridor, dyspnea, use of accessory muscles, dysphagia, and progressive hoarseness have likely sustained significant inhalational injury and require emergent tracheal intubation because of impending airway obstruction (Table 40.1). It is important to note that a patient with minimal airway distress should be questioned as to the events associated with the burn, the patient's name and information, medical history, allergies, surgical history, medications, and other pertinent information prior to manipulation of the airway. Predictive indicators of an inhalation injury include history of a closed-space fire, impaired mental status, loss of consciousness, and associated drug or alcohol use.

The airway can also be assessed by arterial blood gas analysis, chest x-ray, fiberoptic bronchoscopy, fiberoptic and video laryngoscopy, and fiberoptic nasopharyngoscopy used in conjunction with flow-volume curves. A carbon monoxide level of more than 15% strongly suggests smoke inhalation injury.[1] A chest x-ray is rarely helpful initially, because the lung pathology of inhalation injury often lags by 6–24 hours, but it is good for a baseline examination of the patient's lungs.[4] In one study, it was found that in patients with obvious serious

Table 40.1 Symptoms and signs of smoke exposure and inhalation injury

Smoke exposure
Soot in nares
Singed facial hair or nasal hair
Carbonaceous sputum
Inhalation injury
Increased respiratory rate
Increased secretions
Stridor
Dyspnea
Use of accessory muscles
Dysphagia
Progressive hoarseness
Facial burns
Abnormal findings on nasopharyngoscopy or bronchoscopy
Airway edema
Abnormal flow-volume loops
Elevated carbon monoxide level > 15%

Information from references 1,2,4,5

Table 40.2 Indications for immediate tracheal intubation

Cardiovascular instability
Central nervous system depression
Massive burns > 60% of total body surface area (TBSA)
Symptoms of impending airway obstruction

Information from reference 1. See also Chapter 39.

Table 40.3 Potential difficult tracheal intubation

Full stomach
Emergency situation
Cervical collar in place
Abnormal anatomy
Physical exam including:

- Thick neck
- Small mouth opening < 4 cm
- Beard
- Poor dentition
- Protruding teeth
- Short muscular neck
- Receding mandible
- Decreased motion of temporomandibular joint (TMJ)
- High arched palate
- Thyromental distance < 6 cm
- Class 3 or 4 Mallampati score
- Large tongue
- Limited neck range of motion

Morbid obesity
Pregnancy

Information from references 11 and 12. See also Chapter 3.

inhalation injury, 84% had an abnormal chest x-ray at 48 hours.[6] The value of bronchoscopy in the early diagnosis of inhalation injury, when combined with histologic findings, has proven to be sensitive and specific for the diagnosis of inhalation injury.[7] A bronchoscopic grading for inhalation injury has been proposed but has not been validated in burn patients.[8] The technique of fiberoptic laryngoscopy has the ability to evaluate the upper airway injury directly and to determine the need for immediate intubation. Often, patients evaluated by fiberoptic laryngoscopy do not require immediate intubation and could be watched serially with multiple fiberoptic examinations, therefore potentially avoiding the complications associated with prolonged intubation.[9] In multiple studies using serial flow-volume curves and fiberoptic nasopharyngoscopy to assess inhalation injury, it has been found that upper airway obstruction decreases inspiratory but not expiratory flow. With more severe injury, inspiratory and expiratory flows decrease. None of the patients with stable or increased flow rates required intubation.[4,10]

Other indications for immediate intubation include cardiovascular instability, central nervous system (CNS) depression, and massive second- or third-degree burns of greater than 60% of total body surface area (TBSA) (Table 40.2).[1] In general, it is usually best to intubate early rather than late. With time and treatment of the patient with massive fluid resuscitation, the likelihood of airway edema significantly increases.[4,11] It is important to evaluate the patient's airway for potential difficulty of intubation prior to any airway manipulation (see

Chapter 3). The following conditions should raise one's suspicions of a potentially difficult airway independent of the burn injury: (1) full stomach, (2) emergency situation, (3) cervical collar in place, (4) abnormal anatomy, and (5) physical exam, including thick neck, small mouth opening < 4 cm, beard, poor dentition, protruding teeth, short muscular neck, receding mandible, decreased motion of temporomandibular joints, high arched palate, thyromental distance < 6 cm, class III or IV Mallampati score, large tongue, and limited neck range of motion (Table 40.3; see also Chapter 3).[11,12] Patients who are morbidly obese can be very difficult to ventilate. The large head and face make it difficult to mask ventilate, and the patient does not tolerate lying supine because of decreased functional residual capacity and decreased respiratory compliance.[11] Also, a pregnant patient is at risk for a difficult intubation because of the anatomic changes that occur with pregnancy (see Chapter 37), including pharyngolaryngeal edema, weight gain, enlarged breasts, full dentition, and the propensity for rapid arterial oxygen desaturation.

Tracheal intubation of a patient with a normal-appearing airway is usually accomplished with rapid sequence induction and intubation (RSI).[4] All induction agents have been used safely in burn patients (see Chapter 7). Succinylcholine is generally considered to be safe in the first 24 hours after a burn (see Chapter 13). Rocuronium is a good alternative to succinylcholine during the initial 24 hours and can also be given safely after this initial period. Preoxygenation is done with 100% oxygen prior to airway manipulation to ensure a good oxygen reserve during the patient's period of apnea.[11] It is important to remember that, if the patient has a cervical collar in place, he or she will require manual in-line stabilization during the airway manipulation. Once the endotracheal tube is in place, it is important for it to be adequately secured. Unfortunately, the burned face often makes this difficult owing to topical wound agents, continual swelling and edema of the face and neck, and fluid extruding through the facial burn.[2] Often, the endotracheal tube is secured with umbilical tape, which must be reevaluated regularly to ensure that it does not get too tight and cause soft tissue necrosis. Patented fixation devices can also be used. Alternatively, the surgeon may wire the endotracheal tube to the patient's jaw and teeth.

Tracheal intubation of a patient with an abnormal airway is often secured with the patient awake.[4] The most important things to remember during an awake intubation are topical anesthesia, proper patient positioning, and supplemental oxygen. Minimal intravenous (IV) opioids are recommended, because excessive opioid sedation may worsen the airway obstruction. The safest technique for endotracheal tube placement depends on the operator's expertise. Alternatives include, but are not limited to, flexible fiberoptic scope, video laryngoscope (e.g., GlideScope), Bullard scope, Wuscope, and intubating laryngeal mask airway (LMA). If the patient will not cooperate with an awake intubation, then taking the patient to the operating room should be considered for either an inhalational induction with continued spontaneous ventilation, or a surgical airway including retrograde techniques, transtracheal jet ventilation, cricothyroidotomy, or tracheostomy.[4,11] Inhalational induction with oxygen and sevoflurane is often necessary for children.

It is important to remember that the burn patient not only has initial airway concerns, but also may have a compromised airway for life. These patients often require frequent reconstructive surgeries long after the initial insult. Patients with healed burns of the neck, face, and chest may develop scar contractures that make direct laryngoscopy difficult. These patients also have a high incidence of laryngeal and tracheal strictures and bronchial stenosis caused by the inhalation injury and prolonged intubation.[11]

Respiratory pathophysiology

The initial concern regarding the respiratory system in a burn patient is the presence of an inhalation injury (Table 40.1). The incidence of inhalation injury in hospitalized patients varies from 5% to 35%.[4]

The first phase of inhalation injury may include asphyxia and acute toxicity. Asphyxia occurs secondary to the lack of oxygen during combustion. Acute toxicity occurs with the inhalation of carbon monoxide and cyanide. In anyone with a burn injury, it should be presumed that the patient will have some degree of carbon monoxide and cyanide poisoning.[1]

Carbon monoxide is a byproduct of combustion. It is responsible for 80% of deaths associated with smoke inhalation and accounts for the majority of deaths that occur at the scene of the fire.[4,5] Carbon monoxide has an affinity for hemoglobin that is 250 times greater than oxygen. Carbon monoxide preferentially binds with the hemoglobin molecule and prevents oxygen from loading onto the molecule. This causes a leftward shift of the oxyhemoglobin dissociation curve, impairing oxygen delivery and unloading at the cellular level. This results in tissue hypoxia and metabolic acidosis.[1,4,5]

Carbon monoxide poisoning can be diagnosed with an arterial blood gas and measurement of carboxyhemoglobin levels with co-oximeter blood analysis.[1,13] The pulse oximeter saturation and arterial oxygen saturation may be normal and misleading. Pulse oximetry interprets the carboxyhemoglobin as oxyhemoglobin, therefore giving a falsely elevated SpO_2.[4,5] Newer-generation pulse oximeters using multi-wavelength instrumentation are able to differentiate carboxyhemoglobin from oxyhemoglobin. Mixed venous oxygen saturation monitoring does not detect the presence of carboxyhemoglobin and progressively overestimates fractional oxyhemoglobin and carboxyhemoglobin increases.[13] It is also important to note that the patient with carbon monoxide poisoning will manifest no signs of peripheral cyanosis, and will have a characteristic "cherry red" appearance.[5] At a carbon monoxide level of less than 15%, the patient rarely has any signs or symptoms, but at 15–20% the patient will likely have a headache, tinnitus, and confusion.[1,4] At 20–40%, the patient will have nausea, fatigue, and disorientation, and at 40–60% he or she will have hallucinations and display combativeness and cardiovascular instability, followed by death when the levels are greater than 60% (Table 40.4). Treatment consists of the administration of 100% oxygen using a face mask or endotracheal tube.[1,5] High

Table 40.4 Signs and symptoms associated with specific carbon monoxide levels

Carbon monoxide level	Sign or symptom
< 15%	Rare
15–20%	Headache, tinnitus, and confusion
20–40%	Nausea, fatigue, and disorientation
40–60%	Hallucination, combativeness, and cardiovascular instability
> 60%	Death

Information from references 1 and 4.

concentrations of oxygen accelerate the dissociation of carboxyhemoglobin by 50% every 30 minutes.[1] This decreases the half-life of carboxyhemoglobin by nearly a factor of four compared with the half-life when breathing room air.[4] Although it is rarely clinically practical, some hospitals have access to hyperbaric oxygen therapy, which is thought to accelerate the dissociation more quickly.[1] Hyperbaric oxygen appears to be most useful in patients who are comatose with carboxyhemoglobin levels greater than 30%, although randomized trials do not establish whether hyperbaric oxygen treatment reduces the incidence of adverse neurologic outcomes.[13] Hyperbaric oxygen treatment is not recommended in patients with greater than 40% TBSA burns if it will delay fluid resuscitation.[4]

Cyanide is produced by the combustion of plastics; polyurethane, polyacrylonitrile, and acrocyanate glue are found in laminates and are inhaled as an aerosol when combusted.[1,4] Cyanide poisoning causes tissue asphyxia by inhibiting intracellular cytochrome oxidase activity. The diagnosis of cyanide poisoning can be difficult. A concentration of 50 ppm produces symptoms of headache, dizziness, tachycardia, and tachypnea. At levels greater than 100 ppm the patient has lethargy, seizures, and respiratory failure.[4] Cyanide poisoning should be suspected in any patient with a persistent anion gap metabolic acidosis or high lactate levels who fails to respond to oxygen administration.[1,4] The treatment of cyanide poisoning consists of two approaches. The first is a "cyanide antidote kit," in which the patient receives inhalation amyl nitrate until IV access is secured, then a combination of IV sodium nitrite and sodium thiosulfate along with 100% oxygen therapy. The second option is intravenous hydroxycobalamin plus 100% oxygen therapy. Hydroxycobalamin is usually the recommended treatment option in burn patients, because it is safer in patients with inhalational injuries.[15]

During the initial smoke inhalation injury the patient is also exposed to other chemical products of combustion, including ammonia, nitrogen dioxide, sulfur dioxide, and chlorine.[4] These chemicals are very irritating to the airway and lead to bronchospasm, edema, and mucous membrane ulceration. As a result, necrosis of the epithelial lining of the trachea and bronchi occurs. This can lead to partial or complete airway obstruction and loss of an important barrier to infection, predisposing the patient to the development of recurrent infections and pneumonia.[4,5] Physiologic effects on the lungs include increased capillary permeability, increased lung water, reduced lung compliance, decreased lung volumes, increased airway resistance, and impairment in surfactant production. These effects lead to worsening of ventilation and perfusion, and increased pulmonary shunting.

The second phase of inhalation injury begins at 24–96 hours after the injury and is the result of pulmonary parenchymal damage that is caused by the chemical irritation of smoke inhalation.[1,2] The second phase is defined by airway edema, tracheobronchitis, pulmonary edema, atelectasis, increased airway resistance, and decreased static lung compliance. The patient often has symptoms of dyspnea, rales, rhonchi, wheezing, and copious tracheal secretions and exudates. The secretions are often very viscous and may contain carbonaceous particles and pieces of mucous membrane. The clinical picture is almost identical to acute respiratory distress syndrome (ARDS). The initial inhalation injury and resultant pneumonias often influence mortality, which increases from 20% with inhalation injury alone to 60% when combined with pneumonia.

Treatment of inhalation injury includes ventilatory support (see Chapter 19), early and aggressive pulmonary toilet, bronchoscopic removal of casts, and nebulization therapy, including acetylcysteine, heparin, and albuterol.[2,5] One study showed that continuous nebulization of albuterol improves pulmonary function secondary to improved airway clearance and decreased fluid flux in a combined burn/smoke inhalation model.[16] These patients are also at a significantly increased risk of pneumonia. It has been found that nearly 95% of all pneumonias in burn patients are endogenous in origin.[17] The primary endogenous organisms include *Staphylococcus aureus*, *Streptococcus pneumoniae*, and *Haemophilus influenzae*. Unfortunately these forms of pneumonia cannot be controlled or prevented by traditionally recommended measures of hand washing and isolation. Therefore, it is recommended that the patients receive prophylactic selective decontamination of the digestive tract, aiming at eradication and prevention of contamination from existing oropharyngeal and gastrointestinal pathogens.

Ventilation can become very difficult because of the patient's increased airway resistance and increased chest wall resistance caused by full-thickness burns of the chest wall.[1] Also, the patients are often hypermetabolic, with increased oxygen consumption and increased carbon dioxide production that require higher minute ventilation.[1] The burn patient also requires high positive end-expiratory pressure (PEEP) to maintain airway patency and oxygenation.[1] Delivery of high PEEP and high minute ventilation may be difficult for older anesthesia machines, although current-generation machines have improved ventilator capabilities, similar to an intensive care unit (ICU). Although inhalation injury is primarily an acute problem, long-term survivors have a gradual collagen deposition that leads to the development of interstitial fibrosis and restrictive lung disease.[5]

Cardiac pathophysiology

In the immediate setting of a major burn, the cardiovascular response is a decrease in cardiac output and an increase in systemic vascular resistance.[1] This phenomenon is referred to as "burn shock."[4] The decrease in cardiac output is secondary to the alteration in microvascular permeability with a resultant shift of intravascular fluid into the interstitial space and also direct myocardial depressant factors.[1,4] Reduced blood flow to the coronary arteries in the postburn period may also contribute to the decrease in cardiac output. Nonsurvivors tend to have a significantly decreased cardiac output, a higher systemic vascular resistance, more metabolic acidosis, and lower oxygen consumption when compared with survivors.[4]

After the initial burn phase and resuscitation, a massive catecholamine release results in hyperdynamic circulation.[5] This hyperdynamic circulation results in tachycardia, increased cardiac output, decreased systemic vascular resistance, and increased myocardial oxygen consumption.[1,5] A study published in 2011 showed that the heart rate, cardiac output, and cardiac index remained significantly increased for up to 2 years in children surviving burns of > 40% TBSA.[18] It is also important to note that the initial burn injury itself primes the patient so that a second insult, such as aspiration pneumonia, will produce significantly greater cardiac abnormalities than those seen with the burn alone.[19]

Cardiovascular resuscitation begins with early fluid resuscitation to prevent shock, prevent and correct hypovolemia, and prevent further physiologic complications.[1,4] It is important to establish good IV access (see Chapter 4), to have a good knowledge of the fluid status, and to avoid myocardial depressants. Vital signs and urine output are the usual parameters for guiding fluid resuscitation. Some studies have shown an advantage to invasive hemodynamic monitoring in patients with major burns who do not respond to the expected fluid resuscitation. In these same studies, there was often no correlation between vital signs/urine output and pulmonary artery catheter readings (oxygen consumption and cardiac index).[4] This suggests that the vital signs may be normal in a patient who is actually hypovolemic. Therefore, in a patient who is not responsive to fluid loading, invasive monitoring and/or echocardiography are indicated to manage fluid and vasoactive drug therapy (see Chapters 9 and 10). The pulmonary artery catheter may also be useful in groups with preexisting cardiac disease.[4] If invasive monitoring is used, it should be discontinued as early as possible to minimize the risk of local and systemic infections.

Hematologic changes

The effects on the hematologic and coagulation parameters depend on the magnitude of the burn and the time from the injury.[4] Immediately after the injury, the hematocrit level increases as the noncellular fluid translocates into the interstitium. Despite large volumes of resuscitative fluids, the hematocrit often remains elevated during the first 48 hours and therefore cannot be used as a meaningful parameter of resuscitation. Patients will rarely require an early erythrocyte transfusion unless they have a preexisting anemia or another associated injury. During the weeks following the patient's initial injury there is a well-documented burn-associated anemia. This anemia is believed to be due to bleeding from the wounds, frequent blood sampling, and surgical excision. The patient will also have a shortened erythrocyte half-life secondary to the thermal injury and other circulating factors. Patients with moderate burn injury rarely require erythrocyte transfusions. An otherwise healthy burn patient will tolerate a

hematocrit of 20 (packed cell volume = 20%) without any problems, and will replenish the erythrocyte mass with iron supplementation only. A 2006 study showed that transfusions outside of the operating room were associated with increased mortality and infectious episodes in patients with major burn injury, and that the utilization of blood products should be reserved for patients with a demonstrated physiologic need or those undergoing excision and grafting in the perioperative setting.[20]

During the resuscitation of moderately to severely burned patients, the platelet count usually decreases.[4] This thrombocytopenia is due to dilutional effects and the formation of microaggregates in the skin and smoke-damaged lung. The platelet count usually returns to normal by the end of the first week and remains normal unless the patient develops sepsis or multisystem organ failure. Platelet transfusion therapy is rarely necessary unless the patient loses greater than one total body blood volume during surgical excision and grafting or has diffuse bleeding.[4,21] Frequent platelet transfusions can lead to antibody formation and ineffectiveness during future transfusions.[4]

After a major burn, both thrombotic and fibrinolytic mechanisms are activated. Clotting factors decrease secondary to dilution and consumption.[4] Disseminated intravascular coagulation (DIC) is a rare but devastating complication of massive burn injury, which should be treated with an infusion of fresh frozen plasma and cryoprecipitate.[4,21] Later in the course of the burn the patient can develop postburn thrombogenicity secondary to a decrease in antithrombin III, protein C, and protein S levels.[4] This can lead to an increased risk of venous thrombosis and pulmonary embolism. Therefore, all patients with a major burn injury require subcutaneous administration of low-dose heparin for thromboembolism prophylaxis.

Liver function

The liver synthesizes circulating proteins, detoxifies the plasma, produces bile, and provides immunologic support.[21] Hepatic injury can occur after a burn injury as a result of hypotension or hypoxia.[1] After a significant burn injury, effective liver blood flow is markedly decreased even with apparently adequate fluid resuscitation.[22] This suggests that the postburn liver requires oxygen values that exceed normal values, and therefore liver function suffers with even the slightest hypoxia. As a result of liver failure, the protein concentrations of the coagulation cascade decrease, the patient becomes coagulopathic, toxins are not cleared, and bilirubin concentrations increase.[21] The associated changes in the liver metabolism can result in increased or decreased drug metabolism due to the altered protein binding and decreased hepatic blood flow.[1]

Gastrointestinal function and nutrition

The patient's gastrointestinal response to burn injury includes mucosal atrophy, changes in digestive absorption, decreased intestinal blood flow, and increased intestinal permeability.[21]

The atrophy occurs within 12 hours of the injury and is believed to be due to increased epithelial cell death by apoptosis. The patient should receive enteral feeding early, on the first day if possible, not only to meet caloric needs of the burn but also to protect and preserve gut mucosal integrity, improve intestinal blood flow and motility, and blunt the hyperdynamic response.[5,23] Studies show that early enteral feedings reduce septic morbidity and prevent failure of the gut barrier.[21] Most patients tolerate enteral feeding well.[5] There is still some controversy as to the optimal delivery route for the enteral nutrition. Patients with intestinal feedings tend to have smaller gastric residual volumes and tend to tolerate the feeding better. In contrast, patients with a percutaneous endoscopic gastrostomy tube found it to be more comfortable and trouble-free, even if placed through an existing burn wound. Prokinetic agents, such as erythromycin and metaclopromide, can be given to enhance gastric tolerance to enteral feedings.[24]

An important part of successful enteral feeding involves the choice of the correct composition and amount to meet specific nutritional needs without overfeeding the patient. Maintenance of body weight is the common goal of nutritional support, but despite proper feeding, the burn patient will often suffer from obligatory loss of lean body mass.[24] A common formula used to estimate caloric need in the adult burn patient for enteral feeding is the Curreri formula, which estimates the patient's needs to be 25 kcal/kg/day plus 40 kcal/percent TBSA burned per day.[5] Pediatric burn patients require a different formula based on their age.[5,21] Ages zero to 12 months of age usually require 2100 kcal/percent TBSA burned per day plus 1000 kcal/percent TBSA burned per day. Ages 1 through 12 years usually require 1800 kcal/percent TBSA per day plus 1300 kcal/percent TBSA burned per day, and ages 12 through 18 years require 1500 kcal/percent TBSA burned per day plus 1500 kcal/percent TBSA burned per day.

The composition of the nutritional supplement is also important. The optimal diet contains 1–2 g/kg/day of protein, and the nonprotein calories can be given as carbohydrates or fat.[21] Albumin supplementation is important in the acute phase, as protein loss is high and hepatic synthesis of proteins is decreased.[5] Early enteral feeding is especially important, because of the associated finding of inadequate gastrointestinal tissue perfusion and multisystem organ failure.[25]

Recent interest has been focused toward the issues of gut-derived inflammation and bacterial translocation as contributors to the inflammatory response seen in burn patients.[24] The patient will therefore require a judicious use of antibiotics to prevent intestinal overgrowth of potential pathogens, which may contribute to the development of sepsis and organ failure in the burned patient.[26]

Patients with major burns are at an increased risk of forming gastric mucosal stress ulcerations, often called Curling's ulcers. These ulcers can be minimized by early enteral feeding and sucralfate or histamine receptor blocker therapy.[4]

Total parenteral nutrition is rarely used in the treatment of burn patients because of the resulting gut muscle atrophy, fatty infiltration of the liver, and septic morbidity from catheter-related infections.[5] Total parenteral nutrition is reserved only for the patient who cannot tolerate enteral feedings.[21]

Metabolism, electrolyte abnormalities, and thermoregulation

After a burn injury, the patient will develop a hypermetabolic response due to a CNS-driven stress response. The patient will develop significantly elevated levels of catecholamines, glucagon, glucocorticoids, vasopressin (antidiuretic hormone), renin, and angiotensin as a result of an increased metabolic rate.[1] This hypermetabolic response is manifested by hyperthermia, hypertension, tachycardia, increased cardiac output, increased oxygen consumption, severe nitrogen losses, and hyperglycemia.[1,21] The hyperdynamic response can be sustained for months in a severely burned patient and can lead to weight loss and decreased strength. It is important to recognize the patient's hypermetabolic phase and not to administer an overdose of narcotics while trying to normalize the patient's vital signs. Much of the morbidity and mortality of a major burn can be attributed to this hypermetabolic process.[27] Techniques used to ameliorate the hypermetabolism and thereby reduce the metabolic rate include propranolol, insulin, and oxandrolone.[24,28] Propranolol markedly reduces the resting heart rate and energy expenditure and improves the net muscle protein synthesis. It also reduces the rate of hepatic fat accumulation, which is important because fatty infiltration of the liver is a common finding in burn patients.[24] Fatty infiltration leads to hepatic dysfunction and systemic sepsis. The effect of a continuous infusion of insulin to maintain blood glucose values between 100 and 140 mg/dL tends to preserve muscle mass, decrease infection rate, and reduce the length of the hospital stay. Oxandrolone, a synthetic testosterone analog, is used to lessen muscle wasting.[24]

The patient may also develop hyponatremia because of excess ADH secretion or overhydration.[1] Most patients with hyponatremia are asymptomatic. Symptoms including headache, lethargy, and nausea do not appear until the plasma sodium level drops below 120 mEq/L. As the sodium level drops, the risk of seizure and coma increases. Hyponatremia in patients with sepsis and respiratory failure is associated with a poor prognosis.[29]

Because of their hypermetabolic response, burn patients often have impaired thermoregulation.[4] Fever in a burn patient may be physiologic and not due to infection.[30]

Immune suppression

After a burn injury, the wound itself releases paracrine factors that lead to local inflammation and edema. With a major burn, the local injury triggers the release of circulating mediators that result in a systemic response. This systemic response results in immune suppression and systemic inflammatory response syndrome (SIRS). Cytokines are the primary mediators of this immune response.[4] Another factor contributing to immune dysfunction seen with burn injury is the reduction in circulating lymphocytes, neutrophils, and macrophages.[21,24]

Endotoxin can often be detected in burn patients by the third day even in patients with no infection. The levels of the endotoxin correlate with the burn size and can be used to predict the development of multiple-organ failure and death.[4]

The burn patient is at a greater risk for a number of infectious complications, including bacterial wound infections, pneumonia, and fungal and viral infections.[21] Central line infections have been a recurring source of complications in the burn patient.[24] Current recommendations include routine catheter changes and strict aseptic technique for all vascular cannulation, because of the burn-associated immune suppression. This same aseptic technique should also be used for wound care and Foley catheter placement.[4,24]

Renal function

The incidence of acute kidney injury varies from 0.5% to 38% in the burn patient, and depends primarily on the severity of the burn. The associated mortality is very high, 73–100%.[4] Burn injury is associated with two stages of acute kidney injury. The first stage occurs early and is due to hypovolemia, decreased cardiac output, decreased renal perfusion, and decreased glomerular filtration.[1,4,23] Hypovolemia decreases renal blood flow and results in filtration failure and tubular dysfunction.[1] Increased levels of catecholamines, angiotensin, aldosterone, and vasopressin can lead to systemic vasoconstriction and contribute to renal impairment.[4] These effects result in oliguria, which, if left untreated, can lead to acute tubular necrosis and renal failure.[21]

The second stage is a late stage that results from sepsis, high myoglobin levels, nephrotoxic drugs, and multiorgan failure.[1,4] The second stage usually appears by about the third week post injury.[1] The hallmarks of the second stage include decreasing urine output, fluid overload, electrolyte abnormalities, metabolic acidosis, azotemia, increased serum creatinine levels, and hyperkalemia.[21] It is important to monitor the burn patient's electrolytes closely. Treatment of acute kidney injury due to burn injury includes early and aggressive efforts to maintain a urine output of at least 1 mL/kg/h and the institution of dialysis.[1] Some indications for dialysis include volume overload and electrolyte abnormalities not amenable to other treatments. Peritoneal and hemodialysis are both effective in the burned patient. Many burn patients will only require dialysis for a short time, until the acute kidney injury resolves.[21] Mannitol can be given IV to increase renal blood flow in hopes of improving renal function.[1]

Preoperative management
History and physical

Successful anesthesia for excision and grafting of a burn requires extensive planning and preparation.[4] This starts with a complete history and physical. It is important to know the patient's age and percent of TBSA burned. This information provides an index of the patient's likely physiologic condition. The current cardiorespiratory status is important for planning intraoperative monitoring, while the extent of the burn wound excision helps with vascular access and blood product requirements. Knowledge of the location of the burn and planned donor graft sites are important for positioning the body during surgery. It is also important to know the hours of fasting prior to the procedure. As discussed previously, if the airway of the patient is not already secured, a thorough airway assessment is necessary prior to airway manipulation.

Preoperative fasting guidelines

Preoperative fasting guidelines are modified for the burn patient, because achieving adequate caloric intake is difficult; therefore, it is recommended to continue, rather than discontinue, the enteral feedings in patients with a secure airway prior to surgery.[4] This improves preoperative nutrition without increasing the risk of aspiration. In an unintubated patient the recommendation is to stop the feedings 4 hours before surgery. One study showed that, in the immediate postburn period, patients tend to have decreased stomach acid production.[4] Also, if patients are at high risk for aspiration, they can be treated preoperatively with histamine receptor antagonists, metoclopramide, and antacids.

Type of burn

Electrical burns (Table 40.5) may be high-voltage, low-voltage, or lightning injuries. Most electrical burn injuries occur in the workplace for adults and in the home for children.[31] Electrical burns in children usually involve the child chewing on extension and electrical cords, which leads to burns involving the oral mucosa, submucosa, muscles, nerves, and blood vessels. The severity of the injury depends on the intensity of the current, the path the current takes through the patient's body, and the duration of contact with the source of the current.[31]

High-voltage burns, considered to be greater than 1000 volts, generate significant heat, reaching several thousand degrees, which can cause deep burns to the skin and muscle.[1,2,31] The hallmarks of electrical burns are the presence of contact points, which are hard, leathery, and sometimes charred, circumscribed lesions.[2] Tissue damage is most severe in the regions immediately around the contact points, with tissue necrosis extending for significant distances. High-voltage burns can be associated with blunt trauma secondary to the force of the voltage and the location of wires at significant heights.[1,2] The patient often experiences immediate cardiac arrest secondary to ventricular fibrillation and respiratory arrest secondary to paralysis of the respiratory muscles, tetanic contractions, or indirect trauma.[1,31] These patients require initial cardiac monitoring to follow and treat any associated arrhythmias, including sinus tachycardia, supraventricular tachycardias, atrial fibrillation, various degrees of heart block,

Table 40.5 Types of burns

Type	Mechanism	Results
Electrical[a]		
High voltage	> 1000 V	Deep burns to skin and muscle Blunt trauma from falls Immediate cardiac arrest (ventricular fibrillation) Delayed or persistent dysrhythmias requiring telemetry Respiratory arrest Paralysis of respiratory muscles Tetanic contractions Indirect trauma
Low voltage	< 1000 V	Superficial skin burns Rhabdomyolysis due to associated muscle contractions Acute dysrhythmias (rare)
Lightning	30×10^6 V	Rare superficial skin burns Asystole Respiratory arrest due to direct central nervous system injury
Chemical[b]	Exposure to acids, alkali, organic compounds	Continued tissue damage until insulting injury is removed
Meth lab[c]	Explosion-associated burn injury	High incidence of inhalation injury Nosocomial pneumonia Respiratory failure Sepsis Large burn size
Grease[d]	High boiling point Low specific heat Low viscosity	Deep burns requiring surgical excision and grafting

[a] References 1, 2, 31.
[b] References 1, 32.
[c] References 33, 34.
[d] Reference 35.

bundle branch blocks, and prolongation of the QT interval.[2,31] The fluid requirements in a high-voltage burn are nearly twice that of a thermal burn because of the soft tissue and visceral injury, and they cannot be calculated based on cutaneous burn requirements.[1,2] These patients are at significant risk for renal failure secondary to myoglobinuria, which is an indicator of deep tissue/muscle damage. Renal failure can be prevented and treated with vigorous hydration.[2]

Electrical burns from lightning have the highest mortality.[31] Lightning burns are usually due to a shock greater than 30×10^6 V. The patient often experiences immediate asystole and respiratory arrest due to direct CNS injury. Burns of the skin are rare and usually superficial; therefore, rhabdomyolysis is uncommon.

Low-voltage burns are more common in children, the mouth being a common site. The burns of the skin, if any, are superficial, but rhabdomyolysis is common due to the associated tetanic muscle contraction in low-voltage burns. Cardiac rhythm disturbances can be produced with relatively low currents, but low-voltage burns rarely require continued cardiac monitoring if the patient shows no sign of dysrhythmia upon arrival to the hospital.[2,31]

Chemical burns are caused by exposure to acids, alkali, or other organic compounds. Worldwide, there are about 6 million known chemicals; between 33,000 and 63,000 are classified as hazardous by one or more US governmental agencies, and more than 300 common chemicals have been classified by the National Fire Protection Association as "extremely hazardous to health" or "too dangerous to expose to fire fighters."[32] Chemical burns are characterized by continued tissue damage until the insulting injury is removed.[1] Chemical burns are often worse than originally appreciated. Hospital caregivers must wear protective gear to protect themselves from the chemical. Treatment includes immediate irrigation with large amounts of tap water.[2] After irrigation, the burns should be covered with saline-soaked pads.[32] All body parts must be thoroughly irrigated, including those not believed to be involved. Neutralization with acid or alkali is not appropriate; soap and water is sufficient.[2] Immediate surgical debridement is often required, and should be repeated often until the chemical has been completely removed.[32]

With the number of illegal methamphetamine laboratories ("meth labs") increasing across the country, burn units are seeing a significantly increased number of associated burn accidents.[33,34] The production of methamphetamine requires an extremely volatile manufacturing process that puts the manufacturers at high risk of explosion and burn injuries. The typical meth lab burn patient is male, Caucasian, unemployed, and a polysubstance abuser. The patients involved in a meth lab explosion have an increased incidence of inhalational injury that corresponds to increased rates of intubation, days on the ventilator, and tracheostomy. This is associated with an increased incidence of nosocomial pneumonia, respiratory failure, and sepsis. Meth lab burn patients have unique injuries, require 1.8 times greater resuscitation requirements, and consume more critical care resources. Meth lab burn patients tend to have larger burn size and increased morbidity when compared with other burn patients. These patients also tend to have poor recovery and follow-up after the injury, because of lack of health insurance.

Toxic epidermal necrolysis is a skin disorder that causes inflammation leading to separation of the epidermis from the dermis, with eventual sloughing comparable to a second-degree burn. This condition is associated with inflammation of the mouth and oral mucosa, leading to lesions of the trachea and larynx. Airway compromise may occur and tracheal intubation may be difficult. These patients are also at risk for aspiration and hypovolemia.[1]

Grease burns or cooking oil burns are a common burn injury in the home and workplace during food preparation.[35] Because of the high boiling point, lower specific heat, and viscosity of the grease, these patients are at increased risk of developing deep burns that often require surgical excision and grafting. Grease burns tend to follow a specific pattern of injury. Most patients have an isolated upper-extremity injury or an upper-extremity injury in combination with a face, trunk, or lower-extremity injury (Table 40.5).

Burns secondary to abuse are common in children and adults with significant handicaps. It is important to evaluate the pattern of the burn, especially with water immersion burns. The absence of splash marks and the presence of spared regions, bilateral symmetry, and well-demarcated water lines may be evidence of abuse. Signs of abuse such as bruises, whip marks, fractures, and head trauma on either the index admission or in previous medical records are also abuse indicators.[2]

Factors contributing to mortality

The mortality of the burn patient is greatly influenced by the type of burn, and it is higher when the extent of the burn is greater than 40% TBSA, in patients over 60 years old, and in the presence of inhalation injury.[1,36–38] Elderly patients tend to have a worse outcome because of their higher incidence of comorbidities (see Chapter 36), atrophic skin with a thinner dermis, and slower epithelial proliferation.[1] Young age has not proved to be a predictor of mortality.[37] In a 2001 study, it was found that women between the ages of 30 and 59 years had an increased adjusted risk of death compared with men of the same age.[36] A 2006 study showed an increased risk of death for women of all age groups between the ages of 10 and 70 years.[39] The development of sepsis and multiorgan failure is an indication of a poor outcome independent of patient age or gender.[40] Patients with limited donor sites and delayed resuscitation have an increased mortality. Morbidity and mortality of the mother and fetus in a pregnant burn patient is primarily dependent on the size of the burn, followed closely by whether there is an inhalation injury.[41] Pregnancy alone does not adversely affect the outcome of the mother (see Chapter 37). Most fetuses survive if the mother survives and she does not have any significant complications such as sepsis, hypotension, or hypoxia. Other health factors that contribute to mortality include morbid obesity, alcohol and substance abuse, neuropsychiatric conditions, diabetes, and other associated traumatic injury (Table 40.6).[1,42–44]

Laboratory tests

The burn patient will require large volumes of fluid and frequent ventilator changes during the perioperative period. Many facilities have utilized specific ordering protocols to account for the amount of lab tests needed.[45] Preoperatively, it is important to have a recent complete blood count,

Table 40.6 Predictive factors that contribute to burn mortality

Predictors	Factors contributing to mortality
Primary predictors	Total body surface area burned > 40% Age > 60 years Associated inhalation injury
Secondary predictors	Women aged 30–59 years Development of sepsis and multiple organ failure Limited donor sites Delayed resuscitation Morbid obesity Alcohol and substance abuse Diabetes Neuropsychiatric conditions Associated traumatic injury

Information from references 1, 36–38, 40, 42–44.

electrolyte panel, renal function panel, glucose, lactate level, and an arterial blood gas. Other lab tests can be ordered on an individual-case basis. Patients with burn injuries are at risk for significant coagulopathies; therefore, it is also important to check a recent coagulation panel prior to anesthesia.[4] These lab tests can be used as a baseline to adjust the anesthetic management throughout the case.

Intravenous access

Establishing vascular access is extremely important prior to excision and grafting procedures (see Chapter 5). In most cases, a minimum of two large-bore peripheral IV lines or one peripheral and one central line is necessary.[4] It is often difficult to place IVs in these patients because of the extent of the burn. Central venous catheters (e.g., 9 Fr, 12 Fr: see Chapter 5) provide excellent routes for rapid fluid administration and the delivery of vasoactive drugs.[4,46] Pulmonary artery catheters are not routinely placed because of the risk of infection, but they can be used for a brief period in patients with burn injury and ischemia or valvular heart disease to guide fluid administration.[1] The internal jugular and subclavian veins are most commonly used for catheterization, but femoral vessels can be used if the burn involves the neck.[4] Traditionally, central venous access was guided only by the anatomic landmarks and arterial pulsations.[46] This blind approach assumes that each patient has the same anatomy and that their veins have no thrombosis. An ultrasound probe can be used to aid in the placement of the central venous line.[4] The use of an ultrasound probe decreases the risk of complications, including pneumothorax, arterial puncture, hemothorax, hematoma, and nerve injury (see Chapters 5 and 12). These complications are the most significant in patients with coagulopathies, mechanical ventilation, poor pulmonary function, chronic IV use, and soft tissue edema, all of which are usually present in a burn patient.[46] If a central

Table 40.7 Current information about central line changes in a burn patient

Infection rates increase with catheters left in situ for more than 10 days.

Central line infections occur at a frequency of 5–6 infections per 1000 catheters. This is twice the Centers for Disease Control and Prevention (CDC) recognized infection rate for central line infections. Therefore, the CDC has established separate guidelines for the burn patient.

The majority of burn units in the United States change central lines every 72 hours to 7 days, every 72 hours for a line that is placed through burned tissue, and every 7 days for a line placed in a site remote from the burn tissue.

No wire changes are performed.

Central line infections (and not the burn wound) are the most common source of bacteremia in a burn patient.

Information from Sheridan RL. Mechanical and infectious complications of central venous cannulation in children: Lessons learned from a 10-year experience placing more than 1000 catheters. *J Burn Care Res* 2006; **27**: 713–18.

venous catheter is not possible, then a small-bore peripheral vein can be dilated to a larger gauge by using specially designed kits.[4] In children, if IV access cannot be achieved in a timely manner, an intraosseous (IO) infusion can be used to deliver drugs, fluids, and blood with a low incidence of complications (see Chapter 34) until an IV can be placed.[47] IV catheters can be safely placed through a burn site if the usual sterile technique is used. IV fluid and blood products are routinely warmed by using high-capacity fluid warmers in the operating room to help prevent further heat loss and avoid iatrogenic hypothermia (see Chapter 14). Table 40.7 summarizes current information relating to central line changes in a burn patient.

Premedication

Burns are often extremely painful, and the patients are often very anxious. The goal of premedication is to provide adequate analgesia and anxiolysis.[4] If a patient does not have a secure airway in place, it is important not to oversedate and risk losing the airway, especially if the patient appears to be a potentially difficult intubation. Patients who present for excision and debridement are often already intubated and sedated. It is important to continue this sedation in the perioperative period.

Preparing appropriate blood products and limiting intraoperative blood loss

Hemostasis is a critical concern during any burn surgery.[4,5] Large amounts of blood can be lost rapidly during the excision of the burn; therefore, it is important to have an adequate supply of blood products available prior to the excision. It is

difficult to keep up once infusion lags behind blood loss. Documented blood loss and transfusion requirements in patients with greater than 10% TBSA burn showed a mean blood loss of 0.3 mL/cm^2 surface area excised.[4] An average of 20 mL of blood will need to be transfused for each percent of TBSA burned. Other studies have shown that 2–3 units of packed red blood cells can be easily lost during skin excision of one hand, and in burns greater than 25% TBSA the patient can exsanguinate.[5]

Perioperative treatment with timely and targeted correction of coagulopathy can reduce transfusion requirements.[48] A point-of-care viscoelastic coagulation test can be used to determine the allogeneic blood product requirements (see Chapter 9).

Many centers use various and multiple techniques to try to limit blood loss during excision, including the use of tourniquets, postoperative compression dressings, topical epinephrine, topical thrombin, and subcutaneous infusion of saline and epinephrine.[4,5] Tourniquets have been found to be the most effective technique.[5] Epinephrine-soaked compresses at a concentration of 1:10,000 have been shown to provide good hemostasis, but their effectiveness at preventing considerable blood loss is questionable.[5] Despite the high levels of catecholamine from the epinephrine-soaked bandages, complications such as dysrhythmias are not common, because of the reduced affinity of the β-adrenergic receptor in the burn patient for ligands and decreased second-messenger production.[4] Topical thrombin (1000 units/mL) helps with hemostasis by forming a clot, but this sheet of clot can prevent graft take and donor healing. Subcutaneous infusion of 0.45% saline with diluted epinephrine (1:300,000) to the donor sites also helps with hemostasis.[5]

Although the extent of the surgical operation is often intentionally limited in most centers to one volume of blood lost, patients frequently lose more than this amount through thrombocytopenia and other coagulation defects.[4] The best intraoperative fluid replacement includes the use of minimal crystalloid and the replacement of losses with packed red blood cells and fresh frozen plasma.[5] It is important that the patient is typed and crossed for an appropriate amount of blood products prior to beginning the surgery, and that the products are immediately available at induction. In most cases the patient should be given blood immediately upon entering the operating room. After the excision and grafting, the burn patient's coagulation factors and platelets return to baseline values faster than those of unburned patients.[4]

Studies have shown that the number of infections per patient increases with each unit of blood transfused.[20] An increased number of transfusions is also associated with increased mortality. This study did not include blood products given in the operating room. Currently, it is agreed that outside the operating room, the patient's blood transfusion should be guided by physiologic need, and that in the operating room, when there is significant blood loss, the patient's primary fluid replacement should be with blood.

Surgery

Topical wound care

Prehospital burn wound care is basic and simple.[21] It requires that the burn be protected from the environment with the application of a clean dry dressing or sheet. A damp dressing should never be used. The patient should be wrapped in blankets to prevent heat loss during transport. The first step in diminishing the patient's pain is to cover the wounds to prevent contact with exposed nerve endings. Even though this approach sounds simple, it is often difficult to enact, which is unfortunate because inadequate first aid care is often associated with poorer patient outcomes.

Once the extent and depth of the wounds are assessed and the wounds are cleaned and debrided, the management phase begins.[21] Each wound should be dressed with the appropriate covering to protect the damaged epithelium, minimize bacterial and fungal colonization, and provide a splinting action to maintain the desired position of function. The dressing should be occlusive to reduce evaporative heat loss and minimize cold stress. The dressing should also provide comfort over the painful wound.

First-degree wounds are minor, with minimal loss of barrier function, and therefore require no dressing and are treated with topical salves to decrease pain and keep the skin moist.[21] Second-degree wounds can be treated with daily dressing changes and topical antibiotics. Alternatively, the wounds can be treated with temporary biologic or synthetic coverings to close the wound. Deep second-degree and third-degree wounds require excision and grafting for sizable burns, and the initial dressing should be aimed at holding bacterial proliferation in check until the initial operation is performed.

The timely and effective use of antimicrobials has revolutionized burn care, decreasing the number of invasive wound infections.[5,21] The topical antibiotics can be divided into two classes: salves and soaks (Table 40.8; see also Chapter 39).

Topical antimicrobial salves used for burn wound care include silver sulfadiazine (Silvadene), mafenide acetate (Sulfamylon), bacitracin, neomycin, polymyxin B, nystatin (Mycostatin), and mupirocin (Bactroban). Silvadene is advantageous because it is painless upon application and has a broad spectrum of efficacy, but it fails to penetrate the eschar and is therefore not adequate for the treatment of deep partial-thickness and full-thickness burns. In contrast, mafenide acetate is more painful on application but it is associated with much better penetration through the eschar; however, it is associated with a metabolic acidosis. Bacitracin, neomycin, and polymyxin B all have an easy painless application but have a limited antimicrobial spectrum. Nystatin is effective at inhibiting most fungal growth, but cannot be used in combination with mafenide acetate. Mupirocin is very effective in staphylococcal coverage.

Antimicrobial soaks include silver nitrate 0.5%, sodium hypochlorite 0.025% solution (Dakin's solution), and acetic acid 0.25%. Silver nitrate provides broad-spectrum coverage,

Table 40.8 Topical antimicrobial salves and soaks

Application	Medication	Advantages/disadvantages of use
Salves	Silver sulfadiazine (Silvadene)	Painless application Broad-spectrum efficacy Poor penetration of eschar
	Mafenide acetate (Sulfamylon)	Painful application Good penetration of eschar Metabolic acidosis
	Bacitracin	Painless application Limited antimicrobial spectrum
	Neomycin	Painless application Limited antimicrobial spectrum
	Polymyxin B	Painless application Limited antimicrobial spectrum
	Nystatin (Mycostatin)	Effective at inhibiting most fungal growth Cannot be used with Sulfamylon
	Mupirocin (Bactroban)	Effective staphylococcal coverage Higher cost
Soaks	Silver nitrate (0.5%)	Broad-spectrum coverage Poor penetration Can inhibit wound healing Methemoglobinemia
	Sodium hypochlorite (0.025%) (Dakin's solution)	Excellent bactericidal activity No adverse effects on wound healing
	Acetic acid (0.25%)	Effective against most organisms Can inhibit epithelialization

Information from references 4 and 21.

but also fails to penetrate and can inhibit wound healing and cause methemoglobinemia. Dakin's solution provides excellent bactericidal activity, without adverse effects on the wound healing. Acetic acid is effective against most organisms, but can inhibit epithelialization.

Escharotomies

When a deep second- or third-degree burn wound encompasses the circumference of an extremity, the peripheral circulation of the limb can be compromised.[21] The generalized edema and the nonyielding eschar can impede venous outflow and eventually affect arterial inflow to the distal beds. This can be diagnosed by the symptoms of increased tingling or limb pain and by checking the capillary refill or using Doppler ultrasound assessment of blood flow. These extremities will require an escharotomy to release the burn wound eschar. This can be done at the bedside by incising the lateral and medial aspects of the extremity with a scalpel or electrocautery unit. Increased muscle compartment pressures may necessitate a fasciotomy. The most common complications from these procedures include blood loss and the release of anaerobic metabolites, which can cause transient hypotension. Constricting truncal eschars can cause a similar problem, except the effect is decreased ventilation because of limited chest wall excursion. The truncal eschar is treated similarly to the extremity eschar.[21]

Grafting and excision

Traditionally, the treatment of a burn would include dressing changes and topical antimicrobial agents until the eschar separates, then the granulating wound would be covered with split-thickness skin graft.[4,49] This process would often take 3–5 weeks. The patients with severe wounds would often die of sepsis, and those who survived would have severe contractures and hypertrophic scars. A burn is considered to be a major source of inflammatory mediators, which play an important role in maintaining the postburn inflammatory response.[49,50] The consequent acute-phase reaction – including changes in vascular permeability, alterations in coagulation, impaired gut function, hypermetabolic response, and immune depression – leads to increased mortality and morbidity after a severe burn.[50] The concept of early excision and grafting is derived from a goal of possibly averting these deleterious changes by excising the wound before the response is maximized.[49,50] Delays in excision and grafting are associated with longer hospitalizations, delayed wound closure, increased rates of invasive wound infection, and sepsis.[24,50] Excision within the first 48 hours (assuming that the patient has had sufficient resuscitation), early nutritional support, infection control, biologic wound covering, and modulation of the hypermetabolic response is recommended for optimal burn patient care.[4,49,50]

Serial excision of the full-thickness burn wound is the current standard of care in many burn centers throughout the world.[4,5] Operations of excision and grafting are often limited to about 20% of TBSA per surgery. With multiple surgical teams and the use of previously described techniques to limit blood loss, larger areas can be excised without increasing the operating time or blood loss. These procedures will be repeated every 2 days until the burn wound excision is complete. The goal is to perform the entire excision of the burn within 10 days of the injury. All of the full-thickness burns should be excised first. This early near-total burn excision has dramatically improved the survival rate in massive burn cases. Facial burns are often treated last, and superficial burns normally heal on their own within 2 weeks.

During the burn wound excision, all dead tissue must be removed.[5] This provides a clean and living wound bed that is necessary to prevent postoperative infection, graft loss, and reoperation. The living tissue will appear as a white, shiny collagen net with punctate bleeding. Burns of less than 30% TBSA can be successfully covered with skin autografts. The skin autograft is usually a split-thickness graft that is taken with a powered dermatome from the same patient. These grafts are rarely rejected, provide long-lasting coverage, and provide the best cosmetic result. In burns greater than 30%

TBSA, alternative skin grafts are required for coverage. The excised area can be covered with homografts for temporary skin coverage, but the patient will need to be taken back to the operating room once these grafts are rejected and replaced with autografts. The hope is that during these few weeks the patient's donor sites will have healed and can be reused.

Alternative skin care management

Alternative management for the patient with extensive burns includes artificial skin substitutes.[4] The superiority of the dermal substitutes to conventional skin has never been demonstrated, but the most important potential for these products is their ability to temporarily cover the excised wounds until permanent coverage can be established.[24] These types of dressings provide stable coverage without painful dressing changes, provide a barrier to evaporative losses, and decrease pain in the wounds.[21] These grafts should be applied within 72 hours of the injury, before bacterial colonization of the wound occurs. These alternative dressings include Integra, Alloderm, and cultured human keratinocytes (Table 40.9).

Integra is a bilaminate membrane of chondroitin sulfate. The outer silicone layer closes the wound, and the inner layer establishes a vascular supply.[4] The outer layer is removed after 2 weeks and replaced with thin autologous skin grafts. The remaining deep layer provides structural support, so only a thin autologous graft is required. This thin graft allows the

Table 40.9 Characteristics of use for alternative skin care management

Alternative skin care management	Characteristics of use
Integra	Bilaminate membrane of chondroitin sulfate Outer silicone layer closes wound Inner layer establishes vascular supply Provides support to thin-skin autograft Graft large wound areas Lacks transmission of viral infection Avoidance of rejection Expensive Lacks immunologic and metabolic benefits of living skin
Alloderm	Acellular dermal matrix Provides support to thin-skin autograft Dermal replacement option for large burns/limited donor sites
Cultured human keratinocytes	Poor skin coverage Requires weeks to grow Very expensive Long-term skin fragility Recurrent open wounds Increased burn scar contractures Necessary for total body surface area burns > 95% to preserve limited donor sites

Information from references 4 and 5.

donor site to be used more frequently for harvesting. Large areas of burn wound can be grafted with the skin substitute.[5] It has an advantage over a homograft because of its lack of transmission of viral infections and avoidance of rejection. The disadvantage of Integra is that it is more expensive than a homograft and lacks the immunologic and metabolic benefits of a living temporary cover.[5]

Alloderm, an acellular dermal matrix, is derived from human homografts and is similar to Interga in that it also provides support to a thin skin autograft.[4,5] Alloderm can be used as a dermal replacement in patients with large burns and limited donor sites. It can also be used as a dermal replacement for wounds extending over the joints, to prevent contractures.

The experimental use of cultured human keratinocytes was initially promising, but they have been found to have poor skin coverage, require weeks to grow, are very expensive, and are associated with long-term skin fragility, recurrent open wounds, and increased rate of burn scar contractures.[4,5] In burns of greater than 95% TBSA, the shortage of donor sites and the absolute need to preserve these small donor sites for later needs make the cultured epithelial autografts necessary for patient survival.

Intraoperative management
Monitors and Foley catheter

Monitoring for a major burn excision and grafting should be based on the knowledge of the patient's medical condition and the extent of the surgery (see Chapter 9).[4] Vital signs and urine output measurement are considered the standard of care in the resuscitation assessment of the burn patient. Invasive monitoring is reserved for the selected high-risk patient and the patient whose resuscitation is failing.[51]

Electrocardiogram monitoring may be done from burned surfaces by using needle electrodes or surgical staples to which an alligator clamp is attached (Fig. 40.1). Standard

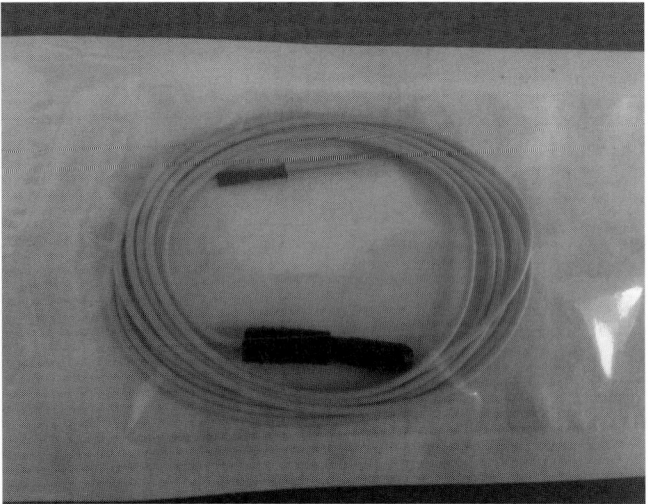

Figure 40.1 Needle electrode for electrocardiogram. (J. Lovich-Sapola.)

electrocardiogram pads may be placed under a dependent part of the body to provide a satisfactory electrocardiographic signal in most patients.[4]

Pulse oximetry has been the standard of care in all patients undergoing anesthesia since the early 1990s.[52] It is a valuable, noninvasive optical monitoring technique that is used for the continuous measurement of arterial blood oxygen saturation. Pulse oximetry usually gives reliable readings of the blood oxygen saturation, but there are times when significant limitations of the accuracy and availability of pulse oximetry occur. When peripheral perfusion is poor (as in states of hypovolemia, hypothermia, vasoconstriction, low cardiac output, and low mean arterial pressure) oxygenation readings become unreliable or cease. Sites for pulse oximeter readings are frequently difficult to find in the burn patient. Standard sites such as fingers and toes may be affected by the burn or rendered unusable due to tourniquet placement.[52] Alternative sites can be used with a standard pulse oximeter probe if the fingers are too severely burned to be used.[4] These sites include the ear, nose, or tongue. Esophageal reflectance pulse oximetry may offer advantages over the standard transmission oximetry if the skin sites for monitoring are limited.[4,52] Ultimately, the physician may have to rely on arterial blood gas analysis.

Arterial blood pressure should be monitored invasively for any large surgical debridement.[4] Indications for an arterial line include arterial blood sampling, continuous real-time monitoring of moment-to-moment blood pressures, failure to take indirect blood pressure measurements, intentional pharmacologic cardiovascular manipulation, and the assessment of supplementary diagnostic clues.[53] Use of an arterial line also allows estimates of systolic pressure and pulse pressure variability and stroke volume (see Chapter 9).

Invasive hemodynamic monitoring is recommended in patients with serious burns who do not respond as expected to fluid resuscitation.[4] This suggests that even if patients have normal vital signs, they can be hypovolemic. Urine output and arterial blood pressure cannot be considered sufficient criteria for fluid resuscitation in patients with preexisting cardiopulmonary or renal disorders and may even provide inaccurate information.[54,55] Echocardiography and assessment of the hemodynamic state may be useful in this regard (see Chapter 10). On occasion, a pulmonary artery catheter may be indicated in patients who do not respond to fluid resuscitation or who have preexisting cardiac disease (see Chapter 9).[4] The pulmonary artery catheter is used to assess the cardiac output, stroke volume, systemic vascular resistance, and calculation of oxygen transport parameters. Central venous pressure and pulmonary capillary wedge pressure have been used as preload indicators to guide volume therapy.[54] The central venous catheter must often be placed through burned tissue, and the catheters should be removed as soon as possible after the excision and grafting procedure to minimize the risk of local and systemic infection.[4] The indication for extended hemodynamic monitoring is frequently present with a burn greater than 50% TBSA.[54] As pulmonary artery catheters are not routinely placed, because of the increased risk of infection, echocardiography can be used to evaluate ventricular function and estimate central venous and pulmonary artery systolic pressure (see Chapter 10).[1]

A catheter should be placed in the patient's bladder to evaluate hourly urine output.[2,4] Even with a severe burn to the genitalia, the catheterization can almost always be performed. The use of silver-impregnated Foley catheters can significantly decrease the rate of urinary tract infection in the burn patient.[56]

Thermal regulation

Temperature monitoring is essential for any burn patient undergoing anesthesia, because hypothermia is common and often difficult to prevent (see Chapter 14).[4] The burn patient develops a hypermetabolic state in proportion to the severity of the burn injury. Ambient temperature has an important effect on the metabolic rate of the burn patient. A burn patient with a thermoneutral ambient temperature of 28–32 °C has a metabolic rate that is 1.5 times greater than in a nonburned control patient. If the burn patient's ambient temperature is decreased to 22–28 °C the metabolic rate is increased in proportion to the burn size. Therefore, in the burn unit and the operating room, the patient's temperature should remain thermoneutral to avoid further increases in the metabolic rate.[4] Hypothermia can also exacerbate coagulopathy and can be potentially devastating during operative debridement of burns.[57] The burn patient is particularly susceptible to hypothermia due to the evaporative heat loss that occurs through his/her wounds.[58] Temperature regulation can be achieved by having the ambient temperature of the operating room higher than 28 °C and having all topical and IV fluids warmed to 38 °C.[4,57,59] When possible, the nonoperative sites should be covered and a forced-air warming device used.[4] If available, over-the-bed warming lamps (radiant heaters) and circulating warm water gel pads can be used.[2,58,59]

Ventilation

Mechanical ventilation is required for patients with more extensive burns, inhalational injury, or respiratory complications.[4] Patients with lung injury often have a substantial increase in dead-space ventilation, so that end-tidal carbon dioxide may not correlate well with arterial carbon dioxide levels. Therefore, arterial blood gases should be measured frequently. For patients with very abnormal ventilation, the standard anesthesia ventilator may be inadequate, and it may be necessary to use the burn unit ventilator. The goal of mechanical ventilation is to provide gas exchange with as little barotrauma as possible (see Chapter 19).[21] Patients with major burn injury frequently develop ARDS.[60] "Permissive hypercapnia" and the current ARDS Network ventilation protocols (Table 40.10) can be used to lower ventilatory rates and volumes and to maintain the arterial pH at greater than 7.25, thereby limiting the positive airway pressures delivered by the ventilator.[21] These techniques include high PEEP and low-volume ventilation.[61] The beneficial

Table 40.10 ARDS Network ventilation protocol

Volume cycled assist control ventilation
Tidal volume of 6 mL/kg presumed body weight
Maximum plateau pressure of 30 cmH$_2$O
PEEP and FiO$_2$ are adjusted in tandem with a PaO$_2$ goal of 55–80 mmHg
Inspiratory flow rates are adjusted to keep the inspiratory: expiratory ratio between 1:1 and 1:3

ARDS, acute respiratory distress syndrome; FiO$_2$, inspired oxygen concentration: PaO$_2$, arterial oxygen tension; PEEP, positive end-expiratory pressure.
Information from Hough CL, Kallet RH, Ranieri VM, *et al.* Intrinsic positive end-expiratory pressure in Acute Respiratory Distress Syndrome (ARDS) Network subjects. *Crit Care Med* 2005; **33**: 527–32.

effects include avoiding lung tissue damage by reducing shearing forces and avoiding alveolar collapse. The high PEEP is also beneficial in helping to avoid pulmonary edema from the massive fluids given during resuscitation. High FiO$_2$ should be avoided if possible, because it can cause lung damage and lead to increased rates of pneumonia.

In addition to the conventional ventilator, new ventilation techniques have been developed in an attempt to improve oxygenation and decrease barotrauma to the lung.[21] One form of ventilation is high-frequency percussive/oscillatory ventilation.[21,60] This method alternates standard tidal volumes and respirations with smaller high-frequency respirations. This technique recruits alveoli at lower airway pressures and has a percussive effect that loosens secretions and improves pulmonary toilet. It has been used successfully in many centers for the management of oxygen failure secondary to ARDS and as a method for intraoperative ventilation to allow surgical burn wound excision despite severe ARDS.[60,62] Another benefit of high-frequency percussive/oscillatory ventilation during burn anesthesia is that hemodynamic instability or compromise in oxygenation is rarely associated with this technique.[62]

Patients with pneumonia or ARDS may require frequent endotracheal suctioning, chest physiotherapy, and bronchodilator therapy.[4,21] Adequate humidification and inhalational therapy, including bronchodilators (Albuterol), nebulized heparin, nebulized acetylcysteine, hypertonic saline, and racemic epinephrine, have all proved effective in clearing the tracheobronchial secretions and decreasing bronchospasm. Bronchoscopy may also be needed to clear the secretions. Steroids have not proved beneficial to the patient with inhalational injury and should not be given unless the patient was steroid-dependent prior to the injury or has bronchospasm that is resistant to standard therapy.

Pharmacokinetics and pharmacodynamics of anesthetics in a burn patient

The pathophysiologic changes that occur after thermal injury alter the pharmacokinetic parameters, including absorption, bioavailability, protein binding, volume of distribution, and clearance.[4] The extent of these changes depends on the magnitude of injury and the time between injury and drug administration. The pharmacokinetic parameters of many drugs will change drastically directly following the injury.[63] The pharmacodynamic changes include changes in the drug–receptor interaction after the burn and appear to account for many of the clinically important alterations in anesthetic pharmacology.[4]

In the hypermetabolic acute phase after the burn injury, organ blood flow is reduced because of hypovolemia and decreased cardiac output, which may affect the dosing requirements of many drugs.[1,4] Changes in blood flow specifically to the kidneys and liver can affect clearance and elimination. Therefore, drugs administered by routes other than IV are likely to show delayed absorption. Plasma albumin concentrations decrease and α-1-acid glycoprotein levels increase. Plasma protein binding of albumin-bound drugs such as benzodiazepines is decreased, resulting in an increase in free fraction. As most anesthetic drugs are not highly protein-bound, and because hemodynamic changes with burns are so marked, the effect of the protein binding on the pharmacologic effects of the anesthetics is minimal. The protein binding of acidic and neutral drugs will decrease and higher amounts of the free fraction will be available, while the basic drugs will exhibit increased protein binding and will probably require an increased dosage to achieve the appropriate pharmacologic effect.[63]

After the initial resuscitation phase, cardiac output increases, as does the internal core temperature, which usually increases drug clearance.[4,63] However, there is wide patient-to-patient variability in renal and hepatic function after the burn, so drug therapy must be tailored to each patient.[4]

Induction and maintenance of anesthesia

General anesthesia with the combination of an opioid, a volatile agent, and a neuromuscular relaxant is the most widely used technique for burn excision and grafting.[4] The induction agents are chosen based on the hemodynamic stability of the patient.[1]

Supplemental opioids are important in burn patients because of the intense pain they experience.[4] Burn patients usually require large doses of opioids to remain comfortable even in the absence of movement or surgical procedures. The increased dose requirement of the burn patient, especially during the hypermetabolic state, is thought to be due to the activation of endogenous pathways during the stress response.[1] Also, because they regularly receive opioids as a part of their daily care, they become tolerant to these drugs.[4]

The choice of volatile anesthetic does not appear to influence the outcome of the anesthesia for burn surgery.[4] Sevoflurane has the advantage of being an ideal agent for inhaled induction of anesthesia in burn patients with abnormal airways. Isoflurane decreases cardiac output and oxygen consumption; however, the reductions parallel one another so that the oxygen supply to the tissue remains sufficient to meet the demands.

Various IV induction agents have been used successfully in burn patients.[1,4] Ketamine offers the advantage of stable hemodynamics and analgesia. It is beneficial for dressing changes and bedside procedures. Its drawbacks include the tendency for dysphoric reactions, which can be decreased with co-administration of benzodiazepines, and the tolerance that develops with repeated use. In a hemodynamically unstable patient, etomidate is a reasonable alternative to ketamine for the induction of anesthesia. Etomidate should not be used for frequent dressing changes, because of the adrenocortical suppressive effects of the drug.[53] In patients who are adequately resuscitated and not septic, propofol may be used.[4]

Depolarizing muscle relaxants, including succinylcholine, have been subject to considerable debate concerning timing and use in burn patients, because of the potential for hyperkalemia and cardiac arrest (see Chapter 13).[1,4] Burn injury results in denervation of the tissue, which causes the entire skeletal muscle membrane, as opposed to the motor endplate only, to develop acetylcholine receptors. On administration of succinylcholine, an exaggerated number of acetylcholine receptors are depolarized, resulting in a massive efflux of potassium from the cell into the extracellular fluid (see Chapter 13). The hyperkalemia cannot be prevented by giving a defasciculating dose of nondepolarizer prior to the administration of succinylcholine. The larger the TBSA of the burn, the higher the likelihood of a hyperkalemic response. The potassium concentration increases within the first minute after succinylcholine administration, peaks within 5 minutes, and starts to decline by 10–15 minutes. Hypersensitivity to succinylcholine begins 48 hours after the burn, and peaks at 1–3 weeks. The hyperkalemic response may persist for up to 2 years. Therefore, succinylcholine is safe for the first 48 hours and is best avoided after that.[1]

Nondepolarizing muscle relaxants (NDMRs) are often used during excision and grafting of burn patients. Patients with thermal injury are usually resistant to the action of NDMRs.[1,4] This effect may take up to a week to develop and may be observed for as long as 18 months after the burn has healed. A marked resistance to NDMRs occurs when the burn is greater than 30–40% TBSA. The mechanism appears to be due to the acetylcholine receptor proliferation that occurs under the burn and at the sites distant from the burn injury. This increase in acetylcholine receptors is usually associated with resistance to NDMRs and an increased sensitivity to depolarizing muscle relaxants. This resistance to NDMRs implies that the burned patient will require larger than normal doses of NDMR to achieve a desired effect and the duration of action will be shorter than normal. Dose requirements can be increased by up to 250–500%. If muscle relaxants are being used, then neuromuscular function should be regularly monitored.

Estimated blood loss and fluid resuscitation during excision and grafting

Excisional treatment of burn wounds is usually associated with a large operative blood loss.[64] Neither the surface area to be excised nor the time from the burn accurately predict the magnitude of the operative blood loss, but an excision performed less than 24 hours after the injury usually has less bleeding than one performed 2–16 days after the injury. Peak hemorrhage appears to occur on days 5 to 12. Percent area of third-degree burn is associated with blood loss, but the percentage of TBSA burned is not. Other operative variables associated with increased blood loss are surgical time, anesthesia preparatory time, and the initial heart rate recorded in the operating room.

Many techniques are used to limit blood loss during excision and grafting, such as tourniquets, multiple surgical teams working simultaneously to decrease the surgical time, epinephrine- and thrombin-soaked gauze, topical vasoconstrictors, compressive dressings, a cell saver, and continuous infusion of vasopressin.[65,66]

In addition to the difficulty in predicting blood loss, estimation of blood loss during excision and grafting can also be difficult. Estimation of blood loss often requires serial hematocrit readings, use of formulas, and, most importantly, constant communication with the burn surgeon.[1] The first formula that can be used is 100–200 mL blood loss per 1% tissue excised; however, this does not take into account the circulating blood volume.[1] A more specific formula used is the percent to be excised × loss of area ratio × estimated blood volume (mL)/100, in which the loss of area ratio is 8 for children and highly vascular areas, and 4 for debridement only and less vascular areas (Table 40.11).

Aggressive fluid resuscitation is imperative to improving mortality, especially in the initial phase of treatment and during operative excision and grafting. Furthermore, the volume of the fluid given during resuscitation may not be as important as the timeliness with which it is given.[5] Blood loss is usually replaced with crystalloids, colloids, packed red blood cells, and fresh frozen plasma.[67] Hemodynamic changes after a burn are significant, and must be managed carefully to optimize intravascular volume, maintain end-organ perfusion, and

Table 40.11 Methods for estimating blood loss during burn excision and grafting

Method 1

EBL = 100 to 200 mL per 1% tissue excised

Method 2

EBL = (% to be excised) × (loss of area ratio) × (EBV in mL)/100

EBL, estimated blood loss; EBV, estimated blood volume.
Loss of area ratio = 8 for children and highly vascular areas.
Loss of area ratio = 4 for debridement only and less vascular areas.
Information from reference 1.

maximize oxygen delivery to the tissues.[5] The initial goal of the cardiovascular resuscitation during excision and grafting is to correct and prevent hypovolemia.[4] IV fluid is usually given in proportion to the percent of TBSA burned and is guided by the clinical assessment, vital signs, and urine output. In a patient with normal renal function, urine output should be at least 0.5 mL/kg/h in adults and 1 mL/kg/h in children.[21] Lactated Ringer's solution is usually the fluid of choice, except in patients younger than 2 years; they should receive 5% dextrose Ringer's lactate.[21] Adequate resuscitation is reflected by stable vital signs and a urine output of 1 mL/kg/h.[2] Changes in the IV fluid should be made on a regular basis, at least hourly, based on the patient's hemodynamic response.[21] The objective of the fluid resuscitation is to replace the fluid losses and therefore maintain adequate tissue perfusion and oxygen delivery to the cells.[2,68] Failure to achieve this goal leads to burn shock, with progressive oxygen debt, anaerobic metabolism, and lactic acidosis.[68]

During the active fluid resuscitation in the operating room, frequent arterial blood samples should be sent to monitor the changing levels of pH and lactate.[68] These lab markers are relevant for impaired cellular perfusion during the resuscitation. Normalization of a previously elevated lactate level indicates improved tissue perfusion at the cellular level, and correction of oxygen debt.[69]

At MetroHealth Medical Center, a modified Parkland (Baxter) formula is used to resuscitate burn patients (Tables 40.12–40.14). As with any resuscitation formula, it serves merely as a guideline to fluid resuscitation. The actual rates must be titrated according to individual patient response. The goal is to give the least amount of fluid necessary to maintain adequate organ perfusion.

Postoperative management
Extubation criteria and tracheotomy placement

Burn patients often receive large volumes of fluid during their resuscitation and therefore develop significant soft tissue edema. Tracheal extubation should be delayed until tissue edema resolves.[4] During general anesthesia, patients often receive large quantities of opioids and NDMRs, which can also delay emergence and extubation. The criteria for extubation should include resolution of intoxication, ability to follow commands, noncombativeness, pain well controlled, appropriate cough and gag, ability to protect the airway from aspiration, no excessive airway edema, adequate tidal volume, normal motor strength, vital capacity greater than 15 mL/kg, negative inspiratory force greater than 20 cm H_2O, PaO_2 greater than 60 mmHg at an FiO_2 of less than 0.50, respiratory rate less than 25/min, A–a gradient less than 200 mmHg, and normothermia without signs of sepsis (Table 40.15).[53,70]

Long-term intubation of a burn patient can be complicated by post-extubation stridor.[4] When planning to extubate the

Table 40.12 Fluid resuscitation protocol for a burn patient at MetroHealth Medical Center, for the first 24 hours

	Estimated fluid volume and rates	Crystalloid	Colloid	Thawed plasma
Adult	1. 4 mL/kg per percent burn for the first 24 hours. 2. Give one-half of the fluid in the first 8 hours post burn. 3. Give the balance over the next 16 hours post burn.	Lactated Ringer's	1. Burns larger than 40% TBSA. 2. Burns requiring > 50% over the calculated fluid requirements.	1. Burns larger than 40% TBSA and those requiring > 50% over the calculated fluid requirement at 12 hours post burn. 2. Give TP at a ratio of one unit (about 250 mL) per every liter of LR.
Child	1. Use the Brooke children's formula: 3 mL/kg/TBSA burn + maintenance. 2. Half of the 3 mL/kg per percent burn is given over the first 24 hours (added to maintenance rate). 3. The other half is given over 16 hours.	D_5LR	Burns larger than 30% TBSA in patients less than age 5 years.	1. Burns larger than 30% TBSA in patients age < 5 years. 2. Run equal volumes of TP and LR at the calculated rate according to the Parkland formula.

D_5LR, 5% dextrose in lactated Ringer's; LR, lactated Ringer's; TBSA, total body surface area burned; TP, thawed plasma. Only deep second-degree and third-degree burns are used in calculating TBSA (see Chapter 39).

Table 40.13 Fluid resuscitation protocol for a burn patient at MetroHealth Medical Center, for the second 24 hours

	Crystalloid	Thawed plasma (TP)
Adults and children	Give half of the total infused during the first 24 hours	Give one unit of TP per liter of crystalloid

Table 40.14 General transfusion requirements at Metro Health Medical Center

Burn patients require packed red cells and/or thawed plasma for the following reasons:
- To maintain adequate plasma volume
- Capillary leak syndrome
- Volume replacement for fevers and dressing changes
- Operating room procedures such as skin grafts, burn debridement, etc.
- Operating room procedures are treated as for a new burn patient for the first 24 hours, afterward needing red blood cells and thawed plasma for volume expansion
- Hematocrit should be between 26% and 30% and/or hemoglobin ≥ 8 g/dL
- Elderly patients or patients with cardiac dysfunction need to have hematocrits > 30%

Table 40.15 Criteria for tracheal extubation

Resolution of intoxication
Ability to follow commands
Noncombative
Pain well-controlled
Appropriate cough and gag
Ability to protect airway from aspiration
No excessive airway edema
Adequate tidal volume
Normal motor strength
Vital capacity > 15 mL/kg
Negative inspiratory force > 20 cmH$_2$O
PaO$_2$ > 60 mmHg at FiO$_2$ < 0.5
Respiratory rate < 25 breaths per minute
Alveolar-arterial oxygen gradient < 200 mmHg
Normothermic
No signs of sepsis

Information from references 53 and 70.

patient's trachea, it is important to wait until an air leak occurs around the endotracheal tube when the cuff is deflated. If the patient appears ready for extubation according to all other criteria and still has no air leak, then direct laryngoscopy may be helpful to determine the extent of residual airway edema. Another effective tool for the trial of extubation on burn patients is the use of a #11 Cook airway exchange catheter (#11 CAEC), which is placed through the endotracheal tube and left in place after the patient is extubated.[70] The CAEC can be used to administer oxygen, which decreases the potential for hypoxia while maintaining the ability to reintubate the trachea, especially in a patient with a potentially difficult airway. Reintubating over the CAEC may be technically difficult in some patients due to the "hang up" of the tube on the epiglottis or other soft tissue, but the ease of intubation can be improved with the use of a Parker endotracheal tube. If reintubation is not possible, then jet ventilation should be initiated. The risk of aspiration, barotrauma, or other airway trauma appears to be low. The CAEC is usually left in the trachea for about 10 hours, and is well tolerated by most patients. Almost all patients are able to vocalize with the CAEC in place. After patients are extubated, they should be monitored closely for progressive airway obstruction during the next 24–48 hours.

Most burn patients' airways can be managed with an endotracheal tube.[4] Performance of a tracheostomy in a recently burned patient is controversial. Concerns include infection, pulmonary sepsis, tracheal stenosis, and tracheoesophageal and tracheoarterial fistulas.[1,4] The risks of associated infection may be limited by delaying the placement of the tracheostomy until after successful neck grafting and by not placing it through an infected burn.[4] Many institutions have developed their own guidelines based on TBSA of the burn and potential for a rapid recovery. Early tracheostomy is almost always required in the following cases: (1) an airway cannot be obtained by using conventional intubation routes, (2) inadvertent extubation of an airway that has maximal edema (reintubation is nearly impossible), (3) acute airway loss, and (4) long-term respiratory failure.[1,4] The advantages of a tracheostomy include easier oral and tracheal hygiene, easier communication (if the patient can mouth words), and easier replacement if dislodged.[4] Although a tracheostomy offers some advantages in terms of patient comfort, the routine performance of early tracheostomies in burn patients does not improve outcomes.[71] The optimal technique and timing of a tracheostomy does not exist; it should be targeted to the individual patient's clinical characteristics.[72] Once the decision to perform a tracheostomy is made, it should be kept in mind that a percutaneous bedside tracheostomy is associated with a lower complication rate than the conventional open tracheostomy.[73]

In a child with a severe burn injury and suspected prolonged intubation, early tracheostomy is recommended, especially if there is facial involvement and inhalation injury. Early tracheostomies have proved to be a safe and effective way to secure the airway and improve ventilator management.[74] The child's trachea is short and has increased risk of endotracheal dislodgement or malposition. The tracheostomy decreases dead-space ventilation, increases laminar flow, and decreases airway resistance. Also, children may not understand why they are intubated and are often unable to stay immobile while intubated. They are unable to communicate and often view the endotracheal tube as punishment. When the burned child has a tracheostomy, it is easier to wean the mechanical ventilation, and the patient will avoid multiple intubations and manipulations of the airway.[74]

Postoperative transport and monitors

Immediately after the surgery the patient will require a period of close ongoing monitoring and treatment in either the postanesthesia care unit (PACU) or the intensive care unit (ICU).[53] The patient should be transported with standard monitors, including pulse oximetry, blood pressure, heart rate, heart rhythm, and respiration. End-tidal CO_2 monitoring is useful if available. The patient should be transferred to the PACU or ICU with the endotracheal tube in place and a full tank of oxygen. It is important to ensure that the patient is receiving good ventilation with hand/bag ventilation prior to leaving the operating room. If there is difficulty with manual ventilation, a transport ventilator may be necessary.

Continued sedation and analgesia

Severe pain is an unavoidable consequence of burn injury.[4] There may be multiple sites of injury involved, the patient may require prolonged care, and there may be complicating psychological and emotional issues and ongoing substance abuse.[53] For these reasons, the burn patient's pain is often difficult to treat. The patient's initial pain is inversely proportional to the depth of the burn.[75] Full-thickness burns are painless because their intrinsic sensory nerves are damaged. Partial-thickness burns, in which the nerves are intact, are extremely painful. The patient's analgesic requirements are often underestimated.[4] The burn patient will require frequent excision, grafting, dressing changes, and physical therapy, all of which will exacerbate the pain. Associated anxiety and depression can also decrease the pain threshold. Pain management in these patients requires an understanding of the type of burn pain (baseline pain, acute pain, or procedure-related pain), frequent assessment of the patient's pain, and ways to address breakthrough pain. It is important to recognize that burn patients tend to develop rapid tolerance to opioids; therefore, individual titration to effect is important.[4] Also, the burn patient tends to develop an increasing number of receptors in response to the ongoing painful stimulus that leads to a "wind up" of the pain over time.[53] An interruption of the upregulation as soon as possible after the injury helps to reduce analgesic requirements over time.

The patient often requires large quantities of opioids to control the pain. Morphine and fentanyl are currently the most widely used drugs for burn pain.[4] Morphine has two pharmacologic advantages for use in burn patients: (1) there is a low amount of protein binding, and (2) the major metabolite is conjugated and removed by glomerular filtration.[75] The respiratory depression caused by the large doses of morphine required for pain control can be reversed with small doses of naloxone.[75] IV fentanyl and oral transmucosal fentanyl citrate are both very effective. Oral transmucosal fentanyl is very effective in children, especially for dressing changes.[76] Postoperatively, benzodiazepines can be useful as an adjunct to the analgesic medication.[4] Meperidine is beneficial in the postoperative period to prevent shivering, which will significantly improve the patient's comfort and reduce the pain associated with excess movement. Meperidine is not recommended for long-term pain control in a burn patient because of the potential for the accumulation of the toxic metabolite normeperidine. IV opioids are recommended early on and in the perioperative period, but if the patient is tolerating enteral feeding, the opioids should be given by this route.[4]

Patient-controlled analgesia (PCA) appears to be an ideal method for opioid administration during acute or procedure-related pain.[4] Overdosing with a PCA is extremely rare, and it is easy to transition from the PCA to oral medications because the patient's daily requirements have been calculated.[53]

Nonopioid analgesia is commonly used for burn patients. Ketamine is ideal for dressing changes because it activates the sympathetic nervous system, increases blood pressure, and causes minimal respiratory depression.[4] Ketamine has the associated risk of prolonged sedation, which can delay the patient's ability to resume oral intake. Studies have shown that ketamine given to burn patients immediately after the diagnosis of sepsis significantly improves survival.[77] This beneficial effect is believed to be due to an interference with the inflammatory cascade. Nitrous oxide can also be used during dressing changes, but it usually requires an operating room because of gas-scavenging requirements and the state of general anesthesia induced when combined with opioids. Patient monitoring must be appropriate for the level of sedation.[4] Dexmedetomidine is an α_2-adrenergic agonist that can be used for sedation, anxiolysis, and analgesia with much less respiratory depression than that which occurs with other sedatives.[78] Dexmedetomidine's sedating and anxiety-reducing effects are useful for prolonged intubation, while the analgesic effects are good for dressing changes. For minor pain, acetaminophen is recommended at doses up to 3–4 g/day.[4,53] Acetaminophen should be avoided in patients with hepatic or renal failure.[53]

Regional anesthesia has several indications in burns, including small burns, burns that are only located below the umbilicus, and burns limited to one extremity (see Chapter 16).[4] An epidural or caudal anesthetic can provide excellent pain relief in a patient with lower-extremity burns. The epidural provides the unique advantage of long-term postoperative analgesia. Epidural anesthesia using local anesthetic agents is relatively contraindicated in patients requiring excessive debridement, owing to the large blood loss in the setting of a sympathectomy. Epidural opioids can be used for this situation. The greatest limitation to regional technique is the extent of the surgical field for debridement and skin graft harvesting. A regional technique should not be performed through burned tissue.

Pain may persist in the burned areas long after they have healed (see Chapter 17). Assessing and managing the persistent pain treatment expectations increases patient satisfaction.[79] Opioids may fail to treat the neuropathic component of the pain.[4] Patients with chronic pain may respond to physical therapy, behavioral therapy, and various drugs, including methadone, antidepressants, anticonvulsants, and IV lidocaine.[4]

Operating room fires

"Approximately 100 operating room fires occur per year in the United States, with 15% resulting in serious injury."[80] A fire requires the presence of three components known as the "fire triad": oxidizer, ignition source, and fuel.[81] In the operating

Table 40.16 Surgical fire risk assessment score

Score	Components
3. High risk	All three components of the "fire triad" are present
2. Low risk with potential to convert to high risk	Thoracic cavity procedure Ignition source is close to a closed oxygen source Ignition source is remote from the oxygen source No supplemental oxygen is used
1. Low risk	Only supplemental oxygen is being used

Information from reference 82.

room the oxidizers are oxygen and nitrous oxide. This oxidizer-enriched environment usually occurs within the closed or semi-closed breathing system. It can be created when the configuration of the drapes and an open oxygen source (mask or nasal cannula) promote trapping or pooling of an oxidizer-enriched atmosphere. The ignition source may be from electrocautery, lasers, heated probes, drills, argon beam coagulators, fiberoptic light cables, and defibrillator pads. Fuel sources include tracheal tubes, drapes, gauze, alcohol-containing solutions, acetone, oxygen masks, patient hair, dressings, ointments, gowns, blankets, and packaging materials.

The Surgical Fire Risk Assessment Score should be used in all operating rooms (Table 40.16).[82] The assessment should be performed by the entire surgical team before the first incision is made. The assessment requires the team to identify the three key elements that are necessary to start a fire: heat, fuel, and oxygen. The team must also identify the three key risks for operating room fires: surgical site above the xiphoid, open oxygen source, and available ignition source.

High-risk procedures are defined as any procedure where the ignition source can come in the proximity of an oxidizer-rich atmosphere.[81] Examples of high-risk procedures include tracheostomy, removal of laryngeal papillomas, cataract or other eye surgery, burr hole, and removal of lesions on the head or neck.

Fire treatment procedures are outlined in Table 40.17. Fire prevention recommendations defined by the American Society of Anesthesiologists (ASA) include the avoidance of ignition sources in the proximity to an oxidizer-enriched atmosphere, configuration of surgical drapes to minimize the accumulation of oxidizers, allowing sufficient drying time for flammable skin-prepping solutions, and moistening sponges and gauze when used in the proximity of an ignition source.[81]

Conclusions

Burn care management has improved significantly over the years, manifested by significant improvements in morbidity and mortality. The final goal in the treatment of a burn patient

Table 40.17 Fire treatment

Airway (immediately, without waiting)

Remove endotracheal tube
Stop the flow of all airway gases
Remove sponges and any other flammable materials
Pour saline into the airway
Re-establish ventilation once fire is out
Examine the tracheal tube to see if any fragments were left behind in the airway
Consider bronchoscopy

Non-airway (immediately, without waiting)

Stop the flow of all airway gases
Remove the drapes and all burning flammable materials
Extinguish burning materials by pouring saline or by other means

If the fire cannot be extinguished

Use a carbon dioxide (CO_2) fire extinguisher
Activate fire alarm
Evacuate the patient
Close the operating room door
Turn off gas supply to the operating room

Information from reference 81.

is to help the person reenter society with maximum function consistent with the injuries sustained.[53] Survivors of massive burns report a good quality of life.[83] The size of the injury, the patient's age, hand function, and the patient's perceived level of social support are all factors that contribute to the patient's perception of his or her quality of life. This information is useful in helping providers to make future decisions about resuscitation, reconstruction, and rehabilitation.

Questions

(1) Which of the following is a limitation of an arterial blood gas (ABG) in assessing the burned patient?
    a. Inaccurate with respect to alveolar oxygen saturation
    b. Inaccurate with respect to carbon monoxide level
    c. Cannot be used in determining possible smoke inhalation injury
    d. Cannot be read within the first 24 hours after a burn

(2) Which of the following is an indication for urgent tracheal intubation in a burn patient with upper airway injury?
    a. Impending signs of airway obstruction
    b. Cardiovascular instability
    c. Central nervous system depression
    d. Massive burn greater than 60% of total body surface area (TBSA)
    e. All of the above

(3) What carbon monoxide level presents with hallucinations, combativeness, and cardiovascular instability?
    a. < 15%

b. 15–20%
c. 20–40%
d. 40–60%
e. > 60%

(4) During the hypermetabolic response that occurs after a burn injury, the patient develops significantly elevated levels of:
    a. Catecholamines
    b. Glucagon
    c. Glucocorticoids
    d. ADH, renin, and angiotensin
    e. All of the above

(5) Which of the following is correct in reference to a typical methamphetamine lab burn patient?
    a. Decreased incidence of inhalational injury
    b. Decreased incidence of nosocomial respiratory failure and sepsis
    c. Often has 1.8 times greater resuscitation requirements
    d. Smaller burn size
    e. Decreased morbidity when compared with other burn patients

(6) The mortality of the burn patient is greatly influenced by:
    a. Type of burn
    b. Extent of the burn (> 40% TBSA)
    c. Patient's age (> 60 years)
    d. Presence of inhalational injury
    e. All of the above

(7) Which of the following choices is true with respect to topical burn wound care?
    a. First-degree wounds require excision and grafting
    b. Second-degree wounds can be treated with daily dressing changes and topical antibiotics
    c. Third-degree wounds are minor and therefore require no dressings and are treated with topical salves
    d. All burn wounds should be left open to the air to minimize bacterial and fungal colonization
    e. An occlusive dressing should never be used, since it tends to hold the heat of the burn in

(8) Which of the following statements is true of depolarizing and nondepolarizing muscle relaxants in burn patients?
    a. Depolarizing muscle relaxants can be used safely for up to 72 hours after the initial burn injury
    b. The hyperkalemic response to succinylcholine given after a burn injury only lasts for about 2 months
    c. Patients with a burn injury are often resistant to the action of nondepolarizing muscle relaxants
    d. The resistance to nondepolarizing muscle relaxants can last for up to 18 years after the burn injury

(9) Which technique can be used during surgical excision and debridement to limit blood loss during surgery?
    a. Tourniquets
    b. Multiple surgical teams working simultaneously

c. Epinephrine- and thrombin-soaked gauze
d. Compressive dressings
e. All of the above

(10) **Which of the following is true with respect to pain in the burn patient?**
a. Analgesic requirements are often overestimated
b. A patient's initial pain is inversely proportional to the depth of the burn
c. Morphine is a poor choice for burn pain
d. Regional anesthesia should never be considered in a burn patient
e. Burn patients using PCA are at significant risk of overdosing

Answers

(1) a
(2) e
(3) d
(4) e
(5) c
(6) e
(7) b
(8) c
(9) e
(10) b

References

1. Blanding R, Stiff J. Perioperative anesthetic management of patients with burns. *Anesthesiol Clin N Am* 1999; **17**: 237–49.

2. Purdue GF, Hunt JL, Burris AM. Pediatric surgical emergencies. *Clin Pediatr Emerg Med* 2002; **3**: 76–82.

3. American Burn Association. *National Burn Repository: 2013 Report*. Chicago, IL: ABA. http://www.ameriburn.org/2013NBRAnnualReport.pdf (accessed September 2014).

4. MacLennan N, Heimbach DM, Cullen BF. Anesthesia for major thermal injury. *Anesthesiology* 1998; **89**: 749–70.

5. Ramzy PI, Barret JP, Herndon DN. Environmental emergencies: thermal injury. *Crit Care Clin* 1999; **15**: 333–52.

6. Peitzman AB, Shires GT, Teixidor HS, *et al.* Smoke inhalation injury: evaluation of radiographic manifestations and pulmonary dysfunction. *J Trauma* 1989; **29**: 1232–8.

7. Masanes MJ, Legendre C, Lioret N, *et al.* Fiberoptic bronchoscopy for the early diagnosis of subglottal inhalation injury: comparative value in the assessment of prognosis. *J Trauma* 1994; **36**: 59–67.

8. Mosier MJ, Pham TN, Park DR, *et al.* Predictive value of bronchoscopy in assessing the severity of inhalation injury. *J Burn Care Res* 2012; **33**: 65–73.

9. Muehlberger T, Kunar D, Munster A, *et al.* Efficacy of fiberoptic laryngoscopy in the diagnosis of inhalation injuries. *Arch Otolaryngol Head Neck Surg* 1998; **124**: 1003–7.

10. Haponik EF, Meyers DA, Munster AM, *et al.* Acute upper airway injury in burn patients. Serial changes of flow-volume curves and nasopharyngoscopy. *Am Rev Respir Dis* 1987; **135**: 360–6.

11. Wilson WC, Benumof JL. Respiration in anesthesia pathophysiology and clinical update. *Anesthesiol Clin N Am* 1998; **16**: 29–75.

12. Barash PG, Cullen BF, Stoelting RK. *Clinical Anesthesia*, 4th edition. Philadelphia, PA: Lippincott, Williams & Wilkins, 2001.

13. Haney M, Tait AR, Tremper KK. Effects of carboxyhemoglobin on the accuracy of mixed venous oximetry monitors in dogs. *Crit Care Med* 1994; **22**: 1181–5.

14. Buckley NA, Juurlink DN, Isbister G, Bennett MH, Lavonas EJ. Hyperbaric oxygen for carbon monoxide poisoning. *Cochrane Database Syst Rev* 2011; (3): CD002041.

15. Hamel J. A review of acute cyanide poisoning with a treatment update. *Crit Care Nurs* 2011; **31**: 72–81.

16. Palmieri TL, Enkhbaatar P, Bayliss R, *et al.* Continuous nebulized albuterol attenuates acute lung injury in an ovine model of combined burn and smoke inhalation. *Crit Care Med* 2006; **34**: 1841–2.

17. de La Cal MA, Cerda E, Garcia-Hierro P, *et al.* Pneumonia in patients with severe burns: a classification according to the concepts of the carrier state. *Chest* 2001; **119**: 1160–5.

18. Williams FN, Herndon DN, Suman OE, *et al.* Changes in cardiac physiology after severe burn injury. *J Burn Care Res* 2011; **32**: 269–74.

19. White J, Thomas J, Maass DL, *et al.* Cardiac effects of burn injury complicated by aspiration pneumonia-induced sepsis. *Am J Physiol* 2003; **285**: H47–58.

20. Palmieri TL, Caruso DM, Foster KN, *et al.* Effect of blood transfusion on outcome after major burn injury: a multicenter study. *Crit Care Med* 2006; **34**: 1602–7.

21. Townsend CM, Beauchamp RD, Evers BM, *et al.* Chapter 22: Burns. In Wolf SE, Herndon DN, eds., *Sabiston Textbook of Surgery*, 17th edition. Philadelphia, PA: Saunders, 2004.

22. Lalonde C, Knox J, Youn YK, *et al.* Relationship between hepatic blood flow and tissue lipid peroxidation in the early postburn period. *Crit Care Med* 1992; **20**: 789–96.

23. Epstein MD, Banducci DR, Manders EK. The role of the gastrointestinal tract in the development of burn sepsis. *Plast Reconst Surg* 1992; **90**: 524–31.

24. Saffle JR. What's new in general surgery: burns and metabolism. *J Am Coll Surg* 2003; **196**: 267–89.

25. Holm C, Horbrand F, Mayr M, *et al.* Assessment of splanchnic perfusion by gastric tonometry in patients with acute hypovolemic burn shock. *Burns* 2006; **32**: 689–94.

26. Magnotti LJ, Deitch EA. Burns, bacterial translocation, gut barrier function, and failure. *J Burn Care Rehabil* 2005; **26**: 383–91.

27. Demling RH, Seigne P. Metabolic management in patients with severe burns. *World J Surg* 2000; **24**: 673–80.

28. Pereira CT, Murphy KD, Herndon DN. Altering metabolism. *J Burn Care Rehabil* 2005; **26**: 194–9.

29. Goh KP. Management of hyponatremia. *Am Fam Physician* 2004; **69**: 2387–94.

30. Cawrse N, Wilson S, Williams M, *et al.* Neuroleptic malignant syndrome in the burns patient? *Burns* 2006; **32**: 647–9.

31. Koumbourlis AC. Electrical injuries. *Crit Care Med* 2002; **30**: S424–30.

32. Barillo DJ, Cancio LC, Goodwin CW. Treatment of white phosphorus and other chemical burn injuries at one burn center over a fifty-one year period. *Burns* 2004; **30**: 448–52.

33. Santos AP, Wilson AK, Hornung CA, *et al.* Methamphetamine laboratory explosions: a new and emerging burn injury. *J Burn Care Rehabil* 2005; **26**: 228–32.

34. Spann MD, McGwin G, Kerby JD, *et al.* Characteristic of burn patients injured in methamphetamine laboratory explosions. *J Burn Care Res* 2006; **27**: 496–501.

35. Klein MB, Gibran NS, Emerson D, *et al.* Patterns of grease burn injury: development of a classification system. *Burns* 2005; **31**: 765–7.

36. O'Keefe GE, Hunt JL, Purdue GF. An evaluation of risk factors for mortality after burn trauma and the identification of gender-dependent differences and outcomes. *J Am College Surg* 2001; **192**: 153–60.

37. Sheridan RL, Weber JM, Schnitzer JJ, *et al.* Young age is not a predictor of mortality in burns. *Pediatric Crit Care Med* 2001; **2**: 223–4.

38. Aldemir M, Kara IH, Girgin S, *et al.* Factors affecting mortality and epidemiological data in patients hospitalised with burns in Diyarbakir, Turkey. *S Afr J Surg* 2005; **43**: 159–62.

39. Kerby JD, McGwin G, George RL, *et al.* Sex differences in mortality after burn injury: results of analysis of the national burn repository of the American Burn Association. *J Burn Care Res* 2006; **27**: 452–6.

40. Wolf SE, Rose JK, Desai MH, *et al.* Mortality determinants in massive pediatric burns. An analysis of 103 children with > = 80% TBSA burns (> = 70% full-thickness). *Ann Surg* 1997; **225**: 554–69.

41. Maghsoudi H, Samnia R, Garadaghi A, *et al.* Burns in pregnancy. *Burns* 2006; **32**: 246–50.

42. Memmel H, Kowal-Vern A, Latenser BA. Infections in diabetic burn patients. *Diabetes Care* 2004; **27**: 229–33.

43. Yanagawa Y, Saitoh D, Sakamoto T, *et al.* Unfavorable outcome of burn patients with neuropsychiatric disorders. *Tohoku J Exp Med* 2005; **205**: 241–5.

44. Hawkins A, MacLennan PA, McGwin G, *et al.* The impact of combined trauma and burns on patient mortality. *J Trauma* 2005; **58**: 284–8.

45. Housinger TA, Warden GD, Shouse J. Ordering of laboratory work in the management of pediatric burn patients: technical note. *J Trauma* 1993; **34**: 139–41.

46. Abboud PC, Kendall JL. Ultrasound guidance for vascular access. *Emerg Med Clin N Am* 2004; **22**: 749–73.

47. Evans RJ, Jewkes F, Owen G, *et al.* Intraosseous infusion: a technique available for intravascular administration of drugs and fluids in the child with burns. *Burns* 1995; **21**: 552–3.

48. Schaden E, Kimberger O, Kraincuk P, *et al.* Perioperative treatment algorithm for bleeding burn patients reduces allogenic blood product requirements. *Br J Anaesth* 2012; **109**: 376–81.

49. Ong YS, Samuel M, Song C. Meta-analysis of early excision of burns. *Burns* 2006; **32**: 145–50.

50. Xiao-Wu W, Herndon DN, Spies M, *et al.* Effects of delayed wound excision and grafting in severely burned children. *Arch Surg* 2002; **137**: 1049–54.

51. Holm C, Mayr M, Tegeler J, *et al.* A clinical randomized study on the effects of invasive monitoring on burn shock resuscitation. *Burns* 2004; **30**: 798–807.

52. Pal SK, Kyriachou PA, Kumaran S, *et al.* Evaluation of oesophageal reflectance pulse oximetry in major burn patients. *Burns* 2005; **31**: 337–41.

53. Miller RD. *Anesthesia*, 6th edition. New York, NY: Churchill Livingstone, 2005.

54. Kuntscher MV, Blome-Eberwein S, Pelzer M, *et al.* Transcardiopulmonary vs. pulmonary arterial thermodilution methods for hemodynamic monitoring of burned patients. *J Burn Care Rehabil* 2002; **23**: 21–6.

55. Holm C, Melcer B, Horbrand F, *et al.* Arterial thermodilution: an alternative to pulmonary artery catheter for cardiac output assessment in burn patients. *Burns* 2000; **27**: 161–6.

56. Newton T, Still JM, Law E. A comparison of the effect of early insertion of standard latex and silver-impregnated latex foley catheters on urinary tract infections in burn patients. *Infect Control Hosp Epidemiol* 2002; **23**: 217–18.

57. Gore DC, Beaston J. Infusion of hot crystalloid during operative burn wound debridement. *J Trauma* 1997; **42**: 1112–15.

58. Sheridan RL, Szyfelbein SK. Trends in blood conservation in burn care. *Burns* 2001; **27**: 272–6.

59. Witkowski W, Maj J. [Pathophysiology and management of perioperative hypothermia.] *Pol Merkuriusc Lek* 2006; **20** (120): 629–34.

60. Cartotto R, Ellis S, Smith T. Use of high-frequency oscillatory ventilation in burn patients. *Crit Care Med* 2005; **33**: 175–81.

61. Wolter TP, Fuchs PC, Horvat N, *et al.* Is high PEEP low volume ventilation in burn patients beneficial? A retrospective study in 61 patients. *Burns* 2004; **30**: 368–73.

62. Walia G, Jada G, Cartotto R. Anesthesia and intraoperative high-frequency oscillatory ventilation during burn surgery. *J Burn Care Res* 2011; **32**: 118–23.

63. Bonate PL. Pathophysiology and pharmacokinetics following burn injury. *Clin Pharmacokinet* 1990; **18**: 118–30.

64. Hart DW, Wolf SE, Beauford RB, *et al.* Determinants of blood loss during primary burn excision. *Surgery* 2001; **130**: 396–402.

65. O'Mara MS, Hayetian F, Slater H, *et al.* Results of a protocol of transfusion threshold and surgical technique on transfusion requirements in burn patients. *Burns* 2005; **31**: 558–61.

66. Gomez M, Logsetty S, Fish JS, *et al.* Reduced blood loss during burn surgery. *J Burn Care Rehabil* 2001; **22**: 111–17.

67. Niemi T, Svartling N, Syrjala M, *et al.* Haemostatic disturbances in burned patients during early excision and skin grafting. *Blood Coagul Fibrinolysis* 1998; **9**: 19–28.

68. Cartotto R, Choi J, Gomez M, *et al.* A prospective study on the implications of a base deficit during fluid

resuscitation. *J Burn Care Rehabil* 2003; **24**: 75–84.

69. Kamolz LP, Andel H, Schramm W, *et al.* Lactate: Early predictor of morbidity and mortality in patients with severe burns. *Burns* 2005; **31**: 986–90.

70. Loudermilk EP, Hartmannsgruber M, Stoltzfus DP, *et al.* A perspective study of the safety of tracheal extubation using a pediatric airway exchange catheter for patients with a known difficult airway. *Chest* 1997; **111**: 1660–5.

71. Saffle JR, Morris SE, Edelman L. Early tracheostomy does not improve outcome in burn patients. *J Burn Care Rehabil* 2002; **23**: 431–8.

72. Pelosi P, Svergnini P. Tracheostomy must be individualized. *Crit Care* 2004; **8**: 322–4.

73. Gravvanis AI, Tsoussos DA, Iconomou TG, *et al.* Percutaneous versus conventional tracheostomy in burned patients with inhalational injury. *World J Surg* 2005; **29**: 1571–5.

74. Palmieri TL, Jackson W, Greenhalgh DG. Benefits of early tracheostomy in severely burned children. *Crit Care Med* 2002; **30**: 922–4.

75. Marx J, Hockberger R, Walls R. *Rosen's Emergency Medicine: Concepts and Clinical Practices*, 6th edition. St Louis, MO: Mosby, 2006.

76. Sharar SR, Bratton SL, Carrougher GJ, *et al.* A comparison of oral transmucosal fentanyl citrate and oral hydromorphone for inpatient pediatric burn wound care analgesia. *J Burn Care Rehabil* 1998; **19**: 516–21.

77. Gurfinkel R, Czeiger D, Douvdevani A, *et al.* Ketamine improves survival in burn injury followed by sepsis in rats. *Anesth Analg* 2006; **103**: 396–402.

78. Walker J, Maccallum M, Fischer C, *et al.* Sedation using dexmedetomidine in pediatric burn patients. *J Burn Care Res* 2006; **27**: 206–10.

79. Browne AL, Andrews R, Schug SA, Wood F. Persistent pain outcomes and patient satisfaction with pain management after burn injury. *Clin J Pain* 2011; **27**: 136–45.

80. Haith LR, Santavasi W, *et al.* Burn center management of operating room fires injuries. *J Burn Care Res* 2012; **33**: 649–53.

81. Apfelbaum JL, Caplan RA, Barker SJ, *et al.* Practice advisory for the prevention and management of operating room fires: an updated report by the American Society of Anesthesiologists Task Force on Operating Room Fires. *Anesthesiology* 2013; **118**: 271–90.

82. Scoring Fire Risk for Surgical Patients. www.surgicalfireorg.fatcow/wp-content/uploads/2012/10/scoring_fire_risks_2.pdf (accessed March 2013).

83. Anzarut A, Chen M, Shankowsky H, *et al.* Quality-of-life and outcome predictors following massive burn injury. *Plast Reconstr Surg* 2005; **116**: 791–7.

Prevention of injuries

James S. Davis and Carl I. Schulman

Objectives

(1) Understand the origins and evolution of the science of injury prevention.

(2) Discuss the challenges and limitations of developing a comprehensive injury prevention program.

(3) Describe two ongoing examples of contemporary injury prevention programs.

Introduction

Traumatic injury ranks among the deadliest and costliest burdens in medicine today. Among patients ages 1–44, it is the most common cause of death, and ranks as the third leading cause of death for all ages. In the United States, injuries account for 30% of total years of life lost due to disease, as well as 42 million emergency department visits and 2 million hospital admissions (see Chapter 1). The estimated total costs for trauma-related injuries is $406 billion annually.[1]

Despite these staggering statistics, trauma has been historically underappreciated. Until as recently as half a century ago, injuries were considered to be "accidents" – unfortunate, capricious events attributable either to God or to human malice. Accordingly, these accidents were felt to be preventable only through prayer and improving human morals.[2] The role of rigorous scientific analysis and systematic intervention was generally ignored.

Today, trauma prevention is vital to any mature trauma and public health system. Anywhere between one-third and one-half of all trauma deaths occur in the field and are considered nonsurvivable. For the deaths occurring en route or in hospital, 98% are also considered nonsurvivable injuries. While it is unlikely that current medical intervention can improve these dire statistics, trauma prevention most certainly can, while lessening the absolute injury number and the burden for those who survive.[3]

This chapter provides an overview of current concepts in trauma prevention. Trauma prevention addresses a vast array of injury mechanisms, and generally involves an overwhelming complement of dry statistics ranging from suicide prevention to side-impact airbags to swimming pool fences. Rather than

dwell on the many details surrounding specific trauma prevention initiatives, this chapter undertakes a more theoretical approach. It will trace the historical arch of trauma prevention from afterthought to its current position of prominence, introducing a theoretical framework for understanding injuries and forming prevention strategies. Then, two injury-prevention programs are analyzed as historical examples of successful and unsuccessful injury prevention applications. Lastly, two contemporary trauma prevention topics, distracted driving and sports-related concussions, will be discussed in detail to provide examples of the depth and importance of specific modes of intervention.

The emergence of injury prevention as a science

Although a scientific approach to trauma prevention is relatively recent, isolated interventions enjoy rich individual histories. In the Bible, Moses instructed the Israelite home builders to install fences on the roof in order to prevent falls from height.[4] A more modern-day example includes John P. Knight's fateful installation of the first traffic light outside the British parliament in 1868, which exploded one year later, killing its operator.[5] Although the merits of traffic control and safety rails are well known today, these early attempts were, at best, isolated, lacking any systematic, deliberate, academic approach.

The first individual credited with approaching trauma prevention from a scientific perspective is Hugh DeHaven.[6] A pilot and engineer, DeHaven survived his own airplane crash in 1919 and spent the next six decades examining whether crash injuries were indeed inevitable. His case-based analysis of falls from height remains among the earliest examples of injury science.[7,8]

Another important figure in the development of injury prevention was the Harvard epidemiologist John Gordon. Gordon asserted that "the biologic principles that govern disease as a community problem are interpreted as holding equally well for injuries."[9] Applying the disease model, he demonstrated how every trauma involved a host, an

Trauma Anesthesia, 2nd Edition, ed. Charles E. Smith. Published by Cambridge University Press. © Charles E. Smith, 2015.

agent, and an environment. Identifying these factors constituted the first step in undertaking systematic trauma prevention.

James Gibson, a behavioral psychologist by trade, took Gordon's concepts further. Gibson expanded the notion that injuries result from an interaction between agent and host, identifying that an energy transfer, in some form, was necessary to cause an injury. Specifically, transfer occurred through one of five modalities: gravitational, mechanical, radiant, thermal, or chemical.[10] Gibson's clear conceptualization enabled subsequent researchers to focus on mode identification, research, and prevention.

These pioneers paved the way for the rapid expansion and institutionalization of scientific injury prevention in the United States. The man chiefly responsible for this change was William Haddon Jr., a public health physician. Haddon recognized that human interactions with environmental hazards can be divided into three distinct phases. In the "pre-event phase," the energy required to cause an injury is generated and becomes unfettered. Next, the energy interaction and transfer occur during the "event phase." Then, in the "post-event phase," a discrete period of time passes when energy forces may be lessened, and damage mitigated. Haddon combined his three-phase overview with the classic three-part public health characterization of risk factors to create a three-by-three matrix.[11] The matrix is extremely versatile, and may be applied to any circumstance of injury. In Table 41.1, Haddon's matrix is applied to a motor vehicle collision (MVC) scenario.

Each individual cell within the matrix suggests opportunities for systematic analysis, targeting, and prevention.

Table 41.1 Haddon's matrix as applied to a motor vehicle collision (MVC) scenario

	Host (driver)	Agent (motor vehicle)	Environment (physical, social)
Pre-event	Driver experience Driver sobriety Seat belt and speed limit compliance	Well-maintained vehicle Functional equipment	Safe road design (sightlines, signals) Speed limits Traffic calming measures
Event	Age, physical fitness to withstand injury	Airbag deployment Vehicle crumple zones	Safe road design (guard rails, breakaway poles, graduated breakdown lanes)
Post-event	Knowledge to respond to injury Physiologic reserve	Protected gasoline tank Automated crash notification	Emergency medical systems Trauma networks

Haddon himself recognized his matrix's utility, and went on to suggest 10 strategies to mitigate the risk factors described within his matrix:[12]

(1) Prevent the initial generation of damaging energy.
(2) Reduce the amount of energy generated.
(3) Prevent the release of the energy.
(4) Modify the rate or spatial distribution of energy release from its source.
(5) Separate, through time or space, the energy released from the susceptible object.
(6) Place physical barriers between the energy released and the object.
(7) Modify the contact surface and basic structure of both energy and object to minimize damage when contact is made.
(8) Strengthen the structure that will receive the energy prior to the event.
(9) Rapidly detect and evaluate the damage and take steps to mitigate/counter its extension.
(10) Stabilize and repair the injured victim to return to long-term viability.

Haddon went on to a decorated career as a public health official. In 1965, Ralph Nader published *Unsafe at Any Speed*,[13] fomenting the necessary political will to create the National Highway Safety Bureau – Haddon served as its first director. Soon thereafter, Congress passed the Occupational Safety and Health Act, and the Consumer Product Safety Act. Federal funding increased for various state injury prevention programs. When the Institute of Medicine published its 1985 report, *Injury in America: a Continuing Public Health Problem*,[14] the science of injury prevention in the USA had come of age.

Injury prevention: application of a science

Haddon's matrix provided a blueprint for subsequent trauma prevention efforts. Further application and practice has demonstrated the multidisciplinary range of professionals needed to design, implement, and monitor an effective trauma prevention campaign.[15] First, certain definitions are helpful when considering current concepts in injury prevention. Active prevention refers to strategies that require human initiation and activity for implementation. Passive prevention requires no such human initiative. In the context of child poisoning, an initiative to place warning labels on the medication bottles is an active strategy – parents must read the labels, and subsequently modify their behavior to prevent children's ingestion.[16] In contrast, legally enforcing child safety caps on all medication bottles is a passive prevention measure.[17] Generally, passive strategies are considered more effective than active ones.

Prevention efforts fall into one of three categories known as the 3 E's: education, engineering, and enforcement. *Education* involves persuading individuals or target populations to alter their behavior in a given way. In New York City's highly successful "Children Can't Fly" campaign, community organizations and media outlets coordinated a massive effort to disseminate statistics and prevention strategies surrounding children falling out of high-rise windows. *Engineering* marshals technology to create automatic protection from injury – for example, installing window guards in high fall-risk areas. Finally, *enforcement* provides for change through legal or administrative measures. Buttressed by significant epidemiological data, New York City amended its health code to require window guards.[18] While not always possible to apply each of the 3 E's to every injury prevention program, each should be implemented to the extent that it is feasible to optimize outcomes.

Initiating a trauma prevention program requires extensive planning that begins with identifying and characterizing a specific problem. National inventories of mortality and injury data, such as the National Vital Statistics System, the National Electronic Injury Surveillance System, and the Health Cost and Utilization Project, provide enormous amounts of retrospective data.[19] The age of electronic records has allowed epidemiologists to compile and link databases, revealing patterns that would otherwise remain elusive. In addition, qualitative surveys of public awareness, behavior patterns, and readiness to change can further shape the size and scope of trauma prevention undertakings. Finally, statistical analysis supplements data collection to determine feasible target demographics. For example, examining injury rates stratified into different age groups may yield little useful information, but those same data divided into socioeconomic groups may yield opportunities for targeted interventions.[20]

Injury prevention efforts must also consider the manner in which specific populations may be targeted. Community-based programs are acknowledged as an acceptable strategy for affecting behavior.[21] Programs using multiple strategies directed towards multiple targets have the greatest chance of achieving long-term success.[22] The Seattle Bicycle Campaign, a program designed to increase bicycle helmet usage among elementary school-aged children, targeted children, parents, and primary care doctors. Prevention communication strategies included television and radio-based public service announcements, community-wide events, and subsidized helmet giveaways.[23] The campaign's success in targeting multiple audiences through a variety of measures provides a blueprint for new trauma prevention programs.

Even when an intervention successfully engages multiple targets, affecting behavioral and cultural change remains a challenge. Coalition and network formation, uniting multiple organizations in support of a common cause, may benefit any trauma prevention campaign through resource conservation, information sharing, expanded outreach, and increased credibility.[24] Some well-recognized examples in the injury prevention field include the Injury Free Coalition for Kids, the National Coalition Against Domestic Violence Injuries, and the Coalition to Stop Gun Violence. Overall, coalitions may provide the critical mass necessary to move a project forward.

Some of the most pervasive and wide-ranging effects result from legislative and public policy enforcement. State seatbelt laws have saved an estimated 255,000 lives since 1975, while mandatory motorcycle helmet laws save 1500 riders annually and $3 billion in associated healthcare costs.[25,26] When direct legislation is untenable, altering local health codes or enforcing already existing legislation may help. Attracting elected officials' attention is often very difficult, but ultimately feasible when supported by sound data, promising cost analyses, and influential coalition partners. Even changing nongovernmental practices of large organizations can have a far-reaching effect. Police institution of field sobriety checkpoints has been credited with saving 15,667 lives between 1975 and 1995.[27] As such, a mixture of governmental and nongovernmental enforcement may dramatically affect the burden of injury.

After planning and implementing a trauma prevention campaign, ongoing evaluation is necessary. Evaluation assumes one of two forms. *Process measures* assess whether the steps of the intervention actually occurred (e.g., were local pools outfitted with child-protective fencing?). *Outcome measures* assess whether the intervention was effective (e.g., did the pool-fencing ordinance reduce drownings?). Sometimes, outcomes may be measured directly. More often, the primary outcome cannot be measured in a meaningful way and surrogate outcomes must be used instead. Dr. Frederick P. Rivara's hierarchical pyramid of outcome measures demonstrates the relative ease and utility of the various outcome measures available (Fig. 41.1).[28] These ongoing evaluations assess a program's efficacy and help justify continued funding and program application.

Overseeing and implementing a trauma prevention program is a major undertaking. Unfortunately, idealism, foresight, and planning alone will not yield success without sufficient funding. Funding is also necessary to cover startup costs, ongoing interventions, and achieving sustainability. Despite the difficulties of fundraising, particularly in a challenging economic climate, trauma prevention has been gaining credibility in recent years, and there are grants available for sound, specific proposals. Private funding from dedicated philanthropic foundations, or smaller donations-in-kind, are also potential funding sources. Local individuals, businesses, and coalition partners can provide some degree of financial support. Meanwhile, the Foundation Center possesses the most comprehensive database of grants and grantmakers in the United States, as well as a rapidly expanding repository for international organizations.[29]

Limitations to developing trauma prevention programs

Designing a trauma prevention program involves the integration of multiple stages. Even with careful design and the best intentions at heart, certain external factors may severely limit any program's effectiveness.

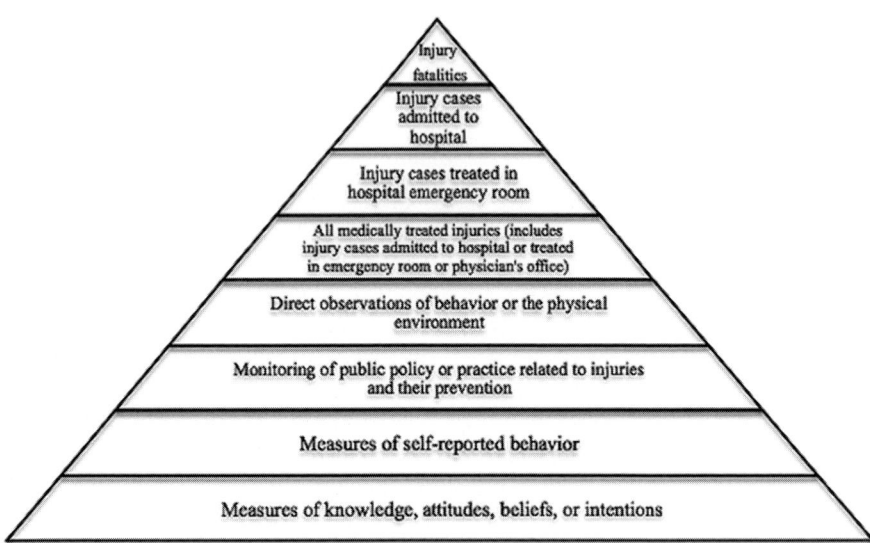

Figure 41.1 Frederick P. Rivara's hierarchy of injury outcome measures.

In the current age of healthcare cost consciousness, trauma prevention proposals invariably require cost-effectiveness. This often includes a calculation of increased productivity, reduced healthcare costs, and even cost of potential lives saved or lost. Placing a dollar value on a human life is complex and problematic, and the pressure to do so can lead to making some very difficult choices when evaluating trauma prevention programs.

Another challenge relates to the competing values of public health and personal autonomy. Trauma prevention initiatives frequently utilize law or rule to alter harmful human behavior. Critics have labeled these efforts "paternalistic," because they are thought to encroach upon an individual's autonomy. This issue is particularly sensitive in the United States, where the individualist tradition dates back to the colonial era and continues to thrive today.

The public traditionally makes much greater allowances for restricting autonomy among specific target populations. Children, the elderly, and the mentally infirm lack the capacity to make rational choices, and society generally accepts public health measures restricting their freedoms. Among these target populations, restrictive public health measures comprise a so-called "weak" paternalism. In contrast, similar efforts aimed at fully capable adults are more likely to be resisted as "strong" paternalism.

Generally, the US courts have defended prevention efforts for activities that negatively affect society as a whole. For example, drunk-driving victims include sober drivers, passengers, and pedestrians – US laws are designed to prevent such collateral damage. A similar approach applies to nonfatal activities, where costs to society include lost worker productivity, partially subsidized hospitalizations, and a drain on communal resources. However, determining what constitutes a legitimate shared societal cost is subjective and contentious. The more tenuous the connection between individual actor and societal harm, the more resistant the anti-paternalists become.

Ethical concerns aside, trauma prevention advocates must account for political aspects that are likely to enter any public health measure. The debate over the Second Amendment to the US Constitution (the part of the United States Bill of Rights that protects the right to bear arms) provides a case in point. For decades, strong evidence exists that increased firearm proliferation, firearm ownership, and firearm storage within the home all correlate with a rise in gun violence.[30] From a trauma prevention perspective, it is clear that gun control should be part of any gun violence prevention program. However, all discussion about firearm prevention is inextricably tied to debates over the Second Amendment. The National Rifle Association has stridently opposed all efforts to limit firearm proliferation, even by convicted criminals, and provides sizable financial support to political figures on all levels of government. Ostensibly, firearm prevention has moved from the realm of trauma prevention to that of constitutional law and politics.

Injury prevention in action

Numerous examples of trauma prevention exist in the public health literature. Every mechanism of injury that exists is potentially reportable, quantifiable, analyzable, and possibly preventable. Instead of a dry list of trauma prevention methods, below are two case studies that illustrate the methods, interventions, and evaluations available when participating in a trauma prevention initiative. The first case, Project WalkSafe, is largely regarded as an example of a successful intervention. The second case, Project Burn Prevention, provides an example an endeavor that failed to accomplish its stated goals.

Project WalkSafe

Pedestrian injuries are an important, yet occasionally overlooked, aspect of traffic safety. In 2000 alone, approximately 25,000 children ages 0–15 were struck by motor vehicles in the US. Researchers at the University of Miami further noted that Florida had the third-highest pedestrian mortality rate in the country. Within the state, Miami-Dade County ranked worst. Analyzing the trauma data further, researchers noted that a significant proportion of pedestrian mortalities were late-afternoon collisions involving children walking in areas nearby schools. These findings provided the impetus for Project WalkSafe.[31,32]

Project WalkSafe is a pedestrian safety program that targets middle school children through multilayered interventions. First, local teachers helped write a school-based curriculum that the Miami-Dade School Board subsequently approved. Teachers implemented the curriculum in a target school district as daily 30-minute lessons over a 5-day period. The curriculum included classroom-based instruction, street-crossing simulation, and a poster competition. In addition, researchers interviewed concerned parties to learn about the most pressing engineering and traffic enforcement problems near target schools. Researchers generated and submitted a list of engineering modifications to the Dade County Public Works Department for consideration. Similarly, traffic enforcement suggestions were provided to the relevant police departments.

Observation and analysis were conducted on multiple axes. Within the district, some schools were selected for the Walk-Safe interventions while others were designated controls. Students received pre- and post-tests for knowledge assessment, video cameras were posted at local intersections to record actual street-crossing behaviors, and the requested engineering modifications were tracked for their departmental approval and implementation. The initial study results demonstrated knowledge increases among all age groups that were retained over a 3-month time period. The Public Works Department approved a majority of the proposed engineering modifications, as well. Unfortunately, information regarding traffic citations and videotaped behaviors, where available, did not conclusively effect driver or pedestrian behavioral change.

Encouraged by the initial promising findings, Project WalkSafe's organizers continued their efforts in Miami-Dade County schools. Over time, several modifications were made. A letter and consent form were sent home with students to engage parents in the initiative, an official kick-off event was added, and the curriculum was streamlined and moved to earlier in the school year. Through the local public television station, researchers made the educational content freely available in order to facilitate program sustainability and implementation.[33]

Despite these positive steps, Project WalkSafe has not been a complete success. When the WalkSafe curriculum was applied in New Jersey, the educational gains present at 3 months among school children did not persist over the longer term. More generally, the project's primary objectives were to lower school-age pedestrian injury and fatality rates. It remains debatable whether the outcome measured (test knowledge) will translate into altered pedestrian behavior, much less lowered fatality rates. Ultimately, Project WalkSafe demonstrates both a positive example and extant challenges in designing a community-based trauma prevention initiative.

Project Burn Prevention

Project Burn Prevention was initiated in 1975 through the US Product Safety Commission, with the stated goal of reducing burn incidence and severity through public educational campaigns. There were two major reasons for the project. First, burn injuries were acknowledged as a small but significant source of morbidity and mortality in the US. Secondly, the project attempted to gauge the efficacy of burn prevention-directed educational campaigns.[34,35]

Three types of interventions targeted discrete metropolitan areas: a media-based campaign, a school-based educational intervention in addition to the media-based campaign, and a community-based intervention in addition to the media-based campaign. Media-based campaigns included television commercials, discussion on television and radio shows, and poster displays on public transportation. The school-based intervention enlisted the support of local principals, teachers, and the school superintendent. The entire school district supported and implemented a classroom-based burn prevention curriculum. Finally, the community-based campaign involved a broad coalition of public and private figures active in community affairs, including the Mayor, the Commissioner of Public Health, police and fire departments, the city public library, parent–teacher associations, and the local Rotary Club. Burn prevention presentations were held at local organizational meetings, "apartment parties," and a community health fair.

The three intervention-based metropolitan areas were matched and compared to comparable control metropolitan areas that received no interventions. Process evaluation proceeded with straightforward counting: raw numbers of public service announcements, community-based prevention sessions, classroom-based prevention lessons, and educational materials distributed. In addition, intervention and control subjects took pre- and post-tests to assess how well they retained burn prevention messages. Lastly, local burn injuries were tabulated before, during, and after the campaign.

Ultimately, Project Burn Prevention did not accomplish its stated goal. The educational intervention produced incremental knowledge gains, but similar gains were not noted in the media or community-based campaigns. Moreover, none of the campaigns resulted in lasting reductions in burn incidence or severity. Project Burn Prevention formally discontinued all interventions in May 1978, and data collection concluded 1 year thereafter.

Study organizers cited several reasons for the campaign's lack of success. First, it addressed too many burn prevention messages. The study targeted 13 different behavioral objectives for the school-based lessons, 11 for community-based lessons, and 4 for a 30-second television commercial. More focused core messages, even at the expense of intervention breadth, may have helped impart one or two points more effectively.

Project Burn Prevention was further limited by its grant and contractual relationship with its funding agency. Implementing all three campaigns in one location may have produced a greater impact, but grant contracts placed severe limitations on the study design. Additional study design measures, such as extending the study and follow-up period, and tracking additional outcome measures, were similarly infeasible due to financial constraints.

Project Burn Prevention provides an instructive example of an unsuccessful trauma prevention campaign. Multiple factors from study design, to outcome assessment, to funding constraints may doom an intervention to failure. Sometimes, specific types of interventions simply have less impact than others. Legislation and grassroots campaigns targeting equipment modifications, such as smoke detector installation, have been proven effective.[36,37] To date, few burn prevention educational programs have shown such promise.[38]

Current challenges in trauma prevention

As long as traumatic injuries exist, so will trauma prevention. Many of today's most pressing trauma prevention topics are not new – gunshot wounds, suicides, and burns have long presented challenges to the public health community. As technology evolves, new trauma mechanisms emerge, and the discipline expands to meet the challenge. The following section discusses two contemporary issues in trauma prevention that have achieved a share of notoriety.

Distracted driving

During the 1990s, cellular phones evolved from an expensive technological luxury to a major mode of communication throughout the world. In the United States alone, the number of cell-phone subscribers increased from 5 million in 1990 to 100 million in 2000, and 300 million by 2010. Increasingly, cell-phone communication has included both traditional talking and text messaging. Unfortunately, the boon to interpersonal interaction comes with the additional risk of distracted driving. In 2010, 3092 people were killed and 416,000 injured in motor vehicle collisions (MVCs) involving a distracted driver. Talking while driving is associated with four times the risk of getting into an accident, and text messaging creates a 23-fold risk. Distracted driving has truly reached epidemic proportions.[39]

The trauma prevention community has mobilized to respond.[40] National figures and organizations have supported public service campaigns to increase distracted driving awareness. Meanwhile, many local and state governments have outlawed distracted driving, some with an accompanying enforceable penalty. At latest count, 44 states, the District of Columbia, Puerto Rico, Guam, and the US Virgin Islands ban text messaging for drivers of all ages. Lastly, mobile device architecture and design provides a means to prevent distracted driving.

Currently, most of the interventions have had minimal impact. The role of public service campaigns has not been thoroughly evaluated. Evaluations from legislative interventions indicate that laws alone appear to have little impact on driver attitude or behavior. Legislative content also differs markedly from state to state. Some states ban mobile devices for a select population, while others impose a blanket ban but without allowing for primary enforcement. Technological alterations may one day help decrease distracted driving, but any such efforts are in their infancy and will face strong opposition from anti-paternalists.

One recent initiative that provides reason for optimism is the National Highway Traffic Safety Administration's "Phone in One Hand, Ticket in the Other" program.[41] Supported jointly by federal and state funds, the program emphasizes public awareness through media and print in Hartford, Connecticut, and Syracuse, New York. Thereafter, police increased enforcement of existing distracted driving restrictions over four separate time periods. Results indicated a 33–75% decrease in mobile device use while driving, and subsequent pilot programs covering Delaware and California demonstrated comparable decreases. Based on these findings, the NHTSA initiated its first national advertising and focused law enforcement campaign in April 2014, called "U drive U text U pay." Results were still pending at press time. Ideally, the three-part formula – legislation, enforcement, and continuing public awareness – will successfully reduce distracted driving throughout the US.

Sports-related head trauma

Another timely issue in trauma prevention is sports-related head injuries. Forty-four million children and adolescents participate in organized sports throughout the US. Recreational activities account for 1.6–3.8 million concussions annually, although the true incidence is thought to be much higher. Groups exposed to greater risk include boys, the sport of football, and playing in game situations.

In one respect, preventing sports-related head trauma is not new. In 1975, the National Operating Committee for Sports and Athletics Equipment published football helmet standards that became accepted within the US. However, recently emerging factors have combined to reorient public discourse regarding head trauma. An emerging body of evidence suggests that chronic traumatic encephalopathy (CTE), a dementia-like condition, is far more prevalent than originally suspected. Multiple ex-professional athletes have reported progressing dementia, and a few high-profile individuals have committed suicide; on autopsy their brains were found to bear the hallmarks of CTE. Given football's station as the most popular and most-played youth sport in the US, there has been renewed focus on sports-related head trauma.

Chronic traumatic encephalopathy may be attributed to one severe hit, but is often a chronic process resulting from multiple concussive and subconcussive head impacts over time. Treatment for concussions is rudimentary at best, and primary prevention is the optimal strategy in dealing with this issue. Determining who has experienced a concussion is itself a challenge, and athlete and coach knowledge and awareness of concussions remains suboptimal. Current concussion numbers are likely underreported.[42]

Trauma prevention researchers are undertaking several strategies to characterize and address the problem, all reflecting the 3-E's paradigm of education, engineering, and enforcement. Clear, universal definitions of concussions and return-to-play guidelines are necessary for epidemiology and management. Guidelines are now disseminated through focused classes for athletes, parents, coaches, and officials. In some states, classes are prerequisites for coaches and officials to participate in scholastic athletics. Besides education, direct rule changes may help decrease traumatic exposures. Limits to the number of full-contact practices, along with in-game rule changes to penalize helmet-to-helmet collisions, are designed to reduce the number of concussions. Finally, continuing improvement in helmet technologies may mitigate the damage when head-on collisions do occur.

The above interventions, while promising, must be rigorously evaluated in controlled settings. A paucity of good evidence exists related to sports injury and prevention.[43] Randomized controlled trials of interventions must assess both attitude changes and real concussion reductions to demonstrate true efficacy. There is a great need for continued research, and broad potential for novel interventions.

Conclusions

Trauma prevention is a necessary and vital aspect of any trauma system. Methods initially pioneered by DeHaven and Haddon have saved thousands of lives, and as technology evolves, new challenges and prevention methods will arise. However, the discipline is not only meant for epidemiologists, public health professionals, and policy experts. The clinician stands at the center of trauma-related care. As acknowledged and respected voices of authority, it behooves trauma physicians to assume active roles in trauma prevention within their respective communities.

Acknowledgments

We thank Elizabeth Kelly and Juliet J. Ray for their help with manuscript preparation.

Questions

(1) Who is considered to be the first person to approach trauma and injury from a scientific perspective?
   a. William Haddon
   b. Joseph P. Knight
   c. John Gibson
   d. Hugh DeHaven

(2) William Haddon's schematic for assessing injuries is called:
   a. Haddon's equation
   b. Haddon's theory
   c. Haddon's matrix
   d. Haddon's schema

(3) The "three E's" associated with injury prevention are:
   a. Education, engineering, and enforcement
   b. Education, execution, and evaluation
   c. Engineering, execution, and enforcement
   d. Extirpation, entitlement, and exegesis

(4) Which of the following is *not* a significant potential obstacle to developing a comprehensive trauma research program?
   a. Political limitations
   b. Cost
   c. Adequate documentation
   d. Public health versus personal autonomy

(5) Which of the following most accurately describes Project Walksafe?
   a. A project to encourage geriatric ambulation and fitness
   b. A project to limit patient falls in hospitals
   c. A project to encourage safe pedestrian habits among elementary school children
   d. A study of human factors and behavior in crowded locations to prevent stampedes and trampling deaths

(6) Which of the following most accurately describes Project Burn Prevention?
   a. A project to encourage fire safety and limit forest fires
   b. A mass campaign to encourage sun-screen application and raise the awareness of skin cancer
   c. A project designed to reduce burn incidence and severity through fire safety simulation
   d. A project designed to reduce burn incidence and severity through public educational campaigns

(7) Project Burn Prevention's failure was most attributable to:
   a. Multiplicity of messages
   b. Multiplicity of targets
   c. Lack of funding
   d. Lack of interest

(8) The "Phone in One Hand, Ticket in the Other" campaign is an example of:
   a. Trauma prevention executed through public education
   b. Trauma prevention executed through legislation and enforcement
   c. Trauma prevention executed through technological means
   d. Trauma prevention executed through vigilante justice

(9) What is CTE?
   a. Chronic traumatic encephalopathy
   b. Continuous traumatic encephalopathy
   c. Chronic temporal encephalopathy
   d. Concussive traumatic encephalopathy

(10) Which of the following is *not* a major source of epidemiologic data for scientists studying injury prevention?
   a. The National Vital Statistics System
   b. The National Electronic Injury Surveillance System

c. The Health Cost and Utilization Project

d. The Accident Oversight and Reporting System

Answers

(1) d
(2) c
(3) a

(4) c
(5) c
(6) d
(7) a
(8) b
(9) a
(10) d

References

1. Centers for Disease Control and Prevention. Web-based Injury Statistics Query and Reporting System (WISQARS). Injury prevention and control: data and statistics, 2012. Atlanta, GA: US Department of Health and Human Services, 2012. http://www.cdc.gov/injury/wisqars (accessed January 2013).

2. Bonnie RJ, Guyer B. Injury as a field of public health: achievements and controversies. *J Law Med Ethics* 2002; **30**: 267–80.

3. Maier RV, Mock C. Injury prevention. In Feliciano DV, Mattox KL, Moore EE, eds., *Trauma*. New York, NY: McGraw Hill, 2008, p. 41.

4. King James Bible. Deuteronomy, Chapter 22, Verse 8.

5. Day L, McNeil I. *Biographical Dictionary of the History of Technology*. New York, NY: Taylor and Francis, 1995, pp. 404–5.

6. Christoffel T, Gallagher SS. *Injury Prevention and Public Health: Practical Knowledge, Skills, and Strategies*, 2nd edition. Sudbury, MA: Jones and Bartlett, 2006, p. 41.

7. Winston FW. Editor's comment. *Inj Prev* 2006; **6**: 62.

8. DeHaven H. Mechanical analysis of survival in falls from heights of fifty to one hundred and fifty feet. *War Med* 1942; **2**: 586–96.

9. Gordon JE. The epidemiology of accidents. *Am J Public Health Nations Health* 1949; **39**: 504–15.

10. Gibson JJ. The contribution of experimental psychology to the formulation of the problem of safety: a brief for basic research. In Jacobs HH, Suchnam EA, Fox BH, *et al. Behavioral Approaches to Accident Research*. New York, NY: Association for the Aid of Crippled Children, 1961, pp. 77–89.

11. Haddon W. A logical framework for categorizing highway safety phenomena and activity. *J Trauma* 1972; **12**: 193–207.

12. Haddon W. On the escape of tigers: an ecologic note. *Am J Public Health Nations Health* 1970; **60**: 2229–34.

13. Nader R. *Unsafe at Any Speed: the Designed-in Dangers of the American Automobile*. New York, NY: Grossman, 1965.

14. Institute of Medicine. *Injury in America: a Continuing Public Health Problem*. Washington, DC: National Academy Press, 1985.

15. Stout NA, Linn HI. Occupational injury prevention research: progress and priorities. *Inj Prev* 2002; **8**: iv9–14.

16. Fergusson DM, Horwood LJ, Beautrais AL, *et al.* A controlled field trial of a poisoning prevention method. *Pediatrics* 1982; **69**: 515–20.

17. Arena JM. Safety closure caps: safety measure for prevention of accidental drug poisoning in children. *J Am Med Assoc* 1959; **169**: 1187–8.

18. Spiegel CN, Lindaman FC. Children can't fly: a program to prevent childhood morbidity and mortality from window falls. *Inj Prev* 1995; **1**: 194–8.

19. Corso P, Finkelstein E, Miller T, *et al.* Incidence and lifetime costs of injuries in the United States. *Inj Prev* 2006; **12**: 212–18.

20. National Committee for Injury Prevention and Control. *Injury Prevention: Meeting the Challenge*. New York, NY: Oxford University Press, 1989, pp. 49–62.

21. Nilsen P. What makes community based injury prevention work? In search of evidence of effectiveness. *Inj Prev* 2004; **10**: 268–74.

22. Aldoory L, Bonzo S. Using communication theory in injury prevention campaigns. *Inj Prev* 2005; **11**: 260–3.

23. DiGuiseppi CG, Rivara FP, Koepsell TD, *et al.* Bicycle helmet use by children: evaluation of a community-wide helmet campaign. *JAMA* 1989; **262**: 2256–61.

24. Cohen L, Baer N, Satterwhite P. Developing effective coalitions: an eight-step guide. *Injury Awareness and Prevention Center News* 1991; **4**: 10.

25. Community Preventive Services Task Force. Guide to community preventive services. Use of safety belts: enhanced enforcement programs. 2012. http://www.thecommunityguide.org/mvoi/safetybelts/enforcementprograms.html (accessed January 2013).

26. Center for Disease Control and Prevention. Motorcycle safety guide: helmet laws save lives and money. 2012. http://www.cdc.gov/motorvehiclesafety/mc/guide/save.html. (accessed January 2013).

27. Bonnie RJ, Fulco CE, Liverman CT. *Reducing the Burden of Injury: Advancing Prevention and Treatment*. Washington, DC: National Academy Press, 1999, p. 25.

28. Rivara FP. Personal communication with authors. Cited in *The National Committee for Injury Prevention and Control. Injury Prevention: Meeting the Challenge*. New York, NY: Oxford University Press, 1989, p. 70.

29. Foundation Center. http://foundationcenter.org (accessed January 2013).

30. American Public Health Association. American Public Health Association applauds President Obama for taking bold steps for toward reducing gun violence. 2012. http://www.apha.org/about/news/pressreleases/2013/White+House+plan+on+gun+violence.htm (accessed January 2013).

31. Hotz GA, Cohn SM, Nelson J, *et al.* Pediatric pedestrian trauma study: a pilot project. *Traffic Inj Prev* 2004; **5**: 132–6.

32. Hotz G, Cohn S, Castelblanco A. WalkSafe: a school-based pedestrian

safety intervention program. *Traffic Inj Prev* 2004; **5**: 382–9.

33. Hotz G, de Marcilla AG, Lutfi K, *et al.* The WalkSafe Program: developing and evaluating the educational component. *J Trauma* 2009; **66**: S3–9.

34. MacKay AM, Rothman KJ. The incidence and severity of burn injuries following Project Burn Prevention. *Am J Public Health* 1982; **72**: 248–52.

35. McLoughlin E, Vince CJ, Lee AM, *et al.* Project Burn Prevention: outcome and implications. *Am J Public Health* 1982; **72**: 241–7.

36. McLoughlin E, Marchone M, Hanger L, *et al.* Smoke detector legislation: its effect on owner-occupied homes. *Am J Public Health* 1985; **75**: 858–62.

37. Katcher ML, Landry GL, Shapiro MM. Liquid-crystal thermometer use in pediatric office counseling about tap water burn prevention. *Pediatrics* 1989; **83**: 766–71.

38. Rivara FP, Grossman DC, Cummings P. Injury prevention. Second of two parts. *N Engl J Med* 1997; **337**: 613–18.

39. Distraction.gov. What is distracted driving? 2012. http://www.distraction. gov/content/get-the-facts/facts-and-statistics.html (accessed January 2013).

40. Jacobson PD, Gostin LO. Reducing distracted driving: regulation and education to avert traffic injuries and fatalities. *JAMA* 2010; **303**: 1419–20.

41. Distraction.gov. Phone in one hand, ticket in the other. 2012. http://www. distraction.gov/content/dot-action/ enforcement.html (accessed January 2013).

42. Rosenbaum AM, Arnett PA. The development of a survey to examine knowledge about and attitudes toward concussion in high-school students. *J Clin Exp Neuropsychol* 2010; **32**: 44–55.

43. MacKay M, Liller K. Behavioral considerations for sports and recreational injuries in children and youth. In Gielen AC, Sleet DA, DiClement RJ, eds., *Injury and Violence Prevention: Behavioral Science Theories, Methods, and Applications*. San Francisco, CA: Jossey-Bass, 2006, pp. 257–73.

Chapter

42

Trauma systems, triage, and transfer

John J. Como

Objectives

(1) Define the concept of and the need for trauma systems.
(2) Relate the history and development of trauma systems in the United States.
(3) Discuss the role of the various trauma centers within the trauma system.
(4) Explain the principles of trauma patient triage.
(5) Describe the principles involved in transfer of the injured patient between institutions.

Trauma systems

The cost to society due to trauma is enormous. Trauma is the leading cause of death for Americans 44 years of age and younger.[1] Traumatic injuries were estimated to be responsible for more than 180,000 deaths in the United States in 2010. In addition to mortality, trauma is significant for number of years of productive life lost and prolonged or permanent disability. In 2010, there were more than 31 million nonfatal injuies reported in the United States.[1] The problem of injury has a profound effect on individuals, families, hospitals, and society at large because it causes tremendous medical, psychosocial, and financial burdens.

Because of this, the prevention of traumatic injury and the treatment of the acutely injured patient are public services central to the mission of public health agencies. Trauma systems and trauma centers are essential to providing these public services. A trauma system is a preplanned, comprehensive, and coordinated statewide and local injury response network that includes all facilities with the capability to care for the injured.[2] It is an organized approach to patient care in acutely injured patients in a defined geographical system that provides full and comprehensive care and is fully integrated with the regional emergency medical services (EMS) system.[3] Its major goal is to enhance the health of the community. Such a system should decrease the risk and burden of traumatic disease to society in general and to individuals in particular. This occurs through public health assessment, policy development, and assurance (Fig. 42.1).

Both prevention programs and the performance of emergent and definitive care of the acutely injured patient are integral components of the trauma system. As more than half of trauma deaths occur within minutes of injury and are never able to be addressed by acute care, prevention is of paramount importance.[4] Injury prevention activities are practiced in the majority of trauma centers in the United States.[5] Disaster preparedness is also an important function of a trauma system.[6,7] The needs of all trauma patients must be met wherever they are injured and wherever they receive care. No facility can provide all of the resources needed by the trauma patient in all situations. Because of this, emphasis should be placed on the need for developing a trauma system instead of developing only individual trauma centers.

All trauma centers in a particular area must participate in the planning, development, and operation of the regional trauma system. A number of studies have suggested that treatment at a trauma center or within a trauma system may be associated with fewer preventable deaths and improved survival among the seriously injured.[8–11] These studies, however, have been inconclusive and hampered by study design limitations. There is thus a substantial variation across states in the number and geographic distribution of trauma centers.[12–14] MacKenzie *et al.* examined differences in mortality between Level I trauma centers and nontrauma centers and found that the in-hospital mortality rate was significantly lower at the trauma centers (7.6% vs. 9.5%) as was the 1-year mortality rate (10.4% vs. 13.8%).[15]

It is the system's inclusiveness, or range of preplanned trauma center and nontrauma center resource allocation, that offers the public a cost-effective plan for injury treatment.[2] An *inclusive trauma system* includes all the components needed to optimize trauma care, including prevention, access, acute hospital care, rehabilitation, and research activities.[16] An *exclusive trauma system* focuses only on the major trauma center. In the inclusive trauma system, the needs of the patient will be matched to the capability of the receiving center. This approach provides the best use of resources and matches patient needs to the level of care provided. Severely injured

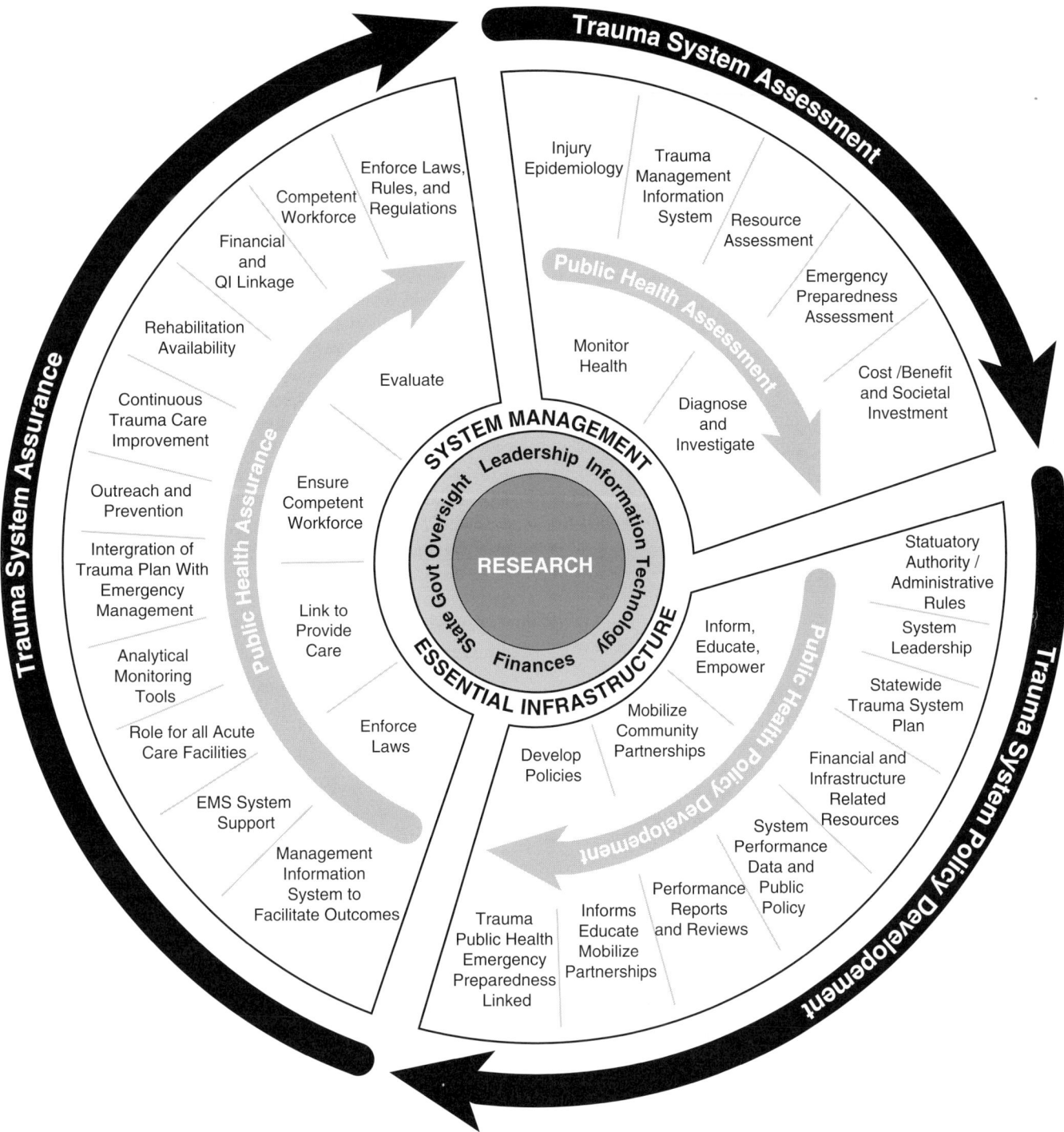

Figure 42.1 The public health approach to trauma system deployment. (From US Department of Health and Human Services, Health Resources and Services Administration, Trauma-Emergency Medical Services Systems Program: Model Trauma Systems Planning and Evaluation.)

patients may have a greater inpatient survival in inclusive trauma systems.[17]

There are a number of important events that have led to the development of modern trauma systems (Table 42.1). A paper by the National Academy of Sciences and the National Research Council entitled *Accidental Death and Disability: the Neglected Disease of Modern Society* was published in

1966.[18] This manuscript publicly announced trauma care as a political issue. In 1973, the Emergency Medical Services Systems Act provided federal guidelines and funding for the development of regional EMS systems.[16]

The guideline *Optimal Hospital Resources for the Care of the Seriously Injured* was first developed by the American College of Surgeons Committee on Trauma in 1976 and is

Table 42.1 Important events leading to the development of modern trauma systems in the US

1966	The National Academy of Sciences and the National Research Council published *Accidental Death and Disability: the Neglected Disease of Modern Society.*
1973	The Emergency Medical Services Systems Act provided federal guidelines and funding for the development of regional Emergency Medical Services systems.
1976	The guideline *Optimal Hospital Resources for the Care of the Seriously Injured* was first developed by the American College of Surgeons Committee on Trauma.
1980	The Advanced Trauma Life Support (ATLS) course was developed by the American College of Surgeons Committee on Trauma.
1987	The American College of Emergency Physicians published *Guidelines for Trauma Care Systems.*
1992	The Division of Trauma and Emergency Medical Services within the Health Resources Services Administration published the *Model Trauma Care System Plan*, meant to aid states in the development of inclusive trauma systems.
2014	The most recent version of the American College of Surgeons Committee on Trauma guidelines, entitled *Resources for Optimal Care of the Injured Patient*, was published.

Table 42.2 Components of an ideal trauma system

Injury prevention
Injury control
Access to care
Prehospital care
Acute hospital care
Rehabilitation
Research

revised periodically.[19] The most recent version of the American College of Surgeons Committee on Trauma guidelines, entitled *Resources for Optimal Care of the Injured Patient*, had been published in 2006,[16] and an updated version has just been issued in late 2014. This document establishes criteria for prehospital and hospital personnel and emphasizes the need for ongoing quality improvement. In 1987, the American College of Emergency Physicians published *Guidelines for Trauma Care Systems*, which established essential criteria for trauma systems, with an emphasis on prehospital care.[20] In 1992 the Division of Trauma and Emergency Medical Services within the Health Resources Services Administration published the *Model Trauma Care System Plan*, which was intended to aid states in the development of inclusive trauma systems.[21] The Advanced Trauma Life Support (ATLS) course was developed by the American College of Surgeons Committee on Trauma in 1980 and has trained over 1 million physicians in 63 countries.[22]

Civilian trauma systems were originally designed for timely and appropriate treatment of the most seriously injured, and emulated military models for treating acutely injured servicemen.[10] It was felt that patient outcomes would improve by ensuring the timely transfer of seriously injured patients to centers having the necessary personnel and the resources needed to treat the patient's injuries. Several studies have shown an improvement in patient outcomes when experience and resources are concentrated in a defined number of facilities.[23] In-hospital mortality from trauma is significantly reduced in urban areas with implementation of a trauma system. The introduction of trauma systems has led to improved outcomes after injury.[15] Even so, there is a great variability in the number of trauma centers per million population throughout the United States. Also, much of the United States remains uncovered by an organized trauma system.[13]

Trauma centers are designated according to the level of care provided and resources available. The trauma system is a network of various levels of definitive care facilities that provide a spectrum of care for all injured patients. Trauma centers are evaluated and verified within the trauma system to verify that they meet certain standards. Each effective trauma system must have one lead hospital. This hospital should be of the highest level available in that particular trauma system. A combination of levels of designated trauma centers will coexist with other acute-care facilities. The commitment to care is expected to be the same at every trauma center level; the different levels should only be differentiated by resource depth.

An ideal trauma system includes all the components associated with optimal care of the injured patient, which include injury prevention and control, access to care, prehospital care, acute hospital care, rehabilitation, and research (Table 42.2).[16] The presence of a large, resource-rich trauma center is central to such a system. Such a center optimally should include the immediate presence of board-certified emergency physicians, anesthesiologists, general surgeons, orthopedic surgeons, and neurosurgeons. Other board-certified specialists should be available within a short period of time if needed.

A trauma center should require a certain number of trauma admissions per year, including the most seriously injured patients in the system, to obtain and maintain a sufficient degree of experience and expertise.[11] Injuries that occur infrequently should be concentrated in the center to ensure that they are properly treated and studied. This center should be responsible for assessing not only the care provided within its own trauma program, but also in the system as a whole. It should also serve as the comprehensive resource for any trauma issues occurring throughout the system. Surgical commitment and leadership is essential for a properly functioning trauma center. A surgeon should be the full-time director of the trauma program, and other surgeons should take an active role at this center in all aspects of taking care of the injured patient, including a performance program. The American College of Surgeons Committee on Trauma has developed a trauma center classification that is intended to assist a region in the development (Table 42.3).[16]

A Level I trauma center usually serves as the lead hospital for the system and is the tertiary care center central to the system.[16] In large urban areas more than one Level I trauma center may be needed. This type of facility must have the capability of taking the lead in all aspects of trauma care, from prevention to rehabilitation. These centers also have the responsibility of providing leadership in education, research, and system planning. Research and prevention programs are essential for a Level I trauma center. This center must have a surgically directed intensive care unit and participate in the training of residents. Qualified general surgeons are expected to participate in the decision making, resuscitation, and operations needed for the acutely injured patient. A Level I trauma center must admit at least 1200 trauma patients per year or have 240 patients with an Injury Severity Score (ISS) of more than 15 or an average of 35 patients with an ISS of more than 15 for all general surgeons taking trauma calls. The ISS is a grading scale that provides a score for patients with multiple injuries. Each individual injury is assigned a measure of severity of trauma – the Abbreviated Injury Scale (AIS) score (range 0–6, based on the severity of the injury), allocated to each of six body regions (head, face, chest, abdomen, extremities, and external). The ISS is then calculated by taking the sum of the squares of the three highest AIS scores. An ISS of 15 or more is commonly used to define major trauma.[24]

A Level II trauma center may provide care in two distinct situations. The first is generally in the urban environment, and this center will then act as a supplemental center to the nearby Level I center. The two centers should then work together to optimize resources available for the care of the injured patient. In a more rural environment, the Level II trauma center may act as the lead center for the geographic area when no Level I center is close. This hospital will then have an outreach program that encompasses the smaller hospitals in the area. Qualified general surgeons must participate in major therapeutic decisions, be involved in resuscitations, participate in operations, and be actively involved in the critical care of the injured patient.

A Level III trauma center should have the capability to perform the initial management of the majority of trauma patients and have transfer agreements with the Level I and Level II trauma centers if the needs of the patients exceed its resources. At a Level III trauma center, a general surgeon continues to take the lead in establishing the trauma team.

Table 42.3 Differences between Levels I–IV trauma centers

Level I	Lead hospital and tertiary care center central to the system
	Leads in all aspects of trauma care, from prevention to rehabilitation
	Must admit at least 1200 trauma patients per year or have 240 patients with an Injury
	Injury Severity Score (ISS) > 15 or an average of 35 patients with ISS > 15 for all general surgeons taking trauma calls
	Either an attending surgeon or a resident at the postgraduate year 4 or 5 must be in-house 24 hours a day
	Resident may begin resuscitation but may not substitute for the surgeon
	Expected that the attending surgeon will be in the emergency department within 15 minutes of patient arrival
	Hospital must document the presence of the attending surgeon at least 80% of the time
	While on call, surgeon must be dedicated only to that center and can have no responsibilities at another center
	Backup call schedule must be available
Level II	Must be 24-hour in-house availability of the attending surgeon
	Resident at the postgraduate 4 or 5 year or an attending emergency physician who is part of the trauma team may begin the resuscitation, but cannot substitute for the surgeon
	Expected that the attending surgeon will be in the emergency department within 15 minutes of patient arrival
	Hospital must document the presence of the attending surgeon at least 80% of the time
	While on call, the surgeon must be dedicated only to that center and can have no responsibilities at another center
	Backup call schedule must be available
Level III	On-call surgeon must be available in the emergency department within 30 minutes of patient arrival
	Must demonstrate a commitment to injury prevention, outreach activities to the local community, and education to all providers involved in the care of the injured patient
Level IV	Located in a rural setting
	Provides initial evaluation of injured patients
	24-hour emergency coverage must be available by a physician
Nontrauma center	Delivers and regularly provides care to less severely injured patients
	Exists within the trauma system

General surgeons on the trauma panel must respond to trauma team activations and remain knowledgeable in trauma principles, whether treating patients locally or transferring patients to a higher level of care. Level III trauma centers must also demonstrate a commitment to injury prevention, outreach activities to the local community, and education to all providers involved in the care of the injured patient.

Level IV trauma centers are located in the rural setting and supplement care within a larger trauma system. These centers provide initial evaluation of injured patients, but most of these will require transfer to a higher level of care. Twenty-four-hour emergency coverage must be available by a physician, and a well-organized resuscitation team is important. Well-designed transfer agreements are essential.

Many "nontrauma centers" that are prepared to deliver and regularly provide care to less severely injured patients exist within the trauma system. If a patient with major injuries is incorrectly triaged to one of these hospitals, transport agreements must be in place to transport the patient to an appropriate center.

Rehabilitation is as important as prehospital and hospital care. It is often the longest and most difficult phase of recovery for the injured person. The role of the rehabilitation center is an important component of an effective trauma system.

A trauma system must monitor its performance over time and identify areas in which improvement is needed. A systemwide trauma registry is essential in ensuring that this process is possible. A systemwide quality improvement program must monitor the quality of care from the time of injury through discharge from rehabilitation, and identify problems and offer solutions.

Trauma triage

Triage refers to the initial evaluation of patients and the determination of priorities and levels of medical care needed.[3] The purpose of triage is to match patients with the optimal resources necessary to adequately and efficiently manage their injuries. The principles of modern prehospital care of the acutely injured patient are derived from concepts developed in the military setting. The management of these patients requires the identification in the field of injuries and mechanisms of trauma that are likely to lead to severe injuries, to allow correct triage to an appropriate facility. Triage protocols should be arranged so that patients are transferred to the most appropriate trauma facility. The goals of the prehospital providers are to prevent further injury, to initiate resuscitation, and to provide safe and rapid transport of the injured patient. The patient should be taken to the trauma center within the system that has the most appropriate resources to deal with the specific injuries the patient may have.

The EMS system is responsible for the initial care of the injured patient, and EMS providers are responsible for deciding which patients warrant transport to a trauma center, which may involve bypassing a closer nontrauma hospital. If medical direction of prehospital trauma care is provided by physician-directed voice communication, this is referred to as *on-line medical direction*.[16] If this is done by preexisting protocol, it is referred to as *off-line medical direction*. Treatment of injured patients in the prehospital setting consists of assessment, extrication, initiation of resuscitation and stabilization, and rapid transport to the nearest appropriate facility. The essential components of resuscitation in the field should be limited to the establishment of an airway, provision of ventilation, control of hemorrhage, stabilization of fractures, and immobilization of the entire spine. Additional time-consuming interventions should in general be avoided. For example, an intravenous line may be started en route to the hospital.

A trauma system should establish and monitor acceptable rates of trauma overtriage and undertriage.[16] *Overtriage* refers to a triage decision in which a minimally injured patient is transported to a higher-level trauma center when retrospective analysis suggests that this was not needed, whereas *undertriage* refers to a triage decision in which a severely injured patient is transported to a lower-level trauma center than required. The viability of the trauma system thus depends on appropriate triage, as undertriage may result in preventable mortality and morbidity due to delays in the provision of definitive care, and overtriage, while having minimal adverse consequences for the individual patient, may result in excessive burden for higher-level trauma centers and thus impair the availability of care to those who are injured most severely. In mass casualty and disaster situations, overtriage may result in adverse outcomes and should be minimized.

The Centers for Disease Control and Prevention (CDC) recently sponsored a committee to review evidence and formulate national standards for prehospital trauma triage, and published an algorithm (Fig. 42.2) based on one that had been published in *Resources for Optimal Care of the Injured Patient*.[16,25,26] This scheme is a four-step evaluation process that entails (1) assessment of vital signs and Glasgow Coma Scale score (see Table 35.1 in Chapter 35); (2) evaluation for critical injury patterns; (3) assessment of high-energy mechanisms of trauma; and (4) assessment of special patient considerations, including the extremes of age, pregnancy, anticoagulation, burns, and end-stage renal disease. This algorithm should be used by each trauma system to assess its own regional guidelines, ensuring that they are evidence-based and addressing local transport challenges.

Another area of controversy involves those trauma patients who can be declared dead in the field, thus avoiding excess use of resources and risk to providers in transporting a nonsalvageable patient. A joint position statement of the National Association of Emergency Medical Services Physicians and the American College of Surgeons Committee on Trauma regarding guidelines for withdrawal or termination of resuscitation in prehospital traumatic cardiopulmonary arrest was published in 2003 (Table 42.4).[27] In summary, these guidelines recommend that resuscitation efforts be withheld from victims of blunt trauma found to be apneic, pulseless, and without

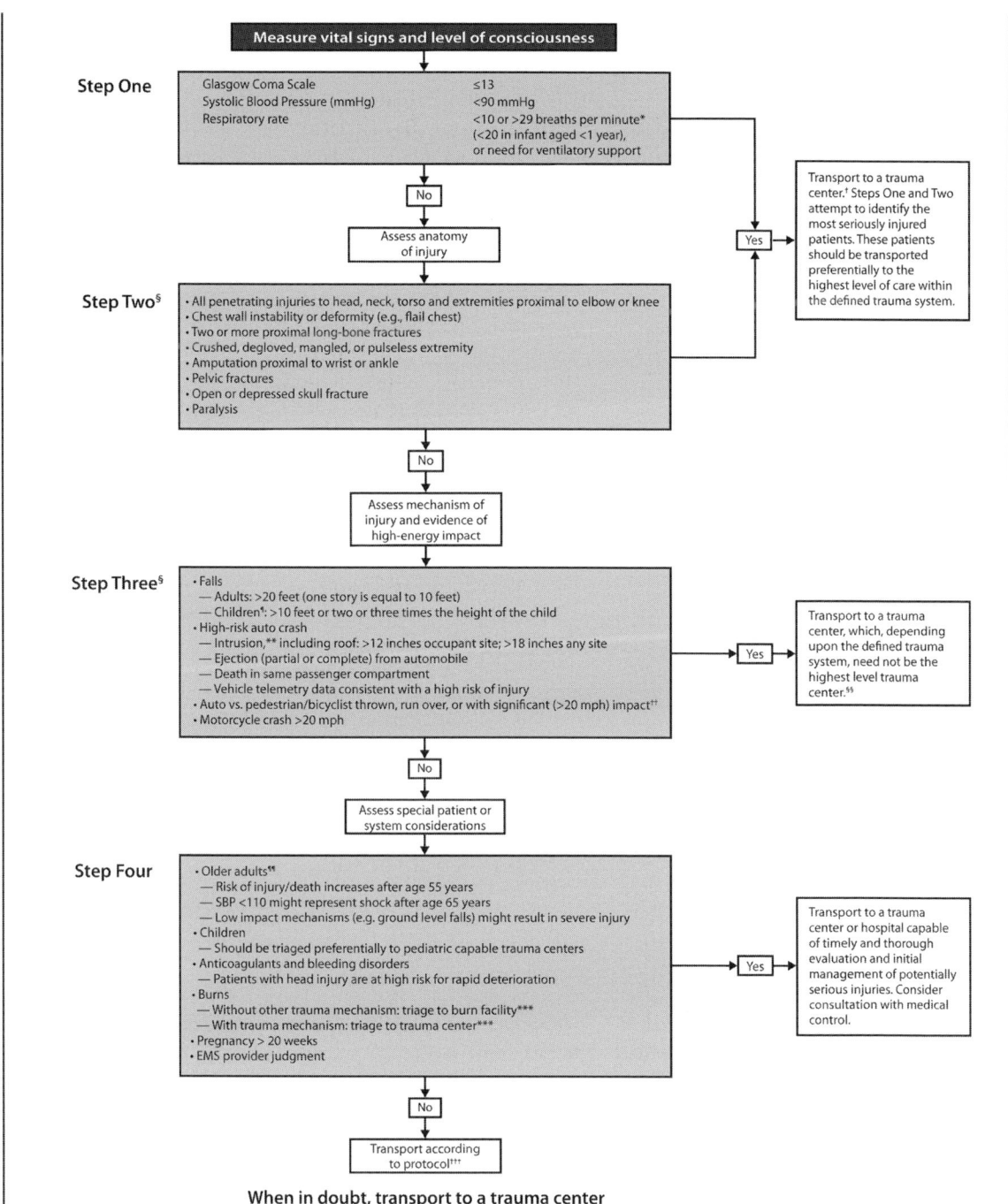

Figure 42.2 Guidelines for field triage of injured patients; United States, 2011. (Reprinted from Sasser *et al.* 2012,[25] with permission from Centers for Disease Control and Prevention.)

* The upper limit of respiratory rate in infants is > 29 breaths per minute to maintain a higher level of overtriage for infants.

† Trauma centers are designated Level I–IV. A Level I center has the greatest amount of resources and personnel for care of the injured patient and provides regional leadership in education, research, and prevention programs. A Level II facility offers similar resources to a Level I facility, possibly differing only in continuous availability of certain subspecialties or sufficient prevention, education, and research activities for Level I designation; Level II facilities are not required to be resident or fellow education centers. A Level III center is capable of assessment, resuscitation, and emergency surgery, with severely injured patients being transferred to a Level I or II facility. A Level IV trauma center is capable of providing 24-hour physician coverage, resuscitation, and stabilization to injured patients before transfer to a facility that provides a higher level of trauma care.

§ Any injury noted in Step Two or mechanism identified in Step Three triggers a "yes" response.

¶ Age < 15 years.

** Intrusion refers to interior compartment intrusion, as opposed to deformation which refers to exterior damage.

†† Includes pedestrians or bicyclists thrown or run over by a motor vehicle or those with estimated impact > 20 mph with a motor vehicle.

§§ Local or regional protocols should be used to determine the most appropriate level of trauma center within the defined trauma system; need not be the highest-level trauma center.

¶¶ Age > 55 years.

*** Patients with both burns and concomitant trauma for whom the burn injury poses the greatest risk for morbidity and mortality should be transferred to a burn center. If the nonburn trauma presents a greater immediate risk, the patient may be stabilized in a trauma center and then transferred to a burn center.

††† Patients who do not meet any of the triage criteria in Steps One through Four should be transported to the most appropriate medical facility as outlined in local EMS protocols.

Table 42.4 NAEMSP/ACSCOT guidelines for withholding or termination of resuscitation in prehospital traumatic cardiopulmonary arrest

1. Resuscitation efforts may be withheld in any blunt trauma patient who, based on out-of-hospital personnel's thorough primary patient assessment, is found apneic, pulseless, and without organized electrocardiogram (ECG) activity upon the arrival of emergency medical services (EMS) at the scene.
2. Victims of penetrating trauma found apneic and pulseless by EMS, based on their patient assessment, should be rapidly assessed for the presence of other signs of life, such as pupillary reflexes, spontaneous movement, or organized ECG activity. If any of these signs are present, the patient should have resuscitation performed and be transported to the nearest emergency department or trauma center. If these signs of life are absent, resuscitation efforts may be withheld.
3. Resuscitation efforts should be withheld in victims of penetrating or blunt trauma with injuries obviously incompatible with life, such as decapitation or hemicorporectomy.
4. Resuscitation efforts should be withheld in victims of penetrating or blunt trauma with evidence of significant time lapse since pulselessness, including dependent lividity, rigor mortis, and decomposition.
5. Cardiopulmonary arrest patients in whom the mechanism of injury does not correlate with clinical condition, suggesting a nontraumatic cause of the arrest, should have standard resuscitation initiated.
6. Termination of resuscitation efforts should be considered in trauma patients with EMS-witnessed cardiopulmonary arrest and 15 minutes of unsuccessful resuscitation and cardiopulmonary resuscitation (CPR).
7. Traumatic cardiopulmonary arrest patients with a transport time to an emergency department or a trauma center of more than 15 minutes after the arrest is identified may be considered nonsalvagable, and termination of resuscitation should be considered.
8. Guidelines and protocols for traumatic cardiopulmonary arrest (TCPA) patients who should be transported must be individualized for each EMS system. Consideration should be given to factors such as the average transport time within the system, the scope of practice of the various EMS providers within the system, and the definitive care capabilities (that is, trauma centers) within the system.
9. Special consideration must be given to victims of drowning and lightning strikes and in situations where significant hypothermia may alter the prognosis.
10. EMS providers should be thoroughly familiar with the guidelines and protocols affecting the decision to withhold or terminate resuscitative efforts.
11. All termination protocols should be developed and implemented under the guidance of the system EMS medical director. On-line medical control may be necessary to determine the appropriateness of termination of resuscitation.
12. Policies and protocols for termination of resuscitation efforts must include notification of the appropriate law enforcement agencies and notification of the medical examiner or coroner for final disposition of the body.
13. Families of the deceased should have access to resources, including clergy, social workers, and other counseling personnel, as needed. EMS providers should have access to resources for debriefing and counseling as needed.
14. Adherence to policies and protocols governing termination of resuscitation should be monitored through a quality review system.

ACSCOT, American College of Surgeons Committee on Trauma; NAEMSP, National Association of Emergency Medical Services Physicians.

organized electrocardiogram (ECG) activity on the arrival of EMS at the scene. In penetrating trauma victims found apneic and pulseless by EMS, rapid assessment should be performed to assess other signs of life, such as pupillary reflexes, spontaneous movement, or organized ECG activity. If these signs of life are absent, resuscitative measures may be withheld. Termination of resuscitative efforts should be considered in trauma patients with EMS-witnessed cardiopulmonary arrest and 15 minutes of unsuccessful efforts or if the transport time to a trauma center is more than 15 minutes. Some of these guidelines have been challenged, however, by Pickens and colleagues, who reported rare survivors with more than 15 minutes of cardiopulmonary resuscitation and with a transport time longer than 15 minutes.[28]

Transfer

Many patients who live in rural communities do not have immediate access to a major trauma center or a regional trauma system. These patients are therefore taken to a local community hospital and may need to be transferred from this center to a regional trauma center. For this reason, an essential component of a trauma system is the development of agreements for transfer of patients between institutions.[16] These agreements should be drafted well in advance of the need for them and should detail the process for transfer of patients and the means for doing so. It is essential that once the decision for transfer has been made, no time should be spent performing tests or procedures that have no impact on the resuscitation or transfer process. For example, there is no need to perform computed tomography of the brain in a patient with a suspected brain injury if there is no neurosurgeon available to treat this patient at the initial center. Outcome may be improved by minimizing the time from injury to definitive care. A regional trauma system improves the efficiency of transfer of patients by having transfer agreements in place that deal with the issue prior to acute patient need.

Once the decision to transfer has been made, it is the responsibility of the referring physician to initiate resuscitation measures within the capabilities of the transferring hospital.[16] Resuscitation should be done according to ATLS principles. Direct physician-to-physician contact is essential. The accepting trauma surgeon should review the physiologic status of the patient and discuss the optimal timing of the transfer.

For example, it may be advantageous for the patient with acute intraabdominal hemorrhage to undergo laparotomy at the transferring hospital to stabilize the patient prior to transfer if a qualified surgeon and operating room resources are available at this center.

Transferring physicians have the responsibility to identify patients needing transfer, to initiate the transfer process by direct contact with the receiving trauma surgeon, to initiate resuscitation measures within the capabilities of the facility, to determine the appropriate mode of transportation in consultation with the receiving surgeon, and to transfer all records, test results, and radiologic evaluations to the receiving facility.[16] Receiving physicians must ensure that resources are available at the receiving facility, provide consultation regarding specifics of the transfer, additional evaluation, or resuscitation before transport, clarify medical control once transfer of the patient is established, and identity a performance improvement and patient safety process for transportation, allowing feedback from the receiving trauma surgeon to the transport team directly or at least to the medical direction for the transport team.

Transfer of the trauma patient should be arranged such that the risk to the patient is minimized throughout the transport process. During transport, qualified personnel and equipment should be available to meet anticipated contingencies. Sufficient supplies should accompany the patient during transport, such as intravenous fluids, blood, and medications, as appropriate. Vital signs should be monitored frequently, and vital functions, such as ventilation, hemodynamics, central nervous system, and spinal protection, should be supported. Records should be kept during transport, and communication should be maintained with online medical direction. The trauma system should ensure prompt transfer once a trauma decision has been made, review all transfers for performance improvement and patient safety, and ensure transportation commensurate with the patient's severity of injury.

The Consolidated Omnibus Budget Reconciliation Act (COBRA) of 1987 imposes civil penalties on individual practitioners and hospitals that fail to provide emergency care in a timely fashion.[16] The Emergency Medical Treatment and Labor Act (EMTALA, 1986) was designed to prevent the transfer of patients based solely on the patient's ability to pay. Additional elements of the Emergency Medical Treatment and Labor Act that are relevant to the transfer of the trauma patient include the need to identify a facility with available space and qualified personnel that has agreed to accept the patient before beginning the transfer; not transferring patients in hemodynamically unstable condition, except for medical necessity and only after providing medical treatment within the facility's capacity that minimizes risks to the patient's health; providing appropriate transportation with a vehicle augmented with life support equipment and staff to meet the anticipated contingencies that may arise during transportation; sending all records, test results, radiologic studies, and other relevant reports or data with the patient to the referring facility

unless delay would increase the risks of transfer, and then sending the information as soon as possible; and issuing a physician transfer certificate and consent for transfer to accompany the patient.

There seems to be a trend toward overtriage of patients who might have easily been treated in an initial hospital. This tends to overburden the Level I centers, the trauma system, and the healthcare system in general. Esposito and colleagues found a disproportionate increase in the transfer of patients between facilities in comparison with the general increase in trauma patients in the state of Illinois from 1999 to 2003.[29] This trend did not seem to be accounted for by any significant increases in injury severity or changes in payor mix. This seemed to suggest either a reluctance or an inability on the part of the initial hospitals to care for patients that they theoretically should be capable of treating. This may be due to low reimbursement and a perceived increase in medicolegal risk. When higher-level centers are overburdened with less severely injured patients, they may be limited in their ability to allocate the appropriate medical care and other resources to the trauma patients who need this most. The overutilization of interfaculty transfer, whatever the cause, will jeopardize patient care and efficient trauma system function. This trend must be recognized and reversed in the near future, recognizing issues related to the supply and demand for services, the idea of "back transfer" or repatriation, liability risk, insurance, and commensurate reimbursement and provider lifestyle issues.

Summary

The mortality and morbidity attributable to trauma is recognized as one of the most important public health problems encountered in the United States. Trauma centers exist as part of regional trauma systems to treat the injured patient. The major goal of the trauma system is to enhance the health of the community. Because no facility can provide all the resources needed by the trauma patient in all situations, the need for developing a trauma system instead of developing only individual trauma centers is apparent. Such a system decreases the risk and burden of traumatic disease both to individuals and to society in general. Both prevention programs and the performance of emergent and definitive care to the acutely injured patient are essential to the function of this system. Appropriate triage and interhospital transfer are also essential in ensuring optimal care for the injured patient. Patient outcome after injury is significantly improved with a regional system of trauma care.

Questions

(1) **Which of the following statements about trauma is *incorrect*?**
    a. Trauma is the leading cause of death in the first four decades of life
    b. Trauma is recognized as one of the most important public health problems encountered in the United States today

c. All trauma centers in a particular area must participate in regional trauma system planning, development, and operation

d. Treatment of the acutely injured patient, but not prevention of injury, is central to the mission of public health agencies

e. The cost to society due to trauma is enormous

(2) Identify the *incorrect* statement regarding trauma systems:

a. The major goal of a trauma system is to enhance the health of the community

b. Disaster preparedness is an important function of trauma systems

c. Only a Level I trauma center can provide all the resources needed by the trauma patient in all situations

d. An inclusive trauma system includes prevention, access, acute hospital care, rehabilitation, and research activities

e. A trauma system should be fully integrated with the regional emergency medical services (EMS) system

(3) Which of the following statements regarding the development of modern trauma systems is *incorrect*?

a. In 1973, the Emergency Medical Services (EMS) Systems Act provided federal guidelines and funding for the development of regional EMS systems

b. The National Academy of Sciences and the National Research Council published a manuscript entitled *Accidental Death and Disability: the Neglected Disease of Modern Society* in 1966

c. The latest American College of Surgeons Committee on Trauma guidelines entitled *Resources for Optimal Care of the Injured Patient* were published in 2014

d. The Advanced Trauma Life Support (ATLS) course was developed by the American College of Surgeons Committee on Trauma in 1980 and has been taken by more than 450,000 healthcare providers

e. The guideline *Optimal Hospital Resources for the Care of the Seriously Injured* was first developed by the American College of Surgeons Committee on Trauma in 1996

(4) Which of the following statements regarding trauma systems is true?

a. Several studies have shown worsened patient outcomes when experience and resources are concentrated in a defined number of facilities

b. Civilian trauma systems originally emulated military models for treating acutely injured servicemen

c. According to the 2002 National Assessment of State Trauma System Development, all 50 states had at least one critical element in place for a trauma system

d. The introduction of trauma systems, although important, has led to no significant reduction in the number of preventable deaths after injury

e. In-hospital mortality from trauma is not significantly reduced in urban areas with implementation of a trauma system

(5) Which of the following statements regarding trauma centers is true?

a. The commitment to care of the trauma patient will vary depending on the trauma center level

b. It is preferable but not essential that a surgeon be the full-time director of a trauma program

c. Research and prevention programs are not essential for a Level I trauma center

d. A Level I trauma center must have a surgically directed intensive care unit and participate in the training of residents

e. A Level I trauma center must admit at least 1800 trauma patients per year

(6) Which of the following statements about trauma triage is *incorrect*?

a. The purpose of triage is to match the patient with the optimal resources necessary to adequately and efficiently manage their injuries

b. The patient should be taken to the trauma center within the system that has the most appropriate resources to deal with the specific injuries the patient may have

c. If medical direction of prehospital trauma care is provided by physician-directed voice communication, this is referred to as on-line medical direction

d. The essential components of resuscitation in the field should be limited to establishment of an airway, provision of ventilation, control of hemorrhage, stabilization of fractures, and immobilization of the spine

e. Undertriage has minimal adverse consequences for the patient

(7) A victim of penetrating trauma is found apneic and pulseless by EMS. The presence of which of the following would *not* mandate resuscitation and immediate transport to a trauma center?

a. Pupillary reflexes
b. Organized ECG activity
c. Gag reflex
d. Spontaneous movement
e. Decapitation

(8) For which of the following trauma patients should resuscitative efforts be withheld?

a. Any blunt trauma patient who is apneic, without a pulse, and without organized ECG activity

b. Any penetrating trauma patient who is apneic, without a pulse, and without organized ECG activity

c. Penetrating trauma victim with pulseless electrical activity

d. Apneic and pulseless penetrating trauma patient with spontaneous movement

e. EMS-witnessed cardiopulmonary arrest and 5 minutes of unsuccessful cardiopulmonary resuscitation

(9) Which of the following statements about trauma transport is *incorrect*?

   a. Once the decision for transfer has been made, no time should be spent performing tests or procedures that have no impact on the resuscitation or transfer process

   b. Outcome may be improved by minimizing the time from injury to definitive care

   c. A regional trauma system improves the efficiency of transfer of patients by having transfer agreements in place that deal with the issue prior to acute patient need

   d. Once the decision to transfer has been made, it is the responsibility of the referring.physician to initiate resuscitation measures within the capabilities of the transferring hospital

   e. Even if a qualified surgeon and operating room resources are available at the transferring hospital, the patient with acute intraabdominal hemorrhage should never undergo laparotomy prior to transfer

(10) Which of the following statements about trauma transport is *incorrect*?

   a. The Emergency Medical Treatment and Labor Act (EMTALA) is designed to prevent the transfer of patients based solely on the patient's ability to pay

   b. The Consolidated Omnibus Budget Reconciliation Act (COBRA) of 1987 imposes civil penalties on individual practitioners and hospitals that fail to provide emergency care in a timely fashion

   c. EMTALA specifies that a facility with available space and qualified personnel agrees to accept the patient before beginning the transfer

   d. EMTALA does not allow for the transfer of patients in hemodynamically unstable condition under any circumstances

   e. EMTALA mandates appropriate transportation with a vehicle augmented with life support equipment and staff to meet anticipated contingencies that may arise

Answers

(1) d
(2) c
(3) e
(4) b
(5) d
(6) e
(7) e
(8) a
(9) e
(10) d

References

1. Centers for Disease Control and Prevention. Web-based Injury Statistics Query and Reporting System (WISQARS). Injury prevention and control: data and statistics, 2012. Atlanta, GA: US Department of Health and Human Services, 2012. http://www.cdc.gov/injury/wisqars (accessed July 2014).

2. US Department of Health and Human Services, Health Resources and Services Administration. Trauma-EMS Systems Program: Model Trauma Systems Planning and Evaluation. http://www.hrsa.gov/trauma/model.htm (last accessed May 28, 2007).

3. Hoyt DB, Coimbra R. Trauma systems. *Surg Clin N Am* 2007; **87**: 21–35.

4. Potenza B, Hoyt D, Coimbra R, *et al.* The epidemiology of serious and fatal injury in San Diego County over an 11-year period. *J Trauma* 2004; **56**: 68–75.

5. McDonald EM, MacKenzie EJ, Teitelbaum SD, *et al.* Injury prevention centers in U.S. trauma centers: Are we doing enough? *Injury* 2007; **38**: 538–47.

6. Champion HR, Mabee MS, Meredith JW. The state of US trauma systems. Public perceptions versus reality: implications for US response to terrorism and mass casualty events. *J Am Coll Surg* 2006; **203**: 951–61.

7. Mann NC, MacKenzie E, Anderson C. Public health preparedness for mass-casualty events: A 2002 state-by-state assessment. *Prehosp Disast Med* 2004; **19**: 245–55.

8. Jurkovich GJ, Mock C. Systematic review of trauma system effectiveness based on registry comparisons. *J Trauma* 1999; **47**: S46–55.

9. MacKenzie EJ. Review of evidence regarding trauma system effectiveness resulting from panel studies. *J Trauma* 1999; **47**: S34–41.

10. Mullins RJ, Mann NC. Population-based research assessing the effectiveness of trauma systems. *J Trauma* 1999; **47**: S59–66.

11. Nathens AB, Jurkovich GJ, Maier RV, *et al.* Relationship between trauma center volume and outcomes. *JAMA* 2001; **285**: 1164–71.

12. Branas CC, MacKenzie EJ, Williams JC, *et al.* Access to trauma centers in the United States. *JAMA* 2005; **293**: 2626–33.

13. MacKenzie EJ, Hoyt DB, Sacra JC, *et al.* National inventory of hospital trauma centers. *JAMA* 2003; **289**: 1515–22.

14. Nathens AB, Jurkovich GJ, MacKenzie, *et al.* A resource-based assessment of trauma care in the United States. *J Trauma* 2004; **56**: 173–8.

15. MacKenzie EJ, Rivara FP, Jurkovich GJ, *et al.* A national evaluation of the effect of trauma-center care on mortality. *N Engl J Med* 2006; **354**: 366–78.

16. American College of Surgeons Committee on Trauma. *Resources for Optimal Care of the Injured Patient.* Chicago, IL: ACS, 2006.

17. Utter GH, Maier RV, Rivara FP, *et al.* Inclusive trauma systems: Do they improve triage or outcomes of the severely injured? *J Trauma* 2006; **60**: 529–37.

18. Committee on Trauma, and Committee on Shock, Division of Medical Sciences, National Academy of Sciences/National Research Council (US). *Accidental Death and Disability: the Neglected Disease of Modern Society.* Washington, DC: National Academy of Sciences, 1966.

19. Committee on Trauma, American College of Surgeons. Optimal hospital resources for care of the seriously injured. *Bull Am Coll Surg* 1976: **61**: 15–22.

20. American College of Emergency Physicians. Guidelines for trauma care systems. *Ann Emerg Med* 1987; **16**: 459.

21. Health Resources and Services Administration. *Model Trauma Care System Plan*. Rockville, MD: Department of Health and Human Services, 1992.

22. American College of Surgeons Committee on Trauma. *Advanced Trauma Life Support Program Student Course Manual*, 9th edition. Chicago, IL: ACS, 2012.

23. Mann NC, MacKenzie E, Teitelbaum SD, *et al.* Trauma care structure and viability in the current healthcare environment: a state-by-state assessment. *J Trauma* 2005; **58**: 136–47.

24. Hoyt DB, Coimbra R, Potenza BM. Trauma systems, triage, and transport. In Moore EE, Feliciano DV, Mattox KL, eds., *Trauma*. New York, NY: McGraw-Hill, 2004.

25. Sasser SM, Hunt RC, Faul M, *et al.*; Centers for Disease Control and Prevention (CDC). Guidelines for field triage of injured patients: recommendations of the National Expert Panel on Field Triage, 2011. *MMWR Recomm Rep* 2012; **61** (RR-1): 1–20.

26. Bulger EM, Maier RV. Prehospital care of the injured: what's new? *Surg Clin N Am* 2007; **87**: 37–53.

27. Hopson LR, Hirsh E, Delgado J, *et al.* Guidelines for withholding or termination of resuscitation in prehospital traumatic cardiopulmonary arrest: joint position statement of the National Association of EMS Physicians and the American College of Surgeons Committee on Trauma. *J Am Coll Surg* 2003; **196**: 106–12.

28. Pickens JJ, Copass MK, Bulger EM. Trauma patients receiving CPR: predictors of survival. *J Trauma* 2005; **58**: 951–8.

29. Esposito TJ, Crandall M, Reed RL, Gamelli RL, Luchette FA. Socioeconomic factors, medicolegal issues, and trauma patient transfer trends: is there a connection? *J Trauma* 2006; **61**: 1380–8.

Chapter

43

Trauma team training and simulation: creating safer outcomes

Paul Barach

Objectives

(1) Discuss the unique competencies that enable teams to perform reliably.
(2) Understand experiential learning and training tools such as simulation in enhancing the learning of trauma providers.
(3) Learn how team training and simulation can enable safer and more reflective trauma healthcare providers.
(4) Explore the role of microsystems in health care.
(5) Explore the role of rehearsal and simulation in training and assessment of trauma care providers.

Introduction

The role of effective teamwork in accomplishing complex tasks is well accepted in many domains. Similarly, there is good evidence that trauma care outcomes depend on effective and well-coordinated trauma team performance. Teamwork during trauma care can be deficient in a number of different ways (Table 43.1), and multiple deficiencies may interact to impair team success, distract team focus, and alter patient

Table 43.1 Problems and pitfalls in trauma teamwork

Difficulties coordinating conflicting actions
Poor communication among team members
Failure of members to function as part of a team
Reluctance to question the leader or more senior team members
Failure to prioritize task demands
Conflicting occupational cultures
Failure to establish and maintain clear roles and goals
Absence of experienced team members
Inadequate number of dedicated trauma team members
Failure to establish and maintain consistent supportive organizational infrastructure
Leaders without the "right stuff"

Modified from Schull et al. 2001,[1] and others.

outcomes. This chapter focuses on understanding, assessing, and improving trauma team performance.

The need to train and evaluate the performance of trauma teams has emerged as an important topic over the last decade.[2] Deficiencies in communication and teamwork have long been cited as frequent contributors to adverse events.[3] Conversely, team training and debriefing have been shown to reduce mortality by 18%.[4] Precise estimates of the extent of the problem are difficult to make, given definitional issues, as well as reporting and measurement problems. However, a variety of studies support the notion that teamwork and communication are critical components of safe healthcare systems. Previous reviews have reported linkages between various aspects of teamwork (e.g., situational monitoring, communication, leadership, trust, and shared mental models) and clinical performance.[5]

Excellent and consistent trauma quality requires an iterative evaluation that must include a review of secondary management, including careful delineation of team structure, command and control tools, thorough and ongoing team training, effective support structures, and continuous quality improvement. Valuable tools for trauma team training and performance improvement, discussed in this chapter, include microsystem-based assessment, process mapping, careful task analysis, reflective learning, rehearsal, debriefing, simulation, and videotape-based analysis.

Background

Higher education methods have shifted from *providing* instruction to *facilitating* successful learning opportunities that focus on engaging the learner. Interactive simulation environments support learner-focused, constructivist approaches that would be unethical, inefficient, and infeasible in actual trauma care situations. Team training has a long history in aviation and the military and, more recently, these experiences have been translated to health care. Studies of aviation teams reveal failures of coordination, communication, and workload management, loss of group situation awareness, and inability to use available resources effectively.[6–8] In thoroughly investigated adverse events, whether patient- or aviation-related, causes of failure were similarly multifactorial, team-based, and complex.[9–13]

Nearly all of health care is provided by interdisciplinary teams, either in the same or disparate locations. Individuals with diverse specialized skills focus on a common task in a defined period of time and space, and must respond flexibly together to contingencies and share responsibility for outcomes. This is particularly true of trauma care. Traditional specialty-centric clinical education and training are remiss because they assume that individuals acquire adequate competencies in teamwork passively without any formal training or rehearsal. Reviews of malpractice claims indicate that communication problems are major contributing factors in 24% of cases.[14] Substantial evidence suggests that teams routinely outperform individuals and are required to succeed in today's complex work arenas where information, cognition, and resources are widely distributed, technology is becoming more complicated, and workload is increasing.[15] Other studies using root cause analysis to examine contributing factors have found teamwork and communication issues as one of the main root causes in two-thirds of process failures and adverse events.[13] Our understanding of how medical teams coordinate in real-life situations, especially during time-constrained and crisis situations, remains incomplete.

Teams and teamwork
What is a team?

One must distinguish between a group of individuals sharing a common task (e.g., a jury) and a team (e.g., a marching band or a football team). A team is defined as "a small number of people with complementary skills who are committed to a common purpose, performance goals, and approach for which they hold themselves mutually accountable."[15] Weick and Roberts define medical teams as "a loosely coupled system of mutually interacting interdependent members and technology with a shared goal of patient care."[16] Katzenbach and Smith argue that any performance situation that warrants a team effort must meet three criteria: (1) collective work products must be delivered in real time by two or more people; (2) leadership roles must shift among the members; and (3) both mutual and individual accountability is necessary.[15] They go on to assert that teams must have a specific team purpose (distinct from that of its individual members), shared performance goals, and a commonly agreed-on working approach, and, in general, must make use of the team's collective work products to regularly evaluate the team's performance. Others have suggested that smaller teams (5–10 members) are generally more effective than larger ones, partially because of familiarity and loyalty, more cross-checking, and high interdependence of team members' roles.

Billington's 5 C's, as adapted by Barach and Weinger, identify five themes associated with effective teams (the 5 C's): Commitment, Common goals, Competence, Consistency (of performance), and Communication.[17,18] The effective team is committed to the achievement of specified goals. Team competence is measured across multiple dimensions and includes technical, non-technical decisional, and interpersonal skills. The diversity of team members with complementary skills is a hallmark of many effective teams, particularly when the team is required to adapt to complex and changing circumstances. Acute-care medical teams, including trauma teams, typically excel at the first two C's (i.e., commitment and common goals) and explicitly strive for competence, but may be much less successful in their consistency of performance (i.e., ability to sustain best practice reliably at all times) and effectiveness of communication between team members.[19] The very best trauma teams maintain an intuitive understanding and situational awareness of the evolving processes of events (see discussion below of team situation awareness), appreciate and anticipate the behaviors of others, prepare for the unknown with back-up plans, and exhibit a high level of trust and respect between members.[20]

Importance of conflict

Conflicts among members are inevitable in every team, and many experts believe that conflict, *and its successful resolution*, are essential to attaining maximal team performance.[1,21,22] The natural tendency, especially among healthcare professionals, is to avoid or gloss over conflicts. However, doing so may sow the seeds of impaired team performance when the conflicts arise. There are four primary conflicts inherent in teamwork.[23] First, there are tensions between individuals and the team as a whole in terms of goals, agenda, and the need to establish a coherent team identity. Second, to attain optimal team performance, one needs to foster both support and confrontation among team members. If team members are unwilling or unable to challenge each others' decisions respectfully, then there is a real risk of poor team outcomes – a team devoid of conflict leads to "group think"[24] and the acceptance of suboptimal team decisions. Third, daily team activities must balance moment-to-moment performance against the need to continually enhance team learning and individual member development. Finally, the team leader must find a balance between managerial authority, on the one hand, and individual team member autonomy and independence, on the other.

Team structure in the medical domain

The surgical trauma resuscitation microsystem is one of the most complex in health care and is centered around very ill patients, a large and diverse range of healthcare providers, sophisticated equipment, and severe time constraints.[18] The trauma team, which assembles rapidly at unpredictable times, must attempt to manage a sudden unique and chaotic situation involving one or more patients presenting with unknown injuries.

The successful management of trauma requires effectively coordinated prehospital care and information management followed by transfer to a well-organized and well-prepared emergency department or dedicated trauma facility. During the trauma resuscitation, the team typically adheres to hospital protocols based on Advanced Trauma Life Support (ATLS) principles. In most mature trauma teams, multiple team members have dedicated roles and simultaneously perform individual patient care tasks.[25,26] While more efficient and effective in achieving rapid resuscitation, this kind of horizontal structure requires team coordination, leadership, and organizational structure.[27] Studies in advanced trauma units have highlighted the difficulties of attaining effective teamwork, noting team breakdowns under dynamic and distracting conditions such as when a patient presents with multiple trauma injuries, or when dealing with numerous patients with traumatic injuries.

Trauma teams typically consist of 5–10 individuals from several clinical disciplines. Traumatologists, usually general surgeons or emergency medicine physicians, serve as team leaders; however, some programs – such as at the Toronto General Hospital and the Shock Trauma Center in Baltimore – have trained team leaders who may also be anesthesiologists.[28] Airway management is commonly performed by anesthesiologists or emergency physicians. Specialized trauma nurses as well as pharmacists, radiologic technicians, and other ancillary personnel (e.g., laboratory technician, orderlies, etc.) may round out the team together with residents in training and medical students. Predefined roles (specific task allocation) and even the marking of the physical location around the trauma patient in the trauma bay are commonly prescribed.

Medical teams, often consisting of a multidisciplinary group of members, might come together for a single clinical event (e.g., a specific surgical procedure) or be together for a short defined period (typically a month or so). Not infrequently, some team members are consistent and have well-defined roles (e.g., the intensive care unit team) while others join on an ad hoc or an as-needed basis (e.g., respiratory therapists, nurses, pharmacists, and anesthesiologists). Thus, a specific group of individuals does not have the opportunity to work together as a fixed team for long periods of time, hampering their learning. Further, trauma care is often provided in academic medical centers, where the trainees who make up much of the trauma team rotate on and off the team on a regular basis, which can lead to inconsistent care. Unfortunately, research in aviation shows that non-fixed or "rostered" teams (constantly changing personnel) are less effective than more stable "fixed" teams.[29] Additionally, Simon *et al.* have demonstrated that rostered teams are less likely than ad hoc teams to call each other out when safety infractions occur, but the rostered teams are more resilient and have better outcomes than non-rostered teams when challenged.[30]

The trauma team leader

The team leader's functions may include the performance of specific tasks such as the conduct of the primary and secondary surveys (Table 43.2). However, given sufficient personnel, the team leader must assume, as quickly as possible, a supervisory role, prioritizing and delegating tasks, and reviewing and overseeing the team's (and patient's) progress throughout

Table 43.2 The trauma team leader's responsibilities

Know the job (e.g., know ATLS guidelines expertly)

Communicate clearly and effectively, and enhance the team's communication

Foster teamwork attitudes through tangible behaviors

Keep the goals and approach relevant and focused

Enhance the team's knowledge and shared expectations

Build commitment, confidence, and trust

Remain positive and supportive, especially under adverse conditions

Acknowledge and manage your own limitations, and those of the team

Strengthen the skills of each team member, and of the team as a whole across all performance dimensions: technical, functional, problem solving, decision making, interpersonal, and teamwork

Manage relationships with outsiders and remove obstacles

Create opportunities for others to grow into leadership roles

Lead by personal example

Reward team performance and discourage individualism that detracts from team performance

Provide constructive feedback and opportunities for reflection and learning

Modified from Cooper and Wakelam 1999,[27] and others.
ATLS, Advanced Trauma Life Support.

the resuscitation.[31] Studies suggest that trauma teams are less effective when the team leader spends significant time performing procedures than when he or she delegates procedures to other team members. The team leader is most effective when anticipating problems and system breakdowns (maintaining feedforward abilities), to successfully improve the team's capability and response to distractions or disturbances in their workflow. However, the team leader should have recognized expertise in treating trauma patients, and should be willing and able to intercede when other team members are not performing to acceptable standards or are unable to perform a necessary procedure, or should the patient deteriorate.

The team leader is also responsible for formulating (or at least approving) the definitive treatment plan. Thus, the team leader must quickly assimilate a large amount of disparate information from other team members with his or her own observations and at times make a command decision. This leads to an overall assessment, which includes decisions about therapeutic and diagnostic interventions, communicating with other team members, coordinating consultations, making triage decisions, and ensuring that all team members are aware of the evolving situation.[32]

Although skill and experience are valuable for every member of the team, it is particularly critical for the trauma team leader. Studies suggest that the presence of a single

Table 43.3 Team leader personality types

"Right stuff"	"Wrong stuff"	"No stuff"
Active	Authoritarian	Unassertive
Self-confident	Arrogant	Low self-confidence
Interpersonal warmth/empathy	Limited warmth/empathy	Moderate warmth/empathy
Competitive	Impatient and irritable	Noncompetitive
Prefers challenging tasks	Prefers challenging tasks	Low desire for challenge
Strives for excellence	Strives for excellence	Doesn't strive for excellence

identified trauma resuscitation team leader leads to a better secondary survey, ATLS guideline adherence, and team coordination.[33] Additionally, the personality of the team leader has a large impact on team performance. Work by Chidester and colleagues,[33] based on studies by Foushee and Helmreich,[6] led to a broad classification of three personality types of team leaders: "right stuff," "wrong stuff," and "no stuff" (Table 43.3). Teams led by individuals with the "right stuff" performed better than others. Team-oriented behaviors do not come naturally in a culture that rewards individualism above teamwork, and that does not hold teams accountable for their outcomes, but these skills can be learned and practiced.

Acquiring expertise in the trauma setting

Data from over 100 surgical root cause analysis investigations in Australia demonstrate a number of recurrent themes that are relevant in understanding and improving trauma care.[13] These themes (Table 43.4) represent a mixture of the outcomes of clinical care (e.g., procedural complications) and explanations relating to complex and emerging problems in the clinical environment (e.g., skill mix of the surgical team, distractions, ineffective handoffs, and missed diagnoses).

The expert performance approach

The expert performance approach offers a systematic framework for examining issues related to improving patient safety.[34] It is based on an analysis of health provider superior performance and traces the acquired processes responsible for the development of high-level skills. The focus on measurable performance avoids documented shortcomings of traditional methods of identifying and studying experts, such as those based on the accumulation of knowledge, experience, and/or peer nomination. The expert performance approach proposes that learning and improvement in performance are not merely a passive accumulation of professional experience. Such gains are mediated by user engagement in goal-directed, self-regulated learning in a way that is quantitatively and qualitatively different from the mere accumulation of experiences.[35]

Table 43.4 Themes and issues identified from surgery-related root cause analysis

Theme	Issues identified
Failure to recognize or respond appropriately to the deteriorating patient within the required time frame	Postprocedure complications Infections Hypothermia
Workforce availability and skills	Orientation, training and supervision of new or junior members of the surgical team, especially outside of normal working hours
Transfer of patients for surgery	Difficulty in organizing an operating room for surgery Failure to hand over information about patient acuity
The management of trauma	Coordination and response of trauma teams Clinical decision making process for trauma patients Coordination of care between multiple clinicians
Access to emergency OR	Hemorrhage and emergency bleeding Urgent orthopedic procedure Urological complications requiring urgent OR Lack of trauma scheduling or lack of back up teams
Missed diagnosis	Thoracolumbar fracture in a trauma patient Subarachnoid hemorrhage thought to be drug overdose
Unexpected procedural complications	Airway obstruction Failed intubation
Sentinel events	Wrong level procedure – chest tube thoracostomy at wrong level Retained surgical products requiring surgical removal

The analysis is derived from a metropolitan health service, Sydney, NSW, Australia. Personal communication, Deputy Director for Clinical Governance, January 2007.

Research shows that experienced and knowledgeable individuals do not always outperform naive individuals.[36] Highly experienced financial, medical, and psychology professionals often fail to make superior forecasts or implement interventions that lead to enhanced treatment outcomes when compared with less-qualified and less-experienced professionals. Experts are typically identified on the basis of peer nomination, the degree of knowledge each seemingly possess, or their length of experience within the domain. In medicine, researchers have reported that the length of professional experience is often unrelated, and sometimes negatively related, to the quality of performance and treatment outcomes.[37] Ericsson and Smith suggest that researchers interested in studying expertise should focus on trying to empirically capture performance with reliable and objective measures.[38] They recommend a three-step approach known as the *expert performance approach.*

First, researchers must recreate the task(s) in the laboratory with sufficient fidelity to elicit the requisite expertise. Second, the antecedents of, and processes responsible for, superior performance should be identified using experimental manipulations and process tracing measures. Third, activities that lead to performance improvement need to be identified so that the path to excellence is clearly delineated and is targeted for training and improvement.[39]

In the 1980s, researchers began to study the way experienced people make decisions in their natural environments or in simulations that preserve key aspects of their environments (naturalistic decision theory).[40] These studies showed that, in contrast to "normative decision theory," experts make real-world decisions through a serial evaluation and application ("trying on") of options that seem appropriate to the apparent situation. The naturalistic decision-making (NDM) theory argues then that, especially under time pressure in complex task domains (e.g., flight landing, trauma units), experts recognize patterns of events in situations, or their integral components, as typical or familiar, and then respond to each specific situation with appropriate preprogrammed, patterned responses. Choosing the first acceptable response that comes to them is called "recognition-primed decision making."[40,41] Thus, competent decision makers in complex domains are very concerned about quickly assessing and reassessing the situation, always maintaining awareness of the current clinical situation. They key is to make rapid decisions and assess how the system responds to the purported decision and actions while being prepared to change course as needed.

Expertise is more than simply having extensive factual knowledge – it also includes complementary skills and attitudes and the ability to deploy these skills in a timely, measured, and precise manner. Experts have specific psychologic traits (e.g., self-confidence, excellent communication skills, adaptability, and risk tolerance) and cognitive skills (e.g., highly developed attention, sense of what is relevant, ability to identify exceptions to the rules, flexibility to changing situations, effective performance under stress, and ability to make decisions and initiate actions quickly based on incomplete data). Clinical experts use highly refined decision strategies such as dynamic feedback, decomposing and analyzing complex problems, and prethinking solutions to tough situations.[42]

A key attribute of expertise in trauma care is the ability to anticipate or to predict what might happen to a patient given his or her injuries and the resources available. Mental simulation including rehearsal, whereby individuals *or teams* envision (simulate) a possible future clinical event or clinical action before it happens, is essential to gaining the expertise to make diagnoses and to perform or function during an evolving or future real event. When expert clinicians simulate situations and actions mentally before they undertake them in real life, the evidence suggests that they save time and improve performance in crucial situations (see simulation section below).[43]

Human factors in the trauma environment

Human factors research on team decision making in complex task environments is of relevance to trauma team performance. One must carefully consider the impact of the many "performance-shaping factors" that can degrade human capabilities (Table 43.5).

Table 43.5 Examples of performance-shaping factors affecting trauma care

Performance-shaping factor	Example
Individual factors	Clinical knowledge, skills, and abilities Cognitive biases Risk preference [a] State of health Fatigue (including sleep deprivation, circadian)
Task factors	Task distribution Task demands Workload Job burnout Shiftwork
Team/communication	Teamwork/team dynamics Interpersonal communication (clinician–clinician and clinician–patient) Interpersonal influence Groupthink [b]
Environment of care	Noise Lighting Temperature and humidity Motion and vibration Physical constraints (e.g., crowding) Distractions
Equipment/tools	Device usability Alarms and warnings Automation Maintenance and obsolescence Protective gear
Organizational/cultural	Production pressure Culture of safety (vs. efficiency) Policies and procedures Documentation requirements Staffing cross coverage Hierarchical structure Reimbursement policies Training programs

[a] Tendency to choose a risky or less risky option
[b] Desire for conformity in the group resulting in an incorrect or deviant decision-making outcome.

Situation awareness

One of the most important decision-making skills in trauma care is to decide what to devote attention to and what can wait. Where data overload is the rule and the patient's status changes continually, the ability to recognize clinical cues quickly and completely, to detect patterns, and to set aside distracting or unimportant data can be life-saving. Situation awareness (or situation assessment) is a comprehensive and coherent representation of the (patient's) current state that is continuously updated based on repetitive assessment.[44] Situation awareness appears to be an essential prerequisite for the safe operation of any complex dynamic system or complex team interaction. In the case of trauma care, establishing and maintaining a "mental model" of the state of the trauma patient and the associated trauma unit facilities, equipment, and personnel is essential to effective situation awareness. Successful team situation awareness requires constant communication that enables members to converge around a shared mental model of the situation and course of action and quickly course-correct as needed.[45] Effective teams adapt to changes in task requirements, anticipate each other's actions and needs, monitor the team's ongoing performance, and offer constructive feedback to other team members.[46] When team members share a common mental model of the team's ongoing activities, they all may "instinctively" know what each of their teammates will do next (and why), and they often communicate their intentions and needs nonverbally (sometimes called implicit communication).

A systematic approach to the evaluation of teamwork training

Assessing team performance is key to developing and implementing methods to improve team performance, patient safety, and patient outcomes (Table 43.6). There is an ongoing argument in the literature that team *process* and *outcomes* must be distinguished.[47] Process is defined by the activities, strategies, responses, and behaviors employed by the team during task accomplishment, while outcomes are the clinical outcomes of the patients cared for by the team. Process measures are important for training, when the purpose of performance measurement is to diagnose performance problems and to provide feedback to trainees. Until recently, the medical community has focused more on outcomes than on process. Medical educators have begun to appreciate the competencies that define effective team processes and lead to entrustment by other colleagues.[13,48] The key is to identify and measure processes that are directly related to patient outcomes (e.g., successful resuscitation). Perhaps most importantly, the results of the assessment must be translatable into specific feedback that will enhance team learning and performance.[49]

There is a variety of methods to support the team's ability to authentically reflect and evaluate their team performance, including debriefing with or without the use of videotaping,

Table 43.6 Questions to ask when assessing or auditing the performance of a trauma team

Is the team the right size and composition?
Are there adequate levels of complementary skills?
Is there a shared goal for the team?
Does everyone understand the team goals?
Has a set of performance goals been agreed upon?
Do the team members hold one another accountable for the group's results?
Are there shared protocols and performance ground rules?
Is there mutual respect and trust between team members?
Does the team leader instill trust and mutual respect by the team members?
Do team members communicate effectively?
Do team members know and appreciate each other's roles and responsibilities?
When one team member is absent or not able to perform his or her assigned tasks, are other team members able to pitch in or help appropriately?

simulation with or without standardized patients, and the use of trained observers. Although metrics are available in non-medical domains, there are few well-defined validated metrics to assess competency in complex clinical team activities such as trauma resuscitation. No rigorous evaluation studies have been undertaken that relate the training experience to actual clinical outcomes, thereby validating metrics for assessing team performance.

Simulations that use pre-scripted learner-focused scenarios not only ensure that relevant competencies are being assessed, but also ease the assessment process because instructors know when key events will occur.[50] Evaluation, both formative and summative, must provide a basis for diagnosing skill deficiencies. In other words, it is not enough that a simulation captures performance outcomes; it must also evaluate the process of moment-to-moment actions and reactions to help design more effective care.

Video analysis of trauma care

Videotaping team performance can be a tremendously valuable training tool, because it ascertains what transpired, and helps both trainees and seasoned clinicians to clearly visualize their performance. Coaches can record voice-over analysis for team members, draw notes on the clips to illustrate the exact goals of each skill, and view videos side by side.

These tools (Ubersense is an app that does this similarly in sports) can be used as a permanent record or as an archive for future educational activities. Beginning with the experience of Hoyt *et al.* in the late 1980s,[51] videotaping and review of resuscitations has become a standard quality assurance method for many trauma centers. Subsequent work has confirmed the benefits from improved team education and training, more efficient and accurate quality assurance (QA) processes, interventions to improve care processes, and better patient survival.[33,52] In a study of simulated anesthetic crises, trainees' review of videotape of the events led to decreases in "time to treat" and workload in subsequent simulations.[53] Scherer *et al.* found that video-based feedback of trauma resuscitations reduced patient disposition time by 50%.[54]

However, videotaping of patient care requires overcoming substantial obstacles, including consent and privacy issues, medicolegal concerns, confidentiality, logistical and resource issues, and analytical limitations.[55,56] Nevertheless, the ability of multiple raters/experts to score performance from videotape allows the evaluation of the inter-rater reliability of performance assessment metrics. In a simulation-based study, investigators used videotape to develop and assess a systematic rating system of behavioral and clinical markers with the objective of creating effective team-training and assessment programs – they found a high correlation among different observers.[57]

Simulation for trauma team training and assessment

There are substantial ethical and educational limitations to the use of patients for the clinical training of individuals and teams. The opportunities to learn and practice desired responses to uncommon events or types of injuries can be quite limited, even in a busy trauma center.[58] In fact, actual trauma resuscitations are not optimal training opportunities, because patient care takes precedence over teaching. Meaningful learning occurs after events, when there is time to review those events and reflect on what worked well. Moreover, trauma resuscitations may occur in an uncontrolled environment under time-pressure constraints. Societal and regulatory pressures will increasingly limit the use of real patients, especially critically ill ones, for hands-on clinical training.[59]

High-fidelity simulators – medical simulators – allow educators to provide repeatable, controlled clinical scenarios without jeopardizing patient health.[60] The simulation environment allows concurrent assessment of response processes while increasing competency training. Simulation training enables trainees to become proficient before treating patients.[61] The fidelity offered by simulators provides the best approximation of the novelty that may be encountered when performing other complicated clinical procedures in real life on real patients. Although access to simulation tools and approaches is rapidly expanding, there is no general agreement about optimal processes, simulator device specifications, metrics to evaluate curricula or their effectiveness, standardized performance measures, or validated simulator protocols for training.

Simulation has been widely touted as a tool to improve clinical care through enhanced training and evaluation. Simulations can include patient actors (e.g., standardized

Table 43.7 Essential skills in trauma crew resource management courses

Adaptability

Prioritization of tasks

Shared situation awareness and distribution of the workload

Team communication before and after patient arrival

Mobilization and use of all resources in the trauma care that extends to the operating room, intensive care unit, and diagnostic facilities

Performance monitoring and crosschecking of data and team functions

Command, communication, and coordination of feedback

Leadership and management of the team members ability to accept leadership

Willingness to challenge each other and resolve conflict

Adapted, in part, from *The Role of the Team Leader*, Team Training Series, Book 3. Orlando, FL: Naval Air Warfare Center Training Systems Division, and others.[64]

patients),[62] personal computer (PC)-based partial task trainers,[61] or full-scale realistic patient simulation (discussed below).[60] Simulation is an essential training tool in almost every other high-risk domain including aviation, space flight, military operations, nuclear and hydroelectric power generation, ground and sea transportation, and chemical process control.[63]

There are many benefits of medical simulation and crew resource management (Table 43.7). Simulations can permit clinicians to learn new or to improve old techniques safely and economically without posing harm to patients or to trainees.[60,63] Simulations can be controlled and modulated according to a team's needs.[58] Decision-making skills can be embedded into the scenario to train for reasoning, metacognition (thinking about thinking, or an appreciation of what one already knows), risk assessment skills, and responsiveness to adverse events.[59] Guided practice with video-based feedback that incorporates measures of performance can be considered managed experience.[65] Lessons taught in a realistic simulation environment may be retained better, due to ability to review events again and again, the active learning and focused concentration, and the direct association with real-world clinical events. Thus, trauma teams using simulation can train, evaluate, and credential providers before letting them join clinical activities.

The literature has begun to provide evidence for the value of realistic patient simulation (RPS) to train and evaluate trauma teams.[66] A study by Holcomb *et al.* evaluated 10 three-trainee teams before and after a 1-month trauma center rotation using RPS scenarios.[67] The teams showed significant improvement on multiple measures of technical and nontechnical skills, supporting the face validity of RPS-based technical performance assessment. Lee *et al.* conducted a prospective randomized controlled trial of surgical interns' trauma assessment and management skills after using either RPS or moulage practice training sessions.[68] RPS-trained interns scored higher on trauma assessment skills and on the management of an acute neurologic event.

Rehearsal and warm-up: new and evolving concepts

Rehearsal and warm-up aim to improve both operator and team performance by improving manual dexterity, mental agility, confidence, communication, and workflow. Rehearsal is considered the practice of technical and nontechnical skills specific to a procedure, while warm-up is defined as "the act or process of warming up for a contest, by light exercise or practice."[69] In health care, warm-up may be considered the practice of motor or mental exercises not specific to a procedure, when undertaken immediately prior to the task being performed. For example, the use of a high-fidelity simulator by the operator to place virtual stents, prior to performing a coronary artery angiogram, is considered rehearsal, while practicing manual dexterity skills using a low-fidelity simulator prior to arterial cannulation is considered a warm-up. Rehearsal and warm-up are gaining increasing recognition as important processes in enhancing team performance and improving patient safety, whether for acquiring competencies or for maintaining procedural and technical proficiency.[70,71] However, more work needs to be done to assess how best to use these methods for assessing expertise.

Realistic patient simulation (RPS)

Realistic patient simulators are fully interactive physical simulations in which the device's responses to clinical interventions are scripted to be realistic. In the highest-fidelity simulators, the mannequin's response is based on detailed physiologic and pharmacologic computer models. The goal is for the simulator to respond to clinical interventions similarly to how a patient would respond. Thus, the participant interacts with a realistic cognitive and physical representation of the full acute-care environment and thereby experiences emotional and physiologic responses similar to those experienced in real patient-care situations.[72]

Realistic patient simulators consist of a computer-controlled system and a plastic patient mannequin that generates physiologic signals such as electrocardiogram, invasive and noninvasive blood pressure, lung sounds, and palpable pulses, which allows for realistic airway management.[60,72] The mannequin's head contains a speaker so that the participant can converse with the patient when contextually appropriate. Participants can query the operator as needed concerning physical signs not reproduced by the mannequin, such as skin color and diaphoresis. There are multiple technical, financial, and methodologic issues that affect the design and implementation of RPS-based training programs.[63,73] Nonetheless, patient simulators have facilitated study of the response to critical incidents, the occurrence of medical error, the role of teamwork, and the effects of other factors on clinical performance.

Scenario design

Oser and colleagues have outlined specific steps for developing simulated scenarios for eliciting team behaviors.[74] First, skill inventories and historical performance data are reviewed to identify what needs to be measured (cognitive task analysis). Identifying the core measurement objectives builds content validity into the scenario. Second, scenario events are created that provide specific reproducible opportunities to observe performance related to the objectives chosen. Third, performance measures are developed that accurately and reliably assess performance of the objectives. Measures should have the ability to describe *what* happened (i.e., outcome measures) in addition to describing *why* certain outcomes were or were not attained (i.e., process measures).

Simulation training and debriefing

A typical simulation-based training course will include a pretest, preparatory didactics (lecture, web, or hands-on demonstrations), the performance of one or more standardized scripted scenario(s) that are videotaped, postsimulation videotape-based debriefing, and a posttraining evaluation of both the trainee and the training experience. The debriefing is the most important experience, especially when doing multidisciplinary team training.[75] Debriefing should occur immediately after each simulation scenario and not uncommonly can last longer than the scenario itself. However, there are surprisingly few papers in the peer-reviewed literature to illustrate how to effectively debrief, how to teach or learn to debrief, or which is the best of three models of debriefing and how effective they are at achieving learning objectives and goals (Table 43.8).

Debriefing is the most important component of the clinical simulation experience, because it allows learners to reflect on and interpret their performance. At the conclusion of each simulation scenario, participants are given the opportunity to review their experience and will benefit by obtaining feedback from their peers and faculty. Skilled instructors may choose to utilize digital recordings of scenarios to enhance the debriefing process. This can be accomplished using simultaneous digital recording to DVD, Quicktime, and Flash formats using multiple video cameras strategically placed in each lab. Faculty are able to annotate and timestamp the videos as each scenario unfolds so that during the debriefing the exact spot in the case can be accessed without delay. Participants are able to review the digital recordings for purposes of self-evaluation and in order to obtain immediate constructive feedback.

The organizational context
The role of clinical microsystems

Teams exist within the context of a system. A system is a set of interacting, interrelated, or independent elements that work together in a particular environment to perform the functions that are required to achieve a specific aim.[76] A clinical

Table 43.8 Three debriefing models

Thatcher and Robinson model

1. Identifying the impact of the experience
2. Identifying and considering the processes which developed
3. Clarifying the facts, concepts, and principles
4. Identifying the ways in which emotion was involved
5. Identifying the different views which each of the participants formed

Lederman model

1. Introduction to the systematic reflection and analysis
2. Intensification and personalization of the analysis of the experience
3. Generalization and application of the experience

Petranek model

1. Events
2. Emotions
3. Empathy
4. Explanations and analysis
5. Everyday applicability
6. Employment of information
7. Evaluation

From Thatcher DC, Robinson MJ. *An Introduction to Games and Simulations in Education*. Hants: Solent Simulations, 1985; Lederman LC. Differences that make a difference: intercultural communication, simulation, and the debriefing process in diverse interaction. Presented at the Annual Conference of the International Simulation and Gaming Association, Kyoto, Japan, July 15–19, 1991; Petranek C. Maturation in experiential learning: principles of simulation and gaming. *Simul Gaming* 1994; 513–22.

Table 43.9 Ten dimensions of clinical microsystems

1. Leadership
2. Organizational support of clinicians
3. Staff focus
4. Education and training
5. Interdependence of team members
6. Patient focus
7. Community and market focus
8. Performance results
9. Process improvement
10. Information and information technology

microsystem is a group of clinicians and staff working together with a shared clinical purpose to provide care for a population of patients.[77] The clinical purpose and its setting define the essential components of the microsystem, which include clinicians, patients, and support staff; information and technology; and specific care processes and behaviors that are required to provide care. The best microsystems evolve over time, as they respond to the needs of their patients and providers, as well as to the external pressures such as regulatory requirements. They often coexist with other microsystems within a larger (macro) organization, such as a hospital.[78]

The conceptual theory of the clinical microsystem is based on ideas developed by Deming and others.[79] Deming applied systems thinking to organizational development, leadership, and improvement. The seminal idea for the clinical microsystem stems from the work of James Quinn.[80] Quinn's work is based on analyzing the world's best-of-best service organizations, such as FedEx, Mary Kay Cosmetics, McDonald's, and Nordstrom. Quinn focused on determining what these extraordinary organizations were doing to achieve consistent, high-quality, explosive growth, high margins, and robust consumer loyalty. He found that these leading service organizations were organized around, and continually engineered, the front-line relationships that connected the needs of customers with the organization's core competency. Quinn called this front-line activity that embedded the service delivery process the *smallest replicable unit* or the *minimum replicable unit*. This

smallest replicable unit, or the microsystem, is the key to implementing a reliable, effective strategy to provide safe and consistent outcomes.

Teams make up a microsystem that also includes knowledge, equipment, and work tasks. The microsystem concept is based on an understanding of systems theory coupled with Quinn's theory of a smallest replicable unit.[80] Nelson and his colleagues have described the essential elements of a microsystem as (1) a core team of healthcare professionals; (2) a defined population they care for; (3) an information environment to support the work of caregivers and patients; and (4) support staff, equipment, and the work environment.[81] Linking performance and outcome data to the microsystem model provides a helpful way to identify potential areas for improvement that does not focus on the individual, but instead on the system that is enabling or inhibiting the processes and outcomes of care.[78,82]

In the late 1990s, Donaldson and Mohr investigated high-performing clinical microsystems.[83] The research was based on a national search for the highest-quality clinical microsystems. Forty-three clinical units were identified using a sampling methodology. Semistructured interviews were conducted with leaders from each of the microsystems. Additional research built on the Donaldson and Mohr study collected 20 case studies of high-performing microsystems, included on-site interviews with every member of the microsystems, and analyzed individual microsystem performance data.[84] The analysis of the interviews suggested that 10 dimensions, shown in Table 43.9, were associated with effective and successful microsystems.

Teamwork protocols and patient transitions

The most common factor cited as a cause of failure in teamwork is lack of effective and meaningful communication between team members, feedback, and ongoing learning. One issue that deserves investigation is the extent to which standardized communication protocols, similar to those used in military and aviation environments, can enhance teamwork and improve patient safety. In observations focused on patient handoffs from the intraoperative to postoperative team,[85] as well as intensive care unit handoffs from operating room team members,[86] there was no constancy in the information that was transferred or in the order in which it was transferred. The result was that important information was sometimes omitted.[87] Recipients did not detect the missing information because they did not have the cognitive scaffolding that a standard briefing protocol with an expected set of parameters would provide. Recent papers on the power of surgical checklists to reduce several intraoperative adverse events reinforce this point.[88] Issues raised by these studies include the need for organizing research into the types of errors that providers are susceptible to during the sign-out process, roles of personality, experience, and cultural factors. These factors may affect the incoming provider's inquisitiveness, and the potential impact on patient care depending on the methods of signing out. A standardized handoff protocol could decrease the cognitive burden of the information on the handoff recipients and induce fewer errors and ultimately better and safer care.[89,90]

The wider organizational environment

Teams do not exist in isolation. The performance of an individual team, as well as the team's attitudes toward patient safety, is a function of the milieu, or the culture, in which the team is required to function. Thus, the effectiveness of any particular team cannot be properly assessed without considering the larger system within which the team functions. In a hospital environment, small teams, such as operating teams, coordinate with other teams within the perioperative microsystem environment that are involved in patient care, and these teams are embedded within larger teams that are directly and indirectly involved in patient care. When looking at the effectiveness of teamwork training for patient safety, one must know how training is supported and reinforced by the organizational culture, the leadership, and the overall sense of psychogical safety in which the team works.

Factors that need to be addressed include:[85]

- Organizational climate. Does the organizational culture support striving for patient safety? Does it allow for nonpunitive reporting of problems and near misses? Do staff members feel safe to speak up about their concerns?
- Organizational support. Is time for training provided whereby trainees and/or staff are temporarily relieved of their regular duties? Is training viewed as more than just a necessary checkmark? Is teamwork training widespread and rewarded across the organization?
- Extent of training. Does the organization only train isolated teams? Does the training of trauma teams incorporate the "wider" team members (e.g., blood bank, radiology, transport, rehab, hospital and unit management)?

Training approach and quality

There are a number of factors that impact on the effectiveness of team training, including:

- Training protocol. How is training achieved? What methods are used to impart knowledge? How are practice and feedback incorporated into training?

- Trainer skill. Is the individual who is in charge of leading the training and providing feedback adequately trained?
- Practice medium and method. How is team practice carried out? What simulation environment is used (e.g., mannequin, virtual, video)? How much practice is given? It is possible that a teamwork training program that does not yield improvements in teamwork may be pedagogically sound, but may require more opportunities for practice and feedback in order to show quantitatively detectable improvements?
- Training intensity. Is it more effective to conduct training over a short time period (e.g., 1–2 days) or to conduct training over a longer time period (e.g., 2–3 hours per week for several weeks)? Which is less disruptive for the trainees and for the system in which they work?

Research recommendations

Team performance measures must be grounded in team pedagogical theory, account for individual and team-level performance, capture team process and outcomes, adhere to standards for reliability and validity, and address real or perceived barriers to measurement.[5] A number of guidelines and recommendations for research on teamwork training effectiveness can be made. The recommendations are organized into those that can be achieved in nearer-term (1–2 years) research and those that can be considered after the initial research phase is well under way (3–5 years).

Nearer-term recommendations

- Clearly specify the training objectives. What knowledge, skills, and attitudes (KSAs) are being trained based on local practice?
- Design scenarios that link scenario events to training objectives. These scenarios could be developed from reported team errors or near misses in which specified teamwork skills were lacking. Ensure that the scenario includes events that trigger trainees to perform the specific competencies targeted for training in that scenario.
- Describe a set of scenarios that can be used to evaluate the effectiveness of varying training programs. Specify the training objectives that each scenario is suitable for evaluating.
- Develop and apply observer-based measures of teamwork process to medical teams. This will allow researchers to assess whether and, if so, which teamwork KSAs improve with training.
- Support multiple research studies in which training is evaluated using a common set of scenarios and common measurement instruments.
- Support training oriented to multidisciplinary teams so that medical team members train in the teamwork context in which they work.
- Train intact teams. Strive to train organic teams, and study whether training carries over to participation in newly formed teams.

Longer-term considerations

- Introduce declarative and procedural knowledge related to the critical components of teamwork early, and reinforce this knowledge throughout the healthcare professional's curriculum and professional development.

- Study the effect of incorporating into training communication protocols (such as readback and a standardized communication form for handoffs) for enhancing communication and team situation awareness.

- Carry out similar training in multiple environments to assess the effects of human factors, environmental factors (e.g., noise, distractions), and organizational factors on training effectiveness and uptake.

- Research training factors (such as amount of practice and quality of feedback) that impact the degree to which teamwork training is effective in promoting high-quality patient care and patient safety.

- Develop a licensure and certification process to assess and regulate healthcare providers' teamwork-related competence.

- Assess the role of simulation in advancing team training and patient safety.

Conclusions

Effective teams make consistently fewer mistakes than do individuals, especially when each team member knows his/her responsibilities, as well as those of the other team members. However, simply bringing individuals together to perform a specified task does not automatically ensure that they will function as a team. The role of the clinical microsystem as the unit of training and measurement is key.[91] Trauma teamwork depends on a willingness of clinicians from diverse backgrounds to cooperate toward a shared goal, communicate, work together effectively, and improve.

Each team member must be able to: (1) anticipate the needs of the others and ideally develop trust in their competencies; (2) adjust to others' actions and to the changing environment; (3) monitor others' activities and distribute the workload dynamically; and (4) have a shared understanding of accepted processes, and how events and actions should proceed (shared mental model).

Teams outperform individuals especially when performance requires multiple diverse skills, judgment, and experience under time constraints. Nevertheless, most people in health care overlook team-based opportunities for improvement because training and infrastructure are designed around individuals and incentives are all individual-based. Teams with clear goals and effective communication strategies can adjust to new information with speed and effectiveness to enhance real-time problem solving. Individual behaviors among team members are more readily amenable to change, perhaps because team identity is less threatened by change than are individuals.

Future work should continue to evaluate the impact and sustainability of team training. This includes evaluating the impact of team training on patient safety outcomes, evaluating team training in other settings (e.g., primary care and outpatient dialysis care settings), examining the comparative effectiveness of different methods for delivering team training, and examining implementation methods to support sustaining behavior changes achieved through training. For example, there is little evidence available to date that provides insight into the frequency of retraining or dedicated practice needed to develop and maintain effective teamwork skills. Additionally, there is a need to examine how dynamic team composition (i.e., changes in team membership, absence of key members) moderates team processes and the effects of team training.

Turning trauma care experts into expert trauma teams requires substantial planning and practice. There is a natural resistance to move beyond individual roles and accountability to the team mindset. One can facilitate this commitment by: (1) fostering a shared awareness of each member's tasks and role on the team through cross-training and other team-training modalities; (2) training members in specific teamwork skills such as communication, situation awareness, leadership, "followership," resource allocation, and adaptability; (3) conducting team training in simulated scenarios with a focus on both team behaviors and technical skills; (4) training trauma team leaders in the necessary leadership competencies to build and maintain effective teams; and (5) establishing reliable and trust-building methods of team performance evaluation and rapid feedback.

The roadmap for future research must include how teamwork training should be structured, delivered, and evaluated to optimize patient safety in the perioperative setting. For teamwork skills to be assessed and have credibility, team performance measures must be grounded in team theory, account for individual and team-level performance, capture team process and outcomes, adhere to standards for reliability and validity, and address real or perceived barriers to measurement. The interdisciplinary nature of work in the trauma environment and the necessity of cooperation among the team members play an important role in enabling patient safety and avoiding errors.

Acknowledgments

This chapter is partially based on Barach P, Weinger M. Trauma team performance. In Wilson WC, Grande CM, Hoyt DB, eds. *Trauma: Resuscitation, Anesthesia, and Critical Care*. New York, NY: Marcel Dekker, 2006; and on Entin EB, Lai F, Barach P. Training teams for the perioperative environment: a research agenda. *Surg Innov* 2006; **13**: 170–8.

Questions

(1) Which statement concerning the identification of medical errors and adverse events is true?

    a. Machines consistently identify medical errors better than human reporting

    b. Voluntary reporting of adverse events is known to underreport the incidence and severity of these events

    c. Fear of consequences is the likely cause of most underreported adverse events

d. All of the above are true

(2) **Which of the following is an example of a simulator?**
    a. Autopsy
    b. Computer-controlled anesthesia mannequin
    c. Screen-based flight simulator
    d. All of the above

(3) **The following has been proved about simulators:**
    a. Practicing in a simulator improves clinical outcomes
    b. Practicing in a simulator saves lives
    c. Practicing in a simulator improves performance in a simulator

(4) **Disasters are fun to analyze because:**
    a. We keep finding new ways to create disasters
    b. They make great shows on National Geographic and the Learning Channel
    c. Analyzing them helps us identify patterns of mistakes

(5) **Computerized physician order entry is advocated for patient safety because the physicians who actively enter data into a computer:**
    a. Can have immediate access to electronic medical references during data entry
    b. Can be presented with patient care reminders that reduce errors of omission
    c. Can be offered real-time decision support during data entry to reduce errors
    d. All of the above

(6) **Medication errors are a blend of:**
    a. Human error and human fallibility
    b. Human error and system error
    c. System error and cybernetic failures
    d. Human error, system error, and design failure

(7) **Medication errors:**
    a. Account for at least 7000 deaths annually
    b. Account for more than 7000 deaths annually
    c. Account for fewer than 7000 deaths annually
    d. Are the most frequent medically adverse event and account for more than 7000 deaths annually

(8) **Choose one theme that is *not* associated with effective teams.**
    a. Commitment
    b. Common goals
    c. Corporate goals
    d. Competence
    e. Communication

(9) **When assessing a trauma team's performance, which of the following is *not* essential to look for:**
    a. Is the team the right size and composition?
    b. Has a set of performance goals been agreed upon?

    c. Is there mutual respect and trust between team members?
    d. Do team members communicate effectively?
    e. Do the team members get paid enough?

(10) **The presence of a well-qualified trauma team leader enhances trauma team performance. Concerning the trauma team leader's responsibilities, which of the following are *incorrect*? Choose *two answers*.**
    a. Know the job (e.g., know ATLS guidelines cold)
    b. Be attractive
    c. Communicate clearly and effectively, and enhance the team's communication
    d. Foster teamwork attitudes through tangible behaviors
    e. Build commitment, confidence, and trust
    f. Remain positive and supportive, especially under adverse conditions
    g. Acknowledge and manage your own limitations, and those of the team
    h. Manage relationships with outsiders and remove obstacles
    i. Be the physically strongest member

(11) **Trauma teams make up a clinical microsystem working to achieve optimal patient outcomes. Which of the following are *not* essential dimensions of a trauma clinical microsystem? Choose *two answers*:**
    a. Organizational support
    b. Staff focus
    c. Education and training
    d. Interdependence
    e. Doctorate-level training
    f. Patient focus
    g. Performance results
    h. Information and information technology
    i. Great location

Answers

(1) d
(2) d
(3) c
(4) c
(5) d
(6) d
(7) d
(8) c
(9) e
(10) b, i
(11) e, i

References

1. Schull MJ, Ferris LE, Tu JV, *et al.* Problems for clinical judgement, 3. Thinking clearly in an emergency. *CMAJ* 2001; **164**: 1170–5.

2. Khetarpal S, Steinbrunn BS, McGonigal M, *et al.* Trauma faculty and trauma team activation: Impact on trauma system function and patient outcome. *J Trauma* 1999; **47**: 576–81.

3. Weaver SJ, Rosen MA, DiazGranados D, *et al.* Does teamwork improve performance in the operating room? A multilevel evaluation. *Jt Comm J Qual Patient Saf* 2010; **36**: 133–42.

4. Neily J, Mills PD, Young-Xu Y, *et al.* Association between implementation of a medical team training program and surgical mortality. *JAMA* 2010; **304**: 1693–700.

5. Baker D, Battles J, King H, Salas E, Barach P. The role of teamwork in the professional education of physicians: current status and assessment recommendations. *Jt Comm J Qual Patient Saf* 2005; **31**: 185–202.

6. Foushee HC, Helmreich RL. Group interaction and flight crew performance. In Wiener EL, Nagel DC, eds., *Human Factors in Aviation*. San Diego, CA: Academic Press, 1988, pp. 189–227.

7. Jones DG, Endsley MR. Sources of situation awareness errors in aviation. *Aviat Space Environ Med* 1996; **67**: 507–12.

8. Kanki BG, Lozito S, Foushee HC. Communication indices of crew coordination. *Aviat Space Environ Med* 1989; **60**: 56–60.

9. Reason J. *Human Error*. Cambridge: Cambridge University Press, 1990.

10. Reason J. Understanding adverse events: human factors. *Qual Health Care* 1995; **4**: 80–9.

11. Perrow C. *Normal Accidents: Living with High-Risk Technologies*. New York, NY: Basic Books, 1984.

12. Kletz T. *Learning from Accidents*, 2nd edition. Oxford: Butterworth-Heinemann, 1994.

13. Cassin BR, Barach PR. Making sense of root cause analysis investigations of surgery-related adverse events. *Surg Clin North America* 2012; **92**: 101–15.

14. Rogers SO, Gawande AA, Kwaan M, *et al.* Analysis of surgical errors in closed malpractice claims at 4 liability insurers. *Surgery* 2006; **140**: 25–33.

15. Katzenbach JR, Smith DK. *The Wisdom of Teams: Creating the High Performance Organization*. Cambridge, MA: Harvard Business School Press, 1993.

16. Weick KE, Roberts KH. Collective mind in organizations: heedful interrelating on flight decks. *Admin Sci Q* 1993; **38**: 357–81.

17. Billington J. The three essentials of an effective team. *Harvard Business School Management Update.* 1997; **2**: 1–4.

18. Barach P, Weinger M. Trauma team performance. In Wilson WC, Grande CM, Hoyt DB, eds., *Trauma: Resuscitation, Anesthesia, & Critical Care*. New York, NY: Marcel Dekker, 2006.

19. Donchin Y, Gopher d, Olin M, *et al.* A look into the nature and causes of human errors in the intensive care unit. *Crit Care Med* 1995; **23**: 294–300.

20. Weick K. Prepare your organization to fight fires. *Harvard Business Review* 1996; #96311.

21. . Lenconi P. *The Five Dysfunctions of a Team*. San Francisco, CA: Jossey-Bass, 2002.

22. Aram JD. Individual and group. In *Dilemmas of Administrative Behavior*. Englewood Cliffs, NJ: Prentice-Hall, 1976, pp. 75–95.

23. Hill LA. Managing your team. *Harvard Business School Teaching Note.* March 28, 1995; 9–494–081.

24. Janis IL. *Groupthink: Psychology Today*. New York, NY: Ziff-Davis, 1971.

25. Driscoll PA, Vincent CA. Organizing an efficient trauma team. *Injury* 1992; **23**: 107–10.

26. Alexander R, Proctor H. *Advanced Trauma Life Support Course*. Chicago, IL: American College of Surgeons, 2001.

27. Cooper S, Wakelam A. Leadership of resuscitation teams: "light-house leadership". *Resuscitation* 1999; **42**: 27–45.

28. Hoff WS, Reilly PM, Rotondo MF, *et al.* The importance of the command-physician in trauma resuscitation. *J Trauma* 1997; **43**: 772–7.

29. Woody JR, McKinney EH, Barker JM, Clothier CC. Comparison of fixed versus formed aircrews in military transport. *Aviat Space Environ Med* 1994; **65**: 153–6.

30. Simon R, Morey JC, Rice, MM, *et al.* Reducing errors in emergency medicine through team performance: the MedTeams project. In Scheffler AL, Zipperer L, eds., *Enhancing Patient Safety and Reducing Errors in Health Care*. Chicago, IL: National Patient Safety Foundation, 1998, pp. 142–6.

31. Sugre M, Seger M, Kerridge R, *et al.* A prospective study of the performance of the trauma team leader. *J Trauma* 1995; **38**: 79–82.

32. Barach P. Team based risk modification program to make health care safer. *Theoretical Issues in Ergonomic Science* 2007; **8**: 481–94.

33. Chidester TR, Helmrieich RL, Gregorich SE, Geis CE. Pilot personality and crew coordination: implications for training and selection. *Int J Aviat Psychol* 1991; **1**: 25–44.

34. Ericsson, KA, Starkes J. *Expert Performance in Sport*. Champaign, IL: Human Kinetics, 2003.

35. Ericsson KA, Krampe RT, Tesch-Römer C. The role of deliberate practice in the acquisition of expert performance. *Psychological Rev* 1993; **100**: 363–406.

36. Ericsson KA, Lehmann AC. Expert and exceptional performance: Evidence on maximal adaptations on task constraints. *Annu Rev Psychol* 1996; **47**: 273–305.

37. Choudhrey NK, Fletcher RH, Soumerai SB. Systematic review: the relationship between clinical experience and quality of health care. *Ann Intern Med* 2005; **142**: 260–73.

38. Ericsson KA, Smith J. *Toward a General Theory of Expertise: Prospects and Limits*. New York, NY: Cambridge University Press, 1991.

39. Harris KR, Tashman L, Ward P, *et al.* Planning, evaluation, and cognition: exploring the structure and mechanisms of expert performance in a representative dynamic task. 28th Annual Conference of the Cognitive Science Society, Vancouver, BC, 2006.

40. Klein G. *Sources of Power: How People Make Decisions*. Cambridge, MA: MIT Press, 1998.

41. Klein GA. Recognition-primed decisions. *Adv Man-Machine Syst Res* 1989; **5**: 47–92.

42. Shanteau J. Competence in experts: the role of task characteristics. *Organ Behav Hum Decision Proc* 1992; **53**: 252–62.

43. O'Leary JD, O'Sullivan O, Barach P, Shorten GD. Improving clinical performance using rehearsal or warm-up: an advanced literature review of randomized and observational studies. *Acad Med* 2014; **89**: 1416–22.

44. Sarter NB, Woods DD. Situation awareness: a critical but ill-defined phenomenon. *Int J Aviat Psychol* 1991; **1**: 45–7.

45. Endsley MR. Measurement of situation awareness in dynamic systems. *Human Factors* 1995; **37**: 65–84.

46. Cannon-Bowers JA, Salas E, Converse S. Shared mental models in expert team decision making. In Castellan NJ, ed., *Individual and Group Decision Making: Current Issues*. Hillsdale, NJ: Lawrence Erlbaum Associates, 1993, pp. 221–46.

47. Cannon-Bowers JA, Salas E. A framework for developing team performance measures in training. In Brannick MT, Salas E, Prince C, eds., *Team Performance Assessment and Measurement*. Mahwah, NJ: Lawrence Erlbaum Associates, 1997, pp. 45–62.

48. Baker DP, Gustafson S, Beaubien JM, Salas E, Barach P. Medical team training programs in health care. In *Advances in Patient Safety: From Research to Implementation: Vol 4, Programs, Tools, and Products*. AHRQ Publication No. 05-0021-4. Rockville, MD: Agency for Healthcare Research and Quality. 2005.

49. Naval Air Warfare Center Training Systems Division. *Performance Measurement in Teams*. Team Training Series, Book 2. Orlando, FL: Naval Air Warfare Center.

50. Christansen U., Hefferman D, Barach P. Microsimulators in medical education: an overview. *Simul Gaming* 2001; **32**: 250–62.

51. Hoyt DB, Shackford SR, Fridland PH, *et al.* Video recording trauma resuscitations: an effective teaching technique. *J Trauma* 1988; **28**: 435–40.

52. Michaelson M, Levi L. Videotaping in the admitting area: a most useful tool for quality improvement of the trauma care. *Eur J Emerg Med* 1997; **4**: 94–6.

53. Byrne AJ, Sellen AJ, Jones JG, *et al.* Effect of videotape feedback on anaesthetists' performance while managing simulated anaesthetic crises: a multicentre study. *Anaesthesia* 2002; **57**: 169–82.

54. Scherer L, Chang M, Meredith J, Battistella F. Videotape review leads to rapid and sustained learning. *Am J Surg* 2003; **185**: 516–20.

55. Ellis DG, Lerner EB, Jehle DV, *et al.* A multi-state survey of videotaping practices for major trauma resuscitations. *J Emerg Med* 1999; **17**: 597–604.

56. Weinger MB, Gonzales DC, Slagle J, Syeed M. Video capture of clinical care to enhance patient safety: the nuts and bolts. *Qual Saf Health Care* 2004; **13**: 136–44.

57. Gaba DM, Howard SK, Flanagan B, *et al.* Assessment of clinical performance during simulated crises using both technical and behavioral ratings. *Anesthesiology* 1998; **89**: 8.

58. Barach P, Fromson J, Kamar R. Ethical and professional concerns of simulation in professional assessment and education. *Am J Anesth* 2000; **12**: 228–31.

59. Barach P, Satish U, Streufert S. Healthcare assessment and performance. *Simul Gaming* 2001; **32**: 147–55.

60. Gaba DM. Human work environment and anesthesia simulators. In Miller RD, ed., *Anesthesia*, 5th edition. New York, NY: Churchill Livingstone, 2000, pp. 2613–68.

61. Schwid HA, Rooke GA, Ross BK, Sivarajan M. Use of a computerized advanced cardiac life support simulator improves retention of advanced cardiac life support guidelines better than a textbook review. *Crit Care Med* 1999; **27**: 821–4.

62. Swanson DB, Stillman P. The use of standardized patients for teaching and assessing clinical skills. *Eval Health Prof* 1990; **13**: 79–80.

63. Tekian A, McGuire C, McGaghie W. *Innovative Simulations for Assessing Professional Competence*. Chicago, IL: University of Illinois, 1999.

64. Naval Air Warfare Center Training Systems Division. *The Role of the Team Leader*. Team Training Series, Book 3. Orlando, FL: Naval Air Warfare Center.

65. Holzman RS, Cooper JB, Gaba DM, *et al.* Anesthesia crisis resource management: real-life simulation training in operating room crises. *J Clin Anesthiol* 1995; **7**: 675–87.

66. Hammond J, Bermann M, Chen B, Kushins L. Incorporation of a computerized human patient simulator in critical care training: a preliminary report. *J Trauma* 2002; **53**: 1064–7.

67. Holcomb JB, Dumire RD, Crommett JW, *et al.* Evaluation of trauma team performance using an advanced human patient simulator for resuscitation training. *J Trauma* 2002; **52**: 1078–86.

68. Lee SK, Pardo M, Gaba DM, *et al.* Trauma assessment training with a patient simulator: a prospective, randomized study. *J Trauma* 2003; **55**: 651–7.

69. Harnett MJ, Shorten GD. Address rehearsal. *Eur J Anaesthesiol* 2011; **28**: 675–7.

70. Satava RM, Hunter AM. The surgical ensemble: choreography as a simulation and training tool. *Surg Endosc* 2011; **25**: 30–5.

71. O'Leary JD, O'Sullivan O, Barach P, Shorten GD. Improving clinical performance using rehearsal or warm-up: an advanced literature review of randomized and observational studies. *Acad Med* 2014; **89**: 1416–22.

72. DeAnda A, Gaba DM. Unplanned incidents during comprehensive anesthesia simulation. *Anesth Analg* 1990; **71**: 77–82.

73. Devitt JH, Kurrek, MM, Cohen, MM, *et al.* Testing internal consistency and construct validity during evaluation of performance in a patient simulator. *Anesth Analg* 1998; **86**: 1160–4.

74. Oser RL, Salas E, Merket DC, Bowers CA. Applying resource management training in naval aviation: A methodology and lessons learned. In Salas E, Bowers CA, Edens E, eds., *Improving Teamwork in Organizations: Applications of Resource Management Training*. Mahwah, NJ: Lawrence Erlbaum Associates, 2001, pp. 283–301.

75. Christansen U, Barach P. Simulation in anesthesia. In Romano E, ed., *Anesthesia Generale Speciale: Principles Procedures and Techniques*, 2nd edition. Turin: Pergamon Press, 2004.

76. Bertalanffy LV. *General System Theory: Foundations, Development, Applications*. New York, NY: George Braziller, 1968.

77. Batalden PB, Nelson EC, Mohr JJ, *et al.* Microsystems in health care: part 5. How leaders are leading. *Jt Comm J Qual Saf* 2003; **29**: 297–308.

78. Mohr J, Barach P, Cravero JP, *et al.* Microsystems in health care: part 6. Designing patient safety into the microsystem. *Jt Comm J Qual Saf* 2003; **29**: 401–8.

79. Deming WE. *Out of the Crisis*. Cambridge, MA: Massachusetts Institute of Technology Center for Advanced Engineering Study, 1986.

80. Quinn JB. *The Intelligent Enterprise*. New York, NY: Free Press, 1992.

81. Nelson EC, Batalden PB, Mohr JJ, Plume SK. Building a quality future.

Front Health Serv Manage 2000;
15: 3–32.

82. Wasson JH, Godfrey, MM, Nelson EC, Mohr JJ, Batalden PB. Microsystems in health care: part 4. Planning patient-centered care. *Jt Comm J Qual Saf* 2003; **29**: 227–37.

83. Donaldson MS, Mohr JJ. *Improvement and Innovation in Health Care Microsystems. A Technical Report for the Institute of Medicine Committee on the Quality of Health Care in America.* Princeton, NJ: Robert Wood Johnson Foundation, 2000.

84. Batalden PB, Mohr JJ, Nelson EC, *et al.* Continually improving the health and value of health care for a population of patients: the panel management process. *Qual Manage Health Care* 1997; **5** (3): 41–51.

85. Entin EB, Lai F, Dierks M, Roth E. *Perioperative Readiness Information Management System: Technical Report.* Woburn, MA: Aptima, Inc., 2004.

86. Sharit J, Barach P. The role of patient hand-offs in health care. *Proceedings of the Society of the Human Factors* 2005; pp. 754–62.

87. Toccafondi GG, Albolino S, Tartaglia R, *et al.* The collaborative communication model for patient handover at the interface between high-acuity and low-acuity care. *BMJ Qual Saf* 2012; **21** (Suppl 1): i58–66.

88. Haynes AB, Weiser TG, Berry WR, *et al.* A surgical safety checklist to reduce morbidity and mortality in a global population. *N Engl J Med* 2009; **360**: 491–9.

89. Arora V, Johnson J, Lovinger D, Humphrey HJ, Meltzer DO. Communication failures in patient sign-out and suggestions for improvement: a critical incident analysis. *Qual Saf Health Care* 2005; **14**: 401–7.

90. Philibert I, Barach P. Balancing scientific rigor, context and trust in a multi-nation program to improve patient handovers. *BMJ Qual Saf* 2012; **21** (Suppl 1): i1–i6.

91. Mohr JJ, Batalden PB, Barach P. Inquiring into the quality and safety of care in the academic clinical microsystem. In McLaughlin K, Kaluzny A, eds., *Continuous Quality Improvement in Health Care*, 3rd edition. Frederick, MD: Aspen Publishers, 2005, pp. 407–23.

Index

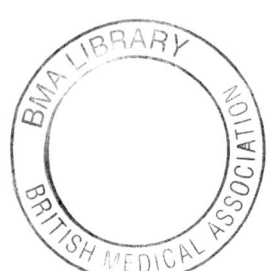

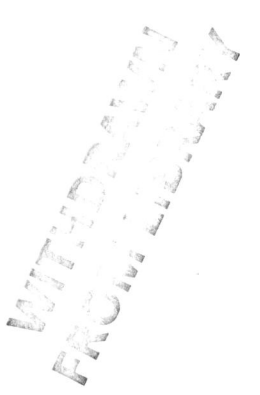